Nursing Diagnosis
Application to Clinical Practice

Nursing Diagnosis

Application to Clinical Practice

Fourth Edition

Lynda Juall Carpenito, R.N., M.S.N.

Nursing Consultant, Mickleton, New Jersey

with 32 additional contributors

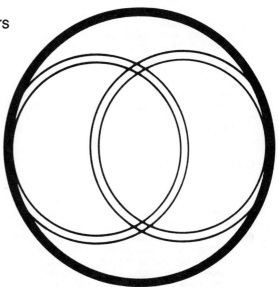

J. B. Lippincott Company Philadelphia

New York   London   Hagerstown

Sponsoring Editor: Donna Hilton
Editorial Assistant: Susan Perry
Project Editor: Tom Gibbons
Design Coordinator: Kathy Kelley-Luedtke
Cover: Louis Fuiano
Indexer: Ellen Murray
Production Manager: Helen Ewan
Production Supervisor: Maura Murphy
Compositor: Circle Graphics
Printer/Binder: R.R. Donnelley & Sons Company

6 5 4 3 2 1

Library of Congress Cataloging-in-Publication Data

Carpenito, Lynda Juall.
    Nursing diagnosis: application to clinical practice / Lynda Juall
  Carpenito, with 32 additional contributors.—4th ed.
      p.   cm.
  Includes bibliographical references and index.
  ISBN 0-397-54890-7
  1. Nursing diagnosis.   I. Title.
  [DNLM: 1. Nursing Diagnosis—outlines.   2. Patient Care Planning—
outlines.   WY 18 C294n]
  RT48.6.C39   1992
  616.07'5'024613—dc20
  DNLM/DLC
  for Library of Congress   91-17531
                                                                              CIP

To Richard, my husband
Through bright and dark you are there, thank you again.

It was such a pretty day we decided
   to take a walk,
And we had not gone ten steps
   before I knew
That you and I are long past the point
   of no return.

Hand in hand we go.
Still close, still loving
Still looking and overlooking
The flaws we hide from others.

Side by side we move,
Sometimes closer, sometimes farther apart.
Because of ways we read and talk,
Agree and disagree.

Step by step we advance
Against the cynics
Those all-knowing unknowings who
   honestly think
Marriage is dead.

—Lois Wyse, "I Still Love You"

Contributors

Rosalinda Alfaro-LeFevre, R.N., M.S.N., President, NDNP Consultants, Malvern, Pennsylvania; Adjunct Instructor, Delaware County Community College, Media, Pennsylvania; Staff Nurse, Critical Care Units, Paoli Memorial Hospital, Paoli, Pennsylvania

(High Risk for Altered Respiratory Function; Ineffective Airway Clearance; Ineffective Breathing Patterns; Diversional Activity Deficit; Impaired Verbal Communication; Fluid Volume Deficit; Fluid Volume Excess; High Risk for Altered Body Temperature and Hyperthermia/Hypothermia)

Virginia Arcangelo, R.N., Ed.D., Assistant Professor, School of Nursing, Thomas Jefferson University, Philadelphia, Pennsylvania

(Altered Sexuality Patterns, Second Edition)

Cynthia Balin, R.N., M.S.N., Chatsworth, California

(Altered Nutrition: Less Than Body Requirements; Altered Nutrition: More Than Body Requirements; Powerlessness; and Impaired Swallowing, Second Edition)

Eleanor A. Bell, B.S., C.N.A., Director of Nursing, Bryn Mawr Rehabilitation Hospital, Malvern, Pennsylvania

(Self-Care Deficit, Second Edition)

Christine Cannon, R.N., M.S.N., Coordinator of Patient Education, Wilmington Medical Center, Wilmington, Delaware

(Altered Health Maintenance [selected sections, First Edition])

Nancy Conrad, R.N., M.S.N., Assistant Professor, Director of Nursing, Rutgers University, Camden, New Jersey

(Fear, Second Edition)

Nancy Eppich, R.N., M.S.N., Clinical Instructor, Nursing Care of Children, Frances Payne Bolton School of Nursing, Case Western Reserve University, Cleveland, Ohio

(Altered Parenting and Parental Role Conflict)

Judy A. Hartmann, Director of Nursing, Kansas Rehabilitation Hospital, Topeka, Kansas

(Altered Patterns of Urinary Elimination; Unilateral Neglect, Third Edition)

Sandra Jansen, R.N., A.C.C.E., A.S.P.O., Certified Childbirth Educator, AASECT Sex Educator, Los Angeles, California

(Ineffective Breast-feeding and Altered Patterns of Sexuality related to changes in body function or image during and after pregnancy)

Susan Kitchell, R.N., M.S., Pediatric Clinical Nurse Specialist, San Francisco, California
(Selected sections of Parental Role Conflict related to Hospitalized Child, Second Edition)

Deborah Lekan-Rutledge, M.S.N., R.N.C., Nursing Consultant
(Selected Gerontological Principles and Rationale)

Morris A. Magnan, R.N., B.S.N., Doctoral Student, Wayne State University; Clinical Nurse Specialist/Case Manager, Surgical Patient Services, Harper Hospital, Detroit Medical Center, Detroit, Michigan
(Activity Intolerance)

Jo Ann Maklebust, M.S.N., R.N., C.S., Case Manager, Surgical Patient Services, Harper Hospital, Detroit Medical Center, Detroit, Michigan
(Impaired Tissue Integrity; High Risk for Altered Health Maintenance related to lack of knowledge of ostomy care; Impaired Skin Integrity; Altered Comfort: Pruritus; and Altered Oral Mucous Membrane)

Glenda S. McGaha, Ph.D., R.N., Department of Nursing, Southeast Missouri State University, Cape Girardeau, Missouri
(Altered Growth and Development)

Janet Hoffman Mennies, R.N.C., M.S.N., Adult Nurse Practitioner
(Noncompliance; Altered Health Maintenance; Selected sections of Altered Family Processes; Ineffective Individual Coping; and Health-Seeking Behaviors)

Margaret C. Metcalfe, R.N., M.S., Ph.D. Candidate, Assistant Professor, College of Nursing, University of Delaware, Newark, Delaware
(Altered Sexuality Patterns)

Linda C. Mondoux, R.N., M.S.N., Clinical Nurse Specialist, Bolsford Hospital, Farmington Hills, Michigan
(Gerontological Considerations for Activity Intolerance; Grieving; Impaired Home Maintenance Management; Spiritual Distress; Impaired Communications; Diversional Activity Deficit; Powerlessness; and Impaired Tissue Integrity)

Kathe H. Morris, R.N., M.S.N., Educational Consultant, West Chester, Pennsylvania
(Rape Trauma Syndrome)

Nancy J. Morwessel, R.N., M.S.N., C.P.N.P., Pediatric Cardiovascular Clinical Nurse Specialist, Children's Hospital Medical Center, Cincinnati, Ohio
(Altered Comfort in Children)

Nursing Diagnosis Discussion Group, Nancy A. Eppich, Chairwoman, Rainbow Babies and Children Hospital, University Hospitals of Cleveland, Cleveland, Ohio
(Parental Role Conflict, Third Edition)

Mary M. Owen, R.N., B.S.N., P.H.N., Epidemiology Specialist, Irvine Medical Center, Santa Ana, California
(Potential for Infection and Potential for Infection Transmission)

Rhonda Panifilli, R.N., M.S.N., Case Manager, Surgical Patient Services, Harper Hospital, Detroit Medical Center, Detroit, Michigan

(Altered Health Maintenance related to Increased Food Consumption)

Mary Sieggreen, M.S.N., R.N., C.S., Clinical Nurse Specialist/Case Manager, Surgical Patient Services, Harper Hospital, Detroit Medical Center, Detroit, Michigan

(Altered Peripheral Tissue Perfusion and High Risk for Injury related to Effects Secondary to Orthostatic Hypotension)

Deborah Soholt, R.N., M.S.N., Clinical Director, Medical Services, St. Luke's Midland Regional Medical Center, Aberdeen, South Dakota

(Decisional Conflict)

Katsuko Tanaka, R.N., M.S., C.S., Staff Nurse, Alcohol and Drug Dependent Treatment Program, Seattle Veterans Administration Medical Center, Seattle, Washington

(Post-Trauma Response)

Laura A. Terrill, R.N., M.S.N., Director of Nursing Education, Wilmington Medical Center, Wilmington, Delaware

(Disturbance in Self-Concept and Social Isolation, First Edition)

Carol Van Antwerp, R.N., M.S.N., Pediatric Nurse Clinician, Children's Health Center, Battle Creek, Michigan

(High Risk for Injury related to Maturational Age, Pediatric Considerations)

Bonnie McDonald Wakefield, R.N., M.A., Quality Assurance/Research, Nursing Service, Veterans Administration Medical Center, Iowa City, Iowa

(Selected sections of Altered Health Maintenance, Third Edition)

Julie Waterhouse, R.N., M.S., Assistant Professor, College of Nursing, University of Delaware, Newark, Delaware

(Spiritual Distress, Altered Sexuality Patterns)

Janet R. Weber, R.N., M.S.N., Instructor, Southeast Missouri State University, Cape Girardeau, Missouri

(Hopelessness)

Anne E. Willard, R.N., M.S.N., Associate Professor, Cumberland County College, Vineland, New Jersey

(Anxiety; High Risk for Violence; Ineffective Family Coping; Altered Thought Processes; High Risk for Self-Harm; Impaired Social Interactions; Self-Esteem Disturbance; Defensive Coping; Ineffective Denial; Chronic Low Self Esteem; and Situational Low Self Esteem)

Anna Mae Spaniolo, R.N., B.S.N., M.S.N., Nurse Educator, Bronson Methodist Hospital School of Nursing, Kalamazoo, Michigan

(High Risk for Injury related to Maturational Age, Pediatric Considerations)

Anna Mae died after a long illness in March 1991. Her contributions to this book are evidence of her expertise in pediatric nursing. Her compassion and spirit for others will continue to live in each of us. We all grieve her loss but celebrate her life!

Consultants

Carol Bechtold, R.N., M.S.N., Assistant Administrator/Education, Department of Nursing, The Hospital Center at Orange, Orange, New Jersey

Jane Bloom, R.N., M.S.N., Clinical Nurse Specialist, Medical Respiratory Intensive Care Unit, Thomas Jefferson Hospital, Philadelphia, Pennsylvania

Michele Clements, R.N., Nurse Manager Labor and Delivery, Women's Health Care, Victoria Hospital, London, Ontario, Canada

Ann Delengowski, R.N., M.S.N., Oncology Clinical Nurse Specialist, Thomas Jefferson University Hospital, Philadelphia, Pennsylvania

Mary Ann Ducharme, R.N., M.S.N., Case Manager, Intensive Care, Harper Hospital, Detroit, Michigan

Cissy Englebert-Passanza, R.N., M.S.N., Clinical Nurse Educator, Mercy Catholic Medical Center, Darby, Pennsylvania

Benjamin M. Evans, R.N., O.N.P., M.S.C., Nurse Consultant, Cincinnati, Ohio

Ann Feins, R.D., Assistant Professor, Saint Anselm College, Manchester, New Hampshire

Jean W. Fitzgerald, R.N., E.T., Enterostomal Therapist, Wilmington Medical Center, Wilmington, Delaware

Debra J. Lynn-McHale, R.N., M.S.N., C.C.R.N., Clinical Nurse Specialist, Surgical Cardiac Care Unit, Thomas Jefferson University Hospital, Philadelphia, Pennsylvania

Morris Magnum, R.N., M.S.N., Graduate Student, Staff Nurse, Harper Hospital, Detroit, Michigan

Kathleen A. Michalski, R.N., B.S.N., C.C.R.N., Clinical Nurse III, Surgical Cardiac Care Unit, Thomas Jefferson University Hospital, Philadelphia, Pennsylvania

Susan Ross, R.N., M.S., Assistant Professor, American International College, Springfield, Massachusetts

Rebecca Rush, M.Ed., Cognitive Therapist, The Center at Plaza Medical, Camden, New Jersey

Ann Smith, R.N., M.S.N., C.C.R.N., Clinical Nurse Specialist, Surgical Intensive Care Unit, Thomas Jefferson University Hospital, Philadelphia, Pennsylvania

Linda H. Snow, R.N., M.S., Assistant Professor, American International College, Springfield, Massachusetts

Jackie Sullivan, R.N., M.S.N., Clinical Nurse Specialist, Neurological Intensive Care Unit, Thomas Jefferson University Hospital, Philadelphia, Pennsylvania

Fe Ayalin Tamparong, R.N., M.A., Director of Education, AMI Circle City Hospital, Corona, California

Carl K. Wyckoff III, D.D.S., Private Practice, Wenonah, New Jersey

Preface

The practice of nursing often interfaces with the practices of the other health care providers.* Sometimes the nurse sees the client problems that require referral for treatment and ignores or fails to detect the problems that she can treat independently. *Nursing Diagnosis: Application to Clinical Practice* focuses on the diagnosis and treatment of client situations that the nurse can and should treat, legally and independently. It provides a condensed, organized outline of clinical nursing practice designed to communicate creative clinical nursing. It is not meant to replace textbooks of nursing, but rather to provide nurses in a variety of settings with the information they need without requiring a time-consuming review of the literature.

From assessment criteria to specific interventions, the book focuses on nursing. It will assist students in transferring their theoretical knowledge to clinical practice; it can also be used by experienced nurses to recall past learning and to intervene in those clinical situations that previously went ignored or unrecognized.

The author agrees that nursing needs a classification system to organize its functions and define its scope. Use of such a classification system would expedite research activities and facilitate communication between nurses, consumer, and other health care providers. After all, medicine took over 100 years to develop its taxonomy. Our work, at the national level, was only begun in 1973 and is still in an early stage. It is hoped that the reader will be stimulated to participate at the local, regional, or national level in the utilization and development of these diagnostic categories.

Since the first edition was published, the use of nursing diagnosis has increased markedly throughout the United States, Canada, and Europe. Practicing nurses vary in experience with nursing diagnosis from just beginning to full practice integration for over 10 years. With such a variance in use, questions posed from the neophyte, such as

- What does the label really mean?
- What kinds of assessment questions will yield nursing diagnoses?
- How do I differentiate one diagnosis from another?
- How do I tailor a diagnosis for a specific individual?
- How should I intervene after I formulate the diagnostic statement?
- How do I care-plan with nursing diagnoses?

differ dramatically from such questions from experts as

- Should nursing diagnoses represent the only diagnoses on the nursing care plan?
- Can medical diagnoses be included in a nursing diagnosis statement?
- What is the difference between high risk and possible nursing diagnoses?
- What kind of problem statement should I write to describe a person at risk for hemorrhage?
- What kind of nursing diagnosis should I use to describe a healthy person?

---

*The model of interlocking circles on the cover depicts this relationship. The common area represents those situations in which nurses and physicians collaborate; the rest denotes the dimensions for which each professional prescribes definitive interventions to prevent or treat.

This fourth edition seeks to continue to answer these questions.

Section I begins with a chapter on the historical etiology of nursing diagnosis and the work of the North American Nursing Diagnosis Association (NANDA). The concepts of nursing diagnosis, classification and taxonomic issues are explored. The fourth edition discusses the review process of NANDA and describes the evolving taxonomy of NANDA's Human Response Patterns.

Chapter 2 differentiates among actual, high risk, and possible nursing diagnoses. A discussion of wellness and syndrome diagnoses also is presented. Guidelines for writing diagnostic statements and avoiding errors are outlined. In this edition, Chapter 2 also covers the use of non–NANDA-approved diagnoses and ethical considerations associated with nursing diagnoses.

Chapter 3 describes the Bifocal Clinical Practice Model. This edition includes a more detailed discussion of nursing diagnoses and collaborative problems, covering their relationship to assessment, goals, interventions, and evaluation.

Chapter 4 focuses on assessment and diagnosis, covering data interpretation and assessment format and concluding with a case study to illustrate clinical applications.

Chapter 5 describes the process of care planning and discusses various care planning systems. Topics covered include priority identification, nursing goals versus client goals, and nursing accountability. Interventions for nursing diagnoses and collaborative problems are differentiated. This edition also clarifies evaluation, distinguishing evaluation of nursing care from evaluation of the client's condition. A discussion of multidisciplinary care is presented, as is a three-tiered care planning system aimed at increasing the clinical use of care plans without increasing writing. Samples of nursing records appear throughout the chapter.

Section II compiles the nursing diagnoses accepted by NANDA along with additional clinically useful diagnoses. The fourth edition includes 113 diagnoses (104 NANDA-approved and 9 added by the author). Besides the new nursing diagnoses, this edition also presents new information on such topics as bed rest deconditioning, bowel incontinence, elder abuse, elder care, Dysfunctional Grieving, Self-Care Deficit Syndrome, Instrumental Self-Care Deficit, sexuality, and spirituality.

Each nursing diagnosis group is discussed under the following subheads:

- Definition
- Defining Characteristics or Risk Factors
- Related Factors
- Diagnostic Considerations
- Errors in Diagnostic Statements
- Focus Assessment
- Principles and Rationale for Nursing Care
    Generic Considerations
    Pediatric Considerations
    Gerontologic Considerations

In this edition, the addition of the two new subheads Diagnostic Considerations and Errors in Diagnostic Statements is designed to help the nurse understand the concept behind the diagnosis, differentiate one diagnosis from another, and avoid diagnostic errors. Pediatric and gerontologic considerations for all relevant diagnoses provide additional pertinent information.

Each nursing diagnosis is followed by one or more specific nursing diagnoses that relate to familiar clinical situations. These specific diagnoses are defined by subjective and objective assessment data. Outcome criteria for the diagnosis are provided with the related interventions, which represent activities in the independent domain of nursing derived from the physical and applied sciences, pharmacology, nutrition, mental health, and nursing research.

This fourth edition also contains a new Section III, Manual of Collaborative Problems. In this section, each of the eight generic collaborative problems is explained under the subheads:

- Physiologic Overview
- Definition
- Diagnostic Considerations
- Focus Assessment Criteria
- Significant Laboratory Assessment Criteria

Discussed under their appropriate problems are 37 specific collaborative problems, covering:

- Definition
- High-Risk Populations
- Nursing Goals
- Interventions

By adding Section III, the fourth edition of *Nursing Diagnosis: Application to Clinical Practice* addresses both types of situations that nurses are responsible for treating. The clarification of the focus of nurses is intended to assist them in addressing clients' human needs, with the expectation that—as more "nursing" is added to nursing—the profession, the nurse, and, most importantly, the client will reap the rewards.

The author invites comments or suggestions from readers. Correspondence can be directed to the publisher or to the author's address: 66 East Rattling Run Road, Mickleton, NJ 08056.

Lynda Juall Carpenito, R.N., M.S.N.

Acknowledgments

When immersed in a manuscript, I seem able to meet only basic needs: air, food, elimination, and safety. I am grateful for all my good friends who don't wait for me to call them. It's these friends who help me meet my other needs—love, belonging, trust—to approach self-actualization. Thank you, Ginny, Pati, and Ronnie.

My publisher, J. B. Lippincott, has provided me with professional marketing, editorial support, and creative freedom. My new editor, Donna Hilton, nudged me to pursue new approaches with my work. Manuscript editor Kevin Law has a unique ability to quickly absorb and integrate the philosophy of my work; he does it so well that I think he must have been a nurse in a previous life. Thank you also to Diana Intenzo, Susan Perry, and Tom Gibbons.

Since the first edition, hundreds of nurse colleagues have shared their experiences with nursing diagnoses and have challenged me to grow, learn, and change. I am grateful for their challenges. Also, thank you to those departments of nursing and schools of nursing that have shared their success stories after integration of the Bifocal Clinical Nursing Model.

At last, I would like to thank Laura Terrill for her moral and professional support while I wrote the first edition; the group in Detroit (Jo Ann Maklebust, Mary Sieggreen, Linda Mondoux) for our late-night talks; Rosalinda Alfaro-LeFevre, who recognized the need for the book and sought to make it a reality; and lastly, a very special person—my son, Olen Juall Carpenito, who has learned to appreciate that his mom's accomplishments require an intense work schedule. Of all my accomplishments, he's the one I treasure most.

Contents

Nursing Diagnosis
Application to Clinical Practice

Section I

Nursing Diagnosis in the Nursing Process

Introduction

Nursing is primarily assisting individuals (sick or well) with those activities contributing to health or its recovery (or to a peaceful death) that they perform unaided when they have the necessary strength, will, or knowledge; nursing also helps individuals carry out prescribed therapy and to be independent of assistance as soon as possible.*

Individuals are open systems who continually interact with the environment, creating individual interaction patterns. These patterns are dynamic and interact with life processes (physiologic, psychologic, sociocultural, developmental, and spiritual) to influence the individual's behavior and health. A person becomes a client not only when an actual or potential alteration in this interaction pattern compromises his health but also when the person desires assistance to achieve a higher level of health.

The use of the term *client* in place of the term *patient* to identify the health care consumer suggests an autonomous person who has freedom of choice in seeking and selecting assistance. The client is no longer a passive recipient of services but an active participant who assumes responsibility for his choices and also for the consequences of those choices. *Family* is used to describe any person or persons who serve as support systems to the client. *Group* is used to describe support systems as well as communities such as senior citizen centers. Societal health needs have changed in the last decade; so must the nurse's view of the consumers of health care (individual, family, community).†

Health is the state of wellness as defined by the client; it is no longer defined as whether or not a biologic disease is present. Health is a dynamic, ever-changing state influenced by past and present interaction patterns. The individual is an expert on himself and is responsible for seeking or refusing health care.

The Bifocal Clinical Practice Model describes the unique responsibilities of nursing in two components. *Nursing diagnoses* address the responses of clients, families, or groups to situations for which the nurse can prescribe interventions for outcome achievement. In contrast, *collaborative problems* describe certain physiologic complications that nurses manage using both nurse- and physician-prescribed interventions. No other discipline but nursing can treat nursing diagnoses and also manage collaborative problems.

The Bifocal Clinical Practice Model provides nurses with a classification system to describe the health status of an individual, family, or community and the risk for complications. Using this system, nurses can describe the health status of individuals or groups concisely and systematically, while also addressing the unique aspects of each situation.

---

*Henderson, V., & Nite, G. (1960). *Principles and practice of nursing* (5th ed.). New York: Macmillan.

† Carpenito, L. J., & Duespohl, T.A. (1985). *A guide to effective clinical instruction* (2nd ed.). Rockville, MD: Aspen Systems.

1

Nursing Diagnosis: Development

Nursing diagnosis provides a useful mechanism for structuring nursing knowledge in an attempt to define the unique role and domain of nursing. The quest to define nursing and its functions began with the writings of Nightingale. In her words, the purpose of nursing is "to put the patient in the best condition for nature to act upon him." In the early 20th century, attempts to differentiate nursing from medicine stemmed from the need to define each of these disciplines for legislative and educational purposes. V. Henderson in 1955 and F. Abdellah in 1960 proposed organizing nursing curricula according to nursing problems or patient needs rather than medical diagnoses.

Why Nursing Diagnoses?

Why does nursing need a classification system, or taxonomy? Although perceived reasons will vary according to the individual nurse's focus, nursing in general needs a classification system to describe and develop a sound scientific foundation to fulfill one of the criteria for professional status. The requisites commonly demanded of an occupational group seeking to claim professional status are listed by Styles as follows:

- An extensive university education
- A unique body of knowledge
- An orientation of service to others
- A professional society
- Autonomy and self-regulation

A classification system for nursing will define the body of knowledge for which nursing will be held accountable. The relationship of nursing diagnosis to accountability and autonomy can be expressed as follows:

Nursing Diagnosis → Clearer identification → Greater accountability → Greater
of the body of nursing professional
knowledge autonomy

Using a classification system to identify nursing's domain provides nurses with a common frame of reference. Historically, nurses have been educated to use medical diagnoses to describe the nursing focus. Since medical terminology provides an easy, convenient solution, some nurses have resisted other, more nursing-oriented terminology. Clinicians would rather use terms like "congestive heart failure," "asthma," and "placenta previa" than "social isolation," "impaired skin integrity," and "self-care deficit."

The need for a common, consistent language for a profession was identified over 200 years ago by medicine. If physicians had elected to use just any word to describe their clinical situations then:

- How could they communicate with each other? With nurses?
- How would research be organized?
- How would new practitioners be educated?
- How could quality assurance be achieved if the diagnoses could not be retrieved systematically?

For example, prior to the formal labeling Acquired Immunodeficiency Syndrome (AIDS), it was difficult or perhaps impossible to define or study the disease. Often, medical records would have a variety of diagnoses or causes of death such as sepsis, cerebral hemorrhage, or Kaposi's sarcoma that were listed to describe the individual with AIDS.

A unified system of terminology establishes a common language to help direct nurses to assess selected data and identify a potential or an actual client problem. Nurses can then refer to the list of terms to assist them in describing the problem. Consistent terminology makes oral and written communication easier and more efficient. In addition, identifying definitive nursing functions increases the nurse's accountability in assessing the client, determining the diagnosis, and providing the treatment called for by the diagnosis. Knowledge of the unique responsibilities of nursing in turn stimulates nurses to acquire new knowledge and skills to use as they intervene to solve these problems.

From the viewpoint of health care delivery, a classification of nursing diagnoses establishes a system suitable for computerization. With the potential for computer use, nursing diagnosis can:

- Provide nurses with a system for retrieving client records using nursing, not medical, diagnoses
- Provide an opportunity for nurses to develop or be included in a computerized health care information system that would collect, analyze, and synthesize nursing data for practice, literature, and research
- Provide a mechanism for the reimbursement of nursing activities related to nursing diagnoses, not medical diagnoses

Clarifying nursing for nurses, employers, the public, and third-party payers can only serve to strengthen and enrich the profession.

The trend to focus nursing education on the principal functions of nursing rather than on medicine continues today with the development of nursing models. During the late 1960s and '70s, nurses sought to organize nursing knowledge and practice through the construction of theoretical or conceptual frameworks. Examples of such frameworks are Roy's adaptation model, Johnson's behavioral system model, Orem's self-care concept of nursing, Rogers's life process theory, and Newman's health systems model. The work of these theorists can help distinguish nursing phenomena within the broad field of health care.

Criticism of most theories and frameworks usually arises from difficulty in applying them to clinical practice. In a critique of theory development in nursing, Kritek (1978) submits that most nursing theories "describe how nursing should be, not how it is in reality." She notes that the use of poorly defined or confusing terms by theorists only limits professional application of these theories. Kritek advocates beginning with a theory that is operational in nature, one that describes "what we see and what we do," rather than with one that appears sophisticated but is obscure.

Nursing diagnosis can provide a solution to the quest of nursing because it serves to:

- Define nursing in its present state
- Classify the domain of nursing
- Differentiate nursing from medicine
- Identify nursing knowledge for students

Basic Concepts

The word *diagnosis* evokes many responses in nurses—some positive, some negative. Because nurses have historically linked the word diagnosis exclusively with medicine, some may tend to overlook the fact that teachers diagnose learning disabilities, hair-dressers diagnose hair problems, and mechanics diagnose automotive disorders. In addition, many nurses were taught to avoid making definitive statements when documenting and were advised to use terms such as "seems to be" or "appears to be." This socialization process rewarded nurses for *not* diagnosing.

By dictionary definition, diagnosis is the careful, critical study of something to determine its nature. The question is not *whether* nurses can diagnose but *what* nurses can diagnose.

In 1953 the term *nursing diagnosis* was introduced by V. Fry to describe a step necessary in developing a nursing care plan. For the next 20 years, references to nursing diagnosis appeared only sporadically in the literature. However, from 1973 (when the first meeting of the National Group for the Classification of Nursing Diagnosis was held) to the present, attention in the literature has increased tenfold, and various definitions of nursing diagnosis have appeared. Four of these definitions follow, describing nursing diagnosis as problems, responses, evaluation, or judgment.

Definitions of Nursing Diagnosis

- An independent nursing function; an evaluation of a client's personal responses to his human experiences throughout the life cycle, be they developmental or accidental crises, illness, hardships, or other stresses (Bircher, 1975)
- Actual or potential health problems that nurses, by virtue of their education and experience, are able and licensed to treat (Gordon, 1982)
- A clinical judgment about an individual, family, or community that is derived through a deliberate, systematic process of data collection and analysis. It provides the basis for prescriptions for definitive therapy for which the nurse is accountable (Shoemaker, 1984)
- A statement that describes the human response (health state or actual/ potential altered interaction pattern) of an individual or group which the nurse can legally identify and for which the nurse can order the definitive interventions to maintain the health state or to reduce, eliminate, or prevent alterations (Carpenito)

In 1973, the American Nurses Association (ANA) published the Standards of Practice; they were followed in 1980 by the ANA Social Policy Statement, which defined nursing as follows:

Nursing is the diagnosis and treatment of human response to actual or potential health problems.

Most state nurse practice acts describe nursing in accordance with the ANA definition.

In March 1990, at the Ninth Conference of the North American Nursing Diagnosis

Association (NANDA), the General Assembly approved an official definition of nursing diagnosis.

Nursing diagnosis is a clinical judgment about individual, family, or community responses to actual or potential health problems/life processes. Nursing diagnosis provides the basis for selection of nursing intervention to achieve outcome for which the nurse is accountable (NANDA, 1990).

Nursing Diagnosis: Process or Outcome?

A review of the literature reveals that, over time, the term nursing diagnosis has been used in three contexts:

1. *As the second step of the nursing process.* In the second step of the nursing process, the data collected during the assessment of the client's health status is analyzed and problems are identified. Some of the conclusions resulting from data analysis will lead to nursing diagnoses, but others will not. It is important to recognize that the outcome of this process can include problems that are primarily treated by nurses and problems that require treatment by several disciplines. For example, while assessing a particular client, the nurse may record observations that point to the medical problems of seizures, hypoglycemia, and hypertension, as well as the nursing diagnosis of *High Risk for Injury.* Using the term *nursing diagnosis* to designate the second step of the nursing process can be confusing and may have the undesirable effect of leading nurses to try to state all conclusions or problems as nursing diagnoses.

2. *As a list of diagnostic labels or titles.* After the first conference on nursing diagnosis in 1973, the term *nursing diagnosis* was applied to specific labels describing health states that nurses could legally diagnose and treat. The purpose of establishing these labels was to define and classify the scope of nursing. These labels are concise descriptors of a cluster of signs and symptoms, such as *Anxiety* or *Altered Family Processes* or of increased vulnerability, such as *High Risk for Infection.*

3. *As a two-part or three-part statement.* Nurses use the term *nursing diagnosis* to describe a two-part or three-part statement about an individual's, a family's, or a group's response to a situation or a health problem.

Thus, it has become necessary to indicate clearly whether the term *nursing diagnosis* is being used in the context of problem identification (critical thinking), a classification system of diagnostic labels (such as that developed by NANDA), or an individualized statement.

To avoid misuse and confusion, the author recommends using the following terms:

- For the second step of the nursing process: diagnosis
- For the list of diagnostic labels or titles: diagnostic *label* or *nursing diagnosis*
- For the diagnostic statement: *nursing diagnosis*

Nursing diagnosis is a statement describing one specific type of problem or situation that nurses identify. It should not be used to label all the problems nurses can ascertain, since such usage will not emphasize the unique role of the nurse. For the purpose of clarity, the use of the term in this book will be restricted to describing the two-part or three-part statement.

The North American Nursing Diagnosis Association (NANDA)

When the first conference on nursing diagnosis was held in 1973, its purpose was to identify nursing functions and to establish a classification system suitable for computerization. From this conference developed the National Group for the Classification of Nursing Diagnosis. This group is composed of nurses from different regions of the United States and Canada, representing all elements of the profession: practice, education, and research. From 1973 to the present, the National Group has met nine times and formulated a list of nursing diagnoses. These diagnostic labels are listed in Table 1-1.

Table 1-1 **Nursing Diagnostic Categories Grouped Under Functional Health Patterns***

1. Health Perception–Health Management

    Growth & Development, Altered

    Health Maintenance, Altered

    Health Seeking Behaviors

    Noncompliance

    High Risk for Injury

        High Risk for Suffocation

        High Risk for Poisoning

        High Risk for Trauma

2. Nutritional–Metabolic

    Body Temperature, High Risk for Altered

        Hypothermia

        Hyperthermia

        Thermoregulation, Ineffective

    Fluid Volume Deficit

    Fluid Volume Excess

    Infection, High Risk for

    ‡Infection Transmission, High Risk for

    Nutrition, Altered: Less than Body Requirements

    Nutrition, Altered: More than Body Requirements

    Nutrition, Altered: High Risk for More than Body Requirements

    † Breastfeeding, Effective

        Breastfeeding, Ineffective

        Swallowing, Impaired

    †Protection, Altered

        Tissue Integrity, Impaired

            Oral Mucous Membrane, Altered

            Skin Integrity, Impaired

3. Elimination

    †Bowel Elimination, Altered

        Constipation

        Colonic Constipation

        Perceived Constipation

        Diarrhea

        Bowel Incontinence

(continued)

Table 1-1 **Nursing Diagnostic Categories Grouped Under Functional Health Patterns*** (continued)

3. Elimination (continued)

Urinary Elimination, Altered Patterns of
Urinary Retention
Total Incontinence
Functional Incontinence
Reflex Incontinence
Urge Incontinence
Stress Incontinence
‡ Maturational Enuresis

4. Activity–Exercise

Activity Intolerance

Cardiac Output, Decreased

Disuse Syndrome, High Risk for

Diversional Activity Deficit

Home Maintenance Management, Impaired

Mobility, Impaired Physical

‡Respiratory Function, Potential Altered
Ineffective Airway Clearance
Ineffective Breathing Patterns
Impaired Gas Exchange

Self-Care Deficit Syndrome
(Specify) ‡(Instrumental, Feeding, Bathing/Hygiene, Dressing/Grooming, Toileting)

Tissue Perfusion, Altered (Specify Type) (Cerebral, Cardiopulmonary, Renal, Gastrointestinal, Peripheral)

5. Sleep–Rest

Sleep Pattern Disturbance

6. Cognitive–Perceptual

‡Comfort, Altered
Pain
Chronic Pain

Decisional Conflict

Dysreflexia

Knowledge Deficit (specify)

High Risk for Aspiration

Sensory–Perceptual Alterations: (Specify) (Visual, Auditory, Kinesthetic, Gustatory, Tactile, Olfactory)

Thought Processes, Altered

Unilateral Neglect

7. Self-Perception

Anxiety

Fatigue

Fear

Hopelessness

Powerlessness

†Self-Concept Disturbance
Body Image Disturbance
Personal Identity Disturbance
Self-Esteem Disturbance
Chronic Low Self-Esteem
Situational Low Self-Esteem

(continued)

Table 1-1   **Nursing Diagnostic Categories Grouped Under Functional Health Patterns*** (continued)

8. Role–Relationship

‡Communication, Impaired
   Communication, Impaired Verbal
Family Processes, Altered
‡Grieving
   Grieving, Anticipatory
   Grieving, Dysfunctional
Parenting, Altered
Parental Role Conflict
Role Performance, Altered
Social Interaction, Impaired
Social Isolation

9. Sexuality–Reproductive

Sexual Dysfunction
Sexuality Patterns, Altered

10. Coping–Stress Tolerance

Adjustment, Impaired
Coping, Ineffective Individual
   Defensive Coping
   Ineffective Denial
Coping: Disabling, Ineffective Family
Coping: Compromised, Ineffective Family
Coping: Potential for Growth, Family
Post Trauma Response
   Rape Trauma Syndrome
‡Self-Harm, High Risk for
Violence, High Risk for

11. Value–Belief

Spiritual Distress

* The Functional Health Patterns were identified by M. Gordon in *Nursing diagnosis: Process and application* (New York, McGraw-Hill, 1982) with minor changes by the author.
† These diagnoses were accepted by the North American Nursing Diagnosis Association in 1990.
‡ These diagnoses are not currently on the NANDA list but have been included for clarity and usefulness.

At its first meeting in 1973, the National Group also appointed a task force to:

1. Gather information and disseminate it through the Association (North American Nursing Diagnosis Association, 3525 Caroline St., St. Louis, MO 63104).
2. Encourage educational activities at regional and state levels to promote the implementation of nursing diagnoses. These activities include conferences to organize nurses to identify additional diagnostic labels and workshops to teach nurses about nursing diagnoses.
3. Promote and organize activities to continue the development, classification, and scientific testing of nursing diagnosis. These activities include planning national conferences, identifying criteria for accepting diagnoses, surveying current research activities, and exploring varied methods for classification.

A proposal from the task force for a more formal organization was approved at the fifth national conference, and the group was renamed the North American Nursing Diagnosis Association. NANDA has elected officers, a board of directors, and standing committees.

Breu et al (1987) describe assimilation of scientific advances like nursing diagnosis into practice as, usually, a three-step process. Initially, the research question is formulated and the research conducted. Next, the research findings are disseminated at scientific meetings and in journals. The third step is the incorporation of the relevant findings into clinical practice. This process is usually linear with little feedback.

NANDA has taken a different approach to the scientific assimilation of nursing diagnosis into practice. It involves three concurrent activities: consensus development, research, and infiltration occurring in an open system (Breu, Dracup & Walden, 1987). As nursing diagnoses are being identified, clinical research using selected designs (Gordon, Sweeney, Fehring) test and refine assumptions.

Clinicians utilize the nursing diagnoses accepted by NANDA for clinical testing and submit revisions to NANDA. Integration of nursing diagnosis into nursing curricula and literature serves to further disseminate the work of NANDA. Figure 1-1 contrasts the traditional method and NANDA's method of incorporating scientific advances into practice.

In December 1986, an advisory panel on Classification for Nursing Practice of the ANA met with liaisons from NANDA. Their purpose was to formally submit a nursing system to the World Health Organization (WHO) for possible inclusion in the tenth revision of the International Code of Diseases (IDC). The document that was submitted represented a compilation of the work of NANDA, the Omaha Classification System, and the Psychiatric-Mental Health Council of the ANA. In August 1987, as the result of collaborative work of the ANA and NANDA, a replacement document was sent to the WHO. This document represents the classification system of NANDA. Also, at this time the ANA officially sanctioned NANDA as the organization to govern the development of a classification system of nursing diagnoses. The Councils of the ANA have been advised to submit proposed nursing diagnoses to NANDA. This timely and significant action by the ANA will facilitate a uniform classification system for the nursing profession.

In March 1990, the first issue of *Nursing Diagnosis,* the official journal of NANDA, was published. This journal aims to promote the development, refinement, and applica-

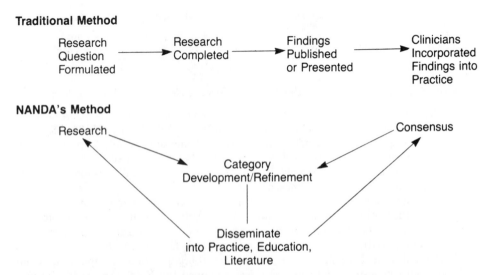

Fig. 1-1   Traditional method versus NANDA's method of incorporating scientific advances into practice.

tion of nursing diagnoses and to serve as a forum for issues pertaining to development and classification of nursing knowledge. It includes a section on news related to board and committee activities.

Evolving Nursing Diagnoses

According to Maas, Hardy, and Craft (1990), "for the science of a practice discipline to progress, the concepts that describe subject matter of the field must be identified, defined, and empirically validated."

Classification systems for other professions (such as physicians, biologists, and pharmacists) developed over hundreds of years and continue to change and evolve. For example, AIDS did not appear in the IDC 10 years ago. But now, after the disorder was added to the IDC and given the label AIDS, all physicians are required to use this diagnostic label. Standardization gives users the expectation of, as Gordon (1990) states, "established usage and meaning for each diagnostic label."

The process of establishing usage and meaning for diagnostic labels in nursing has been both exciting and frustrating. From 1973 to 1984, nursing diagnoses approved by NANDA were developed by groups of nurses invited to participate at the National Conferences. At these conferences, nurses with various clinical and educational experience collaborated to identify and describe health problems that nurses diagnose and treat. These nurses drew on their clinical experience on related literature to identify those clinical phenomena that occur in various states of health, then developed defining characteristics to describe these states. It was expected that this approach initially would yield fairly general nursing diagnoses that most nurses could use. The process for generating and accepting nursing diagnoses changed in 1984, when NANDA established a Diagnostic Review Committee (DRC) to develop a process for review and approval of proposed changes to the list of approved diagnoses. With each subsequent review cycle, the documentation requirements for submitting a proposed change have increased appreciably, owing in large part to the need for a thorough literature investigation of the change. Since 1980, published (and unpublished) research studies on nursing diagnosis have increased greatly. In 1990, the Cumulative Index of Nursing and Allied Health (CINAHL) began indexing all NANDA diagnosis-related articles. Currently, the index contains more than 1300 citations, including nursing dissertations, research and clinical application reports, and conference proceedings.

Avant (1990) describes the need to apply both art and science in developing nursing diagnoses. First, a creative force is necessary to stimulate the exploration of concepts and the development of inventive diagnostic labels and taxonomic structures—the art. Next comes the need for systematic validation of concepts, nursing diagnoses, and the taxonomic structures—the science. In most cases, a single nurse simply is not qualified to bring both art and science to diagnosis development. As Avant (1990) explains, "teams of researchers and clinicians working together would result in much more creative, precise, and useful concepts."

Concept Development and Formalization

Each nursing diagnosis represents a concept that nurses "claim as an area of accountability for research on the phenomena" (Gordon, 1990). In nursing practice, such concepts provide a guiding structure for identifying, naming, and finally diagnosing. As Gordon (1990) explains, "we see what we are ready to see, and perceptual readiness (or cue sensitivity) depends to a large degree on the availability and accessibility of concepts within the structure of long-term memory." Ignorance of basic concepts can interfere with good nursing care. For example, a beginning student reports that a client is drinking a lot of fluid, urinating frequently, and reporting constant hunger. The student likely would recognize these symptoms as abnormal but might not know that, as a cluster, they represent a concept (in this case, a medical disorder)—diabetes mellitus.

Unfortunately, many current NANDA-approved diagnoses are too abstract—such as *Altered Thought Processes*—or overlap unnecessarily with other diagnoses—for example, *Altered Family Processes* and *Ineffective Family Coping: Compromised*. Unclear and imprecise concepts in the literature increase the risk of diagnostic error in clinical situations. To address these problems, NANDA's strategic plan for 1990–1993 contains six priorities. Table 1-2 presents the NANDA priority for refinement and validation.

Concept formalization requires research validation using qualitative and/or quantitative methods. Gordon (1990) recommends a qualitative method when the focus is on concept generation, followed by quantitative methods to validate clinical data, such as signs, symptoms, and risk factors. Two excellent resources for more information on nursing diagnosis research methods are NANDA's *Monograph on Research Methods for Validating Nursing Diagnosis,* which discusses selected research methodologies (qualitative, quantitative, and mixed), and Avant and Walker's *Strategies for Theory Construction in Nursing,* which provides in-depth exploration of concept development and validation.

The Diagnostic Review Process

Developing a complete classification system for nursing diagnosis has proven to be a slow and difficult process involving extensive review and evaluation. Obviously, nursing cannot stop and wait until its classification system is complete, so practice continues while the system evolves.

As outlined in Appendix I, NANDA Guidelines for Submission, a proposal for accepting a new diagnosis or for revising or deleting an existing diagnosis is submitted to NANDA's Diagnostic Review Committee (DRC).

First, the proposal is reviewed by the DRC chairperson for completeness. Once a proposal is deemed complete, it is then reviewed by the entire DRC committee. Based on its review, the committee makes one of three recommendations:

- Accepting it for expert advisory panel review
- Returning it to the originator for revisions

Table 1-2   **Priority 4—NANDA Strategic Plan, 1990–1993**

4. *Continue To Refine The Diagnostic Labels and Components Through Research*
   a. Evaluate the approved diagnoses for consistency and accuracy according to NANDA's nursing diagnosis definition.
   b. Identify gaps in defining characteristics that require further development.
   c. Evaluate developed diagnoses and components in relationship to changes inherent in Taxonomy II, *e.g.,* axes.
   d. Generate research questions for proposal and facilitate focused research groups.
   e. Establish a plan for the development of a research data bank.
   f. Direct research activities for validation of approved diagnoses.
   g. Disseminate monograph of 1989 research conference. Consider a plan for a 1991 conference in combined effort with DRC, Taxonomy and Research.
   h. Develop a plan to facilitate NANDA's involvement in integration of nursing diagnoses into information systems with retrieval capabilities.

Table 1-3 **Reasons for Proposed Nursing Diagnosis "Not Accepted"
for Expert Advisory Panel Review**

• Represents a medical diagnosis
• Represents a treatment or procedure
• Did not represent a human response
• Defining characteristics for actual nursing diagnosis are not cues or signs/symptoms
• Defining characteristics for high-risk nursing diagnosis are not high risk factors

• Not accepting it (see Table 1-3 for various rationales the DRC committee can cite for rejecting a proposal)

A group of selected nurses with expertise in a clinical specialty or concept, the expert advisory panel advises the DRC on the development and utility of the proposed diagnosis. An accepted diagnosis is forwarded to the NANDA Board, then to the General Assembly for the next round of approval, and finally to the entire NANDA membership for a mail-in vote on final acceptance. Figure 1-2 diagrams this diagnosis review process.

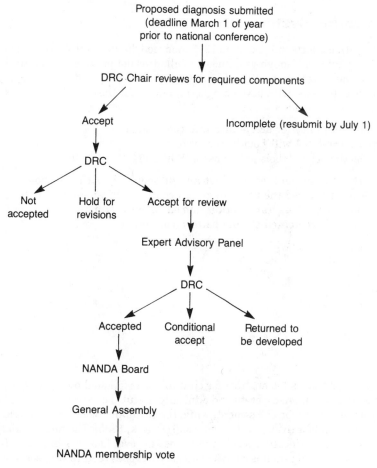

Fig. 1-2 The diagnosis review cycle.

This review process has come under attack on various fronts. As the requirements for developing and submitting a diagnosis to NANDA become ever more rigorous, the need for a membership vote to secure final acceptance seems unwieldy and outmoded. Concluding a scientific exploration with a vote on its findings seems to make little sense. Avant, for one, describes this voting requirement as "unwise and scientifically unsound" (1990).

Beyond the review and approval process, NANDA's list of nursing diagnoses itself also has come under criticism. Some nurses have criticized the list for being too broad or too restrictive, and certain diagnoses as being too medical, too abstract, or too unfamiliar. Some nurses are philosophically opposed to the use of such diagnoses as *Noncompliance* or *Knowledge Deficit*.

Disagreement with particular items in any classification system can be expected. However, the individual has always had the prerogative of simply not using those items. For example, in medicine a physician may disagree with the diagnosis *schizophrenia* and will refrain from using it in his practice. This physician does not reject the entire medical classification system, only one diagnosis. Furthermore, systems change. When the medical classification system was still evolving, dropsy was listed as an accepted diagnosis; years later, however, it was removed.

Classification Systems

The classification efforts that began in 1973 produced diagnoses that are listed alphabetically. The alphabet, although well known to all, does not provide a theoretical basis for the work of classification. In 1976, Sister Callista Roy proposed convening a group of nurse theorists to assist with developing a framework for the classification system. This framework would provide:

- Rules for eligibility for acceptance into the system
- The place the label will hold in the system
- Rules for the set of labels and subsets (Roy, 1984)

The work of the initial theorist group and subsequently of the taxonomic committee of NANDA has produced the beginnings of a conceptual framework for the diagnostic classification system. This framework is named NANDA Nursing Diagnosis Taxonomy I; the taxonomy is composed of nine patterns of human response:

- Exchanging
- Communicating
- Relating
- Valuing
- Choosing
- Moving
- Perceiving
- Knowing
- Feeling

Each pattern that is too abstract for clinical use is followed by two or more levels of abstraction that are more concrete and clinically useful. The second level could become the category structure for assessment, while the third and below levels would serve as the diagnostic label for the individual or group (Kritek, 1986). The nursing diagnoses at level five are more clinically specific than those at level four. For example, *Ineffective Individual Coping* still remains a useful category but does require very specific etiologic

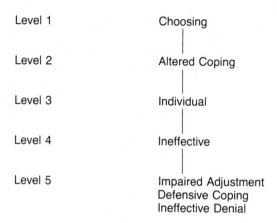

Level 1	Choosing
Level 2	Altered Coping
Level 3	Individual
Level 4	Ineffective
Level 5	Impaired Adjustment Defensive Coping Ineffective Denial

Fig. 1-3   Diagram showing one set of multiple levels of abstraction associated with tHe human response pattern of choosing.

or contributing factors to determine nursing prescriptions for treatment. Figure 1-3 illustrates the levels of abstraction related to one of the human response patterns—choosing.

For further discussion of the diagnostic classification system and for material on the concept of the unitary person, the reader is referred to the proceedings of the fifth, sixth, seventh, and eighth NANDA conferences.

Summary

The development of a classification system for nursing diagnoses has been ongoing since 1973. During this period, the initial question—"Does nursing really need a classification system?"—has been replaced by "How can such a system be developed in a scientifically sound manner?" The ANA has designated NANDA as the official organization to develop this classification system. Despite problems, through the concerted effort of many fine clinical nurses, nurse researchers, and other nursing professionals and organizations, this evolving classification system increasingly reflects both the art and science of nursing.

References

Avant, K. C. (1990). The art and science in nursing diagnosis development. *Nursing Diagnosis, 1*(2), 51–56.

Bircher, A. (1975). On the development and classification of nursing diagnoses. *Nursing Forum, 14,* 10–29.

Breu, C., Dracup, K., & Walden, J. (1987). Integration of nursing diagnoses in the critical care literature. *Heart Lung, 16,* 605–616.

Editorial (1990). NANDA definition. *Nursing Diagnosis, 1*(2), 50.

Gordon, M. (1990). Toward theory-based diagnostic categories. *Nursing Diagnosis, 1*(1), 511.

Gordon, M. (1982). Historical perspective: The National Group for Classification of Nursing Diagnoses. In Kim, M. J. & Moritz, D. A. (Eds.). *Classification of nursing diagnoses.* New York: McGraw-Hill.

Kritek, P. B. (1978). The generation and classification of nursing diagnoses: Toward a theory of nursing. *Image, 10*(2), 33–40.

Maas, M., Hardy, M., & Craft, M. (1990). Some methodologic considerations in nursing diagnoses. *Nursing Research, 1*(1), 24–30.

Roy, C. (1984). Framework for classification systems development: Progress and issues. In Kim, M. J., McFarland, G., & McFarlane, A. (Eds.). *Classification of nursing diagnoses.* New York: McGraw-Hill.

Shoemaker, J. K. (1984). Essential features of a nursing diagnosis. In Kim, M. J., McFarland, G., & McLane, A. (Eds.). *Classification of nursing diagnoses.* New York: McGraw-Hill.

Styles, M. M. (1982). *On nursing: Toward a new endowment.* St. Louis: C. V. Mosby.

2

Nursing Diagnosis: Types and Components

As discussed in Chapter 1, nursing diagnosis involves both a structure and a process. The structure of a nursing diagnosis—its components—depends on its type: actual, high risk, possible, wellness, or syndrome.

Actual Nursing Diagnoses

An actual nursing diagnosis represents a state that has been clinically validated by identifiable major defining characteristics. This type of nursing diagnosis has four components: label, definition, defining characteristics, and related factors.

Label

The qualifying term (such as an adjective) beginning an actual nursing diagnosis, the label should be descriptive of the diagnosis definition and defining characteristics (Gordon, 1990). Whenever possible, it should be a precise qualifier, such as "altered," "impaired," "deficit," "ineffective," or "dysfunctional," rather than a more subjective and vague modifier, such as "maladaptive," "poor," or "inappropriate." The term "actual" is not part of the label in an actual nursing diagnosis.

Definition

By expressing a clear, precise meaning of the diagnosis, the definition helps differentiate a particular diagnosis from similar diagnoses. The definition should be conceptual and consistent with the label and defining characteristics (Gordon, 1990).

Defining Characteristics

In an actual nursing diagnosis, defining characteristics refer to clinical cues—subjective and objective signs or symptoms that, in a cluster, point to the nursing diagnosis.

Before 1986, all defining characteristics were listed together without regard for criticalness to the diagnosis. When attempts were made to differentiate critical cues from other listed cues, critical usually was defined as "must be present 100% of the time"—which proved to be an unwieldy and ultimately unworkable restriction.

Defining characteristics are now separated into major and minor designations. In NANDA's revised Guidelines for Submission (see Appendix I), major defining characteristics are defined as critical indicators present 80%–100% of the time; minor defining characteristics, as supporting indicators, occur 50%–79% of the time. For an example of this differentiation, see Table 2-1, which lists major and minor defining characteristics for the nursing diagnosis *Defensive Coping*.

Through the use of research designs such as Fehring's diagnostic content validity (DCV) scores, the category can be researched to differentiate between major and minor.

All the categories accepted by NANDA are approved for clinical testing, but many have not been clinically tested. This author uses the consensus of experts to differentiate between major and minor. The consensus method is more valid if major is defined as "must be present (100%)." Thus, when clinical validation studies identify the major as between 80% and 100%, this author will reflect the major as 80%–100% instead of 100%.

Table 2-1 **Frequency Scores for Defining Characteristics of Defensive Coping**

Defining Characteristics

Major (80%–100%)

Denial of obvious problems/weaknesses	0.866
Projection of blame/responsibility	0.88
Rationalizes failures	0.836
Hypersensitive to slight criticism	0.858
Grandiosity	0.0795

Minor (50%–79%)

Superior attitude toward others	0.76
Difficulty in establishing/maintaining relationships	0.744
Hostile laughter or ridicule of others	0.707
Difficulty in testing perceptions against reality	0.625
Lack of follow through or participation in treatment or therapy	0.56

(Norris, J. & Kunes-Connell, M. (1987). Self-esteem disturbance: A clinical validation study. In McLane, A. (Ed). *Classification of nursing diagnoses: Proceedings of the seventh NANDA national conference*. St. Louis: C. V. Mosby)

In this edition, the following categories use 80%–100%, not 100%, as the criterion for major:

Hypothermia	Situational Low Self-Esteem
Colonic Constipation	Chronic Low Self-Esteem
Perceived Constipation	Self-Esteem Disturbance
Fatigue	Defensive Coping
Decisional Conflict	Altered Protection

Related Factors

In actual nursing diagnoses, related factors are etiologic or other contributing factors that have influenced the health status change. Such factors can be grouped into four categories: pathophysiologic (biologic or psychologic), treatment-related, situational (environmental, personal), and maturational. Table 2-2 lists examples of these factors.

The following example illustrates the components of an actual nursing diagnosis, in this case the diagnosis *Situational Low Self-Esteem*.

Definition

Situational Low Self-Esteem: The state in which an individual who previously had positive self-esteem experiences negative feelings about self in response to an event (loss, change).

Defining Characteristics*

Major (80%–100%)

- Episodic occurrence of negative self-appraisal in response to life events in a person with a previous positive self-evaluation
- Verbalization of negative feelings about self (helplessness, uselessness)

*Source: Norris, J. & Kunes-Connell, M. (1987). Self-esteem disturbance: A clinical validation study. In McLane, A. (Ed). *Classification of nursing diagnoses: Proceedings of the seventh NANDA national conference*. St. Louis: C. V. Mosby.

Table 2-2 **Examples of Related Factors**

Pathophysiologic (biologic or psychologic)
  Compromised immune system
  Inadequate peripheral circulation

Treatment-related
  Medications
  Diagnostic studies
  Surgery
  Treatments

Situational
  Environmental
    Home
    Community
    Institution
  Personal
    Life experiences
    Roles

Maturational
  Age-related influences

Minor (50%–79%)

- Self-negating verbalizations
- Expressions of shame/guilt
- Evaluates self as unable to handle situations/events
- Difficulty making decisions

Related Factors

Pathophysiologic

    Loss of body parts
    Loss of body function(s)
    Disfigurement (trauma, surgery, birth defects)

Situational (personal, environmental)

    Hospitalization
    Loss of job or ability to work
    Death of significant other
    Separation from significant other
    Increase/decrease in weight
    Pregnancy
    Unemployment
    Financial problems
    Relationship problems
      Marital discord   Step-parents
      Separation   In-laws
    Failure in school
    Legal difficulties

Institutionalization
  Mental health facility   Orphanage
  Jail   Halfway house
Cultural influences
  Ethnic group   Minority
Drug/alcohol abuse by self or family member

Maturational
School-age
  Loss of significant others
  Failure to achieve grade level objectives
  Loss of peer group
Adolescent
  Loss of independence and autonomy
  Disruption of peer relationships
  Disruption in body image
  Interruption of intellectual achievement
  Loss of significant others
  Career choices
Middle age
  Signs of aging
  Menopause
  Career pressures
Elderly
  Losses (people, function, financial, retirement)

Even with defining characteristics and etiologic factors for each nursing diagnosis, nurses continue to have difficulty in using nursing diagnoses, as is illustrated by the questions cited in the Preface:

- What does the label really mean?
- What kinds of assessment questions will yield nursing diagnoses?
- How do I tailor a nursing diagnosis for a specific individual?
- How should I intervene after I formulate the diagnostic statement?
- How do I develop a care plan with nursing diagnoses?

To assist the nurse in using nursing diagnoses, Section II of this book, Manual of Nursing Diagnoses, has been designed so that each nursing diagnosis is described in terms of

- Definition
- Etiologic, contributing, and risk factors (related factors)
- Defining characteristics
- Focus assessment criteria (subjective and objective)
- Principles and rationale for nursing care

Each diagnostic category is further described in terms of one or more specific nursing diagnoses within the category. For example, take the diagnostic category *Impaired Tissue Integrity*. A specific diagnosis under this category would be *Impaired Skin Integrity*.

Each specific diagnosis is explained in terms of

- Assessment data (subjective and objective)
- Outcome criteria
- Nursing interventions

Thus, Section II provides an explanation of each nursing diagnosis, along with related interventions that will assist the nurse in applying nursing diagnoses in clinical practice.

High Risk Nursing Diagnoses

As defined by NANDA, a high risk nursing diagnosis is "a clinical judgment that an individual, family, or community is more vulnerable to develop the problem than others in the same or similar situation." Currently, all potential nursing diagnoses begin with the phrase "Potential for," as in *Potential for Infection*. Beginning in 1992, however, all potential nursing diagnoses will start with "High Risk for." In anticipation of this change, in this book all potential diagnoses will be labeled as "High Risk for."

This change in terminology and philosophy regarding vulnerability is important and timely. All clients are at risk for infection and injury in the hospital, long-term facility, or the community—however, some are at higher risk than others. In light of a health care delivery system that, for financial reasons, passes on sicker clients to nurses and allows less time for interventions, high risk nursing diagnoses provide nurses with a valuable means of identifying clients most vulnerable to problems.

For example, one postoperative client has been assigned a nursing diagnosis of *High Risk for Infection related to loss of protective barrier secondary to incision*. This generic diagnosis for all surgical clients is routine and as such is not included on this client's care plan but instead is part of the unit's standard of care. (See Chapter 5 for a discussion of standards of care.) In contrast, on the same unit is a diabetic client who underwent emergency surgery for a perforated duodenal ulcer. This client has a nursing diagnosis of *High Risk for Infection related to surgical incision and impaired healing secondary to diabetes mellitus and blood loss*. Unlike the generic diagnosis, this diagnosis is included in the client's individualized care plan because the client with diabetes is at *high* risk for infection, whereas the former client is merely at risk.

The validation to support an actual diagnosis is signs and symptoms, whereas the validation to support a high risk diagnosis is risk factors. For example:

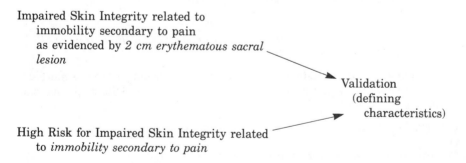

Impaired Skin Integrity related to
  immobility secondary to pain
  as evidenced by *2 cm erythematous sacral
  lesion*

Validation
(defining
  characteristics)

High Risk for Impaired Skin Integrity related
  to *immobility secondary to pain*

Label

In a high risk nursing diagnosis, the concise description of the client's altered health status is preceded by the term "High Risk for".

Definition

As in an actual nursing diagnosis, in a high risk nursing diagnosis the definition expresses a clear, precise meaning of the diagnosis. It should be conceptual and consistent with the label and risk factors, to enable differentiation from similar diagnoses.

Risk Factors

Risk factors for high risk nursing diagnoses represent those situations that increase the vulnerability of a client or group. These factors differentiate high-risk clients and groups from all others in the same population who are at some risk. Before 1990, the term "defining characteristics" was used to describe risk factors for potential nursing diagnoses. But the 1990 NANDA revisions now call for use of defining characteristics only in association with actual nursing diagnoses.

Related Factors

The related factors for high risk nursing diagnoses are the same risk factors previously explained. The components of a high risk nursing diagnostic statement will be discussed later in this chapter.

Possible Nursing Diagnosis

Possible nursing diagnoses are statements describing a suspected problem for which additional data are needed. It is unfortunate that many nurses have been socialized to avoid appearing tentative. In scientific decision-making, a tentative approach is not a sign of weakness or indecision but an essential part of the process. One must reserve judgment until the necessary information has been gathered and analyzed to arrive at a sound scientific conclusion. Physicians demonstrate tentativeness with the statement *rule-out (R/O)*. Nurses should also adopt a tentative attitude until data collection and evaluation have been completed and they are able to confirm or rule out. The word *possible* is used in nursing diagnoses to describe problems that may be present but that require additional data to be confirmed or ruled out. *Possible* serves to alert nurses to the need for additional data. With a possible nursing diagnosis, the nurse has some data to support a confirmed diagnosis but it is insufficient. Possible nursing diagnoses are two-part statements:

- The Possible Nursing Diagnosis
- The "related to" data that leads you to suspect the diagnosis

For example:

> Possible Self-Concept Disturbance Related to Recent Loss of Role Responsibilities Secondary to Exacerbation of MS

When a nurse records a possible nursing diagnosis, other nurses are now alerted to assess for more data to support or refute the tentative diagnosis. After additional data collection, the nurse may:

- Confirm the presence of major signs and symptoms, thus labeling an actual diagnosis or
- Confirm the presence of potential risk factors, a high risk or
- Rule out the presence of a diagnosis (actual or high risk) at this time

A decision tree to be used in differentiating among actual, high risk, and possible nursing diagnoses is shown in Figure 2-1.

Wellness Nursing Diagnoses

According to the NANDA definition, a wellness nursing diagnosis is "a clinical judgment about an individual, group, or community in transition from a specific level of wellness to

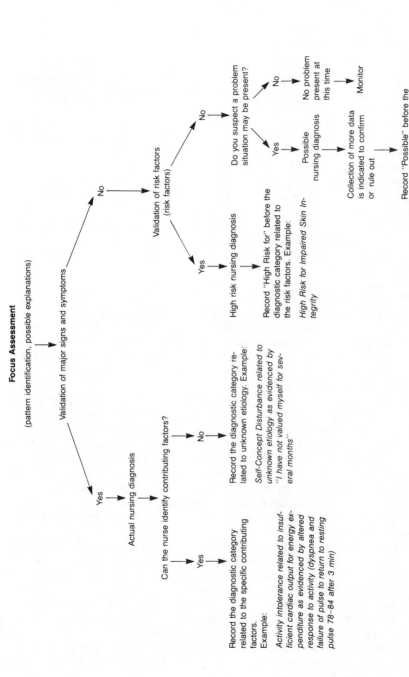

Fig. 2-1 Decision tree for differentiating actual, high risk, and possible nursing diagnoses. (© Lynda Juall Carpenito)

a higher level of wellness." For an individual or group to have a wellness nursing diagnosis, two cues should be present:

- Desire for a higher level of wellness
- Effective present status or function

Diagnostic statements for wellness nursing diagnoses are one-part statements containing the label only. The label for wellness nursing diagnoses begins with "Potential for Enhanced" followed by the higher level wellness that the individual or group desires, for example, *Potential for Enhanced Family Processes.*

Wellness nursing diagnoses do not contain related factors. Inherent in these diagnoses is a client or group who understands that higher level functioning is available if desired or capable. The nurse can infer capability based on the client's or group's expressed desire for or pursuit of health teaching.

As you know, a nursing diagnosis is a clinical judgment derived from observable and/ or reportable cues. Until wellness nursing diagnoses are investigated in the clinical setting, it may be advisable for the nurse to rely on reportable rather than observable cues. In other words, rather than to try and judge whether a client's or group's present health status or function is effective or ineffective, the nurse should rely on reports. Of course, as in all diagnostic reasoning, any clear evidence that refutes the reported data calls for further assessment.

Wellness and Nursing Diagnosis

Since 1973, many nurses have expressed concern that the NANDA list primarily represents alteration or dysfunction (Popkess-Vawter, 1984; Gleit, 1981). Many nurses practice with healthy clients, for example, new parents and school-age children, as well as clients of college health services and well-baby clinics. Nurses also help ill clients to pursue optimal health through interventions such as stress management, exercise programs, and nutritional counseling.

It is important to distinguish the focus of nursing's accountability to a client or group in the area of health and positive functioning. For example, is this focus on assisting a client with a poor diet to achieve better nutrition or on assisting a client with good nutrition to achieve optimal nutritional intake or to prevent inadequate intake? Of course, it is true that almost everyone can improve his or her nutritional status; however, in many cases the focus of nursing is not on changing effective functioning to optimal functioning, but rather on improving areas of compromised functioning. In this situation, the nurse would conclude that the client is exhibiting effective or positive functioning without assuming the responsibility for assisting the client to achieve a higher level of functioning at this time.

Table 2-3 illustrates statements that describe strengths for each of the eleven functional health patterns. These statements are also incorporated into the case study application in Chapter 4. When the nurse and client conclude that there is positive functioning in a functional health pattern, this conclusion is an assessment conclusion but by itself is not a nursing diagnosis. The nurse utilizes these data to help the client reach a higher level of functioning or uses the identified strengths in planning interventions for altered functioning or at-risk for altered functioning.

One could incorporate positive functioning assessment statements under each functional health pattern on the admission assessment tool. Figure 2-2 illustrates an example under the Sleep Rest Pattern.

For example, after assessing a client's role and relationship patterns, the nurse determines that the client exhibits positive functioning. If this client has recently received a diagnosis of cancer of the breast, the nurse can use the client's strength to assist her in dealing with the diagnosis. Another example would be a young couple who

Table 2-3 **Positive Functioning Assessment Statements Grouped Under the Functional Health Patterns**

Functional Pattern	Positive Functioning Assessment Statements
1. Health perception–health management pattern	1. Positive health perception Effective health management
2. Nutritional–metabolic pattern	2. Effective nutritional–metabolic pattern
3. Elimination pattern	3. Effective elimination pattern
4. Activity–exercise pattern	4. Effective activity–exercise pattern
5. Sleep–rest pattern	5. Effective sleep–rest pattern
6. Cognitive–perceptual pattern	6. Positive cognitive–perceptual pattern
7. Self-perception pattern	7. Positive self-perception problem
8. Role–relationship pattern	8. Positive role–relationship pattern
9. Sexuality–reproductive pattern	9. Positive sexuality–reproductive pattern
10. Coping–stress intolerance pattern	10. Effective coping–stress tolerance pattern
11. Value–belief pattern	11. Positive value–belief pattern

recently became parents. They report positive functioning in the role-relationship pattern. The nurse could use this information and the addition of a new baby to the family unit to assist the family to maintain effective role-relationship patterns. The diagnosis *High Risk for Altered Family Processes related to insufficient knowledge of stressors associated with new parenthood* could be used to describe the situation for which the nurse would teach specific interventions to deal with stressors of new parenthood.

Imagine that, 6 years later, this same couple reports a continued positive marital relationship and desires a higher level relationship. In this case, the nurse could use the diagnosis *Potential for Enhanced Marital Relationship* to describe the situation. In this situation, the couple's motivation is to improve on good function, not to prevent poor function, as was the case with the previously mentioned diagnosis *High Risk for Altered Family Processes*. Until the "Potential for Enhanced" diagnoses are developed, the nurse should continue to use *Health-seeking Behaviors (Specify)*.

Figure 2-3 illustrates a decision tree that the nurse can use to differentiate among positive/effective functioning and actual, high risk, and wellness nursing diagnoses.

Syndrome Nursing Diagnoses

A syndrome diagnosis comprises a cluster of actual or high risk nursing diagnoses that are predicted to be present because of a certain event or situation. Table 2-4 lists the related nursing diagnoses associated with the diagnosis *Disuse Syndrome*. When a nurse utilizes a syndrome diagnosis, the associated nursing diagnoses are clustered together to

Sleep/Rest Pattern

Habits: 8 hr/night _____ <8 hr _X_ >8 hr _____ AM nap _____ PM nap

Feel rested after sleep _X_ Yes _____ No

Problems: _X_ None _____ Early waking _____ Insomnia _____ Nightmares

☒ Effective Sleep/Rest Pattern

Fig. 2-2 Positive functioning statements related to sleep/rest pattern.

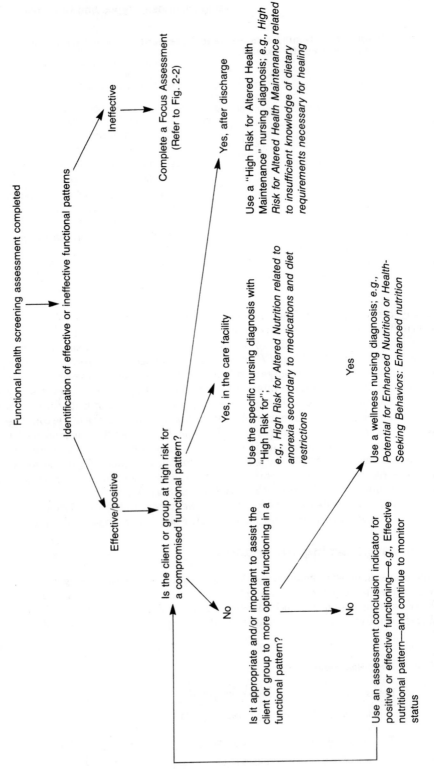

Functional health screening assessment completed

Identification of effective or ineffective functional patterns

Effective/positive

Ineffective → Complete a Focus Assessment (Refer to Fig. 2-2)

Is the client or group at high risk for a compromised functional pattern?

No

Yes, in the care facility → Use the specific nursing diagnosis with "High Risk for"; e.g., *High Risk for Altered Nutrition related to anorexia secondary to medications and diet restrictions*

Yes, after discharge → Use a "High Risk for Altered Health Maintenance" nursing diagnosis; *e.g., High Risk for Altered Health Maintenance related to insufficient knowledge of dietary requirements necessary for healing*

Is it appropriate and/or important to assist the client or group to more optimal functioning in a functional pattern?

No → Use an assessment conclusion indicator for positive or effective functioning—*e.g., Effective nutritional pattern*—and continue to monitor status

Yes → Use a wellness nursing diagnosis; *e.g., Potential for Enhanced Nutrition or Health-Seeking Behaviors: Enhanced nutrition*

Fig. 2-3 Decision tree for differentiating among positive/effective functioning and actual, high risk, and wellness nursing diagnoses.

Table 2-4 *Disuse Syndrome and Associated Nursing Diagnoses*

Disuse Syndrome
  High Risk for Constipation
  High Risk for Altered Respiratory Function
  High Risk for Infection
  High Risk for Thrombosis
  High Risk for Activity Intolerance
  High Risk for Injury
  Impaired Physical Mobility
  High Risk for Altered Thought Processes
  High Risk for Body Image Disturbance
  High Risk for Powerlessness
  High Risk for Impaired Tissue Integrity

emphasize the broad impact of the situation and to allow efficient intervention without using many separate diagnoses. Syndrome nursing diagnoses are one-part diagnostic statements because the etiology or contributing factors for the diagnosis are contained in the diagnostic label—for example, *Rape Trauma Syndrome.*

Types of Diagnostic Statements

Describing the health status of a client or group, diagnostic statements can have one, two, or three parts. One-part statements contain only the diagnostic label, as in wellness and syndrome nursing diagnoses. Two-part statements contain the label and the factors that have contributed or could contribute to a health status change, as in possible nursing diagnoses. Used for actual nursing diagnoses, three-part statements contain the label, the contributing factors, and the signs and symptoms of the health status alteration. Table 2-5 lists types of diagnostic statements with examples. The following section discusses three-part statements.

Three-Part Statement

Actual nursing diagnoses consist of three parts.

Diagnostic label + contributing factors + signs and symptoms

Example:

Grieving Related to Recent Loss of Job, as Evidenced by Statements of Anger at Coworkers and Sadness about Loss of Routine

The presence of signs and symptoms (defining characteristics) provides the clinical validation needed to confirm an actual diagnosis. Statements of high risk or possible diagnoses do not have a third part because in those situations signs and symptoms do not exist.

The third part of an actual nursing diagnosis can be documented using one of several methods including the PES format, the SOAPIE format, or focus charting.

Table 2-5 **Types of Diagnostic Statements**

One-part Statements
- Wellness Nursing Diagnosis, *e.g.,*
  Potential for Enhanced Parenting
  Potential for Enhanced Nutrition
- Syndrome Nursing Diagnoses, *e.g.,*
  Disuse Syndrome
  Rape Trauma Syndrome

Two-part Statements
- High Risk Nursing Diagnoses, *e.g.,*
  High Risk for Injury related to lack of awareness of hazards
- Possible Nursing Diagnoses, *e.g.,*
  Possible Body Image Disturbance related to reports of husband of isolating behaviors postsurgery
- Actual Nursing Diagnoses (when SIS are recorded outside the diagnostic statement, such as in a SOAP note), *e.g.,*
  Impaired Skin Integrity related to prolonged immobility secondary to fractured pelvis

Three-part Statement
- Actual Nursing Diagnoses, *e.g.,*
  Impaired Skin Integrity related to prolonged immobility secondary to fractured pelvis, as evidenced by a 2-cm sacral lesion

PES Format

Gordon identified the following format for recording the signs and symptoms of an actual diagnosis: problem, etiology, and symptom (PES).

Problem	Etiology	Symptom
↓	↓	↓
related to	as evidenced by	
Diagnostic	Contributing	Signs and
category	factors	symptoms

This format cannot be used for high risk or possible diagnoses because signs and symptoms are not present in those instances.

SOAPIE Format

The SOAPIE format of documentation is a systematic method for recording some events. The acronym refers to the following elements:

S = Subjective data
O = Objective data
A = Analysis or diagnosis
P = Plan
I = Implementation
E = Evaluation

The following is an example of the SOAPIE format for a newly validated nursing diagnosis:

S = "I am afraid something terrible will happen."
    "My neighbor had a myelogram and suffered with a headache for a month afterward."
O = N/A

A = Fear related to possible negative effects secondary to scheduled myelogram
P = Refer to care plan

If the nurse uses the SOAPIE format, the initial recording of the diagnosis will reflect the signs and symptoms. It is then unnecessary for the nurse to use the PES method.

Focus Charting

Lampe developed focus charting to provide a concise systematic method for recording client status and/or response. Focus charting uses the acronym DAR to record data. The following is an example of focus charting used to record a newly validated nursing diagnosis.

Focus: Fear related to possible negative effects secondary to scheduled myelogram

Data = Stated, "I am afraid something terrible will happen."
"My neighbor had a myelogram and suffered with a headache for a month afterward."
Action = Initiate care plan
Response = N/A

Writing Diagnostic Statements

Related to

In two- and three-part diagnostic statements, the phrase *related to* reflects a relationship between the first and the second parts of the statement. It is important that the nurse not link the statements with words implying liability, because such a relationship can result in legal or professional difficulty. Examples of such errors are:

- *Impaired Skin Integrity related to infrequent turning*
- *Potential for Injury related to the mother's frequently leaving the children at home unsupervised*

On the other hand, using the diagnostic label by itself without a *related to* etiologic or contributing factor can result in a vaguely stated problem that is not specific enough to direct individualized interventions.

The more specific the second part of the statement, the more specialized the interventions can be. The linking of the diagnostic label with contributing factors also assists the nurse in validating the diagnosis. For example, the diagnosis *Noncompliance* when stated by itself usually conveys the negative implication that the client is not cooperating. When the nurse relates the noncompliance to a factor, this diagnosis can transmit a very different message. For example:

- *Noncompliance: related to the negative side-effects of the drug (reduced libido, fatigue), as evidenced by "I stopped my B/P medicine."*
- *Noncompliance related to inability to understand the need for weekly blood pressure measurements, as evidenced by "I don't keep my appointments if I am busy."*

If the defining characteristics of a nursing diagnosis category are present, but the etiologic and contributing factors are unknown, the statement can be written as:

- *Fear related to unknown etiology, as evidenced by rapid speech, pacing, and "I am worried."*

The use of the term *unknown etiology* alerts the nurse and other members of the nursing staff to assess for contributing factors at the same time that they intervene for the present problem.

If the nurse suspects that certain factors are present or that there is a relationship between certain factors and the nursing diagnosis, the term "possible" can be used—for example, *Anxiety related to possible marital discord.*

Syndrome diagnoses that may represent an exception to the need to use the phrase "related to" are *Rape Trauma Syndrome* and *Disuse Syndrome.* As more specific diagnostic categories evolve, it may become unnecessary for the nurse to write "related to" statements. Instead, many nursing diagnoses of the future may be single-part statements, such as *Functional Incontinence* or *Unilateral Neglect.*

In an attempt to prevent nurses and students from using incorrect "related to" statements, some have recommended using only NANDA-approved labels as related factors for example, *Anxiety related to chronic pain.* This practice is problematic for several reasons, including:

• NANDA labels lack the specificity to direct interventions.
• Many contributing or risk factors cannot be described with a NANDA label, *e.g., Anxiety related to fear of unsatisfactory pain relief.*
• NANDA labels should be reserved for describing specific "clinical judgments," not used for related factors.

So, for example, instead of writing *Impaired Skin Integrity related to Disuse Syndrome,* diagnostic preciseness would encourage the nurse to use *Disuse Syndrome* only as a label. As a result, the nurse would more properly write a diagnosis of *Impaired Skin Integrity related to immobility secondary to pain.*

Directions for Care

The literature has specified that the nurse will direct interventions toward reducing or eliminating etiologic or contributing factors (Bulechek, Gordon). Specifically, if the nurse cannot treat the contributing factors, then the nursing diagnosis is considered incorrect. This is problematic.

As the diagnostic labels evolve into more specific labels, the nurse may encounter nursing diagnoses with contributing factors that are not treatable by nursing. Example:

High Risk for Infection Related to Compromised Immune System

The nurse does not prescribe for compromised immune system, but the nurse can prevent infection in some of these individuals. It is unnecessary to force the nurse to rewrite the contributing factors to reflect direction for treatment as

High Risk for Infection Related to Susceptibility to Environmental Contagions Secondary to Compromised Immune System.

In some instances, the label directs the interventions, and the etiologic or contributing factors are not involved.

Examples of such categories are:

• *Impaired Swallowing*
• *Functional Incontinence*
• *High Risk for Infection*

Figure 2-4 illustrates this relationship.

The nurse should be able to prescribe the definitive therapy for the nursing diagnosis. In the sample diagnosis *Sensory–Perceptual Alteration: Visual related to progressive loss of vision,* the nurse cannot prescribe the definitive interventions to achieve a client goal. The nurse should rewrite the diagnosis or reevaluate; perhaps the category is incorrect and would be better stated as *Fear related to progressive loss of vision.*

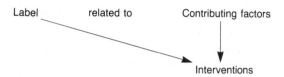

Fig. 2-4 Deriving interventions from the nursing diagnosis. (The author wishes to acknowledge the authors of this diagram as clinical nurse specialists at Harper Division of Detroit Medical Center.)

A thorough discussion of types of interventions for various types of diagnoses is presented in Chapter 3.

Non—NANDA-Approved Diagnoses

The issue of whether nurses should use only NANDA-approved diagnoses continues to spark debate. Some agencies and schools of nursing mandate use of only NANDA-approved diagnoses, whereas others do not support these restrictions.

Several authors, including Alfaro (1990), Gordon (1990), and Carpenito (1990), have made recommendations on using non-NANDA nursing diagnoses. Agencies and schools of nursing should have an approved list containing all NANDA-approved nursing diagnoses as well as any others approved for use by the agency or school. This list would help nurses avoid using unknown and possibly confusing labels.

Nurses, faculty members, or students could submit a non—NANDA-approved diagnosis to be considered for inclusion on the agency or school list for further clinical development. Of course, any proposed diagnosis should contain all its appropriate components, depending on its type. Including non—NANDA-approved diagnoses on agency or school lists can help encourage orderly, scientific development of nursing diagnoses while avoiding terminologic chaos.

Avoiding Errors in Diagnostic Statements

As discussed earlier, the nursing diagnostic statement reflects some change in the client's or group's health status related to factors that have contributed to or could contribute to its development, or a healthy state that may be threatened or achieved. Like any other skill, writing diagnostic statements takes knowledge and practice. To increase the accuracy and usefulness of diagnostic statements (and also to reduce the nurse's frustration), several common errors should be avoided.

Common Statement Errors

Nursing diagnoses are *not* new terms for:

- Medical diagnoses—*e.g.,* diabetes mellitus
- Medical pathology—*e.g.,* decrease in cerebral tissue oxygenation
- Treatments or equipment—*e.g.,* hyperalimentation, Levin tube
- Diagnostic studies—*e.g.,* cardiac catheterization

The nurse, however, may assess for the client's response to a situation and may validate a nursing diagnosis such as

High Risk for Altered Health Maintenance Related to Lack of Knowledge of Relationship of Activity to Insulin and Diet Requirements in Diabetes Mellitus

Nursing diagnostic statements should not be written in terms of:

- Cues—*e.g.,* crying, hemoglobin level
- Inferences—*e.g.,* dyspnea
- Goals—*e.g.,* should perform own colostomy care
- Client needs—*e.g.,* needs to walk every shift; needs to express fears
- Nursing needs—*e.g.,* change dressing; check blood pressure

Avoid legally inadvisable or judgmental statements, such as:

- *Fear related to frequent beatings by her husband*
- *Ineffective Family Coping related to mother-in-law's continual harassment of daughter-in-law*
- *High Risk for Altered Parenting related to low IQ of mother*
- *Noncompliance related to failure to return for follow-up visits*

A nursing diagnosis should not be related to a medical diagnosis. For example:

Self-Concept Disturbance Related to Multiple Sclerosis or Anxiety Related to Myocardial Infarction

If the use of a medical diagnosis adds clarity to the diagnosis, it can be linked to the statement with a *secondary to* (2°), as follows:

Self-Concept Disturbance Related to Recent Losses of Role Responsibilities Secondary to Multiple Sclerosis, as Evidenced by, "My Mother Comes Every Day to Run My House," "I Can No Longer Be the Woman in Charge of My House."

Each nursing diagnosis in Section II contains a section presenting examples of common statement errors followed by an explanation with the corrected example.

Ethical Considerations in Nursing Diagnosis

Nurses and other health professionals commonly are privy to significant personal concerns of clients under their care. According to the ANA Code of Ethics, "the nurse safeguards the client's right to privacy by judiciously protecting information of a confidential nature." However, the professional mandate to apply the nursing process for all clients sometimes places the nurse in a position of conflict. Certain information recorded in assessments and diagnostic statements may compromise a client's right to privacy, choice, and/or confidentiality. Nursing diagnostic statements should never be used to influence others to view or treat an individual, family, or group negatively. Great caution must be taken to ensure that a nursing diagnosis does no harm!

Nurses have a responsibility to make nursing diagnoses and to prescribe nursing treatment. Inherent in the diagnostic process and planning of care is the responsibility to ascertain that there is permission to write the diagnosis, treat the diagnosis, and/or refer the diagnosis as appropriate.

When a client shares personal information or emotions with the nurse, does this information automatically become part of the client's record or care plan? The nurse has two basic obligations to a client: to address applicable nursing diagnoses and to protect the client's confidentiality. The nurse is *not* obligated to pass on all of a client's nursing diagnoses to other nurses, as long as the nurse can ensure that all diagnoses are addressed. Consider the following example: Ms. Jackson, age 45, is hospitalized for treatment of ovarian cancer. At one point, she states to the nurse "the God I worship did this to me, and I hate him for it." Further discussion validates that Ms. Jackson is disturbed about her feelings and changes in her previous beliefs. Based on this assessment data, the nurse develops the nursing diagnosis *Spiritual Distress related to conflict between disease occurrence and religious faith* for Ms. Jackson. But what should the nurse do with the information, which Ms. Jackson makes clear she considers confidential? The nurse can assist Ms. Jackson with this nursing diagnosis through several different avenues, including:

1. Apprising her of available community resources for follow-up assistance in dealing with her spiritual distress
2. Continue assisting her to explore her feelings and using the nurse's notes to reflect discussions (without using quotation marks to denote her actual words)
3. Recording the nursing diagnosis *Spiritual Distress* on the care plan and developing appropriate interventions
4. Referring her to an appropriate spiritual advisor

Analysis of Options

Option 1 returns the problem to the client for management after discharge. Sometimes the nature of a problem and its priority among the client's other problems makes providing the client or family with information on available resources for use after discharge the most appropriate option. The nurse should, however, be cautioned against using this option merely to "wash one's hands" of a problem.

Option 2 allows the nurse to continue a dialogue with the client about the problem but without divulging the problem specifically. The problem with this option is that the client's care plan will not reflect this problem as a nursing diagnosis on the active list. As a result, should the client's nurse become unable to care for the client for some reason, this diagnosis likely would not be addressed.

Option 3 incorporates the problem, as a nursing diagnosis, into the client's care plan, where it can be addressed by the entire nursing staff. To help protect the confidentiality of very sensitive disclosed information, the nurse should make a few modifications, such as not quoting the client's statements exactly.

Documenting the nursing diagnosis on the care plan raises another possible dilemma. What if the primary nurse whom the client or family has confided in will not be able to follow the diagnosis full-time? How can the primary nurse involve others in addressing this diagnosis without violating the client's confidentiality? The primary nurse should encourage the client to allow another nurse to intervene in his or her absence. If the client refuses referral or another nurse, the nurse should document this in the progress notes, continuing to protect the client's confidentiality, for example:

> *Discussed with Ms. Jackson the feasibility of another nurse intervening with her regarding her spiritual concerns in my absence. Ms. Jackson declined involvement of another nurse. Instructed her on whom to contact if she changes her mind.*

This note documents the nurse's responsibility to the client as well as the nurse's accountability.

It is also important to note that, in most cases, the nurse should not share confidential information with family members without the client's permission. However, exceptions to preserving confidentiality "may be necessary if the information the client shares with the nurse contains indications of a threat to the lives of the patient or others" (Curtin & Flaherty, 1982).

Option 4 is a commonly chosen action for clients with spiritual conflicts. Before referring a client, however, the nurse should ascertain the client's receptivity to such a referral. To assume receptivity without first consulting the client can be problematic.

The client chose to share very personal information with a particular nurse, who then is obligated to assist the client with the problem. If the nurse believes that a religious leader or another professional would be beneficial to the client, the nurse should approach the client with the option. An example of such a dialogue follows:

> *Ms. Jackson, we've been discussing your concerns regarding your illness and how it has changed your spiritual beliefs. I know someone who has been very helpful for persons with concerns similar to yours. I'd like to ask her to visit you. What do you think about this?*

Such a dialogue clearly designates the choice as Ms. Jackson's. Just as nurses have an obligation to inform clients and families of available resources, clients have the right to accept or reject these resources.

Summary

On the surface, nursing diagnosis appears to be a convenient, simple solution to some of professional nursing's problems. This impression has led many nurses to use nursing diagnoses; however, many still do not integrate diagnosis into their nursing practice. Integrating nursing diagnosis into nursing practice is a collective and personal process. Collectively, the nursing profession has developed the structure of nursing diagnosis and continues to identify and refine specific diagnoses. Individually, each nurse struggles with diagnostic reasoning and confirmation as well as with related ethical implications. Collectively and individually, these struggles will continue.

References

Alfaro, R. (1990). *Applying nursing diagnosis and nursing process: A step-by-step guide* (2nd ed.). Philadelphia: J. B. Lippincott.

Bircher, A. (1975). On the development and classification of nursing diagnoses. *Nursing Forum, 14,* 10–29.

Breu, C., Dracup, K., & Walden, K. (1987). Integration of nursing diagnosis in the critical care literature. *Heart Lung, 16*(6), 605–616.

Bulechek, G., & McCloskey, J. (1985). *Nursing interventions: Treatments for nursing diagnoses.* Philadelphia: W. B. Saunders.

Carpenito, L. J. (1983). *Nursing diagnosis: Application to clinical practice* (3rd ed.). Philadelphia: J. B. Lippincott.

Carpenito, L. J. (1984). Is the problem a nursing diagnosis? *American Journal of Nursing, 84,* 1418–1419.

Carpenito, L. J. (1987). Impact of nursing diagnosis on practice and outcomes. *Heart Lung, 16*(6), 595–600.

Curtin, L., & Flaherty, M. J. (1982). *Nursing ethics.* Bowie, MD: Brady Communications.

Fehring, R. J. (1986). Validating diagnostic labels: Standardized methodology. In Hurley, M. (Ed.). *Classification of nursing diagnoses: Proceedings of the sixth NANDA conference.* St. Louis: C. V. Mosby.

Fry, V. S. (1953). The creative approach to nursing. *American Journal of Nursing, 53,* 301–302.

Gebbie, K. (1982). Toward the theory development of nursing diagnoses classification. In Kim, M. J. & Moritz, D. A. (Eds.). *Classification of nursing diagnoses.* New York: McGraw-Hill.

Gleit, C. & Tatro, S. (1981). Nursing diagnoses for healthy individuals. *Nursing Health Care, 2,* 456–457.

Gordon, M. (1990). Towards theory-based diagnostic categories. *Nursing Diagnoses, 1*(1), 5–11.

Gordon, M. (1982). *Nursing diagnosis: Process and application.* New York: McGraw-Hill.

Gordon, M. (1982). Historical perspective: The National Group for classification of nursing diagnoses. In Kim, M. J. & Moritz, D. A. (Eds.). *Classification of nursing diagnoses.* New York: McGraw-Hill.

Gordon, M. & Sweeney, M. A. (1979). Methodological problems and issues in identifying and standardizing nursing diagnoses. *Advances in Nursing Science, 2,* 1–15.

Kiley, M. L. (1987). Nursing complexity of two groups of surgical ICU patients. Presented at the Nursing Diagnosis in Critical Care Conference, Milwaukee, WI, March 1987.

Kritek, P. B. (1978). The generation and classification of nursing diagnoses: Toward a theory of nursing. *Image, 10*(2), 33–40.

Kritek, P. (1986). Development of a taxonomic structure for nursing diagnosis. In Hurley, M. (Ed.). *Classification of nursing diagnoses: Proceedings of the sixth NANDA national conference.* St. Louis: C. V. Mosby.

Maas, M., Hardy, M., & Craft, M. (1990). Some methodologic considerations in nursing diagnoses. *Research, 1*(1), 24–30.

Maryland Nurse Practice Act, July, 1986.

McCourt, A. & Carroll-Johnson, R. M. (Eds.) (In press). *Classification of nursing diagnoses: Proceeding of the ninth NANDA national conference.* Philadelphia: J. B. Lippincott.

McLane, A. (1987). Measurement and validation of diagnostic concepts: A decade of progress. *Heart Lung, 16,* 616–624.

Norris, J. & Kunes-Connell, M. (1987). Self-esteem disturbance: A clinical validation study. In McLane, A. (Ed.). *Classification of nursing diagnoses: Proceedings of the seventh NANDA national conference.* St. Louis: C. V. Mosby.

Popkess-Vawter, S. (1984). Strength-oriented nursing diagnoses. In Kim, M. J., McFarland, G., & McLane, A. (Eds.). *Classification of nursing diagnoses.* St. Louis: C. V. Mosby.

Roy, C. (1984). Framework for classification systems development: Progress and issues. In Kim, M. J., McFarland, G., & McLane, A. (Eds.). *Classification of nursing diagnoses.* St. Louis: C. V. Mosby.

Shoemaker, J. K. (1984). Essential features of a nursing diagnosis. In Kim, M. J., McFarland, G., & McLane, A. (Eds.). *Classification of nursing diagnoses.* St. Louis: C. V. Mosby.

Styles, M. M. (1982). *On nursing: Toward a new endowment.* St. Louis: C. V. Mosby.

3

The Bifocal Clinical Practice Model

The official NANDA definition of nursing diagnosis, as discussed in Chapter 1, specifically links nursing diagnosis to nursing interventions. But what about other clinical situations—those not covered by nursing diagnoses—that necessitate nursing intervention? Where do they fit in the scope of nursing practice?

Along with independent nursing diagnoses and interventions, the practice of nursing also often involves a collaborative relationship with other health care disciplines. In many cases, such collaboration provides nurses with additional interventions to add to the nursing care plan. As in any collaborative relationship, functions and activities sometimes overlap.

In 1983, Carpenito introduced a model for practice that describes the clinical focus of professional nurses. This *bifocal clinical practice model* identifies the two clinical situations in which nurses intervene—independent practice and collaboration with other disciplines. This model not only organizes the focus of nursing practice but also helps to distinguish nursing from other health care disciplines.

As you know, nursing's theoretical knowledge derives from various fields, including the natural, physical, and behavioral sciences, the humanities, and nursing sciences. The major differences between nursing and the other health care disciplines with which it interacts lie in nursing's greater depth and breadth of focus as compared with other disciplines. Certainly, the nutritionist has more expertise in the field of nutrition, and the pharmacist in the field of therapeutic pharmacology, than any nurse has. Every nurse, however, brings a knowledge of nutrition and pharmacology to client interactions that is sufficient for most clinical situations. (And when a nurse's knowledge is insufficient for a situation, nursing practice calls for consultation with appropriate disciplines.) No other discipline has this wide knowledge base, possibly explaining why past attempts to substitute other disciplines for nursing have proved costly and ultimately unsuccessful.

Thus, any workable model for nursing practice must encompass all the varied

Pathophysiologic

Myocardial infarction
Borderline personality
Burns

Treatment-related
Anticoagulants
Dialysis
Arteriogram

Personal
Dying
Divorce
Relocation

Environmental

Overcrowded school
No handrails on stairs
Rodents

Maturational
Peer pressure
Parenthood
Aging

Fig. 3-1 Examples of pathophysiologic, treatment-related, personal, environmental, and maturational situations.

situations in which nurses intervene, while also identifying situations in nursing that nonnursing personnel must address. These situations can be organized into five categories: pathophysiologic, treatment-related, personal, environmental, and maturational, as shown in Figure 3-1. Keep in mind that, unlike medicine, nursing does not prescribe for and treat such situations; rather, it prescribes for and treats client *responses* to the situations. The bifocal clinical practice model in Figure 3-2 identifies these responses as either *nursing diagnoses* or *collaborative problems*. Together, nursing diagnoses and collaborative problems comprise the range of responses that nurses treat and as such define the unique nature of nursing. Table 3-1 describes the basic assumptions on which the bifocal clinical practice model rests.

Developing specific nursing diagnoses to describe all situations in which nurses intervene would result in a huge, unwieldy list. Attempting to attach a nursing diagnosis to every facet of nursing practice likewise would lead to misuse of nursing diagnoses and clinical dilemmas, including:

- Using nursing diagnoses without validation, *e.g.,* applying the nursing diagnosis *Altered Nutrition: Less than Body Requirements* for NPO clients

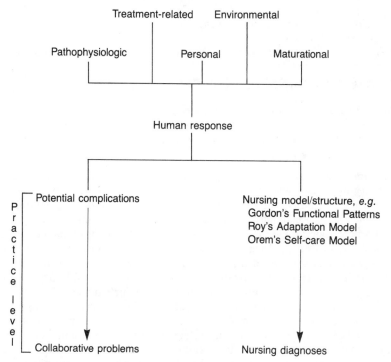

Fig. 3-2 Bifocal clinical nursing model. (© 1985, Lynda Juall Carpenito)

- Renaming medical diagnoses using nursing diagnosis terminology, *e.g., Decreased Cardiac Output* for myocardial infarction
- Omitting problem situations in documentation, when such situations cannot be described through the list of nursing diagnosis labels

Classifying certain situations as collaborative problems has helped minimize these problems while further refining the scope of nursing practice.

Table 3-1   **Major Assumptions in Bifocal Clinical Practice Model**

Client
- Refers to an individual, group, or community
- Continually interrelates with the environment
- Makes decisions according to individual priorities
- Is a unified whole, seeking balance
- Has individual worth and dignity
- Is an expert on his or her own health

Health
- Is dynamic, ever-changing state
- Is defined by the client
- Is an expression of optimum level of well-being
- Is the responsibility of the client

Environment
- Involves physiologic, treatment-related, physical and ecologic environment, external and internal personal stressors, and maturational factors

Nursing
- Promotes optimal health or a peaceful death
- Restores optimal functioning
- Reduces or eliminates internal or external factors that can or do cause compromised functioning

Understanding Collaborative Problems

Collaborative problems are certain physiologic complications that nurses monitor to detect onset or changes in status. Nurses manage collaborative problems utilizing physician-prescribed and nursing-prescribed interventions to minimize the complications of the events.

Unlike medical diagnoses, however, they represent situations that are the primary responsibility of nurses, who diagnose onset and manage changes in status. When a situation no longer requires nursing management, the client is discharged from nursing care. In some cases, a collaborative problem can revert to a medical diagnosis after discharge from nursing care; *e.g., Potential Complication: Ascites* could become a medical diagnosis of ascites. And certain physiologic complications are actually nursing diagnoses—*e.g.,* pressure ulcers (*Impaired Skin Integrity*)—because nurses can prescribe the definitive treatment. To illustrate this difference, Table 3-2 lists possible nursing diagnoses and collaborative problems for a client with pneumonia.

For a collaborative problem, nursing management focuses on monitoring for onset or change in status of physiologic complications and responding to any such changes with physician- and nurse-prescribed nursing interventions. The nurse makes independent decisions for both collaborative problems and nursing diagnoses. The difference is that with nursing diagnoses, nursing prescribes the definitive treatment to achieve the desired outcome; with collaborative problems, prescription for definitive treatment comes from both nursing and medicine.

Differentiating Nursing Diagnoses from Collaborative Problems

Both nursing diagnoses and collaborative problems involve all steps of the nursing process: assessment, diagnosis, planning, implementation, and evaluation. However, the nurse approaches these steps differently for a nursing diagnosis as compared with a collaborative problem. Figure 3-3 presents a graphic depiction of these different approaches. This section discusses some of the important differences in approach; refer to Chapters 4 and 5 for more detailed information on each aspect of the nursing process.

Assessment and Diagnosis

In nursing diagnoses, assessment involves data collection to determine the presence of signs and symptoms of actual nursing diagnoses or risk factors for high risk nursing diagnoses. In contrast, assessment for collaborative problems focuses on determining the status of the problem.

The nurse identifies the diagnosis of a collaborative problem when:

- Certain situations are present that increase the client's vulnerability for the complication, or
- The client has experienced the complication

Figure 3-4 provides examples illustrating this difference.

The nature of collaborative problems is that they occur or probably will occur in association with a specific pathology or treatment. For example, all postoperative abdominal surgery clients will be at some risk for certain problems, such as hemorrhage and hypoxia. Expert nursing knowledge is required to assess a particular client's specific risk for these problems and to identify the problems at an early stage to prevent morbidity and mortality.

In contrast, nursing diagnoses sometimes can be predicted or expected with a high degree of certainty but often require repeated assessments for validation. Because of the uniqueness of individual clients, identifying nursing diagnoses often is more difficult than identifying collaborative problems. This does not mean, however, that nursing diagnoses are more important.

Table 3-2 **Collaborative Problems and Nursing Diagnoses Grouped Under the Medical Diagnosis *Pneumonia****

PNEUMONIA
Collaborative Problems
PC: Septic shock
PC: Paralytic ileus
PC: Respiratory insufficiency

Nursing Diagnoses
Activity Intolerance related to compromised respiratory function
High Risk for Altered Oral Mucous Membrane related to mouth breathing and frequent expectorations
High Risk for Fluid Volume Deficit related to increased insensible fluid loss secondary to fever and hyperventilation
High Risk for Altered Nutrition: Less than Body Requirements, related to anorexia, dyspnea, and abdominal distention secondary to air swallowing
Ineffective Airway Clearance related to pain, tracheobronchial secretions, and exudate
High Risk for Infection Transmission related to communicable nature of the disease
High Risk for Altered Body Temperature related to body's response to infectious process
Altered Comfort related to hyperthermia, malaise, and pulmonary pathology
High Risk for Impaired Skin Integrity related to prescribed bed rest

Carpenito, L. J. (1990). *Handbook of nursing diagnosis* (4th ed.). Philadelphia: J. B. Lippincott)

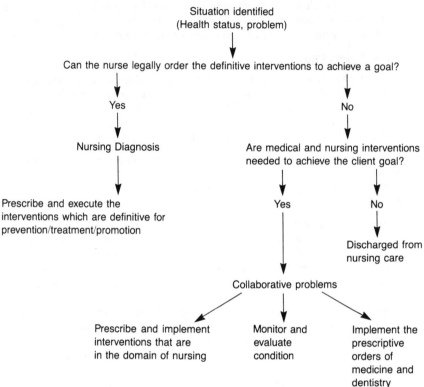

Differentiating Nursing Diagnoses from Other Client Problems

Fig. 3-3   Differentiation of nursing diagnoses from collaborative problems. (© 1990, 1988, 1985, Lynda Juall Carpenito)

Goals

Nursing diagnoses and collaborative problems have different implications for expected outcomes. Bulechek and McCloskey define goals as "guideposts to the selection of nursing interventions and criteria in the evaluation of nursing interventions." These authors continue by saying that "readily identifiable and logical links should exist between the diagnoses and the plan of care, and the activities prescribed should assist or enable the patient to meet the identified expected outcome." Thus, outcome criteria and interventions may be critical to differentiating nursing diagnoses from collaborative problems that nurses treat.

For example, if the following diagnosis is formulated:

High Risk for Fluid Volume Deficit related to loss of fluid during surgery and possible hemorrhage postop

the following client outcome may be written:
The client will demonstrate continued fluid balance, as evidenced by

• Absence of bleeding
• B/P and pulse within normal limits

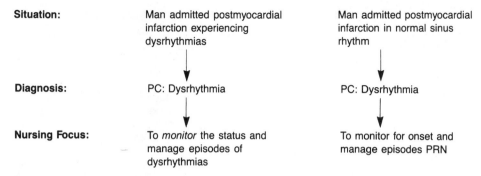

Situation:	Man admitted postmyocardial infarction experiencing dysrhythmias	Man admitted postmyocardial infarction in normal sinus rhythm
Diagnosis:	PC: Dysrhythmia	PC: Dysrhythmia
Nursing Focus:	To *monitor* the status and manage episodes of dysrhythmias	To monitor for onset and manage episodes PRN

Fig. 3-4 Examples of types of collaborative problems.

Client goals are used to determine the success or appropriateness of the nursing care plan. If the goals are not achieved or progress to achievement is not evident, then the nurse must:

• Reevaluate and
• Revise the plan

In the above example, if the client shows evidence of bleeding, is it appropriate for the nurse to change the goals? What changes in the nursing care plan would the nurse make to stop the bleeding?

Neither action is appropriate. The nurse would confer with the physician for delegated orders to treat the bleeding.

When the nurse writes client outcomes that require delegated medical orders for goal achievement, the situation is not a nursing diagnosis but a collaborative problem.

High Risk for Fluid Volume Deficit related to loss of fluid during surgery and possible hemorrhage postop would be better described as Potential Complication: Bleeding.

Client outcome criteria are inappropriate for collaborative problems. They represent criteria that cannot be used to evaluate the effectiveness or appropriateness of nursing interventions. Figure 3-5 illustrates the relationship of goals to nursing diagnoses and collaborative problems.

Intervention

According to Bulechek and McCloskey (1989), nursing interventions are "any direct care treatment that a nurse performs on behalf of a client. These treatments include nurse-initiated treatments resulting from nursing diagnoses, physician-initiated treatments resulting from medical diagnoses and performance of the daily essential functions for the client who cannot do these." Nursing interventions can be categorized into two types: independent (nurse-prescribed) and delegated (physician-prescribed). Regardless of type, all nursing interventions require astute nursing judgment, for the nurse is legally accountable for implementing them appropriately.

In 1987, Carpenito wrote that the relationship of diagnosis to nursing interventions is a critical element in defining nursing diagnosis. Many definitions of nursing diagnosis—including the 1990 NANDA definition—focus on the relationship of selected interventions to nursing diagnosis. The type of intervention helps distinguish a nursing diagnosis from a collaborative problem.

For both nursing diagnoses and collaborative problems, the nurse makes independent decisions regarding nursing interventions. The nature of these decisions differs,

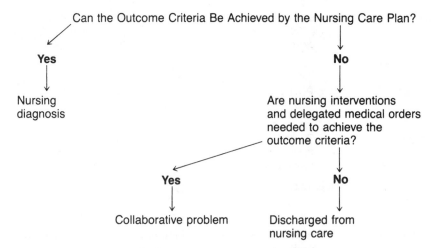

Fig. 3-5   Relationship of goals to nursing diagnosis and collaborative problems.

however. For nursing diagnoses, the nurse independently prescribes the definitive treatment for outcome achievement. In contrast, for collaborative problems, the nurse confers with a physician and implements physician-prescribed nursing interventions as well as nurse-prescribed interventions.

Some physiologic complications, such as pressure ulcers and infection from invasive lines, are problems that nurses can prevent. Prevention is different from detection. Nurses do not prevent hemorrhage or paralytic ileus but, instead, can detect its presence early to prevent greater severity of illness or even death. Physicians cannot treat collaborative problems without nursing's knowledge, vigilance, and judgment. For collaborative problems, nurses institute orders in addition to monitoring, such as ordering position changes, patient teaching, or specific protocols.

Figure 3-5 is a diagram designed to assist the nurse in differentiating a collaborative problem from a nursing diagnosis. As nursing's body of knowledge evolves, some of the collaborative problems of today may be nursing diagnoses tomorrow. Nurses are cautioned not to try to make a collaborative problem a nursing diagnosis simply because the latter is perceived as having greater value.

Evaluation

The nurse evaluates a client's status and progress differently for nursing diagnoses versus collaborative problems. When evaluating nursing diagnoses, the nurse:

- Assesses the client's status
- Compares this response to the outcome criteria
- Concludes whether or not the client is progressing toward outcome achievement

The nurse can record this evaluation on a flow record or on a progress note. In contrast, to evaluate collaborative problems, the nurse:

- Collects selected data
- Compares the data to established norms
- Judges whether the data are within an acceptable range

The nurse records the assessment data for collaborative problems on flow records or on progress notes if findings are significant. (On progress notes, the nurse should follow assessment data with documentation of the nursing management provided.)

Thus, evaluation of nursing diagnoses focuses on progress toward achieving client goals, whereas evaluation for collaborative problems focuses on the client's condition compared with established norms. Evaluation is discussed further in Chapter 5.

Collaborative Problem Diagnostic Statements

All collaborative problems begin with the diagnostic label "Potential Complication" (or PC), for example:

Potential Complication: Hypokalemia
Potential Complication: Sepsis
Potential Complication: Asthma

This label indicates the nursing focus for collaborative problems: to reduce the severity of certain physiologic factors or events.

For example, when a nurse reads on a problem list or care plan the diagnosis *Potential Complication: Hypertension,* the nurse knows that this client is either experiencing hypertension or is at high risk for hypertension. In either case the nurse will receive a report on the status of the collaborative problem and/or will proceed to acquire baseline data on the client's blood pressure. Changing the terminology to distinguish whether the client is actually hypertensive or simply at risk is not necessary or realistic, given the fluctuating condition of most clients.

If the nurse is managing a cluster or group of complications, the collaborative problems may be recorded together, for example:

Potential Complications: Cardiac
Potential Complications of pacemaker insertion

The nurse also can word the collaborative problem to reflect a specific cause, *e.g., Potential Complication: Hyperglycemia related to long-term corticosteroid therapy.* In most cases, however, such a link is unnecessary.

When writing collaborative problem statements, the nurse must make sure not to omit the stem "Potential Complication." This stem designates that nurse-prescribed interventions are required for its treatment. Without the stem, the collaborative problem could be misread as a medical diagnosis, in which case nursing involvement becomes subordinate to the discipline primarily responsible for the diagnosis and treatment of medical diagnoses—medicine.

Case Study Examples

Using the criteria questions from Figure 3-5, the nurse can differentiate collaborative problems from nursing diagnoses, as is illustrated in the following case study vignettes.

Case Study 1

Mr. Smith is a 35-year-old male admitted for a possible concussion after a car accident, with a physician's order for

• Clear liquid diet
• Neurologic assessment q 1 hour

On admission the nurse records

- Is oriented and alert
- Pupils at 6 mm, equal and reactive to light
- BP 120/72, pulse 84, resp 20, temp 99° F

Two hours later the nurse records

- Vomiting
- Restlessness
- Pupils at 6 mm, equal, with a sluggish response to light
- BP 140/60, pulse 65, resp 12, temp 99° F

Problem: Possible increased intracranial pressure (ICP)

Now apply the criteria questions to Case Study 1.

Q. Can the nurse legally order the definitive interventions to achieve the client goal (which would be a reversal of the increasing intracranial pressure)?

A. No, nurses do not definitively treat or prevent increased intracranial pressure. They collaborate with the physician for definitive treatment.

Q. Are medical and nursing interventions needed for goal achievement?

A.   Yes
                                       ↓
                         Collaborative Problems
                  PC: Increased Intracranial Pressure

| Prescribes and implements interventions that are in the domain of nursing | Monitors and evaluates condition | Implements the prescriptive orders of medicine and dentistry |

In this situation, the nurse would monitor to detect ICP or increasing levels of ICP. The nurse also prescribes interventions that reduce ICP, but these interventions are not considered definitive alone and must be accompanied by treatments prescribed by physicians. This problem is the joint responsibility of medicine and nursing.

Case Study 2

Mr. Green is a 45-year-old male with a cholecystectomy incision (10 days postop). The incision is not healing, and there is continual purulent drainage. The nursing care consists of

- Inspecting and cleansing the incision and the surrounding area q 8 hours
- Applying Stomahesive and drainage pouch to contain drainage and protect skin
- Promoting optimal nutrition and hydration to enhance healing

Problem: Adjacent skin at risk for erosion.

Now apply the criteria questions to Case Study 2.

Q. Can the nurse legally order the definitive interventions to achieve the goals (which would be continued intact surrounding tissue)?

↓

A. Yes, nurses do prescribe the interventions that will prevent skin erosion from occurring as a result of wound drainage.

↓

Nursing Diagnosis

↓

High Risk for Impaired Skin Integrity related to draining purulent wound

In this situation the nurse would prescribe the interventions to preserve adjacent skin area. No collaboration with medicine is warranted.

Since each individual is unique, it is difficult to develop exclusive criteria that will always differentiate nursing diagnoses from other client problems. Ultimately, the decision to use or not to use the diagnostic label will rest with the individual nurse until more refined defining characteristics for each category are developed and tested.

Learning to formulate nursing diagnoses is a skill that requires knowledge and practice. The nurse needs to familiarize herself with the nursing diagnoses and their components. Certain ones such as *Altered Bowel Elimination* and *Altered Nutrition* are familiar to most nurses and thus will be easier to use. Section II provides specific information on each category to increase a working knowledge of the various diagnoses.

Summary

According to Wallace and Ivey (1989), "understanding which nursing diagnoses are most effective and the situations in which the term collaborative problem is best applied helps group the mass of data the nurse must consider." The bifocal clinical practice model provides a structure for forming this understanding. In doing so, it uniquely distinguishes nursing from other health care professions, while providing nurses with a logical description of the focus of clinical nursing.

References

Alfaro, R. (1990). *Applying nursing diagnosis and nursing process: A step-by-step guide* (2nd ed.). Philadelphia: J. B. Lippincott.

Bulechek, G. & McCloskey, J. (1985). *Nursing interventions: Treatments for nursing diagnoses.* Philadelphia: W. B. Saunders.

Bulechek, G. & McCloskey, J. (1989). Nursing interventions: Treatments for potential nursing diagnoses. In Carroll-Johnson, M. (Ed.). *Classification of nursing diagnosis: Proceedings of the eighth national conference.* Philadelphia: J. B. Lippincott.

Carpenito, L. J. (1989). *Nursing diagnosis: Application to clinical practice* (3rd ed.). Philadelphia: J. B. Lippincott.

Carpenito, L. J. (1991). *Nursing care plans and documentation: Nursing diagnoses and collaborative problems.* Philadelphia: J. B. Lippincott.

Field, L. & Winslow, E. H. (1985). Moving to a nursing model. *American Journal of Nursing, 85,* 1100–1101.

Gordon, M. (1982). *Nursing diagnosis: Process and application.* New York: McGraw-Hill.

Ledy, S. & Pepper, J. M. (1985). *Conceptual bases of professional nursing.* Philadelphia: J. B. Lippincott.

Riehl, J. & Roy, C. (1980). *Conceptual models for nursing practice.* New York: Appleton-Century-Crofts.

Wallace, D. & Ivey, J. (1989). The bifocal clinical nursing model: Descriptions and application to patients receiving thrombolytic or anticoagulant therapy. *Journal of Cardiovascular Nursing, 4*(1), 33–45.

4

Deriving Nursing Diagnoses: Assessment and Diagnosis

Nursing diagnosis cannot be taken out of the context of the nursing process. To do so would result in a misuse of the concept and would lead to premature labeling or stereotyping. This, in turn, would interfere with accurate and careful observations and result in inappropriate nursing interventions.

Each client is an autonomous and precious person who interacts in a unique manner with the environment and must be assessed within the context of his uniqueness. Because nursing diagnoses are derived from these assessments and because people are continually interacting with their environment, the nurse must apply the process in a continuous round of assessment, diagnosing, planning, implementing, and evaluating.

Figure 4-1 illustrates the cyclic relationship of each step of the nursing process to the other steps and to the whole. Each step depends on the accuracy of the step preceding it. Assessment and evaluation are related to diagnosis, planning, and implementation. For example, when implementing the plan, the nurse also is assessing the client's current condition and evaluating response to the interventions. Thus, the separation of five steps is for explanation purposes; in reality, the process is continuous as collecting data, analysis, and diagnosing.

The Nursing Process

After a client has entered the health care setting (home, office, clinic, hospital), the nurse uses systematic observational and problem-solving techniques to identify his functional status: Is it positive or altered, or is the client at risk for altered functioning? The nurse and client collaborate on appropriate interventions and on the evaluation of the effectiveness of these interventions. The nursing process describes this method, for through its five components—assessment, diagnosis, planning, intervention, and evaluation—it sets the practice of nursing in motion.

The professional acknowledgment that the nursing process is pivotal to nursing is made evident by the fact that it is included in the definition of nursing in most nurse practice acts and in the conceptual framework of most curricula. Despite this emphasis, many nurses fail to apply the process systematically in their practice. The expertise and efficiency of nursing interventions depend on the accurate utilization of the nursing process. A nurse who is expert in this problem-solving technique can intervene in a skillful and successful manner with clients in a variety of settings.

The depth and breath of the knowledge of the individual nurse will directly influence the suitability and relevance of the care given. Students with a limited knowledge base can learn the nursing process by focusing initially on a selected area. As they gain more knowledge and experience, they can then increase their process skills. Experienced nurses can enhance their process skills by identifying areas that were previously avoided or misunderstood.

Assessment

Assessment, the first phase of the nursing process, is the deliberate and systematic collection of data to determine a client's current health status and functional status and

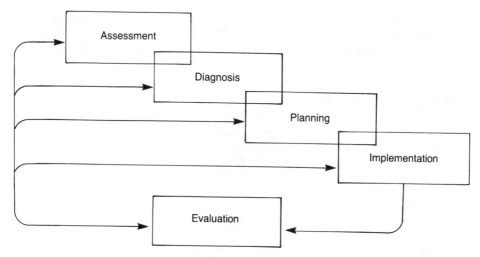

Fig. 4-1 Relationships between the steps of the nursing process. (Alfaro, R. (1990). *Application of nursing process: A step-by-step guide.* Philadelphia: J. B. Lippincott)

to evaluate the client's present and past coping patterns. Data are obtained by five methods:

- Interview
- Physical examination
- Observation
- Review of records and diagnostic reports
- Collaboration with colleagues

Data collection focuses on identifying the client's

- Present and past health status
- Present and past coping patterns (strengths and limitations)
- Present and past functional status
- Response to therapy (nursing, medical)
- Risk for potential problems
- Desire for a higher level of wellness

Nurses collect data to determine the need for nursing service and to assist other professionals (pharmacists, nutritionists, social workers, physicians) in determining their activities. It is therefore important that health care professionals freely exchange data about their clients to increase the quality and the validity of health care. For example, a nurse assesses the signs of orthostatic hypotension in a client. The problem is referred to the physician to investigate the cause and determine the treatment. The nurse plans nursing activities to help the client reduce those factors that contribute to the vertigo and also to prevent injury.

Unfortunately, many nurses primarily gather physiologic data for other professionals to use and ignore the other life processes, those that involve psychologic, sociocultural, developmental, and spiritual considerations. From a holistic view, an understanding of the interaction patterns in all five areas is needed to identify the client's strengths and limitations and help him achieve an optimal level of health. Ignoring any of the life processes can result in frustration and failure for all concerned.

Like the other components of the nursing process, the assessment process is dynamic and ongoing. During every nurse–client interaction, the nurse is continually processing data. The types of data gathered depend on the nurse's knowledge base, experience, and philosophy.

Data Collection Formats

Data collection usually consists of two formats, the nursing baseline interview and the focus assessment, each of which can be used either alone or in conjunction with the other.

Historically, the assessment forms used by nurses were organized under a body system format. Information collected under a body system model is useful to nursing but is incomplete because it does not include data on the areas of sleep, activity, spirituality, and so on. In an attempt to focus data collection on concerns that are more relevant to nursing, the body system model was discarded and replaced by a nursing model. Unfortunately, the nursing model alone failed to provide the nurse with complete data about physiologic functioning.

As was discussed in Chapter 2, nurses encounter, diagnose, and treat two types of human responses—those that can be described by nursing diagnoses and those that represent collaborative problems. Each type requires a different assessment focus.

Initial Assessment

An initial, or baseline, assessment involves collecting a predetermined set of data during the initial contact with the client, *e.g.,* on admission or first home visit. This assessment serves as a tool for making broad prediagnostic hypotheses or inferences or, as Gordon (1982) describes it, "narrowing the universe of possibilities." During this assessment, the nurse interprets data as significant or insignificant. This process is covered later in this chapter.

Assessment Framework

As discussed earlier, nursing assessment should focus on collecting data that validate nursing diagnoses. Gordon's system of functional health patterns provides an excellent, relevant format for nursing data collection.

Functional Health Patterns. To direct the nurse in collecting data to determine an individual's or group's health status and functioning. Gordon has developed a system for organizing a nursing assessment based on function. After data collection is complete, the nurse and client can determine positive functioning, altered functioning, or at-risk status for altered functioning. Altered functioning is defined as functioning that is perceived as a negative change or as undesirable by the client (individual or group). These functional health patterns include:

1. Health perception–health management pattern
2. Nutritional–metabolic pattern
3. Elimination pattern
4. Activity–exercise pattern
5. Sleep–rest pattern
6. Cognitive–perceptual pattern
7. Self-perception pattern
8. Role–relationship pattern
9. Sexuality–reproductive pattern
10. Coping–stress tolerance pattern
11. Value–belief pattern

This standardization of assessment data should not interfere with the nurse's theoretical or philosophical beliefs. It simply directs the nurse to the data that should be collected, not to the approach that should be used in interpreting the data or determining the interventions. Thus, the nurse who subscribes to Roy's adaptation framework, Orem's self-care model, or Rogers's life process model can use the functional health pattern framework developed by Gordon to gather baseline data, then apply his or her individual philosophy or framework for subsequent assessments.

The initial assessment presented in Figure 4-2 is organized according to functional health patterns. It is designed to assist the nurse in gathering initial data. Should questions arise concerning a pattern, the nurse is instructed to gather more data about the diagnostic category by using the assessment criteria under the category. This additional data is based on a focus assessment, a procedure that will be discussed later in this chapter.

Physical Assessment. In addition to functional pattern assessments, the nurse also collects data related to body system functioning. Physical assessment is the collection of objective data concerning the client's physical status. The techniques used include questioning, inspection, palpation, percussion, and auscultation. Physical assessment incorporates the examination of an individual from head to toe with a focus on the body systems.

To determine the purpose of the physical exam from a nursing perspective, we must ask the following question: What can a staff nurse do with the data acquired from performing a data-base physical assessment? If the answer is only to report the findings to the physician, perhaps the nurse should leave that portion of the examination to the physician. The important thing is to stress the assessment skills that are crucial for the nurse generalist. For example, the nurse needs to be able to assess signs of increased intracranial pressure but not necessarily to perform an entire neurologic exam. However, this does not mean that advanced skills should not be learned by nurses who routinely screen, case-find, and treat selected problems.

Table 4-1 lists those areas of physical assessment in which nurses should be proficient. The examination of these areas by the nurse can yield valuable data from which nursing care can be planned. Physical assessment as determined by nurses should be clearly "nursing" in focus. The diagnosis of pathophysiology should be left to the physician. The individual nurse must decide how important it is to his own practice to learn to palpate livers, auscultate murmurs, or use an ophthalmoscope. By examining her philosophy and definition of nursing, the nurse should seek to develop expertise in those areas that will enhance her nursing practice.

Keep in mind that separation of functional health patterns from physical assessment is done for organizational purposes only. No useful nursing assessment framework can restrict actual data collection in such a manner. Because human beings are open systems, positive or altered functioning in one functional health pattern invariably influences body system functioning and/or functioning in another functional health pattern.

Although functional health patterns provide a useful framework for organizing data collection and nursing diagnoses (see Table 1-1 for nursing diagnoses listed under functional health patterns), the nurse should not view these patterns as isolated. Rather, the patterns overlap—as do assessment data and nursing diagnoses. The following case study illustrates this concept.

Mr. Gene, age 61, is admitted for neurologic surgery. He has a history of peripheral vascular disease and Parkinson's disease. The nurse's initial assessment reveals the following findings under the functional health pattern "Activity–Exercise Pattern" and physical assessment of musculoskeletal function:

ACTIVITY–EXERCISE PATTERN
SELF-CARE ABILITY:

0 = independent	1 = Assistive device	2 = Assistance from others
3 = Asssistance from person and equipment		4 = Dependent/Unable

	0	1	2	3	4
Eating/Drinking	✓				
Bathing			✓		
Dressing/Grooming			✓		
Toileting			✓		
Bed Mobility			✓		
Transferring			✓		
Ambulating		✓			
Stair Climbing	✓				
Shopping					✓
Cooking					✓
Home Maintenance					✓

ASSISTIVE DEVICES: ____ None ____ Crutches ____ Bedside commode ✓ Walker
____ Cane ____Splint/Brace ____Wheelchair ____ Other ____

PHYSICAL ASSESSMENT
MUSCULAR–SKELETAL
Range of Motion: ✓ Full ____ Other _____
Balance and Gait: ____ Steady ✓ Unsteady
Hand Grasps: ✓ Equal ✓ Strong ____ Weakness/Paralysis (____ Right ____ Left)
Leg Muscles: ____ Equal ____ Strong ✓ Weakness/Paralysis (✓ Right ____ Left)

Depending on associated findings, these data could support various nursing diagnoses, such as *Self-Care Deficit, High Risk for Disuse Syndrome,* and *High Risk for
Injury.* Two of these diagnoses—*Self-Care Deficit* and *High Risk for Disuse Syndrome*—
are grouped under the functional health pattern Activity–Exercise, whereas *High Risk
for Injury* is listed under Health Perception–Health Maintenance Patterns.

Abnormal or otherwise significant physical assessment data can support various
nursing diagnoses or collaborative problems. For example, if inspection of Mr. Gene's feet
revealed a lesion on his left instep, the nurse would assign the primary nursing diagnosis
of *Impaired Skin Integrity.* If further questioning reveals that Mr. Gene doesn't understand why his feet are vulnerable and why daily foot care and inspection are necessary,
the nurse would identify another nursing diagnosis for him: *Altered Health Maintenance
related to insufficient knowledge of peripheral vascular disease and its effects on the feet.*

Assessment Format

The format of an initial assessment should be organized to permit systematic, efficient
data collection. The assessment form in Figure 4-2 illustrates the use of checking or
circling options, which can help save time when documenting findings. Of course, the
nurse can always elaborate with additional questions and comments. Certain functional
areas are better assessed using open-ended questions, such as family concerns regarding

Table 4-1 **Physical Assessment by Nurse Generalists**

Physical System	Criteria	
Sensory–Perceptual	Mental status Vision and appearance of eyes Hearing Touch Taste and smell	
Skin	Condition (color, turgor, character) Lesions Edema Hair distribution Breast	
Respiratory	Rate, character Breath sounds Cough	

Cardiovascular	Pulses (rate, quality, rhythm)
	  Apical
	  Carotid
	  Brachial
	  Femoral
	Blood pressure
	Circulation (mucous membranes, nail beds)
		Radical
		Dorsalis pedis
		Posterior tibial

Neurologic	Pupillary reactions Orientation Level of consciousness Grasp strength	
Gastrointestinal	Mouth, gums, teeth, and tongue (color and condition) Gag reflex Bowel sounds Presence of distention, impaction, hemorrhoids (external)	
Genitourinary	Presence of reaction Discharge (vaginal, urethral) Uterine response (pregnancy, postpartum) External genitalia	
Musculoskeletal	Muscle tone, strength Gait, stability Range of motion	

hospitalization. A printed data assessment form should be viewed as a guide for the nurse, not a mandate. All data-base forms should have a provision for allowing the nurse to defer the collection of selected data. Before requesting information from a client, the nurse should ask herself, What am I going to do with the data? If certain information is useless or irrelevant for a particular client, then its collection is a waste of time and often distressing to clients. Asking a terminally ill man how much he smokes or drinks, for example, is inexcusable unless the nurse has a specific goal. If a client will be NPO for an

(*Text continues on page 55*)

NURSING ADMISSION
DATA BASE

Date _____ Arrival Time _____ Contact Person _____ Phone _____
ADMITTED FROM: ____ Home alone   ____ Home with relative   ____ Long-term care
                ____ Homeless   ____ Home with _____   facility
                ____ ER   (Specify)   ____ Other _____
MODE OF ARRIVAL: ____ Wheelchair   ____ Ambulance   ____ Stretcher
REASON FOR HOSPITALIZATION: _____
_____

LAST HOSPITAL ADMISSION: Date _____ Reason _____
_____

PAST MEDICAL HISTORY: _____
_____

MEDICATION (Prescription/Over-the-Counter)	DOSAGE	LAST DOSE	FREQUENCY

HEALTH MAINTENANCE-PERCEPTION PATTERN
USE OF:
    Tobacco: ____ None ____ Quit (date) ____ Pipe ____ Cigar ____ <1 pk/day
                  ____ 1–2 pks/day ____ >2 pks/day Pks/year history _____
    Alcohol: ____ None ____ Type/amount ____ /day ____ /wk ____ /month
    Other Drugs: ____ No ____ Yes Type _____ Use _____
    Allergies (drugs, food, tape, dyes): _____ Reaction _____
_____

ACTIVITY/EXERCISE PATTERN
SELF-CARE ABILITY:
    0 = Independent   1 = Assistive device   2 = Assistance from others
    3 = Assistance from person and equipment   4 = Dependent/Unable

	0	1	2	3	4
Eating/Drinking					
Bathing					
Dressing/Grooming					
Toileting					
Bed Mobility					
Transferring					
Ambulating					
Stair Climbing					
Shopping					
Cooking					
Home Maintenance					

ASSISTIVE DEVICES: ____ None ____ Crutches ____ Bedside commode ____ Walker
                      ____ Cane ____ Splint/Brace ____ Wheelchair ____ Other ____

CODE: (1) Non-applicable (2) Unable to acquire
       (3) Not a priority at this time (4) Other (specify in notes)

Side One

Fig. 4-2 Assessment form. (© 1990, 1988, Lynda Juall Carpenito)

NUTRITION/METABOLIC PATTERN
Special Diet/Supplements _____
Previous Dietary Instruction: ____ Yes ____ No
Appetite: ____ Normal ____ Increased ____ Decreased ____ Decreased taste sensation
              ____ Nausea ____ Vomiting ____ Stomatitis
Weight Fluctuations Last 6 Months: ____ None _____ lbs. Gained/Lost
Swallowing Difficulty (Dysphagia): ____ None ____ Solids ____ Liquids
Dentures: ____ Upper (_ Partial _ Full) ____ Lower (_ Partial _ Full)
              With Patient ____ Yes ____ No
History of Skin/Healing Problems: ____ None ____ Abnormal Healing ____ Rash
                                       ____ Dryness ____ Excess Perspiration

ELIMINATION PATTERN
Bowel Habits: ____ # BMs/day ____ Date of last BM ____ Within normal limits
                  ____ Constipation ____ Diarrhea ____ Incontinence
                  ____ Ostomy: Type ____ Appliance ____ Self-care ____ Yes ____ No
Bladder Habits: ____ WNL ____ Frequency ____ Dysuria ____ Nocturia ____ Urgency
                  ____ Hematuria ____ Retention
Incontinency: ____ No ____ Yes ____ Total ____ Daytime ____ Nighttime
                  ____ Occasional ____ Difficulty delaying voiding
                  ____ Difficulty reaching toilet
Assistive Devices: ____ Intermittent catheterization
                       ____ Indwelling catheter ____ External catheter
                       ____ Incontinent briefs ____ Penile implant type _____

SLEEP/REST PATTERN
Habits: ____ hrs/night ____ AM nap ____ PM nap
           Feel rested after sleep ____ Yes ____ No
Problems: ____ None ____ Early waking ____ Insomnia ____ Nightmares

COGNITIVE–CONCEPTUAL PATTERN
Hearing: ____ WNL ____ Impaired (_ Right _ Left) ____ Deaf (_ Right _ Left)
             ____ Hearing Aid ____ Tinnitus
Vision: ____ WNL ____ Eyeglasses ____ Contact lens
            ____ Impaired ____ Right ____ Left
            ____ Blind ____ Right ____ Left
            ____ Cataract ____ Right ____ Left
            ____ Glaucoma
            ____ Prothesis ____ Right ____ Left
Vertigo: ____ Yes ____ No
Discomfort/Pain: ____ None ____ Acute ____ Chronic ____ Description _____
_____
Pain Management: _____

COPING STRESS TOLERANCE/SELF-PERCEPTION/SELF-CONCEPT PATTERN
Major concerns regarding hospitalization or illness (financial, self-care): _____
_____
Major loss/change in past year: ____ No ____ Yes _____
_____

CODE: (1) Non-applicable (2) Unable to acquire
          (3) Not a priority at this time (4) Other (specify in notes)

Side Two

Fig. 4-2 (continued)

SEXUALITY/REPRODUCTIVE PATTERN
LMP: _____
Menstrual Problems: ____ Yes ____ No _____
Last Pap Smear: _____
Monthly Self-Breast/Testicular Exam: ____ Yes ____ No
Sexual Concerns R/T Illness: _____
_____

ROLE-RELATIONSHIP PATTERN
Occupation: _____
Employment Status: ____ Employed ____ Short-term disability
                   ____ Long-term disability ____ Unemployed
Support System: ____ Spouse ____ Neighbors/Friends ____ None
                ____ Family in same residence ____ Family in separate residence
                ____ Other _____
Family concerns regarding hospitalization: _____
_____

VALUE-BELIEF PATTERN
Religion: ____ Roman Catholic ____ Protestant ____ Jewish ____ Other
Religious Restrictions: ____ No ____ Yes (Specify) _____
Request Chaplain Visitation at This Time: ____ Yes ____ No

PHYSICAL ASSESSMENT (Objective)

1. **CLINICAL DATA**
   Age _____ Height _____ Weight _____ (Actual/Approximate)
   Temperature _____
   Pulse: ____ Strong ____ Weak ____ Regular ____ Irregular
   Blood Pressure: Right Arm ____ Left Arm ____ Sitting ____ Lying ____

2. **COGNITIVE-EMOTIONAL**
   Language Spoken: ____ English ____ Spanish ____ Other _____
   Ability to Read English: ____ Yes ____ No _____
   Ability to Communicate ____ Yes ____ No _____
   Ability to Comprehend ____ Yes ____ No _____
   Level of Anxiety ____ Mild ____ Moderate ____ Severe ____ Panic
   Interactive Skills ____ Appropriate ____ Other _____

3. **RESPIRATORY/CIRCULATORY**
   Rate _____
   Quality: ____ WNL ____ Shallow ____ Rapid ____ Labored ____ Other _____
   Cough: ____ No ____ Yes/Describe _____
   Auscultation:
     Upper rt lobes ____ WNL ____ Decreased ____ Absent ____ Abnormal sounds _____
     Upper lt lobes ____ WNL ____ Decreased ____ Absent ____ Abnormal sounds _____
     Lower rt lobes ____ WNL ____ Decreased ____ Absent ____ Abnormal sounds _____
     Lower lt lobes ____ WNL ____ Decreased ____ Absent ____ Abnormal sounds _____
   Right Pedal Pulse: ____ Strong ____ Weak ____ Absent
   Left Pedal Pulse: ____ Strong ____ Weak ____ Absent

4. **METABOLIC-INTEGUMENTARY**
   SKIN:
     Color: ____ WNL ____ Pale ____ Cyanotic ____ Ashen ____ Jaundice ____ Other ____
     Temperature: ____ WNL ____ Warm ____ Cool
     Turgor: ____ WNL ____ Poor
     Edema: ____ No ____ Yes/Description/location _____
     Lesions: ____ None ____ Yes/Description/location _____
     Bruises: ____ None ____ Yes/Description/location _____
     Reddened: ____ No ____ Yes/Description/location _____
     Pruritus: ____ No ____ Yes/Description/location _____
     Tubes: Specify _____
   MOUTH:
     Gums: ____ WNL ____ White plaque ____ Lesions ____ Other _____
     Teeth: ____ WNL ____ Other _____
   ABDOMEN:
     Bowel Sounds: ____ Present ____ Absent

Side Three

Fig. 4-2 (continued)

5. NEURO/SENSORY

Mental Status: ___ Alert ___ Receptive aphasia ___ Poor historian
___ Oriented ___ Confused ___ Combative ___ Unresponsive
Speech: ___ Normal ___ Slurred ___ Garbled ___ Expressive aphasia
Spoken language_____ Interpreter _____
Pupils: ___ Equal ___ Unequal

Left: • • • • • • • ●

Right: • • • • • • • ●

Reactive to light:
Left: ___ Yes ___ No/Specify _____
Right: ___ Yes ___ No/Specify _____

Eyes: ___ Clear ___ Draining ___ Reddened ___ Other _____

6. MUSCULAR-SKELETAL

Range of Motion: ___ Full ___ Other _____
Balance and Gait: ___ Steady ___ Unsteady
Hand Grasps: ___ Equal ___ Strong ___ Weakness/Paralysis (_ Right _ Left)
Leg Muscles: ___ Equal ___ Strong ___ Weakness/Paralysis (_ Right _ Left)

DISCHARGE PLANNING

Lives: Alone ___ With _____ No known residence _____
Intended Destination Post Discharge: ___ Home ___ Undetermined ___ Other _____
Previous Utilization of Community Resources:
___ Home care/Hospice ___ Adult day care ___ Church groups ___ Other _____
___ Meals on Wheels ___ Homemaker/Home health aide ___ Community support group
Post-discharge Transportation:
___ Car ___ Ambulance ___ Bus/Taxi
___ Unable to determine at this time
Anticipated Financial Assistance Post-discharge?: ___ No ___ Yes _____
Anticipated Problems with Self-care Post-discharge?: ___ No ___ Yes _____
Assistive Devices Needed Post-discharge?: ___ No ___ Yes _____
Referrals: (record date)
Discharge Coordinator _____ Home Health _____
Social Service _____ V.N.A. _____
Other Comments: _____
_____

SIGNATURE/TITLE _____ DATE _____

Side Four

Fig. 4-2 (continued)

unlimited period of time, it is probably unnecessary for the nurse to collect data on nutritional patterns. The assessment will be indicated when the person resumes a diet.

If the client is extremely stressed, the nurse should collect only necessary data and defer the collection of functional patterns to another time or day. A stressed person may not be the best source of data because memory is often clouded.

The admission interview form can be structured to allow for deferring or not collecting certain data. The following codes illustrate the options:

1 = N/A, not applicable: applies to sections that are not suitable.
2 = Unable to acquire: applies to items or sections that need to be assessed but cannot be addressed at this time. For example, a confused patient may be unable to provide the needed information.
3 = Not a priority: applies to items or sections that are not appropriate to assess at this time.

4 = Other: applies to items or sections that are not assessed for reasons other than 2 or 3. For example, the admission interview may be discontinued to transport the patient for emergency surgery. This option requires an explanatory note in the chart.

If desired, the admission assessment form can be marked to indicate selected items that must always be assessed, unless, of course, the situation is an Option 2—unable to acquire.

When each question on the assessment form has either an answer or an answer code of 1, 3, or 4, the form should be viewed as complete. When the answer code of 2 is used, the form can be viewed as incomplete. If the information is collected later, the nurse should enter it on the form, then date and initial it, as shown on the following sample:

HEALTH MAINTENANCE–PRESCRIPTION PATTERN

USE OF: *7/8 ∠ ∅ C*
2 Tobacco: ✓ None ____ Quit (date) ____ Pipe ____ Cigar ____ <1 pk/day
                    ____ 1–2 pks/day ____ >2 pks/day Pks/year history _____
2 Alcohol: 7/8   ✓ None ____ Type/amount ____ /day ____ /wk ____ /month
2 Other Drugs: 7/8 ✓ No ____ Yes Type _____ Use _____
2 Allergies (drugs, food, tape, dyes): *none known* Reaction _____
_____   *7/8 ∠ ∅ C*

In an acute care setting, initial assessment should be completed as soon as possible after admission, preferably within 8 hours. In other care settings (such as community health, rehabilitation, mental health, and extended care facilities), performing a baseline assessment may be more appropriate at later client contacts rather than on initial contact. Obviously, a nurse–client relationship that evolves over weeks or months will allow a more detailed baseline assessment than can be obtained in an acute care setting. Keep in mind, however, that if complete baseline assessment is delayed, the nurse still should perform an abbreviated initial assessment of critical functions, such as elimination, self-care ability, and respiratory status. See Appendices II, III, IV, and V for sample initial assessment forms appropriate for mental health care settings, pediatric clients, extended care settings, and maternal clients, respectively.

Focus Assessment

Focus assessment is the acquisition of selected or specific data as determined by the nurse and the client or family or by the condition of the client. A focus assessment can take a few minutes or a longer period of time. The nurse who assesses the condition of a new postoperative client (vital signs, incision, hydration, comfort) is performing a focus assessment.

A focus assessment can also be carried out during the initial interview if the data collected suggest a possible problem area that needs to be validated or ruled out. For example, during the data-base interview, the nurse suspects that certain data (S_1, S_2) may represent a nursing diagnosis. The nurse considers a possible or tentative diagnosis. The nurse then collects additional data (focus assessment) to confirm or rule out the tentative diagnosis. This process can be depicted as:

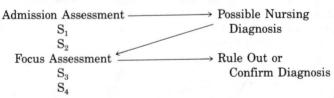

Admission Assessment ⟶ Possible Nursing
        S_1 Diagnosis
        S_2
Focus Assessment ⟵ ⟶ Rule Out or
        S_3 Confirm Diagnosis
        S_4

The nurse initiates focus assessment after reported or observed data provide a diagnostic cue—a finding to which the nurse assigns significance (Gordon, 1982). In a focus assessment, the nurse asks additional questions and/or performs further physical examination aimed at uncovering more cues to form an inference.

Designating data as a diagnostic cue is a complex cognitive activity; grouping a set of cues as a diagnosis is even more difficult (Gordon, 1982). For example, a client's unkempt hair, dirty fingernails, and shabby clothes could be clustered as "poor grooming," an inference that, with other cues, could support a nursing diagnosis of *Self-Care Deficit.* Although a nurse may be able to infer that these assessment data reflect poor grooming, she or he may not understand the possible relationship between the client's poor grooming and the inability to perform self-grooming, lack of desire to perform self-grooming, or a lifelong habit of poor grooming. In some cases, apparently significant data may in fact have no diagnostic significance, *e.g.,* if this client stated, "I'm sorry for my appearance. I rushed here from my work at the gas station." Interpreting data is discussed later in this chapter.

In Section II, each nursing diagnosis is described in terms of focus assessment criteria to identify specific data that may need to be collected to confirm or rule out the diagnosis. These focus assessment criteria can be used in conjunction with the baseline interview or in an isolated situation requiring additional information. Focus assessments can yield collaborative problems (*e.g., Postoperative Hypovolemia*) or nursing diagnoses (*e.g., Anxiety*).

The Assessment Process

To perform an accurate assessment, the nurse must have the ability to

- Communicate effectively
- Observe systematically
- Interpret data accurately

Communicating Effectively

All nurse–client interactions are based on communication. The term *therapeutic communication* is used to describe techniques that provide an opportunity for the client or family to share views and feelings openly. The technique incorporates verbal and nonverbal skills, as well as empathy and a sense of caring. Verbal techniques include asking closed- and open-ended questions, exploring the answers, and summarizing the content for the client. Nonverbal techniques include active listening, the use of silence, touch, and eye contact. Active listening, which is most vital in data collection, is also the most difficult skill to learn. Few people listen objectively; most tend to concentrate on their own forthcoming responses rather than on what the other person is saying. The elements of active listening are:

- Channeling attention to the sender and staying quiet within oneself
- Reducing or eliminating barriers
- Maintaining eye contact
- "Squaring off" eye-to-eye, shoulder-to-shoulder (positioning one's body in alignment with the other person's body)
- Avoiding interruptions

Barriers to active listening are always present, and the professional nurse must take the appropriate measures to eliminate them or their influence on an interaction. Figure 4-3 illustrates the barriers to active listening.

Learning effective communication skills requires knowledge of self and of communi-

1. Internal
    -   The person's views are different from the nurse's perceptions.
    -   The person's appearance or accent is different or distracting.
    -   The person is in pain or is anxious.
    -   The person is telling the nurse something that he or she does not want to hear.
    -   The nurse feels a dislike toward the person.
    -   The nurse is thinking of something else.
    -   The nurse is planning the next statement.
    -   The nurse is anxious or apprehensive.
    -   The nurse is in a hurry.

2. External
    -   Noise from equipment, speakers, television, radio, etc.
    -   Lack of privacy
    -   Physical hindrances such as desks, equipment, space, etc.
    -   Verbal remarks such as clichés, trite comments, or interruptions

Fig. 4-3   Barriers to active listening. (Carpenito, L. J & Duespohl, T. A. (1986). *A guide to effective clinical instruction* (2nd ed.). Rockville, MD: Aspen Systems Co.)

cation and learning theory, as well as continuous practice. Above all, it calls for the determination to retain sensitivity, which can be lost as one develops more advanced communication skills (Ramackers, 1979).

Observing Systematically

The ability to observe systematically depends on the nurse's knowledge base. With increased knowledge about human interaction, the nurse will look for specific data. Knowing what contributes to or causes a particular problem enables the nurse to explore these areas with the client. If the nurse does not know what a problem looks like, she will be unable to recognize and diagnose it. For example, if the nurse does not know the signs and symptoms of *Self-Concept Disturbance,* she may overlook the presence of this response. Systematic observations can be enhanced when written guidelines are used. Such guidelines are invaluable because they identify the specific types of data that need to be collected. Once one becomes familiar with the guidelines, one can gather the data without referring to a written guide.

For each diagnostic category listed in Section II, a focus assessment is presented to direct the nurse in gathering data to confirm or rule out the nursing diagnosis. Each specific nursing diagnosis has its assessment signs and symptoms to further assist in diagnosing.

Interpreting Data Accurately

To interpret data accurately, the nurse must acquire a method of identifying that information. Little and Carnevali (1976) have identified such a process as cue identification and inferencing.

A *cue* is information that one acquires through the use of the five senses (taste, touch, smell, hearing, and sight). Primary sources of cues are the subjective statements of the client and the objective facts observed by the nurse. Secondary sources are family, other health care providers, and diagnostic studies. An *inference* is the nurse's judgment or interpretation of these cues. Inferences are always subjective and are influenced by the knowledge base, values, and experiences of the nurse. For example:

Cue	*Corresponding Inference*
Hgb 9.1	Abnormal
Crying	Possible fear, sadness
5 ft 1 in, 220 lb	Obesity

Differentiating between inferences and cues is important. Although an inference is a subjective judgment, nurses will frequently report it as a fact or fail to gather sufficient cues to confirm it or rule it out. Inferences made with fewer or no supporting cues can result in inappropriate and sometimes dangerous care, especially when invalid inferences are passed on to other members of the health team.

As mentioned before, during data collection the nurse is simultaneously validating and interpreting the data. Validating the data with the client will help the nurse avoid making incorrect inferences. If, for example, a client is observed crying in her room, the nurse familiar with the client's recent medical diagnosis of breast cancer may quite logically connect the crying (cue) with the diagnosis. That the nurse initially makes this inference is not wrong, but problems could result if the nurse doesn't validate this inference with the client. To validate, the nurse should say something like "I see that you're crying; would you like to talk about your feelings?" By doing so, the nurse may in fact discover that the client's crying is related to something other than her diagnosis, such as missing her loved ones.

Validation sometimes involves clarifying vague or ambiguous data with the client (Gordon, 1982). For example, a nurse assessing a client who states "I feel drained" could interpret this statement in various ways, *e.g.,* as evidence of fatigue or stress. For validation, the nurse should ask the client to elaborate on the statement and provide more specific information.

Interpreting data involves two cognitive activities:

- Recognizing the cue or inference as significant
- Assigning meaning to the significance

A nurse recognizes the significance of data based on certain knowledge that denotes these data as abnormal or diagnostic. This knowledge can come from memory of similar past experiences or from other nurses, nursing faculty, and professional books and journals.

Past experiences or knowledge from other sources also can alert the nurse to the significance of certain cues found in pre-encounter data—information available to the nurse before the initial assessment, such as age, racial or ethnic background, and medical diagnosis. Consider the following example: When assessing a 45-year-old woman with diabetes mellitus who has been admitted for abdominal surgery, the nurse finds a new lesion on the client's foot. When questioned, the client states that "It must be from my new shoes." Based on prior knowledge of the client's diabetes gained from pre-encounter data, the nurse would assign this assessment finding more significance than it might warrant in another client.

To sum up, data to support a nursing diagnosis must be a cluster of cues that are documented to represent the condition. By carefully validating observations and client complaints, the nurse can avoid or minimize potentially harmful inaccuracies in data interpretation.

Diagnosis

Nurses make judgments regarding a variety of assessment data. Some of these judgments are nursing diagnoses, some are not. When a nurse concludes that a certain ECG pattern is abnormal, the nurse has made a diagnosis. When the nurse labels certain tonic–clonic movements a seizure, the nurse has made a diagnosis. In both of these situations the nurse had diagnosed, but neither one is a nursing diagnosis. Both of these situations require nursing and medical interventions for successful outcomes to be achieved. The reader is referred to Chapter 3 for an in-depth discussion of nursing diagnoses versus collaborative problems.

Diagnosis involves complex thinking about the data gathered from the client, family, records, and other health care providers. This thinking, combined with relevant information stored in the nurse's memory, is used to generate possible explanations for the data. These intellectual (cognitive) activities are difficult to teach and learn; many nurses who acquire expertise in assessment often flounder when asked to synthesize the data and identify a pattern. Aspinall and Tanner (1981) found that nurses take various approaches to problem identification, ranging from systematic testing of several possible explanations to the quick generation of one explanation. However, if the nurse does not take an approach that considers more than one explanation, the validity and effectiveness of the plan of care are jeopardized. According to Aspinall and Tanner, potential problems that can result when alternative explanations are not considered and tested include:

- Overvaluing the probability of one explanation
- Failing to include the accurate diagnosis in the initial hypothesis
- Failing to consider all the data because of the narrow focus
- Reaching an incorrect diagnosis because of speed, bias, or assumptions based on experience

To assist in identifying alternative explanations and in confirming or ruling out alternatives, the nurse should supplement her own memory-stored information by consulting references on the subject or by talking with other members of the health team. Unfortunately, nurses do not always utilize the most valuable resource available to them—other nurses.

Nursing staff conferences on client care are a nonthreatening and productive method for helping staff members identify alternative solutions to problems and interventions. After the background of the problem has been shared with the group, the members are asked to think of possible explanations for the data. These explanations are then written on a blackboard, after which the group considers what data are needed to confirm or rule out each possibility. Explanations that have been ruled out are crossed off. The nurse caring for the client will then proceed to confirm or rule out the remaining explanations while caring for the client.

As the nurse gains more knowledge and experience, she will need less time to think of alternative explanations. However, this step should never be eliminated. Identifying alternatives is also important when determining interventions, to avoid failure, stereotyping, and monotony.

Assessment Conclusions

Nurses collect data to determine the need for nursing service and to provide other professionals with data. After the data have been gathered and interpreted and alternative explanations tested and ruled out, the nurse will reach one of the following three conclusions:

- No nursing diagnosis evident at this time; continue to monitor
- Collaborative problem
- Actual, high risk, possible, or wellness nursing diagnosis

See Figure 2-3 in Chapter 2 for a decision tree illustrating how to differentiate between actual, high risk, and possible nursing diagnoses.

Identifying Nursing Diagnoses

After collecting the necessary data, the nurse then clusters or organizes the information according to various areas of functioning and determines the client's *pattern of functioning* in each area (positive functioning, altered functioning, or at-risk-for-altered functioning).

During the assessment, the nurse elicits data that reflect the client's past and present functional patterns. As discussed earlier the nurse must be careful not to diagnose patterns with isolated data. Isolated data may be important in the content of the usual pattern, but the usual pattern must be determined before analysis can take place. The following is an example of this error.

Mrs. F is a 33-year-old woman. In response to a 24-hour recall of her diet, she reports:

Breakfast: coffee (1 cup)
Morning break: coffee (1 cup)
Lunch: yogurt
Afternoon break: pound cake (1 slice)
Dinner: pizza, salad, coffee (2 cups)

The inference drawn from this data could be: Inadequate intake of basic four food groups. The nurse should ask Mrs. F, "Is this your usual daily intake?" Mrs. F's response will help the nurse determine the reason for the diet, *e.g.,* financial factors, lack of knowledge of nutrition, unusual circumstances.

If the nurse determines a diagnosis of *High Risk for Altered Nutrition related to inadequate consumption of the four basic food groups,* she then looks to other assessment data to validate the existence of the altered state, *e.g.,* skin, bowel elimination, weight/ height ratio.

If the nurse is uncertain of what data are needed to confirm the nursing diagnosis, she can refer to the specific diagnostic category in Section II for the focus assessment criteria and the defining characteristics.

The nurse also should try to determine whether or not the client's usual pattern presents a risk of contributing to an altered functional pattern. In the case of Mrs. F, if the diet recall presented is her usual state, the nurse can infer that this diet is nutritionally deficient and with additional questions can elicit contributing factors. When the nurse diagnoses the state of risk, she utilizes the diagnosis of: *High Risk for Altered Health Maintenance related to lack of knowledge of implications of inadequate diet and daily nutritional requirements, and the inconvenience of preparing meals for one person*

The following questions may be applied to each area of functioning (listed below) to assist the nurse in formulating a conclusion about the data collected for that category.*

- Is there a problem (actual), or is there a high risk for developing a problem in this area of functioning?
- Do the data collected lead one to suspect a problem (possible) in this area?
- Is there an area in which a higher level of wellness is desired?

*Copyright 1985, Lynda Juall Carpenito

1. Health perception–health management
     Health practices?
     Compliance?
     Injuries?
     Unhealthy life-style?
2. Nutritional–metabolic
     Nutrition?
     Fluid intake?
     Peripheral edema?
     Infection?
     Oral cavity health?
3. Elimination
     Bowel elimination?
     Incontinence?
4. Activity–exercise
     Activities of daily living?
     Leisure activities?
     Home care?
     Respiratory function?
5. Sleep–rest
     Sleep?
6. Cognitive–perceptual
     Decisions?
     Comfort?
     Knowledge?
     Sensory input?
7. Self-perception
     Anxiety/fear?
     Control?
     Self-concept?
8. Role–relationship
     Communication?
     Family?
     Loss?
     Parenting?
     Socialization?
     Violence?
9. Sexuality–reproductive
     Sexuality?
10. Coping–stress tolerance
     Coping?
11. Value–belief
     Spirituality?

Identifying Collaborative Problems

Prior to actual assessment, the nurse may obtain information about the client's medical diagnosis and treatment. During the assessment, the nurse will acquire data regarding medical history and treatment. With this information the nurse can predict physiologic complications for which the client is at risk and for which the nurse must monitor.

For example, a client admitted for elective surgery who also has diabetes mellitus will be monitored for blood sugar fluctuations under the collaborative problem of

Potential Complication: Hypo/hyperglycemia. (See Chapter 3 for a complete discussion of collaborative problems.)

To help identify collaborative problems, nurses may ask themselves the following question:

In any of the following body systems, is a physiologic complication present, or is there a *high* risk for one developing because of a disease, treatment, diagnostic study, or medication that requires monitoring and joint management by you and a physician?

- Cardiac, circulatory
- Immune, hematopoietic
- Respiratory
- Renal
- Neurologic
- Muscular, skeletal
- Reproductive
- Endocrine, metabolic
- Gastrointestinal, hepatic, biliary

Summary

Assessment encompasses data collection, interpretation, clustering, and analysis. This complex cognitive activity requires knowledge gained from personal experience and from other sources. At some point, assessment data become diagnostic cues that support diagnostic statements—nursing diagnoses and collaborative problems.

The nurse must approach this first step of the nursing process cautiously to reduce the risk of erroneous assumptions and interpretations. Errors in assessment will result in invalid diagnoses and ineffective interventions, which can cause harm to clients and lead to inefficient use of nursing resources.

References

Alfaro, R. (1990). *Application of nursing process: A step-by-step guide* (2nd ed.). Philadelphia: J. B. Lippincott.

Aspinall, M. J. & Tanner, C. (1981). *Decision-making in patient care.* New York: Appleton-Century-Crofts.

Bellack, J. P. (1984). *Nursing assessment: A multidimensional approach.* Monterey, CA: Wadsworth.

Block, G. J. & Nolan, J. W. (1986). *Health assessment for professional nursing: A developmental approach* (2nd ed.). New York: Appleton-Century-Crofts.

Fuller, J., & Schaller-Ayres, J. (1990). *Health assessment: A nursing approach.* Philadelphia: J. B. Lippincott.

Gordon, M. (1976). Nursing diagnosis and the diagnostic process. *American Journal of Nursing, 76,* 1298–1300.

Gordon, M. (1982). *Nursing diagnosis: Process and application.* St. Louis: McGraw-Hill.

Gordon, M. (1990). Toward theory-based diagnostic categories. *Nursing Diagnosis, 1*(1), 5–11.

Little, D. & Carnevali, D. (1976). *Nursing care planning.* Philadelphia: J. B. Lippincott.

Miskowski, C. & Nielson, B. (1985). A cancer nursing assessment tool. *Oncology Nursing Forum, 12*(6), 37–42.

Ramachers, M. J. (1979). Communication blocks revisited. *American Journal of Nursing, 79,* 1079–1081.

Smith, V. N. & Bass, T. (1979). *Communication for health professionals.* Philadelphia: J. B. Lippincott.

5

Application to Care Planning

To become a full profession, nursing must identify its unique focus and demonstrate accountability in terms of that focus. As discussed in Chapter 3, the bifocal clinical practice model is a mechanism for identifying the domain of nursing, and care planning is the mechanism for demonstrating accountability. Care plans communicate to the nursing staff the specific problems of the client and the prescribed interventions for directing and evaluating the care given. To prepare a care plan, the nurse must deliberately and systematically engage in problem-solving.

Care Plans

Care plans have two professional purposes—administrative and clinical. The administrative purposes of care plans are:

- To define the nursing focus for the client or group
- To differentiate the accountability of the nurse from that of other members of the health team
- To provide the criteria for reviewing and evaluating care (quality improvement)
- To provide the criteria for patient classification and financial reimbursement

The care plan serves the following clinical purposes:

- Represents the priority set of diagnoses (collaborative problems and nursing diagnoses) for a client
- Provides a blueprint to direct charting
- Communicates to the nursing staff what to teach, what to observe, and what to implement
- Provides outcome criteria and nursing goals for reviewing and evaluating care
- Directs specific interventions for the individual, family, and other nursing staff members to implement

To direct and evaluate nursing care, the care plan should include the following:

- Diagnostic statement
    Collaborative problems
    Nursing diagnoses
- Outcome criteria (client goals) or nursing goals
- Nursing actions or interventions
- Evaluation (status of plan)

Some institutions require that the nursing care plan include only nursing diagnoses and not collaborative problems. However, since nurses treat clients with other problems in addition to those designated by nursing diagnoses, this restriction creates a dilemma. Where is the nurse to record the planned interventions for collaborative problems? Faced with this situation, nurses have tended to respond by rewording all problems as nursing diagnoses, a practice that further confuses the issue and dilutes the effectiveness of nursing as a whole.

Nurses need a system for recording the nursing actions that address problems not covered by nursing diagnoses. Since nurses often find it difficult to separate the collaborative from the independent dimension of nursing, it would be best to use a system that provides a way to designate and include both collaborative problems and nursing diagnoses. Complex collaborative problems and nursing diagnoses could be recorded with the related interventions on the care plans, while routine problems could be addressed on the standard of care. This type of documentation will be explained later in this chapter.

The Process of Care Planning

After the actual or high risk problems have been identified, the nursing activities to monitor, prevent, reduce, or eliminate the problems need to be formulated. Thus, the planning phase of the nursing process is activated. Care plans represent the planning of care, not the delivery of care. The planning phase has three components:

1. Establishing a priority set of diagnoses
2. Designating outcome criteria and nursing goals
3. Prescribing the nursing interventions

Priority Set of Diagnoses

Realistically, a nurse cannot hope to address all, or even most, of the nursing diagnoses and collaborative problems that can apply to an individual, family, or community. By identifying a priority set—a group of nursing diagnoses and collaborative problems that take precedence over other nursing diagnoses or collaborative problems—the nurse can best direct resources toward goal achievement.

How does the nurse identify a priority set? In an acute care setting, the client enters the hospital for a specific purpose, such as surgery or other treatment for acute illness. In such a situation, certain nursing diagnoses or collaborative problems requiring specific nursing interventions commonly apply. Carpenito (1991) uses the term *diagnostic cluster* to describe such a group. Thus, different clients recovering from abdominal surgery will share the same diagnostic cluster. Each of their problem lists will contain the diagnostic cluster diagnoses, along with additional (addendum) diagnoses added to their priority set on the problem list.

How are other diagnoses not on the diagnostic cluster selected for the client's problem list? Selection is aided by:

- The client's identification of a problem or situation necessitating nursing intervention
- The nurse's identification of a problem or situation that necessitates prompt treatment to avoid causing further harm

Limited nursing resources and increasingly reduced client care time mandate that nurses identify nursing diagnoses that can be addressed at a later time and thus do not need to be included on the client's problem list. For example, for a client hospitalized after myocardial infarction who is 50 pounds overweight, the nurse eventually would want to explain the effects of obesity on cardiac function and refer the client to community resources for a weight reduction program after discharge. The discharge summary record would reflect the teaching and the referral; a nursing diagnosis related to weight reduction would not need to appear on the client's problem list.

Numbering the diagnoses on a problem list does not indicate priority but, rather, the order in which the nurse entered them on the list. Assigning absolute priority to nursing diagnoses or collaborative problems can create the false assumption that number 1 is automatically first priority. As you know, in the clinical setting priorities can change rapidly as the client's condition changes. For this reason, the nurse must view the entire problem list as the priority set, with priorities shifting within the list periodically.

Nursing Goals Versus Client Goals

Sometimes referred to as objectives, expected outcomes, or outcomes, goals of care planning are based on client criteria and/or nursing criteria.

Client goals and nursing goals are standards or measures used to evaluate the client's progress (outcome) or the nurse's performance (process). According to Alfaro (1990), "client goals are statements describing a measurable behavior of client, family, or group which denote a favorable status (changed or maintained) after nursing care has been delivered." Nursing goals, on the other hand, are statements describing measurable actions that denote the nurse's accountability for the situation or diagnosis. As discussed in Chapter 3, nursing diagnoses have client goals; collaborative problems have nursing goals.

Bulechek and McCloskey (1985) define client goals as "guideposts to the selection of nursing interventions and criteria in the evaluation of nursing interventions." These authors go on to state that "readily identifiable logical links should exist between the diagnosis and the plan of care, and the activities prescribed should assist or enable the patient to meet the identified expected outcome."

Thus, client goals serve as the criteria for measuring the effectiveness of a care plan. Because these outcome criteria for nursing diagnoses represent favorable statuses that can be achieved or maintained through nursing-prescribed (independent) interventions, they can help differentiate nursing diagnoses from collaborative problems. Outcomes for nursing diagnoses will not serve to evaluate the effectiveness of nursing interventions if physician-initiated interventions are also needed.

The NANDA definition of nursing diagnosis states that it "provides the basis for selection of nursing interventions to achieve outcomes for which the nurse is accountable." Nurses are intricately involved in the diagnosis and treatment of many different problems and situations for which they are not professionally accountable. For instance, a nurse can diagnose disorders such as cardiac dysrhythmias, cerebrovascular accident, and Lyme disease but cannot assume accountability for treatment of these disorders. Rather, physician-initiated interventions are required.

Certain situations may call for involvement of several disciplines. For example, in a client experiencing extreme anxiety, the physician may prescribe an antianxiety medication, an occupational therapist may provide diversional activities, and a nurse may institute nonpharmacologic anxiety-reducing measures, such as relaxation exercises and more effective problem-solving strategies. According to Gordon (1982), "saying a nursing diagnosis is a health problem a nurse can treat does not mean that non-nursing consultants cannot be used. The critical element is whether the nurse-prescribed interventions can achieve the outcome established with the client."

Client goals should be specific and realistically achievable. In several care planning books, the authors often present client outcomes with nursing diagnoses that could prove problematic. Table 5-1 provides selected examples of these. Examine the goals outlined in the table and imagine caring for a client with one or more of the listed goals, for example: "Will not experience cardiac dysrhythmias" or "Vital signs within normal limits for the patient." What if this client developed premature ventricular contractions or a decrease in blood pressure or pulse rate—how should the nurse respond? Should the nurse add or correct any nursing orders to address the problem? Should the nurse change a goal because it proves unachievable? No, the nurse should do neither but rather either initiate delegated orders from medicine (protocols, standing orders) or contact the

Table 5-1 **Literature Examples of Client Goals**

- ABGs are within patient's normal limits (p. 26)
- Blood sugar/electrolytes are within acceptable limits (p. 243)
- Blood loss from mediastinal or pleural tubes is within acceptable limits (p. 23)
  (From Moorhouse, Geissler, Doenges)

- Will not develop paralytic ileus (p. 23)
- Will not experience cardiac dysrhythmias (p. 253)
- Will not experience uremia (p. 420) (From Ulrich, Canale, Wendell)

- Blood pressure will not increase more than 30 mm Hg systolic or 15 mm Hg diastolic (p. 112)
- The causative organism will respond to treatment (p. 116)
- Will progress through labor and delivery without incident or severe fluid deficit, hemorrhage and/or shock (p. 124) (From Aukamp)

- Cardiac rhythm and rate are stable and within normal limits for patient (p. 252)
- No signs and symptoms of hypothermia (p. 251) (From Kim, McFarland, McLane)

physician for delegated orders. Changing nursing orders will not address the client's problem.

If a client goal is not achieved or if progress toward achievement is not evident, the nurse must reevaluate the attainability of the goal and/or review the nursing care plan, asking the following questions (Carpenito, 1991):

- Is the diagnosis correct?
- Has the goal been set mutually? Is the client participating?
- Is more time needed for the plan to work?
- Does the goal need to be revised?
- Does the plan need to be revised?
- Are physician-prescribed interventions needed?

Goals for Collaborative Problems

As discussed earlier, identifying client goals for collaborative problems is inappropriate and can incorrectly imply accountability for nurses. Rather, collaborative problems involve nursing goals, which reflect nursing accountability in situations requiring physician-prescribed interventions. This accountability includes:

- Monitoring for physiologic instability
- Consulting standing orders and protocols or a physician to obtain orders for appropriate interventions
- Performing specific actions to manage and reduce the severity of an event or situation

Nursing goals for collaborative problems can be written as either "_____ will be managed and minimized" or "The nurse will manage and minimize _____." Table 5-2 presents examples of collaborative problems and corresponding nursing goals.

Table 5-2 **Collaborative Problems with Corresponding Nursing Goals**

Potential Complication: Dysrhythmias
The nurse will manage and minimize dysrhythmic episodes.

Potential Complication: Fluid/Electrolyte Imbalances
Fluid and electrolyte imbalances will be managed and minimized.

Goals for Nursing Diagnoses

Client goals, or outcome criteria, can represent resolution of a problem, evidence of progress toward resolution of a problem, progress toward improved health status, or continued maintenance of good health or function. Outcome criteria are used to:

- Direct interventions to achieve the desired changes or maintenance
- Measure the effectiveness and validity of the interventions

Outcome criteria can be formulated to direct and measure positive and negative outcomes.

Positive outcome criteria seek to direct interventions to provide the client with:

1. An improvement in health status by increasing comfort (physiologic, psychologic, social, spiritual) and coping abilities
   - Example: The client will discuss relationship between activity and carbohydrate requirements and walk unassisted to end of hall four times a day.
2. Maintenance of present optimal level of health
   - Example: The client will relate the signs, symptoms, and associated interventions for angina.
3. Optimal levels of coping with significant others
   - Example: The client will relate an intent to discuss with her husband her concern about returning to work.
4. Optimal adaptation to deterioration of health status
   - Example: The client will visually scan the environment while walking, to prevent injury.
5. Optimal adaptation to terminal illness
   - Example: The client will consume protein and high-calorie supplements (800 ml/day) to compensate for periods of anorexia and nausea.
6. Collaboration and satisfaction with health care providers
   - Example: The client will ask questions concerning the care of his colostomy.

Negative outcome criteria seek to direct interventions to prevent negative alterations in the client, such as:

1. Complications
   - Example: The client will not develop the complications of imposed bed rest.
2. Disabilities
   - Example: The client will elevate left arm on pillow and exercise fingers on sponge ball to reduce edema.
3. Unwarranted death
   - Example: The infant will be attached to an apnea monitor at night.

Components of Outcome Criteria. The essential characteristics of outcome criteria are as follows. Outcome criteria should:

- Be long-term or short-term
- Have measurable behavior
- Be specific in content and time
- Be attainable

Client goals can be *long-term* or *short-term goals*. They may be defined as follows:

- Long-term: An objective that is expected to be achieved over a longer period of time, usually over weeks or months.

- Short-term: An objective that is expected to be achieved in a short period of time, usually in less than a week (Alfaro, 1990).

Sometimes short-term goals are objectives for care.

Previously, when hospital stays were frequently longer than a week, it was appropriate to formulate short-term and long-term goals. With current schedules, this is no longer necessary for many hospitalized clients.

Long-term goals are appropriate for clients in long-term care facilities, rehabilitation units, mental health units, community nursing settings, and ambulatory services.

The following represents a long-term goal with the associated short-term goals for an individual at home (Scherman, p. 118).

Long-term: The client will perform activities of daily living independently in 8 weeks.
Short-term: The client will:

1. Feed self after 3 RN visits
2. Dress self after 6–8 RN visits
3. Toilet self after 5–6 RN/PT visits
4. Ambulate with a cane after 6–10 RN/PT visits

Measurable verbs are verbs that describe the exact behavior of the client/family that you expect will occur when the goal has been met. The action/behavior must be such that the nurse can validate it by seeing or hearing.

The other senses—touch, taste, and smell—can also be used to measure goal achievement, but their use is infrequent.

If the verb used does not describe a result that can be seen or heard, as in:

The client *will experience* less anxiety,

the nurse can change the verb to a behaviorally measurable one, as in:

The client *reports* less anxiety.

Examples of verbs that are *not* measurable by sight or sound are:

- Accepts
- Knows
- Appreciates
- Understands

Examples of verbs that are measurable include:

- States
- Performs
- Identifies
- Has a decrease in
- Has an increase in
- Has an absence of
- Specifies
- Administers

Measurement of goal achievement can be made easier by:

- Using the phrase *as evidenced by* to introduce measurable evidence of a reduction in signs and symptoms, as in:
    The client will experience less anxiety, as evidenced by a reduction in signs and symptoms of racing, rapid pulse > 90.

1. Write the activity or behavior that the client and the nurse desire to occur after nursing care has been delivered.
2. Can you see or hear the activity or behavior happen?

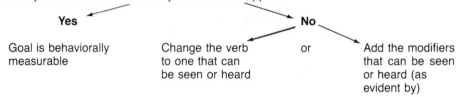

Yes		**No**
Goal is behaviorally measurable	Change the verb to one that can be seen or heard	or Add the modifiers that can be seen or heard (as evident by)

Fig. 5-1 Steps to formulate behaviorally measurable goals.

and in:

> The client will demonstrate tolerance to activity, as evidenced by a return to resting pulse 76, 3 min postactivity.

- Adding the expression *within normal limits (WNL),* as in:

> The client will demonstrate healing WNL, as evidenced by absence of redness, purulent discharge, or edema.

Figure 5-1 represents the process of writing measurable goals.

The outcome criteria should describe the *specific response* planned. Three elements add to the specificity of a goal: content, modifiers, and achievement time.

The *content* area indicates what the client is to do, experience, or learn (usually a verb), such as drink, walk, cough, or verbalize.

Associated with the verb are *modifiers,* which add the specifics or individual preferences to the goal. Modifiers are usually adjectives or adverbs; they explain what, where, when, and how. For example: drink (what and when), walk (where and when), learn (what), and cough (how and when).

The *time for achievement* of a goal can be added to the goal using one of three options:

- By discharge (Will relate an intent to discuss with wife by discharge fears regarding diagnosis.)
- Continued (Will demonstrate continued intact skin.)
- By date (Will walk ½ of hallway with assistance by Friday A.M.).

Often, the nurse has limited data when initial care plans are formulated. Thus, the goals and interventions may lack specificity. As the nurse interacts with the client, more data will be collected. The longer the nurse–client interactions, the more specific the plan would be.

The outcome criteria for each nursing diagnosis in Section II are stated in measurable terms but must be made specific to each client by adding modifiers. These outcome criteria guide the nurse in the areas that need to be observed and measured. The following is an example of outcome criteria for the diagnosis *Pain* that has been rewritten to reflect the goal for a particular client on a rehabilitation unit.

Outcome Criteria	*Individualized Outcome Criteria*
The client will report a reduction in pain and improve mobility by discharge	The client will: 1. Complete his bath without assistance 2. Relate a reduction of pain and request less medication (<250 mg/24 hr) 3. Remain out of bed from 11 A.M. to 2 P.M. and 5 P.M. to 9 P.M.

The nurse must ask himself, How will I measure that the client is experiencing less pain and has increased mobility? For this particular client, the goals stated above will serve as measurements. As this client's mobility increases, the nurse may have to revise the goals to reflect the client's changing status.

Goals for Possible Nursing Diagnoses. Many students and nurses have been instructed to write only client goals (outcome criteria) for the problem statements on the care plan. Since outcome criteria refer to the expected change in the client's status after he has received nursing care, it is inappropriate for the nurse to formulate outcome criteria for collaborative problems and for possible nursing diagnoses. Take a look at the following sample nursing diagnosis and associated outcome criteria:

- Diagnosis: *Possible Feeding Self-Care Deficit related to IV in right hand*
- Outcome criteria: The client will feed himself.

As one can easily see, this goal is problematic. How can a client goal be written for a possible nursing diagnosis if it is not known whether or not the client actually has the problem? Thus, goals for possible nursing diagnosis are omitted because they are not indicated.

Nursing Interventions

As previously discussed in Chapter 3, there are two types of nursing intervention, nurse-prescribed (independent) and physician-prescribed (delegated). Independent interventions are those prescriptions formulated by nurses for themselves or other nursing staff to implement. Delegated interventions are prescriptions formulated by physicians for nursing staff to implement.

Both types of interventions require independent nursing judgment, because legally the nurse must determine whether it is appropriate to initiate the action (independent or delegated). Table 5-3 shows a sample nursing care plan with both types of interventions.

It is important to note that nurses can and should consult with other disciplines, such as social workers, nutritionists, and physical therapists, as appropriate. However, this relationship is consultative only; if interventions for nursing diagnoses result from this consultation, the nurse will write these orders on the nursing care plan for other nursing staff to implement. (A discussion of other disciplines and their role in nursing care plans is included later in this chapter.)

Bulechek and McCloskey (1989) define nursing interventions as "any direct care treatment that a nurse performs on behalf of a client. These treatments include nurse-initiated treatments resulting from nursing diagnoses, physician-initiated treatments resulting from medical diagnoses, and performance of essential daily functions for the client who cannot do these." Bulechek and McCloskey have identified six basic types of nursing interventions. Figure 5-2 lists these interventions (with this author's changes) and illustrates their relationship to nursing diagnoses and collaborative problems.

As discussed in Chapter 3, the major focus of interventions differs for actual, high risk, and possible nursing diagnoses and collaborative problems.

For *actual nursing diagnoses,* the interventions will seek to:

- Reduce or eliminate contributing factors
- Promote a higher level of wellness
- Monitor status

For *high risk nursing diagnoses,* the interventions will seek to:

- Reduce or eliminate risk factors
- Prevent occurrence of the problem
- Monitor for onset

Table 5-3   **Types of Interventions**

Standard of Care

Potential Complication: Increased Intracranial Pressure
I   1. Monitor for signs and symptoms of increased intracranial pressure
         • Pulse changes: Slowing rate to 60 or below; Increasing rate to 100 or above
         • Respiratory irregularities: Slowing rate with lengthening periods of apnea
         • Rising blood pressure or widening pulse pressure with moderately elevated
           temperature
         • Temperature rising
         • Level of responsiveness: Variable change from baseline (alert, lethargic, comatose)
         • Pupillary changes (size, equality, reaction to light, movements)
         • Eye movements (doll's eyes, nystagmus)
         • Vomiting
         • Headache: Constant, increasing in intensity; aggravated by movement/standing
         • Subtle changes: Restlessness, forced breathing, purposeless movements and mental
           cloudiness
         • Paresthesia, paralysis
I   2. Avoid:
         • Carotid massage
         • Prone position
         • Neck flexion
         • Extreme neck rotation
         • Valsalva maneuver
         • Isometric exercises
         • Digital stimulation (anal)
I   3. Maintain a position with slight head elevation
I   4. Avoid rapidly changing positions
I   5. Maintain a quiet, calm environment (soft lighting)
I   6. Plan activities to reduce number of interruptions
I   7. Intake and output; use infusion pump to ensure accuracy
I   8. Consult for stool softeners
Del   9. Maintain fluid restrictions as ordered (may be restricted to 1000 mL /day for a few days)
Del   10. Administer fluids at an even rate as prescribed
Del   11. Administer medications (osmotic diuretics, *e.g.,* mannitol, and corticosteroids, *e.g.,*
          dexamethasone, methylprednisolone if administered)

       (Del = Delegated; I = Independent)

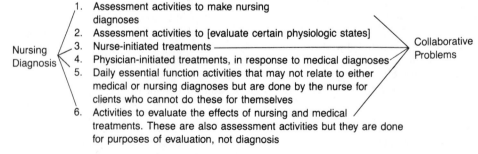

Fig. 5-2 Relationship of nursing interventions to nursing diagnosis and collaborative problems. (Bulechek, G. & McCloskey, J. (1989). Nursing interventions: Treatments for potential nursing diagnoses. In Carroll-Johnson, M. (Ed.). *Classification of nursing diagnosis: Proceedings of the eighth national conference.* Philadelphia: J.B. Lippincott. Brackets indicate changes made by author.)

For *possible nursing diagnoses,* the interventions will seek to collect additional data to rule out or confirm the diagnosis.

For *collaborative problems,* interventions will seek to:

- Monitor the client for changes in status
- Manage changes in status
- Initiate nurse- and physician-prescribed interventions

The specific directions for nursing, *nursing orders,* are composed of the following:

- Date
- Directive verb
- What, when, how often, how long, where
- Signature (Carnevali 1983)

The objective of the nursing order is to direct individualized care to a client. Nursing orders differ from nursing actions, which are broad interventions that can apply to any number of individuals sharing a similar problem. Examples of nursing actions are:

- Increase fluid intake
- Ambulate client
- Reassure client
- Monitor for dysrhythmias

To translate the nursing action into a nursing order, the nurse must have data from the client to answer the following: what, when, how often, how long, and where?

The following example illustrates the translation of a nursing action to a nursing order.

Nursing Action	*Nursing Order*
Increase fluid intake	Increase fluids to at least 2500 mL/24 hr
	1000 mL 7–3
	700 mL 3–11
	100 mL 11–7
	Likes orange and apple juice
	Dislikes carbonated beverages
	Do not count coffee or tea in the 2500 mL

This nursing order reflects the need to hydrate a client with tenacious secretions, considers preferences, and indicates that coffee and tea are permitted, although not as part of the measured increase, since they act as diuretics.

The nursing interventions outlined in Section II for each nursing diagnosis are guidelines for the nurse. The nurse rewrites these interventions considering the components of a nursing order: What, when, how often, how long, and where? The example below illustrates the rewriting of a nursing intervention from Section II as a nursing order.

Nursing Diagnosis: Sleep Pattern Disturbance related to decreased daytime activity level

Nursing Action	*Individualized Nursing Order*
Promote a well-scheduled daytime program of activity	Assist to dining room for each meal
	Have another resident accompany him on a daily afternoon walk around grounds

As with outcome criteria, the nurse must have specific knowledge of the client in order to write nursing orders. Student nurses can write care plans for clients they are yet to meet based on information from their instructors, but it must be specified that they are writing guidelines for care, not nursing orders. After caring for the client, the student can revise the plan with specific orders.

As a nurse increases her knowledge about a client, she may need to revise the nursing orders to reflect changes or to make them more specific. The following example illustrates a nursing order that underwent such revisions.

Nursing Diagnosis: Fear related to uncertain future

Initial order (Day 1)	Provide opportunities to ventilate concerns
Order Day 2	Encourage client to share her concerns
	Explore with husband his concerns for the future
Order Day 4	Reinforce necessity for preserving present function (refer to problem *Impaired Physical Mobility*)
	Discuss a plan for increasing self-care activities
	Assess the communication pattern between husband and wife
	Provide the husband with a time to talk outside wife's room

Implementation

The implementation component of the nursing process involves applying the skills needed to implement the nursing order. The skills and knowledge necessary for the implementation of nursing care usually focus on:

- Performing the activity for the client or assisting the client
- Performing nursing assessments to identify new problems and determine the status of existing problems
- Performing teaching to help clients gain new knowledge concerning their own health or the management of a disorder
- Counseling clients to make decisions about their own health care
- Consulting with and referring to other health care professionals to obtain appropriate direction
- Performing specific treatment actions to remove, reduce, or resolve health problems
- Assisting clients to perform activities themselves
- Assisting clients to identify risks or problems and to explore options available (Alfaro, 1990)

The nurse not only must possess these skills, but must also assess, teach, and evaluate them in any nursing personnel she manages. Often, the nurse is responsible for planning the care but not for its actual implementation. This requires that the nurse also possess the management skills of delegation, assertion, evaluation, and knowledge of change and motivational theory. The nurse should consult the appropriate literature on these topics.

Evaluation

This final component of the nursing process involves three different operations or considerations:

- Evaluation of the client's status
- Evaluation of the client's progress toward goal achievement
- Evaluation of the care plan's status and currentness

The nurse is responsible for evaluating the client's status regularly. Some clients require daily evaluation; others, such as those with neurologic problems, need hourly or constant evaluation. The nurse approaches evaluation differently for nursing diagnoses and collaborative problems.

Evaluation of Nursing Diagnoses

Outcome criteria or client goals are needed to evaluate a nursing diagnosis. After the nurse and client mutually set client goals, the nurse will:

- Assess the client's status
- Compare this response to the outcome criteria
- Conclude whether or not the client is progressing toward outcome achievement

Figure 5-3 presents a decision tree for evaluating nursing diagnoses. The following example illustrates the evaluation process:

Goal: The client will walk unassisted half the length of the hall by 6/5.

To evaluate this goal, the nurse observes the client's response to interventions, asking "How far did the client walk?" and "Was assistance needed?" The nurse then compares the client's response after intervention with the established outcome criteria.

The nurse can record the client's response on flow charts or progress notes. Flow charts can be used to record clinical data such as vital signs, skin condition, presence or absence of side effects, and wound assessments. Progress notes should be used to record specific responses that are not appropriate for flow charts, such as response to counseling, response of family members to the client, and any unusual responses.

Evaluation of Collaborative Problems

Because collaborative problems do not have client goals, the nurse evaluates them differently from nursing diagnoses. For collaborative problems, the nurse will:

- Assess the client's status
- Compare the data to established norms
- Judge whether the data fall within acceptable ranges

The nurse can record the assessment data for collaborative problems on flow records and use progress notes for significant or unusual findings, along with nursing management of the situation.

Evaluating the Status and Currency of the Care Plan

This type of evaluation relies on the conclusions derived from the evaluation of the client's progress. After examining the client's response, the nurse will ask the following questions:

- *Nursing diagnosis*
  - Does the diagnosis still exist?
  - Does a high risk diagnosis still exist?
  - Has the possible diagnosis been confirmed or ruled out?
  - Does a new diagnosis need to be added?
- *Goals*
  - Have they been achieved?
  - Do they reflect the present focus of care?
  - Can more specific modifiers be added?

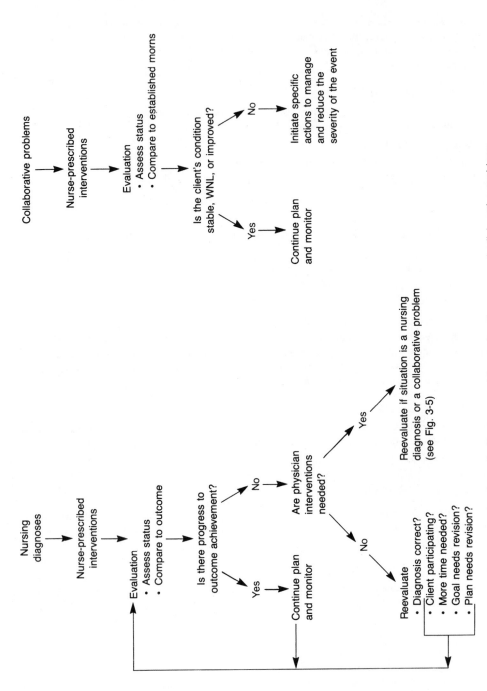

Fig. 5-3 Decision trees representing the evaluation processes for nursing diagnoses and collaborative problems.

- *Interventions*
  - Are they acceptable to the client?
  - Are they specific to the client?
  - Do they provide clear instructions for the nursing staff?
- *Collaborative Problems*
  - Is continuing monitoring indicated?

In reviewing the problems and interventions, the nurse will record one of the following decisions in the evaluation column at the time prescribed for evaluation.

Continue: The diagnosis is still present, and the goals and interventions are appropriate.

Revised: The diagnosis is still present, but the goals or nursing orders require revision. The revisions are then recorded.

Ruled out/confirmed: A possible diagnosis has been confirmed or ruled out by additional data collection. Goals and nursing orders are written.

Resolved: The goal has been achieved, and that portion of the care plan is discontinued.

Reinstate: A diagnosis that had been resolved returns.

An evaluation like that above is appropriate only when the nurse–client relationship will be long-term (over weeks or months), as in long-term care facilities and rehabilitation units. Care plans representing short-term nurse–client relationships should have a status column instead of an evaluation column to reflect diagnoses that have been resolved, discontinued, or ruled out. The nurse can then indicate which sections of the plan are no longer active. An example of a status column is presented later in this chapter.

Students who care for clients for only a short time (less than 2 weeks) usually incorporate this evaluation into the evaluation of the client's response. Both are then recorded on the care plan in the evaluation section. It is, however, important that students recognize that practicing nurses record client response on the flow record or nursing note, not on the care plan.

Minor revisions can be made daily on a care plan by the nurse caring for or directing the care of the client. A yellow felt-tip marker (Hi-Liter) is an excellent pen with which to revise a plan, marking out those areas that are no longer being used. Because it is still possible to read through the yellow marking, the nurse can always refer to what was planned previously. In addition, the marking will not interfere with photocopying. (Documentation examples of evaluation are presented later in this chapter.)

Evaluation of nursing care is a process to measure the client's progress or lack of progress toward the goal. The problem list is examined for its current relevancy, and the prescribed interventions are assessed for their appropriateness and acceptance by the client.

Planning Conferences

Client care conferences are an excellent way to help nurses with planning care. These conferences can be held daily and should be restricted to 15 to 20 minutes. If you are initiating conferences, it is sometimes advantageous to begin with weekly sessions and move gradually to daily or three-times-a-week sessions. Planning conferences should not be restricted to the day shift. They should also be conducted on evening and night shifts. The client or clients discussed can be those who are new admissions, those who have complex problems or conflicts with the staff, or those who are difficult to diagnose from a nursing diagnosis standpoint. The conference time provides nurses with an opportunity to share assessment data, feelings, problems, and knowledge (theory and practice). It can provide nurses who are reluctant to care-plan with an opportunity for collaboration.

Planning conferences should include all levels of nursing staff. Other members of the health team (therapists, social workers) may attend when appropriate. It is not appropriate for other health care professionals to coordinate or conduct these conferences. The planning of nursing care such as discharge planning should be coordinated by the professional nurse. Other disciplines can be consulted as indicated.

When conferences are being initiated, their success can be influenced positively if the following guidelines are considered:

- Manage the conference time judiciously by starting and ending on time
- Include all levels of nursing personnel and encourage their participation when appropriate
- Have personnel rotate covering unit during conferences
- Discourage interruptions
- Select an experienced group leader for beginning sessions
- Introduce inexperienced group leaders only after the conferences are firmly established

Multidisciplinary Care

Care of individuals, families, or groups commonly is provided by at least two disciplines, sometimes more. Good coordination of this care is critical to promote optimum use of resources and to prevent duplication of care. Based on overall knowledge level and time spent with clients, the nurse typically is in the best position to coordinate this care. The case management model subscribes to this philosophy (Cronin & Maklebust, 1989).

Agencies take various steps to promote coordinated multidisciplinary care and/or meet state or federal regulations to demonstrate evidence of multidisciplinary planning. Strategies include:

- Conducting regular multidisciplinary planning conferences
- Creating multidisciplinary problem lists
- Creating multidisciplinary care plans

Some of these strategies can be problematic for nurses, however. As discussed earlier in this chapter, care plans serve as directions for nursing staff in providing patient care. Should staff from other disciplines—physical therapy, social services, nutrition, and others—write on nursing care plans? If so, should they write interventions for nurses to follow or write interventions specific to their discipline?

When the services of another discipline are needed, the physician orders a consultation or the services. Staff from the needed discipline then create a plan of care with goals and interventions relating specifically to their discipline, not to nursing. Should this plan be a part of a multidisciplinary client care plan? Yes, but only if the plan clearly designates which sections apply only to specific disciplines.

Should other disciplines add interventions to the nursing care plan? By law, there are two types of nursing interventions—nurse-prescribed and physician-prescribed. Physician-prescribed interventions are transferred from the chart to appropriate documents, such as medication administration records, treatment records, and Kardexes. It is not necessary to enter physician-prescribed interventions on nursing care plans.

A nurse is accountable for following the interventions prescribed by other professional nurses. If a nurse disagrees with another nurse's care plan, the two nurses should consult and discuss the disagreement. If this is impossible, then the disagreeing nurse can delete or revise the existing nursing orders. Professional courtesy dictates that this nurse leave a note to the previous nurse explaining the change, if it could be problematic.

When a discipline other than nursing or medicine has suggestions for nursing management of a nursing diagnosis, the nurse should view these suggestions as expert advice. The nurse may or may not incorporate these suggestions into the nursing care plan. This situation is similar to that of a consulting physician, who may make recommendations but does not write medical orders for another physician's patient.

When a nurse enters an intervention on the care plan based on a suggestion from another discipline, professional courtesy mandates that the nurse credit the order to the discipline. For example:

Gently perform passive ROM to arms after meals and at 8 to 9 P.M., as suggested by C. Levy, RPT.

Alternatively, the nurse could designate a column on the care plan for "Discipline consulted" and document the information as follows:

Intervention	**Discipline consulted**
Gently provide passive ROM on arms after meals and at 8 to 9 P.M.	C. Levy, RPT

Either option maintains the nurse as the coordinator and prescriber of nursing care while also acknowledging the contribution of consulting disciplines.

Multidisciplinary problem lists can be used to illustrate all disciplines involved in a client's care. This author has never read a multidisciplinary problem list generated in an inpatient facility in which nursing was not involved in every problem. A sample multidisciplinary problem list could read:

CVA	Phys., nsg.
Impaired swallowing	Nsg., Speech T.
Self-care deficit	Nsg., PT
Pot. impaired home maintenance management	Nsg., Social Services

Another approach involves directing other disciplines to record the problem and management on the problem list, while nurses place nursing diagnoses and collaborative problems on the care plan. The following statement would be preprinted on the bottom of the problem list:

Refer to the nursing care plan for nursing diagnoses and collaborative problems.

Multidisciplinary conferencing provides an excellent means of reviewing and evaluating a client's, family's, or group's status and progress. In some facilities, such conferencing is required for all applicable clients.

Care Planning Systems

For years, practicing nurses have held an ambivalent view of care planning. Staff nurses' common oppositions to written care plans include:

- Most nurses don't have enough time to write them.
- They are not necessary except for JCAHO accreditation.
- They are not used after they are written (Carpenito, 1991).

Supporters of care planning in nursing cite these benefits:

- Care plans provide written directions to nursing staff rather than relying on verbal communication.
- They help ensure continuity of care for a client.
- They direct nurses to intervene in the priority set of problems for a particular client.
- They provide a means of reviewing or evaluating care.
- They demonstrate the complex role of professional nurses to validate their position in health care settings (Carpenito, 1991).

Since care plans usually contain only routine interventions (because including too much detail is a burden in a manual system), nurses often do not use them. Obviously, a care plan that is not used is not revised. As a result, the care plan that a nurse reads often does not represent the most current plan for the client. To update the staff on the care that the client requires, the nurse then uses oral communication. This type of communication makes the delivery of nursing care very inefficient and costly. An efficient, professional, and useful care planning system, encompassing standards of care, client problem lists, and standardized and addendum care plans, is possible.

Standards of Care

Standards of care are detailed guidelines that represent the predicted care indicated in specific situations. They do not direct nurses to provide medical interventions but rather provide an efficient method for retrieving generic (general) nursing interventions. Standards of care identify a set of problems (actual or high risk) that typically occur in a particular situation—a diagnostic cluster.

Keep in mind that standards of care should represent the care that nurses are responsible for providing, not an ideal level of care. As discussed earlier, the nurse cannot hope to address all—or, usually, even most—of the problems that a client may have. Rather, the nurse must focus on the client's most serious or most important problems. Problems that will not be addressed in the health care facility should be referred to both the client and family for interventions after discharge. Referrals to community agencies, such as weight loss or smoking cessation programs and psychologic counseling, may be indicated after discharge. Nurses must create realistic standards based on client acuity, length of stay, and available resources. Unrealistic, ideal standards merely frustrate nurses and hold them legally accountable for care that they cannot provide.

A care planning system can be structured with three tiers or levels of care:

- Level I—General unit standard of care
- Level II—Diagnostic cluster or single diagnosis standardized care plan
- Level III—Addendum care plans

Level I—Unit Standards of Care

Level I standards of care represent the predicted generic care required for all or most clients on a unit. These standards contain nursing diagnoses and/or collaborative problems (the diagnostic cluster) applicable to the specific situation. Table 5-4 presents a sample diagnostic cluster for standards of care in a general medical unit. All units—orthopedics, oncology, pediatrics, surgical, postanesthesia, neonatal, emergency, mental health, and so on—should have a generic unit standard of care.

Level I standards can be laminated and placed in each client care area as a reference for nurses. Because these standards apply to all clients, the nurse does not have to write the nursing diagnoses or collaborative problems associated with the generic standard of care on an individual client's care plan. Instead, institutional policy can specify that the generic standard will be implemented for all clients.

Table 5-4   **Generic Diagnostic Cluster for Hospitalized Adults
with Medical Conditions**

Collaborative Problems
Potential Complication: Cardiovascular
Potential Complication: Respiratory

Nursing Diagnosis
Anxiety related to unfamiliar environment, routines, diagnostic tests and treatments, and loss of
control
High Risk for Injury related to unfamiliar environment and physical/mental limitations secondary to
condition, medications, therapies, and diagnostic test
High Risk for Infection related to increased microorganisms in environment, the risk of person-to-
person transmission, and invasive tests and therapies
Self-Care Deficit related to sensory, cognitive, mobility, endurance, or motivation problems
High Risk for Altered Nutrition: Less Than Body Requirements related to decreased appetite
secondary to treatments, fatigue, environment, and changes in usual diet, and increased
protein/vitamin requirements for healing
High Risk for Constipation related to change in fluid/food intake, routine and activity level, effects
of medications, and emotional stress
Sleep Pattern Disturbance related to unfamilar, noisy environment, change in bedtime ritual,
emotional stress, and change in circadian rhythm
High Risk for Spiritual Distress related to separation from religious support system, lack of privacy,
or inability to practice spiritual rituals
Altered Family Process related to disruption of routines, change in role responsibilities, and fatigue
associated with increase workload and visiting hour requirements

To document Level I standards of care, the nurse should use flow chart notations
unless unusual data are found or significant incidents occur. Although standards of care
do not have to be part of the client's record, the record should specify what standards have
been selected for the client. The problem list, representing the priority set of nursing
diagnoses and collaborative problems for an individual client, serves this purpose.

Level II—Standardized Care Plans

Preprinted care plans that represent care to be provided for a client, family, or group in
addition to the Level I unit standards of care, Level II standardized care plans are
supplements to the generic unit standard. Thus, a client admitted to a medical unit will
receive nursing care based on both Level I unit standards and the Level II standardized
care plan for the specific condition that led to admission.

A Level II standardized care plan contains either a diagnostic cluster or a single
nursing diagnosis or collaborative problem, such as *High Risk for Impaired Skin
Integrity* or *PC: Fluid/electrolyte imbalances.* Figure 5-4 presents a Level II standardized
care plan for the collaborative problem *PC: Hypo/Hyperglycemia.*

Level III—Addendum Care Plans

An addendum care plan lists additional interventions beyond the Level I and Level II
standards that an individual client requires. These specific interventions may be added
to a standardized care plan or may be associated with additional priority nursing
diagnoses or collaborative problems not included on the Level II standardized care plan
or Level I unit standards.

For many hospitalized clients, the nurse can direct initial care responsibly using
standards of care. Assessment information obtained during subsequent nurse—client
interactions may warrant specific additions to the client's care plan to ensure outcome
achievement. The nurse can add or delete from standardized plans or handwrite or free-
text (via computer) an addendum diagnosis with its applicable goals and interventions.

POTENTIAL COMPLICATION: HYPO/HYPERGLYCEMIA

Nursing Goal: The nurse will manage and minimize hypo- or hyperglycemia episodes.

1. Monitor for signs and symptoms of hypoglycemia:
   a. Blood glucose <70 mg/dL
   b. Pale, moist, cool skin
   c. Tachycardia, diaphoresis
   d. Jitteriness, irritability
   e. Headache, slurred speech
   f. Incoordination
   g. Drowsiness
   h. Visual changes
   i. Hunger, nausea, abdominal pain
2. Follow protocols when indicated, *e.g.,* concentrated glucose (oral, IV).
3. Monitor for signs and symptoms of ketoacidosis:
   a. Blood glucose >300 mg/dL
   b. Positive plasma ketone, acetone breath
   c. Headache
   d. Kussmaul's respirations
   e. Anorexia, nausea, vomiting
   f. Polyuria, polydipsia
4. If ketoacidosis occurs, follow protocols, *e.g.,* initiation of IV fluids, insulin IV.
5. If episode is severe, monitor vital signs, urine output, specific gravity, ketones, blood sugar, electrolytes q 30 mins or PRN.
6. Document blood glucose findings and other assessment data on flow record. Document unusual events or responses on progress notes.

Fig. 5-4   Level II standardized care plan for Potential Complication: Hypo/Hyperglycemia.

Problem List/Care Plan

As discussed earlier, a problem list represents the priority set of nursing diagnoses and collaborative problems that the nursing staff will manage for a particular client. When appropriate, the term *diagnostic* is used in place of problem (*i.e.,* diagnostic list/care plan) to accommodate wellness diagnoses.

The problem list is a permanent chart record that identifies both the nursing diagnoses and/or collaborative problems receiving nursing management and also the source for interventions: standard of care, standardized care plan, or addendum care plan. Figure 5-5 illustrates a sample nursing problem list/care plan for a client with a history of insulin-dependent diabetes mellitus who is admitted to a medical unit for treatment of pneumonia. This sample includes the client's priority set of diagnoses as well as addendum interventions that the nurse has added to the standardized care plan under the diagnosis *Altered Comfort.*

The Concept of Standardization

Like any concept or system, standardized care planning forms have both advantages and disadvantages. Their advantages include:

- Eliminate the need to write routine nursing interventions
- Illustrate to new employees or transferred personnel the unit standard of care
- Direct nursing staff to selected documentation requirements
- Provide the criteria for a quality improvement program
- Allow the nurse to spend more time on delivering care than on documenting care

NURSING PROBLEM LIST/CARE PLAN

NURSING DIAGNOSIS/ COLLABORATIVE PROBLEM	STATUS	STAND -ARD	ADDENDUM	EVALUATION OF PROGRESS				
Med Unit Standard	9/28 A	✓		7/21 S/LJC	9/22 S/PW	7/23 S-GA		
PC: Hyperthermia	9/20			S/LJC	S/PW	S-GA		
PC: Hyper/Hypoglycemia	9/20 A	✓						
Altered Comfort	9/20 A	✓	✓					

STATUS CODE: A=Active   R=Resolved   RO=Ruled-out
EVALUATION CODE: S=Stable, I=Improved, *W=Worsened, U=Unchanged
           *P=Not Progressing, P=Progressing

Reviewed With Client/Family __9/21 LJC__, _____, _____, (Date)

ADDENDUM CARE PLAN

Nsg Dx/ Coll Prob	Client/Nursing Goals	Date/ Initials	Interventions
Altered Comfort	—	7/23 LJC	1. Provide a gentle back rub in evening
			2. leave blanket at foot of bed for easy access

Initials/Signature			
1. LJC Lynda Carpenito		5.	7.
2. PW Pati Wychoff	4. 6. Arcangelo	6.	8.

Abridged

Fig. 5-5 Sample problem list/care plan.

The disadvantages are:

- May take the place of a needed individualized intervention
- May encourage nurses to focus on predictable problems instead of additional ones

Many nurses experienced the above disadvantages when standardized care plans were introduced into their clinical setting.

When these problems were experienced, the solution was to eliminate standardized care plans. When they were eliminated, care plan audits revealed that the nurses were writing what previously was contained on the standard of care, for example, turn q 2 hours or administer pain relief medication.

Nurses have also been socialized to view standardization as mediocre nursing—unprofessional. Standards of care or standardized care plans should represent responsible nursing care that is predicted to be needed in certain situations. Nurses should view these predictions as scientific. When problems arise with the use of standardized forms, the solution is not to change the forms but to address the nurse's misuse of the forms.

To minimize the disadvantages of standardized care plans, certain strategies can be implemented. Standardized care plans should be formulated only for certain client problems that direct a set of common nursing interventions, for example, for a post-femoral arteriogram or total hip replacement (pre- and postoperatively).

Interposed in Level II standardized care plans can be spaces where the nurse can add specific points to the nursing interventions. This will help avoid the problem of the staff's ignoring the printed care plans. For example, next to the intervention for increased fluid intake, space is allocated for the amount taken within a certain time span.

Increase fluid intake to: _____ per 24 hours

_____ mL 7 A.M.–3 P.M.   Likes _____

_____ mL 3 P.M.–11 P.M.   Dislikes _____

_____ mL 11 P.M.–7 A.M.

In addition, the nurse who initiates the plan will cross out all sections that do not apply to her particular client. However, with clinical use, in time it may prove unnecessary to require additions to all standardized care plans. The staff may find it more efficient to use the Kardex to communicate minor variations, such as in frequency or quantities. Other interventions not appropriate for a Kardex can be entered on an addendum care plan to indicate that additional interventions have been added to a standardized plan. This will prevent the experienced nurse from having to read through known standardized interventions to find addendum interventions.

The documentation of implementation does not take place on a care plan but requires a separate form. Several formats are available—flow chart, graphic chart, or nursing progress notes—depending on the types of data being recorded. Figure 5-6 diagrams the nursing process with the related documentation.

Flow charts are excellent formats for recording treatments, activities of daily living, selected teaching, and observations. Figure 5-7 is an example of a flow chart. Flow charts should be used cautiously to record interactions in the spiritual, cultural, social, and psychologic domains. These responses may need to be recorded in the progress notes, as in explanations and counseling given to clients and families and unusual or unexpected situations (*e.g.*, injuries, clinical emergencies). If the nurses are recording the same data over and over in the progress notes, it may be possible to adapt a flow sheet to accommodate these data more efficiently.

Case Study Applications of Care Planning

The following two case studies and related documentation illustrate care planning for the individuals discussed. Functional health patterns are used in organizing the assessment and the analysis of the data.

Case Study 1

Mrs. Gates, a 42-year-old woman, is admitted with metastatic carcinoma of the breast (recently diagnosed).

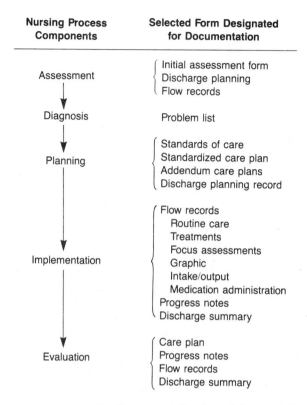

Nursing Process Components	Selected Form Designated for Documentation
Assessment	Initial assessment form Discharge planning Flow records
Diagnosis	Problem list
Planning	Standards of care Standardized care plan Addendum care plans Discharge planning record

Implementation	Flow records
	  Routine care
	  Treatments
	  Focus assessments
	  Graphic
	  Intake/output
	  Medication administration
	Progress notes
	Discharge summary

Evaluation	Care plan Progress notes Flow records Discharge summary

Fig. 5-6 Nursing process components with corresponding form of documentation.

Medical History

Mrs. Gates went to see her medical doctor because of a lump she discovered under her left arm. After a biopsy confirmed a diagnosis of metastatic carcinoma of the breast, Mrs. Gates was admitted for further diagnostic studies. A mammogram revealed a lesion in the left breast. Mrs. Gates is scheduled for a left lower quadrant resection of the breast and node dissection on Thursday 3 days away).

Medical Plan

Present

    Schedule for surgery on Thursday 9/20
        Schedule bone scan, liver scan, chest x-ray
        Complete blood count and urinalysis
        SMA 24 blood studies
        ECG

Future

    Dr. Drong discussed with Mrs. Gates that approximately 3 weeks after surgery he will begin a course of chemotherapy to last 8 months, followed by radiation.

(*Text continues on page 88*)

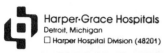

Harper·Grace Hospitals
Detroit, Michigan
☐ Harper Hospital Division (48201)

NURSING SHIFT ASSESSMENT

CODE: LOC = LEVEL OF CONSCIOUSNESS   + = POSITIVE
      NA = NOT APPLICABLE   - = NEGATIVE
      NP = NO PROBLEM   x = TIMES

INITIAL ASSESSMENT	2300-0700	0700-1500	1500-2300
NUTRITION/ METABOLIC PATTERN	Skin: ☐ NP ☐ Edema ☐ Pressure Areas: ____ Other ____	Skin: ☐ NP ☐ Edema ☐ Pressure Areas: ____ Other ____	Skin: ☐ NP ☐ Edema ☐ Pressure Areas ____ Other ____
RESPIRATION/ CIRCULATION PATTERN	Breath Sounds: ☐ Normal ☐ Abnormal ____ ☐ NA Cough: ☐ YES ☐ NO ☐ Productive ☐ Non-productive Peripheral Pulses: ☐ NA ☐ + ☐ - Other ____	Breath Sounds: ☐ Normal ☐ Abnormal ____ ☐ NA Cough: ☐ YES ☐ NO ☐ Productive ☐ Non-productive Peripheral Pulses: ☐ NA ☐ + ☐ - Other ____	Breath Sounds: ☐ Normal ☐ Abnormal ____ ☐ NA Cough: ☐ YES ☐ NO ☐ Productive ☐ Non-productive Peripheral Pulses: ☐ NA ☐ + ☐ - Other ____
ELIMINATION PATTERN	☐ Nausea ☐ Vomiting ☐ Diarrhea ☐ NP Abdomen: ☐ Distended ☐ Non-Distended Bowel Sounds ☐ + ☐ - ☐ NA Other ____	☐ Nausea ☐ Vomiting ☐ Diarrhea ☐ NP Abdomen: ☐ Distended ☐ Non-Distended Bowel Sounds ☐ + ☐ - ☐ NA Other ____	☐ Nausea ☐ Vomiting ☐ Diarrhea ☐ NP Abdomen: ☐ Distended ☐ Non-Distended Bowel Sounds ☐ + ☐ - ☐ NA Other ____
COGNITIVE/ PERCEPTUAL PATTERN	LOC: ☐ Person ☐ Place ☐ Time Responds appropriately to questions: ☐ Yes ☐ No Discomfort ☐ + ☐ - Type: ____ Location: ____ Other: ____	LOC: ☐ Person ☐ Place ☐ Time Responds appropriately to questions: ☐ Yes ☐ No Discomfort ☐ + ☐ - Type: ____ Location: ____ Other: ____	LOC: ☐ Person ☐ Place ☐ Time Responds appropriately to questions: ☐ Yes ☐ No Discomfort ☐ + ☐ - Type: ____ Location: ____ Other: ____
ONGOING ASSESSMENT	Time:	Time:	Time:
HEALTH PERCEPTION/ HEALTH MANAGEMENT PATTERN	Safety: Siderails x ____ ☐ Equipment ____ ☐ Restraints ____ ☐ Special Precautions ____ Other ____	Safety: Siderails x ____ ☐ Equipment ____ ☐ Restraints ____ ☐ Special Precautions ____ Other ____	Safety: Siderails x ____ ☐ Equipment ____ ☐ Restraints ____ ☐ Special Precautions ____ Other ____
NUTRITION/ METABOLIC PATTERN	Supplement/Tube Feeding ____ ☐ NPO Other ____	Diet ____ Breakfast ☐ 100% ☐ 75% ☐ 50% ☐ 25% ☐ Refused ☐ NPO Lunch ☐ 100% ☐ 75% ☐ 50% ☐ 25% ☐ Refused ☐ NPO Supplement ____ Other ____	Diet ____ Dinner ☐ 100% ☐ 75% ☐ 50% ☐ 25% ☐ Refused ☐ NPO Supplement ____ Other ____
ELIMINATION PATTERN	Bowel Movement X ____ ☐ Incontinent of stool Urine ☐ NP ☐ Incontinent of Urine Devices ____ Other ____	Bowel Movement X ____ ☐ Incontinent of stool Urine ☐ NP ☐ Incontinent of Urine Devices ____ Other ____	Bowel Movement X ____ ☐ Incontinent of stool Urine ☐ NP ☐ Incontinent of Urine Devices ____ Other ____
ACTIVITY/EXERCISE PATTERN	Hygiene ☐ Complete ☐ Partial ☐ Self-Care ☐ NA Skin Products ____ Mouth Care ____ Ambulated x ____ Chair x ____ ☐ Bedrest Positioned x ____ Other ____	Hygiene ☐ Complete ☐ Partial ☐ Self-Care ☐ NA Skin Products ____ Mouth Care ____ Ambulated x ____ Chair x ____ ☐ Bedrest Positioned x ____ Other ____	Hygiene ☐ Complete ☐ Partial ☐ Self-Care ☐ NA Skin Products ____ Mouth Care ____ Ambulated x ____ Chair x ____ ☐ Bedrest Positioned x ____ Other ____
SLEEP/REST PATTERN	☐ Restless ☐ Sleeping at Intervals ☐ Awake ☐ None Other ____	☐ Restless ☐ Sleeping at Intervals ☐ Awake ☐ None Other ____	☐ Restless ☐ Sleeping at Intervals ☐ Awake ☐ None Other ____
SIGNATURE & TITLE			

300955 (3/90)

(continued)

Fig. 5-7 Sample flow chart. (Courtesy of Harper Hospital, Detroit, Michigan)

Harper-Grace Hospitals
Detroit, Michigan
☐ Harper Hospital Division (48201)

NURSING TREATMENTS/PROCEDURES

TREATMENTS

	Time/Initials			Time/Initials			Time/Initials		
Date:			Date:			Date:			
Start Date	2300-0700	0700-1500	1500-2300	2300-0700	0700-1500	1500-2300	2300-0700	0700-1500	1500-2300

SPECIMENS

Date									

PROCEDURES: TO OTHER DEPARTMENTS

Initials	Date	Department	Mode of Transportation	Time

Initials	Signature & Title	Initials	Signature & Title

3-90

Fig. 5-7 (continued)

Admission Data Base

Assessment Conclusions:
- *Positive Functioning*
- *Collaborative Problems*
- *Nursing Diagnoses (actual, high risk, possible)*

Health History

Past unusual childhood diseases
Appendectomy at age 21
Menarche at age 13 with a 28-day cycle

Health Perception–Health Management Pattern

Does not smoke
Drinks 1 glass of wine with dinner
Does not exercise regularly
States she "just signed up for an exercise dance class but will have to cancel now"

Altered Health Maintenance related to insufficient exercise

Nutritional-Metabolic Pattern

(24-hour diet recall)
Breakfast: 2 eggs, 1 slice toast, orange juice, coffee
Lunch: Yogurt or cottage cheese with fruit, water
Dinner: Meat, potatoes, vegetable, salad, water, 1 glass wine
Other: 2–3 cups coffee, 1–2 pieces fruit, 1 serving ice cream/cake, cookies
Water: 2 glasses/day

Effective nutritional pattern

Elimination Pattern

Chronic constipation, which she treats with over-the-counter laxatives
Bowel movement q 3–4 days

Colonic Constipation related to possible inadequate water intake, insufficient exercise as evidenced by reports of BM q 3–4 days

Activity-Exercise Pattern

Works full-time as a librarian
Spends most of her free time sewing, gardening, and in activities with husband (plays, day trips)

Refer to Health Perception Pattern

Sleep–Rest Pattern

Sleeps 7–8 hours a night
Retires at 11 P.M., awakens at 6 A.M.
Falls asleep easily

Effective sleep–rest pattern

Cognitive–Perceptual Pattern

Master's degree

Effective cognitive–perceptual pattern

Self-Perception Pattern

States she "hoped that their relationship would not change after the
surgery."

High Risk for Self-Concept Disturbance related to change in appearance from surgery

Role—Relationship Pattern

Married 22 years
Relies on husband for daily support
Married sister with 2 children (ages
12 and 14) lives 20 minutes away;
they talk q.o.d. (every other day)
on telephone and usually have
Saturday or Sunday dinner together

Positive role—relationship pattern

Sexuality—Reproductive Pattern

No children: "I never got pregnant, so
we both accepted it as God's will."
States that both she and her husband
are very happy and satisfied with
their sex life
Engages in intercourse approximately
5 times/month

Positive sexuality pattern

Coping—Stress Management Pattern

Is worried what her husband will do
without her at home (*e.g.*, meals)
Expressed concern about getting sick
with chemotherapy
Related that her cousin, who had chemotherapy for leukemia, vomited
all the time and lost all her hair
but has been doing well for 5
years now

Fear related to cancer diagnosis, uncertainty about treatments and future
High Risk for Impaired Home Maintenance Management related to uncertainty about husband's ability
to manage household

Value—Belief Pattern

Is active in her church (Lutheran)
Teaches Sunday school each week

Positive value—belief pattern

Present Medical Status

Left lower quadrant resection of left
breast and node dissection surgery
9/20

Postoperative Potential Complications:
Bleedings
Paralytic ileus

Figure 5-8 is the problem list for Mrs. Gates 1 day after surgery. It contains the priority nursing diagnoses and collaborative problems for this client, with the status of each, and also indicates evaluation of progress.

The two diagnoses, *Colonic Constipation* and *Fear*, have both standardized and addendum interventions, as indicated by a check in each column (Standard, ACP). The diagnosis *High Risk for Self-Concept Disturbance* has interventions that are represented exclusively on the addendum care plan.

Nursing Diagnosis/ Collaborative Problem	Status	Standard of Care	ACP (Addendum Care Plan)	Evaluation of Progress
1. Standard Postoperative Plan	A 9/20	✓		
2. High Risk for Fluid Volume Excess: left arm related to effects of mastectomy and dependent positions	A 9/20	✓		
3. Colonic constipation related to possible inadequate water intake, insufficient exercise as evidenced by reports of bowel movements q 3–4 days	A 9/20	✓	✓	
4. High Risk for Self-Concept Disturbance related to fears that change in appearance will influence relations with spouse	A 9/21		✓	
5. Fear related to cancer diagnosis, uncertainty about treatments and future as evidenced by expressions of concern about chemotherapy and its success	A 9/21	✓	✓	
6. High Risk for Altered Health Maintenance related to lack of knowledge of arm exercises, self-breast exams, hazards to affected arm, community services	A 9/20	✓		

Code: A = Active   R = Resolved   RO = Ruled-out

Fig. 5-8 Nursing problem list/care plan for Mrs. Gates 1 day postoperatively, showing priority nursing diagnoses and collaborative care problems, the status of each, and evaluation of progress.

Case Study 2

While wrestling with her 15-year-old brother, 11-year-old JS sustained a fracture of her left tibia. She was admitted to the pediatric floor and placed in Buck's extension traction with a boot.

Medical Plan

Continuous traction for 5 weeks
Diazepam (Valium) 2 mg PO q 8 hours
Meperidine (Demerol) 50 mg PO q 4 hours
Regular diet

Medical Diagnosis

Pathologic fracture due to a benign cyst
Plan to discharge in 5 weeks in body cast; duration of body cast approximately 10 weeks

Medical History

Systems review unremarkable
1–2 episodes of upper respiratory infection each winter

Health Maintenance–Health Perception Pattern

Up-to-date with immunizations
Dental checkup q 6 months

Nutritional–Metabolic Pattern

Reports a usual daily intake of:
>Breakfast: Pancakes or cereal, orange juice
>Lunch: Sandwich, hot dog or pizza, ice cream, milk
>Dinner: Meat, potatoes, vegetables (carrots, peas, corn only)
>Snacks: Cookies, popcorn
>Water: 4 glasses

Elimination Pattern

Reports a soft, formed BM qd

Activity–Exercise Pattern

Reports:
>She is well liked in school
>Enjoys sports (soccer)
>Likes to cook
>Likes school (excels in math and science, has to work at her reading skills)
>States she is bored in the hospital

Sleep–Rest Pattern

Retires at 9:00 P.M. on weekdays
Awakens at 7:00 A.M.
Bedtime ritual: Bath, oral hygiene, reads a short story

Cognitive–Perceptual Pattern

Three days postadmission:

- JS experiences intermittent leg spasms that were visible the first 2 days. She continues to complain of spasms that are no longer visible. She responds to the spasms by screaming.
- JS is placed in private room at the end of the hall, and the door is kept closed to muffle her screams.
- JS's mother arrives at 10:30 A.M. and remains until 6:30 P.M. Her husband arrives at 6:30 P.M. and stays until 8:30 or 9:00 P.M.
- JS spends her day watching TV, conversing with her mother, and experiencing spasms. Her contact with the nursing staff is limited to hygiene needs and medications.
- JS complains that her pain meds are often late, and then her spasms are "really bad."

Self-Perception Pattern

Reports she is well liked in school
Expects to be "as good as before, after the fracture heals"

Role–Relationship Pattern

Has a 15-year-old brother
Mother is a former librarian
Father is a pharmacist who teaches at the local university
Reports her family has a good time together

Sexuality–Reproductive Pattern

Reports she learned about sexuality, pregnancy, and menses "from her mom and dad before the health teacher had a class"

Coping–Stress Management Pattern
Says when she is sad, she talks to her mother, father, or brother depending on the reason

Value–Belief Pattern
Attends Catholic church every Sunday
Believes in God and prays for assistance and to say, "Thank you"

You are a part-time nurse caring for JS today.

1. Examine the preceding data. For each of the following functional patterns, are there data to support:
   positive functioning?
   altered functioning?
   at high risk for altered functioning?*
   A. Health Perception–Health Management Pattern
      Health practices
      Compliance?
      Injuries?
      Unhealthy life-style?
   B. Nutritional–Metabolic Pattern
      Nutrition?
      Fluid intake?
      Peripheral edema?
      Infection?
      Oral cavity health?
   C. Elimination Pattern
      Bowel elimination?
      Incontinence?
   D. Activity–Exercise Pattern
      Activities of daily living?
      Leisure activities?
      Home care?
      Respiratory function?
   E. Sleep–Rest Pattern
      Sleep?
   F. Cognitive–Perceptual Pattern
      Comfort?
      Knowledge?
      Sensory input?
   G. Self-Perception Pattern
      Anxiety/fear?
      Control?
      Self-concept?
   H. Role–Relationship Pattern
      Communication?
      Family?
      Loss?
      Parenting?
      Socialization?
      Violence?

*Copyright 1985, Lynda Juall Carpenito

I. Sexuality–Reproductive Pattern
    Knowledge of?
    Sexuality?
J. Coping–Stress Tolerance Pattern Coping?
K. Value–Belief Pattern Spirituality?

2. Is there a physiologic complication present, or is there a *high* risk for one developing because of a disease, treatment, diagnostic study, or medication that requires monitoring and joint management by you and a physician?
    Cardiac, circulatory
    Immune, hematopoietic
    Respiratory
    Renal
    Neurologic
    Muscular, skeletal
    Reproductive
    Endocrine, metabolic
    Gastrointestinal, hepatic, biliary

3. After you have determined which functional patterns are altered or at risk for altered functioning, review the list of nursing diagnostic categories under that pattern and select the appropriate diagnosis.*

A. If you select an actual diagnosis
    Do you have signs and symptoms to support its presence? (Refer to Section II of Manual of Diagnostic Categories under the selected diagnosis.)
    Write the actual diagnosis in three parts:
    (1) label (2) related to contributing factors (3) as evidenced by signs and symptoms

B. If you select a high risk diagnosis
    Do you have risk factors present?
    Write the high risk diagnosis in two parts:
    (1) label (2) related to risk factors

C. Check each nursing diagnosis with the following review questions:*
    1. Is the statement clearly stated?
    2. Is the terminology correct?
    3. Is there a two-part statement?
    4. Does the second part of the statement reflect the specific factors that have contributed or may contribute to the development of the nursing diagnosis?
    5. Is there documentation of validation (signs and symptoms) for actual diagnoses?
    6. Does the nursing diagnosis statement reflect a situation for which a nurse can order the definition interventions to treat or prevent? (If medical orders are needed for outcome achievement, refer to IV.)
    7. *Do you need additional client contact to individualize the diagnostic statement?*

4. After you have identified which physiologic complications should be monitored for, list them as:
    Potential Complications: (list here)

5. A. Write short-term outcome (client goals) for each actual and high risk nursing diagnosis. Write nursing goals for collaborative problems.

    B. Check each client goal with the following review questions:*
      1. Is the goal a client goal or a nursing goal?
      2. Is the goal realistic and attainable?
      3. Is it measurable? (Can the nurse validate it by seeing or hearing?)
      4. Are the verbs measurable (states, demonstrates) or not measurable (knows, understands, experiences)?
      5. Has the content been clearly specified (how much, when, where)?
      6. Can a time for achievement be realistically identified?
      7. *Do you need additional client contact to individualize the goals?*

6. A. Write interventions for both the nursing diagnoses and the collaborative problems.
   B. Check each intervention with the following review questions:*
      1. Are the nursing orders clear (what, when, how often, how long, and where)?
      2. Do the nursing orders reflect creativity (and current practice)?
      3. *Do you need additional client contact to individualize the interventions?*

Now review the following care plan (Fig. 5-9) which represents the priority problems for JS.

(*Text continues on page 100*)

NURSING PROBLEM LIST/CARE PLAN

NURSING DIAGNOSIS/ COLLABORATIVE PROBLEM	STATUS	STAND - ARD	ADDENDUM	EVALUATION OF PROGRESS				
Pediatric Unit Standard	5-1 A	✓						
Pain related to	5-1 A	✓	✓					
ineffective relief of								
muscle spasms								
High Risk for impaired	5-1 A	✓						
skin integrity r.t.								
- imposed bedrest								
- Traction equipment								
High Risk for Colonic	5-1 A	✓						
Constipation r.t.								
- Dietary patterns (low								
fiber)								
- Embarrassment								
Potential Complication	5-1 A	✓						
Neurovascular Comp.								
Diversional Activity	5-2 A		✓					
Deficit r.t. Imposed								
bedrest and imitation								

STATUS CODE: A=Active   R=Resolved   RO=Ruled-out
EVALUATION CODE: S=Stable, I=Improved, *W=Worsened, U=Unchanged
           *P=Not Progressing, P=Progressing

Reviewed With Client/Family _5/1 xfc_ , _5/4 Lfc_ _____ , (Date)

Fig. 5-9 Care plan for Case Study 2.

NURSING PROBLEM LIST/CARE PLAN

NURSING DIAGNOSIS/ COLLABORATIVE PROBLEM	STATUS	STAND -ARD	ADDENDUM	EVALUATION OF PROGRESS					
High Risk for Impaired Home Maintenance Management r.t. discharge with body cast to home for 10 weeks.	5-4 A		✓						
Potential Complication: Impaired Circulation	5-4 A	✓							
STATUS CODE: A=Active R=Resolved RO=Ruled-out EVALUATION CODE: S=Stable, I=Improved, *W=Worsened, U=Unchanged *P=Not Progressing, P=Progressing									
Reviewed With Client/Family _____ , _____ , _____ , (Date)									

Fig. 5-9 (continued)

ADDENDUM CARE PLAN

Nsg Dx/ Coll Prob	Client/Nursing Goals	Date/ Initials	Interventions
Pain r.t. ineffective relief of muscle spasm as manifested by frequent reports of inadequate relief	1. Report less pain 2. Practice selected distraction techniques during pain episodes	5- JW	1. Teach her rhythmic abdominal breathing to practice during muscle spasms. 2. Coach her to practice breathing during episodes of spasms 3. Administer pain med on time. 4. Encourage her to use her radio with earphones during episodes of spasm and to increase the volume as pain increases
Diversional Activity Deficit r.t. imposed bedrest, isolation as manifested by statements of boredom	1. occupy her time with activities other than TV viewing	5-2 PW	1. Consult with recreational therapist for appropriate activities 2. Encourage other children on floor to visit and play cards with her. 3. Encourage her to read stories to small children
Initials/Signature 1. Joann Woolsey RN 2. Pati Wyckoff RN	3. 4.	5. 6.	7. 8.

Fig. 5-9 (continued)

ADDENDUM CARE PLAN

Nsg Dx/ Coll Prob	Client/Nursing Goals	Date/ Initials	Interventions
			on unit in her room
			4. Arrange for Tutoring
			with school district
			5. Try to stimulate her To
			do something other Than
			watching T.V. e.g. Hook
			rug, electronic games.
			6. Allow her opportunities
			To share her feelings
			of loneliness.
N. R. Impaired		5/4 pw	1. Allow parents To share
home maintenance			Their concern about care
r.t. discharge			of daughters after
with body cast			discharge.
To home for			2. Assure them that
10 weeks (appx			They will have an
discharge			opportunity To care for
date 6/10)			daughter under supervision
			in hospital.
			3. Discuss and Teach
			each of the following
			when indicated.
Initials/Signature 1.	3.	5.	7.
2.	4.	6.	8.

Fig. 5-9 (continued)

ADDENDUM CARE PLAN

Nsg Dx/ Coll Prob	Client/Nursing Goals	Date/ Initials	Interventions
			Cast care
			Hygienic measures
			Nutrition (↑ calcium reqts)
			Elimination
			Diversional activities
			Tutoring
			Relief periods for
			parents from care.
Initials/Signature			
1.	3.	5.	7.
2.	4.	6.	8.

Fig. 5-9 (continued)

References

Alfaro, R. (1990). *Applying nursing diagnosis and nursing process: A step-by-step guide* (2nd ed.). Philadelphia: J. B. Lippincott.

Brown, K. & Dunn, K. (1987). Nursing diagnosis and process evaluation: Implications for continuing education. *Journal of Continuing Education in Nursing, 18*(5), 172–178.

Bulechek, G. & McCloskey, J. (1985). *Nursing interventions: Treatments for nursing diagnoses.* Philadelphia: W. B. Saunders.

Burke, L. & Murphy, J. (1988). *Charting by exception.* New York: John Wiley & Sons.

Carnevali, D. L. (1983). *Nursing care planning: Diagnosis and management* (3rd ed.). Philadelphia: J. B. Lippincott.

Carpenito, L. J. (1991). *Nursing care plans and documentation: Nursing diagnoses and collaborative problems.* Philadelphia: J. B. Lippincott.

Cronin, C. J. & Maklebust, J. (1989). Case-managed care: Capitalizing on the CNS. *Nursing Management, 20*(3), 38–47.

Deane, D., McElroy, M. J., & Alden, S. (1986). Documentation: Meeting requirements while maximizing productivity. *Nursing Economics, 4*(4), 176.

Gamberg, D., Hushower, G., & Smith, N. (1981). Outcome charting. *Nursing Management, 12*(1), 37.

Gordon, M. (1982). *Nursing diagnosis: Process and application.* New York: McGraw-Hill.

Lampe, S. S. (1985). Focus charting: Streamlining documentation. *Nursing Management, 16*(7), 43.

McFarland, G. & Wasli, E. (1986). *Nursing diagnosis and process in psychiatric-mental health nursing.* Philadelphia: J. B. Lippincott.

McNally, J., Stair, J., & Somerville, E. (Eds.). (1985). *Guidelines for cancer nursing practice.* Orlando: Grune & Stratton.

Miller, E. (1989). *How to make nursing diagnosis work.* Norwalk, CT: Appleton-Lange.

Scherman, S. (1985). *Community health nursing care plans.* New York: John Wiley & Sons.

Wesorik, B. (1990). *Standards of nursing care.* Philadelphia: J. B. Lippincott.

Section II

Manual of Nursing Diagnoses

Introduction

The *Manual of Nursing Diagnoses* consists of 98 nursing diagnoses. Each diagnosis is described with the three NANDA-required elements first, followed by four additional components:

- Definition
- Defining characteristics, signs and symptoms, or risk factors of the diagnosis
- Related factors, organized according to pathophysiologic, treatment-related, situational, and maturational factors that may contribute to or cause the altered state
- Diagnostic Considerations—discussion of the diagnosis to clarify its concept and clinical use
- Errors in Diagnostic Statements—various incorrect diagnostic statements presented with corresponding explanations of the problem and examples of correct diagnoses
- Focus assessment criteria, subjective and objective, which serve to guide the nurse to specific data collection to help confirm or rule out the diagnosis
- Principles and Rationale for Nursing Care—scientific explanations about the diagnosis and interventions presented under Generic Considerations, Specific age-related considerations, under Pediatric Considerations and Gerontologic Considerations.

Each diagnostic group is then further explained by one or more specific nursing diagnoses. These specific diagnoses were selected because of their frequency in nursing and do not in any respect represent exclusive categories. For example, *High Risk for Injury* has four specific contributing factors:

- Related to sensory/motor deficits
- Related to lack of awareness of environmental hazards
- Related to maturational age of hospitalized child
- Related to vertigo secondary to orthostatic hypotension

But the nurse can utilize this diagnosis to describe other client situations, for example:

High Risk for Injury Related to Unstable Gait Secondary to Total Hip Replacement

Some diagnoses are listed with no specific "related to's", for example: *Anxiety, Fear, Hopelessness, High Risk for Self-Harm*. Instead, each of these categories has one group of interventions that focuses on the treatment associated with the diagnostic label, regardless of the etiologic and contributing factors.

Each specific nursing diagnosis is further explained with:

- Assessment data: the subjective and objective signs and symptoms of the specific diagnosis
- Outcome criteria: the goals for clients with the diagnosis
- Interventions, which specifically direct the nurse to:
  - The assessment of causative and contributing factors
  - The reduction or elimination of the factors
  - The promotion of selected activities
  - Health teaching
  - Referrals

Each diagnosis concludes with a bibliography containing books and periodicals in which the nurse can obtain more information about the diagnosis. Pertinent literature and organizations for the consumer are also cited when appropriate. Several of the diagnoses represent broad categories under which more specific diagnoses fall. As the taxonomic work of NANDA continues, more specific diagnoses will evolve, making the broader diagnoses no longer clinically useful. For example, the addition of the seven diagnoses (six NANDA-approved) related to incontinence.

- *Functional Incontinence*
- *Reflex Incontinence*
- *Stress Incontinence*
- *Total Incontinence*
- *Urge Incontinence*
- *Urinary Retention*
- *Maturational Enuresis* has made *Altered Patterns of Urinary Elimination* too broad for clinical use.

Readers of this manual are encouraged to become familiar with all of the nursing diagnoses and collaborative problems in order to incorporate them into their nursing practice. Until you become familiar with the nursing diagnoses and their defining characteristics or risk factors and collaborative problems, the following guidelines are suggested:

1. Collect data, both subjective and objective, from client, family, other health care professionals, and records.
2. Examine the data described above. For each of the following functional patterns, are there data to support
   positive functioning?
   altered functioning?
   at high risk for altered functioning?*
   - Health perception–health management pattern
     Health management?
     Compliance?
     Injuries?
     Self-care?
   - Nutritional–metabolic pattern
     Nutrition?
     Fluid intake?
     Peripheral edema?
     Infection?
     Oral cavity health?
   - Elimination pattern
     Bowel elimination?
     Incontinence?
   - Activity–exercise pattern
     Activities of daily living?
     Leisure activities?
     Home care?
     Respiratory function?
   - Sleep–rest pattern
     Sleep

*Copyright 1985, 1990, Lynda Juall Carpenito

- Cognitive–perceptual pattern
    Decisions?
    Comfort?
    Knowledge?
    Sensory input?
- Self-perception pattern
    Anxiety/fear?
    Self-concept?
- Role–relationship pattern
    Communication?
    Family?
    Loss?
    Parenting?
    Socialization?
    Violence?
- Sexuality–reproductive pattern
    Knowledge of?
    Sexuality?
- Coping–stress tolerance pattern
    Coping?
- Value–belief pattern
    Spirituality?

3. After you have selected which functional patterns are altered or present a risk for altered functioning, review the list of nursing diagnoses under that pattern and select the appropriate diagnosis (see pages 7–9).
4. If you select an actual diagnosis:
    Do you have signs and symptoms to support its presence? (Refer to Section II, Manual of Nursing Diagnoses, under the selected diagnosis.)
    Write the actual diagnosis in three parts:
    Label; related to (contributing factors); as evidenced by (signs and symptoms)
5. If you select a high risk diagnosis,
    Are risk factors present?
    Write the high risk diagnosis in two parts:
    High Risk for (specify label) related to (risk factors)
6. If you need assistance in writing the nursing diagnosis, refer to Chapters 2 and 4 for guidelines.
7. If you suspect a problem but have insufficient data, refer to the focus assessment data under the category and gather the additional data to confirm or rule out the diagnosis. If this additional data collection needs to be done at a later time or by other nurses, label the diagnosis *Possible . . .* on the care plan. (Refer to Chapter 2 for a discussion of possible nursing diagnoses.)
8. For the nursing diagnoses that you have validated, refer to that category and review the outcome criteria. Rewrite the outcome criteria adding the individualized criteria for the specific client. (Refer to Chapter 5 for specific guidelines.)
9. Review the interventions under the category and select those that are appropriate. Rewrite the interventions, adding individualization when needed. Add other interventions as indicated.
10. Is a physiologic complication present, or is there a high risk of one developing because of a disease, treatment, diagnostic study, or medication that you want to monitor for? (collaborative problem)

a. Cardiac, circulatory
b. Metabolic, hematopoietic
c. Respiratory
d. Renal
e. Genitourinary
f. Neurologic
g. Muscular
h. Skeletal
     i. Endocrine, immune
j. Gastrointestinal, hepatic, biliary
k. Reproductive

11. After you have selected which physiologic complications or collaborative problems are indicated to be monitored for or managed, list them as *Potential Complication: (Specify)*.

12. Initiate a standard care plan or write the collaborative problem on the care plan and add the appropriate interventions that direct nurses to monitor for the problems and intervene accordingly. (Refer to Section III, Manual of Collaborative Problems, for more information.)

Activity Intolerance

- *Related to* **(Specify)**
- *Related to* **Insufficient Knowledge of Adaptive Techniques Needed Secondary to Chronic Obstructive Pulmonary Disease**
- *Related to* **Insufficient Knowledge of Adaptive Techniques Needed Secondary to Impaired Cardiac Function**
- *Related to* **Bed Rest Deconditioning**

DEFINITION

Activity Intolerance: A reduction in one's physiologic capacity to endure activities to the degree desired or required (Magnan, 1987).

DEFINING CHARACTERISTICS

Major (must be present)

An altered physiologic response to activity (*e.g.*)

Respiratory
    Dyspnea   Excessive increase in rate
    Shortness of breath   Decrease in rate

Pulse
    Weak pulse
    Decrease in rate
    Excessive increase in rate
    Rhythm change
    Failure to return to preactivity level after 3 minutes

Blood pressure
    Failure to increase with activity
    Increase in diastolic > 15 mm Hg

Minor (may be present)
    Weakness
    Fatigue
    Pallor or cyanosis
    Confusion
    Vertigo

RELATED FACTORS

Any factors that compromise oxygen transport, lead to physical deconditioning, or create excessive energy demands that outstrip the person's physical and psychologic abilities can cause activity intolerance. Some common factors are listed below.

Pathophysiologic

Cardiac
  Congestive heart failure
  Myocardial infarction
  Cardiomyopathies
  Idiopathic hypertrophic subaortic
    stenosis
  Congenital heart disease
  Angina

  Valvular disease
  Dysrhythmias

Pulmonary
  Atelectasis
  Chronic obstructive pulmonary disease
  Bronchopulmonary dysplasia
Circulatory
  Anemia
  Hypovolemia
  Peripheral arterial disease
Acute or chronic infections
Endocrine or metabolic disorders
Chronic diseases
  Renal
  Hepatic
  Inflammatory

  Musculoskeletal
  Neurologic

Nutritional disorders
  Obesity
  Malnourishment
  Inadequate diet
Electrolyte imbalance
Malignancies

Treatment-Related

Surgery
Diagnostic studies
Nature and frequency of treatments
Prolonged bed rest
Chemotherapy
Irradiation therapy
Medications
  Antihypertensives
  Minor tranquilizers
  Hypnotics

  Antidepressants
  Antihistamines
  Beta blockers

Situational (personal, environmental)

Personal
  Sedentary life-style
  Extreme stress
  Pain
  Depression

  Lack of motivation
  Chronic fatigue
  Sleep disturbances

  Assistive equipment that requires strength (walkers, crutches, braces)

Environmental

Environmental barriers (*e.g.,* stairs)
Climatic extremes (especially hot humid climates)
Air pollution (*e.g.,* smog)
Atmospheric pressure (*e.g.,* recent relocation to high altitude living)

Maturational

The elderly may experience decreased muscle strength and flexibility, as well as sensory deficits. All of these can undermine body confidence and may contribute directly or indirectly to Activity Intolerance.

Diagnostic Considerations

Activity Intolerance is a diagnostic judgment that describes a person with compromised physical conditioning. This person can engage in therapies that increase strength and endurance. *Activity Intolerance* differs from *Fatigue* in that it is relieved by rest. In *Activity Intolerance,* moreover, the goal is to increase tolerance to activity; with *Fatigue,* in contrast, the goal is to assist the person to adapt to the fatigue, not to increase endurance.

Errors in Diagnostic Statements

Activity Intolerance related to dysrhythmic episodes in response to increased activity secondary to recent MI

The goal for this client at this time would not be to increase tolerance to activity, but rather to monitor cardiac response to activity and to prevent decreased cardiac output. This situation would be more appropriately labeled as a collaborative problem: *Potential Complication: Decreased Cardiac Output.*
Activity Intolerance related to fatigue secondary to chemotherapy

The fatigue associated with chemotherapy is not improved by rest and is not amenable to interventions to increase endurance. The following diagnosis would be correct: *Fatigue related to anemia and chemical changes secondary to toxic effects of chemotherapy.*

Focus Assessment

Assessing for activity intolerance is a dynamic process that starts before the onset of activity, proceeds continuously throughout the activity, and terminates in a postactivity evaluation. During preactivity assessment, the nurse establishes baseline "at rest" measurements of blood pressure, pulse, and respiration. The nurse also assesses incentives for activity and the person's perceived capabilities for activity, as well as factors that may decrease tolerance for activity. If a known pathology exists in a particular organ system, then assessment during activity will focus on signs and symptoms indicating intolerance in that system (*e.g.,* exertional dyspnea and/or cyanosis in pulmonary disease, angina in cardiac disease, increased spasticity or decreased coordination in neuromuscular disease). During postactivity assessment, the nurse assesses recovery time, which provides an index for judging physiologic tolerance for activity.

Subjective Data

Assess person's feelings and thoughts about participating in activity. For example, does person report:

- Lack of incentive?
- Disinclination to participate in activities?
- Lack of confidence in ability to perform activity?
- Fear of injury or aggravating disease as a result of participating in activity?
- Difficulty performing activities of daily living because of decreased energy or a lack of strength?
- Pain that interferes with performance of activities?

Does the person complain of:
- Weakness?
- Fatigue?
- Dyspnea?
- Lack of sleep and/or rest?

Objective Data

1. Assess for the presence of contributing factors.
   Situational
       Personal
           Coping strategies focusing on avoidance
           Inadequate social support
       Environmental
           Social isolation   Sensory deprivation
           Sensory overload   Climatic conditions
           Insufficient rest and sleep
               periods
   Disease-related
       Cardiopulmonary disorders   Nutritional deficiencies
       Musculoskeletal disorders   Neurologic disorders
       Fluid/electrolyte imbalance   Chronic diseases
   Treatment-related
       Bed rest/imposed immobility   Diagnostic studies
       Medications   Treatment schedule
       Diet   Surgery
       Caregivers' expectations
       Assistive equipment that requires
           strength
2. Assess strength and balance, evaluate person's ability to:
       Reposition self in bed
       Maintain body alignment
       Assume and maintain sitting position
       Rise to standing position
       Maintain erect posture
       Perform Romberg test
       Ambulate
       Perform activities of daily living
3. Assess response to activity.
       Take resting vital signs (Table II-I)
           Pulse (rate, rhythm, quality)
           Blood pressure
           Respirations (rate, depth, effort)
       Have person perform the activity
       Take vital signs immediately after the activity

Table II-1. **Physiologic Response To Activity (Expected and Abnormal)**

	Pulse	Blood Pressure	Respiration
Resting			
Normal	60–90	<140/90	<20
Abnormal	>100	>140/90	>20
Immediately After Activity			
Normal	↑ Rate	↑ Systolic	↑ Rate
	↑ Strength	Decrease or no change in sys-	↑ Depth
Abnormal	↓ Rate	tolic	Excessive
	↓ Strength		↓ Rate
	Irregular rhythm		
3 Minutes After Activity			
Normal	Within 6 beats of resting pulse		
Abnormal	>7 beats of resting pulse		

Have person rest for 3 minutes; take vital signs again
Assess for presence of:

Pallor   Confusion
Cyanosis   Vertigo

Principles and Rationale for Nursing Care

Generic Considerations

1. Nursing interventions for activity intolerance promote participation in activities to achieve a level of activity desired by the person or required by the therapeutic regimen.
2. Persons use cognitive processing of many types and various sources of information to make decisions about their actions and to exercise control over their environment (Gortner, Miller, & Jenkins, 1988).
3. A person's decision to engage in a particular activity is influenced by knowledge, values, beliefs, and perceived capability for action (Magnan, 1987).
4. Nursing interventions are planned to facilitate engagement in activity based on an understanding of the person's knowledge of activity demands, valuation of activity, beliefs about activity, and perceived capability for activity.
5. The ability to continue a specified task is known as *endurance;* the inability to continue a specified task, *fatigue.* Conceptually, fatigue is the reciprocal of endurance (DeLateur, 1987). Nursing interventions are directed at delaying the onset of task-related fatigue by maximizing the efficient use of muscles that control motion, movement, and locomotion.
6. The ability to maintain a given level of performance depends on personal factors: strength, coordination, reaction time, alertness, and motivation; and on activity-related factors: frequency, duration, and intensity of activity.
7. Tolerance for activity develops cyclically through adjusting frequency, duration, and intensity of activity until the desired level is achieved. Increasing activity frequency precedes increasing duration and intensity (work demand). Increased intensity is offset by a reduction in duration and frequency. As tolerance for more intensive activity of short duration develops, frequency is once again increased.

8. A person's response to activity can be evaluated by comparing preactivity blood pressure, pulse and respiration to postactivity blood pressure, pulse, and respiration. These, in turn, are compared to recovery time—the amount of time required for blood pressure, pulse, and respiration to return to preactivity levels.

9. The symptoms of activity intolerance are relieved by rest. The daily schedule is planned to allow for alternating periods of activity and rest, and coordinated to reduce periods of excess energy expenditure.

Activity Intolerance and Chronic Obstructive Pulmonary Disease

1. Persons with obstructive lung disease can increase their ability to withstand breathlessness, participate in the therapeutic regimen, and perform activities of daily living.

2. Tolerance for activity is maximized through an integrated program that incorporates the principles of physical relaxation, pulmonary hygiene, controlled breathing, and adequate nutrition and hydration.

3. Persons with obstructive lung disease are instructed in techniques of physical relaxation to minimize muscle tension. Relaxation is an essential preliminary step in teaching controlled breathing to eliminate wasteful and unproductive motions of the upper chest, shoulders, and neck.

4. In normal persons, the work of breathing is very limited. In persons with obstructive lung disease, however, the work of breathing may be increased 5 to 10 times above normal. Under such conditions, the amount of oxygen required *just for breathing activities* may be a large fraction of total oxygen consumption.

5. Clearing and defense of the airways are of utmost importance to meeting tissue demands for increased oxygen during periods of rest and periods of increased activity.

6. Persons with pulmonary disease can benefit from specific breathing exercises, which involve retraining of breathing patterns, and from general exercise programs that support normal daily activities (Sinclair, 1984).

7. Specific exercises aimed at retraining breathing should be viewed in terms of what can be realistically expected from them (Sinclair, 1984):
   a. Expending excessive effort to improve should be avoided because it will compress the airways and increase breathlessness.
   b. The oxygen cost of breathing can be reduced by improving the efficient use of accessory muscles.
   c. Controlled increased expiration can reduce gross hyperinflation, which requires increased inspiration air for alveoli exchange.
   d. Airway opening is improved by relaxed breathing; forced breathing compresses airways.
   e. The sensation of breathlessness can be reduced due to decreased neural input from muscle and joint receptors caused by increased diaphragmatic excursion with reduced thoracic movements.
   f. Controlled patterns of breathing can, at least theoretically, alter the distribution of inspired gases and thus improve the efficiency of gas exchange.

Activity Intolerance and Cardiac Disorders

1. Persons with impaired cardiac function often are able to increase both level of activity and tolerance for activity through adaptations in life-style, modifications in approach to activities, and careful monitoring of response to activity.

2. Tolerance for activity is maximized through an integrated program of medically supervised exercise, dietary restriction, stress management, and limited exposure to environmental extremes.

3. Persons with impaired cardiac function can achieve some immediate gains in activity tolerance by modifying their approach to activities, *e.g.,* pacing activities, avoiding isometric work, and limiting the duration of dynamic work by taking frequent rests.
4. All persons with impaired cardiac function should be instructed in self-monitoring techniques, *e.g.,* pulse-taking and recognizing and interpreting symptoms of intolerance.
5. Required reduction in the level of personal activity may result in role identification conflict and disruption of division's of labor within the family unit.

Bed Rest Deconditioning

1. The effects of bed rest deconditioning develop rapidly and may take weeks or months to reverse.
2. All persons confined to bed are at risk for activity intolerance as a result of bed rest-induced deconditioning.
3. Repeated confinement to bed rest and advanced age (over 65) are thought to have an additive effect on the deconditioning process (Bartz, 1982; LeBlanc, Gogia, Schneider, 1988), which may predispose the chronically ill and the elderly to activity intolerance as result of bed rest deconditioning.
4. Loss of skeletal muscle mass, changes in neurohumoral mechanisms and associated general decreases in body metabolic needs are major contributors to the deconditioning process of bed rest (LeBlanc, Gogia, & Schneider, 1988).
5. The deconditioning effects of bed rest lead to a decreased physical capacity for work in the supine position, as a result of changes occurring in the cardiac, circulatory, and musculoskeletal systems. The lack of exposure to orthostatic stress during bed rest leads to further decreases in the physical capacity for work in the upright position (Hung, Goldwater, & Convertino, 1983).
6. Some muscle groups seem to be more vulnerable to the deconditioning effects of bed rest than others, resulting in difference in the rate and degree of muscle atrophy (LeBlanc, Gogia, & Schneider, 1988).
7. During bed rest leg muscles tend to lose strength about twice as fast as arm muscles (Greenleaf, Wade, & Leftheriotis, 1989).
8. A onefold loss of muscle mass in plantar flexors of the lower legs (*e.g.,* gastrocnemius and soleus muscles) is associated with a twofold loss in muscle strength (LeBlanc, Gogia, & Schneider, 1988).
9. Exercises targeted at muscle groups that are more susceptible to bed rest deconditioning may be a more effective countermeasure for deconditioning than general exercise regimens (LeBlanc, Gogia, & Schneider, 1988).
10. Exercises performed in an upright position, against gravitational strain, are of greater value in overcoming the effects of bed rest deconditioning than exercises performed in a supine position.

Pediatric Considerations

1. Children at special risk for activity intolerance include those with respiratory conditions, cardiovascular conditions, anemia, and chronic illnesses, such as nephrosis (Scipien, Chard, Howe, & Barnard, 1990).
2. A child's response to activity can be evaluated through physiologic parameters and engagement in age-appropriate activities. For example, the nurse should assess the infant's sleep–rest cycle, motor activities, and eating behavior (Daberkow, 1989). The nurse should assess these parameters in a toddler, preschooler, and school-age child, as well as the child's involvement in play activities.
3. Play activities are important even for the hospitalized child with activity intolerance.

Play normalizes the child's experience in the hospital and reduces stress. The nurse must continually assess the child's fatigue and/or readiness to engage in more vigorous activity (Whaley & Wong, 1989).

Gerontologic Considerations

1. Some studies have shown a decrease in cardiac output from about 6.5 L/min at age 20 to 3.9 L/min at age 80, a decline of 1%. Stroke volume declines from 85 mL to 60 mL during this same age span. These studies probably did not exclude hidden cases of coronary artery disease, stress response to invasive procedures, or deconditioned status of individuals studied (Fleg, 1986; Gerber, 1990; Matteson & McConnell, 1988).

2. Studies have demonstrated an average age decline of 5–10% per decade in Maximum Oxygen Consumption (VO_2 max) from age 25 to age 75, or approximately 0.28 mL/kg/yr. Individuals who have been very athletic still have declines in VO_2max; however, it is only half of the 10% decade decline that is exhibited in less athletic individuals. There seems to be either decreased efficiency in mobilizing blood to exercising muscles or increased difficulty for muscles in extracting and utilizing oxygen because of decreased muscle mass. (*Note:* VO_2max is very difficult to obtain in older adults because of multiple subjective factors such as muscle fatigue, perceived exhaustion, and motivation to be tested. Often, leg muscles fail the individual before VO_2max can be achieved [Fleg, 1986; Gerber, 1990; Posner, Gorman, Klein, & Woldow, 1986].)

3. By age 75, only 10% of the pacemaker cells in the SA node remain, which could account for the slowed conduction during exercise (Gerber, 1990).

4. Aging brings a general decline in physical activity, which has a significant effect on cardiac performance both at rest and during exercise (Fleg, 1986; Abrams & Berkow, 1990).

5. Coronary artery disease is found on autopsy in 50–60% of the general population. The highest prevalance, based on signs and symptoms, documented in a population over age 75 was approximately 30% (Fleg, 1986).

6. Prolonged immobility and inactivity through self-imposed restrictions, mental status changes, and/or pathophysiologic changes can result in decreased tolerance to activity (Bortz, 1982; Matteson & McConnell, 1988).

7. Decreased muscle mass leads to decreased strength which in turn leads to decreased endurance. Muscle strength which is maximal between ages 20 and 30 drops to 80% of that value by age 65 (Fleg, 1986; Harris, 1982; Matteson & McConnell, 1988).

8. Increased chest wall rigidity with aging leads to decreased lung expansion, resulting in decreased tissue oxygenation. This has immediate effects on activity tolerance.

■ Activity Intolerance
Related to (Specify)

Outcome Criteria

The person will
- Identify factors that aggravate activity intolerance
- Identify methods to reduce activity intolerance
- Progress activity to (specify level of activity desired/required)
- Maintain blood pressure, pulse, and respirations within predetermined ranges during activity

---

Interventions

The following interventions apply to most individuals with activity intolerance, regardless of the etiology.

A. Identify any factors that contribute to activity intolerance (see *Related Factors*)

B. Reduce or eliminate contributing factors if possible
  1. Inadequate rest or sleep periods
    a. Determine adequacy of sleep. (Refer to *Sleep Pattern Disturbance* for additional information.)
    b. Plan rest periods according to the person's daily schedule. (Rest periods should occur throughout the day and between activities.)
    c. Encourage person to rest during the first hour following meals. (Rest can take many forms: napping, sitting and watching TV, or sitting with legs elevated.)
  2. Pain: Evaluate pain and the effectiveness of the present treatment regimen (refer to *Altered Comfort* for specific assessment criteria and interventions)
  3. Treatment-related factors
    a. Medications
      - Assess for side-effects of medication
      - Reduce side-effects, if possible (*e.g.,* for diuretic-induced hypokalemia, teach person to increase dietary potassium—oranges, tomatoes, bananas, dried fruit; for antibiotic-induced diarrhea, instruct person to consume yogurt two or three times a day).
    b. Daily schedule
      - Assess the person's daily schedule; consider treatments, diagnostic studies, etc.
      - Adjust schedule to reduce energy expenditure when possible (*e.g.,* cancel morning shower or bath when a diagnostic study is scheduled for the morning).
  4. Lack of incentive to participate in activity
    a. Identify factors that undermine person's confidence (*e.g.,* fear of falling, perceived weakness, visual impairment).

b. Promote a sincere "can do" attitude to provide a positive atmosphere that encourages increased activity; convey the belief that increasing level of activity and tolerance for activity is possible.

c. Explore possible incentives with the person and the family; consider what the person values, *e.g.:*
- Playing with grandchildren
- Returning to work
- Going fishing
- Performing a task, such as a craft

d. Allow person to set activity schedule and functional activity goals. If his goal is too low, contract with him, *e.g.,* "If you walk halfway up the hall, I'll let you nap for an hour."

e. Plan a purpose for the activity, such as sitting up in a chair to eat lunch, walking to a window to see the view, or walking to the kitchen to get some juice.

f. Help person to identify progress made. Do not underestimate the value of praise and encouragement as an effective motivational technique. In selected cases, it may be helpful to have the patient keep a record of his own progress.

C. Monitor the individual's response to activity

1. Take resting pulse, blood pressure, and respirations.
2. Consider rate, rhythm, and quality (if signs are abnormal—*e.g.,* pulse above 100—consult with physician about advisability of increasing activity).
3. Have person perform the activity.
4. Take vital signs immediately after activity. (Strenuous activity may increase the pulse by 50 beats. Such a rate is still satisfactory, as long as it returns to the resting pulse within 3 minutes.)
5. Have person rest for 3 minutes; take vital signs again.
6. Discontinue the activity if the individual responds to the activity with:
   a. Complaints of chest pain, vertigo, or confusion
   b. Decrease in pulse rate
   c. Failure of systolic blood pressure to increase
   d. Decrease in systolic blood pressure
   e. Increase in diastolic blood pressure by 15 mm Hg
   f. Decrease in respiratory response
7. Reduce the intensity or duration of the activity if:
   a. The pulse takes longer than 3–4 minutes to return to within 6 beats of the resting pulse rate
   b. The respiratory rate increase is excessive after the activity

D. Progress the activity gradually

1. Increase the person's tolerance for activity by having him perform the activity more slowly, or for a shorter period of time with more rest pauses, or with more assistance.
2. Minimize the deconditioning effects of prolonged bed rest and imposed immobility:
   a. Begin range of motion (ROM) at least b.i.d.
      If the person is unable, the nurse should perform passive ROM.
      If the person is able, have him perform active ROM.
   b. Encourage isometric exercise.
   c. Encourage the person to turn and lift himself actively unless contraindicated.

3. Promote optimal sitting balance and tolerance by increasing muscle strength.
   a. Gradually increase sitting tolerance by starting with 15 minutes for the first time out of bed.
   b. Have the person get out of bed 3 times a day, increasing the time out of bed by 15 minutes each day.
   c. Practice transfers. Have the person do as much active movement as possible.
4. Promote ambulation with or without assistive devices
   a. Provide support when the person begins to stand.
   b. If the person is unable to stand without buckling his knees, he is not ready for ambulation; have him practice standing in place with assistance.
   c. Choose a gait that is safe for the individual. (If his gait appears awkward but he has stability allow him to continue; stay close by and give clear coaching messages, *e.g.,* "Look straight ahead, not down.")
5. Allow the person to gauge the rate of ambulation.
6. Provide sufficient support to ensure safety and prevent falling.
7. Encourage the person to wear comfortable walking shoes (slippers do not support the feet properly).

E. Discuss with the person his perceptions of his condition and the effects it will have on role responsibilities, occupation, and finances

F. Provide opportunities for person to discuss limitations of activity tolerance in relation to sexuality
   1. Keep in mind that people tend to retain a high interest in sexuality regardless of limitations imposed by disease or disability.
   2. Sexual information and advice should be provided in a progressive fashion according to the needs of the patient and the ability of the health care provider.

G. Provide family with an opportunity to share their concerns
   1. Assess their knowledge of the condition, treatment, and prognosis.
   2. Encourage them to share their concerns about the future and about role responsibilities.

H. Initiate health teaching and referrals as indicated
   1. Teach the person safety precautions to prevent falls (see *High Risk for Injury*).
   2. Teach the person the proper use of walking aids (crutches, walkers, canes) and ensure the proper fit of such devices.
   3. Consult with a physical therapist for assistance in increasing activity tolerance.

■ Activity Intolerance
Related to Insufficient Knowledge of Adaptive Techniques Needed Secondary to Chronic Obstructive Pulmonary Disease

Assessment

During focus assessment for this diagnosis, the nurse seeks to identify etiology-related factors that contribute to the problem of activity intolerance.

Subjective data

The person reports an inability to participate in or complete desired or required activities due to:
Persistent shortness of breath
Dyspnea on exertion
Anxiety associated with an overwhelming sense of breathlessness
Early onset of task-related fatigue

Objective Data

As a result of activity, the person demonstrates:
Tachypnea or bradypnea
Arrhythmic breathing
Abnormal flow rate; increased I/E ratio
Increased use of accessory muscles of respiration
Gasping before or during speech
Reluctance to speak or inability to speak or cry due to breathlessness
Orthopnea
Mouth breathing
Nasal flaring
Increased cough
Central cyanosis
Peripheral cyanosis

Outcome Criteria

The person will
• Maintain/achieve optimal activity level (specify level)
• Demonstrate methods of controlled breathing to conserve energy
• Demonstrate ability to coordinate controlled breathing with activity

---

Interventions

The following interventions apply to persons experiencing activity intolerance due to a known cause: chronic obstructive pulmonary disease. These interventions are used in conjunction with the interventions identified for general cases of activity intolerance (see Interventions, pp. 114 through 116.)

A. Identify related factors that contribute to the problem. Consider adequacy of:
1. Knowledge of the therapeutic regimen
2. Pulmonary hygiene
3. Breathing techniques
4. Activity level
5. Nutritional intake
6. Health-related behaviors

B. Eliminate or reduce contributing factors
1. Lack of knowledge
   a. Assess person's understanding of the prescribed therapeutic regimen; proceed with health teaching, using simple, clear instructions and including family members.
   b. Specifically assess knowledge of:
      • Pulmonary hygiene
      • Adaptive breathing techniques
2. Inadequate pulmonary hygiene routine
   a. Explain the importance of adhering to daily coughing schedule for clearing the lungs and that this is a lifetime commitment.
   b. Teach the proper method of coughing:
      • Breathe deeply and slowly while sitting up as upright as possible.
      • Use diaphragmatic breathing.
      • Hold the breath for 3–5 seconds and then slowly exhale as much of this breath as possible through the mouth. (Lower rib cage and abdomen should sink down with exhaling.)
      • Take a second deep breath, hold, and cough forcefully from deep in the chest (not from the back of the mouth or throat); use two short, forceful coughs.
      • Rest after coughing sessions.
   c. Instruct person to practice controlled coughing four times a day, ½ hour before meals and at bedtime. Allow 15–30 minutes rest after coughing session and before meals.
   d. Consider use of inhaled humidity, postural drainage, and chest clapping before coughing session. (Assess for use of prescribed aerosol bronchodilators to dilate airways and thin secretions.)
3. Suboptimal breathing techniques
   a. Encourage conscious controlled breathing techniques (pursed-lip and diaphragmatic breathing) for use during periods of increased activity and emotional and physical stress.
   b. It often is helpful to initiate instruction in physical and mental relaxation techniques before teaching controlled breathing (see Appendix X).
   c. Instruct the person by demonstrating the desired breathing technique, then directing the person to mimic your breathing pattern.
   d. For pursed-lip breathing, the person should breathe in through the nose, then breathe out slowly through partially closed lips while counting to seven and making a "pu" sound. (Often, this is learned naturally by persons with progressive lung disease.)
   e. For diaphragmatic breathing:
      • Place your hands on the persons' abdomen below the base of the ribs and keep them there while the person inhales.
      • To inhale, the person relaxes the shoulders, breathes in through the nose,

and pushes the stomach outward against your hands. The person holds the breath for 1–2 seconds to keep the alveoli open, then exhales.
- To exhale, the person breathes out slowly through the mouth while you apply slight pressure at the base of the ribs.
- Have the person practice this breathing technique several times with you; then, the person should place his own hands at the base of the ribs to practice on his own.
- Once the person has learned the technique, have him practice it a few times each hour.

4. Insufficient level of activity
  a. Assess the person's current activity level. Consider:
    - Current pattern of activity/rest
    - Distribution of energy demand over course of day
    - Person's perceptions of most demanding required activities
    - Person's perceptions of areas where increased participation is desired or required
    - Efficacy of current adaptive techniques
  b. Identify physical barriers at home and at work (*e.g.*, number of stairs) that seem insurmountable and/or limit participation in activities.
  c. Identify ways of reducing the work demand of frequently performed tasks (*e.g.*, sitting rather than standing to prepare vegetables; keeping frequently used utensils on a countertop to avoid unnecessary overhead reaching or bending).
  d. Identify ways of alternating periods of exertion with periods of rest to overcome barriers (*e.g.*, place a chair in the bathroom near the sink so the person can rest during daily hygiene).
  e. Keep in mind that a plan including frequent short rest periods during an activity is less demanding and more conducive to completing the activity than a plan that calls for a burst of energy followed by a long period of rest.

5. Inadequate nutritional intake
  a. Recommend that the person brush teeth and use mouthwash before meals (and especially after coughing session, because there is frequently an associated bad taste in the mouth, causing a decreased appetite and tasting ability).
  b. Encourage smaller, more frequent meals. (Large portions require more oxygen/energy to digest and also limit the downward movement of the diaphragm during inspiration.)
  c. Choose foods that are easy to chew and swallow. (Food that must be chewed extensively will require more work, causing fatigue.)
  d. Assist in food preparation (*e.g.*, cutting meat) if person is prone to fatigue easily).
  e. Avoid gas-producing foods or liquids.
  f. Discourage talking while eating; encourage thorough chewing and slow eating.
  g. Encourage drinking 2–3 quarts of liquid a day (minimum) if fluids are unrestricted. (Consult physician for desired daily fluid intake.)

6. Health-related behaviors
  a. Teach person to avoid factors that aggravate symptoms and advance disease (excessive allergens, pollution).
  b. Discourage smoking.
  c. If person chooses to smoke, discourage smoking before meals and activity.
  d. If person wishes to reduce or stop smoking, see further interventions under *Altered Health Maintenance related to tobacco use.*

C. Monitor the individual's response to activity
1. See Interventions, p. 115.
2. While monitoring the response to activity, observe for signs and symptoms of respiratory intolerance:
   a. Markedly increased respiratory rate
   b. Aggravated dyspnea
   c. Pallor
   d. Cyanosis
   e. Loss of ability to maintain rhythmic controlled breathing
   f. Use of accessory muscles.

D. Gradually increase activity
1. Reassure person that some increase in daily activity is possible.
2. Instruct person in controlled breathing techniques.
3. Encourage the person to use controlled breathing techniques to decrease the work of breathing during activities.
4. After the person masters controlled breathing in relaxed positions, begin to increase activity.
5. Teach person to maintain controlled breathing pattern while sitting or standing.
6. Progress person to maintaining controlled breathing during bed-to-chair transfers and walking.
7. Many patients can learn to maintain rhythmic breathing during walking by using a simple 2:4 ratio; 2 steps during inspiration and 4 steps during expiration.
8. Do not progress the person to more demanding activity until breathing is well controlled during less demanding activities.

E. Discuss with person his perceptions of his condition and the effects it will have on role responsibilities, occupation, and finances

F. Provide opportunities for the person to discuss the impact of limited activity tolerance on sexuality
1. Promote an atmosphere of openess, understanding, and acceptance.
2. Some persons with obstructive lung disease may fear that sexual activity will increase dyspnea and, therefore, avoid it altogether. Others may simply give up before or during sexual activity due to shortness of breath and associated frustration.
3. Providing some commonsense information may be all that is needed for persons to resume satisfying sexual relations.
4. Explain that attempting lovemaking while fatigued, during a chest infection, following a large meal, or after indulgence in large amounts of alcohol increases the likelihood of failure.
5. Suggest that planned lovemaking during midday or early evening when energy levels are highest may be more satisfying than late-night relations when the person is already fatigued.
6. Many persons with obstructive lung disease have the mistaken belief that if they rush through an activity it can be accomplished before the onset of shortness of breath. Nothing could be further from the truth. Encourage patients to approach lovemaking in a slow and deliberate manner.
7. Sources of additional (and more detailed) information on sexual counseling for persons with obstructive lung disease are listed in the reference section.

G. Initiate health teaching
1. Teach person to observe his sputum, note changes in color, amount, and odor, and seek professional advice if sputum changes.
2. Explain that the person with chronic pulmonary disease is susceptible to infection and must detect symptoms early and consult with physician for treatment (frequently, early antibiotic therapy is necessary).
3. Discuss the need for annual immunizations against flu. (The utility of one-time-only pneumococcal vaccinations has recently been questioned; therefore, administration should be on an individual basis.)
4. Instruct person to wear warm dry clothing; avoid crowds, heavy smoke, fumes, and irritants; avoid exertion in cold, hot, or humid weather; and balance work, rest, and recreation to regulate energy expenditure.
5. Emphasize the importance of maintaining a good wholesome diet (high calorie, high vitamin C, high protein, and 2–3 quarts of liquid a day, unless on fluid restriction).
6. Evaluate the person's knowledge of the care, cleansing and use of inhalatory equipment.
7. If using oxygen therapy, especially at home, evaluate awareness of fire hazards; explain need for home extinguisher.

H. Make referrals as indicated
1. Refer to community nurse for follow-up.
2. Consult physical therapist for a more comprehensive exercise program tailored to the needs of persons with obstructive pulmonary disease.
3. Refer to community support groups (*e.g.,* Better Breathers) and pertinent literature for persons with lung disorders.

■ Activity Intolerance
Related to Insufficient Knowledge of Adaptive Techniques Needed Secondary to Impaired Cardiac Function

Assessment

Subjective Data
During activity, the person reports:
Chest pain or chest discomfort
Dyspnea or shortness of breath
Dizziness
Exertional fatigue

Objective Data
Rapid pulse
Labored or rapid breathing
Diaphoresis

Dysrhythmias
Cyanosis

Outcome Criteria

The person will
- Identify factors that increase cardiac workload
- Describe adaptive techniques needed to perform activities of daily living
- Demonstrate tolerance for increased activity by maintaining pulse, respirations, and blood pressure within predetermined ranges

---

Interventions

The nursing interventions for this diagnosis represent interventions for individuals experiencing activity intolerance as a result of impairment in cardiac function. These interventions are not applicable to all clients who are activity-intolerant as a result of impaired cardiac function. The physician should be consulted regarding if or when the client can increase activity. To develop an individualized plan of care, the exact nature and extent of the underlying cardiac pathology must be known. The following interventions are used in conjunction with the interventions identified for general cases of activity intolerance (see Interventions, p. 114).

A. Identify related factors that contribute to the problem, consider:

1. Knowledge of the therapeutic regimen
2. Activity level
3. Smoking
4. Overweight/obesity

B. Eliminate or reduce contributing factors if possible

1. Specifically assess knowledge and behavior related to the four "E's":
   Eating
   Exertion
   Exposure
   Emotional stress (adapted from Day, 1984)
   a. Eating
      - Assess knowledge of restricted diet.
      - Explain importance of adhering to prescribed salt-restricted diet.
      - Explore alternatives for seasoning foods to taste using natural herbs and spices (*e.g.,* Mrs. Dash).
      - Encourage a light meal in the evening to promote a more comfortable night's rest.
      - Initially provide easily digestible and chewable foods.
      - Schedule meals to avoid interfering with other activities.
      - Offer food preferences, avoiding dislikes.
      - Consider sociocultural influences.
   b. Exertion
      - Teach person to modify approaches to activities to regulate energy expenditure and reduce cardiac workload (*e.g.,* take rest periods during activities, at intervals during the day, and for 1 hour after meals;

sit rather than stand when performing activities, unless this is not feasible; when performing a task, rest every 3 minutes for 5 minutes to allow the heart to recover; stop an activity if exertional fatigue or signs of cardiac hypoxia [*e.g.*, markedly increased pulse rate, dyspnea, chest pain] occurs).

- Instruct person to avoid certain types of exertion: isometric exercises, *e.g.*, using arms to lift himself, carry objects, and Valsalva maneuver; *e.g.*, bending at the waist in a sit-up fashion to rise from bed, straining during a bowel movement.

c. Exposure
- Instruct person to avoid unnecessary exposure to environmental extremes.
- Exertion during hot humid weather or extreme cold weather places additional demands of the heart and should be avoided.
- Instruct person to dress warmly during cold weather, *e.g.*, create a barrier to cold weather by wearing layers of clothing.

d. Emotional stress
- Assist person to identify emotional stressors (*e.g.*, at home, at work, social).
- Discuss his usual response to emotional stress (*e.g.*, anger, depression, avoidance, discussion).
- Explain the effects of emotional stress on the cardiovascular system (*e.g.*, increased heart rate, increased blood pressure, increased respirations)
- Discuss various methods for stress management/reduction (*e.g.*, deliberate problem-solving [see Appendix VII], relaxation techniques [see Appendix X], yoga or meditation, biofeedback, regular exercise).

2. Activity level
   a. Assess person's current activity level; consider:
   - Current pattern of activity/rest
   - Distribution of energy demand over course of day
   - Person's perceptions of most demanding required activities
   - Person's perceptions of areas where increased participation is desired or required.
   b. Identify person's symptoms of cardiac intolerance.
   c. Evaluate effectiveness of adaptive techniques to manage symptoms (*e.g.*, pacing activities, frequent rest pauses, use of nitrates before planned exertion).
   d. Organize inhospital care to allow for periods of undisturbed rest.

3. Smoking
   a. Discuss with person the effects of smoking on the cardiovascular system (*e.g.*, vasoconstriction increases workload of the heart).
   b. Teach person when not to smoke before an activity and immediately after an activity.
   c. Discuss methods that can help reduce the amount of cigarettes smoked (see *Altered Health Maintenance related to tobacco use*).

4. Overweight/obesity
   a. Assess whether the person is overweight or obese by measuring height and weight and comparing findings with a standardized height-weight chart, or use anthropometric measurements (see *Altered Nutrition: More than Body Requirements* for charts of weight for height and anthropometric norms).

C. Monitor the individual's response to activity (see Interventions, p. 115) and teach him self-monitoring techniques:

1. Take resting pulse
2. Take pulse during activity or immediately after
3. Take pulse 3 minutes after cessation of activity
4. Instruct person to stop activity and report:
   a. Decreased pulse rate during activity
   b. Pulse rate > 112 beats/min
   c. Irregular pulse
   d. Pulse rate that does not return to within 6 beats of resting pulse after 3 minutes
   e. Dyspnea
   f. Chest pain
   g. Palpitations
   h. Perceptions of exertional fatigue.

D. Gradually increase activity

1. Allow for periods of rest before and after planned periods of exertion, such as treatments, ambulation, meals.
2. Encourage gradual increases in activity and ambulation to prevent a sudden increase in cardiac workload.
3. Assess person's perceived capability for increased activity.
4. Assist person in setting short-term activity goals that are realistic and achievable.
5. Reassure person that even small increases in activity will have the effect of lifting his spirits and restoring his self-confidence.

E. Discuss with person his perceptions of his condition and the effects it will have on role responsibilities, occupation, and finances

F. Provide opportunities for the person to discuss the impact of limited activity tolerance in relation to sexuality

1. Individualized sexual counseling can occur only when the nature and extent of cardiac pathology are known. The client's physician or cardiologist should be consulted before proceeding with sexual counseling.
2. In general, persons with impaired cardiac function who are ready to resume sexual activities are advised to (Day, 1984):
   a. Choose a time when he feels relaxed and rested, and avoid sex when emotionally upset; the first thing in the morning might be a good time.
   b. Wait 2–3 hours after drinking excessive amounts of alcohol or eating a heavy meal.
   c. Avoid having sex immediately before or after strenuous exercise or a hot shower.
   d. Keep the room temperature comfortable.
   e. Experiment with positions that place less strain on the heart, *e.g.*,
      • Lying with the partner on top
      • Sitting with the partner on top
      • Lying side-by-side
   f. Notify the physician if sex brings on chest discomfort, dizziness, shortness of

breath, rapid or irregular heartbeat that lasts 15 minutes or more after intercourse.

G. Provide the family with an opportunity to share their concerns

1. Assess their knowledge of the condition, treatment, and prognosis.
2. Encourage them to share their concerns about the future and about role responsibilities.

H. Initiate health teaching and referrals as indicated

1. Instruct the person to consult his physician and physiatrist for a long-term exercise program or to contact the American Heart Association for available local cardiac rehabilitation programs.
2. Explain dietary restrictions to the person and family. Give them written instructions or refer them to pertinent literature on preparation of food for restricted diets.
3. Explain prescribed drug therapy (*e.g.*, diuretics, vasodilators): dosage, side-effects, administration, and storage.

■ Activity Intolerance
Related to Bed Rest Deconditioning

Assessment

During focus assessment for this diagnosis, the nurse seeks to identify etiology-related factors that contribute to the problem of activity intolerance. It often is helpful to relate elements of the assessment to functional status to establish a record of performance. By keeping a record of performance, the nurse can determine the person's current status, monitor progress, and determine the person's status at the conclusion of therapy.

Subjective Data

Person reports an inability to participate in desired or required activities or an inability to complete activities due to:
Weakness
Early onset of task-related fatigue
Dizziness, nausea, diaphoresis, or syncope associated with postural changes

Objective Data

Bed rest
Skeletal muscle atrophy
Skeletal muscle weakness
Tremor
Swaying during ambulation
Orthostatic hypotension
Confusion, disorientation, or decreased attention span

Outcome Criteria

The person will
- Identify factors that contribute to deconditioning
- Participate in planned therapies to minimize or reverse the effects of deconditioning
- Demonstrate sufficient energy and strength to participate in and complete desired or required activities

Interventions

The nursing interventions for this diagnosis focus on overcoming the deleterious effects of bed rest-induced deconditioning through a planned program of reconditioning. These interventions are used in conjunction with the interventions identified for general cases of activity intolerance (see pp. 114 through 116).

A. Identify related factors that contribute to the problem; consider:
1. Prolonged or recurrent confinement to bed rest
2. Disturbances of motor function
3. Adequacy of positioning, repositioning and ROM regimens
4. Orthostatic intolerance
5. Adequacy of nutritional intake

B. Eliminate or reduce contibuting factors if possible
1. Prolonged or recurrent confinement to bed rest
   a. Assess history of bed or bed-chair confinement (*e.g.,* short-term, long-term, repeated).
   b. Is bed or chair confinement prescribed by the medical plan of care, self-imposed, or imposed by expectations/limitations of caregivers?
   c. Evaluate bed mobility. (Persons without independent bed mobility may be more accurately diagnosed with *Disuse Syndrome.*)
2. Assess for motor function disturbances. (Note: A comprehensive motor assessment includes evaluation of muscle bulk, muscle tone, muscle strength, coordination, and involuntary movements [Bates, 1987]. What constitutes a minimally acceptable assessment will depend on the extent and severity of involvement and the assessment abilities of the nurse.)
   a. Muscle atrophy and strength
      When assessing for muscle atrophy, inspect the pelvic and shoulder girdles, hands, and extremities. Muscle wasting in the extremities may give the appearance of excessively large joints. Measuring the circumference of an extremity does not provide reliable information about muscle atrophy since it is unclear what is being measured. Comparable body parts can be compared for symmetry; however, the dominant extremities are often larger than their nondominant counterparts.
      Assess muscle strength around each major joint. Strength is conventionally expressed using the Lovett six-grade scale (Bates, 1987):
      0 (Zero)   No contraction
      1 (Trace)   Some contraction; no motion
      2 (Poor)   Unable to move against gravity

3 (Fair)   Can move against gravity only
4 (Good)   Moves against moderate resistance
5 (Normal) Moves against full resistance

b. Spasticity
   • Determine the degree of spasticity or abnormally increased muscle tone.
   • Spasticity increases the energy costs of activities, can seriously limit functional independence, and interferes with gait training, orthotic prescription, and contracture prevention.
   • The extent and severity of spasticity will often vary in a given individual, depending on time of day, previous activity, posture, and tactile and kinesthetic stimuli.
   • Designate spasticity as mild, moderate or severe.
   • It is often helpful to relate spasticity to functional aspects of the patient's activities (*e.g.,* mild spasticity of lower extremities that progresses to severe spasticity after walking 20 feet on a level grade).

c. Coordination
   • Impaired motor coordination may interfere with completion of many tasks (*e.g.,* feeding or sitting and standing) due to poor balance.
   • By convention, two tests of coordination are generally performed: rapid alternating movements and point-to-point testing.
   • Assess coordination of both upper and lower extremities.
   • The most effective therapy for improving coordination is repeated practice beginning with simple exercises and progressing to more complex tasks. Patients who are confused, inattentive, or have poor memory may have considerable difficulty in acquiring coordination skills necessary for completion of therapeutic and self-care activities.

3. Assess adequacy of positioning, repositioning, and ROM regimens.
   a. Positioning for comfort and pressure relief should be done at least every 2 hours.
   b. If not contraindicated, the repositioning regimen should include periods of upright positioning (*e.g.,* high Fowler's position or up in chair).
   c. Periods of therapeutic positioning where muscles are fully stretched should be included in the repositioning regimen, to prevent muscle shortening, since shortened muscles atrophy quicker.
   d. Prolonged stretching for 20 minutes using moderate force is much more effective than application of brief vigorous stretches to prevent muscle shortening and contractures.
   e. Evaluate need for dorsiflexion orthotics to protect plantar flexors of lower extremities from shortening and accelerated atrophy.
   f. Evaluate ROM of all major joints; express ROM in degrees.
   g. Assess adequacy of ROM exercises. Consider thoroughness, frequency, and resistance (*e.g.,* passive or active).

4. Assess for orthostatic intolerance.
   a. Refer to *High Risk for Injury related to vertigo secondary to postural hypotension.*

5. Assess adequacy of nutritional intake.
   a. Evaluate calorie-nitrogen intake. Nitrogen intake must be sufficient for protein synthesis. Enough nonnitrogen calories must also be taken in to ensure that protein calories will not be metabolized to meet energy needs. A malnourished or stressed patient requires almost double the amount of nitrogen as a healthy individual.

    b. If inadequate nutritional intake is suspected, keep a daily record of foods eaten and consult a dietician.

    c. See *Altered Nutrition: Less than Body Requirements* for specific interventions.

C. Monitor response to activity

1. See Interventions, p. 115.
2. Rapid onset of task-related fatigue is an early indicator of intolerance in deconditioned individuals.
3. While monitoring the response to activity, assess for signs and symptoms of orthostatic intolerance (tachycardia, nausea, diaphoresis, and syncope). (See *High Risk for Injury related to orthostatic hypotension* for specific interventions.)

D. Gradually increase activity

1. Plan strategies to increase bed mobility (*e.g.*, use of overhead trapeze).
2. Implement a planned exercise program that includes lower extremity exercises against resistance.
3. Progress patient to exercise in upright positions against gravitational strain as early as possible.
4. Begin weight bearing at earliest possible date to minimize atrophy of plantar flexors in lower legs.
5. Promote independence in ADLs. Activities that the person can perform independently should be performed by the patient rather than the nurse or caregiver.

E. Initiate health teaching and referrals

1. Instruct patient and caregivers in ROM and therapeutic exercises.
2. Consult physical therapist for an exercise program tailored to the individual's needs.
3. Consult dietician for dietary evaluation and nutritional counseling.

References/Bibliography

General

Abrams W. B. & Berkow, R. (Eds.) (1990). *The Merck manual of geriatrics*. Rahway NJ: Merck & Co.

Adams, C. E., & Leverland, M. B. (1985). Environmental and behavioral factors that can affect blood pressure. *Nurse Practitioner, 10*(11), 39–50.

Aistars, J. (1987). Fatigue in the cancer patient: A conceptual approach to a clinical problem. *Oncology Nursing Forum, 14*(6), 25–30.

Alexy, B. J. (1978). Monitoring cardiovascular status with noninvasive techniques. *Nursing Clinics of North America, 13*(3), 423–435.

Allen, S. R., & Moschak, V. (1981). Step by step: Renew a patient's interest in life with an ambulation incentive program. *Nursing 81, 11*(8), 56–57.

Basmajian, J. V. (1984). *Therapeutic exercise* (4th ed.). London: Williams & Wilkins.

Bortz, W. M. (1982). Disuse and aging. *JAMA, 248*(10), 1203–1208.

Bulechek, G. M., & McCloskey, J. C. (Eds.). (1985). *Nursing interventions: Treatments for nursing diagnoses*. Philadelphia: W. B. Saunders Co.

Cameron, C. (1973). A theory of fatigue. *Ergonomics, 16*(5), 633–648.

Daberkow, E. (1989). Nursing strategies: Altered cardiovascular function. In Foster, R. L., Hunsberger, M. M., & Anderson J. J. T. (Eds.). *Family-centered nursing care of children*. Philadelphia: W. B. Saunders.

de Lateur, B. J. (1984). Exercise for strength and endurance. In Basmajian, J. V. (Ed.). *Therapeutic exercise*. Baltimore: Williams & Wilkins.

Fitzmaurice, J. B. (1987). Nurse's use of cues in the clinical judgment of activity intolerance. In McLane, A. M. (Ed.). *Classification of nursing diagnosis: Proceedings of the seventh conference.* St. Louis: C. V. Mosby.

Fleg, J. L. (1986). Alterations in cardiovascular structure and function with advancing age. *American Journal of Cardiology, 5*(7), 33C–44C.

Gerber R. M. (1990). Coronary artery disease in the elderly. *Journal of Cardiovascular Nursing, 4*(4), 23–34.

Gilman, A. G., Goodman, L., & Gilman, A. (1980). *The pharmacological basis of therapeutics* (6th ed.). New York: Macmillan.

Gordon, M. (1976). Assessing activity tolerance. *American Journal of Nursing, 76*(1), 72–75.

Gordon, M. (1987). *Manual of nursing diagnosis.* New York: McGraw-Hill.

Gordon, M. (1987). *Nursing diagnosis: Process and application* (2nd ed.). New York: McGraw-Hill.

Gortner, S. R., Miller, N. G., & Jenkins, L. S. (1988). Self-efficacy: A key to recovery. In Jillings, C. R. (Ed.). *Cardiac rehabilitation nursing.* Rockville, MD: Aspen Publications.

Gould, M. T. (1983). Nursing diagnoses concurrent with multiple sclerosis. *Journal of Neurosurgical Nursing, 15*(6), 339–345.

Hagberg, J. M., Graves, J. E., Limacher, M., et al. (1989). Cardiovascular responses of 70- to 79-year-old men and women to exercise training. *Journal of Applied Physiology, 66*(6), 2589–2594.

Halfman, M. A., & Hojnacki, L. G. (1981). Exercise and maintenance of health. *Topics in Clinical Nursing 3,* 1–10.

Harris, R. (1982). Exercise and sex in the aging patient. *Medical Aspects of Human Sexuality,* 152–157.

Kim, M. J., McFarland, G. K., & McLane, A. M. (1984). *Classification of nursing diagnoses: Proceedings of the fifth national conference.* St. Louis: C. V. Mosby.

Kreuger, D. W. (Ed.). (1984). *Emotional rehabilitation of physical trauma and disability.* New York: SP Medical & Scientific Books.

Louis, M. C., & Pouse, S. M. (1980). Aphasia and endurance: considerations in the assessment and care of the stroke patient. *Nursing Clinics of North America, 15*(2), 265–282.

Magnan, M. A. (1987). Activity intolerance: Toward a nursing theory of activity. Paper presented at the Fifth Annual Symposium of the Michigan Nursing Diagnosis Association, Detroit, September 1987.

Matteson, M. A. & McConnell, E. S. (1988). *Gerontological nursing: Concepts and practices.* Philadelphia: W. B. Saunders.

McLean, S. L. (1989). Activity intolerance: Cues for diagnosis. In Carroll-Johnson, R. M. (Ed.). *Classification of nursing diagnosis: Proceedings of the eighth conference.* Philadelphia: J. B. Lippincott.

Mitchell, C. A. (1986). Generalized chronic fatigue in the elderly: Assessment and intervention. *Journal of Gerontological Nursing, 12*(4), 19–23.

Muir, B. L. (1988). *Pathophysiology: An introduction to the mechanisms of disease* (2nd ed.). New York: John Wiley & Sons.

Pender, N. J. (1982). *Health promotion in nursing practice.* Norwalk, CT: Appleton-Century-Crofts.

Piper, B. F. (1986). Fatigue. In Carrieri, V. K., Lindsey, A. M., & West, C. M. (Eds.). *Pathophysiological phenomena in nursing: Human responses to illness.* Philadelphia: W. B. Saunders.

Posner, J. D., Gorman, K. M., Klein, H. S., & Woldow, A. (1986). Exercise capacity in the elderly. *American Journal of Cardiology,* 57:52C–58C.

Potempa, K., Lopez, M., Reid, C., & Lawson, L. (1986). Chronic fatigue. *Image, 18*(4), 165–169.

Price, S. A., & Wilson, L. M. (1982). *Pathophysiology: Clinical concepts of disease processes* (2nd ed.). New York: McGraw-Hill.

Schlant, R. C. (1982). Physiology of exercise. In Fletcher, G. F. (Ed.). *Exercise in the practice of medicine.* Mount Kisco, NY: Futura Publishing.

Scipien, G. M., Chard, M. A., Howe, J., & Barnard, M. U. (1990). *Pediatric nursing care.* St. Louis: C. V. Mosby.

Sculco, C. D. (1978). The need for activity. In Yura, H. & Walsh, M. (Eds.). *Human needs and the nursing process.* New York: Appleton-Century-Crofts.

Whaley, L. F., & Wong, D. L. (1989). *Essentials of pediatric nursing* (3rd ed). St. Louis: C. V. Mosby.

Ziegler, J. C. (1980). Physical reconditioning for the convalescent patient. *Nursing, 10*(8), 67–69.

Pulmonary

Hodgkin, J. E., & Petty, T. L. (1987). *Chronic obstructive pulmonary disease: Current concepts.* Philadelphia: W. B. Saunders.

Nett, L. M., & Petty, T. L. (1985). Managing the COPD patient and family at home. In Petty, T. L. (Ed.). *Chronic obstructive pulmonary disease.* New York: Marcel Dekker.

Selecky, P. A. (1987). Sexuality and the COPD patient. In Hodjkin, J. E. & Petty, T. L. (Eds.). *Chronic obstructive pulmonary disease.* Philadelphia: W. B. Saunders.

Sinclair, J. D. (1984). Exercise in pulmonary disease. In Basmajian, J. V. (Ed.). *Therapeutic exercise.* Baltimore: Williams & Wilkins.

Williams, J. H. (1986). Pneumococcal vaccine and patients with chronic lung disease. *Annals of Internal Medicine, 104,* 106–109.

Cardiac

American Heart Association, The Committee on Exercise. (1975). *Exercise testing of individuals with heart disease or at high risk for its development.* Dallas: American Heart Association.

Cantwell, J. D. (1984). Exercise and coronary heart disease: Role in primary prevention. *Heart & Lung, 13,*(1), 6–13.

Day, N. R. (1984). *After your heart attack.* Daly City, CA: Krames Communications.

Ellestad, M. H. (1986). *Stress testing: Principles and practice* (3rd ed.). Philadelphia: F. A. Davis.

Froelicher, V. F. (1987). *Exercise and the heart: Clinical concepts.* Chicago: Year Book Medical Publishers.

Guyatt, G. H., Sullivan, M. J., & Thompson, P. J. (1985). The 6-minute walk: A new measure of exercise capacity in patients with chronic heart failure. *Canadian Medical Association Journal, 132*(4), 919–923.

Jenkins, L. S. (1987). Self-efficacy: New perspectives in caring for patients recovering from myocardial infarction. *Progress in Cardiovascular Nursing, 2,* 32–35.

Jillings, C. R. (Ed.). (1988). *Cardiac rehabilitation nursing.* Rockville, MD: Aspen Publications.

Kavanagh, T. Exercise and coronary artery disease. In Basmajian, J. F. (Ed.). *Therapeutic exercise.* Baltimore, Williams & Wilkins.

Parmley, W. W. (1986). Position report on cardiac rehabilitation. *Journal of the American College of Cardiology, 7*(2), 451–453.

Sanderson, R. G., & Kurth, C. L. (1983). *The cardiac patient: A comprehensive approach.* Philadelphia: W. B. Saunders.

Deconditioning

Bartz, W. M. (1982). Disuse and aging. *JAMA, 248,* 1203–1208.

Bates, B. (1987). *A guide to physical examination and history taking* (4th ed.). Philadelphia: J. B. Lippincott.

Brandstater, M. E., & Basmajian, J. V. (Eds.). (1987). *Stroke rehabilitation.* Baltimore: Williams & Wilkins.

Convertino, V. A., Hung, J., Goldwater, D., et al. (1982). Cardiovascular responses to exercise in middle-aged men after 10 days of bedrest. *Circulation, 65,* 134–142.

Fisher, S. V., & Gullickson, G. (1978). The energy costs of ambulation in health and disability: A literature review. *Archives of Physical Medicine and Rehabilitation, 59*(3), 124–133.

Harper, C. M., & Lyles, Y. M. (1988). Physiology and complications of bed rest. *Journal of American Geriatric Society, 36*(11), 1047–1054.

Greenleaf, J. E., Wade, C. E., & Leftheriotis, G. (1989). Orthostatic responses following 30-day bed rest deconditioning with isotonic and isokinetic exercise training. *Aviation, Space and Environmental Medicine, 6,* 537–542.

Hung, J., Goldwater, D., & Convertino, V. A. (1983). Mechanisms for decreased exercise capacity after bed rest in normal middle-aged men. *The American Journal of Cardiology, 51*(1), 344–348.

LeBlanc, A., Gogia, P., & Schneider, V. (1988). Calf muscle area and strength changes after five weeks of horizontal bed rest. *The American Journal of Sports Medicine, 16*(2), 624–629.

Sandler, H., Popp, R. L., & Harrison, D. (1988). The hemodynamic effects of repeated bed rest exposure. *Aviation, Space and Environmental Medicine, 11,* 1047–1054.

Adjustment, Impaired

■ *Related to* **(Specify)**

DEFINITION

Impaired Adjustment: The state in which the individual is unwilling to modify his/her life-style/behavior in a manner consistent with a change in health status.

DEFINING CHARACTERISTICS

Major (must be present)

Verbalization of nonacceptance of health status change or inadequate capacity to be involved in problem-solving or goal-setting.

Minor (may be present)

Lack of movement toward independence; extended period of shock, disbelief, or anger regarding health status change; lack of future-oriented thinking.

RELATED FACTORS

Adjustment impairment can result from a variety of situations and health problems. Some common sources are listed below.

Pathophysiologic

Spinal cord injury
Paralysis
Loss of limb
Cerebrovascular accident (CVA)
Myocardial infarction
Progressive neurologic diseases
Cancer
Chronic obstructive pulmonary disease (COPD)

Treatment-related

Dialysis

Situational (personal, environmental)

Inadequate support systems
Unavailable support systems
Impaired cognition
Depression
Loss (object, person, job)
Divorce

Maturational

Child/adolescent: chronic disease, disability
Adult: loss of ability to practice vocation, role reversal
Elderly: sensory losses, functional losses, retirement

Diagnostic Considerations

This diagnosis can apply to persons in varied settings: in-patient, rehabilitation, long-term care, and community. Many other nursing diagnoses can coexist or overlap with *Impaired Adjustment, e.g., Grieving, Ineffective Coping, Anxiety,* and *Fear.* This diagnosis may prove most clinically useful during the initial adjustment phase, *e.g.,* the first 3–4 months. Prolonged resistance to change may be more appropriately described as *Ineffective Individual Coping.* At some point, the nurse and person may agree that the choice is not to modify behavior.

It is also important to differentiate the diagnosis *Impaired Adjustment* from *Noncompliance* and *Ineffective Denial. Impaired Adjustment* applies to a person who chooses not to participate in the modifications needed as the result of limitations associated with a health condition or disability. A person with *Noncompliance* desires to comply but factors interfere with his ability to do so. *Ineffective Denial* describes an individual who maintains that a situation detrimental to his health is actually not detrimental.

Errors in Diagnostic Statements

Impaired Adjustment related to denial of problem

If the denial of a problem is an acute response, it represents a normal response to loss. The appropriate nursing diagnosis for this individual would be: *Grieving related to perceived negative effects of disability on life-style and goals.*

If the denial is prolonged and failure to participate in changes in life-style proves detrimental to health, then the nursing diagnosis would be: *Ineffective Denial related to inadequate internal resources to manage the situation.*

Impaired Adjustment related to refusal to participate in muscle-strengthening exercises

The above-related factors represent signs and symptoms, not contributing factors. The correct diagnostic statement would be something like: *Impaired Adjustment related to unrealistic high feelings of self-efficacy, as evidenced by refusal to participate in program and statements of "I always got better in the past."*

Focus Assessment Criteria

The following assessment is indicated for a person who has resisted or refused interventions or modifications in his life-style.

Subjective

Present response
Since you are not participating in prescribed plan, would you share why?
Do you have an alternative plan?
Self-esteem
What personal achievements have given you the most satisfaction?
What do others like most about you?

Control/Decision-making

How much control do you have over your present situation?

How much control do you expect to have?

How would you describe your usual method of decision-making?

Coping styles

What problem situations have you experienced in your life?

How did you deal with the situation? (Problem focused or emotion focused)

Resources

Financial

Religious beliefs/participation

Recreational activities

Social support

To whom do you turn to for help when you have a problem?

Recent life events

Besides the present situation, have you experienced other distressful situations (financial, health, family, friends)?

Objective

Physical appearance

Grooming (appropriate, poor)

Hair (styled, groomed)

Eye contact (appropriate, averts eyes)

Social contact

Initiates interactions

Avoids Contacts

Motivation

Actively seeks information/involvement

Needs encouragement

Reluctant to participate

Refuses to participate

Expresses lack of interest

Principles and Rationale for Nursing Care

Generic Considerations

1. Individuals have a concept of self that includes feelings about self, worth, attractiveness, lovability, and capabilities (Peretz, 1970). One's mental image of one's own body and person is assaulted after a physical injury. This injury or loss involves the grieving process.
2. The grieving process in response to a recent disability has been described as (Friedman-Campbell & Hart, 1984):
   a. Shock-denial
      - Denies injury or severity of the injury
      - Minimally allows self to think of loss to protect self
      - Intellectually accepts the loss but denies it emotionally
   b. Developing awareness
      - Realizes the impact of the loss on self
      - Experiences acute somatic feelings of loss
      - Displaces anger
      - Is preoccupied with guilt and blaming

- Mourns the loss and withdraws
- Shuns change and clings to routines

c. Managing loss of body function
- Begins to deal with the impact of the loss on self
- Frees self slowly from the bondage of the loss
- Readjusts to changed environment
- Invests in new relationships

3. Physically disabled persons are faced with many challenges that require adjustments and change. Everyday stressors challenge the physically disabled more profoundly, *e.g.,* food preparation, time management (Swanson, Cronin-Stubbs, & Sheldon, 1989).

4. Personal and environmental factors influence how a person will cope with a disability. Research findings have supported that motivation and morale are affected by social support, self-concept, locus of control, and hardiness (Evans & Halar, 1985; Kobasa, 1982; Matson & Brooks, 1982; Russell, 1981; Sinyor, Amato, Kaloupek, Becker, Goldenburg, & Coopersmith, 1986).

5. An individual's response to stressful events depends on the personal resources available at the time of the event (Whitborne, 1985).

6. Research has shown that younger adults can cope more effectively if there is higher income, higher self-efficacy, high occupational status, a marriage partner, the availability of a confidant, a large social network, and commitment to and involvement in religious beliefs (Simons & West, 1984–85).

7. Simons and West (1984–85) found older adults differed from younger adults in coping. Higher occupational status and high feelings of self-efficacy impeded effective coping. These characteristics were usually helpful to an older adult except during times of significant life changes.

8. Everyone has implicit or explicit goals. Through experience, patterns of successful behavior in achieving these individual goals are developed. The person then regularly uses this behavior to achieve goals.

9. Goals are established to maintain:
   a. Physical well-being
   b. Self-esteem
   c. Productive satisfying interactions with others

10. The behavior of individuals is such that:
   a. People act to meet needs and achieve goals
   b. Relatively stable patterns of behavior are developed
   c. Behavior is disrupted when both needs and goals are threatened

11. Coping attempts to remove the threats to meeting needs and achieving goals. Lazarus and Monat (1977) state that coping refers to efforts to master conditions of harm, threat, or challenge when a routine or automatic response is not available.

12. Successful coping with physical injury or loss (Hamburg & Adams, 1953)
   a. Reduces stress to manageable limits
   b. Maintains feelings of personal worth
   c. Restores relationships with significant others
   d. Seeks recovery of physical functions
   e. Initiates a situation that is a positive contribution
   f. Initiates a situation (project, job, tasks) after maximum recovery that is viewed as socially acceptable and personally valued
   g. Gains pleasure from mastery

13. A person who is ill or disabled continues to have needs and goals. Previous coping patterns, if effective, may assist the individual to achieve goals and meet needs.

14. Responses to illness, disability or treatments are influenced by:
    a. Attitude toward event (punishment, weakness, challenge, etc.)
    b. Developmental level or age
    c. The extent of interference of the diability in goal-directed activity and the significance of the goal
15. Recognize that gender, level of intelligence, social and cultural background, value systems, and the cognitive and behavioral style of the person falling ill may importantly influence his/her coping style.
16. Crisis is defined by Miller (1983) as "the experiencing of an acute situation where one's repertoire of coping responses is inadequate in effecting a resolution of the stress." For an individual it usually represents a turning point in his/her life and a reorganization of some of the important aspects of his/her psychologic structure.
17. An individual crisis can be described in four sequential stages: shock, defensive retreat, acknowledgment, and adaptation.
18. Optimal intervention can occur only when the defensive attempts have failed and the person has begun a self-examination of the current situation.
19. Adaptation is the process whereby an individual strives to achieve comfortable and effective functioning in the environment. Adaptation is not static; it is an ongoing process.

Pediatric Considerations

1. Children who have difficulty adjusting to their chronic illness or disability may experience problems with functioning at home, at school, and in peer relationships (Whaley & Wong, 1989).
2. Also refer to Pediatric Considerations in *Ineffective Individual Coping*.

Gerontologic Considerations

1. Refer to Items 2 and 3 under Generic Considerations; see also Gerontologic Considerations in *Ineffective Individual Coping*.
2. Older adults with feelings of high self-efficacy may suffer greater when challenged by a disability (Simons & West, 1984–85).
3. Financial stability enhances coping in older adults (Simons & West, 1984–85).
4. Miller (1990) has identified the following factors as risks for high levels of stress and poor coping in older adults: diminished economic resources, an immature developmental level, the occurrence of unanticipated events, the occurrence of several daily hassles at the same time, the occurrence of several major life events in a short period of time, high social status, and high feelings of self-efficacy in situations that cannot change.

■ Impaired Adjustment
Related to (Specify)

Assessment

See Defining Characteristics

Outcome Criteria

The individual will:
- Identify the temporary and long-term demands of the situation
- Differentiate coping behavior that is effective versus ineffective

Interventions

1. Assess and identify the person's:
   a. Premorbid life-style
   b. Premorbid coping style
   c. Amount and type of resources available
   d. Extent of current disruption on life-style
   e. Current level of stress
   f. Current coping methods and their effectiveness
2. Identify factors that interfere with or delay effective adjustment:
   a. Unmanageable level of stress (see *Anxiety*)
   b. Inability to identify the problem or ineffective problem solving (see Appendix VII)
   c. Lack of mastery of developmental tasks for age
   d. History of patterns of ineffective coping and unresolved conflicts
   e. Inadequate or unavailable resources
      - Faith (see *Hopelessness*)
      - Knowledge about illness/disability
      - Finances
      - Support system
      - Skills to manage illness/disability
3. Assess the family's or significant other's response to situation:
   a. Perception of the effects (long-term and short-term) of the illness or disability
   b. Past family dynamics
   c. Present family dynamics (verbal, nonverbal)
4. Promote self-esteem (Miller, 1990):
   a. Provide as much privacy as possible.
   b. Allow a choice between two alternatives, even if there is only a minor difference in the choices, *e.g.,* both at 10:00 or 10:30.
   c. Encourage expression of individuality in room decorations and dress.
   d. Avoid all terms that are associated with babies, *e.g.,* baby food, diapers.
   e. Ask about family pictures, greeting cards, family members, etc.
   f. Explore past accomplishments and life events.
   g. If physical impairments are present, focus on nonphysical attributes, *e.g.,* significant relationships, personality traits.
   h. Assist in improving appearance, *e.g.,* grooming, hair styling, makeup.
5. Facilitate maximum independence (Miller, 1990).
   a. Ensure that necessary assistive aids are available.
   b. Evaluate the person's use of assistive aids.
   c. Allow the person to perform tasks at his own pace.
   d. Avoid unnecessary dependency for efficiency.
   e. Ensure that the environment is adapted to promote independence.
   f. Provide opportunities for the person to observe others who have successfully adapted to a change in function.

6. Assist the family and significant others to cope:
   a. Explore with them their perception of how the situation will progress.
   b. Identify behaviors that facilitate adaptation.
   c. Stress the importance of trying to maintain usual roles and behavior.
   d. When appropriate, include the affected individual in family decision-making.
   e. Discuss the reality of everyday emotions—anger, guilt, jealousy—and relate the hazards of denying these feelings.
   f. Discuss the hazards of trying to minimize the grief and trying to distract the grievers from grieving.
   g. Review progress and lack of progress. Allow for questions.
   h. Ask about family's health and leisure activities.
   i. Stress importance of caring for themselves.
7. Promote positive family visits (Harkulich & Calamita, 1986)
   a. Relate a positive experience that you have observed that represents a strength or individuality of the person.
   b. Encourage the person to be well dressed and groomed for visits.
   c. Encourage activities that the person enjoys, *e.g.*, walking, crafts, card games.
   d. If appropriate, share the weekly schedule of activities.
   e. Elicit suggestions from family for unmet needs.
8. Assess for the presence of denial as a coping mechanism:
   a. Focus on present situation.
   b. Accept denial as an initial response.
   c. Give feedback about current reality: identify positive achievements regardless of how minor.
9. Establish an active constructive relationship with the individual and family by acknowledging the person's increased dependence and initiating a collaborative approach to care (Friedman-Campbell & Hart, 1984).
   a. Give permission to the person to express feelings, if desired. For example: "It must be very hard to have someone wash you."
   b. Share your perception of injury.
10. Identify dysfunctional coping mechanisms, *e.g.*, use of chemical substances, avoidance, morbid preoccupation with the disability.
11. When appropriate, begin health teaching (Friedman-Campbell & Hart, 1984):
    a. Share your perceptions of the injury and the person's response to it.
    b. Explain the nature of the illness or injury.
    c. Discuss the anticipated changes in life-style.
    d. Teach health behaviors that need to be learned to adapt to a new life-style.
12. Explore goals with individual and also with family:
    a. Career
    b. Relationships
    c. Recreation
    d. Compare premorbid goals with post-injury/illness goals.
13. Assist the person to anticipate the effects of events on functioning and life-style
    a. Explore with individual his/her fears. Role-play fearful or stressful situations.
    b. Emphasize that although the person may need some assistance from others, he also can support others with praise, gratitude, and empathic listening to their problems.
14. Assist the person to determine the most appropriate strategies.
    a. Help the person to accurately appraise whether a situation is changeable or not.
    b. Explain the use of problem-focused strategies to change or alter situations, *e.g.*:
       • Treating functional incontinence with bladder retraining

> - Engaging in upper limb muscle strengthening to facilitate use of walker
> - Treating fatigue with energy-conservation techniques
>
> c. Explain the use of emotion-focused strategies to regulate emotional response to the event, *e.g.*:
>   - Performing relaxation exercises to cope with pain
>   - Acknowledging the anger in response to the situation

15. Initiate referrals as indicated
    a. Identify resources available: community, financial, counseling, role models, self-help groups.
    b. Refer individuals and family to appropriate self-help literature (see Literature for Consumer).

References/Bibliography

Beglinger, J. E. (1983). Coping tasks in critical care: Patient and families. *Dimensions in Critical Care Nursing, 2*(2), 80–89.

Burgess, A. W. & Baldwin, B. A. (1981). *Crisis intervention: Theory and practice.* Englewood Cliffs, NJ: Prentice-Hall.

Cheney, R. J. Emotional adaptation to disability. (1984). *Rehabilitation Nurse, 9*(5), 36–37.

Evans, R. L., & Halar, E. M. (1985). Cognitive therapy to achieve personal goals: Results of telephone group counseling with disabled adults. *Archives of Physical Medicine and Rehabilitation, 66,* 693–696.

Fink, S. L. (1967). Crisis and motivation: A theoretical model. *Archives of Physical Medicine and Rehabilitation,* November, 592–597.

Friedman-Campbell M., & Hart, C. A. (1984). Theoretical strategies and nursing interventions to promote psychological adaptation to spinal cord injuries and disability. *Journal of Neurosurgical Nursing, 16* (6), 335–342.

Hamburg, D. A., & Adams, J. E. (1953). A perspective on coping behavior. *Archives of General Psychiatry, 17,* 1–20.

Harkulich, J., & Calamita, B. (1986). *A manual for caregivers of Alzheimer's disease clients in long-term care* (2nd ed.). Beachwood, OH: Nursing Home Training Center, Menorah Park Center for the Aged.

Kobasa, S. C. (1982). Commitment and coping in stress-resistance among lawyers. *Journal of Personality and Social Psychology, 42,* 707–711.

Larsen, P. (1990). Psychosocial adjustment in multiple sclerosis. *Rehabilitation Nursing, 15* (5), 242–247.

Lazarus, R. S., & Monat, A. (1977). *Stress and coping: An anthology.* New York: Columbia University Press.

Marks, S., & Millard, R. (1990). Nursing assessment of positive adjustment for individuals with multiple sclerosis. *Rehabilitation Nursing, 15* (3), 147–151.

Matson, R. R., & Brooks, N. A. (1982). Social-psychological adjustment to multiple sclerosis: A longitudinal study. *Social Science and Medicine, 16,* 2129–2135.

Miller, C. A. (1990). *Nursing care of older adults: Theory and practice.* Glenview, IL: Scott Foresman.

Miller, P. (1983). Family health and psychosocial response to cardiovascular diseases. *Health Values, 7* (6), 10–15.

Peretz, D. (1970). Reaction to loss. In Carr, A. C., & Peretz, D. (Eds). *Loss and grief: Psychological management in medicine.* New York: Columbia University Press.

Oberst, M. T. et al. (1985). Going home: Patient and spouse adjustment following cancer surgery. *Topics in Clinical Nursing, 7* (1), 46–57.

Ott, C. R. et al. (1983). A controlled randomized study of early cardiac rehabilitation: The sickness impact profile as an assessment tool. *Heart Lung, 12* (2), 162–170.

Russell, R. A. (1981). Concepts of adjustment to disability: An overview. *Rehabilitation Literature, 42,* 330–338.

Simons, R. L., & West, G. E. (1984–85). Life changes, coping resources, and health among the elderly. *International Journal of Aging and Human Development, 20* (3), 173–189.

Sinyor, D., Amato, P., Kaloupek, D. G. Becker, R., Goldenberg, M., & Coopersmith, H. (1986). Poststroke depression: Relationship to functional impairment, coping strategies, and rehabilitation outcome. *Stroke, 17,* 1102–1107.

Swanson, B., Cronin-Stubbs, R., & Sheldon, J. (1989). The impact of psychosocial factors on adapting to physical disability: A review of the research literature. *Rehabilitation Nursing, 14* (2), 64–68.

Whaley, L. F. & Wong, D. L. (1989). *Essentials of pediatric nursing* (3rd ed.). St. Louis: C. V. Mosby.

Whitbourne, S. K. (1985). The psychological construction of the life span. In Birren, J. E., & Schaie, K. E. (Eds.). *Handbook of the psychology of aging.* New York: Van Nostrand Reinhold.

Resources for the Consumer

Literature

COPE: Living with Cancer (magazine), PO Box 54679, Boulder, CO 80322
Accent on Living (magazine), PO Box 700, Bloomington, IL 61702

Anxiety

■ *Related to* **(Specify)**

■ *Related to* **Insufficient Knowledge of Preoperative Routines, Postoperative Exercises/Activities, Postoperative Alterations/ Sensations**

DEFINITION

Anxiety: A state in which the individual/group experiences feelings of uneasiness (apprehension) and activation of the autonomic nervous system in response to a vague, nonspecific threat.

DEFINING CHARACTERISTICS

Major (must be present)

Manifested by symptoms from each category—physiologic, emotional, and cognitive. Symptoms vary according to the level of anxiety.

Physiologic

Increased heart rate
Elevated blood pressure
Increased respiratory rate
Diaphoresis
Dilated pupils
Voice tremors/pitch changes
Trembling
Palpitations
Nausea and/or vomiting
Frequent urination
Diarrhea

Insomnia
Fatigue and weakness
Flushing or pallor
Dry mouth
Body aches and pains (especially chest, back, neck
Restlessness
Faintness/dizziness
Paresthesias
Hot and cold flashes

Emotional

Person states that he has feelings of
Apprehension
Helplessness
Nervousness
Fear
Lack of self-confidence
Person exhibits
Irritability/impatience
Angry outbursts
Crying
Tendency to blame others
Startle reaction

Losing control
Tension or being "keyed up"
Inability to relax
Unreality
Anticipation of misfortune

Criticism of self and others
Withdrawal
Lack of initiative
Self-depreciation

Cognitive

Inability to concentrate
Lack of awareness of surroundings
Forgetfulness
Rumination
Orientation to past rather than to present or future
Blocking of thoughts (inability to remember)
Hyperattentiveness

RELATED FACTORS

Pathophysiologic

Any factor that interferes with the basic human needs for food, air, comfort, and security

Situational (personal, environmental)

Actual or perceived threat to self-concept
Change in status and prestige	Loss of valued possessions
Lack of recognition from others	Ethical dilemmas
Failure (or success)	

Actual or perceived loss of significant others
Death	Moving
Divorce	Temporary or permanent
Cultural pressures	separation

Actual or perceived threat to biologic integrity
Dying	Invasive procedures
Assault	Disease

Actual or perceived change in environment
Hospitalization	Safety hazards
Moving	Environmental pollutants
Retirement	

Actual or perceived change in socioeconomic status
Unemployment	Promotion
New job	

Transmission of another person's anxiety to the individual

Maturational (threat to developmental task)

Infant/child: Separation, mutilation, peer relationships, achievement
Adolescent: Sexual development, peer relationships, independence
Adult: Pregnancy, parenting, career development, effects of aging
Elderly: Chronic diseases, financial problems, retirement

Diagnostic Considerations

The nursing diagnoses of anxiety and fear have been examined by several researchers (Jones & Jacob, 1984; Taylor-Loughran, O'Brien, LaChapelle, & Rangel, 1989; Yokom, 1984). Differentiation of these diagnoses focuses on whether or not the threat can be identified. If identification is possible, the diagnosis is fear; if not, it is anxiety (NANDA, 1989). This differentiation has not proved useful for clinicians, however (Taylor-Loughran, O'Brien, LaChapelle, & Rangel, 1989).

Anxiety involves a vague feeling of apprehension and uneasiness in response to threat to one's value system or security pattern (May, 1977). The person may be able to identify the situation—*e.g.*, surgery, cancer—but actually the threat to self relates to the uneasiness and apprehension enmeshed in the situation. In other words, the situation is the source of the threats but is not the threat. In contrast, fear refers to the feelings of apprehension related to a specific threat or danger to which one's security patterns respond—*e.g.*, flying, heights, snakes. When the threat is removed, the fearful feelings dissipate (May, 1977).

Anxiety and fear produce a similar sympathetic response, involving cardiovascular excitation, pupil dilation, sweating, tremors, and dry mouth. Anxiety also involves a parasympathetic response of increased gastrointestinal activity; in contract, fear is associated with decreased GI activity. Behaviorally, the fearful person exhibits increased alertness and concentration with a response of avoidance, attack, or decreasing the risk of threat. The anxious person, on the other hand, experiences increased tension, general restlessness, insomnia, worry, and feelings of helplessness and vagueness regarding a situation that cannot be easily avoided or attacked.

Clinically, both anxiety and fear may coexist in a person's response to a situation. For example, a person facing surgery may be fearful of pain and anxious about a possible cancer diagnosis. According to Yokom (1984), "Fear can be allayed by withdrawal from the situation, removal of the offending object, or by reassurance. Anxiety is reduced by admitting its presence and by being convinced that the values to be gained by moving ahead are greater than those to be gained by escape."

Errors in Diagnostic Statements

Fear related to upcoming surgery

Anticipated surgery can be a source of many threats, including threats to one's security patterns, health, values, self-concept, role functioning, goal achievement, relationships, and security. These threats can produce vague feelings ranging from mild uneasiness to panic. Identifying the threat as merely surgery is too simplistic; these personal threats also are involved. Moreover, although some of the patient's uneasiness may be attributed to fear (which can be eliminated by teachings), the remaining feelings relate to anxiety. Because this situation is inescapable, the nurse must assist the patient with coping mechanisms for managing anxiety.

Focus Assessment Criteria

Subjective Data

1. History of the individual from client and significant others
    Life-style
        Interests   Strengths, limitations
        Work history   Previous level of functioning,
        Coping patterns (past, present)   handling stress
    Support system
        Availability   Quality of support
    History of medical problems/treatments
        Alcohol and drug abuse   Medications
        Activities of daily living
            Ability to perform   Desire to perform
2. History of unusual sensations (*e.g.*, palpitations, tingling, dyspnea, dry mouth, nausea, diaphoresis)

Precipitating factors
Frequency
Duration
3. Assess for feelings of
Extreme sadness and worthlessness
Guilt for past actions
Apprehension
Rejection or isolation
Living in an unreal world
Mistrust or suspiciousness of others
Manipulation by others
4. Orientation
Person
"What is your name?"
"What is your occupation?"
"Tell me about yourself."
Time
"What season is it?"
"What month is it?"
Place
"Where are you?"
"Where do you live?"
5. Usual coping behavior (Refer to *Ineffective Individual Coping* for further assessment criteria)
"How do you usually handle a particular situation (*i.e.*, anger, disappointment, loss, rejection, etc.)?"
"What did you usually do when you were faced with similar situations in the past?"
"What happens when you do that?"
(relevant coping mechanism)
Assess for:
Level of awareness of behavior
Range of coping behavior
Adaptive/maladaptive
Secondary gains

Routine time of occurrence
Description in individual's own words

Harm from others
Mind being controlled by external agents
Being unable to cope
Falling apart
Thoughts racing
Being held prisoner

Subjective and Objective Data
1. General appearance
Facial expression (*e.g.*, sad, hostile, expressionless)
Dress (*e.g.*, meticulous, disheveled, seductive, eccentric)
2. Behavior during interview
Withdrawn
Hostile
Apathetic
Cooperative
Quiet
3. Communication pattern
Content
Appropriate
Rambling
Suspicious
Denial of problem
Homicidal plans
Suicidal ideas
Sexually preoccupied
Delusions (of grandeur, persecution, reference, influence, control, or bodily sensations)
Hallucinations (visual, auditory, gustatory, olfactory, tactile)

Flow of thought
    Appropriate
    Blocking of ideas (unable to
      finish idea)
    Circumstantial (unable to get
      to point)
    Ideas loosely connected

Jumps from one topic to another
Unable to come to conclusion, be
    decisive
Difficulty concentrating
States he is unable to follow what
is being said
Difficulty grasping circumstances or
    events

Rate of speech
    Appropriate
    Excessive

Reduced
Pressured

Nonverbal behavior
    Affect appropriate/inappropriate to verbal content
    Gestures, mannerisms, facial grimaces
    Posture

4. Interaction skills
    With a nurse
      Inappropriate
      Relates well
      Withdrawn/preoccupied with self

Shows dependency
Demanding/pleading
Hostile

    With significant others
      Relates with all family
        members or with some
      Hostile toward one member/
        all members

Does not seek interaction
Does not have visitors

5. Activities of daily living
    Emotionally capable of caring for self
    Physically capable of caring for self

6. Nutritional status
    Appetite
    Eating patterns

Weight (within normal limits,
    decreased, increased)

7. Sleep–rest pattern
    Recent change
    Sleeps too much/too little

Early wakefulness
Insomnia

8. Personal hygiene
    Cleanliness (body, hair, teeth)
    Grooming (clothes, hair, makeup)

Clothes (condition, appropriateness)

9. Motor Activity
    Within normal limits
    Increased
    Decreased

Agitated
Repetitive

10. Present coping behavior
    "Acting-out" behaviors
      Derogating
      Fighting
      Arguing
      Intimidating
      Ritualistic behavior
      Smoking, alcohol, drugs
      Manipulation of others to do tasks
        he is capable of

Resentfulness
Motor restlessness
Pacing
Physical exertion

Paralysis and retreating behaviors
    Withdrawal
    Depression
    Denial
    Diverts attention
    Sleeping
    Avoids talking about self
    Minimizes signs and symptoms
       Dissociation
       Ritualistic behavior
       Blocking

Somatizing
    Headache
    Dyspnea
    Muscle tension
    Hives, eczema
    Anorexia
    Colitis
       Syncope
       Menstrual disturbance

Constructive action
    Seeks support from others
    Ventilates
    Seeks information
    Uses positive thinking techniques
    Sets realistic goals
    Maintains social activities
    Plans rest periods

Principles and Rationale for Nursing Care

Generic Considerations

1. Anxiety refers to feelings aroused by a nonspecific threat to a person's self-concept that impacts health, assets, values, environment, role functioning, needs fulfillment, goal achievement, personal relationships, and sense of security (Miller, 1990). Anxiety varies in intensity depending on the severity of the perceived threat and the success or failure of efforts to cope with the feelings.
2. A person uses both interpersonal and intrapsychic mechanisms to reduce or relieve anxiety. The effectiveness of coping strategies depends on the individual and the situation, not on the behavior itself.
   Interpersonal patterns of coping include:
   a. Acting-out: converting anxiety into anger that is either overtly or covertly expressed
   b. Paralysis or retreating behaviors: withdrawing or being immobilized by own anxiety
   c. Somatizing: converting anxiety into physical symptoms
   d. Constructive action: using anxiety to learn and problem solve (includes goal setting, learning new skills, and seeking information)
   Intrapsychic mechanisms, often called defense mechanisms, lower anxiety and protect self-esteem. Examples include repression, sublimation, regression, displacement, projection, denial, conversion, rationalization, suppression, and identification.
3. Individuals develop a range of coping behaviors, both adaptive and maladaptive. Maladaptive coping mechanisms are characterized by the inability to make choices, conflict, repetition and rigidity, alienation, and secondary gains.
4. Anxiety refers to both a person's response to a particular situation—*state anxiety*—

and the differences among people's interpretation of threatening situations—*trait anxiety*. Persons with relatively high levels of trait anxiety tend to perceive greater danger in situations that threaten self-esteem than do persons with lower levels, which respond with higher levels of state anxiety (Spielberger & Sarason, 1975).

5. The anxious person tends to overgeneralize and assume and anticipate catastrophe. Resulting cognitive problems include difficulty with attention and concentration, loss of objectivity, and vigilance (Taylor & Arnow, 1988).

6. The effects of anxiety on a person's abilities vary with degree:

   Mild

   Perception and attention heightened; alert

   Able to deal with problem situations

   Can integrate past, present, and future experiences

   Uses learning; can consensually validate; formulates meanings

   Curious, repeats questions

   Sleeplessness

   Moderate

   Perception somewhat narrowed; selectively inattentive, but can direct attention

   Slightly more difficult to concentrate; learning requires more effort

   Views present experiences in terms of past

   May fail to notice what is happening in a peripheral situation; will have some difficulty in adapting and analyzing

   Voice/pitch changes

   Increased respiratory and heart rates

   Tremors, shakiness

   Severe

   Perception greatly reduced; focuses on scattered details; cannot attend to more even when instructed to

   Learning severely impaired; highly distractable, unable to concentrate

   Views present experiences in terms of past; almost unable to understand current situation

   Functions poorly; communication difficult to understand

   Hyperventilation, tachycardia, headache, dizziness, nausea

   Panic

   Perception distorted; focuses on blown-up detail; scattering may be increased

   Learning cannot occur

   Unable to integrate experiences; can focus only on present; unable to see or understand situation; lapses in recall of thoughts

   Unable to function; usually increased motor activity and/or unpredictable responses to even minor stimuli; communication not understandable

   Feelings of impending doom/unreality

Dyspnea	Dizziness/faintness
Palpitations	Trembling
Choking	Paresthesia
Hot/cold flashes	Sweating

7. Persons experiencing panic attacks report that a physical feeling most commonly precipitated episodes of anxiety. Their thoughts are related to loss of control, death, and illness (Taylor & Arnow, 1988).

8. Catastrophic misinterpretation of normal body sensations may lead to a learned response in persons suffering from generalized anxiety disorders and panic attacks (Barlow & Cerny, 1988).

Anger and Aggression

(Note: Refer to *High Risk for Violence* for more information on aggression.)

1. A response to frustration and anxiety, anger can mobilize our physical and psychologic defenses toward problem-solving, or it can activate injurious behaviors (Novaco, 1985).
2. Persons express anger overtly or covertly. Examples of overt expression include hitting or fighting, nonverbal glaring, and verbal attack. Examples of covert expression include somatizing, depression, and suicide. A person may find feelings of anxiety or anger unacceptable, and may respond with avoidance coping mechanisms, such as denial, projection, and rationalization.
3. Anger differs from hostility in that anger is usually short-lived and compatible in relationships. In contrast, hostility is a feeling of antagonism accompanied by a wish to hurt or humiliate others. Hostility usually is the result of frustrated or unfulfilled needs or wishes (*e.g.,* unrealistic expectations of others, unrealistic expectations for self, low self-concept, and feelings of humiliation). The hostile person may respond by repressing his hostility and withdrawing (depression), denying the hostility and overreacting with extreme compliance (politeness), or engaging in overt hostile behavior (verbal or nonverbal).
4. Suppressed anger has been associated with elevated blood pressure, although the mechanism of how transient increases convert to chronically elevated levels is unclear (Novaco, 1985).
5. Aggression is a response to a threat or frustration in which verbal and/or physical aggressive action offers relief to the anxiety experienced. Operationally, the steps are:
   a. The individual experiences a threat or frustration
   b. Anxiety is felt
   c. Feelings of insecurity and helplessness occur
   d. Increasing anxiety is decreased through verbal or physical aggression
6. Aggressive behavior may vary from irritation to rage and may be directed toward self, others, or objects.
7. Limits provide a sense of security. There is a need for predictability about self and environment (Lyon, 1978).

Pediatric Considerations

1. Signs of anxiety in children vary greatly depending on developmental stage, temperament, past experience, and parental involvement (Whaley & Wong, 1989). The most common sign of anxiety in children and adolescents is increased motor activity. Signs of anxiety can be viewed developmentally and may be reflected in the following ways:
   Birth to 9 months: disruption in physiologic functioning (*e.g.,* sleep disorders, colic)
   9 months to 4 years: major source is loss of significant others and loss of love; therefore, anxiety may be seen as anger when parents leave, somatic illnesses, motor restlessness, regressive behaviors (thumb sucking, head banging, rocking), regression in toilet training
   4–6 years: major source is fear of body damage; belief that his bad behavior causes bad things to happen (*e.g.,* illness); somatic complaints of headache, stomachache
   6–12 years: excessive verbalization, compulsive behavior (*e.g.,* repeating a task over and over)
   Adolescence: similar to 6–12 years plus types of negativistic behavior

2. Children's anxiety may be heightened by separation from parents, change in usual routines, strange environments, painful procedures, and parental anxiety (Whaley & Wong, 1989). The nurse should assess for alternations in the functional health patterns to detect the presence of anxiety.
3. Children need opportunities and encouragement to express anger in a controlled, acceptable manner (*e.g.,* choosing not to play a particular game, choosing not to play with a particular person, slamming a door, or voicing anger). Unacceptable expressions of anger include throwing an object, hitting a person, and breaking an object. Children who are not permitted to express their anger may develop hostility and perceive the world as unfriendly.

Gerontologic Considerations

1. Research has not validated any age-related increase in anxiety (Schultz, 1987).
2. Lower levels of anxiety in older adults versus younger adults may be attributed to more effective coping mechanisms acquired through experiences (Jarvik, 1979).

■ Anxiety
Related to (Specify)

Assessment
See Defining Characteristics

Outcome Criteria

The person will
- Describe his own anxiety and coping patterns
- Relate an increase in psychologic and physiologic comfort
- Use effective coping mechanism in managing anxiety, as evidenced by (specify)

Interventions
The nursing interventions for the diagnosis *Anxiety* apply to any individual with anxiety regardless of the etiologic and contributing factors.

A. Assist the person to reduce his present level of anxiety

1. Assess level of anxiety (See Principles and Rationale for Nursing Care for specific differentiation)
   a. Mild
   b. Moderate
   c. Severe
   d. Panic

2. Provide reassurance and comfort
   a. Stay with the person.
   b. Do not make demands or ask him to make decisions.
   c. Support present coping mechanisms (*e.g.,* allow client to walk, talk, cry); do not confront or argue with his defenses or rationalizations.
   d. Speak slowly and calmly.
   e. Be aware of your own concern and avoid reciprocal anxiety.
   f. Convey a sense of empathic understanding (*e.g.,* quiet presence, touch, allowing crying, talking, etc.).
   g. Provide reassurance that a solution can be found.
3. Decrease sensory stimulation
   a. Use short, simple sentences.
   b. Give concise directions.
   c. Focus on the here and now.
   d. Remove excess stimulation (*e.g.,* take person to quieter room); limit contact with others—patients or family—who are also anxious.
   e. If person is hyperventilating, have him take slow, deep breaths and breathe with him.
   f. Attempt to occupy person with a simple, repetitive task.
   g. Consult physician for possible pharmacologic therapy, if indicated.
4. Children can be assisted in coping with anxiety through the following nursing interventions:
   a. Establish a trusting relationship.
   b. Minimize separation from parents.
   c. Encourage expression of feelings.
   d. Involve the child in play.
   e. Prepare the child for new experiences, *e.g.,* procedures, surgery.
   f. Provide comfort measures.
   g. Allow for regression.
   h. Encourage parental involvement in care.
   i. Allay parental apprehension and provide them information (Whaley & Wong, 1989).

B. When anxiety is diminished enough for learning to take place, assist person in recognizing his anxiety to initiate learning or problem-solving
   1. Request validation of your assessment of anxiety (*e.g.,* "Are you uncomfortable now?").
   2. If person can say yes, continue with the learning process; if he is not able to acknowledge anxiety, continue supportive measures until he is able (refer to A).
   3. When able to learn, determine usual coping mechanisms: "What do you usually do when you get upset?"
   4. Assess for unmet needs or expectations; encourage recall and description of what the person experienced immediately prior to feeling anxious.
   5. Assist in reevaluation of the perceived threat by discussing the following:
      a. Were expectations realistic?
      b. Was it possible to meet his expectations?
      c. Where in the sequence of events was change possible?
   6. Encourage the person to recall and analyze similar instances of anxiety.
   7. Explore what alternative behaviors might have been used if coping mechanisms were maladaptive.

8. Encourage the person to recall and analyze similar instances of anxiety.
9. Teach anxiety interrupters to use when stressful situations cannot be avoided:
   a. Look up
   b. Control breathing
   c. Lower shoulders
   d. Slow thoughts
   e. Alter voice
   f. Give self directions (out loud, if possible)
   g. Exercise
   h. "Scruff your face"—change facial expression
   i. Change perspective: imagine watching the situation from a distance (Grainger, 1990)

C. Reduce or eliminate problematic coping mechanisms

1. Depression, withdrawal (see *Ineffective Individual Coping*)
2. Violent behavior (see *High Risk for Violence*)
3. Denial*
   a. Develop an atmosphere of empathic understanding.
   b. Assist in lowering level of anxiety.
   c. Focus on present situation.
   d. Give feedback about current reality; identify positive achievements.
   e. Have person describe events in detail; focus on getting specifics of who, what, when, and where.
4. Numerous physical complaints with no known organic base
   a. Encourage expression of feelings.
   b. Give positive feedback when the person is symptom free.
   c. Acknowledge that the symptoms must be burdensome.
   d. Encourage interest in external environment (*e.g.,* outside activity, volunteering, helping others).
   e. Listen to the complaints.
   f. Evaluate the secondary gains the person receives and attempt to interrupt cycle; see the person on a regular basis, not simply in response to somatic complaints.
   g. Discuss with the person how others are reacting to him; attempt to have him identify his behavior when others react negatively (withdrawal? anger?).
   h. Avoid "doing something" to each complaint; set limits when appropriate (*e.g.,* may refuse to call physician in response to a request for headache medication).
   i. When setting limits, provide an alternative outlet (*e.g.,* redirect to use relaxation technique) (see Appendix X).
5. Anger† (*e.g.,* demanding behavior, manipulation)
   a. With adults
      Identify the presence of anger (*e.g.,* feelings of frustration, anxiety, helplessness, presence of irritability, verbal outbursts).
      Recognize your reactions to an individual's behavior; be aware of your own feelings in working with angry individuals.

---

*Denial serves a protective function and is not always maladaptive.

†Anger is a response to frustration and anxiety. Not all anger is problematic. It can be used for problem-solving.

If person can verbalize feelings, assist in identifying sources of frustration and anger.

Assist in making connections between feelings of frustration and subsequent behavior.

Have person analyze consequences of behavior.

Convey a sense of understanding of those things over which he has little control.

Set limits on manipulative or irrational demands.

State limits clearly; tell person exactly what is expected (*e.g.,* "I cannot allow you to scream [throw objects, etc.]").

When stating an unacceptable behavior, give an alternative (*e.g.,* suggest a quiet room, physical exertion, a chance for one-to-one communication).

State the consequences if limits are violated.

Develop behavior modification strategies; discuss with all personnel involved for consistency.

When discussing a limit with the person, avoid stating it in such a way that it is perceived as a challenge.

Give a brief explanation for the limit; if behavior continues, enforce the limit; encourage the person to express his feelings about the limit.

Structure experiences that the person can do successfully.

Provide positive feedback.

Interact with the person when he is not demanding or manipulative.

Discuss your feelings and the person's behavior with entire team; support each other and provide a consistent approach.

  b. With children

Encourage the child to share his anger (*e.g.,* "How did you feel when you had your injection?" or "How did you feel when Mary would not play with you?").

Tell the child that being angry is okay (*e.g.,* "I sometimes get angry when I can't have what I want").

Encourage and allow the child to express his anger in acceptable ways (*e.g.,* loud talking, hitting a play object, or running outside around the house).

D. Initiate health teaching and referrals as indicated

1. For persons identified as having chronic anxiety and maladaptive coping mechanisms, refer for ongoing psychiatric treatment.
2. Instruct in nontechnical, understandable terms regarding his illness and associated treatments. Repeat explanations, since anxiety may interfere with learning.
3. Instruct in maintenance of physical well-being (*i.e.,* nutrition, exercise, elimination).
4. Instruct (or refer) person for assertiveness training.
5. Instruct person in use of relaxation techniques (see Appendix X).
6. Instruct person in constructive problem-solving (see Appendix VII).
7. Assist parents to respond constructively to age-related developmental needs (see Altered Growth and Development).
8. Provide telephone numbers for emergency intervention:
   a. Hotlines
   b. Psychiatric emergency room
   c. On-call staff if available

■ Anxiety
Related to Insufficient Knowledge of Preoperative Routines, Postoperative Exercises/Activities, Postoperative Alterations/Sensations

Assessment

Subjective Data
The person states that he
Is anxious and fearful of unfamiliar situations
Needs instruction

Objective Data
The person
Exhibits anxious behavior, such as

Increased verbalization	Restlessness
Inability to concentrate and retain information	Sweating palms
	Tremulousness

Behaves in a way that indicates a knowledge deficit, regarding:
Preparation for diagnostic study, examination, surgical procedure
The need for diagnostic study, examination, surgical procedure, or treatment and follow-up medical supervision
What is involved with the diagnostic study, examination, surgery, or treatment prescribed

---

Outcome Criteria

The individual will
- Verbalize, if asked what to expect (routines, environment)
- Demonstrate postoperative exercises, splinting, and respiratory regimen
- Relate less anxiety after teaching

Interventions
1. Before hospitalization, the person's physician should explain
   a. Nature of surgery needed
   b. Reason for and anticipated outcomes of surgery
   c. Risks involved
   d. Type of anesthesia
   e. Expectations regarding length of recovery and limitations imposed during the recovery period
2. Determine level of understanding of surgical procedure.
   Reinforce physician's explanation of surgical procedure. Notify physician if additional explanations are indicated.

3. Assess
   a. Past experiences related to surgery and positive or negative effect on client
   b. Nature of concerns, fears
   c. Factors affecting learning (refer to Related Factors and Focus Assessment Criteria)
4. Document and communicate these data to others involved with care to meet the client's needs and ensure continuity of care.
5. Utilize efficient and effective teaching methods
   a. Give bedside instruction concerning specific type of surgery and sensations and appearances (presence of machines, tubes, etc.) that client and family may encounter postoperatively.
   b. Provide instruction (bedside or group) on general information pertaining to the need for active participation, routines, environment, personnel, postoperative exercises.
      • Give general information, pertaining to most people having surgery, in a group session for patients and families.
      • Present information or reinforce learning with the use of written materials (booklets, posters for room on exercises, instruction sheets) or audiovisual aids (slides of surgical areas, personnel, films, videotapes).
      • Demonstrate and conduct practice session for postoperative exercises.
      • Explain the rationale for routines, focusing on positive aspects. For example, "An enema may be ordered preoperatively, which will decrease your need to use the bedpan for a few days postoperatively."
      • Encourage participation by making person feel (without frightening him) that he will be susceptible to complications if he does not participate.
      • Give feedback on progress, rewarding person frequently.
6. Explain all procedures, the reasons for them, and their importance:
   a. Preoperative
      • Enema
      • NPO
      • Preparation
      • Laboratory work
   b. Postoperative
      • Parenteral fluids
      • Vital signs
      • Dressings
      • Nasogastric and other tubes
      • Indwelling bladder catheter
      • Pain and availability of medications
   c. Teach person, using return demonstration:
      • To turn, cough, and breathe deep, depending on surgical procedure
      • To support incision during coughing
      • To deep breathe hourly postoperatively
      • To exercise actively and how passive ROM exercises will be done
      • To sit up, get up, and ambulate—sitting in a chair should be avoided
      • Importance of progressive care
      • Early ambulation
      • Self-care, as soon as patient is able
7. For children (Smallwood, 1988):
   a. Organize tours for children about 5–7 days before the surgery.

b. Group children with similar problems together.

c. Encourage the participation of parents and siblings to provide added security for the child.

d. Involve as many senses as possible. Explain how it feels and smells and whether or not it will hurt.

e. Using a doll, demonstrate the OR garments, blood sample acquisition.

f. Using a volunteer child, demonstrate the taking of blood pressure, temperature, heart and respiration rate.

g. Take children on OR cart to show them where their parents will be waiting while they're in surgery.

h. Have an OR nurse (fully dressed) explain:
  • The reasons for OR attire
  • Anesthesia machine
  • Anesthesia as "hospital air" or "hospital sleep" to avoid confusion
  • Postanesthesia recovery room

  Explain/demonstrate on doll or child:
  • Straps on OR table
  • Monitoring devices (ECG, pulse)
  • Anesthesia mask (on each child, or on parent if child is frightened)
  • Intravenous lines (inserted after induction; removed after child is eating and drinking)

i. Increase the effectiveness of the teaching program and promote security
  • Use name tags so children can be addressed by name.
  • Involve children in discussion, *e.g.*, ask them the colors of objects; ask them to point to their nose.
  • Do not force any child to do anything.
  • If a child resists, have parent perform the activity and encourage child to help. Allow child to handle equipment.
  • Avoid calling anesthesia gas. It may be confused with gas in a car or gas used in euthanasia of animals.
  • Explain that anesthesia does not affect memories.
  • Allow children to take home masks, hats, and ECG buttons.
  • Encourage child to bring a favorite toy when returning for surgery.

j. If tours are not feasible or child cannot attend, consider using or developing a book for parents to use at home with child which they can receive from their surgeon's office, *e.g., Your Operation Day,* by Margary Doroshow and Deborah London (1984).

8. Discuss purpose of recovery room with patient and family.
  a. Visiting policies
  b. Type of care
  c. Length of stay, if applicable
  d. Possibility of placement in intensive care unit (ICU) if needed or indicated.

9. Explain other hospital policies as indicated
  a. Visiting hours
  b. Number of visitors
  c. Location of waiting rooms
  d. How physician will contact them after operation

10. Evaluate
  a. Person's/family's ability to meet preset, mutually planned learning goals (behaviors)
  b. Need for further teaching and support

References/Bibliography

Barlow, D., & Cerny, J. (1988). *Psychiatric treatment of panic.* New York: Guieford.

Byrne, C., & Hunsberger, M. (1989). Concepts of illness: Stress, crisis, and coping. In Foster, R. L., Hunsberger, M. M., & Anderson, J. J. T. (Eds.). *Family-centered nursing care of children.* Philadelphia: W. B. Saunders.

Chitty, K., & Maynard, C. (1986). Managing manipulation. *Journal of Psychosocial Nursing, 24*(6), 9–13.

Decker, N. (1979). Anxiety in the general hospital. In Fann, W., Karacau, I., Parkorny, A. et al. (Eds.). *Phenomenology and treatment of anxiety.* Jamaica, NY: Spectrum Publications.

Grainger, R. (1990). Anxiety interrupters. *American Journal of Nursing, 90*(2), 14–15.

Grainger, R. (1990). Anger within ourselves. *American Journal of Nursing, 90*(7), 12.

Holderly, R., & McNulty, E. (1979). Feelings, feelings: How to make a rational response to emotional behavior. *Nursing 79, 10*(3), 39–43.

Jarvik, K. L., & Russel, D. (1979). Anxiety, aging and third emergency reaction. *Journal of Gerontology, 34*(1), 110–119.

Jones, P. E., & Jakob, D. F. (1984). Anxiety revisited from a practice perspective. In Kim, M. J., McFarland, G. K., & McLane, A. M. (Eds.). *Classification of nursing diagnoses: Proceedings of the fifth national conference.* St. Louis: C. V. Mosby.

Knowles, R. (1981). Handling anger: Responding vs. reacting. *American Journal of Nursing, 81,* 2196–2197.

Lyon, G. (1978). Limit setting as a therapeutic tool. In Backer, B., Dubbert, P., & Eisenman, E. *Psychiatric/mental health nursing: Contemporary readings.* New York: Van Nostrand Reinhold.

May, R. (1977). *The meaning of anxiety.* New York: W. W. Norton.

Medved, R. (1990). Strategies for handling angry patients and their families. *Nursing 90, 20*(4), 66–67.

Miller, C. A. (1990). *Nursing care of the older adult.* Glenview, IL: Scott Foresman.

NANDA (1989). *Taxonomy I.* St. Louis: North American Nursing Diagnosis Association.

Novaco, R. (1985). Anger and its therapeutic regulation. In Chesney, M., & Roseman, R. (Eds.). *Anger and hostility in cardiovascular* and *behavioral disorders.* Cambridge, MA: Hemisphere.

Schultz, N. R. (1987). Anxiety. In G. L. Maddox (Ed.). *The encyclopedia of aging.* New York: Springer Publishing.

Smallwood, S. (1988). Preparing children for surgery. *AORN Journal, 47*(1), 177–182.

Spielberger, C. & Sarason, I. (Eds.). (1975). *Stress and anxiety* (Vol I.). Washington, DC: Hemisphere.

Stewart, A. (1978). Handling the aggressive patient. *Perspectives on Psychiatric Care, 16,* 5–6.

Taylor, C. B., & Arnow, B. (1988). *The nature and treatment of anxiety disorders.* New York: Free Press.

Taylor-Loughran, A., O'Brien, M., LaChapelle, R., & Rangel, S. (1989). Defining characteristics of the nursing diagnoses fear and anxiety: A validation study. *Applied Nursing Research, 2*(4), 178–186.

Weisinger, H. (1985). *Dr. Weisinger's anger work-out book.* New York: Quill.

Whaley, L. F., & Wong, D. L. (1989). *Essentials of pediatric nursing* (3rd ed.). St. Louis: C. V. Mosby.

Wong, D. L., & Whaley, L. F. (1990). *Clinical manual of pediatric nursing* (3rd ed.). St. Louis: C.V. Mosby.

Yokom, C. J. (1984). The differentiation of fear and anxiety. In Kim, M. J., McFarland, G. K., & McLane, A. M. (Eds.). *Classification of nursing diagnoses: Proceedings of the fifth national conference.* St Louis: C. V. Mosby.

Body Temperature, High Risk for Altered

Hyperthermia

Hypothermia

Thermoregulation, Ineffective

Body Temperature, High Risk for Altered

■ *Related to* **(Specify)**

DEFINITION

High Risk for Altered Body Temperature: The state in which the individual is at risk for failing to maintain body temperature within normal range.

RISK FACTORS

Presence of risk factors (See Related Factors)

RELATED FACTORS

Pathophysiologic

Illness or trauma affecting temperature regulation:
  Coma/increased intracranial pressure
  Brain tumor/hypothalamic tumor/head trauma
  Cerebrovascular accident (CVA)
  Infection
  Integument (skin) injury
  Anemia
  Neurovascular disease/peripheral vascular disease
  Pheochromocytoma (tumor of the adrenal medulla)
  Altered metabolic rate

Treatment-related
  Medications (*e.g.*, vasodilators/vasoconstrictors)
  Sedation
  Parenteral fluid infusion/blood transfusion
  Dialysis
  Surgery

Maturational

Extremes of age (*e.g.*, newborn, elderly)

Diagnostic Considerations

High Risk for Altered Body Temperature is difficult to differentiate from the other diagnoses that focus on body temperature: *Hypothermia, Hyperthermia,* and *Ineffective Thermoregulation.* The risk factors listed above could apply to each of these diagnoses as high risk nursing diagnoses, *e.g., High Risk for Hyperthermia related to the effects of aging on ability to acclimatize to heat.*

Usually, a nurse inclines toward using *High Risk for Altered Body Temperature* for a client who has experienced temperature elevation but is presently afebrile. In this situation, *High Risk for Hyperthermia* would be useful. In acute care situations when a patient experiences fluctuations in temperature, the nursing diagnosis *Altered Comfort related to malaise, chills, and temperature fluctuations* may more appropriately describe the nursing focus.

Errors in Diagnostic Statements

High Risk for Altered Body Temperature related to intraoperative exposure to cool environment, extremes of age, dehydration, and use of medications and anesthetics

This diagnosis mixes a situation that nurses can prevent—intraoperative hypothermia—with a situation that requires rapid detection and medical and nursing management—malignant hyperthermia. The proper nursing diagnosis for this situation would be: *Potential Hypothermia related to intraoperative exposure to cool environment, extremes of age, and dehydration.* The nurse also would identify the collaborative problem *Potential Complication: Malignant hyperthermia* to describe a situation necessitating rapid detection and cotreatment by nurses and physicians.

Hyperthermia

■ *Related to* **(Specify): High Risk for**

DEFINITION

Hyperthermia: The state in which an individual has or is at risk of having a sustained elevation of body temperature of greater than 37.8° C (100° F) orally or 38.8° C (101° F) rectally because of increased vulnerability to external factors.

DEFINING CHARACTERISTICS

Major (must be present)
Temperature greater than 37.8° C (100° F) orally or 38.8° C (101° F) rectally

Minor (may be present)
  Flushed skin
  Warm to touch
  Increased respiratory rate
  Tachycardia
  Shivering/goose pimples
  Dehydration
  Specific or generalized aches and pains (*e.g.,* headache)
  Malaise/fatigue/weakness
  Loss of appetite

RELATED FACTORS

Situational (personal, environmental)
  Exposure to heat, sun
  Inappropriate clothing for climate
  Poverty
  Extremes of weight
  Dehydration
  Vigorous activity

Maturational
  Extremes of age (*e.g.,* newborn, elderly)

Diagnostic Considerations

The nursing diagnoses *Hypothermia* and *Hyperthermia* represent persons with temperature below and above normal, respectively. These abnormal temperature states are treatable by nursing interventions, such as correcting the external causes, *e.g.,* inappropriate clothing, exposure to elements (heat or cold), dehydration. The nursing focus centers on preventing or treating mild hypothermia and hyperthermia. As life-threatening situations that require medical and nursing interventions, severe hypothermia and hyperthermia represent collaborative problems and should be labeled *Potential Complication: Hypothermia* or *PC: Hyperthermia.*

Temperature elevation due to infections, other disorders (*e.g.,* hypothalamic) or treatments (*e.g.,* hypothermia units) requires collaborative treatment. If desired, the nurse could use the nursing diagnosis *Altered Comfort* and the collaborative problem *PC: Hypothermia* or *PC: Hyperthermia.*

Errors in Diagnostic Statements

Hyperthermia related to intraoperative pharmacogenic hypermetabolism
  This situation describes malignant hyperthermia, a life-threatening inherited disorder resulting in a hypermetabolic state related to the use of anesthetic agents and depolarizing muscle relaxants. The collaborative problem *Potential Complica-*

tion: Malignant hypertension would more appropriately describe this situation, which necessitates rapid detection and cotreatment by nursing and medicine.

Hyperthermia related to effect of circulating endotoxins on hypothalmus secondary to sepsis

Nursing care for persons with elevated temperature in an acute care setting focuses on monitoring and managing the fever with nursing and physician orders and or promoting comfort through nursing orders. The nursing diagnosis *Altered Comfort* would more appropriately describe a situation that nurses treat, with the collaborative problem *Potential Complication: Sepsis* representing the physiologic complication that nurses monitor for and manage with nursing- and physician-prescribed interventions.

Focus Assessment Criteria

Subjective Data

1. Assess history of symptoms (cool skin, clouded mentation, headaches, nausea, lethargy, vertigo).

    Onset?

    Associated factors

    Exercise

    Fluid intake

    Exposure to cold, heat

    Symptoms relieved by what?

2. Assess for presence of contributing or causative factors.

    Recent exposure to communicable disease without known immunity (*e.g.,* measles without vaccine or previous illness)

    Recent overexposure to sun heat

    Recent overactivity

    Radiation/chemotherapy/immunosuppression

    Alcohol use

    Home environment:

    Adequate heating?

    Adequate clothing (*e.g.,* socks, hat, gloves)?

    Adequate ventilation?

    Poverty?

    Recent exposure to cold/dampness

    Inactivity

    Impaired judgment

    Medications:

    Diuretics

    Anticholinergics

    Barbiturates

    Antidepressants

    Vasodilators/vasoconstrictors?

    How often taken? Last dose taken when?

    Effect on circulatory system?

3. Note if clothing is appropriate for environment.

4. Assess past history.

    Repeated infections

    Diabetes mellitus

Cardiovascular disorders
Mobility problems
Neurologic disorders

Objective Data

1. Vital signs
    Elevated temperature?
    Tachycardia?
    Tachypnea?
    Abnormal blood pressure?
2. Assess mental status
    Alert/drowsy/confused/oriented/comatose
3. Assess skin and circulation
    Intact?
    Burned (specify degree and site)?
    Injured (specify)?
    Rash (specify type and site)?
    Bites (specify site)?
    Turgor: normal/dehydrated
    Temperature/feel: hot/warm/cold/damp
    Appearance: flushed/pale
    Quality of peripheral pulses (radial, pedal)
4. Assess for signs of dehydration
    Parched mouth/furrowed tongue/dry lips
    Determine fluid intake and output

Principles and Rationale for Nursing Care

Generic Considerations

1. The nursing focus for this diagnosis is on reducing or eliminating risk factors and assisting the person to adapt to risk factors (*e.g.,* wearing a hat when in cold weather, removing clothing when overheated).
2. Body temperature is greatly affected by the environmental temperature; high humidity increases the effect of cold or heat on the body.
3. Exposure of the head, face, hands, and feet can affect body temperature greatly. These are vascular areas where heat is conducted from the blood vessels to the skin and from the skin to the air, and where cold is conducted from the air to the skin and from the skin to the blood vessels.
4. Rectal temperature reading is 1° higher than oral temperature reading. Axillar temperature reading is 1° lower than oral temperature reading.
5. All of the principles listed under hyperthermia and hypothermia can also apply to *High Risk for Altered Body Temperature.*

Hyperthermia

1. Adding clothes or blankets to a person inhibits the body's natural ability to reduce body temperature; removing clothes or blankets enhances the body's natural ability to reduce body temperature.
2. Perspiring is a sign of the human effort to reduce body temperature.
3. Increased metabolic rate increases body temperature, and vice versa (increase in body temperature causes an increased metabolic rate).
4. Shivering causes an increase in metabolic rate and body temperature.

5. Increased calories and fluids are required to maintain metabolic functions when fever is present.
6. Fever is a major sign of onset of infection, inflammation, and disease: treatment with aspirin or acetaminophen without medical consultation may mask important symptoms that should receive medical attention.
7. Fever associated with immunosuppression, stiff neck, rashes, infection, mental confusion, prolonged vomiting, respiratory difficulty, or abdominal tenderness should be referred to the physician.
8. People with fevers often are subject to irritability, generalized aches, pains, and discomfort.
9. Blood is the cooling fluid of the body: low blood volume due to dehydration predisposes one to fever.

Hypothermia

1. Hypothermia reduces blood pressure and contributes to shock.
2. Vasolidation promotes heat loss and predisposes one to hypothermia.
3. The elderly and the very young require more heat to maintain normal body temperature (room temperature should be 70°–74° F).
4. During the immediate postoperative period, patients are prone to hypothermia related to prolonged exposure to cold in the operating room and the infusion of large quantities of cool intravenous fluids.
5. People with known peripheral vascular disease should minimize exposure to cold because hypothermia causes the body to try to conserve heat by means of vasoconstriction (which creates an even greater vascular compromise).
6. Severe hypothermia can cause life-threatening cardiac arrhythmias and must be referred to a physician.
7. Immobility (*e.g.,* surgery) reduces muscle activity, thus producing less heat.

Pediatric Considerations

1. Almost every child will experience a fever of 100°–104° F at some time (Schmitt, 1984).
2. The nurse should consider the child's age when assessing fever:
    a. A neonate can have an infection without fever.
    b. A febrile neonate needs prompt assessment by a physician.
    c. Fever in children under age 2 months (Schmitt, 1984) and medically fragile children requires prompt medical attention (Wong & Whaley, 1990).
3. Normal children usually are not harmed by fever; only approximately 4% of febrile children are susceptible to convulsions (Hunsberger, 1989).
4. Most childhood fevers are caused by viral illness. Acetaminophen is the drug of choice for fever management; use of aspirin during a viral illness is associated with an increased risk of Reye's syndrome (Hunsberger, 1989).
5. Neonates and small infants, diaphoretic infants, and children receiving cool humidified oxygen or cool mist therapy are at special risk for developing hypothermia (Whaley & Wong, 1989).
6. Research comparing rectal, axillary, and inguinal temperature measurement routes in full-term newborn infants suggests that inguinal temperatures may be more reflective of rectal temperatures than of axillary temperatures (Bliss-Holtz, 1989).
7. Research comparing rectal, femoral, axillary, and skin-to-mattress temperatures in stable neonates suggests that it may take less time to register an accurate temperature in the rectal site (optimal placement time = 5 minutes), than in the femoral and

axillary sites (optimal placement time = 11 minutes) and the skin-to-mattress sites (optimal placement time = 13 minutes) (Kunnel, 1988).

8. There is an increase in mortality in children (especially 0–4 years old) associated with *hypothermia* during the winter months.

Gerontologic Considerations

1. Older adults can become hypothermic or hyperthermic in moderately cold or hot environments, as compared to younger adults, who require exposure to severe cold or hot temperatures (Miller, 1990).
2. Age-related changes that interfere with the body's ability to adapt to cold temperature include inefficient vasoconstriction, decreased cardiac output, decreased subcutaneous tissue, and delayed and diminished sweating (Miller, 1990).
3. Older adults have a higher threshold for the onset of sweating and decreased efficiency of sweating when it occurs.
4. Older adults have a dulled perception of cold and warmth and thus may lack the stimulus to initiate protective actions.
5. The thirst mechanism becomes less efficient with aging, as does the kidney's ability to concentrate urine, increasing the risk of heat-related dehydration.
6. Inactivity and immobility increase susceptibility to hypothermia by suppressing shivering and reducing heat-generating muscle activity.
7. Seventy percent (70%) of all heatstroke victims are over 60 years of age (Bafitis & Sargent, 1977).

■ High Risk for Hyperthermia
Related to (Specify)

Assessment

Subjective Data
The person reports history of heat stroke

Objective Data
Presence of risk factors (see Related Factors, *Hyperthermia*)

Outcome Criteria

The person will
- Identify risk factors for hyperthermia
- Relate methods of preventing hyperthermia
- Maintain normal body temperature

Interventions

A. Assess for the presence of contributing risk factors
1. Dehydration
2. Environmental warmth/exercise

B. Monitor body and environmental temperature

C. Remove or reduce contributing risk factors
1. For dehydration:
   a. Monitor intake and output and provide favorite fluids to maintain a balance between intake and output.
   b. Teach the importance of maintaining an adequate fluid intake (at least 200 ml a day of cool liquids unless contraindicated by heart or kidney disease) to prevent dehydration. Explain the importance of not relying on thirst sensation as an indication of the need for fluid.
   c. See also Fluid Volume Deficit.
2. For environmental warmth/exercise:
   a. Assess whether clothing or bedcovers are too warm for the environment or planned activity.
   b. Remove excess clothing and/or blankets (remove hat, gloves, or socks, as appropriate) to promote heat loss. Wear loose cotton clothing to maintain temperature below 85°.
   c. Provide air conditioning, dehumidifiers, fans, or cool baths or compresses as appropriate.
   d. Teach the importance of increasing fluid intake during warm weather and exercise.
   e. Teach to wear a hat during sun exposure.

C. Initiate health teaching as indicated
1. Explain the relationship of age as a risk for hyperthermia.
2. Teach the early signs of hyperthermia or heat stroke:
   | Flushed skin | Headache |
   | Fatigue | Loss of appetite |
3. Teach to take cool baths several times a day in hot temperatures, avoiding soap to prevent skin drying.
4. Teach to apply ice packs or cool wet towels to the body, especially on the axillae and groin.
5. Explain the need to avoid alcohol, caffeine, and large heavy meals during hot weather.

Hypothermia

■ *Related to* **(Specify): High Risk for**

DEFINITION

Hypothermia: The state in which an individual has or is at risk of having a sustained reduction of body temperature of below 35° C (95° F) orally or 35.5° C (96° F) rectally because of increased vulnerability to external factors.

DEFINING CHARACTERISTICS*

Major (80%–100%)

Reduction in body temperature below 35° C (95° F) orally or 35.5° C (96° F) rectally.
   Cool skin
   Pallor (moderate)
   Shivering (mild)

Minor (50%–79%)

   Mental confusion/drowsiness/restlessness
   Decreased pulse and respiration
   Cachexia/malnutrition

RELATED FACTORS

Situational (personal, environmental)

   Exposure to cold, rain, snow, wind
   Inappropriate clothing for climate
   Poverty (inability to pay for shelter or heat)
   Extremes of weight
   Consumption of alcohol
   Dehydration/malnutrition
   Operating suite

Maturational

Extremes of age (*e.g.,* newborn, elderly)

Diagnostic Considerations

See *High Risk for Altered Body Temperature* and *Hyperthermia*

---

*Adapted from Carroll, S. M. (1989). Nursing diagnosis: Hypothermia. In Carroll-Johnson, R. M. (Ed.). *Classification of nursing diagnoses: Proceedings of the eighth conference.* Philadelphia: J.B. Lippincott.

Errors in Diagnostic Statements

See *High Risk for Altered Body Temperature* and *Hyperthermia*

Focus Assessment

See *Hyperthermia*

Principles and Rationale for Nursing Care

See *Hyperthermia*

■ High Risk for Hypothermia
Related to (Specify)

Assessment

Subjective Data

The person reports:
"I get cold easily/I'm always cold."
"I can't afford to pay the heat."
"I don't have the right clothes to go out."
"I have poor circulation."
"My feet are always cold."
"My hands are always cold."

Objective Data

Presence of risk factors (see Related Factors in *Hypothermia*)

Outcome Criteria

The person will
- Identify risk factors for hypothermia
- Relate methods of maintaining warmth/preventing heat loss
- Maintain body temperature within normal limits

Interventions

A. Assess for the presence of risk factors

1. Prolonged exposure to cold environment (either at home or outside)
2. Poverty/inability to pay for adequate heat/shelter
3. Extremes of age (*e.g.,* newborn, elderly)
4. Neurovascular/peripheral vascular disease
5. Malnutrition/cachexia
6. Perioperative experience

B. Monitor body and environmental temperatures.

C. Reduce or eliminate causative or contributing factors if possible
1. For prolonged exposure to cold environment:
   a. Assess room temperatures at home.
   b. Teach the person to keep room temperatures at 70°–75° F or to layer clothing with sweaters.
   c. Explain the importance of wearing a hat, gloves, and warm socks and shoes to prevent heat loss.
   d. Encourage the person to limit going outside when temperatures are very cold.
   e. Acquire an electric blanket, warm blankets, or down comforter and flannel sheets for bed.
   f. Provide a hot bath before the person is cold.
   g. Teach to wear close-knit undergarments to prevent heat loss.
   h. Explain that more clothes may be needed in the morning when body metabolism is lowest.
2. For poverty/inability to pay for heat:
   a. Consult with social service to identify sources of financial assistance/warm clothing/blankets, shelter.
   b. Teach the person the importance of preventing heat loss before body temperature is actually lowered.
   c. Acquire warm socks, sweaters, gloves, and hats.
3. For extremes of age (newborn, elderly):
   a. Maintain room temperature at 70°–74° F.
   b. Have the client wear hat, gloves, and socks if necessary to prevent heat loss.
   c. Explain to family members that newborns, infants, and the elderly are more susceptible to heat loss (see also *Ineffective Thermoregulation*).
4. For neurovascular/peripheral vascular disease:
   a. Keep room temperature between 70°–74° F.
   b. Assess for adequate circulation to extremities (*i.e.,* satisfactory peripheral pulses).
   c. Have the person wear warm gloves and socks to reduce heat loss.
   d. Teach the person to take a warm bath if he is feeling unable to get warm.
5. For children and elderly during intraoperative experience (Burkle, 1988):
   a. Increase ambient temperature of OR room prior to case.
   b. Use a portable radiant heating lamp to provide additional heat during surgery.
   c. Cover person with warm blankets when arriving in OR.
   d. When possible, use a warming mattress.
   e. During prepping and surgery, keep as much of body surface covered as possible.
   f. Warm prep set, blood, fluids, anesthesia, irrigants.
   g. Keep head covered well.
   h. Continue heat-conserving interventions postoperatively.
6. Initiate health teaching if indicated.
   a. Explain the relationship of age as a risk for hypothermia.
   b. Teach the early signs of hypothermia:
      Cool skin
      Pallor, blanching, redness
   c. Explain the need to drink 8–10 glasses of water daily and to consume frequent small meals with warm liquids.
   d. Explain the need to avoid alcohol during periods of very cold weather.

References/Bibliography

Anderson, A. (1988). Parental perception and management of school-age children's fevers. *Nurse Practictioner, 13*(5), 8–9.

Bafitis, H. & Sargent, F. (1977). Human physiological adaptability through the life sequence. *Gerontology, 32*(4), 402–410

Bindler, R.N. & Howry, R.N. (1988). Nursing care of children with febrile seizures. *American Journal of Nursing, 78,* 270–273.

Birdsall, C. (1985). How do you handle heat loss? *American Journal of Nursing, 85*(4), 367.

Bliss-Holtz, J. (1989). Comparison of rectal, axillary, and inguinal temperatures in full-term newborn infants. *Nursing Research, 38*(2), 85–87.

Boyd-Shurett, P.H., & Coburn, C. (1981). Heat and heat related illness. *American Journal of Nursing, 81,* 1298–1301.

Brunner, L.S., & Suddarth, D.S. (1988). *Textbook of medical-surgical nursing* (6th ed.). Philadelphia: J. B. Lippincott.

Bulschek, G., & McCloskey, J. (1985). *Nursing interventions.* Philadelphia: W. B. Saunders.

Burkle, N. (1988). Inadvertent hypothermia. *Journal of Gerontologic Nursing, 14*(6); 26–29.

Carnevali, D., & Patrick, M. (1985) *Nursing management for the elderly.* Philadelphia: J. B. Lippincott.

Carpenito, L. J. (1991) *Handbook of nursing diagnosis* (4th ed.). Philadelphia: J. B. Lippincott.

Castle, M., & Watkins, J. (1979). Fever: Understanding the sinister sign. *Nursing 79, 9*(2), 26–33.

Collins, K. (1988). Hypothermia in the elderly. *Health Vist, 61*(2), 50–51.

Feldman, M. (1988). Inadvertent hypothermia: A threat to homeostasis in the postanesthetic patient. *Journal of Post Anesthesia Nursing, 3*(2), 82–87.

Green, M. (1987). Hypothermia: The chiller that may be missed? ... low body temperature can be triggered by a variety of factors. *Geriatric Nursing Home Care, 7*(12), 20–21.

Greer, P. (1988). Head coverings for newborns under radiant warmers. *JOGNN, 17*(4), 265–271.

Hayes, K. (1984). Dealing with heat injuries. *RN, 47*(7), 41–44.

Hunsberger, M. (1989). Principles and skills adapted to the care of children. In Foster R.L, Hunsberger M.M, & Anderson, J. J. T. (Eds.). *Family-centered nursing care of children.* Philadelphia: W. B. Saunders.

Jacobs, M. & Geels, W. (1985). *Signs and symptoms in nursing.* Philadelphia: J. B. Lippincott.

Jenkins, G. (1987). Safe and warm this winter. *Geriatric Home Care, 7*(11), 9–10.

Jones, S. (1984). The use and misuse of hypothermia blankets. *RN, 47*(3), 55.

Kilman, C. (1987). Parents' knowledge and practices related to fever management. *Journal of Pediatric Health Care, 1*(4), 173–179.

Kilman, C. (1987). Home management of children's fevers. *Journal of Pediatric Nursing, 2*(6), 400–404.

Kunnel, M, (1988). Comparisons of rectal, femoral, axillary, and skin-to-mattress temperatures in stable neonates. *Nursing Research, 37*(3), 162–189.

Miller, C.A. (1990). *Nursing care of older adults.* Glenview IL: Scott, Foresman.

Patrick, M., Woods, S., Craven, R., & Rokosky, J. (1985). *Medical-surgical nursing.* Philadelphia: J. B. Lippincott.

Porth, C. (1990). *Pathophysiology* (2nd ed.) Philadelphia: J. B. Lippincott.

Reeves-Swift, R. (1990). Rational management of a child's acute fever. *American Journal of Maternal-Child Nursing, 15* (2), 82–85.

Robbins, A.S. (1989). Hypothermia and heat stroke: Protecting the elderly patient. *Geriatrics, 44*(1), 73–79.

Schmitt, B. D. (1984). Fever in childhood. *Pediatrics, 74*(5), 929–936.

Taylor, C., Lillis, C. & LeMone, P. (1989). *Fundamentals of nursing: The art and science of nursing care.* Philadelphia: J. B. Lippincott.

Whaley, L. F., & Wong, D. L. (1989). *Essentials of pediatric nursing* (3rd ed.). St. Louis: C. V. Mosby.

Wong, D. L., & Whaley, L. F. (1990). *Clinical manual of pediatric nursing* (3rd ed.). St. Louis: C. V. Mosby.

Thermoregulation, Ineffective

■ *Related to* **Newborn Transition to Extrauterine Environment**

DEFINITION

Ineffective Thermoregulation: The state in which an individual experiences or is at risk of experiencing an inability to maintain a stable core normal body temperature in the presence of adverse or changing external factors.

DEFINING CHARACTERISTICS

Major (must be present)

Temperature fluctuations related to limited metabolic compensatory regulation in response to environmental factors

RELATED FACTORS

Situational (personal, environmental)

Fluctuating environmental temperatures
Cold or wet articles (clothes, cribs, equipment)
Inadequate heating system
Inadequate housing
Wet body surface
Inadequate clothing for weather (excessive, insufficient)

Maturational

Neonate
    Large surface area relative to body mass
    Limited ability to produce heat (metabolic)
    Limited shivering ability
    Increased basal metabolism
Premature
    (Same as neonate but more severe)
Elderly
    Decreased basal metabolism
    Loss of adipose tissue (limbs)

Diagnostic Considerations

Ineffective Thermoregulation is a useful diagnosis for persons who have difficulty maintaining a stable core body temperature over a wide range of environmental temperatures. This diagnosis most commonly applies to elderly persons and neonates.

The nursing focus centers on manipulating external factors (*e.g.*, clothing and environmental conditions) to maintain body temperature within normal limits and on teaching prevention strategies.

Errors in Diagnostic Statements

Ineffective Thermoregulation related to effects of a hypothalamic tumor
Tumors of the hypothalamus can affect the temperature-regulating centers, resulting in body temperature shifts. This situation requires constant surveillance and rapid response to changes with appropriate nursing and medical treatments. Thus, this situation would be better described as a collaborative problem: *Potential Complication: Hypo/hyperthermia*
Ineffective Thermoregulation related to temperature fluctuations
Temperature fluctuations represent a manifestation of the diagnosis, not a related factor. If the fluctuations result from age-related limited compensatory regulation, the diagnosis would be written: *Ineffective Thermoregulation related to decreased ability to acclimatize to heat or cold secondary to age as evidenced by temperature fluctuations*

Focus Assessment Criteria

Subjective
    Tone/activity (neonate)
        Active
        Quiet
        Irritable
    Cry (neonate)
        Vigorous
        High-pitched
        Weak
    History of hypothermia or hyperthermia
    Usual body temperature
    Medications

Objective
    Skin
        Color
        Nailbeds
        Integrity (cord, lacerations)
        Rashes
    Temperature
        Environment (home, infant [ambient, radiant, Isolette])
        Body (adult, child [rectal, oral], newborn [axillary])
    Vital signs
        Respiratory (rate, rhythm, presence of retractions, breath sounds)
        Heart rate

Principles and Rationale for Nursing Care

See *Hyperthermia* for principles on body temperature regulation.

Generic Considerations

1. Thermoregulation involves the balancing of heat production and heat loss.
2. The body responds to cold environments with mechanism aimed at preventing heat loss and increasing heat production
   a. Muscle contraction
   b. Peripheral vasoconstriction
   c. Increased heart rate
   d. Dilation of blood vessels in muscles
   e. Shivering and vasodilation
   f. Release of thyroxine and corticosteroids.
3. The body responds to hot environments by increasing heat dissipation through:
   a. Increased sweat production
   b. Dilation of peripheral blood vessels

Pediatric Considerations

1. The neonate is vulnerable to heat loss because of:
   a. Large body surface area relative to body mass
   b. Increased basal metabolism rate
   c. Less adipose tissue for insulation
   d. Environmental conditions (delivery room, nursery)
2. The neonate with hypoxia or under the influence of drugs (*e.g.,* given to the mother during labor) will have difficulty increasing heat production (Ouimette, 1985).
3. The neonate has limited ability to adapt to environmental temperature changes because of:
   a. Limited ability to produce heat (brown fat synthesis)
   b. Limited shivering ability
4. The newborn loses heat through (Neeson & May, 1986):
   a. Evaporation (loss of heat when water on skin changes to vapor)
   b. Convection (loss of heat when cool air flows over skin)
   c. Conduction (transfer of heat when skin surface is in direct contact with a cool surface)
   d. Radiation (transfer of heat from infant to cooler surfaces without direct contact)
5. Nonshivering thermogenesis is a heat-production mechanism located in brown fat (highly vascular adipose tissue), which is found only in infants. When skin temperature begins to drop, thermal receptors transmit impulses to the central nervous system (Neeson & May, 1986). The following sequence illustrates this mechanism:
   Central nervous system → Stimulates sympathetic nervous system → Release of norepinephrine from adrenal gland and at nerve endings in brown fat → Heat production
6. Calorie requirements are high for newborns (approximately 117 cal/kg body weight/ day).
7. An increased metabolic rate for heat production results in increased demands for oxygen and glucose. With prolonged cold stress or in compromised neonates, acidosis can result (Klaus, Famanroff, & Martin, 1979).
8. Premature or low-birth-weight infants are more susceptible to heat loss because of the reduced metabolic reserves available (*e.g.,* glycogen).
9. Cooling reduces the amount of glucose as well as oxygenation and circulation, which inhibits the production of surfactant.
10. The newborn can also experience overheating from excessive clothing in hot weather. The full-term infant can sweat in response to overheating, but the premature infant cannot.

Gerontologic Considerations
See *Hypothermia*

■ Ineffective Thermoregulation
Related to Newborn Transition to Extrauterine
Environment

Assessment

Objective

Episodes of temperature >37° C. or
Episodes of temperature <36.4° C.

Outcome Criteria

The infant will
• Have a temperature between 36.4° and 37° C.
The parent will
• Explain techniques to avoid heat loss at home

Interventions

A. Assess for contributing factors
    1. Environmental sources of heat loss
    2. Lack of knowledge (caregivers, parents)

B. Reduce or eliminate the sources of heat loss
    1. Evaporation
        a. In the delivery room, quickly dry skin and hair with a heated towel and place infant in a heated environment.
        b. When bathing, provide a warm environment.
        c. Wash and dry baby in sections to reduce evaporation.
        d. Limit time in contact with wet diapers or blankets.
    2. Convection
        a. Reduce drafts in delivery room.
        b. Avoid drafts on infant (air conditioning, fans, windows, open portholes on Isolette).
    3. Conduction
        a. Warm all articles for care (stethoscopes, scales, hands of caregivers, clothes, bed linens, cribs).
        b. Place infant very close to mother to conserve heat (and foster bonding).
    4. Radiation
        a. Place infant next to mother in the delivery room.

    b. Reduce objects in the room that absorb heat (metal).

    c. Place crib or Isolette as far away from walls (outside) or windows as possible.

C. Monitor temperature of newborn (Waechter, Phillips, & Holaday, 1985)

1. Assess axillary temperature initially q ½ hour until stable, then q 4–8 hour.
2. If temperature is less than 36.3° C:
   a. Wrap infant in two blankets
   b. Put stockinette cap on.
   c. Assess for environmental sources of heat loss.
   d. If hypothermia persists over 1 hour, notify physician.
   e. Assess for complications of cold stress: hypoxia, respiratory acidosis, hypoglycemia, fluid and electrolyte imbalances, weight loss.
3. If temperature is >37° C:
   a. Loosen blanket.
   b. Remove cap, if on.
   c. Assess environment for thermal gain.
   d. If hyperthermia persists over 1 hour, notify physician.
4. Assess for signs and symptoms of sepsis every shift:
   a. Respiratory function (rate, rhythm, pattern)
   b. Skin (tone, color, perfusion)
   c. Poor feeding
   d. Irritability
   e. Signs of localized infections (skin, umbilicus, circumcision, eyes, birth lacerations)

D. Initiate health teaching

1. Teach caregiver why infant is vulnerable to temperature fluctuations (cold and heat).
2. Explain sources of environmental heat loss (see section B.)
3. Demonstrate how to conserve heat during bathing.
4. Instruct that it is not necessary to routinely check temperature at home.
5. Teach to check temperature if infant is hot, sick, or irritable as follows:
   a. Shake down the thermometer
   b. Place in femoral fold
   c. Hold in place for 11 minutes
   d. Read at eye level
   e. Report temperature >37.5° C to health care professional

References/Bibliography

Fanaroff, A, & Martin, R. (Eds.). (1983). *Behrman's neonatal-perinatal medicine*. St. Louis: C. V. Mosby.

Klaus, M. Fananroff, A. & Martin R. (Eds.). (1979). *Care of the high-risk neonate*. Philadelphia: W. B. Saunders.

Neeson, J., & May, K. (1986). *Comprehensive maternity nursing*. Philadelphia: J. B. Lippincott.

Ouimette, J. (1985). *Perinatal nursing*. Boston: Jones & Bartlett.

Ruchala, P. (1985). The effects of wearing headcoverings on axillary temperature of infants. *American Journal of Maternal Child Nursing*, 10(4), 240.

Waechter, E., Phillips, J. & Holaday, B. (1985). *Nursing care of children*. Philadelphia: J. B. Lippincott.

Whaley, L.F., & Wong, D. L. (1989). *Essentials of pediatric nursing* (3rd ed.). St. Louis: C. V. Mosby.

Ziegel, E., & Cranley, M. (1984). *Obstetric nursing*. New York: Macmillan.

Bowel Elimination, Altered*

Constipation

Colonic Constipation

Perceived Constipation

Diarrhea

Bowel Incontinence

Bowel Elimination, Altered

DEFINITION

Altered bowel elimination: The state in which an individual experiences or is at high risk of experiencing bowel dysfunction resulting in diarrhea, incontinence, or constipation.

DEFINING CHARACTERISTICS

Major (must be present)

Reports or demonstrates one or more of the following:
  Hard, formed stool
  Painful defecation
  Habitual use of laxatives/enemas
  Bowel movements less than three times a week
  Loose liquid stools
  Increased frequency (more than three times a day)

Minor (may be present)
  Painful defecation
  Abdominal discomfort
  Rectal fullness
  Headache
  Anorexia
  Urgency
  Abdominal cramping
  Increased or decreased bowel sounds

*This diagnostic category is not currently on the NANDA list but has been included for clarity and usefulness.

RELATED FACTORS

See Related Factors under *Constipation* and *Diarrhea*

Constipation

■ *Related to* **Painful Defecation**

DEFINITION

Constipation: The state in which an individual experiences or is at high risk of experiencing stasis of the large intestine resulting in infrequent elimination or hard, dry feces.

DEFINING CHARACTERISTICS

Major (must be present)
  Hard, formed stool and/or
  Defecation occurs less than three times a week

Minor (may be present)
  Decreased bowel sounds
  Reported feeling of rectal fullness
  Reported feeling of pressure in rectum
  Straining and pain on defecation
  Palpable impaction

RELATED FACTORS

Pathophysiologic
  Malnutrition
  Sensory/motor disorders
    Spinal cord lesions   Cerebrovascular accident (stroke)
    Spinal cord injury   Neurologic diseases
    Spina bifida
  Metabolic and endocrine disorders
    Anorexia nervosa   Hypothyroidism
    Obesity   Hyperparathyroidism
  Affective disorders
  Pain (upon defecation)
    Hemorrhoids   Back injury
  Decreased peristalsis related to hypoxia (cardiac, pulmonary)
  Cancer

Treatment-Related

Drug side-effects

Antacids	Calcium
Iron	Anticholinergics
Barium	Anesthetics
Aluminum	Narcotics (codeine, morphine)
Aspirin	Diuretics
Phenothiazines	Antiparkinsonian agents

Surgery
Habitual laxative use

Situational (personal, environmental)

Immobility	Lack of privacy
Pregnancy	Inadequate diet (lack of roughage
Stress	thiamine)
Lack of exercise	Dehydration
Irregular evacuation patterns	Fear of rectal or cardiac pain
Cultural/health beliefs	Faulty appraisal/dementia
	Inability to perceive bowel cues

Maturational

Infant: Formula
Child: Toilet training (*e.g.,* reluctance to interrupt play)
Elderly: Decreased motility of GI tract

Diagnostic Considerations

Altered Bowel Elimination probably is too broad a category for clinical use. This diagnostic category includes five more specific nursing diagnoses: *Constipation, Colonic Constipation, Perceived Constipation, Diarrhea,* and *Bowel Incontinence.*

Two of the three constipation diagnoses contain their etiologic or contributing factors in the diagnostic labels *Colonic* and *Perceived.* Colonic constipation results from delayed passage of food residue in the bowel due to factors that the nurse can treat, *e.g.,* dehydration, insufficient dietary roughage, immobility. Perceived constipation refers to a faulty perception of constipation with self-prescribed overuse of laxatives, enemas, and/or suppositories.

When constipation results from factors other than those related to colonic or perceived constipation and are amenable to nursing interventions, the nursing diagnosis *Constipation* can apply.

Errors in Diagnostic Statements

Constipation related to reports of infrequent hard, dry feces

A report of infrequent hard, dry feces is a validation of constipation, not a contributing factor. If the nurse does not know the cause of constipation, the diagnosis can be written: *Constipation related to unknown etiology, as evidenced by reports of infrequent hard, dry feces.*

Diarrhea related to opportunistic enteric pathogens secondary to AIDS

Diarrhea, sometimes chronic, occurs in 60%–90% of persons with AIDS. Prolonged diarrhea represents a collaborative problem: *Potential Complication: Fluid/ electrolyte/nutritional imbalances related to diarrhea*

Besides cotreating the above collaborative problem with a physician, the nurse will treat other responses to chronic diarrhea such as: *High Risk for Impaired Skin Integrity or High Risk for Social Isolation*

Focus Assessment Criteria

Subjective Data

1. Elimination pattern
    Usual pattern
    Present pattern

    Expectation (appropriate?)
    Laxative use (type? how often?)
    Enema use (type? how often?)

2. History of symptoms
    Onset
    Duration
    Location
    Description

    Frequency
    Precipitated by what?
    Relieved by what?
    Aggravated by what?

3. Associated symptoms/complaints of
    Headache
    Weakness
    Lethargy
    Anorexia

    Thirst
    Pain
    Cramping
    Weight loss/gain

4. Life-style
    Activity level
    Occupation
    Exercise (what? how often?)

    Nutrition
      24-hour recall of foods and
        liquids taken
    Usual 24-hour intake
      Carbohydrates
      Fat
      Protein
      Roughage
      Liquids

5. Current drug therapy
    Antibiotics
    Iron
    Steroids

    Antacids
    CNS depressants

6. Medical-surgical history
    Present conditions
    Past conditions

    Surgical history (colostomy?
    ileostomy?)

7. Awareness of bowel cues

Objective Data

1. Stool

Color	Odor	Consistency
Brown	Normal	Soft, formed
Yellow	Foul	Soft, bulky
Yellow-green		Small, dry
Green		Pasty
Black		Diarrheal
Tan (clay-colored)		Hard
Red		

Size/Shape	*Components Blood*
Narrow	Mucus
Large caliber	Pus
Small caliber	Parasites
Round	Undigested food

2. Nutrition

Food Intake	*Fluid intake*
Type	Type
Amounts	Amounts

3. GI motility (auscultation, light palpation)

Bowel Sounds

High-pitched, gurgling (5/min)	Weak and infrequent
High-pitched frequent, loud, pushing	Absent

Abdominal Distention

None	Moderate
Slight	Severe

Flatulence

None	Frequent
Occasionally	

4. Perianal area/rectal examination

Hemorrhoids	Irritation
Fissures	Impaction
Control of rectal sphincter (presence of anal wink, bulbocavernosus reflex)	Presence/absence of stool in rectum

Principles and Rationale for Nursing Care

Generic Considerations

1. Bowel patterns may be culturally and/or familially determined.
2. Circadian rhythms may be utilized to assist defecation at a regular time.
3. Activity influences bowel elimination by improving muscle tone and stimulating appetite and peristalsis.
4. Factors that influence the characteristics of stool:

Color	*Diet*	*Drugs*	*Disease*
Yellow–yellow green	Breast milk	Antibiotics Senna	Severe diarrhea
Green	Green vegetables	Mercurous chloride Indomethacin Calomel Dithiazanine	Severe diarrhea
Black–dark brown	Cherries	Iron Charcoal Bismuth	Upper GI bleeding Anticoagulants Steroids and salicylates

Color	Diet	Drugs	Disease
Pale–whitish	Milk Meat	Antacids	
Clay-colored	Fat		Common bile duct blockage
Red	Beets	Bromsulphalein Tetracyclines (syrup) Phenolphthalein Pyridium	

5. The odor of the stool varies with the pH and the amount of bacterial fermentation.
6. The normalcy of one's bowel patterns is determined by the individual.
7. Psychologic discomfort and inadequate coping can produce elimination alterations.
8. Intestinal elimination is controlled by neural innervation from the spinal cord and by the stimulation of neural centers in the lower intestinal wall by fecal contents.
9. Bowel evacuation can be delayed by voluntarily inhibiting the urge to defecate.
10. The gastrocolic reflex and duodenocolic reflex stimulate mass peristalsis two or three times a day, most often following meals.
11. Voluntary contraction of the muscles of the abdominal wall aid in the expulsion of feces.

Nutrition

1. Sufficient fluid intake, at least 2 L daily, is necessary to maintain bowel patterns and promote proper stool consistency.
2. A well-balanced diet high in fiber content stimulates peristalsis. Foods high in fiber should be avoided during episodes of diarrhea. These include:
   Whole grains and nuts (bran, shredded wheat, brown rice, whole wheat bread)
   Raw and coarse vegetables (broccoli, cauliflower, cucumbers, lettuce, cabbage, turnips, Brussels sprouts)
   Fresh fruits, with skins
3. Bulk and consistency of stool are influenced by dietary and fluid patterns. High vegetable diet produces soft, bulky stools. High meat diet produces small, dry, hard stools.
4. Diets high in unrefined fibrous food produce large soft stools that decrease the colon's susceptibility to disease.
5. Diets low in fiber and high in concentrated refined foods produce small hard stools that increase the colon's susceptibility to disease.
6. Fiber that is not digested absorbs water, which adds bulk and softness to the stool, speeds up the passage through the intestines, and slows down the rapid transit (Schuster, 1983).
7. Fiber without adequate fluid can aggravate, not facilitate, bowel function.

Laxative Abuse

1. Chronic laxative abuse is one of the major causes of constipation in the elderly (Schuster, 1983).
2. Laxatives and enemas are not components of a bowel management program, but are for emergency use only (Ellickson, 1988).
3. Lactose intolerance can cause gas formation and bloating. These responses may be confused with constipation with a subsequent response of laxative use.

Pediatric Considerations

1. As the infant ages, the stomach enlarges to hold a greater amount of food, and the rapid peristaltic activity of the GI tract slows down. As a result, stools change in color, consistency, and frequency with maturation (Whaley & Wong, 1989).
2. Constipation refers to the passage of hard, pebbly, rocklike stools; it is not related to the frequency of bowel movements, straining or grunting, or the number of days between movements (Chow, Durand, Feldman, & Mills, 1984).
3. Voluntary withholding (functional constipation) is the most common cause of constipation beyond the neonatal period. Conflicts in toilet training or pain on defecation may lead to stool retention (Byrne, 1990).
4. Encopresis (fecal incontinence) may occur secondary to constipation. It is not the result of a physical disorder but is commonly associated with other somatic problems such as antisocial-aggressive behaviors and social withdrawal (Whaley & Wong, 1989).
5. Diarrhea is an increase in the number and decrease in the consistency of stools. Diarrhea may be acute or chronic (Whaley & Wong, 1989).
6. Various factors predispose children to diarrhea and its physiologic consequences (Whaley & Wong, 1989), including
   a. Younger children are more susceptible to diarrhea and more likely to experience a severe episode.
   b. Children debilitated from disease and malnourished children are at increased risk.
   c. Children who live in warm environments and in conditions of poor sanitation and refrigeration, and children who live in crowded and substandard environments are at risk of eating contaminated food.
7. Normally, breastfed babies have soft, unformed—but not watery—stools (Anderson, 1989).
8. Rotaviruses are the major cause of vial diarrhea in young children (Hunsberger & Issenman, 1989).

Gerontologic Considerations

1. Older adults experience reduced mucus secretion in the large intestines and decreased elasticity of the rectal wall (Miller, 1990). However, no research validates that elderly persons are at higher risk for constipation because of age-related changes.
2. The elderly are prone to constipation due to such factors as decreased activity, insufficient dietary fiber and bulk, insufficient fluid intake, side effects of medications, and laxative abuse (Miller, 1990).

■ Constipation
Related to Painful Defecation

Assessment

Subjective Data

The person reports:

Pain on defecation
Rectal itching
Straining at stool

Objective Data

Hard consistency of stool
Hemorrhoids
Impaction palpated on rectal examination
Irritated or excoriated perianal area

Outcome Criteria

The person will
- Relate less pain on defecation
- Describe causative factors when known
- Describe rationale and procedure for treatments

Interventions

A. Assess causative factors

Fecal impaction/constipation
Hemorrhoids
Anal fissures
Pregnancy
Surgery that reduces ability to
  bear down

Pilonidal cyst
Anorectal abscess
Lower intestinal obstruction
Enlargement of prostate gland

B. Reduce rectal pain, if possible, by instructing person in corrective measures

1. Increase fluid intake.
2. Increase dietary intake of high-fiber foods.
3. Increase daily exercise.
4. Gently apply a lubricant to anus to reduce pain on defecation.
5. Apply cool compresses to area to reduce itching.
6. Take sitz bath or soak in tub or warm water (43°–46° C) for 15-minute intervals if soothing.
7. Take stool softeners or mineral oil as an adjunct to other approaches.
8. Consult with physician regarding use of local anesthetics and antiseptic agents.

C. Protect the surrounding skin from breakdown

1. Evaluate the surrounding skin area.
2. Cleanse properly with nonirritating agent (e.g., use gentle motion; use soft tissues following defecation).
3. Suggest a sitz bath following defecation.
4. Gently apply protective emollient or lubricant.

D. Initiate health teaching if indicated

1. Teach the methods to prevent rectal pressure that contributes to hemorrhoids.
2. Avoid prolonged sitting (e.g., stand up every 1 hour for 5–10 minutes to relieve pressure).

3. Avoid straining at defecation.
4. Soften stools (*e.g.,* low roughage diet, high fluid intake) (see Principles and Rationale for Nursing Care).

Colonic Constipation

- ■ *Related to* **Change in Life-style**
- ■ *Related to* **Effects of Immobility on Peristalsis**

DEFINITION

Colonic constipation: The state in which an individual experiences or is at risk of experiencing a delay in passage of food residue resulting in dry, hard stool.

DEFINING CHARACTERISTICS*

Major (80%–100%)
    Decreased frequency
    Hard, dry stool
    Straining at stool
    Painful defecation
    Adominal distention

Minor (50%–79%)
    Rectal pressure
    Headache, appetite impairment
    Abdominal pain

RELATED FACTORS

Pathophysiologic
    Malnutrition
    Sensory/motor disorders
        Spinal cord lesions
        Spinal cord injury
        Spina bifida
    Metabolic and endocrine disorders
        Anorexia nervosa
        Obesity

Cerebrovascular accident (CVA, stroke)
Neurologic diseases

Hypothyroidism
Hyperparathyroidism

*Adapted from McLane, A. M., & McShane, R. E. (1986). Empirical validation of defining characteristics of constipation: A study of bowel elimination practices of healthy adults. In M. E. Hurley (Ed.). *Classification of nursing diagnoses: Proceedings of the sixth conference.* St. Louis: C. V. Mosby.

Affective disorder
Decreased peristalsis related to hypoxia (cardiac, pulmonary)
Cancer

Treatment-Related

Drug side-effects
  Antacids
  Iron
  Barium
  Aluminum
  Calcium
  Anticholinergics
  Anesthetics
  Narcotics (codeine, morphine)
  Aspirin
  Phenothiazines
  Diuretics
  Antiparkinsonian agents
Surgery
Habitual laxative use

Situational (personal, environmental)

Immobility	Lack of privacy
Pregnancy	Inadequate diet (lack of roughage/
Stress	thiamine)
Lack of exercise	Dehydration
Irregular evacuation patterns	Fear of rectal or cardiac pain

Maturational

Infant
  Formula
Child
  Toilet training (reluctance to interrupt play)
Elderly
  Decreased motility of gastrointestinal tract

■ Colonic Constipation
Related to Change in Life-style

Assessment

Subjective Data

The person reports:
  Hard dry stools less than three times a week
  A change in living patterns (*e.g.*)

Altered daily routine	Inadequate fluid intake

Decreased activity
Lack of privacy
Diet reported lacking in sufficient
roughage

Recent illness or hospitalization
Change in regular schedule of
elimination

Objective Data

Hard formed stools
Palpable impaction

Outcome Criteria

The person will
• Describe contributing factors when known
• Describe methods to prevent constipation

Interventions

A. Assess for causative factors

1. Stress
   a. Occupation
   b. Family responsibilities
   c. Financial considerations
2. Sedentary life-style
3. Hospitalization
4. Drug side-effect
5. Debilitation
6. Lack of privacy (at work or at school)
7. Recent or frequent travel
8. Lack of time

B. Promote corrective measures

1. Regular time for elimination
   a. Identify normal defecation pattern prior to constipation.
   b. Review daily routine.
   c. Advise that time for defecation be included as part of daily routine.
   d. Discuss suitable time (based on responsibilities, availability of facilities, etc.).
   e. Provide stimulus to defecation (*e.g.,* coffee, prune juice).
   f. Advise that an attempt to defecate should be made about an hour or so following meal and that it may be necessary to remain in the bathroom a suitable length of time.
   g. Utilize bathroom instead of bedpan if possible.
   h. Offer bedpan or bedside commode if unable to use bathroom.
   i. Assist into position on bedpan or commode.
   j. Provide for privacy (close door, draw curtains around bed, play television or radio to mask sounds, have room deodorizer available).
   k. Provide for comfort (reading material as diversion) and safety (call bell available).
   l. Allow suitable position (sitting, if not contraindicated).

2. Adequate exercise
   a. Review current exercise pattern.
   b. Provide for moderate physical exercise on a frequent basis (if not contraindicated).
   c. Provide frequent ambulation of hospitalized patient when tolerable.
   d. Perform ROM exercises for person who is bedridden.
   e. Teach exercises for increased abdominal muscle tone (unless contraindicated).
      • Contract abdominal muscles several times frequently throughout day.
      • Do sit-ups keeping heels on floor with knees slightly flexed.
      • While supine, raise lower limbs, keeping knees straight.

C. Eliminate or reduce contributing factors

1. Untoward side-effects of current medical regimen.
   a. Administer mild laxative following oral administration of barium sulfate.*
   b. Assess elimination status while on antacid therapy (may be necessary to alternate magnesium-type antacid with other types).*
   c. Encourage increased intake of high-roughage foods and increased fluid intake as adjunct to iron therapy (*e.g.,* fresh fruits and vegetables with skins; bran, nuts, and seeds; whole wheat bread).
   d. Encourage early ambulation, with assistance if necessary, to counter effects of anesthetic agents.
   e. Assess elimination status while receiving certain narcotic analgesics (morphine, codeine) and alert physician if the patient is experiencing difficulty with defecation.
2. Laxative abuse
   a. See *Perceived Constipation.*
3. Stress
   a. See Appendix X for relaxation techniques for stress reduction.
4. Inadequate dietary and fluid intake: see *Altered Nutrition: Less Than Body Requirements.*

D. Conduct health teaching as indicated

1. Explain to person and family the relationship of life-style changes to constipation.
2. Explain interventions that relieve symptoms.
3. Explain techniques to reduce the effects of stress and immobility.

■ Colonic Constipation
Related to Effects of Immobility on Peristalsis

Assessment

Subjective Data

The person reports:

*May require a physician's order.

Hard stools less than three times a week
Inability or difficulty moving bowels

Objective Data

Immobility (*e.g.*, casts, traction, paralysis)
Altered state of consciousness
Altered body position (*e.g.*, legs elevated)

Multiple support equipment (*e.g.*, catheters, IV, arterial lines, respiratior)
Body restraints
Forced bed rest

Outcome Criteria

The person will
* Describe therapeutic bowel regimen
* Relate or demonstrate improved bowel elimination
* Explain rationale for interventions

Interventions

A. Assess causative factors of immobility

Musculoskeletal (*e.g.*, fractures, sprain, contractures, hip replacement)
Reliance on life-support systems
Chronic or acute illness
Trauma (*e.g.*, burns, head injury)
Physical handicap
Inappropriate coping mechanisms
Bed rest
Psychosomatic illness
Degenerative joint changes (arthritis)
Surgery

B. Promote corrective measures

1. Balanced diet
   a. Review list of foods high in bulk.
      * Fresh fruits with skins
      * Bran
      * Nuts and seeds
      * Whole grain breads and cereals
      * Cooked fruits and vegetables
      * Fruit juices
   b. Discuss dietary preferences.
   c. Take into account any food intolerances or allergies.
   d. Include approximately 800 g of fruits and vegetables (about four pieces of fresh fruit and large salad) for normal daily bowel movement.
   e. Suggest use of bran in moderation at first (may irritate GI tract, produce flatulence, cause diarrhea or blockage).
   f. Gradually increase amount of bran as tolerated (may add to cereals, baked goods, etc.). Explain the need for fluid intake with bran.

    g. Consider financial limitations (encourage the use of fruits and vegetables in season).

  2. Adequate fluid intake

    a. Encourage intake of at least 2 L—8–10 glasses—unless contraindicated.

    b. Discuss fluid preferences.

    c. Set up regular schedule for fluid intake.

    d. Recommend a glass of hot water to be taken one-half hour before breakfast that may act as stimulus to bowel evacuation.

  3. Regular time for elimination

    a. Identify normal defecation pattern prior to constipation.

    b. Review daily routine.

    c. Include time for defecation as part of regular routine.

    d. Discuss suitable time (based on responsibilities, availability of facilities, etc.).

    e. Provide stimulus to defecation (*e.g.,* coffee, prune juice).

    f. Suggest that person attempt defecation about an hour or so following meal and remain in bathroom suitable length of time.

    g. Utilize bathroom instead of bedpan if possible.

    h. Offer bedpan or bedside commode if unable to use bathroom.

    i. Assist into position on bedpan or commode.

    j. Provide for privacy (close door, draw curtains around bed, play television or radio to mask sounds, make room deodorizer available).

    k. Provide for comfort (reading material as diversion) and safety (call bell available).

  4. Optimal position

    a. Assist patient to normal semisquatting position to allow optimum usage of abdominal muscles and effect of force of gravity.

    b. Assist onto bedpan if necessary and elevate head of bed to high Fowler's position or elevation permitted.

    c. Use fracture bedpan for comfort if preferred.

    d. Stress the avoidance of straining.

    e. Encourage exhaling during straining.

    f. Place call bell within easy reach.

    g. Maintain safety (siderails).

    h. Provide privacy.

    i. Chart results (color, consistency, amount).

C. Eliminate or reduce contributing factors

  1. Fecal impaction

    a. If fecal impaction is suspected, perform digital examination of rectum: Have client assume position lying on left side. Don glove, lubricate forefinger, and insert; attempt to break up any hardened fecal mass and remove pieces.

    b. If impaction is out of reach of gloved finger:

      • Administer oil retention enema to aid in removal of mass.*

      • Instruct person to retain enema at least 60 minutes or possibly overnight

      • Follow with cleansing enema* (both enemas may need to be repeated; may need to follow with repeated attempt to break up mass digitally).

    c. Make client comfortable and allow to rest.

    d. Client may require temporary use of stool softener or mild cathartic.*

    e. Maintain accurate bowel elimination record.

---

*May require a physician's order.

2. Severe constipation
   a. First day, insert glycerin suppository and have client attempt bowel movement through intermittent straining efforts.
   b. If ineffective, on second day, insert glycerin suppository and follow same routine.
   c. If no results, on third day, request prescription for suppository, which if not effective should be followed by enema.*
   d. To aid in stimulation of reflex, suppository may be followed in 20–30 minutes by digital stimulation of anal sphincter.
   e. Return to first-day routine and follow until pattern is established (may be every 2–3 days).

D. Conduct health teaching as indicated
   1. Explain to person and significant others the interventions required to prevent constipation (*e.g.,* diet, exercise) versus those required to treat it.
   2. Refer to Principles and Rationale for Nursing Care for specifics.

Perceived Constipation

■ *Related to* **(Specify)**

DEFINITION
Perceived constipation: The state in which an individual self-prescribes the daily use of laxatives, enemas, and/or suppositories to ensure a daily bowel movement.

DEFINING CHARACTERISTICS†

Major (80%–100%)
   Expectation of a daily bowel movement with the resulting overuse of laxatives, enemas and suppositories
   Expected passage of stool at same time, every day

---

*May require a physician's order.

†McLane, A. M., & McShane, R. E. (1986). Empirical validation of defining characteristics of constipation: A study of bowel elimination practices of healthy adults. In Hurley, M. E., (Ed.). *Classification of nursing diagnoses: Proceedings of the North American Nursing Diagnoses Association sixth conference.* St. Louis: C. V. Mosby.

RELATED FACTORS

Pathophysiologic
Altered affect caused by change in:
Body chemistry
Tumor
Obsessive-compulsive disorders
CNS deterioration

Situational (personal, environmental)
Cultural/familial health beliefs
Faulty appraisal

Diagnostic Considerations
See *Constipation*

Focus Assessment Criteria
See *Constipation*

Principles and Rationale for Nursing Care
See *Constipation*

■ Perceived Constipation
Related to (Specify)

Assessment
See Defining Characteristics

Outcome Criteria

The person will
• Verbalize acceptance with bowel movement q 2–3 days
• Not use laxatives regularly
• Relate the causes of constipation
• Describe the hazards of laxative use
• Relate an intent to increase fiber, fluid, and exercise in daily life as instructed

Interventions

A. Assess causative or contributing factors
1. Painful defecation (see *Constipation related to painful defecation*)

2. Inadequate diet, fluids and/or exercise
3. Cultural/familial belief
4. Faulty appraisal

B. Explain that bowel movements are needed every 2–3 days, not daily
   1. Be sensitive to his beliefs.
   2. Be patient.

C. Explain the hazards of regular laxative use
   1. Provide only temporary relief
   2. Promote constipation by interfering with peristalsis
   3. In emergencies use rectal suppository instead of oral laxative

D. Plan Corrective Measures
   1. Balanced diet
      a. Review list of foods high in bulk.
         • Fresh fruits with skins
         • Bran
         • Nuts and seeds
         • Whole grain breads and cereals
         • Cooked fruits and vegetables
      b. Discuss dietary preferences.
      c. Take into account any food intolerances or allergies.
      d. Include approximately 800 g of fruits and vegetables (about four pieces of fresh fruit and large salad) for normal daily bowel movement.
      e. Suggest use of bran in moderation at first (may irritate GI tract, produce flatulence, cause diarrhea or blockage).
      f. Gradually increase amount of bran as tolerated (may add to cereals, baked goods, etc.). Explain the need for fluid intake with bran.
      g. Suggest a commercial fiber product if fiber is inadequate in diet.
   2. Adequate fluid intake
      a. Encourage intake of a least 6–10 glasses (unless contraindicated).
      b. Discuss fluid preferences.
      c. Set up regular schedule for fluid intake, increase in hot weather.
      d. Recommend a glass of hot water to be taken one-half hour before breakfast that may act as stimulus to bowel evacuation.
   3. Regular time for elimination
      a. Include time for defecation as part of regular routine (*e.g.,* 15 minutes after eating breakfast).
      b. Discuss suitable time (based on responsibilities, availability of facilities, etc.).
      c. Provide stimulus to defecation (*e.g.,* warm drink, prunes).
      d. Teach not to ignore the urge to defecate.
      e. Provide for privacy (close door, draw curtains around bed, play television or radio to mask sounds, make room deodorizer available).
      f. Provide for comfort (reading material as diversion) and safety (call bell available).
   4. Optimal position
      a. Assist patient to normal semisquatting position to allow optimum usage of abdominal muscles and effect of force of gravity.
      b. Assist onto bedpan if necessary and elevate head of bed to high Fowler's position or elevation permitted.

    c. Use fracture bedpan for comfort if preferred.

    d. Stress the avoidance of straining.

    e. Encourage exhaling during straining.

    f. Place call bell within easy reach.

    g. Maintain safety (siderails).

    h. Provide privacy.

    i. Chart results (color, consistency, amount).

5. Regular exercise

    a. Teach the rationale for increasing activity.

    b. Suggest walking (refer to *Health Maintenance*).

    c. If walking is prohibited

- Teach to lie in bed or sit on chair and bend one knee at a time to chest (10–20 times) each knee 3–4 times/day
- Teach to sit in chair or lie in bed and turn torso from side to side (20–30 times) 6–10 times/day

Diarrhea

■ *Related to* **Untoward Side-effects (Specify)**

DEFINITION

Diarrhea: The state in which the individual experiences or is at risk of experiencing frequent passage of liquid stool or unformed stool.

DEFINING CHARACTERISTICS

Major (must be present)

    Loose, liquid stools and/or

    Increased frequency (more than three times a day)

Minor (may be present).

    Urgency

    Cramping/abdominal pain

    Increased frequency of bowel sounds

    Increase in fluidity or volume of stools

RELATED FACTORS

Pathophysiologic

    Nutritional disorders and malabsorptive syndromes

Kwashiorkor
Gastritis
Peptic ulcer
Diverticulitis
Ulcerative colitis
Metabolic and endocrine disorders
Diabetes mellitus
Addison's disease
Dumping syndrome
Infectious process
Trichinosis
Dysentery
Cholera
Malaria
Cancer
Uremia

Crohn's disease
Lactose intolerance
Spastic colon
Celiac disease (sprue)
Irritable bowel

Thyrotoxicosis

Shigellosis
Typhoid fever
Infectious hepatitis

Treatment-related

Surgical intervention of the bowel
Loss of bowel
Drug side-effects
Thyroid agents
Antacids
Laxatives
Tube feedings

Stool softeners
Antibiotics
Chemotherapy

Situational (personal, environmental)

Stress or anxiety
Irritating foods (fruits, bran cereals)
Travel
Change in bacteria in water
Bacteria, virus, parasite to which no immunity is present
Hot weather
Increased caffeine consumption

Maturational

Infant: Breastfed babies
Elderly: Decreased sphincter reflexes

Diagnostic Considerations

See *Constipation*

Focus Assessment Criteria

Refer to criteria for *Constipation*

Principles and Rationale for Nursing Care

1. Rapid transit of feces through the large intestine results in less water absorption and an unformed, liquid stool.
2. Dehydration and electrolyte imbalance occur if diarrhea continues.

3. Malabsorption results in an increase in the bulk of the colon and stimulates intestinal motility.
4. Diarrheal stool can cause excoriation of the anal area because it is usually acidic and contains digestive enzymes.
5. Hyperperistalsis is the motor response to intestinal irritants.
6. High-solute tube feedings may cause diarrhea if not followed by sufficient amounts of water.
7. Diarrhea may be related to an inflammatory process in which the intestinal mucosal wall becomes irritated, resulting in increased moisture content in the fecal masses.
8. Refer to Principles and Rationale for Nursing Care for *Constipation*.

■ Diarrhea
Related to Untoward Side-effects (Specify)

Assessment

Subjective Data
The person reports:

Loose stools more than three times daily	Cramps
	Weakness
Pain	

Objective Data

Observable signs of dehydration	Frequent stools (more than three
Increased bowel sounds	times daily)
Liquid stools	

Outcome Criteria

The person will
• Describe contributing factors when known
• Explain rationale for interventions
• Report less diarrhea

Interventions

A. Assess causative contributing factors
   1. Tube feedings
   2. Dietary indiscretions/contaminated foods
   3. Food allergies
   4. Foreign travel

B. Eliminate or reduce contributing factors
   1. Administration of tube feeding
      a. Control infusion rate (depending on delivery set).
      b. Administer smaller, more frequent feedings.*
      c. Change to continuous-drip tube feedings.*
      d. Administer more slowly if signs of GI intolerance occur.
      e. Control temperature.
      f. If refrigerated, warm in hot water to room temperature.
      g. Dilute strength of feeding temporarily.*
      h. Follow standard procedure for administration of tube feeding.
      i. Follow tube feeding with specified amount of water to assure hydration.
      j. Be careful of contamination/spoilage (unused but opened formula should not be used after 24 hours; keep unused portion refrigerated).
   2. Contaminated foods (possible sources)
      a. Raw seafood
      b. Shellfish
      c. Excess milk consumption
      d. Raw milk
      e. Restaurants
      f. Improperly cooked/stored food

C. Reduce diarrhea
   1. For adults
      a. Discontinue solids.
      b. Ingest clear liquids (fruit juices, Gatorade, broth).
      c. Avoid milk products, fat, whole grain, fresh fruits and vegetables.
      d. Gradually add semisolids and solids (crackers, yogurt, rice, bananas, applesauce).
   2. For breastfed infants
      a. Discontinue solids.
      b. Offer clear liquid supplements.
      c. Continue breastfeeding.
   3. For formula-fed infant or milk-fed child
      a. Discontinue formula, milk products, and solid foods.
      b. Offer small amounts of clear fluids (sweetened diluted tea, diluted cola, ginger ale, sugar water, diluted Jell-O water) 15–30 mL each one half to 1 hour for first 8 hours.
      c. Increase amount to 60–90 mL every 1–2 hours if number of stools has lessened.
      d. Add plain solids (Jell-O, bananas, rice, cereal, crackers) after 24 hours, if improved.
      e. Gradually return to regular diet (except milk products) after 36–48 hours; after 3–5 days gradually add milk products (half-strength skim to skim milk to half-strength whole milk to whole milk).
      f. Gradually introduce formula (half-strength formula to full-strength formula).

D. Replace fluids and electrolytes
   1. Increase oral intake to maintain a normal urine specific gravity.

*May require a physician's order.

2. Encourage liquids (water, apple juice, flat ginger ale).
3. Children may need administration of commercially prepared solution (*e.g.*, Pedialyte).*
4. Encourage fluids high in potassium and sodium (orange and grapefruit juices, bouillon).
5. Caution against use of every hot or cold liquids.
6. See *Fluid Volume Deficit* for additional interventions.

E. Conduct health teaching as indicated

1. Explain to client and significant others the interventions required to prevent future episodes.
2. Explain the effects of diarrhea on hydration.
3. Teach precautions to take when traveling to foreign lands (Maresca, 1986).
   a. Avoid foods served cold, salads, milk, fresh cheese, cold cuts and salsa.
   b. Drink carbonated or bottled beverages, avoid ice.
   c. Peel fresh fruits and vegetables.
4. Consult with primary health care provider for prophylactic use of bismuth subsalicylate (Pepto-Bismol) 30–60 mL qid during travel and 2 days after return; or antimicrobials, for treatment of traveler's diarrhea.
5. Explain how to prevent transmission of infection
   a. Hand washing
   b. Proper storage, cooking and handling of food
   c. If sexually transmitted (fecal-oral contamination), explain methods to prevent

Bowel Incontinence

■ *Related to* **Lack of Voluntary Sphincter Control secondary to spinal cord injury above T$_{11}$ or involving sacral reflex arc (S$_2$–S$_4$)**

DEFINITION

Bowel incontinence: A state in which an individual experiences a change in normal bowel habits characterized by involuntary passage of stool.

DEFINING CHARACTERISTICS

Major (must be present)

Involuntary passage of stool

RELATED FACTORS

Pathophysiologic

Loss of sphincter control

Progressive dementia

Progressive neuromuscular disorder (*e.g.,* multiple sclerosis)
Inflammatory bowel disease

Situational

Depression
Cognitive impairment
Surgery
    Coloncolostomy

Diagnostic Considerations

Bowel Incontinence describes dysfunction resulting from interruption in the neural pathways due to neurologic disorders such as spinal cord injury, multiple sclerosis, diabetic spinal lesions, cerebrovascular accident, head injuries, and brain tumors. The person may have a loss of cerebral awareness, inability to inhibit defecation, and/or loss of anal sphincter control or sensation (Toth, 1988).

Errors in Diagnostic Statements

Bowel Incontinence related to oozing of stool
    Oozing of stool is not the cause of bowel incontinence, but rather evidence of bowel incontinence. If the etiology is not known, the diagnosis should be written: *Bowel Incontinence related to unknown etiology, as evidenced by oozing of stool.*
    When the etiology is known, the diagnosis should reflect this, *e.g., Bowel Incontinence related to relaxed anal sphincter secondary to S_4 lesion.*

Focus Assessment

See *Constipation*

Principles and Rationale for Nursing Care

Generic Considerations

1. Neurogenic bowel results from interruption of neural pathways that supply the rectum, external sphincter, and accessory muscles for defecation (Toth, 1988).
2. Complete spinal cord injury, spinal cord lesions, neurologic disease, or congenital defects causing an interruption of the sacral reflex arc (at the sacral segments S_2, S_3, S_4) result in an areflexic (autonomous) or flaccid bowel. Flaccid paralysis at this level, known as an LMN lesion, results in loss of the defecation reflex, loss of sphincter control (flaccid anal sphincter), and absence of the bulbocavernosus reflex.
3. Because of an interrupted sacral reflex arc and a flaccid anal sphincter, bowel incontinence can occur without rectal stimulation whenever stool is present in the rectal vault. The stool may leak out if too soft or remain (if not extracted), predisposing the person to fecal impaction or constipation. Some intrinsic contractile abilities of the colon remain, but peristalsis is sluggish, leading to stool retention with contents present in the rectal vault.
4. Complete CNS lesions or trauma occurring above sacral cord segments (S_2, S_3, S_4) (T_{12}–L_1–L_2 vertebral level) result in a reflexic neurogenic bowel. The ascending sensory signals between the sacral reflex center and the brain are interrupted, resulting in the inability to feel the urge to defecate. Descending motor signals from the brain are also interrupted, causing loss of voluntary control over the anal sphincter. Because the sacral reflex center is preserved, it is possible to develop a

stimulation response bowel evacuation program using digital stimulation or digital stimulation devices.

5. Frequency and consistency of stool are related to fluid and food intake. Fiber increases fecal bulk and enhances absorption of water into the stool. Adequate dietary fiber and fluid intake promote firm but soft well-formed stools and decrease the risk of hard, dry constipated stools. Physical activity promotes peristalsis, aids digestion, and facilitates elimination.

6. Laxatives upset a bowel program, because they cause much of the bowel to empty and can cause unscheduled bowel movements. With constant use, the colon loses tone and bowel retaining becomes difficult. Chronic use of bowel aids can lead to inconsistent stool consistency, which interferes with the scheduled bowel program and bowel management. Stool softeners may not be necessary if diet and fluid intake are adequate. Enemas lead to overstretching of the bowel and loss of bowel tone, contributing to further constipation (Toth, 1988).

7. Fecal impaction and constipation may lead to autonomic dysreflexia in a client with injury at T_7 or higher, owing to bowel overdistention. Chronic constipation can lead to overdistention of the bowel, with further loss of bowel tone. Unrelieved constipation may result in fecal impaction. Early intervention in diet and fluid intake, bowel evacuation methods, and schedules helps prevent constipation, further loss of bowel tone, and fecal impaction.

Pediatric Considerations

See *Constipation*

Gerontologic Considerations

See *Constipation*

■ Bowel Incontinence
Related to Lack of Voluntary Sphincter Control secondary to spinal cord injury above T_{11} or involving sacral reflex arc (S_2–S_4)

Assessment

Subjective Data

Previous and current bowel patterns
Awareness of bowel cues
Control of rectal sphincter

Objective Data

Presence of anal wink
Presence of bulbocavernosus reflex

Outcome Criteria

The person will
 • Evacuate a soft formed stool every other day or every third day

Interventions

A. Assess contributing factors
   1. Lack of routine evacuation schedule
   2. Lack of knowledge of bowel elimination techniques
   3. Insufficient fluid and fiber intake
   4. Insufficient physical activity

B. Assess individual's ability to participate
   1. Neurologic status
   2. Functional ability

C. Plan a consistent, appropriate time for elimination:
   1. Institute a daily bowel program for 5 days or until a pattern develops, then move to an alternate-day program (morning or evening).
   2. Provide privacy and a nonstressful environment.
   3. Provide reassurance and protection from embarrassment while establishing the bowel program.

D. Teach effective bowel elimination techniques:
   1. Position a functionally able person in an upright or sitting position. If the person is not functionally able (e.g., quadriplegic), position in left side-lying position.
   2. For a functionally able person, use assistive devices; e.g., dil stick, digital stimulator, raised commode seat, and lubricant and gloves, as appropriate.
   3. For a person with upper extremity mobility and abdominal musculature innervation, teach bowel elimination facilitation techniques as appropriate:
      a. Valsalva's maneuver
      b. Forward bends
      c. Sitting push-ups
      d. Abdominal massage
   4. Assist with or provide equipment needed for hygiene measures, as necessary.
   5. Maintain an elimination record or a flow sheet of the bowel schedule that includes time, stool characteristics, assistive method(s) used, and number of involuntary stools, if any.

E. Explain fluid and dietary requirements:
   1. 8–10 glasses of water daily
   2. Diet high in bulk and fiber
   3. Refer to *Colonic Constipation* for specific dietary instructions.

F. Explain the effects of activity on peristalsis. Assist in determining the appropriate exercises for person's functional ability

G. Initiate health teaching, as indicated:

1. Explain the hazards of using stool softeners, laxatives, suppositories, and enemas.
2. Explain the signs and symptoms of fecal impaction and constipation. (Refer to *Dysreflexia* for additional information.)
3. Initiate teaching of a bowel program before discharge. If the client is functionally able, encourage independence with the bowel program; if not, incorporate assistive devices or attendant care, as needed.

References/Bibliography

Aman, R. A. (1980). Treating the patient, not the constipation. *American Journal of Nursing, 80,* 1634–1635.

Anderson, J. J. (1989). Development and adaptation of the family with an infant. In Foster, R. L., Hunsberger, M. M., & Anderson, J. J. T. (Eds.). *Family-centered nursing care of children.* Philadelphia: W. B. Saunders.

Burkitt, D. P., & Meisner, P. (1979). How to manage constipation with high fiber diet. *Geriatrics, 34*(2), 33–40.

Byrne, W. J. (1990). The gastrointestinal tract. In Behrman, R. E. & Kliegman, R. (Eds.). *Nelson essentials of pediatrics.* Philadelphia: W. B. Saunders.

Chow, M. P., Durand, B. A., Feldman, M. N., & Mills, M. A. (1984). *Handbook of pediatric primary care* (2nd ed.). New York: John Wiley & Sons.

Ellickson, E. (1988). Bowel management plan for the homebound elderly. *Journal of Gerontological Nursing, 14*(1), 16–19.

Hickey, J. (1981). *The clinical practice of neurological and neurosurgical nursing.* Philadelphia: J. B. Lippincott.

Hunsberger, M., & Issenman, R. (1989). Nursing strategies: Altered digestive function. In Foster, R. L., Hunsberger, M. M., & Anderson, J. J. T. (Eds.). *Family-centered nursing care of children.* Philadelphia: W. B. Saunders.

Krause, M. V., & Mahan, L. K. (1979). *Food, nutrition, and diet therapy.* Philadelphia: W. B. Saunders.

Lara, L. L. (1990). The risk of urinary tract infection in bowel incontinent men. *Journal of Gerontological Nursing, 16*(5), 24–26, 40–41.

Maresca, T. (1986). Assessment and management of acute diarrheal illness in adults. *Nurse Practitioner, 11*(11), 15–16.

McShane, R., & McLane, A. (1988). Constipation: Impact of etiological factors. *Journal of Gerontological Nursing, 14*(4), 31–34.

Miller, C. A. (1990). *Nursing care of older adults.* Glenview, IL: Scott, Foresman.

Resnick, B. (1985). Constipation: Common but preventable. *Geriatric Nursing, 6*(4), 213–215.

Rodman, M. J., & Smith, D. W. (1979). *Pharmacology and drug therapy in nursing.* Philadelphia: J. B. Lippincott.

Ross, D. (1990). Constipation among hospitalized elder. *Orthopaedic Nursing, 9*(3), 73–77.

Schuster, M. M. (1983). Fiber deficiency in gastrointestinal disease. In Texter, E. C. (Ed.): *The aging gut.* New York: Masson Publishing.

Toth, L. (1988). *Alterations in bowel elimination in an neuroscience nursing: Phenomena and practice.* Norwalk, CT: Appleton & Lange.

Whaley, L. F., & Wong, D. L. (1989). *Essentials of pediatric nursing* (3rd ed.). St. Louis: C. V. Mosby.

Wright, B., & Staats, D. (1986). The geriatric implications of fecal impaction. *Nurse Practitioner, 11,* 53–66.

Yakabowich, M. (1990). Prescribe with care: The role of laxatives in the treatment of constipation. *Journal of Gerontological Nursing, 16*(7), 4–11, 42–43.

Effective Breast-Feeding

DEFINITION

Effective Breast-feeding: The state in which a mother–infant dyad exhibits adequate proficiency and satisfaction with the breast-feeding process.

DEFINING CHARACTERISTICS

Major (must be present)

Mother's ability to position infant at breast to promote a successful latch-on response
Infant content after feeding
Regular and sustained suckling/swallowing at the breast
Appropriate infant weight for age
Effective mother–infant communication patterns (infant cues, maternal interpretation and response)

Minor (may be present)

Signs and/or symptoms of oxytocin release (let-down or milk ejection reflex)
Adequate infant elimination patterns for age
Eagerness of infant to nurse
Maternal verbalization of satisfaction with the breast-feeding process

Diagnostic Considerations

This diagnosis reportedly represents a newly proposed NANDA wellness diagnosis, defined as "a clinical judgment about an individual, family, or community in transition from a specific level of wellness to a higher level of wellness" (NANDA Guidelines, Appendix VIII). The definition for this diagnosis does not describe a mother–infant dyad seeking higher-level breast-feeding, but rather "adequate proficiency and satisfaction with the breast-feeding process."

In the management of breast-feeding experience, the nurse will encounter three situations covered by the nursing diagnoses

Ineffective Breast-feeding
High Risk for Ineffective Breast-feeding
Potential for Enhanced Breast-feeding

Effective Breast-feeding would be used to describe an evaluation judgment of a mother's and infant's breast-feeding session for both ineffective and potentially ineffective breast-feeding. This evaluation is the result of the nurse observing or the mother reporting those signs and symptoms listed as defining characteristics. These signs and symptoms do not describe higher-level breast-feeding.

If the nurse cares for a mother reporting proficiency and satisfaction with the breast-feeding process and desiring additional teaching to achieve even greater proficiency and satisfaction, the nursing diagnosis of *Potential for Enhanced Breast-feeding* would be appropriate. The focus of this teaching and continued support would not be on preventing ineffective breast-feeding or rather maintaining adequate proficiency and satisfaction, but rather on promoting higher-quality breast-feeding.

This diagnosis is not useful in its present form; instead, the nurse should use *Ineffective Breast-feeding* or *High Risk for Ineffective Breast-feeding*. Nurses desiring to use a wellness nursing diagnosis could use *High Risk for for Enhanced Breast-feeding*. Because this diagnoses is not on the NANDA list, nurses using it should send their experiences to NANDA.

Ineffective Breast-Feeding

■ *Related to* **(Specify)**

DEFINITION

Ineffective breast-feeding: The state in which a mother, infant or child experiences dissatisfaction or difficulty with the breast-feeding process.

DEFINING CHARACTERISTICS

Major (must be present)

Unsatisfactory breast-feeding process

Minor (may be present)

Actual or perceived inadequate milk supply
Infant inability to attach on to maternal breast correctly
No observable signs of oxytocin release
Observable signs of inadequate infant intake
Nonsustained suckling at the breast
Insufficient emptying of each breast per feeding
Persistence of sore nipples beyond the first week of breast-feeding
Insufficient opportunity for suckling at the breast
Infant exhibiting fussiness and crying within the first hour after breast-feeding; unresponsive to other comfort measures
Infant arching and crying at the breast resisting latching on

RELATED FACTORS

Pathophysiologic

Breast anomaly
Infant anomaly/poor sucking reflex cleft lip/palate
Prematurity
Previous breast surgery

Situational

Maternal fatigue
Maternal anxiety
Maternal ambivalence
Inadequate nutrition intake
Inadequate fluid intake
History of unsuccessful breast-feeding
Nonsupportive partner/family
Lack of knowledge
Interruption in breast-feeding
    Ill mother
    Ill infant

Diagnostic Considerations

In managing the breast-feeding experience, the nurse strives to reduce or eliminate factors that contribute to *Ineffective Breast-feeding* or to reduce risk factors that can increase vulnerability for a problem using the diagnosis *High Risk for Ineffective Breast-feeding*.

In the acute setting after delivery, too little time will have elapsed for the nurse to conclude that there is no problem in breast-feeding, unless the mother is experienced. For many mother–infant dyads, the nursing diagnosis *High Risk for Ineffective Breast-feeding related to inexperience with the breast-feeding process* would represent a nursing focus on preventing problems in breast-feeding.

Errors in Diagnostic Statements

Ineffective Breast-feeding related to reports of no symptoms of let-down reflex

When a mother reports or the nurse observes no signs of let-down reflex, the nursing diagnosis *Ineffective Breast-feeding* is validated. If the contributing factors are unknown, the diagnosis could be written as: *Ineffective Breast-feeding related to unknown etiology, as evidenced by reports of no signs of let-down reflex and mother's anxiety regarding feeding.*

If the nurse has validated contributing factors, she or he can add them. The nurse should assess for various possible contributing factors, rather than prematurely focusing on a common etiology that may be incorrect for the specific situation.

Focus Assessment Criteria

Subjective Data

1. History of breast-feeding (self, sibling, friend)
2. Supportive persons (partner, friend, sibling, parent)
3. Source of information on breast-feeding
4. Daily intake:
   Calories
   Calcium
   Vitamin supplement
   Basic food groups
   Fluids
   Medications

Objective Data

Breast condition (soft, firm, engorgement)
   Engorgement
   Soft
Nipples
   Cracks
   Inverted
   Sore

Principles and Rationale for Nursing Care

1. Lactation is the result of a complex process of interacting factors of the health and nutrition status of the mother, the health status of the infant, and breast tissue development under the influence of estrogen and progesterone (Panwar, 1983).

2. Milk production and the let-down reflex is controlled by pituitary hormones, prolactin, and oxytocin and is stimulated by infant sucking and maternal emotions (Panwar, 1983).
3. The nutritional and fluid requirements for a lactating mother are outlined in Table II-2.
4. Many medications are excreted in breast milk. Some are harmful to the infant. Advise the mother to consult with a health care professional (nurse, physician, pharmacist) prior to taking a medication (prescribed or over-the-counter)
5. The advantage of breast-feeding are:
> To infant
>> Easier to digest
>> Meets nutritional needs
>> Reduces allergies
>> Provides antibodies and macrophages for early immunization
>> Fewer gastrointestinal infections, almost no constipation
> To mother
>> Hastens uterine involution and postpartum resolution
>> Reduces risks for breast cancer
>> Allows more time to rest during feedings
>> Less preparation, less cost
>> Faster bonding
6. The disadvantages of breast-feeding are:
> Someone cannot substitute
> Time-consuming
> Environmental pollutants (PCBs, etc.) in breast milk (Note: Pollutants are also present in cow's milk.)

Pediatric Considerations

1. An adolescent's eating habits are influenced by physical and psychosocial pressure. This may put the teenage mother and her infant at risk during the breast-feeding period (Williams, 1985).

■ Ineffective Breast-Feeding
Related to (Specify)

Assessment

See Defining Characteristics

Outcome Criteria

The mother will
- Make an informed decision related to method of feeding infant (breast or bottle)
- Identify activities that deter or promote successful breast-feeding

---

Interventions

A. Assess causative or contributing factors
1. Lack of knowledge
2. Lack of role model
3. Lack of physician's support
4. Discomfort
   a. Leaking
   b. Engorgement
   c. Loss of control of bodily fluid
   d. Nipple soreness
5. Embarrassment
6. Partner's influence
7. Patient's mother's attitudes and misconceptions
8. Social pressure against nursing
9. Change in body image
10. Change in sexuality
11. Feelings of being tied down
12. Presence of stress
13. Lack of conviction regarding decision to nurse
14. Sleepy, unresponsive infant
15. Fatigue

B. Promote open dialogue
1. Assess knowledge.
   a. Has woman taken a class in breast-feeding?
   b. Has she read anything on the subject?
   c. Does she have friends who are nursing their babies?
   d. Did her mother nurse?
2. Explain myths and misconceptions.
   a. Ask her to list difficulties she is anticipating.
   b. Common myths:
      • My breasts are too small
      • My breasts are too large
      • My mother couldn't nurse
      • How do I know my milk is good?
      • How do I know the baby is getting enough?
      • The baby will know that I'm nervous
      • I have to go back to work, so what's the point of nursing for a short time?
      • I'll never have any freedom
      • Nursing will cause my breasts to sag
      • My nipples are inverted, so I can't nurse
      • My husband wouldn't like my breasts any more
      • I'll have to stay fat if I nurse
      • I can't nurse if I have a cesarean section
3. Build on mother's knowledge.
   a. Clarify misconceptions.
   b. Explain process of nursing.
   c. Offer literature.
   d. Show video.

e. Discuss advantages and disadvantages.

f. Bring nursing mothers together to talk about nursing and their concerns.

4. Support her decision to breast-feed or bottle-feed.

C. Assist mother during first feedings

1. Promote relaxation.
   a. Position comfortably.
   b. Use pillows for positioning (especially cesarean-section mothers).
   c. Use foot stool or phone book to bring knees up while sitting.
   d. Use relaxation breathing techniques.
2. Demonstrate different positions.
   a. Sitting
   b. Lying
   c. Football hold: instruct to place supporting hand on baby's bottom and turn his body toward mother's (this promotes security in infant)
3. Demonstrate and explain rooting reflex and show how it can be used to help infant latch on.
   a. Show mother how to grasp breast with fingers under breast and thumbs on top; this way she can point nipple directly at baby's mouth (avoid scissor hold because it constricts milk flow).
   b. Make sure baby grasps a good portion of areola and not just the nipple.
4. Advise mother to increase feeding times gradually, to start at 10 minutes per side and build up over next 3–5 days.
   a. More important than time at the breast is the latch-on. Make sure the infant has a portion of the areola as well as the nipple in his mouth. Observe for bruising following feeding.
5. Instruct mother to offer both breasts at each feeding, alternating the beginning side each time.
6. Demonstrate:
   a. How to use a finger to keep breast tissue from obstructing infant's nose
   b. Use of finger in infant's mouth to break seal before removing from breast
   c. Ways to awaken baby (may be necessary before offering the second breast)
7. Inform mother that burping may not be necessary with breast-fed babies, but if baby grunts and seems full between breasts she should attempt to burp baby, then continue feeding.

D. Provide follow-up support during hospital stay

1. Develop care plan so that other health team members are aware of any problems or needs. Try to establish a consistant plan so the nursing mother does not receive mixed and opposing opinions from her health care providers.
2. Allow for flexibility of feeding schedule; avoid scheduling feedings. Strive for 10–12 feedings/24-hour period according to the infant's size and need. (Frequent feedings help prevent or reduce breast engorgement.)
3. Promote rooming in.
4. Allow for privacy during feedings.
5. Be available for questions.
6. Be positive even if experience is difficult.
7. Reassure mother that this is a learning time for her and the infant and they will develop together as the days go by.

E. Assist mother with specific nursing problems (may need assistance of lactation consultant)

1. Engorgement
   a. Wear well-fitting support brassiere day and night.
   b. Apply warm compresses for 15–20 minutes before nursing.
   c. Nurse frequently.
   d. Use hand expression, hand pump, or electric pump to tap off some of the tension before putting infant to breast.
2. Sore nipple
   a. Decrease nursing time to 5–10 minutes per side. Start baby on nontender side first. Allow for more frequent, short feedings. Suggest alternate positions to rotate infant's grasps. Allow breasts to dry after each feeding.
   b. Keep nursing pads dry.
   c. Coat nipples with breast milk (which has healing properties) and allow to air-dry.
   d. Use breast shield as last measure and remove after milk has let down.
3. Difficulty with baby grasping nipple
   a. Cup breast with fingers underneath.
   b. Position baby for mother's and infant's comfort (turn baby's abdomen toward mother's body).
   c. Stroke infant's cheek for rooting reflex.
   d. Hand-express some milk into infant's mouth.
   e. Roll nipples to bring them out before feeding.
   f. Use a nipple shell between feedings to help extend inverted nipples. Remove shield after letdown occurs.
   g. Assess infant's suck—may need assistance in development of suck. Use lactation consultant if indicated
4. Separation (following cesarean section for stressed infants, premature infants, jaundiced infants)
   a. Encourage visits and bonding as much as possible.
   b. Provide comfortable, private location for nursing during visit.
   c. Provide supportive atmosphere (freedom to ask questions, etc.).
   d. Provide breast pump or make patient aware of availability.
      • Rental of electric pump
      • Battery-operated pump
      • Cylinder-type hand pump (do not use bicycle horn pump)
      • Provide instruction in use of pump and assist mother to integrate breast-feeding into life-style
   e. Many hospitals have a lactation educator or consultant on hand to assist with instruction and support.

F. Explore feelings regarding changes in body

1. Encourage verbal expression of feelings.
   a. Many women dislike leaking and lack of control. Explain that this is temporary.
      • Demonstrate use of nursing pad.
      • With a disposable pad, should not use waterproof backing, to prevent irritation; cotton (washable) seems to reduce occurrence of irritation.
   b. Changes breasts from "sexual objects" to implements of nutrition. This can affect sexual relationship. Husband gets milk if he sucks on nipples. Milk is released with orgasm. Infant suckling is "sensual" feeling—this causes guilt

or confusion in woman. Encourage discussion with other mothers. Include partner in at least one discussion to assess his feelings and how they most affect the nursing experience.

   c. Self-consciousness during feedings. Explore woman's feelings about nursing.
- Where?
- Around whom?
- What is husband's reaction to when and where she nurses?
- Demonstrate use of shawl for modesty, allowing nursing in public.
- Remind her that what she is doing is normal and natural and the best for her child.

G. Assist the family with

1. Sibling reaction
   a. Explore feelings and anticipation of problems. Older child may be jealous of contact with baby. Mother can use this time to read to older child. Older child may want to nurse.
   b. Allow him to try—usually does not like it.
   c. Stress older child's attributes—freedom, movement, and choices.
2. Fatigue and stress
   a. Explore situation.
   b. Encourage mother to make herself and infant a priority.
   c. Encourage to limit visits from relatives for first 4 weeks.
   d. Needs support and assistance during first 4 weeks.
   e. Encourage support person to help as much as possible.
   f. Explain to mother not to try to be "superwoman" but to ask directly for help from friends or relations, or hire someone.
3. Feelings of being enslaved
   a. Allow to express feelings.
   b. Seek assistance.
   c. Pump milk to allow others to feed baby.
   - Can store harvested breast milk for 4 hours at room temperature, 48 hours in a refrigerator, and 4 months in the back of a separate freezer compartment.
     (Note: Never microwave frozen breast milk, which will destroy its immune properties.)
   d. Husband can change baby and bring to bed to nurse.
   e. Remember that time between feedings will get longer (every 2 hours for 4 weeks; then, every 3–4 hours by 3 months).

H. Initiate referrals as indicated

1. Refer to lactation consultant if indicated by:
   a. Lack of confidence
   b. Ambivalence
   c. Problems with infant suck and latch-on
   d. Infant weight drop or lack of urination
   e. Prolonged soreness
   f. Hot tender spots on breast
      Note: Consultant can make follow-up home visits as necessary.
2. Refer to La Leche League.
3. Refer to childbirth educator and childbirth class members.
4. Refer to other breast-feeding mothers.

References/Bibilography

Cahill, M. (1976). *Breast-feeding and working?* (Booklet No. 58). Franklin Park, IL: La Leche League.

Helsing, E., & King, F. S. (1982). *Breastfeeding in practice: A manual for health.* New York: Oxford University Press.

La Leche League International (1978). *The womanly art of breast-feeding.* Franklin Park, IL: Author.

Lawrence, R. (1980) *Breastfeeding: A guide for the health professional.* St. Louis: C. V. Mosby.

Morris, S. E. (1982). *The natural acquisition of oral feeding skills: Implications for assessment and treatment.* Tucson: Therapeutic Skills Builders.

Mason, D., & Ingersol, D. (1986). *Breastfeeding and the working mother.* New York: St. Martin's Press.

Panwar, S. (1983). The postpartum period. In Buckley, K. & Kulb, N. (Eds.). *Handbook of maternal-newborn nursing.* New York: John Wiley & Sons.

Riordan, J. (1983). *Practical guide to breastfeeding.* St. Louis: C. V. Mosby.

Shirago, L. & Bocar, D. (1990). The infant's contribution to breastfeeding. *Journal of Obstetric, Gynecological and Neonatal Nursing, 19*(3), 209–215.

Williams, S. R. (1985). *Nutrition and diet therapy.* St. Louis: C. V. Mosby.

For Parents

Dana, N., & Price, A. (1985). *The working woman's guide to breastfeeding.* New York: Simon & Schuster.

Michaelson, K. R. (1986). *Breastfeeding basics for busy moms and dads: A training manual for lactation educators.* Santa Barbara, CA: Therapeutic Media, Inc.

Videos

The ABC's of breastfeeding, Roman Productions.
Breastfeeding techniques that work, Kitty Franz, Producer.
1. First Attachment (getting the baby to the breast)
2. First Attachment After Cesarean Section
Breastfeeding your baby, A Mother's Guide—Medela.

Decreased Cardiac Output

DEFINITION

Decreased Cardiac Output: A state in which the individual experiences a reduction in the amount of blood pumped by the heart, resulting in compromised cardiac function.

DEFINING CHARACTERISTICS

Low blood pressure	Dysrhythmia
Rapid pulse	Oliguria
Restlessness	Fatigability
Cyanosis	Vertigo
Dyspnea	Edema (peripheral, sacral)
Angina	

Diagnostic Considerations

This nursing diagnosis represents a situation in which nurses have multiple responsibilities. Persons experiencing decreased cardiac output may display various responses that disrupt functioning, (such as activity intolerance, sleep–rest disturbances, and anxiety or fear) and/or may be at risk for developing physiologic complications such as dysrhythmias, cardiogenic shock, and congestive heart failure.

When *Decreased Cardiac Output* is used clinically, the associated outcome criteria are usually written:

Systolic blood pressure is > 100
Urine output is > 30 mL/hr
Cardiac output is > 5
Cardiac rate, rhythm are within normal limits

These outcome criteria do not represent parameters for evaluating nursing care, but rather for evaluating the person's status. Because, they are monitoring criteria that the nurse uses to guide implementation of nursing-prescribed and physician-prescribed interventions, *Decreased Cardiac Output* is not appropriate as a nursing diagnosis. Not using this nursing diagnosis allows the nurse to more specifically describe the related situations that nurses treat as nursing diagnoses or cotreat as collaborative problems. (Refer to *Activity Intolerance related to insufficient knowledge of adaptive techniques needed secondary to impaired cardiac function* and to *Potential Complication: Cardiac/Vascular* [Section III] for more information.)

Errors in Diagnostic Statements

Decreased Cardiac Output related to dysrhythmias

This diagnosis necessitates continuous monitoring, early detection of changes in physiologic status, rapid initiation of medical and nursing interventions, and evaluation of response. Because the nurse manages this situation with nurse-prescribed and physician-prescribed interventions, it is a collaborative problem: *Potential Complication: Decreased cardiac output related to dysrhythmias.*

Decreased Cardiac Output related to vasodilation and bradycardia secondary to spinal shock

As with the previous example, this situation represents a situation for which nurses cannot write outcomes that can be used to measure the effectiveness of nursing interventions. For this reason, this situation should be written as a collaborative problem: *Potential Complication: Spinal Shock.*

A nurse reading this collaborative problem on a care plan knows that this client either is experiencing spinal shock or is at high risk for it. Shift reports and/or initial assessment will determine present status.

Comfort, Altered:

Pain

Chronic Pain

Comfort, Altered:

- *Related to* **(Specify) as Evidenced by Pruritus**
- *Related to* **(Specify) as Evidenced by Nausea and Vomiting**
- *Related to* **Malaise and Body Temperature Fluctuations**

DEFINITION

Altered comfort: The state in which an individual experiences an uncomfortable sensation in response to a noxious stimulus.

DEFINING CHARACTERISTICS

Major (must be present)

The person reports or demonstrates a discomfort

Minor (may be present)

Autonomic response in acute pain
   Blood pressure increased
   Pulse increased
   Respiration increased
   Diaphoresis
   Dilated pupils
Guarded position
Facial mask of pain
Crying, moaning
Abdominal heaviness
Cutaneous irritation

RELATED FACTORS

Any factor can contribute to altered comfort. The most common are listed below.

Pathophysiologic

Musculoskeletal disorders
   Fractures
   Contractures
   Spasms

   Arthritis
   Spinal cord disorders

Visceral disorders
  Cardiac
  Renal
  Hepatic
  Intestinal
  Pulmonary
Cancer
Vascular disorders
  Vasospasm
  Occlusion
  Phlebitis
  Vasodilation (headache)
Inflammation
  Nerve
  Tendon
  Bursa
  Joint
  Muscle
Contagious diseases (rubella, chicken pox)

Treatment-related

Trauma (surgery, accidents)
Diagnostic tests
  Venipuncture
  Invasive scanning (*e.g.*, IVP)
  Biopsy
Medications
Radiation therapy
Chemotherapy

Situational (personal, environmental)

Immobility/improper positioning
Overactivity
Pressure points (tight cast, Ace
  bandages
Pregnancy (prenatal, intrapartum,
  postpartum)
Allergic response
Chemical irritants
Stress

Maturational

Infancy (colic)
Infancy and early childhood (teething, ear pain)
Middle childhood (recurrent abdominal pain, growing pains)
Adolescence (headaches, chest pain, dysmenorrhea)

Diagnostic Considerations

A diagnosis not on the current NANDA list, *Altered Comfort* can represent various uncomfortable sensations, such as pruritus, immobility, and NPO status. For a person experiencing nausea and vomiting, the nurse should assess whether *Altered Comfort, High Risk for Altered Comfort,* or *High Risk for Altered Nutrition: Less than Body Requirements* is the appropriate diagnosis. Short-lived episodes of nausea and/or vomiting (*e.g.*, postoperatively) can be best described with *Altered Comfort related to effects of anesthesia or analgesics.* When nausea/vomiting may compromise nutritional intake, the appropriate diagnosis may be *High Risk for Altered Nutrition: Less than Body Requirements related to nausea and vomiting secondary to (specify).*

Altered Comfort also can be used to describe a cluster of discomforts related to a condition or treatment, such as radiation therapy.

Errors in Diagnostic Statements

Altered Comfort related to immobility

Although immobility can contribute to an altered state of comfort, the nursing diagnosis *Disuse Syndrome* describes a cluster of nursing diagnoses that apply or are at high risk to apply due to immobility. *Altered Comfort* can be included in *Disuse Syndrome;* thus, the diagnosis should be written as *High Risk for Disuse Syndrome.*

Altered Comfort related to nausea and vomiting secondary to chemotherapy

Nausea and vomiting represent signs and symptoms of an altered comfort state, not contributing factors. *Altered Comfort* can be used to describe a cluster of discomforts associated with chemotherapy, *e.g., Altered Comfort related to the effects of chemotherapy on bone marrow production and irritation of emetic center, as evidenced by complaints of nausea, vomiting, anorexia, and fatigue.*

Focus Assessment Criteria

This nursing assessment of pain is designed to acquire data for assessing a person's adaptation to pain, not for determining the cause of pain or whether it exists.

Subjective Data

A. Pain Assessment
1. "Where is your discomfort located; does it radiate?" (Ask child to point to place).
2. "When did it begin?"
3. "Can you relate the cause of this discomfort?" or "What do you think is the cause of your discomfort?"
4. Ask person to describe the discomfort and its pattern.
   a. Time of day
   b. Duration
   c. Frequency (constant, intermittent, transient)
   d. Quality/intensity
5. Ask person to rate his pain: at its best, after pain relief measures, and at its worst. Use consistent scale, language, or set of behaviors to assess pain.
   - For adults, use a numeric scale of 0 to 10 (0 = no pain, 10 = worst pain ever experienced) orally or visually.
   - For children, select a scale appropriate for *developmental* age: can use scale for assessed age or younger; include child in selection. Wong and Baker (1988) found that the favorite scale from age 3 to adolescent was the faces scale.
      3 years and older: use drawings of faces or photographs of faces (Oucher scale) ranging from smiling to frowning to crying with numeric scale (Beyer, 1983).
      4 years and older: use four white poker chips to ask child how many pieces of hurt he is feeling (no hurt = no chips) (Hester, 1979)
      6 years and older: use a numeric scale, 0 to 5 or 0 to 10 (verbally or visually); use blank drawing of body, front and back, and ask child to use three colors of crayons to color where a little bit of pain, a medium amount of pain, and a lot of pain is present (Eland Color Tool).
6. "How do you usually react to pain (crying, anger, silence)?"
7. "Are there any other symptoms associated with your discomfort (nausea, vomiting, numbness)?"
8. "What helps you when you have discomfort (medications [what, route, dosage, how often], heat, cold, activity, rest)?"

9. "Do you talk to others about your discomfort (spouse, friends, doctor, nurse)?"
"Who do you talk to?"
10. Have person indicate the effect of each of the following factors on his discomfort by noting if there is an increase, a decrease, or no effect.*

Liquor	Vibration	Defecation
Stimulants (*e.g.,*	Pressure	Tension
caffeine)	No movement	Bright lights
Eating	Movement/activity	Loud noises
Heat	Sleep, rest	Going to work
Cold	Lying down	Intercourse
Damp	Distraction (*e.g.,* TV)	Mild exercise

Separation from family/friends

Weather changes	Urination	Fatigue
Massage		

11. Ask person what effect pain has had on the following areas or what effect is anticipated.
    a. Work/activity pattern (work/home activities, leisure/play)
    b. Relationships/relating (wanting to be alone, with people)
    c. Sleep pattern (difficulty falling asleep/staying asleep)
    d. Eating pattern (appetite, weight gain/loss)
    e. Elimination patterns (bowel, constipation/diarrhea, bladder)
    f. Menses
    g. Sexual pattern (libido, function)

B. Assessment of pruritus

Onset
Precipitated by what
Site(s)
Relieved by what
History of allergy (individual, family)

C. Assessment of nausea/vomiting

Onset, duration
Frequency
Vomitus (amount, appearance)
Associated with?

Medications	Activity
Meals (specific foods)	Time of day
Position	Pain

Relief measures?

Objective Data (acute/chronic pain)

1. Behavioral manifestations

Mood	*Eye Movements*
Calmness	Fixed
Moaning	Searching
Crying	Open
Grimacing	Closed

*Adapted from the McGill Pain Questionnaire.

Mood

Pacing
Restlessness
Withdrawn
2. Musculoskeletal manifestations

Mobility of Painful Part

Full
Limited/guarded
No movement
3. Dermatologic manifestations
    Color (redness)
    Temperature
4. Cardiorespiratory manifestations

Cardiac

Rate
Blood pressure
Palpations present
5. Neurologic manifestations
Sensory alterations
    Paresthesia
    Dysesthesias
6. Cognitive manifestations
Thought processes
    Appropriate
    Inappropriate
    Cooperative
7. Developmental manifestations

Eye Movements

Perceptions
Oriented to time and place

Muscle Tone

Spasm
Tenderness
Tremors (in effort to hide pain)

Moisture/diaphoresis
Edema

Respiratory

Rate
Rhythm
Depth

Combative
Confused

    Infant: Irritability, changes in eating or sleeping, inconsolability, generalized body movements
    Toddler: Irritability, changes in eating or sleeping, aggressive behavior (kicking, biting), rocking, sucking, clenched teeth
    Preschool: Irritability, changes in eating or sleeping, aggressive behavior, verbal expressions of pain
    School Age: Changes in eating or sleeping, change in play patterns, verbal expressions of pain, denial of pain
    Adolescent: Mood changes, behavior extremes ("acting out"), verbal expressions of pain when asked, changes in eating or sleeping

Principles and Rationale for Nursing Care

Pain

1. Pain is inevitable; life cannot be pain free. One must learn to live with pain, to control it rather than be controlled by it (Carpenito, 1987).
2. Each individual experiences and expresses pain in his own manner, utilizing various sociocultural adaptation techniques.
3. All pain is real, regardless of its causes. Pure psychogenic pain is probably rare, as is pure organic pain. Most bodily pain is a combination of mental events (psychogenic) and physical stimuli (organic).

4. Pain has two components—a sensory component, which is neurophysiologic, and a perceptual or experiential dimension with cognitive and emotional origins. The interaction of these two components determines the amount of suffering (Schechter, 1989a).
5. Pain tolerance is the duration and intensity of pain that an individual is willing to endure. Pain tolerance differs in individuals and may vary in one individual in different situations.
6. Personal factors that influence pain tolerance are
   Knowledge of pain and its cause
   Meaning of pain
   Ability to control pain
   Energy level (fatigue)
   Stress level
7. Social and environmental factors that influence pain are
   Interactions with others
   Response of others (family, friends)
   Secondary gains
   Sensory overload or deprivation
   Stressors
8. If a person must try to convince health care providers that he has pain, he will experience increased anxiety that increases the pain. Both of these are energy depleting.
9. Persons who are prepared for painful procedures by explanations of the actual sensations that will be felt experience less stress than individuals who receive vague explanations of the procedure.
10. Studies have shown that the human brain secretes endorphins, which have opiate-like properties that relieve pain. The release of endorphins may be responsible for the positive effects of placebos and noninvasive pain relief measures.
11. Studies have shown that diagnosed physiological pain does respond to placebos, so a positive response to placebos cannot be used to diagnose pain as psychogenic.
12. The use of noninvasive pain relief measures (*e.g.,* relaxation, massage, distraction) can enhance the therapeutic effects of pain-relief medications.
13. Adults and children who are experiencing pain feel their bodies and their lives are out of control. Attempts must be made to provide some choice or control during their day (Schechter, 1987).
14. Inadequate sleep decreases one's ability to tolerate pain and depletes the energy needed to participate in social activities (Eland, 1988).

Medications, Tolerance, Addiction

1. The preventive approach to pain is to establish a regular schedule for medication administration to treat the pain before it becomes severe rather than follow the PRN approach.
2. The preventive approach may reduce the total 24-hour dose compared with PRN approach; it provides a constant blood level of the drug, it reduces craving for the drug, and it reduces the anxiety of having to ask and wait for PRN relief.
3. The oral route of administration is preferred when possible. Liquid medications can be given to individuals who have difficulty swallowing.
4. If frequent injections are necessary, the IV route is preferred because it is not painful and absorption is guaranteed, but the side-effects ($\downarrow$ respirations, $\downarrow$ BP) may be more profound.

5. Addiction is a psychologic syndrome characterized by compulsive drug-seeking behavior generally associated with a desire for drug administration to produce euphoria or other effects, not pain relief. Addiction is believed to be rare, and there is no evidence that adequate administration of opioids for pain produces addiction.
6. Nurses' fear of precipitating respiratory depression often makes them reluctant to use intravenous medications. Yet a study reported that only 3 of 3263 patients developed respiratory depression from narcotics during an acute hospitalization (Miller, 1990).
7. Nurses' fear of precipitating addiction often makes them reluctant to administer narcotics. Porter and Jick (1980) identified that 4 addicts of 11,000 reported they received Demerol in the hospital.
8. Drug tolerance is a physiologic phenomenon in which, after repeated doses, the prescribed dose begins to lose its effectiveness.
9. Drug dependence is a physiologic state that results from repeated administration of a drug. Withdrawal is experienced if the drug is abruptly discontinued. Tapering down the drug dosage will manage the withdrawal symptoms.

Acute Pain Compared with Chronic Pain

1. Pain can be classified as acute or chronic, according to cause and duration, not intensity.
2. Acute pain is an episode of pain that has a duration of 1 second to less than 6 months. The cause is usually organic disease or injury. With healing, the pain subsides and eventually disappears.
3. Chronic pain is a pain experience that lasts for 6 months or longer. Chronic pain can be described as limited, intermittent, or persistent. *Limited pain* is pain caused by known physical pathology, and an end of the pain will come (*e.g.,* burns). *Intermittent pain* is pain that provides the person with pain-free periods. The cause may or may not be known (*e.g.,* headaches). *Persistent pain* is pain that usually occurs daily. The cause may or may not be known and is usually not a threat to life (*e.g.,* low back pain).
4. The visible signs of pain (physical and behavioral) are determined by the individual's pain tolerance and the duration of the pain, not the pain intensity.
5. The person may respond to acute pain physiologically and behaviorally: physiologically by diaphoresis, an increased heart rate, an increased respiratory rate, and increased blood pressure; behaviorally by crying, moaning, or showing anger.
6. The person with chronic pain usually has adapted to pain, both physiologically and behaviorally, so that visible signs of pain may not be present.
7. The inability to manage pain produces feelings of frustration and inadequacy in the health care providers.
8. The person with chronic pain may respond with withdrawal, depression, anger, frustration, and dependency, all of which can affect the family in the same way.

Pruritus

1. Pruritus (itching) is the most common skin alteration. It can be a response of the skin to an allergen or it can be a sign or symptom of a systemic disease such as cancer, liver or renal dysfunction, or diabetes mellitus.
2. Pruritus, described as a tickling or a tormenting situation, originates exclusively in the skin and provokes the urge to scratch (Branov, Epstein, & Grayson, 1989).
3. Although the same neurons are likely to transmit signals for itching as for pressure, pain, and touch, each of these sensations is perceived and mediated differently (Branov, Epstein, & Grayson, 1989).

4. Pruritus arises as a result of subepidermal nerve stimulation by proteolytic enzymes. These enzymes are released from the epidermis as a result of either primary irritation or secondary allergic responses (Callen, Starviski, & Voorhees, 1980).
5. The same unmyelinated nerves that act for burning pain also serve for pruritus (Callen, Starviski, & Voorhees, 1980).
6. Clinically, burning and pain are allied sensations. As a pruritic sensation increases in intensity, the sensation may become burning (Baer, 1990).
7. The areas immediately surrounding body openings are most susceptible to itching. This apparently is related to a concentration of sensory nerve endings and vulnerability to external contamination (Branov, Epstein, & Grayson, 1989).
8. Pruritus is aggravated by excessive warmth, excessive dryness, rough fabrics, fatigue or stress, and monotony (lack of distractions) (DeWitt, 1990).
9. Methods that interrupt pain also will interrupt pruritus. Local anesthetics, cold, or peripheral nerve resection eliminate both pain and pruritus (Baer, 1990).
10. The psychological influence of stress and anxiety in the itch-scratch-itch cycle is combined with the physical factors. The individual feels an irresistible urge toward self-mutilation, yet itching may only cease when the pain elicited by scratching becomes overpowering (Branov, Epstein, & Grayson, 1989).
11. Damage to the subepidermal network abolishes itch selectively because deep receptors do not exist for itch as they do for pain. If dermatitic skin is severely damaged, there may be damage to the itch receptor. As the skin heals, pruritus may return (Callen, Starviski, & Voorhees, 1980).

Nausea/Vomiting

1. Nausea and vomiting, when determined to have emotional origins, may be the result of developmental adjustment and adaption. A child learns that vomiting is unacceptable and thus learns to control vomiting. The child receives approval for not vomiting. Should childhood situations or conflicts resurface, the adult may experience nausea and vomiting. This adult may use nausea and vomiting to control or get attention.
2. Vomiting serves as a first-line defense against injurious agents ingested. Nausea may precede vomiting.
3. Nausea and vomiting may be a signal of disease, injury, or the normal physiologic adjustment to pregnancy.
4. From 50%–80% of all pregnant women experience "morning sickness" (Ieioro, 1988).
5. Fatigue has been reported to precipitate nausea/vomiting in pregnant women (Voda & Randall, 1982).
6. Voda and Randall (1982) reported that eating a high-protein snack before going to bed at night decreases morning nausea in some pregnant women.
7. Cotanch and Strum (1987) reported that progressive muscle relaxation was most effective in decreasing vomiting in individuals receiving chemotherapy.
8. Nausea and vomiting can be a response to pain in children.
9. In the infant, assess and differentiate between regurgitation, vomiting, gastroesophageal reflux, and pyloric stenosis (*e.g.*, relationship to feedings, position, force of vomiting) when vomiting present.
10. Self-stimulation to produce vomiting can be an effect of environmental and emotional deprivation in a child (particularly toddler and preschool ages).
11. Adolescent girls are at highest risk for anorexia, bulimia, and other eating disorders.

Pediatric Considerations

1. Several studies reported that when adults and children undergo the same surgery, the children are undermedicated (Eland, 1977; Beyer, 1983). In one study, 52% of the children received no analgesic postoperatively, while the remaining 48% received aspirin or acetaminophen predominantly.
2. The response to pain in children is influenced by maturational age, cultural-ethnic background, previous experience with pain, and response from others to the pain.
3. The child's maturational and chronologic age will influence this response to pain.

   Infant: Association of environment with painful experience

   Loud crying and verbal protest long after the stimulus is withdrawn

   Toddler: Fear of body intrusion

   No understanding of rationale for pain or ability to conceptualize the duration of experience even if told

   Seeking out parental figures as a source of comfort

   Preschool: Magical thinking or fantasies (*e.g.,* something they thought or did caused the pain experience)

   Increased verbal skills to communicate pain

   Limited understanding of time

   After pain passes, talking to toys or other children about the pain experience

   Denial of pain, especially if associated with adverse consequences (*e.g.,* injection, ridicule if not brave)

   School-age: Fear of body injury

   Ability to describe the cause, type, quality, and severity of pain

   Ability to rate the severity of pain

   Attempts to relate the pain experience to previous events and gain control over actions

   Denial of pain, especially if associated with adverse consequences (see above)

   Possible influence of presence of parents on child's expression of pain

   Adolescent: Importance of body image

   Overconfidence compensating for fear

   Behavioral responses to pain more "socially acceptable" than younger child's, but fear and anxiety *not* less

   Possible influence of presence of parent on child's expression of pain
4. Consistent pain assessment criteria (*e.g.,* assessment scale, specific behaviors) should be identified and used by nurses, physicians, and parents to assess pain in a child.
5. Verbal communication is usually not sufficient or reliable for explaining pain or painful procedures to children under age 7. The nurse can explain by demonstrating with pictures or dolls. The more senses that are stimulated in the explanations to children, the greater the communication. When possible, include parents in preparation.
6. Because a child may respond more openly to pain when parents are present, the parents' presence should be encouraged to facilitate pain assessment, provide support, and promote trust.
7. The weight of the child, not the age, should be considered when calculating analgesic relief.
8. Children often will deny pain to avoid injections (Eland & Anderson, 1977). Although oral administration of analgesia is the route of choice for children, followed by intravenous administration (Berde, 1989), O'Brien and Konsler (1988) found that 40% of medications for postoperative pain were administered intramuscularly.

Gerontologic Considerations

1. Pain is omnipresent in the elderly and may be accepted by elders and professionals as a normal and unavoidable accompaniment to aging. Unfortunately, many chronic diseases that are common in the elderly, such as osteoarthritis and rheumatoid arthritis, may not be adequately managed regarding pain.
2. Elderly persons may not demonstrate objective signs and symptoms of pain because of years of adaptation and increased pain tolerance. The individual may eventually accept the pain, thereby lowering expectations for comfort and mobility. Pain coping mechanisms cultivated throughout life are important to identify and reinforce in pain management. Effective pain management can greatly improve the overall physical functioning and emotional well-being of the individual.
3. The effects of narcotic analgesics are prolonged in the elderly, because of decreased metabolism and clearance of the drug. Also, side effects seem to be more frequent and pronounced in the elderly, especially anticholinergic effects, extrapyramidal effects, and sedation. It is advised that drugs be started at a lower dosage, and because elderly persons often take multiple drugs, drug interactions should be monitored.

■ Comfort, Altered
Related to (Specify) as Evidenced by Pruritus

Assessment

Subjective Data

The person reports itching/burning sensations and an urge to claw, scratch, or dig at body parts.
The person reports fatigue.

Objective Data

Scratch marks/redness (erythema)
Dermographic streaks
Restlessness, irritability
Rubbing or scratching of body parts
Rash or lesions/thickened skin

Outcome Criteria

The person will
• Verbalize decreased pruritus
• Describe causative factors when known
• Describe rationale and procedure for treatment

Interventions

A. Assess causative and contributing factors
  1. Skin care habits (home remedies)
  2. Exposure to poisonous plants (poison ivy, sumac, oak)
  3. Exposure to a contagious disease (rubella, fungus)
  4. Exposure to chemical irritant (paints, oils, cleaning agents, cosmetics)
  5. Systemic disease (liver disease, diabetes, thyroid dysfunction, collagen disease, renal disease, leukemia, Hodgkin's disease)
  6. Parasites (pinworms, chiggers, ringworm)
  7. Hypersensitivity to drug, food, insect bite
  8. Psychogenic stress (acute or chronic)

B. Reduce or eliminate causative and contributing factors if possible
  1. Maintain hygiene without producing dry skin.
     a. Baths should be given frequently.
     b. Use cool water when acceptable (Baer, 1990).
     c. Use mild soap (castile, lanolin) or a soap substitute.
     d. Blot skin dry; do not rub.
     e. Apply cornstarch lightly to skin folds by first sprinkling on hand (to avoid caking of powder); for fungal conditions, use antifungal or antiyeast powder preparations (mycostatin, nystatin) or Lotrimin cream.
  2. Prevent excessive dryness.
     a. Lubricate skin with Alpha Keri lotion unless contraindicated; pat on by hand or with gauze.
     b. Apply lubrication after bath before skin is dry to help moisture retention.
     c. Apply wet dressings continuously or intermittently to relieve itching and remove crusts and exudate.
     d. Provide 20- to 30-minute tub soaks with temperature of 32° to 38° C; water can contain oatmeal powder, Aveeno, cornstarch, or baking soda (Branov, Epstein, & Voorhees, 1989).
  3. Promote comfort and prevent further injury.
     a. Advise against scratching; explain the scratch-itch-scratch cycle.
     b. Secure order for topical corticosteroid cream for local inflamed pruritic areas; apply sparingly and occlude area with plastic wrap at night to increase effectiveness of cream and prevent further scratching (Baer, 1990).
     c. Secure an antihistamine order if itching is unrelieved.
     d. Utilize mitts (or cotton socks) if necessary on children and confused adults.
     e. Maintained trimmed nails to prevent injury; file after trimming.
     f. Remove particles from bed (food crumbs, caked power).
     g. Use old, soft sheets and avoid wrinkles in bed; if bed protector pads are used, place draw sheet over them to eliminate direct contact with skin.
     h. Avoid using perfumes and scented lotions (Branov, Epstein, & Voorhees, 1989).
     i. Avoid contact with chemical irritants/solutions (Tucker & Key, 1983).
     j. Wash clothes in a mild detergent and put through a second rinse cycle to reduce residue; avoid use of fabric softeners (Branov, Epstein, & Voorhees, 1989).
     k. Prevent excessive warmth by use of cool room temperatures and low humidity, light covers with bed cradle; avoid overdressing.

   l. Apply ointments with gloved or bare hand, depending on type, to lightly cover skin; rub creams into skin.
   m. Utilize frequent, thin applications of ointment rather than one thick application.
4. In children
   a. Explain to child why he should not scratch.
   b. Dress child in long sleeves, long pants, or a one-piece outfit to prevent scratching.
   c. Avoid overdressing child, which will increase warmth.
   d. Give child a tepid bath before bedtime; add two cups of cornstarch to bath water.
   e. Apply caladryl lotion to weeping pruritic lesions; apply with small paint brush.
   f. Use cotton blankets or sheets next to skin.
   g. Remove furry toys that may increase lint and pruritus.
   h. Teach child to press area that itches but not to scratch, or to put cool cloth on the area if permitted.

C. Proceed with health teaching when indicated

1. Explain causes of pruritus and possible methods to avoid causative factors.
2. Explain interventions that relieve symptoms.
3. Explain factors that increase symptoms.
4. Teach person to avoid fabrics that irritate skin (wool, coarse textures).
5. Teach person to wear protective clothing (rubber gloves, apron) when using chemical irritants.
6. Refer for allergy testing if indicated.
7. Provide opportunity to discuss frustrations.
8. For further interventions, refer to *Ineffective Individual Coping* if pruritus is stress-related.

■ Comfort, Altered
Related to (Specify) as Evidenced by Nausea and Vomiting

Assessment
See Defining Characteristics

Assessment

Subjective Data
Person complains of feeling nauseated ("sick to my stomach"), vomiting

Objective Data
Vomiting

Outcome Criteria

The individual will
- Report decreased symptoms
- Describe relief measures during episodes

Interventions

A. Assess nausea and vomiting episodes
   1. Duration
   2. Frequency
   3. Vomitus (amount/appearance)
   4. Associated with
      a. Medications
      b. Meals
      c. Position
      d. Activity
      e. Time of day
      f. Pain (headache, earache, constipation)
      g. Specific foods
   5. Relief measures (medications, food)

B. Institute measures to protect and comfort individual
   1. Protect persons at risk for aspiration (immobile patients, children).
   2. Address the cleanliness of the person and environment.
   3. Provide opportunity for oral care after each episode.
   4. Apply cool damp cloth to person's forehead, neck, and wrists.

C. Reduce or eliminate noxious stimuli
   1. Pain
      a. Plan care so that unpleasant or painful procedures do not take place before meals.
      b. Medicate individual for pain one-half hour before meals according to physician's orders.
      c. Provide pleasant, relaxed atmosphere for eating (no bedpans in sight; do not rush); try a "surprise" (e.g., flowers with meal).
      d. Arrange plan of care to decrease or eliminate nauseating odors or procedures near mealtimes.
   2. Fatigue
      a. Teach or assist individual to rest before meals.
      b. Teach individual to spend minimal energy in food preparation (cook large quantities and freeze several meals at a time; request assistance from others).
   3. Odor of food
      a. Teach him to avoid cooking odors—frying foods, brewing coffee—if possible (take a walk; select foods that can be eaten cold).
      b. Suggest using foods that require little cooking during periods of nausea.

D. Decrease the stimulation of the vomiting center
1. Reduce unpleasant sights and odors.
2. Provide good mouth care after vomiting.
3. Teach person to practice deep breathing and voluntary swallowing to suppress the vomiting reflex.
4. Instruct him to sit down after eating but not to lie down.
5. Encourage him to eat smaller meals and eat slowly.
6. Restrict liquids with meals to avoid overdistending the stomach; also avoid fluids 1 hour before and after meals.
7. If possible, avoid the smell of food preparation.
8. Try eating cold foods, which have less odor.
9. Loosen clothing.
10. Sit in fresh air.
11. Avoid lying down flat for at least 2 hours after eating (an individual who must rest should sit or recline so head is at least 4 in. higher than feet).

E. Promote foods that stimulate eating and increase protein consumption
1. During acute episodes:
   a. Encourage frequent small amounts of ice chips or cool clear liquids (dilute tea, Jell-O water, flat ginger ale or cola) unless vomiting continues (adults 30–60 mL q ½–1 hr; children 15–30 mL q ½–1 hr).
   b. Consider giving medications by suppository rather than by mouth.
2. Maintain good oral hygiene (brush teeth, rinse mouth) before and after ingestion of food.
3. Offer frequent small feedings (six per day plus snacks) to reduce the feeling of a distended stomach.
4. Allow individual to choose food items as close to actual eating time as possible.
5. Arrange to have highest protein/calorie nutrients served at the time individual feels most like eating (*e.g.*, if chemotherapy is in early morning, serve in late afternoon).
6. Encourage significant others to bring in favorite home foods.
7. Instruct person to
   a. Eat dry foods (toast, crackers) upon arising
   b. Eat salty foods if permissible
   c. Avoid overly sweet, rich, greasy, or fried foods
   d. Try clear, cool beverages
   e. Sip slowly through straw (*e.g.*, soda water)
   f. Take whatever he feels he can tolerate
   g. Eat small portions, low in fat, and eat more frequently
   h. Drink peppermint, spearmint, or raspberry tea
   i. Eat yogurt or milk at night or before arising

F. Initiate health teaching and referrals as indicated
1. Teach techniques to individual and family for home food preparation to increase nutritional intake.
   a. Add powdered milk or egg to milkshakes, gravies, sauces, puddings, cereals, meatballs, or milk to increase protein-calorie content.
   b. Add blenderized or baby foods to meat juices or soups.
   c. Use fortified milk (*e.g.*, 1 c instant nonfat milk to 1 qt fresh milk).
   d. Use milk or half and half instead of water when making soups and sauces; soy formulas can also be used.

   e. Add cheese or diced meat whenever able.
   f. Add cream cheese or peanut butter to toast, crackers, celery sticks.
   g. Add extra butter or margarine to soups, sauces, vegetables.
   h. Spread toast while hot.
   i. Use mayonnaise (100 cal/T) instead of salad dressing.
   j. Add sour cream or yogurt to vegetables or as dip.
   k. Use whipped cream (60 cal/T).
   l. Add raisins, dates, nuts, and brown sugar to hot or cold cereals.
   m. Have extra food (snacks) easily available.
   n. Try commercial supplements available in many forms (liquid, powder, pudding); keep switching brands until some are found that are acceptable to individual in taste and consistency.
2. Explain to a person undergoing chemotherapy (Hogan, 1990):
   a. The need to take an aggressive approach to prevent nausea and vomiting if therapy has a high emetogenic potential
   b. That there is a strong likelihood of emetic control with therapy with low emetic potential
   c. To consult with a physician for combination antiemetic therapy (corticosteroids, neurotransmitters, phenothiazines, metoclopramide, butyrophenones, dronabinol, benzodiazepines, antihistamines, serotonin antagonists)
   d. To experiment with eating patterns 12 hours prior to chemotherapy to evaluate its effects on reducing nausea or vomiting, *e.g.,* easily digested foods only, liquids only, complex carbohydrates only
   e. To avoid eating favorite foods during nausea and vomiting periods to prevent associations after therapy
   f. To use headsets to listen to music and look at pictures depicting relaxing scenes during therapy (Frank, 1985)
   g. To try light exercising, *e.g.,* walking or stationary biking, for chronic nausea
   h. That if anticipatory nausea and vomiting are present to practice progressive muscle relaxation (see Appendix VI)
3. Teach that a variety of interventions have been reported to be helpful to control nausea when pregnant.
   a. Avoidance of fatigue
   b. High-protein meals and snack before retiring
   c. Carbohydrates (crackers) on arising
   d. Carbonated beverages, coke syrup, orange juice, ginger ale, and herbal teas
   e. Lying down to relieve symptoms
4. Instruct the pregnant woman to try one food- or beverage-type relief measure at a time (*e.g.,* high-protein meals/bedtime snack); if nausea is not relieved, try another measure.

■ Comfort, Altered
Related to Malaise and Body Temperature
Fluctuations

Assessment

Subjective

Reports of:
  Chills
  Fatigue
  Excessive warmth

Objective

Body temperature below or above normal

Outcome Criteria

The individual will
  • Identify methods to prevent changes in temperature
  • Maintain normal body temperature

Interventions

A. Maintain fluid balance by increasing fluid intake

  1. Remember to account for the increased fluid loss of perspiration.
  2. See *Fluid Volume Deficit.*

B. Increase caloric intake

  1. Explain the need to increase caloric intake because of increased metabolic rate.
  2. Have the person maintain a written record of food intake/caloric intake.
  3. Provide favorite high-calorie snacks

C. Provide for periods of uninterrupted rest

  1. Rest before and after activity (*e.g.,* meals).

D. Maintain good skin care and comfort

  1. Provide frequent sponge baths/cleansing baths in tepid water.
  2. Use alcohol rubs to refresh and cleanse.
  3. Provide frequent change of bedclothes (absorbent cotton is better than silk or nylon) and linens to minimize dampness.
  4. Use powder unless allergic.
  5. Provide for safety.
  6. Monitor mental status closely for confusion.
  7. Keep siderails up.
  8. Assist the person when ambulating.

E. Consult with physician
   1. To determine frequency of assessment of vital signs (monitor temperature, pulse, respirations, blood pressure)
   2. Regarding use of medication (*e.g.*, aspirin) or necessity for cultures, if early symptoms of hyperthermia become evident (*e.g.*, shaking, chills)

Pain

■ *Related to* **(Specify)**

■ **(in Children)** *Related to* **(Specify)**

DEFINITION
Pain: The state in which an individual experiences and reports the presence of severe discomfort or an uncomfortable sensation.

DEFINING CHARACTERISTICS

Subjective
Communication (verbal or coded) of pain descriptors

Objective
Guarding behavior, protective
Self-focusing
Narrowed focus (altered time perception, withdrawal from social contact, impaired thought processes)
Distraction behavior (moaning, crying, pacing, seeking out other people and/or activities, restlessness)
Facial mask of pain (eyes lackluster, "beaten look," fixed or scattered movement, grimace)
Alteration in muscle tone (may span from listless to rigid)
Autonomic responses not seen in chronic stable pain (diaphoresis blood pressure and pulse change, pupillary dilation, increased or decreased respiratory rate)

RELATED FACTORS
See *Altered Comfort*

Diagnostic Considerations
Nursing management of pain presents specific challenges. Is acute pain a response that nurses treat as a nursing diagnosis or as a collaborative problem? Is acute pain

the etiology of another response that better describes the condition that nurses treat? Does some cluster of nursing diagnoses represent a pain syndrome or chronic pain syndrome, *e.g., Fear, High Risk for Ineffective Family Coping, Impaired Physical Mobility, Social Isolation, Altered Sexuality Patterns, High Risk for Colonic Constipation, Fatigue?* McCafferty and Beebe (1989) cite 18 nursing diagnoses that can apply to persons experiencing pain. Viewing pain as a syndrome diagnosis can provide nurses with a comprehensive nursing diagnosis for persons in pain for whom many related nursing diagnoses could apply.

Errors in Diagnostic Statements

Pain related to surgical incision

Viewing incisional pain as an etiology rather than a response may better relate to nursing's focus. For a surgical client, the nurse focuses on reducing pain to permit increased participation in activities and to reduce anxiety, as described by the nursing diagnosis *Imparied Physical Mobility related to fear of pain and weakness secondary to anesthesia and insufficient fluids and nutrients.*

Pain related to cardiac tissue ischemia

The nurse has several responsibilities for a person experiencing chest pain, including evaluating cardiac status, reducing activity, administering PRN medication, and reducing anxiety. Before discharge, the nurse will teach self-monitoring, self-medication, signs and symptoms of complications, follow-up care, and necessary life-style modifications. Because nursing management of chest pain involves nurse-prescribed and physician-prescribed interventions, this situation should be described as the collaborative problem *Potential Complication: Cardiac.*

This collaborative problem would encompass a variety of cardiac complications, *e.g.,* dysrhythmias, decreased cardiac output, angina. In addition, two nursing diagnoses would apply: *Anxiety related to present situation, unknown future, and perceived effects on self and significant others* and *Potential Altered Health Maintenance related to insufficient knowledge of condition, signs and symptoms of complications, risk factors, activity restrictions, and follow-up care.*

Pain
Related to (Specify)

Assessment
See Defining Characteristics

Outcome Criteria

The person will
- Convey that others validate that the pain exists
- Relate relief after a satisfactory relief measure as evidenced by (specify)

Interventions

A. Assess for factors that decrease pain tolerance
1. Disbelief on the part of others
2. Lack of knowledge
3. Fear (*e.g.,* of addiction or loss of control)
4. Fatigue
5. Monotony

B. Reduce or eliminate factors that increase the pain experience
1. Disbelief on the part of others
   a. Relate to the individual your acceptance of his response to pain.
   - Acknowledge the presence of his pain.
   - Listen attentively to him concerning his pain.
   - Convey to him that you are assessing his pain because you want to better understand it (not determine if it is really present).
   b. Assess the family for the presence of misconceptions about pain or its treatment.
   - Explain the concept of pain as an individual experience.
   - Discuss the reasons why an individual may experience increased or decreased pain (*e.g.,* fatigue [increased] or presence of distractions [decreased]).
   - Encourage family members to share their concerns privately (*e.g.,* fear that the person will use his pain for secondary gains if they give him too much attention).
   - Assess whether the family doubts the pain and discuss the effects of this on the person's pain and on the relationship.
   - Encourage the family to give attention also when pain is not exhibited.
2. Lack of knowledge
   a. Explain causes of the pain to the person, if known.
   b. Relate how long the pain will last, if known.
   c. Explain diagnostic tests and procedures in detail by relating the discomforts and sensations that will be felt and approximate the length of time involved (*e.g.,* "During the intravenous pyelogram you might feel a momentary hot flash through your entire body").
   d. Allow person to see and handle equipment if possible.
3. Fear
   a. Provide accurate information to reduce fear of addiction.
   - Explore with him the reasons for the fear.
   - Explain the difference between drug tolerance and drug addiction (refer to Principles and Rationale for Nursing Care).
   b. Assist in reducing fear of losing control.
   - Provide him with privacy for his pain experience.
   - Attempt to limit the number of health care providers who provide care to him.
   - Allow him to share how intense his pain is and express to him how well he tolerated the pain.
   c. Provide information to reduce fear that the medication will gradually lose its effectiveness.
   - Discuss drug tolerance with him.
   - Discuss the interventions for drug tolerance with the physician (e.g., changing the medication, increasing the dose, decreasing the interval).

- Discuss the effect of relaxation techniques on medication effects.
4. Fatigue
    - Determine the cause of fatigue (sedatives, analgesics, sleep deprivation).
    - Explain that pain contributes to stress, which increases fatigue.
    - Assess the person's present sleep pattern and the influence of his pain on his sleep.
    - Provide him with opportunities to rest during the day and with periods of uninterrupted sleep at night (must rest when pain is ↓).
    - Consult with physician for an increased dose of pain medication at bedtime.
    - Refer to *Sleep Pattern Disturbance* for specific interventions to enhance sleep.
5. Monotony
    a. Discuss with the person and family the therapeutic uses of distraction, along with other methods of pain relief.
    b. Emphasize that the degree an individual can be distracted from his pain is not at all related to the existence of or the intensity of the pain.
    c. Explain that distraction usually increases pain tolerance and decreases pain intensity, but after the distraction ceases the individual may experience increased awareness of pain and fatigue.
    d. Vary the environment if possible. If on bed rest:
        - Encourage personnel to wear seasonal pins and bright-colored apparel.
        - Encourage family to decorate room with flowers, plants, pictures.
        - Provide the person with music.
        - Consult with recreational therapist for an appropriate task.
    e. If at home:
        - Encourage individual to plan an activity for each day, preferably outside the home.
        - Discuss the possibility of learning a new skill (*e.g.,* a craft, a musical instrument).
    f. Teach a method of distraction during an acute pain (*e.g.,* painful procedure) that is not a burden (*e.g.,* count items in a picture, count anything in the room, such as patterns on wallpaper or count silently to self); breathe rhythmically; listen to music and increase the volume as the pain increases.

C. **Collaborate with the individual to determine what methods could be used to reduce the intensity of his pain**
    1. Consider the following prior to selecting a specific pain relief method:
        a. The individual's willingness to participate (motivation), ability to participate (dexterity, sensory loss), preference, support of significant others for method, contraindications (allergy, health problem)
        b. The method's cost, complexity, precautions, and convenience
    2. Explain the various noninvasive pain relief methods to the individual and his family and why they are effective (see Appendix VI).

D. **Collaborate with the individual to initiate the appropriate noninvasive pain relief measures (refer to Appendix VI for specific instructions on each method)**
    1. Relaxation
        a. Instruct on techniques to reduce skeletal muscle tension, which will reduce the intensity of the pain.

b. Use pillows and blankets to support the painful part to reduce the amount of muscle tension.

c. Promote relaxation with a back rub, massage, or warm bath (*e.g.,* for a person with a fractured limb, rub the opposite limb over the fractured site).

d. Teach a specific relaxation strategy (*e.g.,* slow, rhythmic breathing or deep breath—clench fists—yawn).

e. Enlist the aid of the family as coaches.

2. Cutaneous stimulation

a. Discuss with the person the various methods of skin stimulation and their effects on pain (see Appendix VI)

b. Discuss the use of heat applications,* their therapeutic effects and when indicated

c. Discuss each of the following methods and the precautions
- Hot water bottle
- Electric heating pad
- Warm tub
- Moist heat pack
- Hot summer sun
- Thin plastic wrap over painful area to retain body heat (*e.g.,* knee, elbow)

d. Discuss the use of cold applications,* their therapeutic effects and when indicated

e. Discuss each of the following methods and the precautions of each
- Cold towels (wrung out)
- Cold water immersion for small body parts
- Ice bag
- Cold gel pack
- Ice massage

f. Explain the therapeutic uses of menthol preparations and massage/back rub

E. Provide the person with optimal pain relief with prescribed analgesics

1. Determine preferred route of administration: po, IM, IV, rectal (refer to Principles and Rationale for Nursing Care).

2. Assess vital signs, especially respiratory rate, prior to administering medication.

3. Consult with pharmacist for possible adverse interactions with other medications (*e.g.,* muscle relaxants, tranquilizers).

4. Use a preventive approach

a. Medicate prior to an activity (*e.g.,* ambulation) to increase participation, but evaluate the hazard of sedation.

b. Instruct the person to request PRN pain medication before the pain is severe.

c. Collaborate with physician to order meds on a 24-hour basis rather than PRN (refer to Principles and Rationale for Nursing Care for information on the preventive approach).

F. Assess the response to the pain-relief medication

1. After administering a pain-relief medication, return in one-half hour to assess effectiveness.

2. Ask person to rate the severity of his pain, prior to the medication, and the amount of relief received.

3. Ask him to indicate when the pain began to increase.

*May require a physician's order.

4. Consult with physician if a dosage or interval change is needed; the dose may be increased by 50% until effective (Twycross & Lack, 1983).

G. Reduce or eliminate common side-effects of narcotics

1. Sedation
   a. Assess whether the cause is the narcotic, fatigue, sleep deprivation, or other drugs (sedatives, antiemetics).
   b. Inform person that drowsiness usually occurs the first 2–3 days and then subsides.
   c. If drowsiness is excessive, consult with physician to try a slight dose reduction.
2. Constipation
   a. Explain the effect of narcotics on peristalsis.
   b. Consult with physician on the use of a stool softener with long-term drug use.
   c. Refer to Constipation for additional interventions.
3. Nausea and vomiting (see also *Nausea/Vomiting*)
   a. Instruct person that nausea will usually subside after a few doses.
   b. Refrain from withholding narcotic doses because of nausea; rather, secure an order for an antiemetic.
   c. Instruct individual to take deep breaths and to voluntarily swallow to decrease vomiting reflex.
   d. If nausea persists, consult with physician for the appropriate antiemetic or for a change of narcotic that produces less nausea (*e.g.,* morphine).
4. Dry mouth
   a. Explain that narcotics decrease saliva production.
   b. Instruct person to rinse mouth often, suck on sugarless sour candies, eat pineapple chunks or watermelon, if permissible, and drink liquids often.
   c. Explain the necessity of good oral hygiene and dental care.

H. Assist the family to respond positively to the individual's pain experience

1. Assess the family's knowledge of and response to the pain experience.
2. Give accurate information to correct family misconceptions (*e.g.,* addiction, doubts about pain).
3. Provide individuals with opportunities to discuss their fears, anger, and frustrations in private; acknowledge the difficulty of the situation.
4. Incorporate family members in the pain relief modality if possible (*e.g.,* stroking, massage).
5. Praise their participation and their concern.

I. Assist the person with the aftermath of pain

1. Inform him when the cause of the pain has been removed or decreased (*e.g.,* spinal tap).
2. Encourage him to discuss his pain experience.
3. Praise him for his endurance and convey to him that he handled his pain well, regardless of how he behaved.
4. Allow person to keep souvenir of his pain, if desired (*e.g.,* gallstones), or a record of repeated procedures (*e.g.,* venipunctures).

J. Initiate health teaching as indicated

1. Discuss with the person and the family noninvasive pain relief measures (relaxation, distraction, massage).

2. Teach the techniques of choice to the person and his family.
3. Explain the expected course of the pain (resolution) if known (*e.g.,* fractured arm, surgical incision).

■ **Pain** (in Children)
Related to (Specify)

Assessment

Subjective Data

Whimpering
Crying
Moaning
Not sleeping

Reduced appetite (poor feeder)
Does not want to be left alone or
  wants to be left alone
Inability to be comforted

Objective Data

Tense body posture
Irritability
Restlessness

Rubbing or pulling body part
Refusal to move body part
Strained facial expression

Outcome Criteria

According to age and ability, the child will
• Identify the source of his pain
• Identify activities that increase and decrease pain
• Describe comfort from others during the pain experience

Interventions

A. Assess for pain experience
  1. Assess the child's pain experience.
    a. Determine the child's concept of the cause of pain, if feasible.
    b. Ask child to point to the area that hurts.
    c. Determine the intensity of the pain at its worst and best.
    d. Use a pain assessment scale appropriate for the child's developmental age. Use the same scale the same way each time, and encourage its use by parents and other health care professionals. Indicate on the care plan which scale to use and how (introduction of scale, language, etc. specific for child); attach copy if visual scale. (See page 213 for a description of pain scales.)
    e. Ask the child what makes the pain better and what makes it worse.
    f. Assess whether fear, loneliness, or anxiety are contributing to pain.

g. Assess effect on sleep and play. *Note:* A child who sleeps and/or plays can be a child in pain (sleep and play can be a type of distraction) or a child adequately medicated for pain.

2. Assess the child and his family for the presence of misconceptions about pain or its treatment.

   a. Explain the pain source to the child using verbal and sensory (visual, tactile) explanations (*e.g.,* allow child to handle equipment or perform treatment on doll) (refer to Appendix IX for specific techniques of play therapy).

   b. Explicitly explain and reinforce to the child that he is not being punished.

   c. Explain to the parents the necessity of good explanations to promote trust.

   d. Explain to the parents that the child may cry more openly when they are present but that their presence is important for promoting trust.

   e. Parents and older children may have misconceptions about pain and analgesia, and may be fearful of narcotic use/abuse. Emphasize that narcotic use for moderate or severe pain does not lead to addiction (Schechter, 1989). Discuss with parents and older children that "say no to drugs" does not apply to analgesia for pain prescribed by physicians and monitored by physicians and nurses.

B. **Promote security with honest explanations and opportunities for choice**

1. Promote open, honest communications

   a. Tell the truth; explain
   - How much it will hurt
   - How long it will last
   - What will help the pain

   b. Do not threaten (*e.g., do not* tell the child, "If you don't hold still you won't go home").

   c. Explain to the child that the procedure is necessary so he can get better and it is important to hold still so it can be done quickly.

   d. Discuss with the parents the importance of truth-telling; instruct parents to
   - Tell child when they are leaving and when they will return
   - Relate to the child that they cannot take away his pain but that they will be with him (except in circumstances when parents are not permitted to remain)

   e. Allow the parents opportunities to share their feelings about witnessing their child's pain and their helplessness

2. Prepare the child for a painful procedure.

   a. Discuss the procedure with the parents; determine what they have told the child.

   b. Explain the procedure in words suited to the child's age and developmental level (see *Altered Growth and Development* for age-related needs).
   - Allow a 2-year-old to watch you taking out sutures from a doll or stuffed animal.
   - Permit the child to hold instruments.

   c. Relate the discomforts that will be felt (*e.g.,* what the child will feel, taste, see or smell).
   - "You will get an injection that will hurt for a little while and then it will stop."
   - Be sure to explain when an injection will cause two discomforts: the prick of the needle and the absorption of the drug.

d. Encourage the child to ask questions before and during the procedure; ask the child to share with you what he thinks is going to happen and why.

e. Share with the child (who is old enough—over 3¹/₂) that:
- You expect that he will hold still and that it will please you if he can.
- It is all right to cry or squeeze your hand if it hurts.

f. Find something to praise after the procedure, even if child was not able to hold still, etc.

g. Arrange to have parents present for procedures (especially for children under 10 years); describe what to expect to parents before procedure, and give them a role during procedure (*e.g.*, hold the child's hand, talk to the child).

3. Reduce the pain during treatments when possible.

a. If restraints must be used, have sufficient personnel available in order not to delay the procedure.

b. If injections are ordered, try to obtain an order for oral or intravenous analgesics instead. If injections must be used:
- Expect the child (over 2¹/₂ or 3) to hold still
- Have the child participate by holding the Band-Aid for you
- Tell the child how pleased you are that he helped
- Pull the skin surface as taut as possible (for IM)
- Comfort the child after the procedure
- Tell child step-by-step what is going to happen right before it is done

c. Offer the child the option of learning distraction techniques for use during the procedure. (The use of distraction without the child's knowledge of the impending discomfort is not advocated because the child will learn to mistrust.)
- Tell a story with a puppet.
- Ask the child to name or count objects in a picture.
- Ask the child to look at the picture and to locate certain objects ("Where is the dog?").
- Ask child to tell you about his pet.
- Ask child to count your blinks.

d. Avoid rectal temperatures in preschoolers; if possible, use electronic oral probes.

e. Provide the child with privacy during the painful procedure; use a treatment room rather than the child's bed.
- The child's bed should be a "safe" place.
- No procedures should be done in the playroom or schoolroom.

4. Provide the child optimal pain relief with prescribed analgesics.

a. Medicate child prior to painful procedure or activity (*e.g.*, ambulation).

b. Consult with physician for a change of the IM route to the IV route.

c. Assess appropriateness of medication, dose, and schedule for cause of pain, child's weight, and child's response.

d. Besides using pain scales to assess pain, observe for behavioral signs of pain (since the child may deny pain); if possible, identify specific behaviors that indicate pain in an individual child.

5. Reduce or eliminate the common side-effects of narcotics.

a. Sedation
- Assess whether the cause is the narcotic, fatigue, sleep deprivation, or other drugs (sedatives, antiemetics).
- If drowsiness is excessive, consult with physician to try a slight dose reduction.

b. Constipation
  - Explain to older children why pain medications cause constipation.
  - Increase roughage in diet (*e.g.,* ask child which fruits he likes; sprinkle 1 teaspoon of bran on cereal).
  - Encourage child to drink 8–10 (8-oz) glasses of liquids each day.
  - Teach child how to do abdominal isometric exercises if activity is restricted (*e.g.,* "Pull in your tummy; now relax your tummy; do this ten times each hour during the day").
  - Instruct child to keep a record of his exercises (*e.g.,* make a chart with a star sticker placed on it whenever the exercises are done).
  - Refer to *Constipation* for additional interventions.
c. Dry mouth
  - Explain to older children that narcotics decrease saliva production.
  - Instruct to rinse mouth often, suck on sugarless sour candies, eat pineapple chunks and watermelon, drink liquids often.
  - Explain the necessity of brushing his teeth after every meal.
6. Assist the child with the aftermath of pain.
  a. Tell the child when the painful procedure is over.
  b. Pick up the small child to indicate it is over.
  c. Encourage the child to discuss his pain experience (draw or act out with dolls).
  d. Encourage the child to perform the painful procedure using the same equipment on a doll under supervision (see Appendix IX for specific interventions).
  e. Praise the child for his endurance and convey to him that he handled the pain well regardless of how he behaved (unless he was violent to others).
  f. Give the child a souvenir of his pain (Band-Aid, badge for bravery).
  g. Teach the child to keep a record of painful experiences and to plan a reward each time he achieves a behavioral goal, *e.g.,* a gold star (reward) for each time he holds still (goal) during an injection. Encourage achievable goals; holding still during an injection may not be possible for every child, but counting or blowing may be possible.
7. Collaborate with child to initiate appropriate noninvasive pain relief modalities.
  a. Encourage mobility as much as indicated, especially when pain is at its lowest level.
  b. Discuss with child and parents activities that are liked and incorporate them in daily schedule (*e.g.,* clay modeling, painting).
  c. Discuss with the child (over 7) that the pain can be less if the child thinks about something else and demonstrate the effects.
    - Ask child to count to 100 (or count your eye blinks).
    - As child is counting, apply gentle pressure to Achilles tendon (pinch back of heel).
    - Gradually increase the pressure.
    - Ask child to stop counting but keep pressure on heel.
    - Ask child if he can feel the discomfort in his heel now and if he felt it when he was counting.
  d. Refer to guidelines for noninvasive pain relief measures (Appendix VI).
8. Assist the family to respond optimally to the child's pain experience.
  a. Assess the family's knowledge of and response to the pain experience (*e.g.,* does the parent support the child who has pain?).
  b. Assure the parents that they can touch or hold their child, if feasible (*e.g.,* demonstrate that touching is possible even in the presence of tubes and equipment).

    c. Give accurate information to correct misconceptions (*e.g.*, the necessity of the treatment even though it causes pain).

    d. Provide parents with opportunities to discuss their fears, anger, frustrations in private.

    e. Acknowledge the difficulty of the situation.

    f. Incorporate the parents in the pain relief modality if possible (*e.g.*, stroking, massage, distraction).

    g. Praise their participation and their concern.

    h. Negotiate goals of pain management plan and reevaluate regularly (*e.g.*, pain-free, decrease in pain).

C. Initiate health teaching and referrals if indicated

1. Provide child and family with ongoing explanations.
2. Utilize the care plan to promote continuity of care for hospitalized child.
3. Utilize available mental health professionals, if needed, for assistance with guided imagery, progressive relaxation, and hypnosis.
4. Refer parents to pertinent literature for themselves and children (see Bibliography).

Chronic Pain

■ *Related to* **(Specify)**

DEFINITION

Chronic pain: The state in which an individual experiences pain that is persistent or intermittent and lasts for more than 6 months.

DEFINING CHARACTERISTICS

Major (must be present)

The person reports that pain has existed for more than 6 months (may be the only assessment data present)

Minor (may be present)
  Discomfort
  Anger, frustration, depression because of situation
  Facial mask of pain
  Anorexia, weight loss
  Insomnia
  Guarded movement
  Muscle spasms
  Redness, swelling, heat
  Color changes in affected area
  Reflex abnormalities

RELATED FACTORS

See *Altered Comfort*

Diagnostic Considerations
See *Altered Comfort*

Errors in Diagnostic Statements
See *Altered Comfort*

Focus Assessment Criteria
See *Altered Comfort*

Principles and Rationale for Nursing Care
See *Altered Comfort*

■ Chronic Pain
Related to (Specify)

Assessment

Subjective Data
The person reports that the following signs have existed for more than 6 months
  Pain (may be the only assessment data present)
  Discomfort
  Anger, frustration, depression about situation

Objective Data

Facial mask of pain
Anorexia, weight loss
Insomnia
Guarded movement
Muscle spasms
Redness, swelling, heat
Color changes in affected area
Reflex abnormalities

Outcome Criteria

The person will
- Relate that others validate that the pain exists
- Practice selected noninvasive pain relief measures to manage his pain
- Relate improvement of pain and an increase in daily activities as evident by (specify)

The child will
- Communicate improvement in pain verbally, by pain assessment scale, or behavior (specify)
- Maintain usual family role and relationships throughout pain experience, as evidenced by (specify)
- Demonstrate coping mechanisms for pain, methods of controlling pain, and the pain cause/disease, as evidenced by an increase in play and usual activities of childhood, and (specify)

Interventions

A. Assess the person's pain experience; determine the intensity of the pain at its worst and best
  1. Ask person to rate his pain using a scale of 0–10 (0 = absence of pain; 10 = worst pain) or a 0–5 scale.
    a. Rate it at its best
    b. Rate it after a pain-relief measure
    c. Rate it at its worst
  2. Collaborate with the individual to determine what methods could be used to reduce the intensity

B. Assess for factors which decrease pain tolerance
  1. Disbelief on the part of others
  2. Fear
  3. Fatigue
  4. Monotony

C. Reduce or eliminate factors that increase the pain experience
  1. Disbelief of others
    a. Relate to the individual your acceptance of his response to pain.
      - Acknowledge the presence of his pain.

- Listen attentively to him concerning his pain.
- Convey to him that you are assessing his pain because you want to better understand it, not determine if it is really present.

  b. Assess the family for the presence of misconceptions about pain or its treatment.
   - Explain the concept of pain as an individual experience.
   - Discuss the reason why an individual may experience increased or decreased pain (*e.g.*, fatigue [increased] or presence of distractions [decreased]).
   - Encourage family to share these concerns privately (*e.g.*, fear that the person will use his pain for secondary gains if they give him too much attention).
   - Assess if the family doubts the pain.
   - Discuss the effects of this on the person's pain and on the relationship.
   - Encourage family to give him attention also when he does not exhibit the pain.

2. Provide person with accurate information to reduce his fears.
  a. Fear of addiction
   - Explore with him the reasons for the fear.
   - Explain the difference between drug tolerance and drug addiction.
  b. Fear of losing control
   - Provide privacy for his pain experience.
   - Attempt to limit the number of health care providers who provide care to him.
  c. Fear that the medication will gradually lose its effectiveness
   - Discuss drug tolerance with him.
   - Explain the use of combining noninvasive pain relief measures with medications.
  d. Fear of family that the person will use his pain for secondary gains
   - Encourage family to share these concerns privately.
   - If the family doubts the pain, discuss the effects of this on the person's pain experience and on their relationship.
   - Encourage family to give him attention also when he does not exhibit pain.

3. Fatigue
   - Determine the cause of fatigue (sedatives, analgesics, sleep deprivation).
   - Explain that pain contributes to stress, which increases fatigue.
   - Assess the person's present sleep pattern and the influence of pain on his sleep.
   - Provide opportunities to rest during the day and periods of uninterrupted sleep at night.
   - Refer to *Sleep Pattern Disturbance* for specific interventions to enhance sleep.

4. Monotony
  a. Discuss with the person and family the therapeutic uses of distraction, along with other methods of pain relief.
  b. Emphasize that the degree to which an individual can be distracted from his pain is not at all related to the existence of or the intensity of the pain.
  c. Explain that distraction usually increases pain tolerance and decreases pain intensity, but after the distraction ceases the individual may experience increased awareness of pain and fatigue.

    d. Vary the environment if possible. If on bed rest:
- Encourage personnel to wear seasonal pins and bright-colored apparel.
- Encourage family to decorate the room with flowers, plants, pictures.
- Provide the person with music.
- Consult with recreational therapist for an appropriate activity.

    e. If at home:
- Encourage individual to plan an activity for each day, preferably outside the home.
- Discuss the possibility of learning a new skill (*e.g.,* a craft, a musical instrument).

D. **Assess the effects of chronic pain on the individual's life, utilizing the person and his family**
1. Performance (job, role responsibilities)
2. Social interactions
3. Finances
4. Activities of daily living (sleep, eating, mobility, sexuality)
5. Cognition/mood (concentration, depression)
6. Family unit (response of members)

E. **Assist the person and his family to reduce the effects of depression on lifestyle**
1. Encourage verbalization of individual and family concerning difficult situations.
2. Listen carefully.
3. Explain the relationship between chronic pain and depression.
4. See *Ineffective Individual Coping* for additional interventions.

F. **Consult with the individual to determine what methods could be utilized to reduce the intensity of his pain**
1. Before selecting a specific noninvasive pain relief method, consider the person's
   a. Willingness to participate (motivation)
   b. Ability to participate (dexterity, sensory loss)
   c. Preference
   d. Support of significant others for method
   e. Contraindications (allergy, health problem)
2. Consider the method's cost, complexity, precautions, and convenience.
3. Explain the various noninvasive pain relief methods to the individual and his family and why they are effective (Appendix VI).

G. **Collaborate with the individual to initiate the appropriate noninvasive pain relief measures (refer to Appendix VI for specific instructions on each method)**
1. Explain relaxation techniques to reduce skeletal muscle tension that will reduce the intensity of the pain.
   a. Use pillows and blankets to support the painful part to reduce the amount of muscle tension.
   b. Promote relaxation with a back rub, massage, or a warm bath* (*e.g.,* for a person with a fractured limb, rub the opposite limb over the fractured site).

*May require a physician's order.

    c. Teach a specific relaxation strategy (*e.g.,* slow, rhythmic breathing or deep breath—clench fists—yawn).

    d. Enlist the aid of the family as coaches.

    e. Discuss other techniques that can be learned (meditation, yoga, biofeedback, guided imagery).

2. Cutaneous stimulation

    a. Discuss with the person the various methods of skin stimulation and their effects on pain (Appendix VI).

    b. Discuss the use of heat applications,* their therapeutic effects and when indicated.

    c. Discuss each of the following methods and their precautions:
- Hot water bottle
- Electric heating pad
- Electric light bulb
- Warm tub
- Moist heat pack
- Hot summer sun
- Thin plastic wrap over painful area to retain body heat (*e.g.,* knee, elbow)

    d. Discuss the use of cold applications,* their therapeutic effects and when indicated.

    e. Discuss each of the following methods and their precautions:
- Cold towels (wrung out)
- Cold water immersion for small body parts
- Ice bag
- Cold gel pack
- Ice massage

    f. Explain the therapeutic uses of:
- Menthol preparations
- Massage/back rub
- Pressure
- Vibration
- Transcutaneous electric nerve stimulation (TENS)

3. Discuss with the person and the family the therapeutic uses of distraction along with other methods of pain relief.

    a. Emphasize that the degree to which an individual can be distracted from his pain is not at all related to the existence or intensity of the pain.

    b. Explain that distraction usually increases pain tolerance and decreases pain intensity, but after the distraction ceases the individual may experience increased awareness of pain and fatigue.

    c. If possible, use modalities that stimulate one or more of the major senses in a rhythmic manner.
- Hearing: music, counting silently to self, being read to
- Vision: television, counting items in a picture or patterns on wallboard, reading (or telling) a story
- Touch and movement: massage, rocking, rhythmic breathing, stroking

    d. Encourage the person to participate in activities that are pleasurable and time-consuming (*e.g.,* arts and crafts).

---

*May require a physician's order.

H. Provide the individual pain relief with prescribed analgesics*

1. Determine preferred route of administration: po, IM, IV, rectal (refer to Principles and Rationale for Nursing Care).

2. Assess the response to the medication.
   a. For admitted persons
      - After administering a pain relief medication, return in one-half hour to assess effectiveness.
      - Ask him to rate the severity of his pain prior to the medication and the amount of relief received.
      - Ask him to indicate when the pain began to increase.
      - Consult with the physician if a dosage or interval change is needed.
   b. For outpatients
      - Ask him to keep a record of when he takes his medication and what kind of relief was received.
      - Instruct him to consult his physician with questions concerning medication dosage.

3. Encourage the use of po medications as soon as possible.
   a. Consult with physician for a schedule to change from IM to po.
   b. Explain to individual and family that oral medications can be as effective as IM.
   c. Explain how the transition will occur:
      - Begin po medication at a larger dose than necessary (loading dose).
      - Continue PRN IM medication.
      - Gradually reduce IM medication dose.
      - Use the person's account of pain to regulate po doses.
   d. Consult with physician for the possibility of adding aspirin or acetaminophen to the medication regime.

I. Reduce or eliminate common side-effects of narcotics

1. Sedation
   a. Assess if the cause is the narcotic, fatigue, sleep deprivation, or other drugs (sedatives, antiemetic).
   b. Inform individual that drowsiness usually occurs the first 2–3 days then subsides.
   c. If drowsiness is excessive, consult with physician to try a slight dose reduction.

2. Constipation
   a. Explain the effect of narcotics on peristalsis.
   b. Consult with physician for the use of a stool softener with long-term drug use.
   c. Instruct person to always use the toilet or commode to have a bowel movement in order to assume the correct position for defecation.
   d. Teach to increase roughage in diet (*e.g.,* add 1–2 tsp of bran to food and increase fruit, whole grain breads, and cereal in diet).
   e. Encourage to drink 8–10 glasses (8-oz) of liquids each day.
   f. Encourage daily exercises (*e.g.,* walking, teach isometric exercises to individuals in bed).

*May require a physician's order.

f. Refer to *Constipation* for additional interventions.
3. Nausea and vomiting
   a. Consult with physician for the appropriate antiemetic or for a change of narcotic that produces less nausea (*e.g.,* morphine).
   b. Instruct person that nausea will usually subside after a few doses.
   c. Refrain from withholding narcotic dose because of nausea; rather, secure an order for an antiemetic.
   d. Encourage small, frequent amounts of ice chips or cool, clear liquids (dilute tea, Jell-O water, flat ginger ale, or Coke) unless vomiting continues (*e.g.,* adults 30–60 mL q ½–1 hr; children, 15–30 mL q ½–1 hr).
   e. Consider giving medications by suppository rather than by mouth.
   f. Decrease the stimulation of the vomiting center by reducing unpleasant sights and odors and providing good mouth care after vomiting.
   g. Instruct person to
      • Practice deep breathing and voluntary swallowing to suppress the vomiting reflex
      • Sit down after eating but not lie down
      • Eat smaller meals; eat slowly
      • Restrict liquids with meals to avoid overdistending the stomach; avoid drinking fluids 1 hour before and after meals
      • If possible, avoid the smell of food preparation
      • Try eating cold foods because they have less odor
      • Avoid sweets and fried or fatty foods
      • Eat salty foods if not contraindicated
      • Loosen clothing
      • Sit in fresh air
4. Dry mouth
   a. Explain that narcotics decrease saliva production.
   b. Instruct to rinse mouth often, suck on sugarless sour candies, eat pineapple chunks or watermelon, and drink liquids often.
   c. Explain the necessity of good oral hygiene and dental care.

J. Assist the family to respond optimally to the individual's pain experience
1. Assess the family's knowledge of pain and of responses to the pain experience.
2. Give accurate information to correct family misconceptions (*e.g.,* addiction, doubt about pain).
3. Provide individuals with opportunities to discuss their fears, anger, frustrations in private; acknowledge the difficulty of the situation.
4. Incorporate the family in the pain relief method if possible (*e.g.,* coaching relaxation, massaging).
5. Encourage family to seek assistance if needed for specific problems, such as coping with chronic pain: family counselor; financial and service agencies (*e.g.,* American Cancer Society).

K. Promote optimal mobility
1. Discuss the value of exercise to strengthen and stretch muscles, decrease stress, and promote sleep.
2. Assist individual to plan daily activities when pain is at its lowest level.

L. Assist the child with chronic pain

1. Assess pain experiences by using developmentally appropriate assessment scales and by assessing behavior. Incorporate child and family in ongoing assessment. Identify potential for secondary gain for reporting pain (*e.g.,* companionship, attention, concern, caring, distraction) and include strategies for meeting identified needs in plan of care.
2. Set goals for pain management with child and family (short- and long-term) and evaluate regularly, *e.g.,* totally relieve pain, partially relieve pain, control behavior or anxiety associated with pain.
3. Promote normal growth and development; involve family and available resources, such as occupational, physical and Child Life Therapists.
4. Promote the "normal" aspects of the child's life: play, school, relationships with family, physical activity.
5. Promote a trusting environment for child and family:
   a. Believe the child's pain.
   b. Encourage child's perception that interventions are attempts to help.
   c. Have child, family, and nurse participate in controlling pain.
6. Provide continuity of care and pain management by health care providers (nurse, physician, pain team) and in different settings (inpatient, outpatient, emergency department, home).
7. Utilize interdisciplinary team for pain management as necessary, *e.g.,* nurse, physician, child life therapist, mental health therapist, occupational therapist, physical therapist, nutritionist.
8. Identify myths and misconceptions about pediatric pain management (*e.g.,* IM analgesia, narcotic use and dosing, assessment) in attitudes of health care professionals and child and family; provide accurate information and opportunities for effective communication.

M. Initiate health teaching and referrals as indicated; discuss with the individual and family the various treatment modalities available

1. Family therapy
2. Group therapy
3. Behavior modification
4. Biofeedback
5. Hypnosis
6. Acupuncture
7. Exercise program

References/Bibliography

Anderson, J. (1982). Nursing management of the cancer patient in pain: A review of the literature. *Cancer Nursing, 5,* 33–41.

Barber, J. (1978). Hypnosis as a psychological technique in the management of cancer pain. *Cancer Nursing, 1,* 361–363.

Beyer, J. E. (1984). *Ultra: A user manual and technical report.* Evanston, IL: Hospital Play Equipment Co.

Beyerman, K.: (1982). Flawed perceptions about pain. *American Journal of Nursing, 82,* 302–304.

Bray, C. A. (1986). Postoperative pain: Altering the patient's experience through education. *AORN Journal, 43*(3), 674–675.

Carpenito, R. (1987). Personal communication.

Copp, L. (1985). Pain coping model and typology. *Image, 17*(3), 69–71.

Coyle, N. (1987). Analgesics and pain—Current concepts. *Nursing Clinics of North America, 22,* 727–741.

Dernham, P. (1986). Phantom limb pain *Geriatric Nursing, 7,* (1), 34–37.

Donovan, M. (1986). Symptom management—The nurse is the key. In McCorkle, R. S. & Hingladarion, J. (Eds.). *Issues and topics in cancer nursing.* Norwalk: Appleton-Century-Crofts.

Eland, J. (1988). Pain management and comfort. *Journal of Gerontology Nursing, 14*(4), 10–15.

Foley, K. (1985). The treatment of cancer pain. *New England Journal of Medicine, 313*(2), 84–95.

Eland, J. M. (1981). Minimizing pain associated with prekindergarten intramuscular injections: Issues in comprehension. *Pediatric Nursing, 5*(5–6), 361–372.

Hansen, B, & Evans, M. (1981). Preparing a child for procedures. *Maternal and Child Nursing Journal, 6,* 392–397.

Hester, N. (1979). The preoperational child's reaction to immunization. *Nursing Research, 28*(4), 250–255.

Jacox, A. K. (Ed.). (1977). *Pain: A source book for nurses and other professionals.* Boston: Little, Brown.

Johnson, J. A., & Repp, E. C. (1984). Nonpharmacologic pain management in arthritis. *Nursing Clinics of North America, 19*(4), 583–591.

Klisch, M. L. (1980). The Simonton method of visualization. *Cancer Nursing, 3,* 295–300.

Krieger, D. (1975). Therapeutic touch: The imprimatur of nursing. *American Journal of Nursing, 75,* 784–787.

Kwentus, J., Harkins, S., Lignon, N. & Silverman, J. (1985). Current concepts of geriatric pain and its treatment. *Geriatrics, 40*(4), 48–57.

McCaffery, M., & Beebe, A. (1989). *Pain: Clinical management for nursing practice.* St. Louis: C. V. Mosby.

McCaffery, M., Meinhart, N. (1983). *Pain: A nursing approach to assessment and analysis.* Norwalk: Appleton-Century-Crofts.

McCafferty, M. (1980). *Nursing management of the patient with pain* (2nd ed.). Philadelphia: J. B. Lippincott.

McGuire, D. B.. (1984). Assessment of pain in cancer inpatients using the McGill Pain Questionaire. *Oncology Nursing* Forum, *11*(6), 32–7, Nov–Dec.

McGuire, D.B. (1984). Selecting an instrument to measure cancer related pain. *Oncology Nursing Forum, 11*(6), 85–87.

Miller, C. A. (1990). *Nursing care of older adults.* Glenview, IL: Scott Foresman.

Mosely, J. R. (1985). Alterations in comfort related to terminal illness. *Nursing Clinics of North America, 20*(2), 427–438.

Perry, S. & Heidrich, G. (1981). Placebos. *America Journal of Nursing, 81,* 721–725.

Porter, J., & Jick, H. (1980). Addiction rate in patients treated with narcotics. *New England Journal of Medicine, 302,* 123.

Silman, J., Diblasi, M., & Washburn, C. J. (1979). The management of pain. *American Journal of Nursing, 79,* 74–78.

Watt-Watson, J. (1987). Nurses' knowledge of pain issues—survey. *Journal of Pain and Symptom Management, 2,* 207–211.

Pruritus

Baer, R.L. (1990). Poison ivy dermatitis. *Cutis, 46*(1), 34–36.

Branov, C.H., Epstein, J.H., & Grayson, L. D. (1989). When pruritus is a diagnostic puzzle. *Patient Care, 23*(15), 41–44, 50–4.

Branov, C.H. Epstein, J. H., & Grayson, L. D. (1989). How to relieve persistent itching. *Patient Care, 23*(16), 107.

Bulechek, G, & McCloskey, J. (1985). *Nursing interventions: Treatments for nursing diagnoses.* Philadelphia: W. B. Saunders.

Callen, J. P., Starviski, M. A., & Voorhees, J. J. (1980). Cutaneous manifestations of systemic illness. In *Manual of Dermatology.* Chicago: Year Book Medical Publishers.

DeWitt, S. (1990). Nursing assessment of skin and dermatological lesions. *Nursing Clinics of North America, 25*(1), 235–245.

Frantz, R. A., & Kinney, C. N. (1986). Variables associated with skin dryness. *Nursing Research, 2,* 98.

Hardy, M. A. (1990). A pilot study of the diagnosis and treatment of impaired skin integrity: Dry skin in older persons. *Nursing Diagnosis, 1*(2), 57–63.

Jacobs, M. & Geels, W. (1985). *Signs and symptoms in nursing: Interpretation and management.* Philadelphia: J. B. Lippincott.

Lisanti, P. (1983). Altered integumentary functioning. In Mahoney, E. A. & Flynn, J. P. (Eds). *Handbook of medical-surgical nursing.* New York: John Wiley & Sons.

Tucker, S. & Key, M. (1983). Occupational skin disease. In Rom, W. M. (Ed). *Environmental and occupational medicine.* Boston: Little, Brown.

Twyeross, R. G., & Lack, S. A. (1983). *Symptom control in far advanced cancer: Pain relief.* Baltimore: Urban and Schwarzenberg.

Nausea/Vomiting

Cotanch, P. & Strum, S. (1987). Progressive muscle relaxation as antiemetic therapy for cancer patients. *Oncology Nursing, 14*(1), 33–37.

Frank, J. M. (1985). The effect of music therapy and guided visual imagery on chemotherapy-induced nausea and vomiting. *Oncology Nursing Forum, 12*(5), 47–52.

Frick, S. B., DelPo, E. G., Keith, J. A., & Davis, M. S. (1988). Chemotherapy-associated nausea and vomiting in pediatric oncology patients. *Cancer Nursing, 11*(2), 118–124.

Hogan, C. M. (1990). Advances in the management of nausea and vomiting. In Miaskowski, C. (Ed.). *Advances in oncology nursing. Nursing Clinics of North America, 25*(2), 475–497.

Ieiorio, C. (1988). The management of nausea and vomiting in pregnancy. *Nurse Practitioner, 13*(5), 23–28.

Morrow, G. R. (1989). Chemotherapy-related nausea and vomiting: Etiology and management. *Cancer, 39*(2), 89–104.

Voda, A. & Randall, M. (1982). Nausea and vomiting of pregnancy. In Norris, C. (Ed). *Concept clarification in nursing.* Maryland: Aspen System.

Wickam, R. (1989). Managing chemotherapy-related nausea and vomiting: The state of the art. *Oncology, 16*(4), 563–674.

Children

Berde, C. (1989). Pediatric postoperative pain management. *Pediatric Clinics of North America, 36*(4), 921–940.

Beyer, J. E., et al.(1983). Patterns of postoperative analgesic use with adults and children following cardiac surgery. *Pain, 17*(9), 71–81.

Broome, M., & Slack, J. (1990). Influence on nurses' managment of pain in children. *American Journal of Maternal-Child Nursing, 15*(3), 158–162.

Ellis, J. (1988). Using pain scales to prevent undermedication. *Maternal-Child Nursing Journal, 13*(3), 180–182.

Eland, J. M., & Anderson, J. (1977). The experience of pain in children. In Jacox, A. K. (Ed). *Pain: A sourcebook for nurses and other health professionals.* Boston: Little, Brown.

Kuttner, L. (1988). Favorite stories: A hypnotic pain-reduction technique for children in acute pain. *American Journal of Clinical Hypnosis, 30*(4), 289–295.

Masek, B., Russo, D., & Varni, J. (1984). Behavioral approaches to the management of chronic pain in children. *Pediatric Clinics of North America, 31*(5), 1113–1131.

O'Brien, S. & Konsler, G. (1988). Alleviating children's postoperative pain. *Maternal-Child Nursing Journal, 13*(3), 183–186.

Puntillo, K. (1988). The phenomenon of pain and critical care nursing. *Heart & Lung, 17*(3), 262–270.

Saderman, J. (1990). Pain relief during routine procedures for children with leukemia. *American Journal of Maternal-Child Nursing, 15*(2), 163–166.

Schechter, N. (Ed.). (1989a). Acute pain in children. *Pediatric Clinics of North America, 36*(4), 781–1045.

Schechter, N. (1989b). Undertreatment of pain in children: An overview. *Pediatric Clinics of North America, 36*(4), 781–794.

Schechter, N. (1987). Pain: Acknowledging it, assessing it, treating it. *Contemporary Pediatrics, 4*(7), 16–46.

Wong, D., & Baker, C. (1988). Pain in children: Comparison of assessment scales. *Pediatric Nursing, 14*(1), 9–17.

Communication, Impaired*

Communication, Impaired Verbal

Communication, Impaired*

- ■ *Related to* **Effects of Hearing Loss**
- ■ *Related to* **Effects of Aphasia on Expression or Interpretation**
- ■ *Related to* **Foreign Language Barrier**

DEFINITION

Impaired communication: The state in which the individual experiences, or is at high risk to experience, a decreased ability to send or receive messages (*i.e.,* has difficulty exchanging thoughts, ideas, or desire).

DEFINING CHARACTERISTICS

Major (must be present)

Inappropriate or absent speech or response

Minor (may be present)

Incongruence between verbal and nonverbal messages
Stuttering
Slurring
Problem in finding the correct word when speaking
Weak or absent voice
Impaired vision
Decreased auditory comprehension
Statements of not understanding or being misunderstood
Deafness or inattention to noises or voices
Confusion
Inability to speak dominant language
Use of sign language

RELATED FACTORS

Pathophysiologic

Cerebral impairment
Expressive or receptive aphasia
Cerebrovascular accident

*Note: This diagnostic category was developed by Rosalinda Alfaro-Lefever and is not currently on the NANDA list, but is here for clarity and usefulness.

Brain damage (*e.g.*, birth/head trauma)
CNS depression/increased intracranial pressure
Tumor (of the head, neck, or spinal cord)
Mental disabilities
Chronic hypoxia/decreased cerebral blood flow
Neurologic impairment
Quadriplegia
Nervous system diseases (*e.g.*, myasthenia gravis, multiple sclerosis)
Vocal cord paralysis
Auditory nerve damage
Respiratory impairment (*e.g.*, shortness of breath)
Auditory impairment (decreased hearing)
Laryngeal edema/infection
Oral deformities
Cleft lip or palate
Malocclusion or fractured jaw
Missing teeth
Dysarthria

Treatment-related

Endotracheal intubation
Tracheostomy/tracheotomy/laryngectomy
Surgery of the head, face, neck, or mouth
Pain (especially of the mouth or throat)
Drugs (*e.g.*, CNS depressants, anesthesia)

Situational (personal, environmental)

Anger, pain, anxiety, fear, or fatigue
Poor timing/poor choice of words
Lack of feedback
Not listening to feedback
Speech pathology
Stuttering
Lisping
Ankyloglossia ("tongue-tie")
Voice problems
Language barrier (unfamiliar language or dialect)/word meaning problems
Lack of privacy/confidentiality
Loss of recent memory recall
No access to hearing aid/malfunction of hearing aid

Maturational

Elderly (auditory losses)
Children developmentally disabled, *e.g.*, muscular dystrophy

Diagnostic Considerations

Impaired Communication and *Impaired Verbal Communication* are diagnoses describing persons who desire to communicate but are encountering problems. *Impaired Communication* may not be useful to describe a person in whom communication problems are a manifestation of a psychiatric illness or a coping problem. If nursing interventions focus on reducing hallucinations, fear, or anxiety, the diagnosis *Fear* or *Anxiety* would be more appropriate.

Errors in Diagnostic Statements

Impaired Communication related to failure of staff to use effective communication techniques

The diagnostic statement should not be used as a vehicle to reveal a problem resulting from incorrect or insufficient nursing intervention. Instead, the nurse should write the diagnosis as *Impaired Verbal Communication relate to effects of tracheotomy on ability to talk*. The care plan would specify the communication techniques to be used. Failure to use the techniques would be a nursing management issue, not a care plan problem.

Focus Assessment Criteria

Subjective Data

1. Note the usual pattern of communication as described by the person or his family

Very verbal	Speaks only when spoken to
Sometimes verbal	Does not speak/respond
Uses sign language	Responds inappropriately
Writes only	Gestures only

   a. Does the person feel he has difficulty hearing or has he ever worn a hearing aid?
   b. Does the person feel he is communicating normally today?
   c. If not, what does he feel may help him to communicate better?
   d. Is there a specific person he would like to talk with or have present to help him express ideas?
2. Does the person feel he can usually express himself well?
3. Does the person feel there are barriers hindering his ability to communicate?
   Lack of privacy
   Fear of uncertain origin
   Fear of being inappropriate or "stupid"
   Not enough time to gather his thoughts and ask questions
   Need for presence of significant other or familiar face
   Language, dialect, or cultural barrier (specify)
   Lack of knowledge of subject being discussed
   Pain, stress, or fatigue

Objective Data

1. Describe the person's ability to form words

Good	Weak (whisper)
Slurred	Absent
Lisping	Language barrier
Stuttering	Difficulty breathing and talking
Slow	

2. Describe the person's ability to comprehend
   Understands simple commands or ideas
   Able to follow complex instructions or ideas
   Sometimes able to follow instructions or ideas
   Not able to follow simple instructions or ideas

Understands only if hearing aid is working
Understands only if he can see your mouth (lip-reads)
Talks, rather than listens
3. What is the person's developmental age?

Child	Adult
Adolescent	Aged

4. Describe the person's ability to make sentences

Good	Unclear ideas	Can make short,
Slow	Nonsensical or	simple sentences
Weak	confused	Language barrier

5. How does the person's affect or manner appear to you?

Nervous	Fearful	Pained
Anxious	Withdrawn	Uncomfortable
Attentive	Flat	Comfortable

6. Does the person maintain eye contact?

Good	Occasional	None	Blind

7. Are there contributing factors that may inhibit the person's ability to communicate (See Related Factors)?

Principles and Rationale for Nursing Care

Generic Considerations

1. Effective communication is an interactive process involving the *mutual exchange* of information (thoughts, ideas, feelings, and perceptions) between two or more people. This process can be hampered by problems with *sending* or *receiving* messages, or both.
2. Speech represents humans' fundamental way of expressing needs, desires, and feelings. Poor communication can cause feelings of frustration, anger, hostility, depression, fear, confusion, and isolation.
3. After survival, perhaps the most basic human need is to communicate with others. Communication provides a sense of security to patients that they are not alone and that there are people who will listen (Beck, 1988).
4. If only one person expresses information, without any feedback from the listener(s), effective communication cannot be said to have taken place.
5. Problems with *sending* information can be caused by any of the following:
   a. Inability or failure to send messages that can be clearly understood by the listener, *e.g.,* due to language problems, word-meaning problems, failure to speak when the listener is ready to listen
   b. Fear of being overheard, judged, or misunderstood, *e.g.,* due to lack of privacy, confidentiality, trust, or nonjudgmental attitude
   c. Concern over the response to what is being said, *e.g.,* "I don't want to hurt anyone's feelings or "make anyone angry at me."
   d. Use of words that "talk down" to the individual receiving the message, *e.g.,* talking to an elderly or handicapped person as if he were a child
   e. Failure to allow sufficient time for listening to or providing feedback
   f. Physical problems that interfere with the ability to see, talk, or move
6. Problems with *receiving* information can be caused by:
   a. Language or vocabulary problems
   b. Fatigue, pain, fear, anxiety, distractions, attention span problems
   c. Nonrealization of the importance of the information
   d. Physical problems that interfere with the ability to see or hear

7. The meaning of messages is affected not only by the choice of words, but also by the loudness and intonation of voice, the proximity of the communicators, and the use of body language, eye contact, and gestures. Words that express *approval or acceptance* can be negated by body language, facial expressions, and eye contact that express *disapproval*.
8. Mutual understanding of communication can be enhanced by the use of both verbal *and* written messages. Important information should be written down, mutually discussed, and made readily available for later reference.
9. Good communicators are also good listeners, who listen for both facts and feelings.
10. "Presencing," or just being present and available, even if little is said or done, can be an effective way of communicating caring for another individual.

Principles For Special Communication Problems

Hearing Loss

1. Speech-reading (or lip-reading) takes a great deal of skill and concentration. Only about 30% of English sounds are visible on the lips (DiPietro, Knight, & Sans, 1981). Pain, stress, or fatigue may impair the ability to read lips.
2. People who suffer from deafness are prone to social isolation because of their difficulty in communicating with people who can hear normally.
3. Many people over 65 suffer from some sort of hearing loss.
4. Hearing aids *all* magnify sounds. Therefore extraneous sounds (*e.g.*, rustling of papers, minor squeaks, etc.) can inhibit understanding of voiced messages.
5. Deafness can disrupt the reciprocal relationship necessary in the health care process (DiPietro, Knight, & Sans, 1981).
6. Deaf individuals are often deprived of the benefits of exposure to discussions of health on TV, radio, at home, work or school (DiPietro, Knight, & Sans, 1981).
7. Many deaf persons do not know their medical histories or medical terminology (DiPietro, Knight, & Sans, 1981).
8. It has been reported that 32.9% of deaf respondents reported that they only understood some or very little of what hospital staff said.
9. Most deaf persons can talk, but many choose not to speak in public.
10. Speech-reading is difficult and fatiguing in the hospital. Unfamiliar terminology, anxiety, and poor lighting all can contribute to errors.
11. Writing messages is slow, causing a tendency to abbreviate messages. Moreover, expressing emotions in writing is difficult.
12. Limited educational experience may compromise a deaf person's ability to read or write. The average prelingually deaf adult reads on only a fourth-grade level (DiPietro, Knight, & Sans, 1981).

Dysarthria/Aphasia

1. Dysarthria is a disturbance in the voluntary muscular control of speech caused by conditions such as Parkinson's disease, multiple sclerosis, myasthenia gravis, cerebral palsy, and CNS damage. The same muscles are used in eating and swallowing. Persons with dysarthria usually do not have problems with comprehension.
2. Aphasia is an altered ability to communicate because of cerebral damage. The alterations can be verbal, gestural, visual, or graphic.
3. Expressive aphasia is a disturbance in the ability to speak, write, or gesture understandably.
4. Receptive aphasia is a disturbance in the ability to comprehend written and spoken language.

5. The person with receptive aphasia may have intact hearing but cannot process or is unaware of his own sounds.
6. People with head trauma or aphasia may have difficulty with retention and memory recall. Old memories may return first, with memory recall of recent events returning last.
7. Emotional lability (swings between crying and laughing) is common to persons with aphasia. This behavior is not intentional and declines with recovery.

Cultural or Foreign Language Barriers

1. Knowledge of a foreign language depends on four elements: the knowledge of how to speak the language in conversation, the ability to understand the language in conversation, the ability to read the language, and the ability to write the language.
2. An answer of "yes" from a foreigner may be an effort to please rather than a sign of understanding what has been said.
3. Even though the nurse cannot speak another's language, she can convey a climate of acceptance by talking in a pleasant tone of voice and using actions to demonstrate meaning (*e.g.*, smiling and motioning to sit down, while saying, "Sit down, please.")
4. An attempt on the nurse's part to communicate over a language barrier encourages a foreign individual to do the same.
5. People should overcome the human tendency either to ignore or shout at people who do not speak the dominant language.
6. Appropriate distance between communicators varies from culture to culture. Some may normally stand face to face, whereas others must stand several feet apart to be comfortable.
7. Communicating through the use of touch or holding varies from culture to culture. For example, some cultures view touching as an extremely familiar gesture, some cultures shy away from touching a given part of the body (a pat on the head may be offensive), and some cultures consider it appropriate for men to kiss each other and for women to hold hands.

Pediatric Considerations

1. Communication with children must take into account developmental stage, language abilities, and cognitive level (Hunsberger, 1989; Whaley & Wong, 1989).
2. Communication with children involves verbal and nonverbal aspects. Although the majority of verbal communication occurs between the nurse and parents, the child's verbal input should not be ignored. Writing, drawing, play, and using body language (facial expressions, gestures) are forms of nonverbal communication used by the child (Whaley & Wong, 1989).
3. In children, receptive language is always more advanced than expressive language; children understand more than they can articulate (Hunsberger, 1989). (See Table II-7 in the diagnostic category *Growth and Development, Altered,* under "Language/ Cognition.")
4. Communication impairment may result from learning disability, speech impairment, or hearing loss (Wong & Whaley, 1990).
5. The child with hearing loss may exhibit alterations in the following responses.
   a. Orientation response, *e.g.*, lack of startle reflex to a loud sound
   b. Vocalizations and sound production, *e.g.*, lack of babbling by age 7 months
   c. Visual attention, *e.g.*, responding more to facial expression than verbal explanation
   d. Social/emotional behavior, *e.g.*, becomes irritable at inability to make self understood (Hunsberger, 1989).

6. Numerous screening tests are available to assist the nurse in detecting communication impairment. Appropriate referrals should be made (Wong & Whaley, 1990).

Gerontologic Considerations

1. Elderly persons are at higher risk for presbycusis, a progressive bilateral, symmetrical hearing loss of high-pitched frequencies. This difficulty can begin in the middle years; however, most persons wait for 5 to 10 years before seeking medical evaluation (Corbin, Reed, Nobbs, Eastwood, & Eastwood, 1985; Matteson & McConnell, 1988; Rappaport, 1984).

2. About 40% of people over age 65 have a significant hearing impairment that interferes with communication in general. Prevalence data probably overestimate hearing impairment due to problems with testing; however, prevalence from 31%– 87% has been documented in the well elderly. About 90% of all nursing home residents over age 65 have a hearing impairment (Matteson & McConnell, 1988; Voeks, Gallagher, Langer, & Drinka, 1990).

3. Community surveys have indicated 20%–30% of the elderly report hearing impairments, but the actual number based on pure-tone audiometry was as high as 60%. Pure-tone threshold sensitivy usually decreases with age, more rapidly in males than in females (Corbin, Reed, Nobbs, Eastwood, & Eastwood, 1985; Thomas, Hunt, Garry, Hood, Goodwin, & Goodwin, 1983).

4. Loss of elasticity in the cartilaginous portion of the pinna and external auditory canal is the most significant change in the ear that occurs as a result of aging. This loss of resilience can occlude the ear canal and affect sound transmission. High-frequency hearing loss occurs (Rappaport, 1984).

5. Six general classes of morphologic changes in the auditory pathways are considered a function of age:
   a. Sensory presbycusis: atrophy and degeneration of cells in the cochlea
   b. Metabolic presbycusis: atrophy of the stria vascularis affects the biochemical and bioelectrical abilities of the cochlea
   c. Mechanical presbycusis: reduction in the vibratory capabilities of the cochlea
   d. Neural presbycusis: loss of neurons of the 8th nerve
   e. Vascular presbycusis: loss of blood supply to cochlea
   f. Central presbycusis: loss of neurons in the auditory pathway of the brain stem and cortex (Rappaport, 1984)

6. Cerumen impaction is increased in the elderly, especially men. A smaller number of ceruminal glands and decreased activity results in production of drier ear wax. Increased coarseness and length of hairs on the lateral external canal impede the natural dislodgment of the cerumen in men (Rappaport, 1984; Moon, 1990).

7. Approximately 34% of elderly persons have never had audiometric testing. Communication problems start to occur when the hearing threshold level is at 40 dB hearing level, which is approaching moderate hearing loss (Moon, 1990; Voeks, Gallagher, Langer, & Drinka, 1990).

8. Hearing loss really does not have significance until it has an effect on the individual's activities of daily living, at which point it is designated as a functional hearing handicap. Older individuals in a protected environment may function adequately with hearing levels above 25 dB, even though levels beyond that are considered abnormal (Voeks, Gallagher, Langer, & Drinka, 1990).

9. Only 18%–20% of older persons with hearing impairments wear hearing aids. Elderly persons who wear hearing aids must be encouraged to use them consistently, clean and maintain them, and replace batteries. They should be assertive in letting significant others know about situations and environmental areas in which they

experience difficulty with enhancement of background noise while wearing the aid (Ayers, 1990; Irvine, 1982; Moon 1990).

10. Aural rehabilitation in the elderly is difficult because visible aids are linked with body image and self-concept, negative experience with an aid which was purchased without audiology work-up, difficulty manipulating controls on the aid, situating the aid properly, and replacing batteries. Poor tolerance of amplification after years of progressive hearing loss is also a factor in adjusting to the aid. Dexterity must be considered when choosing a hearing aid. For a rehabilitation program to be successful, the individual must accept that there is a hearing deficit and be motivated to do something about it (Matteson & McConnell, 1988; Moon, 1990; Rappaport, 1984).

11. There is a social stigma attached to hearing loss that is not associated with vision deficits as evidenced by disguising some aids within eyeglasses (Rappaport, 1984).

12. For loss in hearing sensitivity by audiogram there is a disproportionate decrease in ability to discriminate speech in elderly, hearing-impaired individuals. This difficulty is related to degeneration of the 8th nerve, auditory brain stem, and auditory cortex. The ability to discriminate speech decreases with age. There are two tests that measure speech discrimination. The Speech Reception or Spondee Threshold Test measures ability to discern two-syllable words at frequency ranges made up of the acoustic spectrum. The Word Discrimination Test assesses the ability of an individual to identify words of one syllable at a normal level of speech in a quiet setting (Moon, 1990; Rappaport, 1984).

13. Speech-reading, any visual information provided by the speaker's face or body, is often useful for the hearing impaired in determining the content of a spoken message. Individuals with decreased vision and short-term memory deficits, often found in the elderly, have a greater difficulty with speech-reading. Longer stimulus durations are needed to identify visual forms than in individuals with no memory deficit. A vision-impaired individual is at greater risk of hearing impairment because he depends on visual cues to locate noise direction (Ebersole & Hess, 1990; Irvine, 1982; Moon, 1990).

14. Paranoia is a significant concern because the older hearing-impaired individual often suspects that others are talking about him (Hogstel, 1990; Irvine, 1982).

15. Reduced auditory acuity has a positive correlation with social isolation. Understanding speech in group conversations has been identified as a prime area of hearing difficulty for older individuals. Some older individuals choose to withdraw from social gatherings because of the frustration they feel in asking people to repeat what has been said. Likewise, some friends and family will refrain from entertaining hearing-impaired individuals because they have labeled them as distant because they do not participate in dialogue or turn their heads away during conversation. Others are thought to have mental impairments because of inappropriate comments during conversation and irritability and inattention (Corbin, Reed, Nobbs, Eastwood, & Eastwood, 1985; Vaughn, Lightfoot, & Teter, 1988; Voeks, Gallagher, Langer, & Drinka, 1990).

16. Environmental sounds (*e.g.,* such as rippling water, hum of traffic) help individuals keep in touch with the environment. When these sounds cannot be heard, the older individual is at risk of dissociation from the active world. This can lead to depression (Rappaport, 1984).

17. Excessive environmental noise and dim lighting place the older person at risk for hearing impairment (Voeks, Gallagher, Langer, & Drinka, 1990).

18. Many older persons have been exposed to higher noise levels in occupational settings prior to OSHA requirements for ear protection. Certain medications used in past years have since been found to produce ototoxicity and have been virtually eliminated as treatment regimens or else now require careful dosing and monitoring.

Before immunization was available against measles, many persons suffered resultant hearing loss (Moon, 1990).

19. Limited finances and poor insurance coverage place the older person at risk for not being able to procure appropriate assistive devices and hearing aids.

20. The best predictors of quality of life in women aged 54 and older were found to be social hearing handicap (negative influence), functional social support, and perceived health (positive influences). Individuals who had later onset of hearing loss demonstrated lower perception of quality of life (Magilvy, 1985).

21. Older people have a higher prevalence of chronic conditions that can interfere with speech or understanding of speech. Some of these conditions are Parkinson's disease (1% of individuals over age 60 in the United States), Alzheimer's disease (15% of those over age 65), cerebrovascular accidents (75% of all strokes occur in individuals over age 65), structural changes due to head and neck cancer, and functional voice disorders of inadequate loudness or quality due to vocal abuse (Matteson & McConnell, 1988).

22. Long-term use of certain psychotropic agents can result in dysarthria. The elderly are at increased risk; 75% of persons over age 65 take either prescribed or over-the-counter medications. Psychoactive drugs are commonly among those prescribed (Hogstel, 1990).

■ Impaired Communication
Related to Effects of Hearing Loss

Assessment

Subjective Data

The person reports that he has difficult hearing.
The person reports that he should be wearing a hearing aid.
The person uses sign language/gestures only.

Objective Data

The person wears a hearing aid.
The person does not respond to sound/voices.
The person responds inappropriately to spoken words.
The person is inattentive much of the time.
The person shouts much of the time.

Outcome Criteria

The person will
- Wear a hearing aid (if appropriate)
- Receive messages through alternative methods (*e.g.*, written communication, sign language, speaking distinctly into "good" ear)
- Relate/demonstrate an improved ability to communicate

Interventions

A. Elicit from the person what mode of communication is desired and record on care plan the method to be used by staff and by person:

 1. Writing
 2. Speech-reading (or lip-reading)
 3. Speaking
 4. Sign language

B. Assess the person's ability to receive verbal messages

 1. If he can hear with a hearing aid, make sure that it is on and functioning.
    a. Check batteries by turning volume all the way up until it whistles. (If it does not whistle, new batteries should be inserted.)
    b. Make sure volume is at a level that enhances hearing. (Many people with hearing aids turn the volume down from time to time for peace and quiet.)
    c. Make a special effort to have the patient wear his hearing aid on off-the-unit visits. (For example, the hearing aid should be on when the patient goes for special studies, or to the operating room, and the chart should be flagged so that everyone is aware of this.)
 2. If he can hear with only one ear, speak slowly and *clearly* directly into the good ear. (It is more important to speak *distinctly* than to speak loudly.)
    a. If the person is admitted to the hospital, place him so that his good ear faces the door.
    b. Approach the person from the side on which he hears best (*e.g.*, if he hears better with his left ear, approach him from the left).
 3. If the person can speech-read
    a. Look directly at the person and talk slowly and clearly.
    b. Avoid standing in front of light—have the light on your face so that the person can see your lips.
    c. Minimize distractions that may inhibit the person's concentration.
       • Minimize conversations if the person is fatigued or use written communication.
       • Reinforce important communications by writing them down.
 4. If he can read and write, provide pad and pencil at all times (even when he goes to the radiology department, etc.).
 5. If he can understand only sign language, have an interpreter with him as much as possible. Address all communication to the person not to the interpreter, *e.g.*, do not say "ask Mrs. Jones . . ."
 6. If the person is in a group (*e.g.*, diabetes class), place him in the front of the room near the teacher.

C. Utilize factors that promote hearing and understanding

 1. Talk distinctly and clearly, facing the person.
 2. Minimize unnecessary sounds in the room:
    a. Have only one person talk.
    b. Be aware of background noises (*e.g.*, close the door, turn off the television or radio).
 3. Repeat, then rephrase a thought, if the person does not seem to understand the whole meaning.
 4. Use touch and gestures to enhance communication.
 5. Encourage the person to maintain contact with other deaf people to minimize feelings of social isolation.

6. Write as well as speak all important messages.
7. Validate the person's understanding by asking questions that require more than "yes" or "no" answers. Avoid asking "Do you understand?"

■ Impaired Communication
Related to Effects of Aphasia on Expression or Interpretation

---

Aphasia is a communication impairment—a difficulty in expressing, a difficulty in understanding, or a combination of both—resulting from cerebral impairments.

Assessment

Subjective Data

The person reports:
    An inability to express self
    A difficulty in responding verbally
    History of
        Cerebrovascular accident
        Tumor
        Cerebral trauma/increased intracranial pressure

Objective Data

    Slurred speech
    Unintelligible speech/absent speech
    Inappropriate responses to questions

Outcome Criteria

The person will
  • Demonstrate increased ability to understand
  • Demonstrate improved ability to express himself
  • Relate decreased frustration with communication

Interventions

A. Identify a method the person can use to communicate basic needs
    1. Assess ability to comprehend, speak, read, and write.
    2. Provide alternative methods of communication.
        a. Use pad and pencil, alphabet letters, hand signals, eye blinks, head nods, bell signals.
        b. Make flash cards with pictures or words depicting frequently used phrases (*e.g.*, "Wet my lips," "Move my foot," glass of water, bedpan).

    c. Encourage person to point, use gestures, and pantomime.

    d. Consult with speech pathologist for assistance in acquiring flash cards.

B. Identify factors that promote communication

  1. Create atmosphere of acceptance and privacy.

  2. Provide a nonrushed environment.

    a. Use normal loudness level and speak slowly in short phrases.

    b. Encourage the person to take his time talking and to enunciate words carefully with good lip movements.

    c. Decrease external distractions.

    d. Delay conversation when the person is tired

  3. Assess the individual's frustration level and do not push beyond it.

    a. Estimate 30 seconds of passed time before providing the individual with the word he may be trying to find (except when the person is frustrated or needs the request immediately, *e.g.*, bedpan).

    b. Provide cues through pictures or gestures.

  4. Use techniques to increase understanding.

    a. Face the individual and establish eye contact if possible.

    b. Use uncomplicated one-step commands and directives.

    c. Have only one person talk (it's more difficult to follow a multisided conversation).

    d. Encourage the use of gestures and pantomime.

    e. Match words with actions; use pictures.

    f. Terminate conversation on a note of success (*e.g.*, move back to an easier item).

    g. Validate that message is understood.

C. Use techniques that enhance verbal expression

  1. Make a concerted effort to understand when the person is speaking.

    a. Allow enough time to listen if the person speaks slowly.

    b. Rephrase messages aloud to validate what was said.

    c. Respond to all attempts at speech even if they are unintelligible (*e.g.*, "I do not know what you are saying. Can you try to say it again?").

    d. Acknowledge when you understand and do not be concerned with imperfect pronunciation at first.

    e. Ignore mistakes and profanity.

    f. Do not pretend you understand if you do not.

    g. Observe the person's nonverbal cues for validation (*e.g.*, he answers yes and shakes his head no).

    h. Allow the person time to respond; do not interrupt; supply words only occasionally.

  2. Teach techniques to improve speech.

    a. Ask the person to slow speech down and say each word clearly, while providing the example.

    b. Encourage the person to speak in short phrases.

    c. Explain to the person that his words are not clearly understood (*e.g.*, "I can't understand what you are saying").

    d. Suggest a slower rate of talking or taking a breath prior to speech.

    e. Encourage the person to take his time and concentrate on forming his words.

    f. Ask the person to write down his message, or to draw a picture, if verbal communication is difficult.

g. Encourage the person to speak in short phrases.

h. Ask questions that can be answered with a yes or no.

i. Focus on the present; avoid topics that are controversial, emotional, abstract, or lengthy.

D. Acknowledge the individual's frustration

1. Verbally address the problem of frustration over inability to communicate, and explain that patience is needed for both the nurse and the person who is trying to talk.

2. Maintain a calm, positive attitude (*e.g.*, "I can understand you if we work at it").

3. Use reassurance (*e.g.*, "I know it's hard, but you'll get it"); use touch if acceptable.

4. Maintain a sense of humor.

5. Allow tears (*e.g.*, "It's OK. I know it's frustrating. Crying can let it all out").

6. For the person who has a limited ability to talk (*i.e.*, can make simple requests, but not lengthy statements), encourage writing letters or keeping a diary to ventilate feelings and share concerns.

7. Give the person opportunities to make decisions about his care (*e.g.*, "Do you want a drink? Would you rather have orange juice or prune juice?").

8. Provide alternative methods of self-expression
   a. Humming/singing
   b. Dancing/exercising/walking
   c. Writing/drawing/painting/coloring
   d. Helping (tasks such as opening mail, choosing meals)

E. Identify factors that promote comprehension

1. Assess hearing ability and use of functioning hearing aids.

2. Assess ability to see, and encourage the person to wear his glasses.
   a. Explain to the person that seeing better will increase understanding of what is happening around him.
   b. Even if the person is blind, look at him when talking to "throw" voice in his direction.

3. Provide sufficient light and remove distractions (see *Sensory-Perceptual Alterations*).

4. Speak when the person is ready to listen.
   a. Achieve eye contact, if possible.
   b. Gain the person's attention by a gentle touch on the arm and a verbal message of "Listen to me" or "I want to talk to you."

5. Modify your speech.
   - Speak slowly, enunciate distinctly.
   - Use common adult words.
   - Do not change subjects or ask multiple questions in succession.
   - Repeat or rephrase requests.
   - Do not increase volume of voice unless person has a hearing deficit.
   - Match your nonverbal behavior with your verbal actions to avoid misinterpretation (*e.g.*, do not laugh with a coworker while performing a task).
   - Try to use the same words with the same task (*e.g.*, bathroom vs. toilet, pill vs. medication).
   - Keep a record at bedside of the words to maintain continuity.
   - As the person improves, allow him to complete your sentences (*e.g.*, "This is a . . . [pill]").

6. Use other methods of communication besides verbal.

       a. Use pantomine

       b. Point

       c. Use flash cards

       d. Show him what you mean (*e.g.,* pick up a glass)

       e. Write key words on a card, so he can practice them while you show the object (*e.g.,* paper, toilet)

F. Show respect when providing care

1. Avoid discussing the person's condition in his presence; assume he can understand despite his deficits.
2. Monitor other health care providers.
3. Talk to the person whenever you are with him.

G. Initiate health teaching and referrals if indicated

1. Teach techniques to significant others and repetitive approaches to improve communications.
2. Encourage the family to share feelings concerning communication problems.
   a. Explain the reasons for labile emotions and profanity.
   b. Explain the need to include the person in family decision-making.
3. Seek consultation with a speech pathologist early in treatment regime.

■ Impaired Communication
Related to Foreign Language Barrier

Assessment

Subjective Data

The person states
    "I don't understand . . . [name of language]"
    "I don't speak . . . [name of language]"

Objective Data

Foreign accent
Absence of speech
Body language only means of communication (person only nods or gestures)

Outcome Criteria

The person will
- Be able to communicate basic needs
- Relate feelings of acceptance, reduced frustration and isolation

Interventions

A. Assess the individual's ability to communicate in English.*

1. Assess what language the person speaks best.
2. Assess the person's ability read, write, speak, and comprehend English.

B. Identify factors that promote communication through a language barrier when a translator is not present

1. Face the person and give a pleasant greeting, in a normal tone of voice.
2. Talk clearly and somewhat slower than normal (do not overdo it).
3. If the person does not understand or speak (respond), use an alternative method of communication.
   a. Try writing down message.
   b. Use gestures or actions.
   c. Use pictures or drawings.
   d. Make flash cards that translate words or phrases.
4. Encourage the person to also use the aforementioned methods of communication (try to overcome shyness).
5. Encourage the person to teach others some of the words or greetings of his own language (this helps to promote a feeling of acceptance and a willingness to learn).

C. Be cognizant of possible cultural barriers

1. Be careful when touching the person, for it may not be appropriate in some cultures.
2. Be aware of the different ways that men and women are expected to be treated (cultural differences may influence whether a man speaks to a woman about certain matters, or vice versa).
3. Make a conscious effort to be nonjudgmental about another's cultural differences.
4. Make note of what seems to be a comfortable distance from which to speak.

D. Initiate referrals when needed

1. Use a *fluent* translator when discussing matters of importance (such as taking a health history or signing an operation permit).
2. If possible, allow the translator to spend as much time as the person wishes (be flexible with visitor's rules and regulations).
3. If a translator is not available, try to plan a daily visit from someone who has some knowledge of the person's language (many hospitals and social welfare offices keep a "language" bank with names and phone numbers of people who are willing to translate).

*English will be used as an example of the dominant language.

Communication, Impaired Verbal

■ *Related to* **The Effects of Mechanical Devices or Neurologic Impairment**

DEFINITION

Impaired verbal communication: The state in which the individual experiences, or is at high risk to experience, a decreased ability to speak but can understand others.

DEFINING CHARACTERISTICS

Major (one must be present)
    Inability to speak words but can understand others
    Articulation or motor planning deficits

Minor (may be present)
    Shortness of breath

RELATED FACTORS

See *Impaired Communication*

Focus Assessment Criteria

See *Impaired Communication*

Principles and Rationale for Nursing Care

See *Impaired Communication*

■ ## Impaired Verbal Communication
Related to the Effects of Mechanical Devices or Neurologic Impairment

Assessment

Subjective Data

The person reports inability or difficulty in pronouncing words

Objective Data
    Difficulty in pronouncing words
    Inability to use voice
        Postlaryngectomy   Tracheostomy
        Intubation   Decreased ventilatory capacity

> **Outcome Criteria**
>
> The person will
> - Demonstrate improved ability to express self
> - Relate decreased frustration with communication

Interventions

A. Identify a method by which person can communicate his basic needs

1. Assess ability to comprehend, speak, read, and write.
2. Provide alternative methods of communication.
   a. Use pad and pencil, alphabet letters, hand signals, eye blinks, head nods, bell signals.
   b. Make flash cards with pictures or words depicting frequently used phrases (*e.g.,* "Wet my lips," "Move my foot," glass of water, bedpan).
   c. Encourage the person to point, use gestures, and pantomime.
   d. Consult with a speech pathologist for assistance in acquiring flash cards.

B. Identify factors that promote communication

1. For individuals with dysarthria
   a. Reduce environmental noise to increase the caregiver's ability to listen to words (*e.g.,* radio, TV).
   b. Do not alter your speech or messages, since his comprehension is not affected; speak on an adult level.
   c. Encourage the person to make a conscious effort to slow down his speech and to speak louder (*e.g.,* "Take a deep breath between sentences").
   d. Ask him to repeat words that are unclear; observe for nonverbal cues to help understanding.
   e. If he is tired, ask questions that require only short answers.
   f. If speech is unintelligible, teach the person to use gestures, written messages, and communication cards.
2. For individuals who cannot speak (*e.g.,* endotracheal intubation, tracheostomy)
   - Reassure that his speech will return, if it will.
   - If not, explain what alternatives are available (*e.g.,* esophageal speech, sign language).
   - Do not alter your speech, tone, or type of message, since the person's ability to understand is not affected; speak on an adult level.
   - Read lips for cues.

C. Promote continuity of care to reduce frustration

1. Observe for signs of frustration or withdrawal.
   a. Verbally address the problem of frustration over inability to communicate, and explain that patience is needed for both the nurse and the person who is trying to talk.
   b. Maintain a calm, positive attitude (*e.g.,* "I can understand you if we work at it").
   c. Use reassurance (*e.g.,* "I know it's hard, but you'll get it").
   d. Maintain a sense of humor.
   e. Allow tears (*e.g.,* "It's OK. I know it's frustrating. Crying can let it all out").
   f. For the person who has a limited ability to talk (*e.g.,* can make simple

requests, but not lengthy statements), encourage writing letters or keeping a diary to ventilate feelings and share concerns.

    g. Anticipate needs and ask questions that need a simple yes or no answer.

2. Maintain a specific care plan.

    a. Write the method of communication that is used (*e.g.,* "Uses word cards," "Points to night stand for bedpan").

    b. Record directions for specific measures to reduce communication problems (*e.g.,* allow him to keep urinal in bed).

D. Initiate health teaching and referrals as indicated

1. Teach significant others techniques and repetitive approaches to improve communications.
2. Encourage the family to share feelings concerning communication problems.
3. Seek consultation with a speech pathologist early in the treatment regimen.

References/Bibliography

Communication, Impaired

Anderson, J. (1987). The cultural context of caring. *Canadian Critical Care Nurse Journal, 4*(4), 7–13.

Ayers, R. E. (1990). Getting the job done: Helping hands in geriatric primary care. *Geriatrics, 45*(2), 78.

Beck, C., & Heacock, P. (1988). Nursing interventions for patients with Alzheimer's disease. *Nursing Clinics of North America, 23*(1), 96–99.

Benner, P. (1984). *From novice to expert.* Menlo Park, CA: Addison-Wesley.

Boczko, F. (1987). The talking cure: Communication group in long term care. *Nursing Homes, 36*(6), 26–27.

Bushweller, E. (1984). Bridging the communication gap. *Nursing, (14)*9, 112.

Campbell, S. (1984). Some sound advice for managing a hearing impaired patient. *Nursing, (14)*12, 46.

Conture, E. (1982), *Stuttering.* Englewood Cliffs, NJ: Prentice-Hall.

Cunliffe, P. (1989). Communicating with children in the intensive care unit . . . triadic relationship of child/parent/nurse. *Intensive Care Nurse, 3*(2), 71–77.

DiPietro, L. Knight, C., Sans, J. (1981). Health care delivery for deaf patients: The provider's role. *Annals of the Deaf, 126*(4), 106–112.

Dreber, B. (1981). Overcoming speech and language disorders. *Geriatric Nursing, 2,* 345–349.

Ebersole, P., & Hess, P. (1990). *Toward healthy aging: Human needs and nursing response.* St. Louis: C. V. Mosby.

Faller, H. (1988). A child's perception of the hospital. *American Journal of Maternal-Child Nursing, 13*(1), 38.

Foster, S. (1988). When the message gets garbled. *American Journal of Material-Child Nursing, 13*(5), 367.

Goetler, W. (1986). Nursing diagnoses and interventions with the acute stroke patient. *Nursing Clinics of North America, 21*(2), 309–318.

Hanawalt, A. & Troutman, K. (1984). If your patient has a hearing aid. *American Journal of Nursing, 7,* 900–901.

Heinrich, K. (1988). What's my type? Teaching interviewing skills. *Nursing Education 84*(23), 24–27.

Hogstel, M. O. (1990). *Geropsychiatric nursing.* St. Louis: C. V. Mosby.

Hunsberger, M. (1989). Communicating with children and families. In Foster R. L., Hunsberger M. M. & Andreson J. J. T. (Eds.). *Family-centered nursing care of children.* Philadelphia: W. B. Saunders.

Hunsberger, M. (1989). Nursing strategies: Sensory and communication alterations. In Foster, R. L., Hunsberger, M. M. & Anderson J. J. T. (Eds.). *Family-centered nursing care of children.* Philadelphia: W. B. Saunders.

Irvine, P. W. (1982). The hearing-impaired elderly patient. *Postgraduate Medicine, 72*(4), 115–118.

Jungman, L. (1979). When your feelings get in the way. *American Journal of Nursing, 79,* 1074–1075.

Leonard, R. (1985). Speak for yourself. *Nursing. 15*(11), 30–31.

Lombardino, L., et al. (1987). Evaluating communicative behaviors in infancy. *Journal of Pediatric Health Care, 1*(5), 240–246.

Loveridge, L., et al. (1988). Confirming interactions. *Journal of Gerontological Nursing, 14*(5), 27–30.

Magilvy, J. K. (1985). Quality of life of hearing-impaired older women. *Nursing Research, 34*(3), 140–144.

Matteson, A. M., McConnell, E. S. (1988). *Gerontological nursing: Concepts and practice.* Philadelphia: W. B. Saunders.

McAlvanah, M. (1988). Communication: A two way street. *Pediatric Nurse, 14*(2), 140.

Moon, E. (1990). Otology. In Cassel, C. K., Riesenberg, D. E., Sorensen, L. B., & Walsh, J. R. (Eds.). *Geriatric medicine* (2nd ed.). New York: Springer-Verlag.

Norris, M. L., & Cunningham, D. R. (1981). Social impact of hearing loss in the aged. *Journal of Gerontology, 36*(6), 727–729.

Patry-Lahey, R. (1985). Helping a laryngectomy patient go home. *Nursing, 15*(3), 63–64.

Phillips, A. (1987). Clearing a path to communication: Dementia—how you can help. *Geriatric Nursing Home Care, 7*(11), 16–18.

Rappaport, B. Z. (1984). Audiology. In Cassel, C. K., Walsh, J. R. (Eds.). *Geriatric medicine, medical, psychiatric and pharmacological topics.* New York: Springer-Verlag.

Santopietro, M. (1981). How to get through to a refugee patient. *Nursing, 11*(1), 43–48.

Staff. (1986). Clinical news: The speaking endotracheal tube. *American Journal of Nursing (86), 11,* 1095.

Staffe, D. (1985). More than a touch: Communicating with a blind and deaf patient. *Nursing, 15*(8), 36–39.

Stovsky, B., Rudy, E., & Dragonette, P. (1988). Comparison of two types of communication methods used after cardiac surgery with patients with endotracheal tubes. *Heart & Lung, 17*(3), 281–289.

Thomas, P., Hunt, W., Garry, P. J., Hood, R. B., Goodwin, J. M. & Goodwin, J. S. (1983). Hearing acuity in a healthy elderly population: Effects on emotion, cognitive and social status. *Journal of Gerontology, 38*(3), 321–325.

Van Riper, C. (1982). *Speech correction* (6th ed.). Englewood Cliffs, NJ: Prentice-Hall.

Vaughn, G. R., Lightfoot, R. K., & Teter, D. L. (1988). Assistive listening devices and systems enhance the lifestyles of hearing impaired persons. *American Journal of Otology, 9*(suppl), 101–106.

Voeks, S. K., Gallagher, C. M., Langer, E. H., & Drinka, P. J. (1990). Hearing loss in the nursing home: An institutional issue. *Journal of American Geriatrics Society, 38,* 141–145.

Watkins, S., et al. (1984). Clearing impacted ears. *American Journal of Nursing, 84*(9), 1107.

Weinhouse, I. (1981). Speaking to the needs of your aphasic patient. *Nursing, 11*(3), 34–36.

Whaley, L. F., & Wong, D. L. (1989). *Essentials of pediatric nursing* (3rd ed.). St. Louis: C. V. Mosby.

Wilson, D. (1989). My trips over the language barrier. *American Journal of Nursing, 12,* 1718.

Wong, D. L., & Whaley, L. F. (1990). *Clinical manual of pediatric nursing* (3rd ed.). St. Louis: C. V. Mosby.

Workman, D., et al. (1988). The microcomputer as an aid to written communication. *British Journal of Occupational Therapy, 51*(6), 188–190.

Resources for the Consumer

Organizations

Agency for Hearing Loss, Write: Alexander Graham Bell Association, 3417 Volta Place N.W., Washington, DC 20007

American Annals of Deaf, 814 Thayer Ave, Silver Spring, MD 20910

Resource Guide for Persons with Speech, Language or Hearing Impairments, P.O. Box 2150, Atlanta, GA 30301-2150

Coping, Ineffective Individual

Defensive Coping

Ineffective Denial

Coping, Ineffective Individual

■ *Related to* **Depression in Response to Identifiable Stressors**

DEFINITION
Ineffective individual coping: A state in which the individual experiences, or is at high risk to experience, an inability to manage internal or environmental stressors adequately due to inadequate resources (physical, psychological, behavioral and/or cognitive).

DEFINING CHARACTERISTICS*

Major (one must be present)
> Change in usual communication patterns (if acute)
> Verbalization of inability to cope
> Inappropriate use of defense mechanisms
> Inability to meet role expectations

Minor (may be present)
> Anxiety
> Reported life stress
> Inability to solve problems
> Alteration in social participation
> Destructive behavior toward self or others
> High incidence of accidents
> Frequent illnesses
> Verbalization of inability to ask for help
> Verbal manipulation
> Inability to meet basic needs

RELATED FACTORS

Pathophysiologic
> Changes in body integrity
>> Loss of body part
>> Disfigurement secondary to trauma

*Adapted from Vincent (see Bibliography)

Altered affect caused by changes in body chemistry
   Tumor (brain)
   Injection of mood-altering substance
Physiologic manifestations of persistent stress
Severe or fatal illness (*e.g.,* AIDS, cancer)

Situational (personal, environmental)

Changes in physical environment
   War
   Natural disaster
   Relocation

   Seasonal work (migrant worker)
   Poverty
   Homelessness
   Inadequate finances

Disruption of emotional bonds due to
   Death
   Separation or divorce
   Desertion

   Relocation
   Incarceration

Unsatisfactory support system
Institutionalization
   Jail
   Foster home, orphanage

   Educational institution
   Institution for disabled

Sensory overload
   Factory environment

   Urbanization: crowding, noise
      pollution, excessive activity

Inadequate psychological resources
   Poor self-esteem
   Excessive negative beliefs about
      self

   Helplessness
   Lack of motivation to respond
   Immature developmental level

Culturally related conflicts with life experiences
   Premarital sex
   Abortion
   Unrealistic expectations

Treatment-related

Separation from family and home (*e.g.,* hospitalization, nursing home)
Conflict between need for medical treatment and culture
Disfigurement due to surgery
Altered appearance due to drugs, radiation, or other treatment
Altered affect due to hormonal therapy
Sensory overload due to medical technology (*e.g.,* critical care units)
Early discharge from hospital

Maturational

Child
   Developmental tasks
      (independence vs. dependence)
   Entry into school

   Competition among peers
   Peer relationships

Adolescent
   Physical and emotional changes
   Independence from family
   Heterosexual relationships

   Sexual awareness
   Educational demands
   Career choices

Young adult
    Career choices
    Educational demands
    Leaving home
Middle adult
    Physical signs of aging
    Career pressures
    Child-rearing problems
Elderly
    Physical changes
    Changes in financial status
    Change in residence

Marriage
Parenthood
Intimate relationships

Problems with relatives
Social status needs
Aging parents

Retirement
Response of others to older people
Multiple stressful events

Diagnostic Considerations

Ineffective Individual Coping describes an individual experiencing difficulty in adapting to stressful event(s). Usual effective coping mechanisms may be inappropriate or ineffective for this event, or the person may have a poor history of coping with stressors.

If the event is recent, ineffective individual coping may be a premature judgment. For example, a person may respond to overwhelming stress with a grief response such as denial, anger, or sadness, making a *Grieving* diagnosis appropriate.

Impaired Adjustment may be more useful than *Ineffective Individual Coping* in the initial period following a stressful event. *Ineffective Individual Coping* and its related diagnoses may be more applicable to prolonged or chronic coping problems, *e.g., Defensive Coping* for a person with a long-standing pattern of ineffective coping.

Errors in Diagnostic Statements

Ineffective Individual coping related to perceived effects of breast cancer on life goals, as evidenced by crying and refusal to talk

If this diagnosis was recent, the person's response of crying and refusal to talk would be normal grief responses. Thus, the proper diagnosis would be *Grieving related to perceived effects of breast cancer on life goals*. If this response was prolonged and evidence of "moving ahead" was not present (*e.g.,* initiation of social activities), *Ineffective Individual Coping* would be appropriate.

Ineffective Individual Coping related to reports of substance abuse

Substance abuse is a reportable or observable cue validating a diagnosis. If the person acknowledged the abuse and desires assistance, the diagnosis would be *Ineffective Individual Coping related to inability to manage stressors without drugs*. If the substance abuse was observed but the person denied that it existed or that it was a problem, the diagnosis would be *Ineffective Denial related to unknown etiology as evidenced by lack of acknowledgment of drug dependency*.

Focus Assessment Criteria

Ineffective coping can be manifested in a variety of ways. A person or family may respond with an alteration in another life process (*e.g.,* spiritual distress, altered parenting, potential for violence). The nurse should be aware of this and use assessment data to ascertain the dimensions affected.

Subjective Data

Stressors

- Current/recent stressors (number, type, duration)
- Assess major life events and everyday stresses
- Social—financial change, job pressure, marital/family conflicts, role changes, retirement, pregnancy, marriage, divorce, aging, school, death
- Psychological—anxiety, depression, low self-esteem, lacks interpersonal skills, loneliness
- Environmental—moving, hospitalization, loss of privacy, sensory deprivation/overload
- Physiologic—presence of stress-related symptoms

    Cardiovascular

Headache	Palpitations
Chest pain	Fainting (blackouts, spells)
Increased pulse	Increased blood pressure

    Respiratory

Shortness of breath	Chest discomfort
Smoking history	(pain, tightness, ache)
Increased rate and depth of breathing	

    Gastrointestinal

Nausea	Change in appetite
Vomiting	Change in stool
Abdominal pain (cramps, stomach ache)	Obesity/frequent weight changes

    Musculoskeletal

Pain	Fatigue
Weakness	

    Genitourinary

Menstrual changes	Sexual difficulty (pain,
Urinary discomforts (pain, burning, urgency, hesitancy)	impotence, altered libido, anorgasmia)

    Dermatologic

Itching	"Sweats"
Rash	Ecezma

    Mental health

Phobias	"The blues"
Panic	"Bad nerves"
Insomnia	

- Perception of stressor

    How did you feel when this occurred? (Threatened or challenged?)
    How do you feel now?
    How have these stressors affected you?
    How are the problems working out?

Coping Strategies

- How did you relieve tension in above situation(s)? (Ways of coping adapted from Lazarus & Folkman, 1984)

    Analyzed problem
    Made a plan of action
    Compromised

Stood my ground and fought
Read about the problem and possible solutions
Turned to work (other activities) to take my mind off it
Talked to someone about the problem, sought professional help
Talked to myself about the problem
Ignored it, tried to forget it
Took a vacation
Avoided people/subject/situation
Used alcohol/drugs/medication
Increased or started smoking
Tried something new
Prayed
Kept my feelings to myself
Imagined things were different
Daydreamed
Accepted it, since I could do nothing about it
Changed something about myself/job
Exercised
Compared myself with others
- In similar situations:
  Tried to find a reason
  Blamed myself
  Prepared myself for the worst
  Made light of situation (humor)
  Ate more than usual
  Slept more than usual
  Other (describe)
- Alcohol/drug history
  Types of substance taken? Prescribed? Over-the-counter? Street?
  How often?   How long?
  How much?   Route?
  Time of last dose of each substance?
  Has using this substance presented any problems?

Objective Data

Appearance
    Altered affect ("poker" face)   Poor grooming
    Appropriate   Inappropriate dress
Behavior
    Calm   Tearful
    Hostile   Sudden mood swings
    Withdrawn
Cognitive function
    Altered orientation to time, place, person
    Impaired concentration
    Altered ability to solve problems
    Impaired memory
    Impaired judgment
Abusive behaviors
    To self
        Excessive smoking
        Excessive alcohol intake

Excessive food intake
Drug abuse
Reckless driving
Suicide attempts
Unsafe sexual practices
To others
Does not care
Neglects needs of dependent family members
Is unwilling to listen
Does not communicate
Imposes physical harm on family member (bruises, burns, broken bones)
Unsafe sexual practices

Principles and Rationale for Nursing Care

Generic Considerations

1. Lazarus (1985) defines coping as "constantly changing cognitive and behavioral efforts to manage specific external and/or internal demands that are taxing or exceeding the resources of the person."
2. Effectiveness of coping is influenced by the number, duration, and intensity of the stressors; past experiences; support system; and personality of the individual (Fuller & Schaller-Ayers, 1990).
3. Coping effectively requires successful management of many tasks: maintenance of self-concept, maintenance of satisfying relationships with others, maintenance of emotional balance, and management of stress.
4. Expectations of mastery encourage maturation and persistence. Expectations of failure induce avoidance behaviors (Potocki & Everly, 1989).
5. Coping behaviors fall into two broad categories (Lazarus & Folkman, 1984):
   a. Problem-focused: Efforts to improve the situation by changing things or taking some action
   b. Emotion-focused: Those thoughts or actions that relieve the emotional distress caused by the situation. Emotion-focused coping behaviors do not alter the situation, but do make the person feel better.
   Examples include:

Problem-focused	*Emotion-focused*
Make appointment with the boss to discuss pay raise	Play basketball three times per week
Write out time schedule for homework and adhere to it	Denying anything is wrong
Studying	Using alcohol/drugs to relax
Seeking help	Joking

6. Emotion-focused behaviors include the following:
   a. *Minimization* occurs when the seriousness of a problem is minimized. This may be useful as a way to provide needed time for appraisal, but it may become dysfunctional when it precludes appraisal.
   b. *Projection, displacement,* and *suppression of anger* occur when anger is attributed to or expressed toward a less threatening person or thing, which may reduce the threat enough to allow an individual to deal with it. Distortion of reality and disturbance of relationships may result, which further compound the problem. Suppression of anger may result in stress-related physical symptoms.

    c. *Anticipatory preparation* is the mental rehearsal of possible consequences of behavior or outcomes of stressful situations, which provides the opportunity to develop perspective as well as to prepare for the worst. It becomes dysfunctional when the anticipation creates unmanageable stress, as, for example, in anticipatory mourning.

    d. *Attribution* is the finding of personal meaning in the problem situation, which may be religious faith or individual belief. Examples are fate, the will of the divine, luck. Attribution may offer consolation but becomes maladaptive when all sense of self-responsibility is lost.

7. Problem-focused behaviors include the following:

    a. *Goal-setting* is the conscious process of setting time limitations on behaviors, which is useful when goals are attainable and manageable. It may become stress-inducing if unrealistic or short-sighted.

    b. *Information-seeking* is the process of learning about all aspects of a problem, which provides perspective and, in some cases, reinforces self-control.

    c. *Mastery* is the learning of new procedures or skills, which facilitates self-esteem and self-control: for example, self-care of colostomies, insulin injection, or catheter care.

    d. *Help-seeking* is the reaching out to others for support. Sharing feelings with others provides an emotional release, reassurance, and comfort, as, for example, with Weight Watchers and other self-help and support groups.

8. Persons use various processes to cope with stress. These processes are continually changing as the situation evolves. Any change in the person–environment relationship leads to a reevaluation of the situation, which in turn influences subsequent coping efforts (Lazarus & Folkman, 1984).

9. Coping strategies vary depending on the stage of the event. Each stage requires its own unique processes. During anticipation, the appraisal processes focus on: Will it happen? Can it be prevented? Can it be postponed? During and after impact, thoughts and actions are directed toward: What is the significance? What new challenges are imposed? Have things changed appreciably? (Lazarus & Folkman, 1984).

10. Appraisal is the thought process that evaluates the situation. Constructive realistic appraisal strategies can be facilitated with the following questions: What is at stake? What are the choices? Where is there help? Appraisal and reappraisal are ongoing coping techniques.

11. Cognitive adaptation to threatening events (*e.g.,* illness) focuses on searching for meaning, gaining control over the situation, and comparing one's situation with others (Taylor, 1983). For example, clients adjusting after an acute myocardial infarction attempt to regain control. How these clients perceive the situation depends on the stage of the process; thus, coping mechanisms change throughout the process. Initially, clients distance themselves. Next, they seek causal explanations, minimizing uncertainty by establishing guidelines for living. In the final stage, they accept limitations and refocus from the heart to other areas of life (Johnson & Morse, 1990).

12. The low prevalence of clinical depression in end-stage renal disease clients has been hypothesized to be the result of defensive denial. That is, the situation is simply too threatening to be included in conscious awareness (Bink, Devins, & Orme, 1989).

13. Addictive behavior is a habitual maladaptive way of coping with stress.

14. Interpersonal skill deficits interact with genetic vulnerability and situational demands to interfere with effective coping, leading to alcohol/substance abuse (Monti, Abrams, Kadden, & Cooney, 1989).

15. To facilitate client coping, the nurse must focus on "the thoughts and actions

individuals engage in to overcome threats to health, and deal with life crises encountered, in order to attain or retain optimal health and functioning" (Nyamathi, 1989).

16. Individuals who work through the anticipated event (*e.g.,* retirement, surgery) are more likely to cope more effectively than those who avoid thinking about the upcoming event (Fiske, 1980).

17. According to Miller (1990), individuals "who have a rigid set or narrow range of coping skills are at more risk for impaired coping because of different types of coping strategies are effective in different situations."

Stress

1. Stress may be defined as the nonspecific response of the body to any demand (Selye, 1974).

2. Stress and disease maybe linked in three ways:
   a. Overstimulating a target organ through the neuroendocrine system
   b. Engaging in styles of living that are damaging, such as pressured life-style, poor diet, heavy use of tobacco or drugs
   c. Minimizing the significance of symptoms, leading to neglect or delay in seeking medical care (Monat & Lazarus, 1985).

3. Responses to stress vary among individuals due to personal perceptions of the event. Both positive and negative life events may initiate a stress response.

4. The stress response can initiate growth and learning.

5. The physiologic signs and symptoms of stress result from activation of the neuroendocrine and sympathetic nervous systems (see Physiologic: Presence of stress-related symptoms). In addition, both cognitive and behavioral changes occur (see anxiety principles) (Cotton, 1990).

6. Stress management techniques fall into three categories (Monat & Lazarus, 1985):

Life-style	*Personality/perceptions*	*Biologic responses*
Time management	Assertiveness	Relaxation
Proper nutrition	Thought stopping	Meditation
Exercise	Refuting irrational	Breathing exercises
Stop smoking/drink-	beliefs	Biofeedback
ing, etc.	Stress inoculation	

Refer to Appendix X for a further discussion of these techniques.

Denial

1. Denial is a set of dynamic processes that protect the person from a threat to self-esteem.

2. The cost and/or benefits of denial must be evaluated in terms of the situation and resources available (Lazarus, 1985).

3. Denial is common in the grieving process.

4. When action is essential to change a threatening or damaging situation, then denial is maladaptive; however, when no action is needed or when the outcome cannot be changed, then denial can be positive and can help reduce stress (Lazarus, 1985).

5. Partial, tentative, or minimal denial allows the person to use problem-focused coping skills while reducing the distress (an emotion-focused coping skill) of the situation (Lazarus, 1985).

6. When a particular stress is encountered repeatedly, denial prevents mastery of the situation (Lazarus, 1985).

7. Denial may be valuable in the early stages of coping when resources are not sufficient to manage more problem-focused approaches (Lazarus, 1985).
8. Denial can take several forms:
   a. Denial of relevance to the person
   b. Denial of immediacy of the threat
   c. Denial of responsibility
   d. Denial that threat is anxiety provoking
   e. Denial of threatening information
   f. Denial of any information
9. Denial in alcoholism may include denial of loss of control, of family pain, or of the alcoholic's part in the family problem.
10. Denial of alcohol/drug abuse may also be present among relatives and colleagues, as it is difficult to accept (Sullivan, Bissell, & Williams, 1988).
11. Alcohol and drug abuse is reinforced by the drug itself (*e.g.*, feelings of being high, increased congeniality, gaining attention) or avoiding unpleasant situations. Treatment approaches must be aimed at removing identified reinforcers (Washton, 1989).

Depression

1. Reactive depression occurs as a response to a situational stressor.
2. Endogenous depression, possibly somatic in origin, is a maladaptive response to often unidentifiable causes.

Reactive vs. Endogenous Depression

Element	Reactive Depression	Endogenous Depression
Precipitating event	Identifiable	Unclear
Family history	Unrelated	Familial tendency
Symptoms	Related to grief and anxiety; worse at night	Seemingly unrelated to events; worse in morning
Activity	Diminished motor and cognitive behavior	Agitated, restless
Emotion	Client feels sad	Alternates between sadness and manic gaiety
Cognitive abilities	May be slightly diminished	Retarded psychomotor performance
Orientation	Oriented and responsive to environment	May not be oriented or responsive
Treatment	Responds well to counseling and environmental change	Requires somatic treatment

Pediatric Considerations

1. A child's ability to cope is affected by inborn traits, social support, and family coping (Whaley & Wong, 1989).
2. Children who are more vulnerable to stress and demonstrate poorer coping skills include males, those between age 6 months and 4 years, those with a difficult temperament, and those with below-average intelligence (Whaley & Wong, 1989).
3. As children mature, they develop and expand their coping strategies (Byrne & Hunsberger, 1989).

See Pediatric Considerations for nursing diagnostic category *Adjustment, Impaired.*

Gerontologic Considerations

1. Miller (1990) identified six major psychosocial challenges of older adults: retirement, death of friends, chronic illness, relocation from family, disruption of household, and stereotypes associated with 65th birthday.
2. Folkman, Lazarus, Pimley, & Novacek (1987) reported that younger subjects reported more stressors related to finances and work while older subjects reported stress related to concerns about health, home maintenance, and social and environmental issues.
3. Anticipation and perceived control over circumstances are predictors of the impact of stress for elderly persons (Willis, Thomas, Garry, & Goodwin, 1987).
4. In older adults, coping is facilitated in those with higher incomes, higher occupational status, and feelings of high self-efficacy. However, when significant life changes are necessary, higher occupational status and feelings of high self-efficacy were liabilities, because these individuals bring an unrealistic view of what is controllable (Simons & West, 1984).
5. No one life event has a consistently negative impact on an older adult; rather, a number of events in a short period of time represents the greatest challenge (Miller, 1990).
6. The choice of coping mechanisms depends on the type of stress and the person's level of maturity rather than on age (Folkman, Lazarus, Pimley, & Novacek, 1987).

■ Ineffective Individual Coping
Related to Depression in Response to Identifiable Stressors

Assessment

Subjective Data

The person verbalizes feelings of
Failure ("I should have . . .)
Sadness, blues
Loneliness
Worry, fear

Vague confusion
Helplessness ("I can't . . . ")
Hopelessness, apathy
Preoccupation with self

The person describes symptoms of
Fatigue
Constipation or diarrhea
Insomnia or excessive sleep
Anorexia
Headache
Dry mouth

General pain
Stiffness
Menstrual changes
Dizziness, numbness
Frequent crying episodes (or desire to cry)

Objective Data

Physical symptoms
Rashes
Tachycardia

Lusterless eyes
Weight changes

Emotional symptoms
   Distressed, tearful, sad   Altered affect
Altered cognitive ability
   Inability to concentrate   Difficulty with problem-solving
   Poor memory   Inability to make decisions
Physical appearance
   Poor personal hygiene   Poor nutrition
   Lack of grooming

Outcome Criteria

The person will
 • Verbalize feelings related to his emotional state
 • Identify his coping patterns and the consequences of the behavior that results
 • Identify personal strengths and accept support through the nursing relationship
 • Make decisions and follow through with appropriate actions to change provocative situations in personal environment

---

Interventions

A. Assess causative and contributing factors

   1. Negative self-concept
   2. Moral or ethical conflict (see *Spiritual Distress*)
   3. Disapproval by others
   4. Inadequate problem-solving
   5. Loss-related grief (see *Grieving*)
   6. Sudden change in life pattern
   7. Recent change in health status of self or significant other
   8. Inadequate support system

B. Assess for risk factors for poor coping in older adults (Miller, 1990)

   1. Inadequate economic resources
   2. Immature developmental level
   3. Unanticipated stressful events
   4. Occurrence of several major events in short period of time
   5. Unrealistic goals

C. Assess individual's present coping status

   1. Determine onset of feelings and symptoms and their correlation with events and life changes.
   2. Assess ability to relate facts.
   3. Listen carefully as client speaks, to collect facts and observe facial expressions, gestures, eye contact, body positioning, tone and intensity of voice.
   4. Determine risk of client's inflicting self-harm and intervene appropriately.
      a. Assess for signs of potential suicide.
         • History of previous attempts or threats (overt and covert)
         • Changes in personality, behavior, sexual life, appetite, sleep habits

- Preparations for death (putting things in order, making a will, giving away personal possessions, acquiring a weapon)
- A sudden elevation in mood

   b. Demonstrate to client that you believe him and desire to help.
- Avoid challenging him, minimizing his feelings, arguing, or trying to reason with him.
- Listen attentively and stay close until the danger has passed or help is secured.

   c. Offer support as client talks.
- Reassure him that the feelings he has must be difficult.
- When client is pessimistic, attempt to provide a more hopeful, realistic perspective.

   d. See *High Risk for Self-harm* for additional information on suicide prevention

D. Teach constructive problem-solving techniques

1. Assist the person to problem-solve in a constructive manner.
   a. What is the problem?
   b. Who or what is responsible for the problem?
   c. What are his options? (Make a list.)
   d. What are the advantages and disadvantages of each option?
2. Discuss possible alternatives (*i.e.,* talk over the problem with those involved, try to change the situation, or do nothing and accept the consequences).
3. Assist the individual to identify problems that he cannot control directly and help him to practice stress-reducing activities for control (*e.g.,* exercise program, yoga); see Appendix VII for problem-solving techniques.
4. Instruct client in relaxation techniques; emphasize the importance of setting 15–20 minutes aside each day to practice relaxation. Write down the following guidelines (see Appendix X for additional relaxation techniques).
   a. Find a comfortable position in chair or on floor.
   b. Close eyes.
   c. Keep noise to a minimum (only very soft music if desired).
   d. Concentrate on breathing slowly and deeply.
   e. Feel the heaviness of all extremities.
   f. If muscles are tense, tighten, then relax, each one from toes to scalp.

E. Assist client to develop appropriate strategies based on his personal strengths and previous experiences

1. Have client describe previous encounters with conflict and how he managed to resolve them.
2. Encourage client to evaluate his own behavior.
   a. "Did that work for you?"
   b. "How did it help?"
   c. "What did you learn from that experience?"
3. Be supportive of functional coping behaviors.
   a. "Your way of handling this situation 2 years ago worked well for you then, can you do it now?"
   b. Give options; however, the decision-making must be left to the client.
4. Mobilize the client into a gradual increase in activity.
   a. Identify activities that were previously gratifying but have been neglected: personal grooming or dress habits, shopping, hobbies, athletic endeavors, arts and crafts.

   b. Encourage client to include these activities in daily routine for a set time span ("I will play the piano for 30 minutes every afternoon").
   c. Stress importance of activity in helping one recover from depression; state that depression is immobilizing and that client must make a conscious effort to fight it in order to recover.
5. Find outlets that foster feelings of personal achievement and self-esteem.
   a. Make time for relaxing activities (*e.g.*, dancing, exercising, sewing, woodworking).
   b. Find a helper to take over responsibilities from time to time (get a babysitter).
   c. Learn to compartmentalize (do not carry problems around with you all the time; enjoy free time).
   d. Take longer vacations (not just a few days here and there).
   e. Provide opportunities to learn and use stress management techniques (*e.g.*, jogging, yoga; see also Appendix X).
6. Facilitate emotional support from others:
   a. Seek out people who share a common challenge: establish telephone contact, initiate friendships within the clinical setting, develop and institute educational and support groups.
   b. Establish a network of people who understand your situation.
   c. Decide who is best able to act as a support system (do not expect empathy from people who themselves are overwhelmed with their own problems).
   d. Make time to share personal feelings and concern with coworkers (encourage ventilation; frequently people who share the same circumstances are helpful to one another).
   e. Maintain a sense of humor.
   f. Allow tears.

F. Assist client to cope with a recent diagnosis of cancer, as appropriate:
   1. Encourage ongoing appraisal/reappraisal with client about the meaning of the diagnosis.
      a. Nature of the disease: procedures, sensations associated with diagnostic and treatment modalities, side effects, prognosis
      b. Impact on family relationships, friendships, and professional and recreational activities
      c. Sources of help (see D.6 above)
   2. Maximize self-care at home and at treatment center to encourage independence and mobility, improve self-esteem, and decrease feelings of powerlessness.
      a. Allow flexibility in appointments
      b. Give as many choices possible
   3. Promote hopefulness and setting of realistic goals with client and family.
      a. Demonstrate empathy
      b. Provide ongoing client education
      c. Listen effectively
   4. Encourage use of ambulatory services whenever possible to allow client to remain at home.
   5. Coordinate multidisciplinary activities to serve the client's best interests and provide continuity of care.

G. Initiate health teaching and referrals as indicated
   1. For depression-related problems beyond the scope of nurse generalists, refer to appropriate professional (marriage counselor, psychiatric nurse therapists, psychologist, psychiatrist).

Defensive Coping

■ *Related to* **(Specify)**

DEFINITION
Defensive coping: The state in which an individual repeatedly projects falsely positive self-evaluation as a defense against underlying perceived threats to positive self-regard.

DEFINING CHARACTERISTICS*

Major (80%–100%)
   Denial of obvious problems/weaknesses
   Projection of blame/responsibility
   Rationalizes failures
   Hypersensitive to slight criticism
   Grandiosity

Minor (50%–79%)
   Superior attitude toward others
   Difficulty in establishing/maintaining relationships
   Hostile laughter or ridicule of others
   Difficulty in testing perceptions against reality
   Lack of follow through or participation in treatment or therapy

RELATED FACTORS
See *Chronic Low Self-esteem*

Diagnostic Considerations
See *Ineffective Individual Coping*

Focus Assessment Criteria
See *Ineffective Individual Coping*

Principles and Rationale for Nursing Care
See *Ineffective Individual Coping*

*Source: Norris, J. & Kunes-Connell, M. (1987) Self-esteem disturbance: A clinical validation study. In McLane, A. (Ed.). *Classification of nursing diagnoses: Proceedings of the seventh conference*. St. Louis: C. V. Mosby.

■ Defensive Coping
Related to (Specify)

Assessment
See Defining Characteristics

Outcome Criteria

The person will
- Verbalize a realistic perception of self with strengths and limitations
- Identify consequences of his behavior

Interventions

A. Provide opportunities to channel emotional and physical energy
  1. Provide paper and pen for writing thoughts and feelings.
  2. Encourage noncompetitive activities, avoid activities that require concentration and attention to rules.
  3. Use brief, one-to-one interactions during time when person is easily distracted; increase time as attention span increases.

B. Decrease environmental stimuli
  1. Be aware of how person is responding to stimuli (*e.g.*, increase in loudness, activity, irritability).
  2. Decrease noise, visitors, and other persons in environment.
  3. Avoid group activities when individual is easily distractible.

C. Assist in appropriate expression of thoughts and feelings
  1. Clarify what is being said (*e.g.*, "Who are 'they'?").
  2. Validate your interpretation ("Is this what you mean?").
  3. Refocus conversation so that only one topic at a time is discussed.
  4. Let the person know when you are unable to follow the flow of conversation.

D. Assist person to realistically evaluate his behavior
  1. Direct conversation from a delusional orientation to a reality-based one.
  2. Tactfully express doubt about reality distortions.
  3. Have person examine the consequences of his grandiose/ambitious acts.

E. Provide positive socialization experiences
  1. See *Altered Thought Processes* related to *Inability to Evaluate Reality* for interventions.

F. Be aware of your own reactions
  1. Don't take verbal abuse personally; respond in a matter-of-fact attitude.
  2. Talk over with team members to prevent manipulation.
  3. Be consistent in your approach.

4. Define acceptable behavior.
5. Enforce established limits.

G. Maintain physical safety and health

1. Ensure adequate rest periods.
2. Ensure adequate elimination pattern.
3. Provide high-calorie, high-protein foods.
4. Monitor for weight loss.
5. Use foods and liquids that are easily digested.
6. Observe for signs and symptoms of infections or illness.
7. Assist with grooming.

H. Initiate health teaching

1. Teach
   a. The importance of taking medication even when the patient feels good
   b. Medication side effects, toxic effects and associated care such as routine blood levels
2. Explain that feelings of grandiosity may lead to overspending and personal risks.
3. Describe clues that will indicate the need for professional help (*e.g.,* promiscuity, alcohol/drug overuse, insomnia, euphoria, overspending).

Ineffective Denial

■ *Related to* **Impaired Ability to Accept Consequences of His/Her Behavior as Evidenced by Lack of Acknowledgment of Substance Abuse/Dependency**

DEFINITION

Ineffective denial: The state in which an individual minimizes or disavows symptoms or a situation to the detriment of his health.

DEFINING CHARACTERISTICS*

Major (80%–100%)

Delays seeking or refuses health care attention to the detriment of health
Does not perceive personal relevance of symptoms or danger

---

*Source: Norris, J. & Kunes-Connell, M. (1987). Self-esteem disturbance: A clinical validation study. In McLane, A. (Ed.). *Classification of nursing diagnoses: Proceedings of the seventh conference*. St. Louis: C. V. Mosby.

Minor (50%–79%)

Uses home remedies (self-treatment) to relieve symptoms
Does not admit fear of death or invalidism
Minimizes symptoms
Displaces source of symptoms to other areas of the body
Unable to admit impact of disease on life pattern
Makes dismissive gestures or comments when speaking of distressing events
Displaces fear of impact of the condition
Displays inappropriate affect

RELATED FACTORS

Pathophysiologic

Any chronic and/or terminal illness

Treatment-related

Prolonged treatment with no positive results

Situational/Psychological

Loss of job
Loss of spouse/significant other
Financial crisis
Feelings of negative self-concept, inadequacy, guilt, loneliness, despair, sense of failure
Feelings of increased anxiety/stress, need to escape personal problems, anger and frustration
Feelings of omnipotence
Culturally permissive attitudes toward alcohol/drug use
Religious sanctions

Maturational

Adolescence: peer pressure
Adulthood: job stress, expectation of alcohol/drug use, losses (job, spouse, children)
Elderly: losses (spouse, function, financial), retirement

Biologic/Genetic

Family history of alcoholism

Diagnostic Considerations

This type of denial differs from the denial in response to a loss. The denial in response to an illness or loss is necessary to maintain psychologic equilibrium and is beneficial. Ineffective denial is not beneficial when the individual will not participate in regimens to improve health or the situation (*e.g.*, denial of substance abuse). If the cause of the ineffective denial is not known, *Ineffective Denial related to unknown etiology* can be utilized; for example, *Ineffective Denial related to unknown etiology as evidenced by repetitive refusal to admit barbiturate use is a problem.*

Errors in Diagnostic Statements

See *Ineffective Individual Coping*

Focus Assessment Criteria

See *Ineffective Individual Coping*

Principles and Rationale for Nursing Care

See *Ineffective Individual Coping*

■ Ineffective Denial
Related to Impaired Ability to Accept Consequences of His/Her Behavior as Evidenced by Lack of Acknowledgment of Substance Abuse/Dependency

Assessment

Subjective Data

The person will
    Deny that alcohol/drug use is problematic
    Justify his use of alcohol/drugs
    Blame others for his use of alcohol/drugs
    Verbalize need of daily use
    Report unsuccessful attempts to reduce or stop use
    Express grandiosity, inflated self-esteem
    Express suspiciousness
    Report need for increased amount to achieve same effect (tolerance)
    Frequent complaints of illness and/or marital problems

Objective Data

The person will demonstrate interference in:
    Occupational functioning
        Absenteeism
        Frequent unexplained brief absences
        Elaborate excuses for tardiness/absence
        Daytime fatigue
        Failed assignments
        Loss of job
    Social functioning
        Mood swings
        Isolation (avoidance of others)
        Arguments with mate/friends
        Violence while intoxicated
        Traffic accidents/citations
        Legal difficulties
        Boisterousness/talkativeness
        Impulsiveness
        Poor judgement
        Apathy
        Signs of intoxication, overdose

Physical complications
    Alcohol abuse
        Blackout
        Memory impairment
        Decreased sensation in lower extremities
        Malnutrition
        Impatience
        Unsteady gait
        Liver dysfunction
        Gout symptoms
        Anemia
        Gastritis/gastric ulcers
        Pancreatitis
        Cardiomyopathy
        Withdrawal symptoms (*e.g.,* tremors, nausea, vomiting, increased blood pressure, pulse, sleep disturbances, disorientation, hallucinations, agitation, seizures)
    Opiate abuse
        Drowsiness
        Slurred speech
        Pupillary constriction
        Impaired memory
        Slowed motor movements
        Malnutrition
        Infections (*e.g.,* pneumonia, TB, skin abscesses)
        Liver disease
        Low testosterone levels
        Gastric ulcers
        Respiratory depression
        Constipation
        Tetanus
        Decreased response to pain
        Withdrawal symptoms (*e.g.,* tearing, runny nose, dilated pupils, mild hypertension, tachycardia, nausea, vomiting, restlessness, joint pain)
    Amphetamine and cocaine abuse
        Increased alertness
        Decreased appetite
        Increased heart rate
        Dilated pupils
        Chills
        Nausea and vomiting
        Hepatitis
        Tetanus
        Infections and abscesses associated with self-injections
        CVA
        Hallucinations
        Cardiac dysrhythmias
        Seizures
        Respiratory depression
    Hallucinogen abuse
        Increased heart rate

Sweating
Palpitations
Blurred vision
Tremors
Incoordination
Hallucinations
Flashbacks
Cannabis abuse
Increased heart rate
Conjunctival injection
Increased appetite
Impaired lung structure
Sinusitis
Possible impaired sperm production and chromosomal damage
Barbiturate/sedative/hypnotic abuse
Drowsiness
Impaired memory
Cellulitis
Hepatitis
Endocarditis
Pneumonia
Respiratory depression
Signs of intoxication and withdrawal similar to alcohol abuse

---

Outcome Criteria

The person will
- Admit to an alcohol/drug abuse problem
- Explain the psychologic and physiologic effects of alcohol and/or drug use
- Abstain from alcohol/drug use
- States recognition of the need for continued treatment
- Express a sense of hope
- Use alternative coping mechanisms to cope with stress

Interventions

A. Assist to improve self-esteem

1. Be nonjudgmental.
2. Assist person in gaining an intellectual understanding that this is an illness, not a moral problem.
3. Provide opportunities to perform successfully; gradually increase responsibility.
4. Provide educational information about the progressive nature of substance abuse and its effects on the body and interpersonal relationships.
5. Refer to *Self-Esteem Disturbance* for further interventions.

B. Instill a sense of hope

1. Maintain a positive attitude.
2. Communicate the expectation that person can overcome problems.

3. Set realistic, short-term goals.
4. Facilitate interactions with persons who have recovered or are recovering.
5. Refer to *Hopelessness* for further interventions.

C. Assist in identifying and altering patterns of substance abuse

1. Identify situations when the user is expected to use alcohol/drugs (*e.g.*, at home with TV, after work with friends).
2. Encourage avoidance of situations when alcohol/drugs are being used.
3. Assist person in replacing drinking/smoking buddies with nonusers (AA/NA are helpful alternatives here. Each AA/NA group is unique; encourage person to find a group he is comfortable with.)
4. Assist in organizing and adhering to a daily routine.
5. Have person chart his alcohol/drug use (amount, time, situation); useful with early-stage substance abusers who are resistant to treatment (Metzger, 1988).

D. Assist in meeting physiologic and safety needs

1. Observe for signs of withdrawal.
2. Provide supportive care through the detoxification period.
3. Prevent access to abused substances. Monitor visitors and belongings.
4. Assess for presence of medical consequences of alcohol/drug use.
   a. Prostatitis
   b. Fetal alcohol syndrome (mental retardation, malformations, hyperactivity, growth deficiency, cardiac problems)
   c. WBC, RBC, platelet deficiencies
   d. Bleeding tendencies (decreased vitamin K production)
   e. Peripheral neuropathy, myopathy
   f. Hypertension
   g. Cardiac tissue damage, cardiomyopathy
   h. Gastritis, pancreatitis
   i. Hepatitis (alcoholic) cirrhosis
   j. Vitamin metabolism defects
   k. Esophageal varices, hemorrhoids, ascites
5. Assess potential for violence, refer to *High Risk for Violence* for further interventions
6. Assess for suicide potential, refer to *High Risk for Self-harm* for further interventions
7. Teach side effects and appropriate interventions associated with medications (*e.g.*, disulfiram [Antabuse], methadone, antianxiety drugs [Librium]

E. Assist person to identify effects of substance abuse on his life and significant others

1. In early stages of abstinence, blaming alcohol for problems may be helpful: avoids guilt and blame (Metzger, 1988).
2. As abstinence becomes more secure, assist person to take responsibility for own choices.
3. Discuss reasons for drug/alcohol use.
4. Explore problems that have resulted from substance abuse (marriage, relationships, work).
5. Assess motivation to stop abuse (*e.g.*, What areas of life are important enough to change for—job, family, health? From his point of view, what does he gain/lose? How does he see life in a few years? Will substance abuse interfere?).

F. Discuss alternative coping strategies

1. Teach relaxation techniques and meditation. Encourage use when he recognizes anxiety. Refer to Appendix X for stress management techniques.
2. Teach thought-stopping techniques to use when thoughts about drinking/substance use occur. Instruct him to say vocally or subvocally "STOP, STOP" and to replace that thought with a positive one. The technique must be practiced and the individual may need assistance in identifying replacement thoughts.
3. Assist in anticipating stressful events (*e.g.,* job, family, social situations) in which alcohol/drug use is expected; role-play alternative strategies.
   a. Teach assertiveness skills.

G. Assist person to achieve abstinence

1. Set short-term goals (*e.g.,* stopping one day at a time versus insisting never to drink/use again).
2. Provide structure (Washton, 1989):
   a. Discard supplies.
   b. Break contact with dealers/users.
   c. Avoid high-risk places.
   d. Help to plan free time.
   e. Avoid large blocks of time without activities.
3. Assist in recognizing stressors that lead to substance abuse (*e.g.,* boredom, the drug, interpersonal situations).
4. Assist person in evaluating the negative consequences of the behavior. Visualization may be helpful.
5. When person denies alcohol/drug use, look for nonverbal clues to substantiate facts (*e.g.,* is there verbal and nonverbal congruence, deteriorating appearance, job performance or social skills?).
6. When on firm ground and a trusting relationship has been established, confront his denial.
7. Discourage person from attempting to correct other problems such as obesity and smoking during this time.
8. Do not attempt to probe past history in early abstinence.

H. Assist in resocialization

1. Involve in groups and in establishing an alcohol/drug-free network.
2. Establish a trusting relationship.
3. Involve the family in the treatment process.

I. Initiate health teaching and referral, as indicated

1. Refer to Alcoholics Anonymous, Alanon, AlaTeen.
2. Refer to treatment facility.
3. Teach side-effects of drug usage.
4. Nutritional counseling

References/Bibliography

General

Anderson, J. (1989). The nurse's role in cancer rehabilitation. *Cancer Nursing, 12*(2), 85–94.

Bink, Y., Devins, G., & Orme, C. (1989). Psychological stress and coping in end-stage renal disease. In Neufeld, R. *Advances in the investigation of psychological stress.* New York: Wiley & Sons.

Byrne, C., & Hunsberger, M. (1989). Concepts of illness: Stress, crisis, and coping. In Foster, R. L. Hunsberger, M. M. & Anderson J. J. T. (Eds.). *Family-centered nursing care of children.* Philadelphia: W. B. Saunders.

Cotton, D. (1990). *Stress management.* New York: Brunner/Mazel.

Derdiarian, A. (1989). Effects of information on recently diagnosed cancer patients' and spouses' satisfaction with care. *Cancer Nursing, 12*(5), 285–292.

Dorin, A. (1978). Adolescent sexuality, adolescent depression. *Pediatric Nursing, 3*(4), 49–50.

Faulk, L. & Bellack, J. (1984). Intrapersonal and interpersonal assessment. In Bellack, J. (Ed.). *Nursing assessment.* Bradford, PA: Wadsworth Health Sciences.

Fiske, M. (1980). Tasks and crises of the second half of life: The interrelationship of commitment, coping, and adaptation. In Birren, J. E. and Sloan, R. B. (Eds.): *Handbook of mental health and aging,* pp 337–373. Englewood Cliffs, NJ: Prentice-Hall.

Folkman, S., Lazarus, R., Pimley, S., & Novacek, J. (1987). Age differences in stress and coping processes. *Psychology and Aging, 2*(3), 171–184.

Forchuk, C., & Westwell, J. (1987). *Journal of Psychosocial Nursing, 25*(6), 9–13.

Fuller, J., & Schaller-Ayer, J. (1990). *Health assessment: A nursing approach.* Philadelphia: J. B. Lippincott.

Hymovich, D. P. (1984). Development of the chronicity impact and coping instrument: Parent questionnaire (C1C1: PQ). *Nursing Research, 33*(4), 218–222.

Johnson, J., & Morse, J. (1990). Regaining control: The process of adjustment after myocardial infarction. *Heart & Lung, 19*(2), 126–135.

Lazarus, R. (1985). The costs and benefits of denial. In Monat, A., & Lararus, R. (Eds.). *Stress and coping: An anthology* (2nd ed.). New York: Columbia.

Lazarus, R., & Folkman, S. (1984). *Stress, appraisal and coping.* New York: Springer.

Lazarus, R. & Folkman, S. (1980). An analysis of coping in a middle-aged community sample. *Journal of Health and Social Behavior, 21,* 219–239.

Maxwell, M. (1980). Cancer and suicide. *Cancer Nursing, 3*(2), 33–38.

Metzger, L. (1988). *From denial to recovery.* San Francisco: Jossey-Bass.

Miller, C. A. (1990). *Nursing care of older adults.* Glenview, IL: Scott & Foresman.

Monat, A., & Lazarus, R. (1985). *Stress and coping: An anthology.* New York: Columbia.

Nyamathi, A. (1989). Comprehensive health seeking and coping paradigm. *Journal of Advanced Nursing, 14*(4), 281–290.

Potocki, E., & Everly, G. (1989). Control and the human stress response. In Everly, G. *A clinical guide to treatment of human stress response.* New York: Plenum Press.

Selye, H. (1974). *Stress without distress.* Philadelphia: J. B. Lippincott.

Simons, R. L., & West, G. E. (1984). Life changes, coping resources and health among the elderly. *International Journal of Aging and Human Development, 20*(3), 173–189.

Taylor, S. (1983). Adjustment to threatening events. *American Psychologist, 38,* 1161–1173.

Tulman, L., & Fawcett, J. (1990). A framework for studying functional status after a diagnosis of breast cancer. *Cancer Nursing, 13*(2), 95–99.

Vincent, K. G. (1985). The validation of a nursing diagnosis. *Nursing Clinics of North America, 20*(4), 631–639.

Whaley, L. F., & Wong, D. L. (1989). *Essentials of pediatric nursing* (3rd ed.). St. Louis: C. V. Mosby.

Willis, L., Thomas, P., Garry, P. J., & Goodwin, J. (1987). A prospective study of response to stressful life events in initially healthy elders. *Journal of Gerontology, 42*(8), 627–630.

Wright, T. (1989). Coping strategies and diastolic blood pressure. *Psychological Reports, 65,* 443–449.

Substance Abuse

Bennett, G. (Ed.). (1989). *Treating drug abusers.* New York: Tavistock.

Finley, B. (1981). Counseling the alcoholic client. *Journal of Psychiatric Nursing, 19*(6), 32–34.

Kurose, K., Anderson, T., Bull, W., et al. (1981). A standard care plan for alcoholism. *American Journal of Nursing, 81,* 1001–1006.

Lecues, J., Dana, R. & Blenius, G. (1988). *Substance abuse counseling: An individualized approach.* Pacific Grove, CA: Brooks/Cole Publishing.

Marks, V. L. (1980; 1981). Health teaching for recovering alcoholic patients. *American Journal of Nursing, 80,* 2058–2061; *81,* 755–757.

Monti, P., Abrams, D., Kadden, R. J., & Cooney, N. (1989). *Treating alcohol dependence.* New York: Greatford Press.

Orief, A., & Westermeyer, J. (Eds.). (1988). *Manual of drug and alcohol abuse.* New York: Plenum Press.

Powell, A., & Minick, M. Alcohol withdrawal syndrome, *American Journal of Nursing, 88*(3), 312–315.

Richard, E., & Shephard, A. C. (1981). Giving up smoking: A lesson in loss theory. *A merican Journal of Nursing, 81,* 755–757.

Schucket, M. (1989). *Drug and alcohol abuse: A clinical guide to diagnosis and treatment* (3rd ed.). New York: Plenum Press.

Sullivan, E., Bissell, L., & Williams, E. (1988). *Clinical dependency in nursing.* Menlo Park, CA: Addison-Wesley.

Waititz, J. (1983). *Adult children of alcoholics.* Pompano Beach, FL: Health Communications.

Washton, A. (1989). *Cocaine addiction: Treatment, recovery and relapse prevention.* New York: Norton.

Wilson, J. (1981). The plight of the elderly alcoholic. *Geriatrics, 2*(2), 114–118.

Resources for the Consumer

Literature

Girdano, D., & Everly, G. (1979). *Controlling stress and tension.* Englewood Cliffs, NJ: Prenti e Hall.

Selye, H. (1974). *Stress without distress.* Philadelphia: J. B. Lippincott.

Newman, M., & Berkowitz, B. (1971). *How to be your own best friend.* New York, Ballantine Books.

Mace, D., & Mace, V. (1977). *How to have a happy marriage.* Nashville: Festival Books.

Simonton, O. C., Simonton, S., & Creighton, J. (1978). *Getting well again.* New York: St. Martin's Press.

Woititz, J., (1983). *Adult children of alcoholics.* Pompano Beach, FL: Health Communications.

Organizations

Drug and Alcohol Nursing Association, Inc., Box 371, College Park, MD 20740

Alcohol, Drug Abuse and Mental Health Administration, Office of Communications and Public Affairs, 5600 Fishers Lane, Room 6C-15, Rockville, MD 20857

National Clearinghouse for Mental Health Information, Public Inquiries Section, 5600 Fishers Lane, Room 11A-21, Rockville, MD 20857

American Cancer Society, 777 3rd Avenue, New York, NY 10017

American Heart Association, 7320 Greenville Avenue, Dallas, TX 75231

American Lung Association, 1740 Broadway, New York, NY 10019

National Interagency Council on Smoking and Health, 291 Broadway, Room 1005, New York, NY, 10007

Coping, Ineffective Family: Disabling

- Related to **(Specify) as evidenced by Domestic Abuse (Adults)**
- Related to **(Specify) as evidenced by Child Abuse/Neglect**
- Related to **Multiple Stressors Associated with Elder Care; High Risk for**

DEFINITION

Ineffective family coping, disabling: The state in which a family demonstrates, or is at high risk to demonstrate, destructive behavior in response to an inability to manage internal or external stressors due to inadequate resources (physical, psychologic, cognitive, and/or behavioral).

DEFINING CHARACTERISTICS

Major (one must be present)

Abusive or neglectful care of the client
Decisions/actions that are detrimental to economic and/or social well-being
Abusive or neglectful relationships with other family members

Minor (may be present)

Distortion of reality regarding the client's health problem
Intolerance
Rejection
Abandonment
Desertion
Psychosomaticism
Taking on illness signs of client
Agitation
Depression
Aggression
Hostility
Impaired restructuring of a meaningful life for self
Prolonged overconcerns for client
Client's development of helpless inactive dependence

RELATED FACTORS

Pathophysiologic

Any condition that challenges one's ability for self-care, for fulfilling role responsibilities, and finances can contribute to *Ineffective Family Coping*

Situational

Change in health status (client, family member)
Changing role within family (*e.g.,* getting a job, going back to school)
Differing religions, cultural backgrounds

Isolation from neighbors, relatives
Ill family member
Use of drugs, alcohol
Family addition (childbirth, aging parent)
Loss of job, inadequate income
Requires frequent assistance (*e.g.,* medications, ADLs)
Arguments about sex

Maturational

Low self-esteem
Physical and emotional adolescent changes
Birth of a sibling
Retirement
Failure to progress in school
Inability of a parent to maintain independence (requires assistance with transportation, ADL, finances)

Other

Unrealistic expectations of child by parent
Unrealistic expectations of self by parent
Unrealistic expectations of parent by child
Unmet psychosocial needs of child by parent
Unmet psychosocial needs of parent by child

Diagnostic Considerations

Ineffective Family Coping: Disabling describes a family with a history of overt or covert destructive behavior or response to a stressor with abuse. This diagnosis necessitates long-term care from a nurse therapist with advanced specialized education in family systems and violence.

The use of this diagnosis in this book will focus on nursing interventions appropriate for a nurse generalist in a short-term relationship (*e.g.,* emergency unit, non-psychiatric in-house unit) and for any nurse in the position to prevent *Ineffective Family Coping* through teaching, counseling, or referrals.

Errors in Diagnostic Statements

Ineffective Family Coping: Disabling related to reports of beatings by alcoholic husband

This diagnostic statement is incorrectly formulated and legally inadvisable for a nurse to write. Reported beatings by an alcoholic husband is not the contributing factor to the diagnosis, but rather a diagnostic cue. This diagnosis should be written as *Ineffective Family Coping: Disabling related to unknown etiology, as evidenced by wife reporting "My husband is an alcoholic and beats me frequently."* The quoted statement represents the data as reported by the wife, rather than the nurse's judgment.

Focus Assessment Criteria

Owing to the complexity and variability of this nursing diagnosis, the nurse must determine the type and extent of the assessment needed with each family.

1. Individual coping patterns of adult members: refer to assessment criteria for *Ineffective Individual Coping*
2. Family coping patterns: refer to assessment criteria for *Altered Family Processes*
3. Parenting patterns: refer to assessment criteria for *Altered Parenting*
4. Violence potential: refer to assessment criteria for *High Risk for Violence*
5. Potential Stressors
   Employment status
      Unemployed
      Job satisfaction
   Housing
      Physical space: adequate, crowded   Privacy
      Cleanliness
   Transportation
      Car   Shared
      Bus
      Dependency on other
      Proximity to work/school/shopping
   Financial
      Resources   Medical expenses
      Additional expenses
   Child/elder care provisions
      Who shares burden
   Change in job/school status
   Legal history
   History of criminal/delinquent
      offenses

Principles and Rationale for Nursing Care

Generic Considerations

Refer to *Altered Family Processes* for principles of the family.
1. Domestic violence/abuse is one expression of a dysfunctional family system. There are numerous other ways dysfunction can be expressed, and this will need to be assessed by nurse.
2. Abuse can take several forms: physical assault, which may or may not result in injury; verbal attacks; isolation; theft of money or property; violation of rights including eviction from own home; forced sexual activity; social and emotional neglect.
3. A dysfunctional system is one in which there is interference with mutual need attainment.
4. Abusive families are characterized by:
   a. Poor differentiation of individuals within the family
   b. Lack of autonomy
   c. Family is insulated from the influence of others; socially isolated
   d. Desperate competition for affection and nurturance among members
   e. Feelings of helplessness and hopelessness
   f. Abuse/violence learned as a way to reduce tension
   g. Low frustration tolerance; poor impulse control
   h. Closeness and caring confused with abuse/violence
   i. Communication patterns are characterized by mixed and double messages

    j. High level of conflict surrounding family tasks

    k. Parental coalition is nonexistent

5. Impulse control can be diminished by neurologic impairment or alcohol/drug abuse.
6. The role of the victim is a critical factor in the occurrence of child and spouse abuse. The role is socially learned and characterized by helplessness. This occurs when victims learn over time that they cannot control their lives (Shapiro, 1984).
7. The process of generational inversion creates problems in that some parents have difficulty accepting that their children are adults.
8. Elderly are increasingly vulnerable to abuse as they become economically, physically, socially, and emotionally more dependent and resources of the caretakers are limited.
9. The intensity of the reaction to an abusive experience indicates the degree of critical life issues and may be compounded by previous unresolved conflicts.
10. Guilt reactions are common among victims. They frequently feel responsible for the incident. This helps to protect them against feelings of powerlessness.
11. Elderly individuals are reluctant to report abuse for fear of retaliation, exposure of their child to legal/community censure, and fear of removal from the home.

Spouse Abuse

1. Spouse abuse in the form of beatings occurs in 1% of all families. Fifty percent of American families are disrupted by some form of violence. Fifteen percent of all homicides are spouse killings; 50% of the victims are women. Women usually kill their husbands with guns and knives, while husbands usually beat wives to death.
2. The battered wife syndrome has three major concepts—the cycle of violence (Fig. II-1), learned helplessness, and anticipatory fear (Blair, 1986).
3. Learned helplessness can be the result of childhood experiences, witnessing or receiving abuse, or the outcome of the battering relationship (Blair, 1986).
4. Victims of abuse are "brainwashed by terror." The victim of abuse uses denial and rationalization when she remains in the battering relationship (Blair, 1986).
5. Battered women rarely report the incident to the health care provider, but instead seek assistance with psychosomatic conditions (chest pain, choking sensations, abdominal pain, fatigue, GI disorders and pelvic pain) or with injuries with inappropriate explanations for them (Greany, 1984).
6. The victims seldom report abuse because of (Blair, 1986):
    a. Feelings of guilt and shame
    b. Fear of social stigmatization
    c. Fear of the abuser
    d. View of violence as normal
    e. Lack of alternative resources
7. Violent episodes
    a. Escalate in frequency and severity over time
    b. Require less and less provocation to trigger them
    c. Include verbal as well as physical abuse
    d. Are made more brutal by alcohol use
8. Battering has a distinct cycle, as indicated in Figure II-1.
9. Women who attempt to defend themselves during the tension-building phase often are successful in preventing the beating, while women who attempt to defend themselves during the assaultive phase often sustain a more brutal beating.
10. The abuser's ability to control his spouse directly increases his feelings of autonomy and esteem. Therefore, the fear of loss (and control) of his spouse directly influences his feelings about himself.

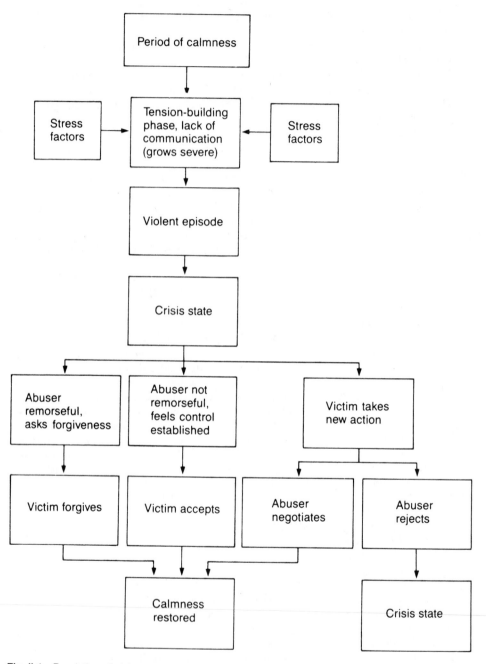

Fig. II-1 Escalation of violence.

11. Battered women who did not witness abuse as children usually remain in the marriage twice as long as women who witnessed abuse as children.
12. Factors contributing to a battered woman's remaining in the marriage are
    a. Belief that children need a two-parent family
    b. Lack of financial support

    c. Lack of a place to go

    d. Belief that the abuse will stop

    e. Fear for her life or her children's lives

    f. Fear of unknown future

13. Personal characteristics of the abuser

    a. No dominant ethnic or socioeconomic characteristics

    b. History of abuse from caregivers or witnessed abuse as a child

    c. Blames outside factors for everything that goes wrong; blames wife for causing him to get angry

    d. Denies the violence or minimizes its severity

    e. Impulsive

    f. Excessively dependent on and jealous of spouse (spouse is usually the only significant relationship he has)

    g. Fears losing her, which can contribute to suicide, homicide, depression, or anger

    h. When not hitting, is often reported to be a good, loving husband

    i. Perceives self as having poor social skills

14. Personal characteristics of the battered woman

    a. Low self-esteem

    b. Easily upset

    c. Belief that she has incited her husband to beat her and is to blame

    d. Raised in families that restricted emotional expression (*e.g.,* anger, hugging)

    e. Subscribes to the feminine sex-role stereotype

    f. Frequently marries to escape restrictive, confining family

    g. Becomes extremely resourceful and self-sufficient in order to survive

    h. Usually was not abused as a child and did not witness abuse

    i. Views herself as a victim with no option but to appease her spouse

15. The likelihood of a woman seeking and utilizing assistance for abuse is increased if (Sammons, 1981):

    a. She has been in the relationship less than 5 years

    b. She is employed

    c. She has friends or relatives who live nearby (within a few miles)

    d. She discussed the abuse with others

    e. The abuse is frequent (daily, weekly), severe (required medical treatment/hospitalization), or increasing in frequency

Pediatric Considerations:

1. About 2.2 million cases of suspected child abuse and neglect were reported in 1987. Of these cases, 40% were substantiated (AHA, 1990). A federally funded study conducted by Westat, Inc. in 1986 estimated that the professionals they surveyed failed to report almost 40% of the sexually abused children they saw, 30% of fatal or serious physical abuse cases, almost 50% of moderate physical abuse cases, and 70% of neglect cases. At the same time, an equally serious problem is a high number of "unfounded" (not indicated) reports of child maltreatment (Besharov, 1990).

2. The discrepancy between the reported cases of child abuse and neglect and the estimated number is related to differences in laws defining abuse/neglect, professionals' failure to recognize the signs, ignorance of the law, fear of court involvement, and lack of faith in child protective services (Thomas, 1989).

3. The nurse should consult the legislation mandating the reporting of child abuse for the specifics of legal definition, penalties for failure to report, reporting procedure, and legal immunity for reporting (Kauffman, Neill, & Thomas, 1986).

4. The nurse may come in contact with an abused child in an emergency room, school, or physician's office or in her personal life (Kauffman, Neill, & Thomas, 1986).

5. The identification of child abuse depends on the nurse's recognizing the physical signs, specific parent behavior, specific child behavior, inconsistencies in the history of the injury, and contributing factors (*e.g.,* familial, environmental) (Kauffman, Neill, & Thomas, 1986).

6. To minimize misdiagnosis of child abuse, health care professionals should be aware that (Hurwitz & Castells, 1987; Wong, 1987):
   a. False allegations of abuse are common
   b. Child abuse may be mistaken for diseases as hemophilia, erythema multiforme, osteogenesis imperfecta, or accidental injuries such as car seat burns.
   c. Child abuse may be used as a charge in custody battles.
   d. Anatomically correct dolls and drawings are tools to help confirm abuse, but they are not confirmation in themselves.
   e. Parents or accused persons may not have been given adequate opportunity to present their account of the incident.

7. The first priority of care for the abused child is preventing further injury (Whaley & Wong, 1989).

8. Child abuse is a symptom of a family in crisis or a family dysfunction. The crisis can be illness, financial difficulties, or any recent change in the family unit (*e.g.,* new members, loss of a member, relocation) (Kauffman, Neill, & Thomas, 1986).

9. Separation of the infant from its parents, as in the case of prematurity, can reduce the attachment and nurturing behaviors of the mother toward her child. A disproportionate number of abused children were premature or ill at birth (Kauffman, Neill, & Thomas, 1986).

10. Children are usually abused by someone they know: a parent, a babysitter, a relative, or a friend of the family. It must be remembered that the majority of people who abuse a child are well-intentioned adults who know the child and care about his or her welfare. The intent was to punish or teach the child a lesson. The abuser usually feels extremely guilty and is often relieved when help is offered. The child also may feel guilt, sensing that he is "bad" and therefore required the discipline (Whaley & Wong, 1989).

11. Factors that contribute to child abuse include (Whaley & Wong, 1989):
   a. Lack of or unavailability of the extended family
   b. Economic conditions (*e.g.,* inflation, unemployment)
   c. Lack of role model as a child
   d. High-risk children (*e.g.,* unwanted, of undesired sex or appearance, physically or mentally handicapped, hyperactive, terminally ill)
   e. High-risk parents (*e.g.,* single, adolescent, emotionally disturbed, alcoholic, drug addicted, physically ill)

12. Characteristic personal patterns of abusers include (Kauffman, Neill, & Thomas, 1986):
   a. No dominant ethnic or socioeconomic characteristics
   b. History of abuse by their parents and lack of warmth and affection from them
   c. Social isolation (few friends or outlets for tensions)
   d. Marked lack of self-esteem, with low tolerance for criticism
   e. Emotional immaturity and dependency
   f. Distrust of others
   g. Inability to admit the need for help
   h. Unrealistic expectations for/of child
   i. Desire for the child to give them pleasure

13. The nonabusing parent, who is usually passive and compliant in the abuse, must be included in the treatment plan (Kauffman, Neill, & Thomas, 1986).

14. The impact of abuse on the parent includes termination of parental rights, relating to large numbers of people/institutions, angry reactions from professionals, court proceedings and court-ordered treatment, reactions of family members and community, and financial obligations (due to medical and legal expenses) (Kaufman, Neill, & Thomas, 1986).

Gerontologic Considerations

1. Elder abuse is defined as maltreatment, intentional or unintentional, resulting from actions or inactions of others, usually caregivers. Types of elder abuse include physical and psychologic mistreatment, misuse of property, and violation of personal rights (Miller, 1990).
2. An estimated 1.5 million elders are abused or mistreated each year (Fulmer, 1989).
3. Multiple, interrelated variables seem to be responsible for elder abuse. Invisibility of the problem and vulnerability of the older person are common to all elder abuse (Miller, 1990).
4. Research on elder abuse has found origins in both the victim and the perpetrator and also in the relationship between the two (Miller, 1990).
5. Steinmetz (1988) reported that caregivers' perceptions of stress and feelings of burden are strong predictors of elder abuse.
6. Abusive caregivers have been associated with factors such as social isolation, recent decline in health, dependency, co-residency, and poor interpersonal relations with elder (Anetzberger, 1987).
7. Abused elders usually will not report abuse because of fear of reprisal or abandonment. Rather, elder abuse must be detected.
8. According to Miller (1990), "Mandatory reporting laws do not require reporters to know that abuse or neglect has occurred, but merely to report it if they suspect its occurrence."

■ Ineffective Family Coping: Disabled
Related to (Specify) as evidenced by Domestic Abuse

Domestic abuse is defined as any action that is intended to harm another person (physical, emotional, financial, social, sexual).

Assessment

Subjective Data

The person relates
Punishments that inflict physical, emotional, financial, social, or sexual harm
Statements indirectly suggesting abuse
"I need help."
"I can't go home."
"I need a friend."

A family history of violence/abuse
   Verbal assaults/threats
   Reports of neglect—elderly without adequate physical care, grooming, nutrition
   Social isolation
   History of forced sexual activity
   Failure to receive medical care—eyeglasses, medications

Objective Data
Bruises or welts
   On face, buttocks, thighs, or upper body
   May appear patterned (by rope, belt, or palm)
   May be different colors from different episodes
   Incompatible with normal injuries
Burns
   From cigarettes (on palms, soles, hands, back, or buttocks)
   Oval-shaped (from immersion in scalding liquids)
   From rope (around neck or extremity)
Fractures or dislocations
Lacerations and abrasions
Miscellaneous injuries
   Nausea and abdominal swelling (from being punched in abdomen)
   Bald patches (from having hair pulled)
   Poisoning
   Gunshot wound
   Malnutrition
   Poor hygiene

Outcome Criteria

The person will
- Discuss the physical assaults
- Identify factors that contribute to violence
- Seek assistance for abusive behavior
- Relate community resources available when help is desired

Interventions
The interventions needed to address the complexity and the magnitude of the problems inherent in domestic violence are usually out of the scope of a nurse generalist. The interventions provided here are to assist the nurse who has a short-term interaction with the individual.

A. Develop rapport
1. Interview in private.
2. Be emphatic.
3. Avoid displaying shock or surprise at the details.
4. If contact is made by phone, find out how to get in touch with victim.

B. Evaluate potential danger to victim and others
   1. Assess actual physical abuse.
      a. Current and past physical/sexual abuse
      b. When did it happen last?
      c. Are you hurt now?
      d. Are the children hurt?
      e. Assess danger to children
   2. Assess support system.
      a. Does she have a safe place to go?
      b. Does she want police called?
      c. Does she need an ambulance?
   3. Assess drug and alcohol use.
      a. Is victim using drugs/alcohol?
      b. Is abuser using drugs/alcohol?

C. Assess for the presence of factors that inhibit victims from seeking aid
   1. Personal beliefs
      a. Fear for safety of self or children
      b. Fear of embarrassment
      c. Low self-esteem
      d. Guilt (punishment justified)
      e. Myths ("It is normal"; "It will stop")
   2. Lack of knowledge of
      a. The severity of the problem
      b. Community resources
      c. Legal rights
   3. Lack of financial independence
   4. Lack of support system

D. Encourage decision-making
   1. Provide an opportunity to validate abuse and talk about feelings; if the acutely injured person is accompanied by spouse/caregiver who is persistent about staying, make an attempt to see the person alone (*e.g.,* tell her you need a urine specimen and accompany her to the bathroom).
   2. Be direct and nonjudgmental (Blair, 1986).
      a. How do you handle stress?
      b. How does your partner or caregiver handle stress?
      c. How do you and your partner argue?
      d. Are you afraid of him?
      e. Have you ever been hit, pushed, or injured by your partner?
   3. Provide options but allow them to make a decision at their own pace.
   4. Encourage a realistic appraisal of the situation; dispel guilt and myths.
      a. Violence is not normal for most families.
      b. Violence may stop but it usually becomes increasingly worse.
      c. The victim is not responsible for the violence.

E. Provide referral information
   1. Provide a list of community agencies available to victim and abuser (emergency and long-term).
      a. Hotlines
      b. Legal services

     c. Shelters

     d. Counseling agencies

  2. Discuss the availability of the social service department for assistance.

  3. Consult with the legal resources in the community and familiarize the victim with the state laws regarding:

     a. Eviction of abuser

     b. Counseling

     c. Temporary support

     d. Protection orders

     e. Criminal law

     f. Types of police interventions

  4. Refer for individual, group, or couples counseling.

F. Assist in developing support system

1. Provide a safe environment, if consenting.
2. Discuss the importance of regular social contacts to provide opportunities to share and to prevent isolation.
3. Assist in arranging respite care and other home health services (hot meals, patient aides) for the elderly.

G. Document findings and dialogue for possible future court use (Blair, 1986)

1. Occurrence, frequency
2. Type of injury
3. Record suspicious injuries when "the pattern of injuries is inconsistent with the history."

H. Initiate health teaching if indicated

1. Teach the community about the problem of spouse/elder abuse.

     a. Parent–school organizations

     b. Women's clubs

     c. Programs for schoolchildren

2. Instruct caregivers in how to properly manage an elderly client at home, transferring to chair, modified appliances, how to maintain orientation.
3. Refer for financial assistance and transportation arrangements.
4. Refer for assertiveness training (see Appendix X).
5. Inform family of senior citizen centers or day-care programs.
6. Refer the abuser to the appropriate community service (only refer men who have asked for assistance or admitted their abuse, for revealing the wife's confidential disclosure may trigger more abuse).
7. To secure additional information, contact:

     National Clearinghouse on Domestic Violence

     P.O. Box 2309

     Rockville, MD 20852

■ Ineffective Family Coping: Disabling
Related to (Specify) as manifested by
Child Abuse/Neglect

Child abuse is an action or inaction that brings injury to a child, including physical and psychological injury, neglect, and sexual abuse.

Assessment

Subjective Data (Heifer & Kempe, 1972)
The parent or caretaker
    Cannot explain the source of injury
    Gives an explanation that is in conflict with the developmental ability of the child
        (*e.g.,* 6-month-old spilled pot on stove)
    Gives an explanation that is inconsistent with injury (*e.g.,* concussion and broken leg
        from falling out of bed)
    Has delayed seeking medical attention
    Describes frequent injuries and accidents
    Blames someone else for causing the injury
    Verbalizes family discord, feelings of inadequacy; says that the child is different in
        some way or that his anger cannot be controlled
The child
    Reports an incident of abuse
    Tells a story that conflicts with the caretaker's story

Objective Data
The parent or caretaker
    Does not comfort the child
    Is detached
    Is out of control or highly controlled
The child
    Has a developmental lag
    Appears poorly cared for
    Is fearful of adults
    Seeks to comfort the parent
    Remains stoic during painful procedures
    Has a lack of social initiative

Findings and reports
Of abuse
    Multiple injuries in various stages of healing
    Injury to genital area
    Gonorrhea
    Marks on skin from straps, buckles, rope, cigarette burns
    Subdural hematoma
    Bruising around the eye
    Contusions
    Ruptured abdominal organs
    Early pregnancy (age 12–14)

Of neglect
　Malnourished
　Unbathed
　Inadequately dressed for weather
　Frequently left unsupervised

Outcome Criteria

The child will
　• Seek comfort from the nurse
　• Be free from injury or neglect
The parent will
　• Seek assistance for the abusive behavior
　• Demonstrate nurturing behavior toward the child

Interventions

A. Identify families at risk for child abuse

　1. Refer to Principles and Rationale for Nursing Care

B. Intervene prior to abuse with families at risk

　1. Establish a relationship with parents that encourages them to share difficulties ("Being a parent is sure hard [frustrating] work, isn't it?").
　2. Provide parents with access to information about parenting and child development (see *Altered Growth and Development*).
　3. Provide anticipatory guidance relative to growth and development (*e.g.*, the need to cry in early months; toilet training).
　4. Stress the importance of support systems (*e.g.*, encourage parents to exchange experiences with other parents).
　5. Encourage parents to allow time for their own needs (*e.g.*, attend an exercise class three times a week).
　6. Discuss with parents how they respond to parental frustrations (share feelings with other parents?) and instruct them not to discipline children when very angry.
　7. Explore other methods of discipline aside from physical punishment.
　8. Refer parents to expert help.
　9. Inform parents of community services (telephone hotlines, clergy).

C. Identify suspected cases of child abuse

　1. Assess for and evaluate
　　a. Evidence of maltreatment (refer to Assessment data)
　　b. History of incident or injury
　　　• Conflicting stories
　　　• Story improbable for age of child
　　　• Story not consistent with injury
　　c. Parental behaviors
　　　• Care sought for a minor complaint (*e.g.*, cold) when other injuries are seen

- Exaggerated or absent emotional response to the injury
- Unavailable for questioning
- Fails to show empathy for child
- Angry or critical of child for being injured
- Demands to take child home if pressured for answers

d. Child behaviors
- Does not expect to be comforted
- Adjusts inappropriately to hospitalization
- Defends parents
- Blames self for inciting parents to rage

D. Report suspected cases of child abuse

1. Know your state's child abuse laws and procedures for reporting child abuse (*e.g.,* Bureau of Child Welfare, Department of Social Services, Child Protective Services).
2. Maintain an objective record
   a. Description of injuries
   b. Conversations with parents and child in quotes
   c. Description of behaviors, not interpretation (*e.g.,* avoid "angry father," instead, "Father screamed at child, 'If you weren't so bad this wouldn't have happened' ")
   d. Description of parent-child interactions (*e.g.,* shies away from mother's touch)
   e. Nutritional status
   f. Growth and development compared to age-related norms

E. Promote a therapeutic environment during hospitalization for child and parent

1. Provide the child with acceptance and affection.
   a. Show child attention without reinforcing inappropriate behavior.
   b. Use play therapy to allow child self-expression.
   c. Provide child with consistent caregivers and reasonable limits on behavior; avoid pity.
   d. Avoid asking too many questions and criticizing parent's actions.
   e. Ensure that play and educational needs are met.
   f. Explain in detail all routines and procedures.
2. Assist child with grieving if foster home placement is necessary.
   a. Acknowledge that child will not want to leave parents despite how severe the abuse was.
   b. Allow opportunities for child to ventilate feelings.
   c. Explain the reasons for not allowing child to return home; dispel belief that this is a punishment.
   d. Encourage foster parents to visit child in hospital.
3. Provide interventions that promote parent's self-esteem and sense of trust.
   a. Tell them it was good that they brought the child to the hospital.
   b. Welcome parents to the unit and orient them to activities.
   c. Promote their confidence by presenting a warm, helpful attitude and acknowledging any competent parenting activities.
   d. Provide opportunities for parents to participate in their child's care (*e.g.,* feeding, bathing).

F. Initiate health teaching and referrals as indicated
1. Provide anticipatory guidance for families at risk.
   a. Assist individuals to recognize stress and to practice techniques to manage stress; see Appendix X (*e.g.,* planning for time alone away from child).
   b. Discuss the need for realistic expectations of the child's capabilities.
   c. Teach about child development and constructive methods for handling developmental problems (enuresis, toilet training, temper tantrums); refer to literature in Bibliography.
   d. Discuss methods of discipline other than physical (*e.g.,* deprive the child of his favorite pastime: "May not ride your bike for a whole day;" "May not play your stereo").
   e. Emphasize rewarding positive behavior.
2. Refer abusive parents to community agencies and professionals for counseling.
3. Disseminate information to the community about the problem of child abuse (*e.g.,* parent-school organizations, radio, television, newspaper).
   a. Discuss with parents and parents-to-be the problems of parenting.
   b. Teach those who are at risk of being future abusers.
   c. Discuss constructive stress management.
   d. Teach the signs and symptoms of abuse and the method for reporting.
   e. Focus on abuse as a problem that results from child-rearing difficulties, not parental deficiencies.
   f. Relay your understanding of stresses but do not condone abuse.
   g. Focus on the parent's needs; avoid an authoritative approach.
   h. Take opportunities to demonstrate constructive methods for working with children (give the child choices; listen carefully to the child).
4. Consider developing parenting classes for parents (preventive, corrective) to increase their skills as nurturers and teachers. Weekly topic examples:
   a. What is parenting?
   b. Child development and play
   c. Discipline and toiling training
   d. Play and nutrition
   e. Safety and health
   f. Discipline and common problems
   g. Parental needs
   h. Expectations versus realities (Seditus & Mock, 1988).

■ High Risk for Ineffective Family Coping: Disabling
Related to Multiple Stressors Associated with Elder Care

Assessment

Presence of high-risk individuals (caregiver, elder) (refer to Intervention A)

Outcome Criteria

The caregiver will
- Discuss the stressors of elder care
- Relate strategies to reduce stressors
- Identify community resources available

The elder will
- Describe methods to increase socialization beyond caregiver
- Identify resources available for assistance

Interventions

A. Identify high-risk individuals (caregiver, elder) for abuse
  1. Caregiver
     a. Social isolation
     b. Dependency on elder (financial, emotional); co-residency
     c. Health problems (physical, mental)
     d. Substance abuse
     e. Poor relationship history with elder
     f. Financial problems
     g. Transgenerational violence
     h. Relationship problems
  2. Elder
     a. Dependent on others for activities of daily living
     b. Isolated
     c. Financially insecure
     d. Impaired cognitive functioning
     e. Depressive personality
     f. History of abuse to caregiver
     g. Incontinence

B. Assist caregivers to reduce stressors
  1. Establish a relationship with caregivers that encourages them to share difficulties.
  2. Encourage them to share experiences with others in same situation.
  3. Evaluate caregiver's ability to provide long-term in-home care.
  4. Explore sources of help (*e.g.,* housekeeping, home delivered meals, day care, respite care, transportation assistance).
  5. Encourage caregiver to discuss sharing responsibilities with other family members.
  6. Discuss alternative sources of care (*e.g.,* nursing home, senior housing).
  7. Discuss how caregiver can allow time for his or her own needs.
  8. Discuss community resources available for help (*e.g.,* crisis hotline, social service, voluntary emergency caregivers).

C. Assist elders to reduce risks of abuse by providing the following suggestions (AARP, 1987):
  1. Keep contact with old friends and neighbors if you relocate with relative.
  2. Plan a weekly contact in person with friend, neighbor.

3. Participate in community activities as much as possible.
4. Take care of own personal needs.
5. Have your own telephone.
6. Acquire legal advice for possible future disability.
7. Do not accept personal care in exchange for transfer of assets or property without legal advice.
8. Do not live with someone who has a history of violence or substance abuse.

D. Identify suspected cases of elder abuse; observe for these signs:

1. Failure to adhere to therapeutic regimens, which can pose threats to life (*e.g.*, insulin administration, ulcerated conditions)
2. Evidence of malnutrition, dehydration
3. Bruises, swelling, lacerations, burns, bites
4. Pressure ulcers
5. Caregiver not allowing nurse to be alone with elder

E. Report suspected cases (Anetzberger, 1987)

1. Consult with supervisor for procedures for reporting suspected cases of abuse.
2. Maintain an objective record, including:
   a. Description of injuries
   b. Conversations with elder and caregivers
   c. Description of behaviors
   d. Nutritional, hydration status
3. Consider the elder's right to choose to live at risk of harm providing he is capable of making that choice.
4. Do not initiate an action that could increase the elder's risk of harm or antagonize the abuser.
5. Respect the elder's right to secrecy and the right for self-determination.

F. Initiate health teaching and referrals as indicated

1. Refer high-risk caregivers for counseling.
2. Disseminate information to community regarding prevention.
   a. Publicize support services.
   b. Seek to assist caregiving families (*e.g.*, companions, respite care, day-care centers).
   c. Seek to establish weekly contact with dependent elderly.
   d. Attempt to reduce isolation of caregivers and elders.
   e. Develop procedures for investigation, public education.

Compromised Family Coping

DEFINITION

Compromised family coping: That state in which a usually supportive primary person (family member or close friend) is providing insufficient, ineffective, or compromised support, comfort, assistance, or encouragement that may be needed by the client to manage or master adaptive tasks related to his or her health challenge.

DEFINING CHARACTERISTICS

Subjective

Client expresses or confirms a concern or complaint about significant other's response to his or her health problem.

Significant person describes preoccupation with personal reactions (*e.g.*, fear, anticipatory grief, guilt, anxiety) to client's illness, disability, or to other situational or developmental crises.

Significant person describes or confirms an inadequate understanding or knowledge base, which interferes with effective assistive or supportive behaviors.

Objective

Significant person attempts assistive or supportive behaviors with less than satisfactory results.

Significant person withdraws or enters into limited or temporary personal communication with the client at time of need.

Significant person displays protective behavior disproportionate (too little or too much) to the client's abilities or need for autonomy.

RELATED FACTORS

See *Altered Family Processes*

Diagnostic Considerations

This nursing diagnosis describes situations that are similar to the diagnostic categories *Impaired Adjustment* and *Altered Family Processes*. Until clinical research differentiates this category from the aforementioned categories, use *Impaired Adjustment* and/or *Altered Family Processes*.

Coping, Family: Potential for Growth

DEFINITION
Family coping, potential for growth: Effective managing of adaptive tasks by family member involved with the client's health challenge, who now is exhibiting desire and readiness for enhanced health and growth in regard to self and in relation to the client.

DEFINING CHARACTERISTICS
Family member attempting to describe growth impact of crisis on his or her own values, priorities, goals or relationships

Family member moving in direction of health-promoting and enriching life-style that supports and monitors maturational processes, audits and negotiates treatment programs, and generally chooses experiences that optimize wellness

Individual expressing interest in making contact on a one-to-one basis or on a mutual-aid group basis with another person who has experienced a similar situation

RELATED FACTORS
See *Health-Seeking Behaviors* and Altered Family Processes

Diagnostic Considerations
This nursing diagnosis describes components that are found in *Altered Family Processes* and *Health-Seeking Behaviors*. Until clinical research differentiates the category from the aforementioned category, use *Altered Family Processes* or *Health-Seeking Behaviors*, depending on the data presented.

References/Bibliography

Aiken, M. M. (1990). Documenting sexual abuses in prepubertal girls. *Journal of Maternal–Child Nursing, 15*(3), 176–177.

Allen, J. & Allen, B. (1981). Violence in the family. *Family and Community Health, 4*(2), 19–33.

Blair, K. (1986). The battered woman: Is she a silent partner? *Nurse Practitioner, 11*(6), 38.

Harris, C. (1981) Women and violence. In Fogel, C., & Woods, N. (Eds.). *Health care of women: A nursing perspective.* St. Louis: C. V. Mosby.

Friedman, M. M. (1981). *Family nursing: Theory and assessment.* New York: Appleton-Century-Crofts.

Greany, G. (1984). Is she a battered woman? A guide for emergency response. *American Journal of Nursing, 84*(5), 725–727.

Greenland, C. (1980). Violence and the family. *Canadian Journal of Public Health, 7*(1), 19–24.

Hymovich, D., & Barnard, M. (Eds). *Family health care,* 2 Vols. New York: McGraw-Hill.

Machling, K. (1988). Battered women and abusive partners: Treatment issues and strategies. *Journal of Psychosocial Nursing, 26*(9), 6–9.

Mercer, R.T. (1980). Teenage motherhood: The first year. *Journal of Obstetrical and Gynecological Nursing, 9*(1), 16–29.

Nelms, B. (1981). What is a normal adolescent? *Maternal–Child Nursing Journal, 6*(6), 402–406.

Petrillo, M., Sagay, S. (1980). *Emotional care of the hospitalized child.* Philadelphia: J. B. Lippincott.

Sammons, L. (1981). Battered and pregnant. *Maternal–Child Nursing Journal, 6,* 246–250.

Senner, A., et al. (1989). Munchausen syndrome by proxy. *Issues of Comprehensive Pediatric Nursing, 12*(5), 345–357.

Shapiro, R. (1984). Therapy with violent families. In Saunders, S. Anderson, A. Hart, C, et al. (Eds.). *Violent individuals and families: A handbook for practitioners.* Springfield, IL: Charles C. Thomas.

Walker, L. (1979). *The battered woman.* New York: Harper & Row.

Woolery, L., Barkley, N. (1981) Enhancing couple relationship during prenatal and postnatal classes. *Maternal–Child Nursing Journal, 6*(3), 184–188.

Child

Besharov, D. J. (1990). Gaining control over child abuse reports. Public agencies must address both underreporting and overreporting. *Public Welfare,* Spring, 34–40.

Hurwitz, A., & Castells, S. (1987). Misdiagnosed child abuse and metabolic diseases. *Pediatric Nursing 13,* 33–36.

Kauffman, C. K., Neill, M. K., & Thomas, J. N. (1986). The abusive parent. In Johnson, S. H. (Ed.) *High-risk parenting: Assessment and nursing strategies for families at risk.* Philadelphia: J. B. Lippincott.

Thomas, B. H. (1989). Nursing strategies: Child abuse and maltreatment. In Foster, R. L., Hunsberger, M. M., & Anderson, J. J. T. (Eds.). *Family-centered nursing care of children.* Philadelphia: W. B. Saunders.

Whaley, L. F., & Wong, D. L. (1989). *Essentials of pediatric nursing* (3rd ed.). St. Louis: C.V. Mosby.

Wong, D. L. (1987). False allegations of child abuse. The other side of the tragedy. *Pediatric Nursing, 13*(5), 329–333.

Abuse

Anderson, C. L. (1987). Assessing parenting potential for child abuse risk. *Pediatric Nursing, 13*(5), 323–327.

American Humane Association (AHA). (1987). *Highlights of official child neglect and abuse reporting 1985.* AHA: Denver, CO.

Elvik, SL. (1987). From disclosure to court: The facets of sexual abuse. *Journal Pediatric Health Care, 1*(6), 136–140.

Elvik, S. L., Berkowitz, C., & Greenberg, C. (1986). Child sexual abuse: The role of the nurse practitioner. *Nurse Practitioner, 11*(1), 15.

Helfer, R. E. & Kempe, C. H. (1972). *Helping the battered child and his family.* Philadelphia: J. B. Lippincott.

Hurwitz, A., & Castells, S. (1987). Misdiagnosed child abuse and metabolic diseases. *Pediatric Nursing, 13,* 33–36.

Mulvihill, D. (1987). Between parent and child. *The Canadian Nurse, 83*(2), 12–15.

Seditus, C., & Mock, D. Interrupting the cycle of child abuse. *Maternal–Child Nursing Journal, 13*(3), 196–198.

Wong, D. (1987). False allegations of child abuse: The other side of tragedy. *Pediatric Nursing, 13*(5), 329–333.

Elder Abuse

Anetzberger, G. J. (1987). *The etiology of elder abuse by adult offspring.* Springfield, IL: Charles C Thomas.

Fulmer, T. T. (1989). Mistreatment of elders. *Nursing Clinics of North America, 24*(3), 707–716.

Miller, C. A. (1990). *Nursing care of older adults.* Glenview, IL: Scott Foresman,

Steinmetz, S. K. (1988). *Duty bound elder abuse and family care.* Newberry Park, CA: Sage.

Resources for the Consumer

Literature

American Association of Retired Persons. (1987). *Domestic mistreatment of the elderly: Towards prevention—some do's and don't's* (pamphlet).

Child Care Manual.

ROCOM Press, P.O. Box 1577, Newark, NJ 07101

Christophersen, E. R. (1977). *Little people: Guidelines for common sense childrearing.* Lawrence, KS: H & H Enterprises.

Forward S. (1986). *Men who hate women and the women who love them.* New York: Bantam Books.

Salk, L., & Kramer, R. (1973). *How to raise a human being.* New York: Warner Books.

Your child from 1 to 6. U.S. Department of Health, Education, and Welfare, Children's Bureau, Publication No. 30, Washington, DC 20014.

Organizations

American Humane Association (AHA), Denver, CO

National Aging Resource Center on Elder Abuse, 810 First St. NE, Suite 500, Washington DC 20002-4205

Parents Without Partners, 7910 Woodmount Avenue, #1000, Washington, DC 20014; also local chapters

LaLeche League International, 9616 Minneapolis Avenue, Franklin Park, IL 60131; also local chapters

Parent Effectiveness Training, 531 Stevens Avenue, Solana Beach, CA 92075

Local Counseling Services

Catholic Charities, Jewish Family Services, Christian Family Services, community agencies, and mental health centers

Decisional Conflict

DEFINITION

Decisional conflict: The state in which an individual/group experiences uncertainty about a course of action when the choice involves risk, loss, or challenge.

DEFINING CHARACTERISTICS*

Major (80%–100%)

Verbalized uncertainty about choices
Verbalization of undesired consequences of alternative actions being considered
Vacillation between alternative choices
Delayed decision-making

Minor (50%–79%)

Verbalized feeling of distress while attempting a decision
Self-focusing
Physical signs of distress or tension (increased heart rate, increased muscle tension, restlessness, etc.) whenever the decision comes within focus of attention
Questioning personal values and beliefs while attempting to make a decision

RELATED FACTORS

Many situations can contribute to decisional conflict, particularly those that involve complex medical interventions of great risk. Any decisional situation can precipitate conflict for an individual; thus, the examples listed below are not exhaustive, but reflective of situations that may be problematic and possess factors that increase the difficulty.

Treatment-related

Surgery	Diagnostics
Tumor removal	Amniocentesis
Cataract	Ultrasound
Laminectomy	X-rays
Orchiectomy	Chemotherapy
Cosmetic	Radiation
Joint replacement	Dialysis
Hysterectomy	Mechanical ventilation
Transplant	Enteral feedings
	Intravenous hydration

*Supporting research from Hiltunen, E. (1989). Nursing diagnosis: Decisional conflict (specify). In R. M. Carroll-Johnson, (Ed.). *Classification of nursing diagnoses: Proceedings of the eighth conference.* Philadelphia: J. B. Lippincott.

Situational
  Personal
    Marriage   Foster home placement
    Separation   Institutionalization (child, parent)
    Divorce   Breast vs. bottle feeding
    Parenthood   Abortion
    Birth control   Sterilization
    Artificial insemination   Nursing home placement
    Adoption
  Work/task
    Career change
    Relocation
    Business investments
    Professional ethics
  Lack of relevant information
  Confusing information
  Disagreement within support systems
  Inexperience with decision-making
  Unclear personal values/beliefs
  Conflict with personal values/beliefs
  Resignation
  Family history of poor prognosis
  Hospital environment—loss of control
  Ethical dilemmas—quality of life
                       cessation of life-support systems
                       do not resuscitate
                       organ donation

Maturational
  Adolescent
    Peer pressure   Use of birth control
    Sexual activity   Whether to continue a relationship
    Alcohol/drug use   College
    Illegal/dangerous situations   Career choice
  Adult
    Career change   Marriage
    Relocation   Parenthood
  Older adult
    Retirement
    Relocation
    Nursing home placement

Diagnostic Considerations

The nurse has an important role in assisting clients and families with decision-making. Since nurses usually do not benefit financially from decisions made regarding treatments and transfers, they are in an ideal position to assist with decisions. Although, according to Davis (1989), "nursing or medical expertise does not enable health care professionals to know the values of patients or what patients think is best for themselves," nursing expertise does enable nurses to facilitate systematic decision-making that considers all possible alternatives and possible outcomes, and takes into account individual beliefs and values. The focus is on assisting with logical decision-making, not on promoting a certain decision.

Errors in Diagnostic Statements

Decisional Conflict related to failure of physician to gain permission for mechanical ventilation from family

If this situation did occur, this statement represents an unprofessional and legally problematic nursing approach to the situation. Failure of the physician to gain permission for mechanical ventilation would be a practice dilemma necessitating formal reporting to the appropriate parties. Should the family have evidence that this treatment was not desired by the client (*i.e.*, a living will), this situation would not be described as *Decisional Conflict*, because there is no uncertainty about a course of action. The nurse should further assess the family for responses fitting other nursing diagnoses, such as *Grieving*.

Decisional Conflict related to uncertainty about choices

Uncertainty about choices validates *Decisional Conflict*; it is not a causative or contributing factor. If the person needed more information, the diagnosis would be *Decisional Conflict related to insufficient knowledge about choices and their effects.*

Focus Assessment

Decisional conflict is a subjective state that the nurse must validate with the individual. The nurse will assess each individual to determine the person's level of decision-making within the present conflict situation. Some of the same cues may be seen in persons with diagnoses of *Powerlessness, Spiritual Distress,* and *Hopelessness.*

Subjective Data

Decision-making patterns
"Tell me about the decisions you need to make."
"How would you describe your usual method of making decisions?"
"In the past, how did you arrive at decisions that had a positive outcome?"
"What decisions have you made that you felt confident about?"
"When you make a decision, do you do it alone or do you like to involve other people? If so, whom do you consult for advice?"

Person may say:
"I simply cannot decide."
"What should I do?"
"What would you do if you were me?"
"Why don't you just tell me what I should do?"

Perception of the conflict
"How does it make you feel when you think about the decision you have to make?"
"Why is this a stressful decision for you?"
"What things make you uncomfortable about deciding?"
"Has there been a change in your sleep patterns, appetite, activity level?"

Person may state:
"The risk is too great for me to decide."
"This whole situation makes me very anxious."
"I can't believe I got myself into this predicament."
"I feel so uptight every time I think about the decision I have to make."
"I feel like I have no control over the decision that needs to be made."

Objective Data
>   Body language
>>   Posture (relaxed, rigid)
>>   Facial expression (calm, annoyed, tense)
>>   Hands (relaxed, rigid, wringing)
>>   Eye contact (appropriate, darting)
>   Motor activity
>>   Within normal limits
>>   Immobile
>>   Increased
>>   Pacing
>>   Agitation
>   Affect
>>   Within normal limits
>>   Labile
>>   Controlled
>>   Flat
>>   Inappropriate

Principles and Rationale for Nursing Care

Generic Considerations

1. Making decisions is a way of life.
2. An antecedent condition of decision-making is a problem. Problems exist when goals are to be attained and there is uncertainty about an appropriate solution. A problem suggests more than one alternative solution.
3. Making a decision is a systematic process—a means, rather than an end (McDevitt-Graham, 1987). Decision-making is a sequential process in which each step builds on the previous one (Lancaster & Lancaster, 1982). Optimal decision-making is more likely to occur when done in systematically, but it does not necessarily have to be a rigid, step-by-step process.
4. The logical steps of decision-making are well identified in clinical practice (Bailey & Hendricks, 1987; Huber, 1980; Lancaster & Lancaster, 1982; Mapanga, 1985; Minogue & Reedy, 1988; Pitz & Riedel, 1984). They can be summarized in the following steps:
   a. Definition of the problem
   b. Listing of the possible alternatives or options
   c. Identification of the probable outcomes of the various alternatives
   d. Evaluation of the alternatives based on actual or potential threats to beliefs/values
   e. Making a decision
5. People usually are not taught a systematic method for making a decision, so frequently they rely on past experiences and intutition (Bailey & Hendricks, 1987). The intuitive mode of decision-making is characterized by interaction and association among ideas that seem to coexist simultaneously (Nugent, 1982).
6. Janis and Mann (1977) see man "not as a rational calculator always ready to work out the best solution, but as a reluctant decision maker—beset by conflict, doubts, and worry. . . ."
7. The decision-making process is complicated when there is a need for a rapid decision (Minogue & Reedy, 1988). Making an intelligent decision during a period of acute

stress is difficult if not impossible. The stress can be enormous if the decision is compounded by a sense of urgency (Valanis & Rumpler, 1985).

8. Mastering content for effective decision-making requires time. Time allows a person to choose the option that provides the most benefit with the least amount of risk.

9. Difficult decisions create stress and conflict. Conflict occurs when values and actions are not in congruence.

10. Decisional conflict occurs when a person has simultaneous opposing tendencies to accept or reject a course of action (Janis & Mann, 1977).

11. Decisional conflict becomes more intense when it involves a threat to status and self-esteem (Zotti, 1987).

12. Decisional conflict is greater when the alternative is good.

13. Conflict can create fears and anxieties that negatively impact the ability to make an effective decision. External resources become very important for the person in decisional conflict who has a low level of confidence in his ability to make an autonomous decision.

Locus of Control

1. There are essentially three decision-making models in health care (Bille, 1987; Burke, 1980; Valanis & Rumpler, 1985):
   a. Paternalism
      - Health care providers make all of the decisions regarding patient care.
      - Based on a perceived need to protect the patient
      - Locus of control is external to the patient and significant others.
   b. Consumerism
      - Health care providers only provide the patient and significant others with the information they request.
      - Based on the premise that the patient "knows best"
      - Locus of control is internal for the patient and significant others.
   c. Humanism/advocacy
      - Health care providers collaborate with the patient and significant others to arrive at a decision.
      - Based on mutual respect for individual dignity and worth
      - Locus of control is shared and all participants have an equal role in decision-making.

2. The most important right that a person possesses in the right of self-determination, the right to make the ultimate decision concerning what will or will not be done to his body (Marsh, 1986). Choice is facilitated when an individual is free to make it (Kohnke, 1980).

3. Ward, Heidrich and Wolberg (1989) studied 22 women regarding the factors they took into account when deciding on the type of surgery for breast cancer. Postsurgery, the women reported that participation in decision-making was important to them. They rated "people" sources of information as more important than written or visual materials.

4. Personal characteristics influence the desire to maintain control over the decision-making process. People who are strongly self-directed and have in the past taken responsibility for their own health practices will be more likely to assume an active role in decision-making.

Values and Decision-making

1. Every decision made and course of action taken is based on consciously or unconsciously held beliefs, attitudes, and values (Simon, Howe, & Kirschenbaum, 1978).

2. Values provide one foundation for decision-making. Experience is a major source for value development. Values involve choice (Coletta, 1978).
3. Value conflicts often lead to confusion, indecision, and inconsistency. Decision-making is more complicated for a person when his goals conflict with those of his significant others. People may decide contradictory to their values if the need to please others is greater than the need to please themselves (Kohnke, 1980).
4. Health care providers' own values will shape their interaction with families facing ethical decisions (Minogue & Reedy, 1988).
5. In a crisis situation, decisions are influenced more by values than by consideration of possible outcomes. Myers (1988) reports that with organ donation decisions, it is essential that there is congruence among the family unit with respect to values to provide the moral foundation necessary to make such an ethical decision.

End-of-Life Decisions

1. Intense stress is experienced when families and health care providers are faced with decisions regarding either the initiation or discontinuation of life-support systems. When there is no indication of the person's wishes or choices for his end of life or the family disagrees, the stress increases (Johnson & Justin, 1988).
2. In a study conducted by Myers (1988) the following characteristics were identified as being reflective of families faced with the required decision of organ donation:
   a. An intense need to be supported by the family network and health professionals
   b. Negative effect on cognitive processing during the decision-making period
   c. Uncertainty and assistance from the health professional in making the required decision
   d. Emotional physical and psychologic family interaction
3. Individuals and families should be encouraged to provide documented directions that can be used to guide future clinical decisions in the event they become incompetent or unable to make them (Johnson & Justin, 1988).
4. Johnson and Justin (1988) reported the following in a sampling of 400 persons who had no current life-threatening disease:
   a. 43% had discussed their feelings regarding end-of-life decisions with others.
   b. 95% had no desire to be kept alive if they would be mentally incompetent.
   c. 93% always wanted to be told the truth about their condition.

Pediatric Considerations

1. In most cases, children do not make major decisions for themselves. A surrogate, usually a parent, must make the decision on behalf of the child (Brunnquell, 1990).
2. A child's ability to understand a situation and make a decision depends on age, developmental level, and past experience. However, understanding should not be confused with legal competence (Brunnquell, 1990).
3. As the adolescent matures, he gains the ability to analyze problems and make decisions (Scott, 1989).
4. Researchers working with children should seek assent from children with a mental age of 7 years or older. Parents must give written informed consent for the child to participate in the study (Whaley & Wong, 1989).

Gerontologic Considerations

1. Decisions are often made for, not with, older adults.
2. Barriers to decision-making by older adults include dementia, depression, long-term passivity regarding decisions, and hearing or other communication problems (Miller, 1990).

3. Reasons why decision-makers exclude elderly persons from involvement in decisions that profoundly affect their lives include beliefs that the elderly are incompetent, not qualified, or not interested and the desire to avoid discussion of sensitive topics, *e.g.*, finances, relocation (Miller, 1990).

Outcome Criteria

The individual/group will
- Relate the advantages and disadvantages of choices
- Share their fears and concerns regarding choices and responses of others
- Make an informed choice

Interventions

A. Assess causative/contributing factors
  1. Lack of experience with or ineffective decision-making
  2. Value conflict
  3. Fear of outcome/response of others
  4. Insufficient/inconsistent information
  5. Controversy with support system
  6. Unsatisfactory health care environment

B. Reduce or eliminate causative or contributing factors
  Internal

  1. Lack of experience with or ineffective decision-making
    a. Review past decisions made by the person and what steps were taken to help him decide. Focus on major life events and what the final outcome was. Capitalize on past decisions that have served the person well.
    b. Facilitate a logical decision-making process.
      - Assist the person in recognizing what the problem is and clearly identify the decision that needs to be made.
      - Generate a list of all the possible alternatives or options.
      - Help identify the probable outcomes of the various alternatives.
      - Aid in evaluating the alternatives based on actual or potential threats to beliefs/values.
      - Encourage the person to make a decision.
    c. Assess the person's usual locus of control (see *Powerlessness)* and support decision-making patterns.
    d. Encourage the person's significant others to be involved in the entire decision-making process.
    e. Suggest that the person use significant others as a sounding board when considering the decision alternatives.
    f. Respect the person as a competent decision-maker—treat decisions and desires with respect.
    g. Be available to review the decision that needs to be made and the various alternatives.
    h. Teach and assist with relaxation techniques (see Appendix X) when the decision causes anxiety and stress.

i. Facilitate refocusing on the decision that needs to be made when the person experiences fragmented thinking during periods of high anxiety.
j. Encourage the person to take time in deciding.
k. With adolescents, focus on the present—what will happen versus what will not. Help identify the important things in their life as they do not have extensive past experiences upon which to base decisions.

2. Value conflict (also refer to *Spiritual Distress*)
a. Explore the whys of how the person is feeling.
b. Assist the individual in exploring personal values and relationships that may have an impact on the decision.
c. Explore obtaining a referral with the person's spiritual leader.
d. Utilize values clarification techniques to assist the person in reviewing the parts of his life that reflect what he believes in.
   • Have the person identify the most prized and cherished activities in his life.
   • Ask reflective statements that lead to further clarification.
   • Review past decisions in which the person needed to make public affirmation of opinions and beliefs.
   • Evaluate stands the person has taken on controversial subjects. Does he view them in black and white terms, or various shades of gray?
   • Identify values the person is proud of. Rank them in order of importance.
e. Encourage the person to base decision on the most important values.
f. Support individual making informed decision—even if decision conflicts with own values
   • Consult own spiritual leader
   • Change patient assignments so person can be cared for by nurse with compatible beliefs.
   • Arrange for discussions among health care team to share feelings.

3. Fear of outcome/response of others (also refer to *Fear*)
a. Provide clarification regarding potential outcomes and correct misconceptions.
b. Explore with the person what the risks of not deciding would be.
c. Encourage expression of feelings.
d. Promote self-worth.
e. Encourage the person to face fears.
f. Encourage the person to share what he fears with significant others.
g. Actively reassure the person that the decision is his to make and that he has the right to do so.
h. Assist the person in recognizing that it is his life; if he feels comfortable with the decision, others will respect the conviction.
i. Reassure the person that individuality is acceptable.

External

4. Insufficient or inconsistent information
a. Provide information in a comprehensive and sensitive manner.
b. Correct misinformation.
c. Give concise information that covers the major points when the decision must be made quickly.
d. Inform the person of his right to know.
e. Enable the person to determine the amount of information that he desires to obtain.

    f. Encourage verbalization to determine the person's perception of choices.

    g. Ensure that the person clearly understands what is involved concerning the decision and the various alternatives—informed choice.

    h. Encourage the person to seek second professional opinions regarding health.

    i. Collaborate with other health care members/significant others to determine appropriate timing for truthfulness.

5. Controversy with support system

    a. Ensure the person that he does not have to give in to pressure from others, whether they are family, friends, or health professionals.

    b. Do not allow others to undermine the person's confidence in making the decision personally.

    c. Identify leaders within the support system and provide information.

    d. Do not support the family's exclusion of the person from decision-making.

6. Unsatisfactory health care environment

    a. Establish a trusting and meaningful relationship that promotes mutual understanding and caring.

    b. Provide a quiet environment for thought; reduce sensory stimulation.

    c. Allow uninterrupted periods with significant others.

    d. Promote accepting, nonjudgmental attitudes.

    e. Reduce the number of small decisions that the person needs to make to facilitate focusing on the decision in conflict.

    f. Avoid using paternalistic/maternalistic attitudes and actions. Foster acceptance of responsibility for the person's own decisions.

    g. Assist family to communicate conflicts with physician; arrange for a meeting, but do not act as an intermediary and do not explain physician's decisions.

C. Initiate health teaching and referrals when indicated

1. Explore with individual and family whether they have discussed and recorded their end-of-life decisions.

2. Describe the possible future dilemmas when these discussions are avoided.

3. Instruct the individual and family members to provide directives in the following areas:

    a. Person to contact in emergency

    b. Person individual most trusts with personal decisions

    c. Decision to be kept alive if individual will be mentally incompetent

    d. Preference to die at home, hospital, no preference

    e. Desire to sign a living will

    f. Decision on organ donation

    g. Funeral arrangements, burial, cremation

    h. Circumstances when information should be withheld from individual

4. Document these decisions and make two copies (retain one and give one to the person who is designated to be the decision-maker in an emergency).

5. Discuss the purpose of a living will. Provide information when requested. To obtain a copy of your state's living will, write to the Society for the Right to Die, 250 West 57th Street, New York, NY 10107.

References/Bibliography

Aberman, S., & Kirchhoff, K. T. (1985). Infant-feeding practices. Mothers' decision making. *Journal of Obstetric, Gynecologic, and Neonatal Nursing, 14*(5), 394–397.

Bailey, J. T., & Hendricks, D. E. (1987). Decisions made easy. *Nursing Life, 7*(4), 18–19.

Bedell, S. E. (1986). "Do you want to be resuscitated?" *Hospital Practice, 21*(3), 6–9.

Bille, D. A. (1987). Locus of decision making in patient and family education: Its effects on promoting wellness. *Nursing Administration Quarterly, 2*(3), 62–65.

Brunnquell, D. (1990). *Difficult decisions: Overcoming factors which make discussion of ethical issues difficult.* Paper presented at the meeting of the Association for the Care of Children's Health, Washington, DC, May 1990.

Bulechek, G., & McCloskey, J. (1985). *Nursing interventions: Treatments for nursing diagnoses.* Philadelphia: W. B. Saunders.

Burke, G. (1980). Ethics and medical decision-making. *Primary Care, 7*(4), 615–624.

Coletta, S. S. (1978). Values clarification in nursing: Why? *American Journal of Nursing, 78*(12), 2057–2063.

Davis, A. J. (1989). Clinical nurses' ethical decision making in situations. *Advanced Nursing Science, 11*(3), 63–69.

Gadow, S. (1981). Advocacy: An ethical model for assisting patients with treatment decisions. In Wong, C. B., & Swazey, J. P. (Eds.). *Dilemmas of dying: Policies and procedures for decisions not to treat.* Boston: G. K. Hall.

Hiltunen, E. (1987). Decisional conflict: A phenomenological description from the points of view of the nurse and the client. In McLane, A. M. (Ed.). *Classification of nursing diagnoses: Proceedings of the seventh conference.* St. Louis: C. V. Mosby.

Hiltunen, E. (1989). Nursing diagnosis: Decisional conflict (specify). In Carroll-Johnson, R. M. (Ed.). *Classification of nursing diagnoses: Proceedings of the eighth conference.* Philadelphia: J. B. Lippincott.

Huber, G. P. (1980). *Managerial decision making.* Glenview, IL: Scott, Foresman.

Janis, I. L., & Mann, L. (1977). *Decision making. A psychological analysis of conflict, choice, und commitment.* New York: The Free Press.

Johnson, R. A., & Justin, R. (1988). Documenting patients end of life decisions. *Nurse Practitioner, 13*(6), 41.

Kohnke, M. F. (1980). The nurse as advocate. *American Journal of Nursing, 80*(11), 2038–2040.

Lancaster, W., & Lancaster, J. (1982). Rational decision making: Managing uncertainty. *Journal of Nursing Administration, 12*(2), 23–28.

Mapanga, M. (1985). Deciding factors. *Nursing Mirror, 161*(12), 31–32.

Marsh, F. L. (1986). Refusal of treatment. *Clinical Geriatric Medicine, 2*(3), 511–520.

McDevitt-Graham, S. M. (1987). Decision-making: The multi-attribute model. *Nursing Management, 18*(3), 18–19.

Miller, C. A. (1990). *Nursing care of older adults.* Glenview, IL: Scott, Foresman.

Minogue, J. P., & Reedy, N. J. (1988). Companioning parents in perinatal decision making. *Journal of Perinatal & Neonatal Nursing, 1*(3), 25–35.

Myers, M. B. (1988). *Conception of a nursing diagnosis: Decision-making, family: Required.* Unpublished master's thesis, University of Illinois, Urbana.

Nugent, P. S. (1982). Management and modes of thought. *Journal of Nursing Administration, 12*(2), 19–25.

Pitz, G. F., & Riedel, S. (1984). The content and structure of value tree representations. *Acta Psychologica, 56*(1–3), 59–70.

Schoene-Seifer, B., & Childress, J. F. (1986). How much should the cancer patient know and decide? *CA–A Cancer Journal for Clinicians, 36*(2), 85–94.

Scott, P. N. (1989). Families with adolescents. In Foster, R. L., Hunsberger, M. M., & Anderson, J. J. T. (Eds.). *Family-centered nursing care of children.* Philadelphia: W. B. Saunders.

Simon, S. B., Howe, L. W., & Kirschenbaum, H. (1978). *Values clarification. A handbook of practical strategies for teachers and students.* New York: A & W Publishers.

Tauer, K. M. (1983). Promoting effective decision making in sexually active adolescents. *Nursing Clinics of North America, 18*(2), 275–292.

Thomas, S. G. (1978). Breast cancer: The psychosocial issues. *Cancer Nursing, 1*(1), 53–60.

Valanis, B. G. & Rumpler, C. H. (1985). Helping women to choose breast cancer treatment alternatives. *Cancer Nursing, 8*(3), 167–175.

Ward, S., Heidrich, S., & Wolberg, W. (1989). Factors women take into account when deciding upon type of surgery for breast cancer. *Cancer Nursing, 12*(6), 344–351.

Whaley, L. F., & Wong, D. L. (1989). *Essentials of pediatric nursing* (3rd ed.). St. Louis: C. V. Mosby.
Zotti, M. E. (1987). Nursing intervention to assist patients' decision making with respect to family planning. *Public Health Nursing, 4*(3), 146–150.

Resources for the Consumer

Literature
Life support: Families speak about hospitals, hospice and home care for the fatally ill. The Institute for Consumer Policy Research, 256 Washington St., Mt. Vernon, NY 10553
Morra, M. & Potts, E. (1987) *Choices: Realistic alternatives in cancer treatment.* New York: Avon
Scully, T., & Scully, C. (1987). *Playing God.* New York: Simon and Schuster
Thinking of having surgery. Department of Health and Human Services, Washington, DC 20201 800-638-6833 (free)
Questions and answers on organ transplantation. Health Resources and Services Administration, 5600 Fishers Lane, Room 17–60, Rockville, MD 20857 (free)

Organizations
Cancer Information Services, 1-800-4Cancer
Society For Right to Die, 250 West 57th St., New York, NY 10107; Information on living will
National Genetics Foundation Inc., 555 West 57th St., New York, NY 10019
Friends and Relatives of Institutionalized Aged, Inc., 440 East 26th St., New York, NY 10010, 212-481-4422
National Information Center for Handicapped Children and Youth, P.O. Box 1492, Washington, DC 20013, 703-522-3332
United Network for Organ Sharing, P.O. Box 13770, Richmond, VA 23225-8770, 1-800-24-DONOR

High Risk for Disuse Syndrome

DEFINITION

High Risk for Disuse Syndrome: The state in which an individual is at risk for deterioration of body systems as the result of prescribed or unavoidable musculoskeletal inactivity.

DEFINING CHARACTERISTICS

Presence of risk factors (see Related Factors)

RELATED FACTORS

Pathophysiological

Decreased sensorium
Unconscious
Neuromuscular impairment
Multiple sclerosis   Muscular dystrophy
Parkinsonism   Partial/total paralysis
Guillain-Barré syndrome   Spinal cord injury
Musculoskeletal
Fractures
Rheumatic diseases
End-stage disease
AIDS   Cardiac
Renal   Cancer
Psychiatric/mental health disorders
Major depression   Severe phobias
Catatonic state

Treatment-related

Surgery (amputation, skeletal)
Traction/casts/splints
Prescribed immobility
Mechanical ventilation
Invasive vascular lines

Situational

Depression
Fatigue
Debilitated state
Pain

Maturational

Newborn/infant/child/adolescent
Down syndrome
Legg-Calvé-Perthes disease
Osteogenesis imperfecta

Cerebral palsy
Spina bifida
Risser-Turnbuckle jacket
Juvenile arthritis
Autism
Mental/physical disability
Elderly
Decreased motor agility
Muscle weakness
Presenile dementia

Diagnostic Considerations

High Risk for Disuse Syndrome describes a situation in which a person is at risk for the adverse effects of immobility. As a syndrome diagnosis, it contains its etiology in the diagnostic label (*Disuse*); a "related to" statement is not applicable. As discussed in Chapter 2, a syndrome diagnosis comprises a cluster of actual or high risk nursing diagnoses predicted to be present because of the situation. Eleven high risk or actual nursing diagnoses are clustered under *High Risk for Disuse Syndrome:*
- *High Risk for Impaired Skin Integrity*
- *High Risk for Constipation*
- *High Risk for Altered Respiratory Function*
- *High Risk for Altered Peripheral Tissue Perfusion*
- *High Risk for Infection*
- *High Risk for Activity Intolerance*
- *High Risk for Impaired Physical Mobility*
- *High Risk for Injury*
- *High Risk for Sensory–Perceptual Alterations*
- *Powerlessness*
- *Body Image Disturbance*

The nurse no longer needs to use separate diagnoses as *High Risk for Altered Respiratory Function* or *High Risk for Impaired Skin Integrity,* for they are incorporated into this syndrome category. However, if an individual who is immobile manifests the signs or symptoms of impaired skin integrity or another diagnosis, the specific diagnosis should be used. The nurse should continue to use *High Risk for Disuse Syndrome* so that deterioration of the other body systems does not occur.

Errors in Diagnostic Statements

High Risk for Disuse Syndrome related to reddened sacral area (3 cm)

A reddened sacral area is evidence of the diagnosis *Impaired Skin Integrity.* Thus, the nurse should use two diagnoses for this person: *Impaired Skin Integrity related to effects of immobility, as evidenced by reddened sacral area (3 cm)* and *High Risk for Disuse Syndrome.*

Focus Assessment Criteria

Subjective Data

History of systemic disorders
Neurologic
CVA, head trauma, increased intracranial pressure

Multiple sclerosis, poliomyelitis, Guillain-Barré, myasthenia gravis
Spinal cord injury, tumor, birth defect
Cardiovascular
Myocardial infarction
Congential heart anomaly
Congestive heart failure
Musculoskeletal
Osteoporosis
Fractures
Arthritis
Respiratory
Chronic obstructive pulmonary disease (COPD)
Orthopnea
Pneumonia
Dyspnea on exertion
Debilitating diseases
Cancer
Endocrine disease
Renal disease
History of symptoms (complaints of)
Pain
Muscle weakness
Fatigue
History of recent trauma or surgery
Fractures
Head injury
Abdominal surgery or injury

Objective Data

Dominant hand

Right	Left	Ambidextrous

Motor function

Right arm	Strong	Weak	Absent	Spastic
Left arm	Strong	Weak	Absent	Spastic
Right leg	Strong	Weak	Absent	Spastic
Left leg	Strong	Weak	Absent	Spastic

Mobility

Ability to turn self	Yes	No	Assistance needed (specify)
Ability to sit	Yes	No	Assistance needed (specify)
Ability to stand	Yes	No	Assistance needed (specify)
Ability to transfer	Yes	No	Assistance needed (specify)
Ability to ambulate	Yes	No	Assistance needed (specify)

Weight-bearing (assess both right and left sides)

Full	As tolerated
Partial	Non-weight bearing

Gait

Stable	Unstable

Assistive devices

Crutches	Walker	Prosthesis
Cane	Wheelchair	Other
Braces		

Restrictive devices

Cast or splint	Ventilator	IV
Traction	Drain	Monitor
Braces	Foley	Dialysis

Range of motion (shoulders, elbows, arms, hips, legs)

Full	Limited (specify)	None

Motivation (as perceived by nurse and/or reported by person)

Excellent	Satisfactory	Poor

Principles and Rationale for Nursing Care

Generic Considerations

1. "Immobility is inconsistent with human life." Mobility provides one control over one's environment; without mobility, one is at the mercy of one's environment (Christian, 1982).
2. Activity, mobility and flexibility are integral to one's life-style. Immobility has a serious impact on one's self-concept and life-style (Christian, 1982).
3. Society values youthfulness, energy, and productivity. Immobility is contradictory to these values.
4. Immobility restricts the person's ability to seek out sensory stimulation. In contrast, immobile persons may be unable to remove themselves from an environment that is too stressful or noisy (Christian, 1982).
5. Musculoskeletal inactivity or immobility has adverse effects on all the body systems. Table II-3 outlines the effects of immobility on body systems.
6. A muscle loses about 3% of its original strength each day it is immobilized.
7. Prolonged immobility has adverse effects on psychologic health, learning, socialization, and ability to cope. Table II-4 illustrates these effects.
8. The more portions of the body immobilized and the longer the immobilization, the greater the adverse effects.
9. Joints without range of motion will develop contractures in 3–7 days because flexor muscles are stronger then extensor muscles.
10. Increased serum calcium resulting from bone destruction caused by lack of motion and weight-bearing increases the coagulability of the blood. This, in addition to circulatory stasis, makes the person vulnerable to thrombosis formation.
11. The peristaltic contractions of the ureters are insufficient when in a reclining position, thus there is stasis of urine in the kidney pelvis.
12. Compression of nerves by casts, restraints, or improper positions can result in ischemia and nerve degeneration. Compression of the peroneal nerve results in footdrop; compression of the radial nerve results in wristdrop.

Pediatric Considerations

1. Mobility is essential for physical growth and development and mastery of developmental tasks (Whaley & Wong, 1989). Restricted movement can thwart achievement of developmental tasks. Refer to Table II-7 in the diagnostic category *Altered Growth and Development*.
2. Physical activity serves as a vehicle for communication and expression for children.
3. The major physiologic consequences of immobility include:
   a. Loss of muscle mass and strength
   b. Bone demineralization
   c. Loss of joint movement, increased risk for footdrop, contractures
   d. Increased activity as a result of anxiety (Whaley & Wong, 1989)

Table II-3   **Adverse Effects of Immobility on Body Systems**

System	Effect
Cardiac	Decreased myocardial performance Decreased heart rate and stroke volume Decreased oxygen uptake
Circulatory	Venous thrombosis Dependent edema Reduced venous return Increased intravascular pressure
Respiratory	Stasis of secretions Impaired cilia Drying of sections of mucous membranes Slower, more shallow respirations
Musculoskeletal	Muscle atrophy Shortening of muscle fiber (contracture) Decreased strength/tone Osteoporosis Joint degeneration Fibrosis of callogen fibers (joints)
Metabolic	Nitrogen excretion Hypercalcemia Anorexia Decreased metabolic rate Obesity Elevated creatine levels
Gastrointestinal	Constipation
Genitourinary	Urinary stasis Urinary calculi Urinary retention
Integumentary	Decreased capillary flow Tissue acidosis to necrosis
Neurosensory	Reduced innervation of nerves damaged by pressure or compromised blood supply

4. The major psychologic/emotional consequences of immobility include:
   a. Sensory deprivation, leading to altered self-perception and environmental awareness
   b. Isolation from peers
   c. Feelings of helplessness, frustration, anxiety, and boredom (Whaley & Wong, 1989; Wright, 1989).
5. Children who are restrained by casts, splints, or straps during the first 3 years of life have more difficulty with language than children whose activities are unrestricted (Whaley & Wong, 1989).
6. Children's responses to immobility may range from active protest to withdrawal and/or regression (Whaley & Wong, 1989; Wright, 1989).

Table II-4 **Psychosocial Effects of Immobility**
(Mammer & Kenan, 1980; Zubek & McNeil, 1967)

	Effect
Psychological	Increased tension
	Negative change in self-concept
	Fear, anger
Learning	Decreased motivation
	Decreased ability to retain, transfer learning
	Decreased attention span
Socialization	Change in roles
	Social isolation
Growth and development	Dependency

Gerontologic Considerations

1. Aging affects muscle functioning due to progressive loss of muscle mass and loss of strength and endurance.
2. Age-related changes in joint and connective tissue include impaired flexion and extension movements, decreased flexibility, and reduced cushioning protection for joints (Whitbourne, 1985).
3. After menopause, women experience an accelerated loss of trabecular and cortical bone: 9%–10% per decade (Miller, 1990).
4. Bed rest can cause an average vertical bone loss of 0.9%/week (Krolner & Toff, 1983).

■ High Risk for Disuse Syndrome

Assessment

Presence of risk factors

Outcome Criteria

The person will demonstrate continued
- Intact skin/tissue integrity
- Maximum pulmonary function
- Maximum peripheral blood flow
- Full range of motion
- Bowel, bladder, and renal functioning within normal limits
- Use of social contacts and activities when possible

The person will
- Explain rationale for treatments
- Make decisions regarding care when possible
- Share feelings regarding immobile state

Interventions

A. Identify causative and contributing factors
   1. Pain; refer also to *Altered Comfort*
   2. Fatigue; refer also to *Fatigue*
   3. Decreased motivation; refer also to *Impaired Adjustment*
   4. Depression; refer also to *Ineffective Individual Coping*

B. Promote optimal respiratory function
   1. Vary the position of the bed, thus gradually changing the horizontal and vertical position of the thorax, unless contraindicated.
   2. Assist to reposition, turning frequently from side to side (hourly if possible).
   3. Encourage deep breathing and controlled coughing exercises five times every hour.
   4. Teach individual to use blow bottle or incentive spirometer every hour when awake (with severe neuromuscular impairment, the person may have to be awakened during the night as well).
   5. For child, use colored water in blow bottle; have him blow up balloons, blow soap bubbles, blow cotton balls with straw.
   6. Auscultate lung fields every 8 hours; increase frequency if altered breath sounds are present.
   7. Encourage small frequent feedings to prevent abdominal distention.

C. Maintain usual pattern of bowel elimination. Refer to *Constipation related to immobility* for specific interventions

D. Prevent pressure ulcers
   1. Utilize repositioning schedule that relieves vulnerable area most often (*e.g.,* if vulnerable area is the back, turning schedule would be left side to back, back to right side, right side to left side, and left side to back); post "turn clock" at bedside.
   2. Turn person or instruct him to turn or shift weight every 30 minutes to 2 hours, depending on other causative factors present and the ability of the skin to recover from pressure.
   3. Frequency of turning schedule should be increased if any reddened areas that appear do not disappear within 1 hour after turning.
   4. Position person in normal or neutral position with body weight evenly distributed.
   5. Keep bed as flat as possible to reduce shearing forces; limit Fowler's position to only 30 minutes at a time.
   6. Use foam blocks or pillows to provide a bridging effect to support the body above and below the high-risk or ulcerated area so that affected area does not touch bed surface; do not use foam donuts or inflatable rings, since they will increase the area of pressure.
   7. Alternate or reduce the pressure on the skin surface with:
      a. Foam mattresses
      b. Air mattresses
      c. Air-fluidized beds
      d. Vascular boots to suspend heels
   8. Utilize enough personnel to lift person up in bed or chair rather than pull or slide skin surfaces; use Heelbo protectors to reduce friction on elbows and heels.

9. To reduce shearing forces, support feet with footboard to prevent sliding.
10. Promote optimum circulation when person is sitting.
    a. Limit sitting time for person at high risk for ulcer development.
    b. Instruct person to lift self using chair arms every 10 minutes if possible or assist person in rising up off the chair every 10–20 minutes, depending on risk factors present.
11. Inspect areas at risk of developing ulcers with each position change
    a. Ears
    b. Occiput
    c. Heels
    d. Sacrum
    e. Scrotum
    f. Elbows
    g. Trochanter
    h. Ischia
    i. Scapula
12. Observe for erythema and blanching and palpate for warmth and tissue-sponginess with each position change.
13. Massage non-reddened, vulnerable areas gently with each position change.
14. Refer to *Impaired Skin Integrity* for additional interventions.

E. Promote factors that improve venous blood flow

1. Elevate extremity above the level of the heart (may be contraindicated if severe cardiac or respiratory disease is present).
2. Avoid standing or sitting with legs dependent for long periods of time.
3. Consider the use of Ace bandages or below-knee elastic stocking to prevent venous stasis.
4. Reduce or remove external venous compression, which impedes venous flow
    a. Avoid pillows behind the knees or get bed that is elevated at the knees.
    b. Avoid leg crossing.
    c. Change positions, move extremities, or wiggle fingers and toes every hour.
    d. Avoid garters and tight elastic stockings above the knees.
5. Measure baseline circumference of calves and thighs daily if individual is at risk for deep venous thrombosis, or if it is suspected.

F. Maintain limb mobility and prevent contractures

1. Increase limb mobility.
    a. Perform ROM exercises (frequency to be determined by condition of the individual).
    b. Support extremity with pillows to prevent or reduce swelling.
    c. Encourage the person to perform exercise regimens for specific joints as prescribed by physician or physical therapist.
2. Position the person in alignment to prevent complications.
    a. Avoid placing pillows under knee; support calf instead.
    b. Point toes and knees toward ceiling when the client is in a supine position.
    c. Use footboard to prevent footdrop.
    d. Avoid prolonged periods of hip flexion (*i.e.*, sitting position).
    e. To position hips, place rolled towel lateral to hip to prevent external rotation.
    f. Keep arms abducted from the body with pillows.
    g. Keep elbows in slight flexion.

    h. Keep wrist in a neutral position, with fingers slightly flexed and thumb abducted and slightly flexed.

    i. Change position of shoulder joints during the day (*e.g.,* abduction, adduction, range of circular motion).

G. Prevent urinary stasis and calculi formation

1. Provide a daily intake of fluid of 2000 mL or greater a day (unless contraindicated); refer to *Fluid Volume Deficit* for specific interventions.
2. Maintain urine pH below 6.0 (acidic) to reduce the formation of calcium calculi with acid ash foods (cereals, meats, poultry, fish, cranberry juice, apple juice).
3. Teach to avoid foods high in calcium and oxalate (* very high) as:
   a. Milk, milk products, cheese
   b. Bran cereals
   c. *Spinach, cranberries, plums, raspberries, gooseberries
   d. Sardines, shrimp, oysters
   e. Legumes, whole-grain rice
   f. *Chocolate
   g. Asparagus, rhubarb, kale, Swiss chard, turnip greens, mustard greens, broccoli, beet greens
   h. Peanut butter, ripe olives

H. Reduce and monitor bone demineralization

1. Monitor for hypercalcemia.
   a. Serum levels
   b. Nausea/vomiting, polydipsia, polyuria, lethargy
2. Provide weight-bearing when possible.
   a. Tilt-table
3. Maintain vigorous hydration.
   a. Adult 2000 mL/day
   b. Adolescents 3000–4000 mL/day

I. Promote sharing and a sense of well-being

1. Encourage to share feelings and fears regarding restricted movement.
2. Utilize play therapy (Appendix IX) to encourage child to share feelings (*e.g.,* put cast on doll).
3. Encourage client to wear own clothes rather than pajamas.
   a. Encourage the wearing of unique adornments as an expression of individuality (*e.g.,* baseball caps, colorful socks)

J. Reduce the monotony of immobility

1. Vary daily routine when possible (*e.g.,* give bath in the afternoon, so that the person can watch a special show or talk with a visitor who drops in to see him).
2. Include the individual in planning schedule for daily routine.
   a. Allow the person to make as many decisions as possible.
   b. Make daily routine as normal as possible (*e.g.,* have the person wear street clothes during the day if feasible).
3. Plan time for visitors.
   a. Encourage person to make a schedule for visitors so everyone does not come at once or at an inconvenient time.
   b. Spend quality time with the person (*i.e.,* not time that is task-oriented; rather, sit down and talk).

4. Be creative; vary the physical environment and daily routine when possible.
   a. Update bulletin boards, change the pictures on the walls, move the furniture within the room.
   b. Maintain a pleasant, cheerful environment (*e.g.*, plenty of light, flowers, conversation pieces).
   c. Place the person near a window if possible.
   d. Provide reading material, radio, television, "books on tape" (if person is visually impaired).
   e. Plan an activity daily to give person something to look forward to; always keep your promises.
   f. Discourage the use of television as the primary source of recreation unless it is highly desired.
   g. Consider using a volunteer to spend time reading to the person or helping with an activity.
   h. Encourage suggestions and new ideas (*e.g.*, "Can you think of things you might like to do?").
5. Plan appropriate activities for children.
   a. Provide an environment with accessible playthings that suit the child's developmental age and see that they are well within reach.
   b. Encourage family to bring in child's favorite playthings, including items from nature that will keep the real world alive (*e.g.*, goldfish, leaves in fall).

K. Provide opportunities for individual to control decisions
1. Allow person to manipulate surroundings, such as deciding what is to be kept where (shoes under bed, picture on window).
2. Keep needed items within reach (call bell, urinal, tissues).
3. Discuss daily plan of activities and allow person to make as many decisions as possible about it.
4. Increase decision-making opportunities as person progresses.
5. Respect and follow individual's decision if you have given him options.
6. Record person's specific choices on care plan to ensure that others on staff acknowledge preferences ("Dislikes orange juice," "Takes shower," "Plan dressing change at 7:30 prior to shower").
7. Keep promises.
8. Provide opportunity for person and family to express feelings.
9. Provide opportunities for person and family to participate in care.
10. Plan a care conference to allow staff to discuss methods of individualizing care; encourage each nurse to share at least one action that she discovered a particular individual liked.
11. Shift emphasis from what one cannot do to what one can do.
12. Set goals that are short-term, practical, and realistic.

References/Bibliography

Baird, S. (1985). Development of a nursing assessment tool to diagnose altered body image in immobilized patients. *Orthopedic Nursing, 4*(3), 47–54.

Bohachick, P. A. (1987). Pulmonary embolism in neurological and neurosurgical patients. *Journal of Neuroscience Nursing, 19*(4), 191–197.

Brower, P., & Hicks, D. (1972). Maintaining muscle function in patients on bed rest. *American Journal of Nursing, 72*(7), 1250–1253.

Carnevali, D., & Brueckner, S. (1970). Immobilization—reassessment of a concept. *American Journal of Nursing, 70*(7), 1502–1507.

Christian, B. J. (1982). Immobilization: Psychosocial aspects. In Norris, C. (Ed.). *Concept clarification in nursing*. Rockville, MD: Aspen Publications.

Downs, F. (1974). Bedrest and sensory disturbances. *American Journal of Nursing, 74*(3), 434–438.

Drayton-Hargrove, S. & Reddy, M. A. (1986). Rehabilitation and long-term management of the spinal cord–injured adult. *Nursing Clinics of North America, 21*(4), 599–610.

Erikson, E. (1959). Identity and the life cycle: Selected papers, *Psychological Issues, 1*(6), 118–146.

Hammer, R., & Kenan, E. (1980). The psychological aspects of immobilization. In Steinberg, F.U. (Ed.): *The immobilized patient: Functional pathology and management*. New York: Plenum Press.

Houk, N.G. (1980). The disabled adolescent: Promoting a positive self-concept by achievement of developmental tasks. In Chinn, P.L., & Leonard, K.B. (Eds.). *Current practice in pediatric nursing*. St. Louis: C. V. Mosby.

Kalafatich, A. (1982). Immobilization in adolescents. In Norris, C. (Ed): *Concept clarification in nursing*. Rockville, MD: Aspen Publications.

Kelly, M. (1986). Exercises for bedfast patients. *American Journal of Nursing, 66*(10), 2209–2213.

Krolner, B., & Toft, B. (1983). Vertical bone loss: An unheeded side effect of therapeutic bedrest. *Clinical Science, 64*(3), 537–540.

Lentz, C. (1981). Selected aspects of deconditioning secondary to immobilization. *Nursing Clinics of North America, 16*(4), 729–737.

Maklebust, J. (1987). Pressure ulcers: Etiology and prevention. In Mondoux, L. (Ed.): *Pressure ulcers*. Philadelphia: W. B. Saunders.

Miller, C. A. (1990). *Nursing care of older adults: Theory and practice*. Glenview, IL: Scott Foresman.

NANDA (1989). *Taxonomy I*. St. Louis: North American Nursing Diagnosis Association.

Ng, L., & McCormick, K. (1982). Position changes and their physical consequences. *Advances in Nursing Science, 4*(4), 13–25.

Olson, E. (1967). The hazards of immobility. *American Journal of Nursing, 67*, 780–797.

O'Neil, R. (1981). Problems associated with disuse syndromes—including the integument. In Beland, I.L., & Passos, J. Y. (Eds.). *Clinical nursing* (4th ed.) New York: Macmillan.

Schaupner, C. (1985). Impaired mobility. In Jacobs, M. & Geels, W. (Eds.). *Signs and symptoms in nursing*. Philadelphia, J. B. Lippincott.

Smith, K. V. & Henry, J.P. (1967). Cybernetic foundations for rehabilitation. *American Journal of Physical Medicine, 46*(2), 379–467.

Tyler, M. (1984). The respiratory effects of body positioning and immobilization. *Respiratory Care 29*, 472–481.

Whaley, L. F., & Wong, D. L. (1989). *Essentials of pediatric nursing* (3rd ed.). St. Louis: C.V. Mosby.

Whitbourne, S. K. (1985). Appearance and movement. In Whitbourne, S. K. (Ed.). *The aging body*. New York: Springer-Verlag.

Wright, S. (1989). Nursing strategies: Altered musculoskeletal function. In Foster, R. L., Hunsberger, M. M., & Anderson, J. J. T. (Eds.). *Family-centered nursing care of children*. Philadelphia: W. B. Saunders.

Zubek, J.P., & McNeil, M. (1967). Perceptual deprivation phenomena: Role of the recumbent position. *Journal of Abnormal Psychology, 72*, 147.

Diversional Activity Deficit

- *Related to* **Monotony of Confinement**
- *Related to* **Post-Retirement Inactivity (Change In Life-Style)**

DEFINITION

Diversional Activity Deficit: The state in which the individual or group experiences or is at risk of experiencing decreased stimulation from, or interest in, leisure activities.

DEFINING CHARACTERISTICS

Major (must be present)

Observed and/or statements of boredom/depression due to inactivity

Minor (may be present)

Constant expression of unpleasant thoughts or feelings
Yawning or inattentiveness
Flat facial expression
Body language (shifting of body away from speaker)
Restlessness/fidgeting
Immobile (on bed rest or confined)
Weight loss or gain
Isolation
Hostility
Physical/emotional handicap

RELATED FACTORS

Pathophysiologic

Communicable disease
Pain

Treatment-related

Long or frequent treatments

Situational (Personal, environmental)

Loss of social network, (*e.g.,* due to relocation)
Monotonous environment
Long-term hospitalization or confinement
Lack of motivation
Loss of ability to perform usual or favorite activities
Excessively long hours of work
No time for leisure activities
Career changes (*e.g.,* teacher to housewife, retirement)
Children leaving home ("empty nest")

Immobility
Decreased sensory perception (*e.g.*, blindness, hearing loss)

Maturational

Infants/children (lack of appropriate toys/peers)
Elderly (sensory/motor deficits)

Diagnostic Considerations

A deficit in diversional activities is expressed by the person, who alone can determine whether types and amounts of activity are problematic. Miller (1990) writes that one's self-concept is affirmed through activities associated with various role supports.

To validate a nursing diagnosis of *Diversional Activity Deficit*, the nurse will need to explore the etiology for factors that are amenable to nursing interventions with the main focus on increasing or improving the quality of leisure activities. For a person with personality problems that hinder relationships and result in decreased social activities with others, the diagnosis *Impaired Social Interactions* would be more valid. The nurse would focus on helping the person identify the behavior as a barrier for socialization.

Errors in Diagnostic Statements

Diversional Activity Deficit related to boredom and reports of no leisure activities
This diagnosis does not reflect the required treatment. Boredom and reports of no leisure activities represent manifestations of the diagnosis, not contributing factors. Thus, the diagnosis should be written as: *Diversional Activity Deficit related to unknown etiology, as evidenced by reports of boredom and no leisure activities.*
Diversional Activity Deficit related to inability to sustain meaningful relationships, as evidenced by "no one calls me to go out"
This diagnosis would focus nursing interventions on enhancing the person's diversional activities. In this situation, the nurse should delay making a formal diagnosis and should collect more data to explore more specifically the meaning of "no one calls me to go out." Other diagnoses may be more applicable, *e.g., Impaired Social Interactions, Self-Concept Disturbance, Ineffective Coping*, and *Defensive Coping*.

Focus Assessment Criteria

Subjective Data

Perception of person's current activity level
Too busy (not enough time for relaxing activities)
Busy but able to find time to do relaxing activities
Bored, trapped, wishes there was more recreational activity
Past activity patterns (type, frequency)
Work
Leisure
Activities the person desires
Availability   Assistance needed
Feasibility   Support system

Objective Data
    Developmental age
    Motivation
        Interested   Withdrawn
        Disinterested   Hostile
    Presence of barriers to recreational activities
    Physical
        Immobility   Pain
        Altered level of consciousness   Sensory deficits (visual, auditory)
        Fatigue   Equipment (traction, IVs)
        Altered hand mobility   Communicable disease/isolation
    Psychologic/cognitive
        Lack of motivation   Depression
        Lack of knowledge   Embarrassment
    Socioeconomic
        Lack of available support system   Financial limitations
        Previous patterns of inactivity   Transportation difficulties
        Language barrier

Principles and Rationale for Nursing Care

Generic Considerations

1. All human beings need stimulation. In the adult, lack of stimulation results in boredom and depression. In the infant or child it causes "failure to thrive" and may stunt growth severely.
2. A significant relationship exists between informal activity and life satisfaction. The quality or type of interaction is more important than the quantity of activity (Lemon, Bengston, & Peterson, 1972).
3. Informal activities promote well-being more than formally structured activities. Solitary activities have little effect on life satisfaction (Longino & Kart, 1982).
4. Boredom paralyzes an individual's productivity and causes a feeling of stagnation. It is often a major contributing factor to substance abuse (overeating, drug abuse, alcoholism, and smoking).
5. The bored person has introspective feelings of being oppressed and trapped, which give rise to conscious or unconscious anger or hostility.
6. Being aware that one is bored allows one to redirect activities to increase stimulation.
7. Nurses who understand the concept of boredom and are aware of their own patterns of reacting to and dealing with boredom are better able to deal with boredom in others.
8. Taking responsibility for doing something about a boring situation is a positive means of dispelling boredom.
9. Music therapy, or "the controlled use of music, its elements, and their influences on the human being to aid the physiologic, psychologic, and emotional integration of the individual during the treatment of an illness or disability" (Munrro & Mount, 1978) can be a valuable intervention in relieving boredom, sparking interest, and assisting individuals in coping with social problems (Buckwalter, Harsock, & Gaffney, 1985).
10. Membership in a group or a support group can boost self-esteem and self-worth, provide a sense of belonging, and encourage activities that the person otherwise may

have shied away from. Support groups can often assist individuals with stressful, costly, or time-consuming problems.

11. Reminiscing, or spending time focusing on recalling significant memories, can be a satisfying and stimulating past time for the bored, ill, confined, or elderly individual (Halmilton, 1985).

Pediatric Considerations:

1. Children at special risk for diversional activity deficit include:
   a. Those who are bored
   b. Those who are immobilized
   c. Those who are hospitalized for long periods of time
   d. Those who are isolated to protect themselves or others
   e. Those who have diminished contact with family and/or friends
2. Age-appropriate activities should be provided to promote mental health and human development (Scipien, Chard, Howe, & Barnard, 1990). Refer to Table 11-7 in the diagnostic category *Altered Growth and Development.*
3. Children who are bored may be at greater risk for injury. Refer to the diagnostic category *High Risk for injury related to Maturational Age of the Hospitalized Child,* for more information.

Gerontologic Considerations

1. The older individual's cultural background strongly influences his use of diversional activities because of the value placed on work versus leisure activities (Matteson & McConnell, 1988).
2. Older, less educated, rural persons tend to place less value on leisure activities (Matteson & McConnell, 1988).
3. Because of functional changes related to age, worsening chronic disease, or change in social networks, many older individuals must restructure use of time (Ebersole & Hess, 1990; Matteson & McConnell, 1988).
4. In our society, retirement generally occurs from age 62–70. About 80% of men and 90% of women over age 65 are identified as being retired. The lost work role for the male can result in a void and subsequent depression, particularly if there has been no preretirement planning (Matteson & McConnell, 1988; McPherson & Guppy, 1979).
5. The aging process is enhanced when the person has cultivated varied interests and activities throughout life (Ebersole & Hess, 1990; Matteson & McConnell, 1988; McPherson & Guppy, 1979).
6. A change in living arrangements or environment might subject the elderly to a diversional activity deficit. For example, an organic gardener in his own private yard moves to a senior high-rise apartment where no land is available for a garden, or an older man who plays the drums moves in with his adult children who have neither the space for his drum set nor the inclination to listen to his drum solos (Matteson & McConnell, 1988).
7. Social isolation resulting from death of a spouse, lack of transportation, hearing impairment, or other physical or psychologic disabilities places the older individual at risk for diversional activity deficit (Hogstel, 1990).
8. Cognitive impairments, musculoskeletal impairment, pain, metabolic abnormality, or sensory deficit may force an elderly person to consider modification of long-time leisure activities or development of new activities. For example, a person who likes to cook but has poor eyesight might obtain large-print cookbooks, have a friend write

favorite recipes in bold print, or tape-record recipes (Harrell, McConnell, Wildman, & Samsa, 1989; Kane, Ouslander, & Abrass, 1984; Matteson & McConnell, 1988).

9. Limited financial resources and a set income might limit or prohibit leisure activities that were meaningful in the person's younger years (Matteson & McConnell, 1988).

10. Relocation might have an impact on recreational activities that a person enjoyed throughout life, *e.g.,* a move from New Hampshire to Florida for a person who loves to ski (Ebersole & Hess, 1990, Matteson 1988).

11. Volunteer activities provide diversion for 21% of individuals aged 55–64 and 14% of those aged 65 and over. Those aged 65 and over volunteered an average of 8 hr/wk. Reasons cited for not volunteering include transportation difficulties, financial concerns, and age discrimination by some community organizations (Ebersole & Hess, 1990; Hogstel, 1990; Matteson & McConnell, 1988).

12. The current generation of elderly persons has not been involved in physical fitness as a leisure activity to the degree as has been seen in the "Baby Boomers." National studies show that as a group the elderly are not physically fit, and only 39% report involvement in a regular exercise program. There seems to be a reluctance to engage in exercise programs, even those geared specifically to the individual, because of feelings that there is no purpose or usefulness to the exercise (Crase & Rosato, 1979; Ebersole & Hess, 1990; Matteson & McConnell, 1988).

■ Diversional Activity Deficit
Related to Monotony of Confinement

Assessment

Subjective Data

The person states
"I'm bored; there's nothing to do"
"I feel trapped"
"I can't do anything"
"I'm tired of being here"
"I have no friends or family"
"I have no one to play with"
"I feel restless"

Objective Data

Inability to move
Confinement to room or building
Limited or no support system
Flat affect or facial expression
Lethargy or sleepiness
Restlessness/fidgeting
Hostility/anger

Outcome Criteria

The person will
- Relate feelings of boredom and discuss methods of finding diversional activities
- Related methods of coping with feelings of anger or depression caused by boredom
- Report an increase in diversional activity

Interventions

A. Assess causative factors

1. Monotony
2. Inability to make decisions concerning his own plan of care (see *Powerlessness*)
3. Diminished socialization (see *Social Isolation*)
4. Lack of motivation/depression

B. Reduce or eliminate causative factors

1. Monotony
   a. Vary daily routine when possible (*e.g.,* give bath in the afternoon, so that the person can watch a special show or talk with a visitor who drops in to see him)
   b. Include the individual in planning schedule for daily routine.
      - Allow the person to make as many decisions as possible.
      - Make daily routine as normal as possible (*e.g.,* have the person wear street clothes during the day if feasible).
   c. Plan time for visitors.
      - Encourage person to make a schedule for visitors so everyone does not come at once or at an inconvenient time.
      - Spend quality time with the person (*i.e.,* not time that is task oriented; rather, sit down and talk).
   d. Be creative, vary the physical environment and daily routine when possible.
      - Update bulletin boards, change the pictures on the walls, move the furniture within the room.
      - Maintain a pleasant, cheerful environment (*e.g.,* plenty of light, flowers, conversation pieces).
      - Place the person near a window if possible.
      - Provide reading material, radio, television "books on tape" (if person is visually impaired).
      - Plan an activity daily to give person something to look forward to and always keep your promises.
      - Discourage the use of television as the primary source of recreation unless it is highly desired.
      - Consider using a volunteer to spend time reading to the person or helping with an activity.
      - Encourage suggestions and new ideas (*e.g.,* "Can you think of things you might like to do?").
      - Recognize that computers and telephones can help the confined become involved.

2. Lack of motivation
   a. Stimulate motivation by showing interest and encouraging sharing of feelings and experiences.
      - Discuss the person's likes and dislikes.
      - Encourage sharing of feelings of present and past experiences.
      - Spend time with the person purposefully talking about other topics (*e.g.,* "I just got back from the shore. Have you ever gone there?").
   b. Help the person to work through feelings of anger and grief
      - Allow him to ventilate.
      - Take the time to be a good listener.
      - See *Anxiety* for additional interventions.
   c. Encourage the person to join a group that might be of interest or help (may have to participate via intercom or special arrangement).
   d. Consider the use of music therapy (Buckwater, Harsock, and Gaffney, 1985) or reminiscence therapy (Halmilton, 1985) as an intervention.
   e. Plan appropriate activities for children.
      - Provide an environment with accessible playthings that suit the child's developmental age and see that they are well within reach.
      - Keep toys in all waiting areas.
      - Encourage family to bring in child's favorite playthings, including items from nature that will help to keep the real world alive (*e.g.,* goldfish, leaves in fall).

■ Diversional Activity Deficit
Related to Postretirement Inactivity
(Change in Life-Style)

Assessment

Subjective Data

The person reports
  "There's nothing to do"
  "I'm too old"
  "I feel useless"
  "No one needs me anymore"
Recent retirement
Empty nest (children gone from home)
Career terminated
Loss of significant others

Objective Data

Flat affect
Lethargy
Anger

Outcome Criteria

The person will
- Relate feelings of improved self-esteem and productivity
- Relate available community services and agencies that can be used for hobbies or recreational activities
- Use his strengths to contribute to himself and others
- Redirect energy toward interests that are personally fulfilling and provide diversional activity

Interventions

A. Assess causative factors
   1. Lack of significant others (loneliness, "empty nest")
   2. Loss of independence (*e.g.,* inability to drive, climb stairs)
   3. Fear of being unwanted or not needed
   4. Retirement
   5. Career termination or changes

B. Identify factors that promote activity and socialization
   1. Encourage socialization with peers and all age groups (frequently the very young and the very old mutually benefit from interaction with each other).
   2. Acquire assistance to increase the person's ability to travel.
      a. Arrange transportation to activities if necessary.
      b. Acquire aids for safety (*e.g.,* wheelchair for going to shopping center, a walker for ambulating in hallways).
   3. Increase the person's feelings of productivity and self-worth.
      a. Encourage person to use his strengths to help others and himself (*e.g.,* give him tasks to perform in a general project).
      b. Acknowledge efforts made by the person (*e.g.,* "You look nice tonight" or "Thank you for helping Mr. Jones with his dinner").
      c. Encourage open communication; value the person's opinion ("Mr. Jones, what do you think about . . . ?").
      d. Encourage the person to challenge himself with learning a new skill or pursuing a new interest.
      e. Refer to *Social Isolation* for additional interventions.

C. Consider the use of music therapy or reminiscence therapy as an intervention

D. Initiate referrals if indicated
   1. Suggest joining AARP (American Association of Retired Persons)
   2. Write the local Health and Welfare Council
   3. Provide a list of associations with senior citizen activities
      YMCA
      Churches
      Golden Age Club
      Encore Club
      MORA (Men of Retirement Age)

Gray Panthers
Sixty Plus Club
XYZ Group (Extra Years of Zest)
Young at Heart Club
SOS (Senior Outreach Services)
Leisure Hour Group

References/Bibliography

Ames, B., (1980). Art and the dying patient. *American Journal of Nursing, 80,* 1094–1096.

Billings, C. (1980). Emotional first aid. *American Journal of Nursing, 80,* 2005–2009.

Brooten, D. (1981). Career guide: To change what needs changing . . . doesn't take Wonder Woman. *Nursing, 11*(3), 81–83.

Buckwalter, K., Harsock, J., & Gaffney J. (1985). Music therapy. In Bulechek, G. *Nursing interventions and treatments.* Philadelphia: W. B. Saunders.

Bulechek, G. & McColskey, J., (1985). *Nursing interventions and treatments.* Philadelphia: W. B. Saunders.

Burnside, I. (1973). *Psychosocial nursing care of the aged.* New York: McGraw-Hill.

Carlson, C. (1979). *Behavioral concepts in nursing.* Philadelphia: J. B. Lippincott.

Carnevali, D., & Patrick, M. (1986). *Nursing management of the elderly.* Philadelphia: J. B. Lippincott.

Carpenito, L. (1991). *Handbook of nursing diagnosis* (4th ed.). Philadelphia: J. B. Lippincott.

Clark, C (1980). Burnout: Assessment and intervention. *Journal of Nursing Administration, 10*(9), 39–43.

Crase, D., & Rosato, F. (1979). Exercise and aging: New perspectives and educational approaches. *Educational Gerontology, 4,* 367–376.

Ebersole, P., & Hess, P. (1990). *Toward healthy aging: Human needs and nursing response* (3rd ed.) St. Louis: C.V. Mosby.

Frye, V., & Peters, M. (1972). *Therapeutic recreation: Its theory, philosophy and practice.* Harrisburg, PA: Stockpole Co.

Hadsell, N. (1974). A sociological theory and approach to music therapy with adult psychiatric patients. *Journal of Music Therapy, 11,* 113–124.

Halmilton, D. (1985) Reminiscence therapy. In Bulechek, G. *Nursing interventions and treatments.* Philadelphia: W.B. Saunders.

Harrell, J. S., McConnell, E. S., Wildman, D. S., & Samsa, G. P. (1989). *Journal of Gerontological Nursing, 15*(10), 13–19.

Hinds, P. (1980). Music: A milieu factor with implications for the nurse therapist. *Journal of Psychiatric Nursing, 18,* 28–33.

Hogstel, M. O. (1990). *Geropsychiatric nursing.* St. Louis: C. V. Mosby.

Jacobs, M., & Geels, W. (1985). *Signs and symptoms in nursing.* Philadelphia: J. B. Lippincott.

Kane, R.L., Ouslander, J. G. & Abrass, I. B. (1984). *Essentials of clinical geriatrics.* New York: McGraw-Hill.

Kauffman, M. (1978). Sharing the patient experience. *American Journal of Nursing, 78,* 860–862.

Kinney, C., Mannetter, R., & Carpenter, M. (1985). Support groups. In Bulechek, G. *Nursing interventions and treatments.* Philadelphia: W. B. Saunders.

Koch, K. (1978). Teaching poetry writing to the old and the ill. *Milbank Memorial Fund Quarterly Health and Society, 56*(1), 113–125.

Kovesces, J. (1980). Burnout doesn't have to happen. *Nursing, 10*(10), 105–110.

Lemon, B. W., Bengston, V. L., & Peterson, J. A. (1972). An exploration of the activity theory of aging: Activity types and life satisfaction among in-movers to a retirement community. *Journal of Gerontology, 27,* 511–523.

Longino, C. F., & Kart, C. S. (1982). Explicating activity theory: A formal replication. *Journal of Gerontology, 37,* 713–722.

Lore, A. (1979). Supporting the hospitalized elderly person. *American Journal of Nursing, 79,* 496–499.

Martin, D. (1981). Enjoyable activity for everyone. *Geriatric Nursing, 2,* 210–213.

Matteson, A. M., & McConnell, E. S. (1988). *Gerontological nursing concepts and practice.* Philadelphia: W. B. Saunders.

McGoran, S. (1978). On developing empathy: Teaching students self-awareness. *American Journal of Nursing, 78,* 859–860.

McPherson, B., & Guppy, N. (1979). Preretirement lifestyle and the degree of planning for retirement. *Journal of Gerontology, 34*(2), 254–263.

Miller, C. A. 19. *Nursing care of older adults.* Glenview, IL: Scott Foresman.

Munro, S., & Mount B. (1978). Music therpy in palliative care. *Canadian Medical Association Journal, 19*(1), 1029–1034.

Newman, M., & Gaudiano, J. (1984). Depression as an explanation for decreased subjective time in the elderly. *Nursing Research, 33*(3), 137.

Piche, J. (1978). Tell a story. *American Journal of Nursing, 78,* 1189–1193,

Rainwater, A., & Christiansen, K. (1984). Wellness/quality of life programs in a long-term care facility. *Journal of Long-Term Care Administration, 12*(4), 13,

Scipien, G. M., Chard, M. A., Howe, J., & Barnard, M. U. (1990). *Pediatric nursing care.* St. Louis: C. V. Mosby.

Travelbee, M. (1971). *Interpersonal aspects of nursing.* Philadelphia: F. A. Davis.

Warnick, M. (1985). Acute care patients can stay active. *Journal of Gerontological Nursing, 11*(12), 31.

Weiner, M. (1978). *Working with the aged.* Englewood Cliffs, NJ: Prentice-Hall.

Resources for the Consumer

Literature

American Association of Retired Persons, 1909 K Street NW, Washington, DC

Technology for Persons with Disabilities, National Support Center for Persons with Disabilities, P.O. Box 2150, Atlanta, GA 30301-2150, 800-426-2133

White House Conference on Aging. (1981). Report of Technical Committee on the Physical and Social Environment and Quality of Life. Washington, DC: US Government Printing Office

Dysreflexia

■ *Related to* **Reflex Stimulation of Sympathetic Nervous System secondary to loss of autonomic control; High Risk for**

DEFINITION

Dysreflexia: The state in which an individual with a spinal cord injury at T7 or above experiences a potential life-threatening uninhibited sympathetic response of the nervous system to a noxious stimulus.

DEFINING CHARACTERISTICS

Major (must be present)

Individual with spinal cord injury (T7 or above) with:
    Paroxysmal hypertension (sudden periodic elevated blood pressure in which systolic pressure is over 140 mm Hg and diastolic is above 90 mm Hg)
    Bradycardia or tachycardia (pulse rate of less than 60 or over 100 beats/minute)
    Diaphoresis (above the injury)
    Red splotches on skin (above the injury)
    Pallor (below the injury)
    Headache (a diffuse pain in different portions of the head and not confined to any nerve distribution area)

Minor (may be present)

    Chilling
    Conjunctival congestion
    Horner's syndrome (contraction of the pupil, partial ptosis of the eyelid, enophthalmos and, sometimes, loss of sweating over the affected side of the face)
    Paresthesia
    Pilomotor reflex
    Blurred vision
    Chest pain
    Metallic taste in mouth
    Nasal congestion

RELATED FACTORS

Pathophysiologic
Visceral stretching and irritation
    Bowel
        Constipation
        Fecal impaction

Bladder
Distended bladder
Urinary calculi
Infection
Cutaneous Stimulation
Tight clothing/sheets
Skin lesions
Temperature extremes

Infection

Stimulation of skin (abdominal, thigh)
Acute abdominal conditions
Spastic sphincter

Treatment-related

Removal of fecal impaction
Clogged or nonpatent catheter
Surgical incision

Situational

Lack of knowledge

Diagnostic Considerations

Dysreflexia represents a life-threatening situation that nurses can prevent or treat through nurse-prescribed interventions. Prevention involves teaching the client to reduce sympathetic nervous system stimulation and avoiding nursing interventions that can cause sympathetic stimulation. When dysreflexia occurs, nursing interventions focus on reducing or eliminating the noxious stimulus, *e.g.,* fecal impaction, urinary retention. If nursing actions do not eliminate the stimuli and resolve symptoms, initiation of medical intervention is critical. When a client requires medical treatment for all or most episodes of dysreflexia, the situation would be labeled as a collaborative problem: *Potential Complication: Dysreflexia*.

Errors in Diagnostic Statements

Dysreflexia related to paroxysmal hypertension
Paroxysmal hypertension is a sign of dysreflexia, not a causative or contributing stimulus. The diagnosis should be restated as *High Risk for Dysreflexia related to possible reflex stimulation by visceral or cutaneous irritation, as evidenced by (specify)*.
Clinically, *High Risk for Dysreflexia* is a more descriptive diagnosis than *Dysreflexia*. The client is in a potential state the majority of the time, with associated nursing responsibilities of prevention, teaching, and early removal of stimulus.

Focus Assessment Criteria

Subjective Data

History of dysreflexia
Triggered by
Bladder distention
Bowel distention

Tactile stimulation
Skin lesion
Sexual activity
Menstruation
Initial symptoms
Headache
Sweating, where?
Chills
Metallic taste in mouth
Nasal congestion
Blurred vision
Numbness
Other _____
Medications used? What? Any recent changes?
Bladder program (type, problems, any recent changes?)
Bowel program (type, problems, any recent changes?)
Knowledge of dysreflexia
Cause
Self-treatment
Medical treatment
Prevention

Principles and Rationale for Nursing Care

Generic Considerations

1. The autonomic nervous system, sympathetic and parasympathetic, is located in the cerebrum, hypothalamus, medulla, brain stem, and spinal cord. With spinal cord injury, the cord activity below the injury is deprived of the controlling effects from the higher centers, which results in poorly controlled responses (Hickey, 1986).

2. When sensory receptors are stimulated below a spinal lesion, sympathetic discharge, medicated by the spinothalamic tract and posterior columns, results. This reflex stimulation of the sympathetic nervous system causes spasms of the pelvic viscera and the arterioles. These spasms cause vasoconstriction below the level of the injury. Baroreceptors in the aortic arch and carotid sinus respond to the hypertensive state with superficial vasodilatation, flushing, diaphoresis, and piloerection (gooseflesh) above the level of the spinal lesion. Vagal stimulation slows the heart rate, but because the cord is severed, vagal impulses to dilate vessels are prohibited (Hickey, 1986).

3. Intravenous pharmocologic intervention may be warranted if the noxious stimuli cannot be removed and/or the hypertension is not reduced. Some medications are: diazoxide (Hyperstat), hydralazine (Apresoline), sodium nitroprusside (Nipride), and ganglionic blocking agents such as phenoxybenzamine (Dibenzyline) and guanethidine sulfate (Ismelin).

4. Failure to reverse dysreflexia can result in status epilepticus, stroke, and death. Uncontrolled hypertension can cause systolic blood pressure to rise as high as 240–300 mm Hg.

■ High Risk for Dysreflexia
Related to Reflex Stimulation of Sympathetic Nervous system secondary to loss of autonomic control

Assessment
See Related Factors

Outcome Criteria

The individual/family will
- State factors that cause dysreflexia
- Describe the treatment for dysreflexia
- Relate when emergency treatment is indicated

Interventions

A. Assess for the presence of causative or contributing factors.

See Related Factors

B. If signs of dysreflexia occur, *raise the head of the bed* and remove the noxious stimuli
   1. Bladder distention
      a. Check for distended bladder
      b. If catheterized
         - Check catheter for kinks or compression
         - Irrigate with only 30 mL saline very slowly
         - Replace catheter if it will not drain
      c. If not catheterized, insert catheter using dibucaine hydrochloride ointment (Nupercainal) ointment and remove 500 mL, then clamp for 15 minutes; repeat cycle until bladder is drained.
   2. Fecal impaction
      a. First apply Nupercainal to the anus and into the rectum for 1 inch (2.54 cm).
      b. Gently check rectum with a well-lubricated glove using index finger.
      c. Insert rectal suppository or gently remove impaction.
   3. Skin irritation
      a. Spray skin lesion that is triggering dysreflexia with a topical anesthetic agent.

C. Continue to monitor blood pressure every 3–5 minutes

D. Immediately consult physician for pharmacologic treatment if symptoms or noxious stimuli are not eliminated

E. Initiate health teaching and referrals as indicated
1. Teach signs and symptoms and treatment of dysreflexia to person and family.
2. Teach when immediate medical intervention is warranted.
3. Explain what situations can trigger dysreflexia (menstrual cycle, sexual activity, bladder or bowel routines)
4. Teach to watch for early signs and to intervene immediately.
5. Teach to observe for early signs of bladder infections and skin lesions (pressure ulcers, ingrown toenails).
6. Advise consultation with physician for long-term pharmocologic management if individual is very vulnerable.

References/Bibliography

Disabato, J., & Wulf, J. (1989). Nursing strategies: Altered neurologic functions. In Foster, R. L., Hunsberger, M. M., & Anderson, J. J. T. (Eds.). *Family-centered nursing care of children.* Philadelphia: W. B. Saunders.

Guttman, L., & Whitteridge, D. (1947). Effects of bladder retention on autonomic mechanisms after spinal cord injuries. *Brain, 70*(4), 361–404.

Head, H., & Riddoch, G. (1917). The autonomic bladder, excessive sweating and some other reflex conditions in gross injuries of the spinal cord. *Brain,* 40, 188–263.

Hickey, J. (1986). *Neurological and neurosurgical nursing* (2nd ed.). Philadelphia: J. B. Lippincott.

Kewalramani, L. S. (1980). Autonomic dysreflexia in traumatic myelopathy. *American Journal of Physical Medicine, 59*(1), 1–19.

Kurnick, N. B. (1956). Autonomic hyperreflexia and its control in patients with spinal cord lesions. *Annals of Internal Medicine, 44,* 678–686.

Lindan, R., et al. (1980). Incidence and clinical features of autonomic dysreflexia in patients with spinal cord injury. *Paraplegia, 18,* 285–292.

Mathias, C. J., et al. (1976). Plasma catecholamines during paroxysmal neurogenic hypertension in quadriplegic man. *Circulation Research, 39*(2), 204–208, 1976

Naftchi, N. E., et al. (1978). Hypertensive crisis in quadriplegic patients. *Circulation, 57* (2), 336–341

Niederpruem, M. S. (1984) Autonomic dysreflexia. *Rehabilitation Nursing, 9,* 29–31.

Family Processes, Altered

■ *Related to* **Impact (specify) of Ill Member On Family System**

DEFINITION
Altered family processes: The state in which a usually supportive family experiences, or is at risk to experience, a stressor that challenges its previously effective functioning.

DEFINING CHARACTERISTICS
Family system cannot or does not:

Major (must be present)
Adapt constructively to crisis
Communicate openly and effectively between family members

Minor (may be present)
Meet physical needs of all its members
Meet emotional needs of all its members
Meet spiritual needs of all its members
Express or accept a wide range of feelings
Seek or accept help appropriately

RELATED FACTORS
Any factor can contribute to altered family processes. Some common factors are listed below.

Pathophysiologic
Illness of family member
    Discomforts related to the illness's symptoms
Trauma
    Surgery

Change in the family member's ability to function

Loss of body part or function

Treatment-related
Disruption of family routines due to time-consuming treatments (*e.g.,* home dialysis)
Physical changes due to treatments of ill family member
Emotional changes in all family members due to treatments of ill family member
Financial burden of treatments for ill family member
Hospitalization of ill family member

Situational (personal, environmental)
Loss of family member
    Death
    Going away to school
    Separation
    Divorce

Incarceration
Desertion
Hospitalization

Gain of new family member

Birth	Marriage
Adoption	Elderly relative

Poverty

Disaster

Relocation

Economic crisis

Unemployment	Financial loss

Change in family roles

Working mother	Retirement

Birth of child with defect

Conflict

Goal conflicts	Cultural conflict with reality
Moral conflict with reality	Personality conflict in family

Breach of trust between members

Dishonesty	Adultery

History of psychiatric illness in family

Social deviance by family member (including crime)

Diagnostic Considerations

Altered Family Processes describes a family that reports usual constructive function but a current challenge from a stressor has altered the family's functioning. The family is viewed as a system, with interdependency between members. Thus, life challenges for individual family members also challenge the family system. Certain situations have the potential to negatively influence family functioning; examples include illness, elderly relative moving in, relocation, separation, or divorce. The diagnosis *High Risk for Altered Family Process* can represent such as situation.

Errors in Diagnostic Statements

Altered Family Process related to family not discussing the situation

A Family's failure to discuss a situation does not represent a related factor, but rather a possible validation of the problem. If this situation is usual for the family, the diagnosis *Ineffective Family Coping: Disabling* should be investigated. If a failure to support each other represents a response to a stressor affecting the family system, the diagnosis *Altered Family Processes related to (specify stressor), as evidenced by report of family not discussing the situation* may be appropriate.

Focus Assessment Criteria

Character of family

Age and sex of members

Ethnic background

Religious background

What is the religious affiliation?

Does the family participate in religious activity?

How often?

Health status

What is the current health status of each member?

Are children within the appropriate range for growth and development?

What is the health history of each family member?

Illness	Accidents
Surgery	Allergies

What preventive measures are practiced?

Immunizations

Health exams

Dental	Eye
General	Gynecologic

Health practices

Family planning	Abstention from or moderate use
Regular exercise (2–3 times	of alcohol
a week for 30 minutes)	Daily dental care
Weight control	Self-breast exam (for women)
Abstention from smoking	Testes exam (for men)

Constructive responses

Relies on each other	Seeks knowledge and resources
Shares feelings, thoughts	Uses support systems
Appraises problem accurately	

Destructive responses

Denial	Abandonment
Exploitation of members	Authoritarianism
(threats, violence, neglect,	
scapegoating)	

Do any adults have a history of ineffective coping patterns (depression, violence, substance abuse)?

What are the strengths of the family?

What are the limitations of the family?

Caregiver assessment (adapted from Given, Collins & Given, 1988):

Prior relationship (type, quality)

Ill person's problematic characteristics

Responsibilities of caregiver (family, work, ill person)

Sources of instrumental support (household members, friends, relatives, formal agencies)

Sources of emotional support (individuals, professional)

- Impact on physical/mental health
- Alternatives (home health care, institutionalization)

Principles and Rationale for Nursing Care

Generic Considerations

1. Each family has a personality to which each member contributes.
2. The family unit may be viewed as a system with
   a. Interdependency between members
   b. Interactional patterns that provide structure and support for members
   c. Boundaries between the family and the environment and between members with varying degrees of permeability
3. Families change with time. They must accomplish specific tasks that originate from the needs of their members. Table II-5 illustrates the tasks of the family.
4. Each family responds to life challenges in ways that reflect experiences in the past and goals for the future.
5. Within a family, members interact in a variety of roles, which result from individual

Table II-5 **Stage-Critical Family Developmental Tasks Through the Family Life Cycle**

Stage of the Family Life Cycle	Positions in the Family	Stage-Critical Family Developmental Tasks
1. Married couple	Wife Husband	Establishing a mutually satisfying marriage Adjusting to pregnancy and the promise of parenthood Fitting into the kin network
2. Childbearing	Wife-mother Husband-father Infant daugher or son or both	Having, adjusting to, and encouraging the development of infants Establishing a satisfying home for both parents and infant(s)
3. Preschool-age	Wife-mother Husband-father Daughter-sister Son-brother	Adapting to the critical needs and interests of preschool children in stimulating growth-promoting ways Coping with energy depletion and lack of privacy as parents
4. School-age	Wife-mother Husband-father Daughter-sister Son-brother	Fitting into the community of school-age families in constructive ways Encouraging children's educational achievement
5. Teenage	Wife-mother Husband-father Daughter-sister Son-brother	Balancing freedom with responsibility as teenagers mature and emancipate themselves Establishing postparental interests and careers as growing parents
6. Launching center	Wife-mother-grandmother Husband-father-grandfather Daughter-sister-aunt Son-brother-uncle	Releasing young adults into work, military service, college, marriage, etc., with appropriate rituals and assistance Maintaining a supportive home base
7. Middle-aged parents	Wife-mother-grandmother Husband-father-grandfather	Rebuilding the marriage relationship Maintaining kin ties with older and younger generations
8. Aging family members	Widow-widower Wife-mother-grandmother Husband-father-grandfather	Coping with bereavement and living alone Closing the family home or adapting it to aging Adjusting to retirement

(Duvall, E.M. [1977]. *Marriage and family development* (5th ed.) Philadelphia: J. B. Lippincott, reproduced with permission)

and group needs: parent, spouse, child, sibling, friend, teacher, and so on. Illness of a family member may cause great changes, putting the family at high risk for maladaptation (Fife, 1985).

6. Communication patterns of the family determine the quality of the family life.
7. Each family member influences the family unit. Thus, the health of an individual will influence the health of the family.

Crisis and Family Coping

1. Stress is defined as the body's response to any demand made on it. Stress has the potential for becoming a crisis when the person or family cannot cope constructively.
2. A crisis is an event that occurs when the person's usual problem-solving methods are inadequate to resolve the situation.
3. The family in response to crisis will do one of the following: return to precrisis functioning, develop a more optimal level of functioning (higher level), or develop a destructive form of functioning (lower level).
4. The goal of crisis management is to assist the family to return to its precrisis functioning. If the precrisis functioning was destructive (*e.g.*, alcoholism), the goal would be to develop a more optimal level of functioning. (See Appendix VII for guidelines for crisis management.)
5. Common sources of family stress are (Minuchin, 1974):
   a. External sources of stress that one member is experiencing (*e.g.*, job- or school-related)
   b. External sources of stress that influence the family unit (*e.g.*, finances, relocation)
   c. Developmental stressors (*e.g.*, child-bearing, new baby, child-rearing, adolescence, new member or members—arrival of older grandparent, marriage of single parents—or loss of spouse)
   d. Situational stressors (*e.g.*, illness, hospitalization, separation)
6. Constructive or functional coping mechanisms of families faced with a stress crisis are (Friedman, 1981).
   a. Greater reliance on each other
   b. Maintenance of a sense of humor
   c. Increased sharing of feeling and thoughts
   d. Promotion of each member's individuality
   e. Accurate appraisal of the meaning of the problem
   f. Search for knowledge and resources about the problem
   g. Utilization of support systems
7. Destructive or dysfunctional coping mechanisms of families faced with a stress or crisis are (Friedman, 1981):
   a. Denial of the problem
   b. Exploitation of one or more of the family members (threats, violence, neglect, scapegoating)
   c. Separation (hospitalization, institutionalization, divorce, abandonment)
      • Authoritarianism (no negotiation)
      • Preoccupation of family or members (who lack affection) to appear close
8. Parenthood is a crisis. Some common problems are
   a. Increase in mate arguments
   b. Fatigue resulting from schedule
   c. Disrupted social life
   d. Disrupted sex life
   e. Multiple losses—actual or perceived (*e.g.*, independence, career, attractiveness, attention)

9. Characteristics of families prone to crisis include
   a. Apathy (resigned to state in life)
   b. Poor self-concept
   c. Low income
   d. Inability to manage money
   e. Unrealistic preferences (materialistic)
   f. Lack of skills and education
   g. Unstable work history
   h. Frequent relocations
   i. History of repeated inadequate problem-solving
   j. Lack of adequate role models
   k. Lack of participation in religious or community activities
   l. Environmental isolation (no telephone, inadequate public transportation)

Illness in the Family

1. Successful coping with illness requires the family to complete the following tasks: acknowledge the problem and seek help, accept the problem and its implications, and adjust as the member begins reconstruction.
2. The family acknowledges the problem by identifying the symptoms as serious enough to warrant investigation, and gaining knowledge of accessible resources.
3. There exists a time lag between identification of symptoms and help-seeking behavior, which may vary between families, depending on previous experience with the health care system, cultural interpretations of health and illness, and financial concerns.
4. The family must face the diagnosis and its implications. This task is multidimensional, including
   a. Experiencing the initial shock
   b. Engaging in open communication between members
   c. Minimizing anxiety and its disabling consequences
   d. Preventing prolonged despair, guilt, blame, hostility
   e. Accepting a valid diagnosis
5. The family must adjust, as the member begins to recover, by
   a. Adapting to new ways of living and making appropriate changes as recovery ensues
   b. Fostering independence of recovering member
   c. Accepting residual disability and making any necessary accommodations
   d. Recognizing depression and anxiety in family member during change from "sick role" to "well role"
6. The family must return to normalcy by returning to previous activities as much as possible and incorporating the recovered member back into the flow of family activities and responsibilities.
7. Factors that positively influence the caregiving environment are "the social supports that the caregiver feels are available, the community services used and the financial conditions imposed by caregiving" (Given, Collins, & Given, 1988).
8. House (1981) describes four basic types of social support: emotional (concern, trust), appraisal (affirms self-worth), informational (useful advice, information for problem-solving), and instrumental (caregiving) assistance or tangible goods (money, help with chores).
9. Caregivers who provide care as the individual deteriorates set in motion a cycle of isolation, sadness, and frustration (Given, Collins, & Given, 1988).
10. Pagel (1985) reported that of 68 family caregivers of persons with Alzheimer's disease, 28 met the criteria for clinical depression.

11. According to Larkin (1987), families that "can come to agreement on what the presence of chronic illness in the family means to them are more likely to avoid the destruction and dissolution of family relationships"
12. Regularly scheduled periods of respite are critical to a caregiver's emotional health (Pallet, 1990).

Pediatric Considerations

1. Two of the most significant stresses a child and family may experience are illness and hospitalization. The stresses of separation from parents, loss of control in a strange environment, and fear of bodily injury and pain make children particularly vulnerable (Whaley & Wong, 1989).
2. Parents share many of the same stresses as hospitalized children. Additionally, they may experience stress if their roles as primary caretakers are taken over by hospital staff. Parents are responsible as well for the care of siblings, who are affected by the crisis of illness and hospitalization (Craft & Craft, 1989).
3. Parents of hospitalized children often are not aware of the number of changes that siblings experience (Craft & Craft, 1989).

Gerontologic Considerations

1. As the population ages, more adult children will be caring for dependent elderly parents.
2. As size of families decreases and population mobility increases, the burden of caregiving may tend to fall more on one adult child.
3. The elder's cognitive and behavioral characteristics, functional ability, and prior relationship with the caregiver will affect caregiver–elder reactions (Given, Collins, & Given, 1988).

■ Altered Family Processes
Related to Impact (specify) of Ill Member On Family System

Assessment

Subjective Data

Family members verbalize fear, anxiety, and anger.

Family members engage in destructive bickering.

Individual family members make direct or subtle appeal for help, such as:

"I can't cry but feel like I need to" (asking for permission to cry).

"I don't want her to know how worried I am" (asking for help with communication).

"I haven't eaten anything since this morning" (asking permission to leave the bedside of ill family member).

"I don't know where I went wrong" (requesting reassurance that illness is not his fault).

Family members are unable to make a decision together.

One or more family members refuse to assist with ill member's care.

Objective Data

Absence of family interaction (both verbally and nonverbally)

Tendency of family members to interfere with necessary nursing and medical interventions

Sudden outburst of emotions without apparent cause and/or emotional liability of family members

---

Outcome Criteria

The family members will

- Frequently verbalize feelings to professional nurse and each other
- Participate in care of ill family member
- Facilitate return of ill family member from sick role to well role
- Maintain functional system of mutual support for each member
- Identify appropriate external resources available

Interventions

A. Assess causative and contributing factors

  1. Illness-related factors

    a. Sudden, unexpected nature of illness

    b. Burdensome problems of a chronic nature

    c. Potentially disabling nature of illness

    d. Symptoms creating disfiguring change in physical appearance

    e. Social stigma associated with illness

    f. Financial burden

  2. Factors related to behavior of ill family member

    a. Refuses to cooperate with necessary interventions

    b. Engages in socially deviant behavior associated with illness: suicide attempts, violence, substance abuse

    c. Isolates self from family

    d. Acts out or is verbally abusive to health professionals and family members

  3. Factors related to the family as a whole

    a. Presence of unresolved guilt, blame, hostility, jealousy

    b. Inability to problem-solve adequately

    c. Ineffective patterns of communication among members

    d. Changes in role expectations and resulting tension

  4. Factors related to illness in family

    a. Lack of family members available for support

    b. Inadequate finances

    c. Lack of knowledge of caregiver

    d. History of poor relationship between caregiver and ill member

    e. Overburdened caregiver

  5. Factors related to health care environment

    a. Intervening professionals lack expertise in crisis intervention, counseling, or basic communication skills.

    b. Not enough health professionals can spend time with the family.

    c. Lack of continuity of care

    d. Lack of physical facilities in institution to ensure privacy or individualized care

  6. Factors related to the community

    a. Lack of support from spiritual resources (philosophical and/or religious)

    b. Lack of relevant health education resources

    c. Lack of supportive friends

    d. Lack of adequate community health care resources (*e.g.,* long-term follow-up care, hospice, respite agency)

B. Acknowledge your feelings about the family and their situation

1. Attempt to resolve these feelings.
    a. Pity
    b. Identifying with own family
    c. Blaming ill person and/or family for circumstances
    d. Judgmental attitude toward family
    e. Practicing punishing behavior (*e.g.,* ignoring people involved)
2. Gain experience in crisis intervention and communication skills.
3. Approach the family with warmth, respect, and support.
4. Avoid vague and confusing advice and clichés such as "Take it easy, everything will be OK."
5. Reflect family emotions to confirm these feelings ("This is very painful for you"; "You are very frightened.").
6. Keep family members abreast of changes in ill member's condition when appropriate.

C. Create a private and supportive hospital environment for family

1. Keep client's door closed if possible.
2. Provide family members with a meeting place alternative to client's room.
3. Make sure family members are oriented to visiting hours, bathrooms, vending machines, cafeteria, etc.
4. If possible, provide pillows/blankets for family members spending the night.

D. Facilitate family strengths

1. Acknowledge these strengths to family when appropriate.
    a. "I can tell you are a very close family."
    b. "You know just how to get your mother to eat."
    c. "Your brother means a great deal to you."
2. Involve family members in care of ill member when possible (feeding, bathing, dressing, ambulating).
3. Involve family members in patient care conferences when appropriate.
4. Encourage family to acquire substitutes to care for the ill person, to provide the family with time away.
5. Promote self-esteem of individual family members ("Your daughter may respond to your drawings if we place them in her crib") (see *Self-Concept Disturbance . . .*).
6. If appropriate help ill member identify how to give support to caregiver, *e.g.,* praise, listening.

E. Intervene when family weaknesses dominate

1. Facilitate communication.
2. Encourage verbalization of guilt, anger, blame, and hostility and subsequent recognition of own feelings in family members.

3. Enlist help of other professionals when problems extend beyond realm of nursing (*e.g.,* social worker, clinical psychologist, nurse therapist, clinical specialist, psychiatrist, child care specialist).

F. Facilitate understanding, in other family members, of how ill member feels

1. Discuss stresses of hospitalization.
2. Describe implications of "sick role" and how it will return to "well role."
3. Aid family members to change their expectations of the ill member in a realistic manner.

G. Assist family with appraisal of the situation

1. What is at stake? Encourage family to have a realistic perspective by providing accurate information and answers to questions.
2. What are the choices? Assist family to reorganize roles at home and set priorities to maintain family integrity and reduce stress.
3. Initiate discussions regarding stressors of home care (physical, emotional, environmental, financial).
4. Emphasize the importance of respites to prevent isolating behaviors that foster depression.
5. Discuss with the non-primary caregivers their responsibilities in caring for the primary caregiver.
6. Where is there help? Direct family to community agencies, home health care organizations, and sources of financial assistance as needed. (See *Impaired Home Maintenance Management* for additional interventions.)

H. Provide the family with anticipatory guidance as illness continues

1. Inform parents of the effects of prolonged hospitalization on children (appropriate to developmental age).
2. Prepare family members for signs of depression, anxiety, and dependency, which are a natural part of the illness experience.
3. If the ill family member is an elderly parent undergoing surgery, inform the children that the patient may be confused or disoriented for a limited period of time following surgery.

I. Discuss the implications of caring for ill family member with all household members; cover:

1. Available resources (finances, environmental)
2. 24-hour responsibility
3. Effects on other household members
4. Likelihood of progressive deterioration
5. Sharing of responsibilities (with other household members, siblings, neighbors)
6. Likelihood of exacerbation of long-standing conflicts
7. Impact on life-style
8. Alternative or assistive options (*e.g.,* community-based health care providers, life care centers, group living, nursing home)

J. Initiate health teaching and referrals as necessary

1. Include family members in group education sessions.
2. Refer families to lay support and self-help groups.
   Al-Anon
   Syn-Anon
   Alcoholics Anonymous

Sharing and Caring (American Hospital Association)
Ostomy Association
Reach for Recovery
Lupus Foundation of America
Arthritis Foundation
National Multiple Sclerosis Society
American Cancer Society
American Heart Association
American Diabetes Association
American Lung Association
Alzheimer's Disease and Related Disorders Association
3. Facilitate family involvement with social supports.
   a. Assist family members to identify reliable friends (clergy, significant others, etc.) and encourage seeking help (emotional, technical) when appropriate.

References/Bibliography

Austin, J. K. (1990). Assessment of coping mechanisms used by parents and children with chronic illness. *Issues in Comprehensive Pediatric Nursing, 15*(2), 98–102.

Burr, B., Good, B. J., & Good, M.D. (1978). The impact of illness on the family. In Taylor, R. B. (Ed): *Family medicine: Principles and practice.* New York: Springer-Verlag.

Christensen, K. E. (1979). Family epidemiology: An approach to assessment and intervention. In Hymovich, D. P., & Barnard, M. V. (Eds.). *Family health care* (2nd ed.). New York: McGraw-Hill.

Clements, D. B. (1990). Critical times for families with a chronically ill child. *Pediatric Nursing, 16*(2), 157–161

Clipp, E. C. (1990). Caregiver needs and patterns of social support. *Journal of Gerontological Nursing, 45*(3), 102–111.

Craft, M. J., & Craft, J. L. (1989). Perceived changes in siblings of of hospitalized children: A comparison of sibling and hospitalized and parent reports. *Children's Health Care, 18*(1), 42–48.

Duvall, E. M: (1977). *Marriage and family development* (5th ed.). Philadelphia: J. B. Lippincott.

Fife, B. L: (1985). A model for predicting the adaptation of families to medical crisis: An analysis of role integration. *Image: Journal of Nursing Scholarship, 18*(4), 108–112.

Friedman, M. (1981). *Family nursing: Theory and assessment.* New York: Appleton-Century-Crofts.

Giacquinta, B. (1977). Helping families face the crisis of cancer. *American Journal of Nursing, 77,* 1585–1588.

Given, C., Collins, C., & Given, B. (1988). Sources of stress among families caring for relatives with Alzheimer's disease. *Nursing Clinics of North America, 23*(1), 69–82.

House, J. S. (1981). *Work stress and social support.* Reading, MA: Addison-Wesley.

Hymovich, D. P., & Barnard, M. V. (Eds.). (1979). *Family health care* (2nd ed.). New York: McGraw-Hill.

Larkin, J. (1987). Factors influencing one's ability to adapt to chronic illness. *Nursing Clinics of North America, 22*(3), 535–542.

McCubbin, M. (1984). Nursing assessment of parental coping with cystic fibrosis. *Western Journal of Nursing Research, 6*(4), 407–418.

Miller, S., Winstead-Fry, P. (1982). *Family systems theory in nursing practice.* Norwalk, CT: Reston Publishing.

Minuchin, A, (1974). *Families and family therapy.* Cambridge: Harvard University Press.

Pagel, M. D., (1985). Loss of control, self-blame, and depression: An investigation of spouse caregivers of Alzheimer's disease patients. *Journal of Abnormal Psychology, 94* (2), 169–182.

Pallet, P. (1990). A conceptual framework for studying family caregivers burden in Alzheimer's type dementia. *Image, 22*(1), 52–57.

Reed, S. (1990). Potential for alterations in family process: When a family has a child with cystic fibrosis. *Issues in Comprehensive Pediatric Nursing, 13*(1), 15–23.

Tilden, V. P. & Weinert, C. (1987). Social support and the chronically ill individual. *Nursing Clinics of North America, 22*(3), 613–620.

Whaley, L. F., & Wong, D. L. (1989). *Essentials of pediatric nursing* (3rd ed.). St. Louis: C. V. Mosby.

Wright, L. M. (1990). Trends in nursing of families. *Journal of Advanced Nursing, 15*(2), 148–154.

Fatigue

■ *Related to* **(Specify)**

DEFINITION

Fatigue: The self-recognized state in which an individual experiences an overwhelming sustained sense of exhaustion and decreased capacity for physical and mental work that is not relieved by rest.

DEFINING CHARACTERISTICS*

Major (80%–100%)

> Verbalization of an unremitting and overwhelming lack of energy Inability to maintain usual routines

Minor (50%–79%)

Perceived need for additional energy to accomplish routine tasks
Increase in physical complaints
Emotionally labile or irritable
Impaired ability to concentrate
Decreased performance
Lethargic or listless
Disinterest in surroundings/introspection
Decreased libido
Accident prone

RELATED FACTORS

Many factors can cause fatigue. Some common factors are:

Pathophysiologic

Acute infections
> Mononucleosis
> Hepatitis
> Viral

Fever
Chronic infection
> Hepatitis
> Endocarditis

Impaired oxygen transport system
> Congestive heart failure
> Chronic obstructive lung disease
> Anemia
> Peripheral vascular disease

---

*Voith, A. M., Frank, A. M., & Pigg, J. S. (1987). Validations of fatigue as a nursing diagnosis. In *Classification of nursing diagnoses: Proceedings of the seventh national conference*. St. Louis: C. V. Mosby.

Endocrine/metabolic disorders
  Diabetes mellitus
  Hypothyroidism
  Pituitary disorders
  Addison's disease
Chronic diseases
  Renal failure
  Cirrhosis
Neuromuscular disorders
  Parkinson's disease
  Arthritis
  Myasthenia gravis
  Multiple sclerosis
Obesity
Electrolyte imbalances
Cancer
Nutritional disorders
Gait disorders
Acquired immunodeficiency syndrome (AIDS)

Treatment-related

Chemotherapy
Radiation therapy
Antidepressants
Drug withdrawal

Situational (personal, environmental)

Depression
Extreme stress
Crisis (personal, developmental, career, family, financial)
Sensory overload (noise, illumination, etc.)
Extreme temperatures
Prolonged excessive role demands

Maturational

Adult
  Pregnancy (first trimester)
  Caregiver (ill child, aging parent)

Diagnostic Considerations

Fatigue is different from tiredness. Tiredness is a transient, temporary state (Rhoten, 1982) caused by lack of sleep, improper nutrition, sedentary life-style, or a temporary increase in work or social responsibilities. Fatigue is a pervasive, subjective, drained feeling that cannot be eliminated, but the individual can be assisted to adapt to fatigue. Activity intolerance is different from fatigue in that the person with activity intolerance will be assisted in increasing endurance to progress and will increase his activity.

The person with fatigue is not focused on increasing endurance. If the cause of fatigue resolves or abates (*e.g.*, acute infection, chemotherapy, radiation), the *Fatigue* diagnosis is discontinued and the diagnosis *Activity Intolerance* can be initiated to focus on improving the deconditioned state.

Errors in Diagnostic Statements

Fatigue related to feelings of lack of energy for routine tasks

When a person reports insufficient energy for routine tasks, the nurse performs a focus assessment and collects additional data to determine whether Fatigue is the appropriate diagnosis or whether fatigue is actually a symptom of another diagnosis, such as *Activity Intolerance, Ineffective Coping, Altered Family Processes, Anxiety,* or *Altered Health Maintenance.* When fatigue is caused by acute or chronic disorders or therapies, the nurse will need to determine whether the person increases endurance (which would call for the diagnosis *Activity Intolerance*) and/or whether energy conservation techniques will be needed to help the person accomplish desired activities.

When fatigue results from ineffective stress management or poor daily health habits, the diagnosis of *Fatigue* or *Activity Intolerance* is not indicated. During data collection to determine contributing factors, the nurse can record the diagnosis as: *Possible Fatigue related to reports of lack of energy.* Labeling the diagnosis as "Possible" indicates the need for additional data collection to rule out or confirm.

Focus Assessment Criteria

Subjective Data

History of fatigue
    Onset?
    Precipitated by what?
    Pattern
        Morning, evening, transient, unfading
    Relieved by rest?
Associated signs and symptoms
    Fever   Dyspnea
    Weight loss   Sleep disorders
    Sleep-seeking behavior   Decreased motivation
    Irritability
Medical history (recent illnesses, chronic disease)
Medications
Effects of fatigue on
    Concentration   Family
    Finances   Marriage
    Occupation   Recreation
    Role responsibilities

Objective Data

Proceed with physical assessment based on the subjective data collected, *e.g.*, general appearance, speech affect, vital signs, ROM, muscle strength, etc.

Principles and Rationale for Nursing Care

Generic Considerations

1. Fatigue can be a simple or complex problem. It is a subjective experience with physiologic, situational, and psychological components.
2. Normal fatigue is an expected response to physical exertion, change in daily activities, additional stress, or inadequate sleep (Kellum, 1985).
3. Fatigue can be (Morris, 1982)
   a. Psychologically caused with resulting psychological and physiologic manifestations
   b. Physiologically caused with resulting psychological and physiologic manifestations
   c. A warning sign of a health disorder
   d. Relieved by prescribed rest (physical and psychological)
4. American society values energy and productivity. Those without energy are viewed as sluggish or lazy. Energy and vitality are valued positively, while fatigue and tiredness are viewed negatively (Rhoten, 1982).
5. Fatigue can result from pathophysiology such as:
   a. Decreased cardiac output
   b. Prolonged circulatory time
   c. Accumulation of metabolic wastes
   d. Decreased oxygen transport
6. Fatigue can be manifested in areas of cortical inhibition such as (Rhoten, 1982):
   a. Decreased attention
   b. Slowed and impaired perception
   c. Impaired thinking
   d. Decreased motivation
   e. Decreased performance in physical and mental activities
   f. Loss of fine coordination
   g. Poor judgment
   h. Indifference to one's surroundings
7. Rest is not defined as lying in bed. Rest is described as a person in an environment where one can relax, mentally and physically. The person replenishes his or her energy supply during this period (Morris, 1982).
8. Depression slows one's thought processes and produces a decrease in physical activities. Work output decreases, and endurance is reduced. The effort to continue activity produces fatigue.
9. Anxiety can interfere with one's thought processes, increase movements, and disturb gastrointestinal function, thus causing fatigue.
10. Hargreaves described a high incidence of "fatigue syndrome" in young married women in moving to a new town. Factors that contributed to the fatigue were increased physical work, changes in support systems, and other stresses in relocation.
11. Reciprocity or returning support to one's support system is vital for balanced and healthy relationships (Tilden & Weinert, 1987). Individuals who are fatigued have difficulty with reciprocity.

Cancer and Fatigue

1. Prolonged stress may be the main cause of chronic fatigue in persons with cancer (Aistars, 1987).

2. The stressors (pathophysiologic, situational, treatment-related) contributing to fatigue in cancer clients are illustrated in Table II–6.

Pediatric Considerations

1. Infants and small children are unable to express fatigue. This information can be elicited by the nurse from interviewing the parents and carefully assessing key functional health patterns, *e.g.*, sleep/rest, activity/exercise (which may reveal respiratory difficulties and/or activity intolerance), and nutrition/metabolic (which may reveal feeding difficulties).
2. Children at risk for fatigue include those with acute or chronic illness, congenital heart disease, and anemia (Daberkow, 1989).
3. Children depend on parents/caregivers to modify their environment to mitigate the effects of fatigue.

Gerontologic Considerations

1. The normal effects of aging do not in themselves increase the risk of or cause fatigue.
2. Fatigue in older adults has basically the same etiologies as in younger adults. The difference lies in the fact that older adults tend to experience more chronic diseases than younger adults. Thus, fatigue in older adults is not due to age-related factors, but rather to such risk factors as chronic diseases, medications, and others.
3. Depression is the most common psychosocial impairment in older adults. Depression-related affective disturbances affect 27% of adults in a community-living setting (Blazer, 1986).
4. Chronic fatigue and diminished energy are functional consequences of late-life depression (Miller, 1990).
5. According to Miller (1990), "the activity theory proposed that older adults would remain psychologically and socially fit if they remained active." One's self-concept is affirmed through participation in activities.

Table II-6 **Fatigue-Contributing Factors in Cancer Clients**

Pathophysiologic (Alstars, 1987)
Hypermetabolic state associated with active tumor growth
Competition between the body and the tumor for nutrients
Chronic pain
Organ dysfunction (*e.g.*, hepatic, respiratory, gastrointestinal)

Treatment-related (Alstars, 1987)
Accumulation of toxic waste products secondary to radiation, chemotherapy
Inadequate nutritional intake secondary to nausea, vomiting
Anemia
Analgesics, antiemetics
Diagnostic tests
Surgery

Situational (personal, environmental)
Uncertainty about future
Fear of death, disfigurement
Social isolation
Losses (role responsibilities, occupational, body parts, function, appearance, economic)
Separation for treatments

6. The quality or type of activity reportedly is more important than the quantity (Lemon, Bengston, & Peterson, 1972). Informal activities promoted well-being the most, followed by formal structured activities, and last by solitary activities, which were found to have little or no effect on life satisfaction (Longino & Kart, 1982).

7. Chronic fatigue, reported by approximately 70% of the elderly, can result in diminished motor activity and muscle tone. Note that anemia, very common in the elderly, is another possible contributor to chronic fatigue complaints (Mitchell, 1986; Matteson & McConnell, 1988).

■ Fatigue
Related to (Specify)

Assessment
See Defining Characteristics

Outcome Criteria

The person will
- Discuss the causes of fatigue
- Share feelings regarding the effects of fatigue on his/her life
- Establish priorities for daily and weekly activities
- Participate in activities that stimulate and balance physical, cognitive, affective, and social domains

---

Interventions
The nursing interventions for this diagnosis are interventions for individuals with fatigue with etiologies that cannot be eliminated. The focus of nursing care is to assist the individual and family to adapt to the fatigue state.

A. Assess causative or contributing factors
1. Lack of sleep, refer to *Sleep Pattern Disturbance*
2. Poor nutrition, refer to *Altered Nutrition*
3. Sedentary life-style, refer to *Health-Seeking Behaviors*
4. Inadequate stress management, refer to *Health-Seeking Behaviors*
5. Physiologic impairment
6. Treatment (chemotherapy, radiation, medications)
7. Chronic excessive role or social demands

B. Explain the causes of his/her fatigue (see Principles for explanations)

C. Allow expression of feelings regarding the effects of fatigue on his life
1. Identify those activities that are difficult
2. Interfere with role responsibilities

3. Frustrations
4. Refer to *Impaired Adjustment* if individual expresses nonacceptance of limitations

D. Assist the individual to identify strengths, abilities, interests
1. Identifying client's values and interests
2. Identifying client's areas of success and usefulness; emphasize his past accomplishments
3. Utilize this information to develop goals with the client.
4. Assist the client to identify sources of hope (*e.g.,* relationships, faith, things to accomplish).
5. Assist the client to develop realistic short-term and long-term goals (progress from simple to more complex; may use a "goals poster" to indicate type and time for achieving specific goals).

E. Assist individual to identify energy patterns and the need to schedule activities
1. Instruct individual to record fatigue levels every 1 hour during a 24-hour period, select a usual day (Aistars, 1987).
   a. Ask client to rate his fatigue 0–10 using the Rhoten fatigue scale (0 = not tired, peppy; 10 = total exhaustion).
   b. Record the activities at the time of each rating.
2. Analyze together the 24-hour fatigue levels.
   a. Times of peak energy
   b. Times of exhaustion
   c. Activities associated with increasing fatigue

F. Assist individual to identify what tasks can be delegated
1. Explore what activities are viewed as important for the individual to maintain self-esteem.
2. Attempt to divide the vital activities or tasks into components; delegate parts of the task but retain certain components, *e.g.,* meal preparation, shopping, storing, preparing food for cooking, cooking, serving, cleaning up.
3. Plan the important tasks during periods of high energy, *e.g.,* prepare all the day's meals in the morning.

G. Explain the purpose of pacing and prioritization (Brunner)
1. Assist individual to identify priorities and to eliminate nonessential activities.
2. Plan each day to avoid energy- and time-consuming nonessential decision-making.
3. Organize work with work items within easy reach.
4. Distribute difficult tasks throughout the week.
5. Rest before difficult tasks and stop before fatigue ensues.

H. Teach energy conservation techniques
1. Modify the environment.
   a. Replace steps with ramps.
   b. Install grab rails.
   c. Elevate chairs 3–4 inches.
   d. Organize kitchen or work areas.
   e. Reduce trips up and down stairs, *e.g.,* put a commode on first floor.

2. Plan small frequent meals to decrease energy required for digestion.
3. Use taxi instead of driving self.
4. Delegate housework, *e.g.*, employ a high school student for a few hours after school.

I. Explain the effects of conflict and stress on energy levels and assist to learn effective coping skills

1. Teach the client the importance of mutuality in sharing concerns.
2. Explain the benefits of distraction from negative events.
3. Teach the client the value of confronting issues.
4. Teach and assist patient relaxation techniques (see Appendix X) prior to anticipated stressful events. Encourage mental imagery to promote positive thought processes (see Appendix X).
5. Allow the client time to reminisce to gain insight into past experiences.
6. Teach the client to maximize esthetic experiences (*e.g.*, smell of coffee, back rub, or feeling the warmth of the sun or a breeze).
7. Teach the client to anticipate experiences he takes delight in each day (*e.g.*, walking, reading favorite book, writing letter).

J. Explain the psychologic and physiologic benefits of exercise and discuss what is realistic

1. Refer to *Health-Seeking Behaviors* for specific information.

K. Provide significant others opportunities to discuss their feelings in private regarding:

1. Changes in the person with fatigue
2. Their care-taking responsibilities
3. Financial issues
4. Changes in life-style, role responsibilities, relationships
5. Refer to *Impaired Home Maintenance Management* for additional strategies for caregivers.

L. Initiate health teaching and referrals as indicated

1. Counseling
2. Community services (Meals-On-Wheels, housekeeper)
3. Financial assistance

References/Bibliography

Aistars, J. (1987). Fatigue in the cancer patient: A conceptual approach to a clinical problem. *Oncology Nursing Forum, 14*(6d), 25–30.

American Psychiatric Association diagnostic and statistical manual of mental disorders. (1980). Washington, DC: APA.

Blazer, D. G. (1986). Depression: Paradoxically a cause for hope. *Generations, 10*(3), 21–23.

Brunner, L., & Suddarth, D. (1988). *Textbook of medical surgical nursing* (6th ed.). Philadelphia: J. B. Lippincott.

Daberkow, E. (1989). Nursing strategies: Altered cardiovascular function. In Foster, R. L., Hunsberger, M. M., & Anderson, J. J. T. (Eds.). *Family-centered nursing care of children.* Philadelphia: W. B. Saunders.

Freal, J. E., Kraft, G. H., & Coryell, J. K. (1963). Principles of prioritizing symptomatic fatigue in multiple sclerosis. *Archives of Physical Medicine and Rehabilitation,* March, 135–137.

Hargreaves, M. (1977). The fatigue syndrome. *Practitioner, 218,* 841–843.

Kellum, M. D. (1985). Fatigue. In Jacobs, M. M., & Geels, W. (Eds.): *Signs and symptoms in nursing.* Philadelphia: J. B. Lippincott.

Lemon, B. W., Bengston, V. L., & Peterson, J. A. An exploration of activity theory of aging. *Journal of Gerontology, 27* (6), 511–523.

Longino, C. F., & Kart, C. S. (1982). Explicating activity theory: A formal replication. *Journal of Gerontology, 37*(8), 713–722.

Matteson, M. A., & McConnell, E. S. (1988). *Gerontological nursing: Concepts and practices.* Philadelphia: W. B. Saunders.

Miller, C. A. (1990). *Nursing care of older adults.* Glenview, IL: Scott Foresman.

Mitchell, C. A. (1986). Generalized chronic fatigue in the elderly: Assessment and intervention. *Journal of Gerontological Nursing, 12*(4), 19–23.

Monroe, L. F. Psychological and physiological differences between good and poor sleepers. *Journal of Abnormal Psychology, 72*(3), 255–264.

Morris, M. (1982). Tiredness and fatigue. In Norris, C. (Ed.): *Concept clarification in nursing.* Rockville, MD: Aspen Systems.

Piper, B. F. (1989). Recent advances in the management of biotherapy related side effects: Fatigue. *Oncology Nursing Forum, 16*(6), 27–34.

Potempa, K., Lopez, M., Reid, C., & Lawson, L. (1986). Chronic fatigue. *Image, 18*(4), 165–169.

Rhoten, D. (1982). Fatigue and the postsurgical patient. In Norris, C. (Ed.): *Concept clarification in nursing.* Rockville, MD: Aspen Systems.

Riddle, P. K. (1982). Chronic fatigue and women: A description and suggested treatment. *Women Health, 7*(1), 37–47.

Tilden, V. P., & Weinert, C. (1987). Social support and the chronically ill individual. *Nursing Clinics of North America, 22*(3), 613–620.

Fear

■ *Related to* **(Specify)**

DEFINITION

Fear: A state in which an individual or group experiences a feeling of physiologic or emotional disruption related to an identifiable source that is perceived as dangerous.

DEFINING CHARACTERISTICS

Major (must be present)

Feeling of dread, fright, apprehension and/or
Behaviors of
  Avoidance
  Narrowing of focus on danger
  Deficits in attention, performance, and control

Minor (may be present)

Verbal reports of panic, obsessions
Behavioral acts of
  Aggression
  Escape
  Hypervigilance
Visceral-somatic activity

Dysfunctional immobility
Compulsive mannerisms
Increased questioning/verbalization

Musculoskeletal

Muscle tightness
Fatigue

Cardiovascular

Palpitations
Rapid pulse
Increased blood pressure

Respiratory

Shortness of breath
Increased rate

Gastrointestinal

Anorexia
Nausea/vomiting
Diarrhea

Genitourinary

Urinary frequency

Skin

Flush/Pallor
Sweating
Paraesthesia

CNS/perceptual

Syncope
Insomnia
Lack of concentration
Irritability
Absentmindness
Nightmares
Pupil dilation

RELATED FACTORS

Fear can occur as a response to a variety of health problems, situations, or conflicts. Some common sources are indicated below.

Pathophysiologic

Loss of body part

Loss of body function

Disabling illness

Long-term disability

Terminal disease

Treatment-related

Hospitalization

Surgery and its outcome

Anesthesia

Invasive procedures

Radiation

Situational (personal, environmental)

Influences of others

Pain

New environment

New people

Crime

Lack of knowledge

Change or loss of significant other

Divorce

Success

Failure

Maturational

Children: age-related fears (dark, strangers), influence of others

Adolescent: school adjustments, social and intellectual competitiveness, independence, authorities

Adult: marriage, pregnancy, parenthood

Diagnostic Considerations

See *Anxiety*

Focus Assessment (Subjective/Objective)

1. Onset

    Have the person tell you his "story" about his fearfulness

2. Manner of communication

    Verbal reports of distress?

    Fear-related behavioral acts?

    Visceral or somatic activity?

3. Thought process and content

    How does person organize his thoughts?

    Are thoughts clear, coherent, logical, confused, or forgetful?

    Can he concentrate or is he preoccupied?

    Do misperceptions interfere with reality testing?

4. Control behaviors

    Does fear interfere with life-style?

    Can the person use several control behaviors or only one persistent behavior?

    What understanding does the person have about his fear?

Do coping mechanisms help solve problems (functional) or do they contribute to further problems (maladaptation)?
5. Emotional state

Is emotional feeling tone appropriate or inappropriate to the situation?

Do facial expressions, voice tone, and body posture correspond to the intensity of the person's verbal expression of fear?
6. Perception and judgment

Is fear still present after stressor is eliminated?

Do only major events lead to fearfulness, or do minor events trigger fears?

Can the person comprehend the present and focus on his actions or is he overwhelmed by future anticipations?

Is the fear a response to a present stimulus or is it distorted by influences in the past?
7. Relatedness to others

Does the person's intensity of fear cause movement away from others?

What or who are his support systems?

Can he accept support from the nurse or others?
8. Children

Is the child's fear normal and expected for his age group?

What actions of the parents contribute to the fear?

What actions of the parents reduce the fear?
9. Assess for the presence of visceral-somatic activity

Musculoskeletal	*Genitourinary*
Muscle tightness	Urinary frequency
Fatigue	
Cardiovascular	*Skin*
Palpitations	Flush/pallor
Rapid pulse	Sweating
Increased blood pressure	Paresthesia
Respiratory	*CNS/perceptual*
Shortness of breath	Syncope
Increased rate	Insomnia
	Lack of concentration
	Irritability
	Absentmindness
	Nightmares
Gastrointestinal	*Visual*
Anorexia	Pupil dilation
Nausea/vomiting	
Diarrhea	

Principles and Rationale for Nursing Care

Generic Considerations

1. Psychologic defense mechanisms are distinctly individual and can be adaptive or maladaptive.
2. Fear differs from anxiety in that fear is the feeling aroused when there is an accurate

perception of an external threat; anxiety is a feeling aroused when the perception is of an imagined danger in response to internal beliefs.

3. Both fear and anxiety lead to disequilibrium.
4. Activity uses energy and dissipates the physical reaction to fear.
5. Anger may be an adaptive response to certain fears.
6. Safety feelings increase when a person identifies with another person who has successfully dealt with a similar fearful situation.
7. A sense of adequacy in confronting danger reduces fear. Fear disguises itself. The expressed fear may be a substitute for other fears that are not socially acceptable. Awareness of factors that cause intensification of fears enhances controls and prevents heightened feelings. Fear is reduced when the safe reality of a situation is confronted.
8. Fear can become anxiety (*e.g.*, fear becomes internalized and serves to disorganize instead of becoming adaptive).
9. Chronic physical reactions to stressors lead to susceptibility and chronic disease.
10. Physiologic responses are manifested throughout the body primarily from the hypothalamus's stimulation of the autonomic and endocrine systems.
11. Individuals interpret the degree of danger from a threatening stimulus. The physiologic and psychologic systems react with equal intensity to the perceived threat ($\uparrow$ BP, $\uparrow$ heart rate, $\uparrow$ respiratory rate).
12. Fear is adaptive and is a healthy response to danger.

Pediatric Considerations

1. Infants and small children experience fear but are unable to verbally identify the threat. Verbal (crying, protesting, *e.g.*, "NO") and nonverbal responses (kicking, biting, holding back) are important indicators of children's fear (Broome, Bates, Lillis, & McGahee, 1990; Hunsberger, 1989).
2. Fear behaviors are *consistent* and *immediate* on exposure or mention of a specific stressor; if the response is erratic, the diagnosis might more accurately be anxiety (Hunsberger, 1989). Refer to Table 11-7 in the diagnostic category *Altered Growth and Developoment* and/or the pediatric considerations for the diagnostic category *Anxiety.*
3. Fears throughout childhood follow a developmental sequence and are influenced by culture, environment, and parental fears (Forman, Hetznecker, & Dunn, 1983).
4. Main fears of different age groups include:
   a. *Infants and toddlers (birth to 2 years):* Fears evolve from physical stimuli, *e.g.*, loud noises, separation from parents/caregivers, strangers, sudden movements (Hunsberger, 1989).
   b. *Preschoolers (3–5 years):* Fears evolve from real or imagined situations, *e.g.*, injury or mutilation, ghosts, devils, monsters, the dark, bathtub and toilet drains, being alone, dreams, robbers (Whaley & Wong, 1989).
   c. *School-agers (6–12 years):* Fears are numerous and include large machines, bodily injury, loss of self-control, not being liked, separation from parents and peers, and failure (Anderson, 1989).
   d. *Adolescents:* Fears can be verbalized and include loss of self-control, disturbance to body image, death, and separation from peers (Hunsberger, 1989; Whaley & Wong, 1989).

■ Fear
Related to (Specify)

Assessment
See Defining Characteristics

Outcome Criteria

The adult will
- Relate increase in psychological and physiologic comfort
- Differentiate real from imagined situations
- Describe effective and ineffective coping patterns
- Identify his own coping responses

The child will
- Discuss his fears
- Relate an increase in psychological comfort

Interventions

The nursing interventions for the diagnosis *Fear* represent interventions for any individual with fear regardless of the etiologic or contributing factors.

A. Assess possible contributing factors

1. Perception of threatening stimulus (realistic)
   a. Unfamiliar environment (new home, hospital admission, new people)
   b. Intrusion on personal space
   c. Life-style change (promotion, marriage, retirement)
   d. Biologic change (dysfunction, rejection)
   e. Self-esteem threat (abandonment, rejection)
2. Distorted perceptions of dangerous stimulus
3. Age-related fears

B. Reduce or eliminate contributing factors

1. Unfamiliar environment
   a. Orient to environment using simple explanations.
   b. Speak slowly and calmly.
   c. Avoid surprises and painful stimuli.
   d. Use soft lights and music.
   e. Remove threatening stimulus.
   f. Plan one-day-at-a-time familiar routine.
   g. Encourage gradual mastery of a situation.
   h. Provide transitional object with symbolic safeness (security blanket, religious medals).
2. Intrusion on personal space
   a. Allow personal space.
   b. Move person away from stimulus.
   c. Remain with him until fear subsides (listen, use silence).

    d. Later, establish frequent and consistent contacts; utilize family members and significant others to stay with him.

    e. Use touch as tolerated (sometimes holding person firmly will help him maintain control).

3. Threat to self-esteem

    a. Support preferred coping style when adaptive mechanisms are used (some prefer details; others, general explanations).

    b. Initially, decrease the person's number of choices.

    c. Use simple direct statements (avoid detail).

    d. Give direct suggestion to manage everyday events.

    e. Encourage expression of feelings (helplessness, anger).

    f. Give feedback about his expressed feelings (support realistic assessments).

    g. Refocus interaction on areas of capability rather than dysfunction.

    h. Encourage normal coping mechanisms.

    i. Encourage sharing common problems with others.

    j. Give feedback of effect his behavior has on others.

    k. Encourage him to face the fear.

4. Distorted perceptions

    a. Encourage responses that reflect reality.

    b. Ask straightforward questions ("Do you feel pain?" "Does my asking you about your feelings make you uncomfortable?").

    c. Provide information to reduce distortions ("No, I will not harm you" "That was only a shadow and not the bogey man").

    d. Encourage specifics and discourage generalizations; have him give details, not vague general assumptions ("Who are you referring to when you say 'they' are trying to kill you?").

    e. Explore superficial interactions.
- Examine the person's reason for avoiding feelings.
- Allow him to know that it is OK to feel.
- Share your reaction to the event ("I can see why you're upset; if that happened to me I would have felt like screaming").

    f. Provide an emotionally nonthreatening atmosphere.
- Provide situations that are predictable.
- Allow for consistency in personnel to enhance comfort and familiarity.
- Announce changes in the environment.

5. Age-related fears (refer to Principles and Rationale for Nursing Care)

    a. Provide child with opportunities to express his fears and to learn healthy outlets for anger or sadness, *e.g.,* play therapy (see Appendix IX for Guidelines for Play Therapy).

    b. Acknowledge illness, death, and pain as real and refrain from protecting children from the reality of their existence; encourage open, honest sharing.

    c. Accept the child's fear and provide him with an explanation, if possible, or some form of control; share with child that these fears are okay.
- Fear of imaginary animals, intruders ("I don't see a lion in your room, but I will leave the light on for you, and if you need me again, please call.")
- Fear of parent being late (establish a contingency plan, *e.g.,* "If you come home from school and Mommy is not here, go to Mrs. S. next door.")
- Fear of vanishing down a toilet or bathtub drain
  - Wait until child is out of tub before releasing drain
  - Wait until child is off the toilet before flushing

Leave toys in bathtub and demonstrate how they do not go down the drain
- Fear of dogs, cats
Allow child to watch a child and a dog playing from a distance
Do not force child to touch the animal
- Fear of death
See Principles and Rationale for Nursing Care for *Grieving*
- Fear of pain
See *Pain in Children*

d. Discuss with parents the normalcy of fears in children; explain the necessity of acceptance and the negative outcomes of punishment or of forcing the child to overcome the fear.

e. Provide child with opportunity to observe other children cope successfully with feared object.

C. Initiate health teaching and referrals as indicated

1. When intensity of feelings has decreased, bring behavioral cues into the person's awareness.
   a. Teach signs that indicate increased fear ("Your face flushes and you clench your fists when we discuss your discharge.").
   b. Indicate adaptiveness of behavior.
2. Explain how expressed fear of one thing may be hidden fear of something else.
3. Teach how to problem-solve.
   a. What is the problem?
   b. Who or what is responsible for the problem?
   c. What are the options?
   d. What are advantages and disadvantages of each option?
4. Teach ways for enhancing control.
   a. Include the person in the treatment process ("Please raise your hand if the procedure causes pain.").
   b. Share test results when appropriate.
   c. Inform ahead of time about tests (time interval depends on ability to cope).
   d. Identify activities that rechannel emotional energy to diffuse intensity.
   e. Use nightlight or flashlight to diffuse fear (child with fear of dark can be given a flashlight to use when needed).
   f. Before tests or surgery, prepare patient as to what to expect, especially sensations, and define this role and how to participate in the role (*e.g.*, breathing exercises postoperatively may take mind off of fears and dissipate physical reaction).
5. Recommend or instruct concerning methods that increase comfort or relaxation (see Appendix X for Guidelines).
   a. Progressive relaxation technique
   b. Reading, music, breathing exercises
   c. Desensitization, self-coaching
   d. Thought stopping, guided fantasy
   e. Yoga, hypnosis, assertiveness training
6. Participate in community functions to teach parents age-related fears and constructive interventions, *e.g.*, parent-school organizations, newsletters, civic groups.

References/Bibliography

Anderson, J. J. (1989). Families with school-age children. In Foster, R. L., Hunsberger, M. M., & Anderson, J. J. T. (Eds.). *Family-centered nursing care of children*. Philadelphia: W. B. Saunders.

Bowlby, J. (1961). Children, mourning and its implications for psychiatry. *American Journal of Psychiatry, 118*, 481–498.

Broome, M. E., Bates, T. A., Lillis, P. P., & McGahee, T. W. (1990). Children's medical fears, coping behaviors, and pain perceptions during a lumbar puncture. *Oncology Nursing Forum, 17*(39), 361–367.

Burke, S. (1981). A developmental perspective on the nursing diagnosis of fear and anxiety. *Nursing Papers, 13*(4), 20, 59–64.

Forman, M. A., Hetznecker, W. H., & Dunn, J. M. (1983). Developmental pediatrics. In Behrman, R. E., Vaughan, V. C., & Nelson, W. E. (Eds.). *Nelson textbook of pediatrics* (12th ed.). Philadelphia: W. B. Saunders.

Hunsberger, M. (1989). Principles and skills adapted to the care of children. In Foster, R. L., Hunsberger, M. M., & Anderson, J. J. T. (Eds). *Family-centered nursing care of children*. Philadelphia: W. B. Saunders.

McFarland, G., & Wasli, E. (1986). *Nursing diagnosis and process in psychiatric mental health nursing*. Philadelphia: J. B. Lippincott.

Petrillo, M., & Sanger, S. (1980). *The emotional care of the hospitalized child*. Philadelphia: J. B. Lippincott.

Ross, D. (1984). Thought-stopping: A coping strategy for impending feared events. *Issues in Comprehensive Pediatric Nursing, 7*, 83–89.

Sadler, A. (1985). Assertiveness training. In Bulechek, G., & McCloskey, J. (Eds): *Nursing interventions: Treatments for nursing diagnoses*. Philadelphia: W. B. Saunders.

Scandrett, S. & Uecker, S. (1985). Relaxation training. In Bulechek, G., & McCloskey, J. (Eds.). *Nursing interventions: Treatments for nursing diagnoses*. Philadelphia: W. B. Saunders.

Yanni, M. (1982). Perceptions of parents' behavior and children's general fearfulness. *Nursing Research, 31*(2), 79–82.

Yocum, C. (1984). The differentiation of fear and anxiety. In Kim, M., McFarland, G., & McLane, A. (Eds): *Classification of nursing diagnoses: Proceeding of fifth national conference*. St. Louis: C. V. Mosby.

Wass, H., & Cason L. (1985). Fears and anxieties about death. *Issues in Comprehensive Nursing, 8*(1/6), 25–45.

Whaley, L., & Wong D. (1979). *Nursing care of infants and children*. St. Louis: C. V. Mosby.

Whaley, L. F., & Wong, D. L. (1989). *Essentials of pediatric nursing* (3rd ed.). St. Louis: C. V. Mosby.

Wieczorek, R., & Natapoff, J. (1981). *A conceptual approach to nursing of children: Health care from birth through adolescence*. Philadelphia: J. B. Lippincott.

Fluid Volume Deficit

- *Related to* **Decreased Oral Intake**
- *Related to* **Abnormal Fluid Loss**

DEFINITION

Fluid Volume Deficit: The state in which an individual who is not NPO experiences or is at risk of experiencing vascular, interstitial, or intracellular dehydration.

DEFINING CHARACTERISTICS

Major (must be present)
> Insufficient oral fluid intake
> Negative intake and output
> Dry skin/mucous membranes

Minor (may be present)
> Decreased urine output or excessive urine output
> Concentrated urine or urinary frequency
> Decreased fluid intake
> Decreased skin turgor
> Thirst/nausea/anorexia

RELATED FACTORS

Pathophysiologic
> Excessive urinary output
>> Uncontrolled diabetes
>> Diabetes insipidus (inappropriate antidiuretic hormone)
> Burns (postacute)
> Fever or increased metabolic rate
> Infection
> Abnormal drainage
>> Wound
>> Excessive menses
>> Other
> Peritonitis
> Diarrhea

Situational (personal, environmental)
> Vomiting/nausea
> Decreased motivation to drink liquids
>> Depression
>> Fatigue

Dietary problems
  Fad diets/fasting
  Anorexia
  High solute tube feedings
Difficulty swallowing or feeding self
  Oral pain
  Fatigue
Climate exposure
  Extreme heat/sun
  Excessive dryness
Hyperpnea
Extreme exercise effort/diaphoresis
Excessive use of
  Laxatives or enemas
  Diuretics or alcohol

Maturational

Infant/child: Decreased fluid reserve, decreased ability to concentrate urine
Elderly: Decreased fluid reserve, decreased sensation of thirst

Diagnostic Considerations

Fluid Volume Deficit frequently is used to describe persons who are NPO, in hypovolemic shock, or experiencing bleeding, as well as persons with insufficient oral fluid intake. The present NANDA-approved defining characteristics contribute to its clinical misuse in cases of hemoconcentration, change in serum sodium, or hypotension. Related factors are listed as active fluid volume loss and failure of regulatory mechanisms.

A validation study of *Fluid Volume Deficit* yielded additional critical indicators: thready pulse, decreased venous filling, and decreased cardiac output; according to the authors, "pinpointing which indicators are most relevant can help the practitioner collect and interpret data when researching and assessing fluid volume status" (Gershan, 1990). Should the nursing diagnosis *Fluid Volume Deficit* be used to represent such clinical situations as shock, renal failure, or thermal injury?

Errors in Diagnostic Statements

High risk for Fluid Volume Deficit related to increased capillary permeability, protein shifts, inflammatory process, and evaporation secondary to burn injuries

This diagnosis does not represent a situation for which nurses could prescribe interventions for outcome achievement (e.g., "The client will have stable vital signs and adequate urine output [0.5–1.0 mL/kg]"). Because both nurse- and physician-prescribed interventions are needed to accomplish this outcome, this situation is actually the collaborative problem. *Potential Complication: Fluid/Electrolyte Imbalance* with the nursing goal of: The nurse will manage and minimize fluid and electrolyte imbalances.

Fluid Volume Deficit related to effects of NPO status

Managing fluid balance in an NPO client is a nursing responsibility involving both nurse- and physician-prescribed interventions. Thus, this situation is best described with the collaborative problem. *Potential Complication: Fluid/Electrolyte Imbalance.* If the nurse desires to specify etiology, the diagnosis can be written:

Potential Complication: Fluid/Electrolyte Imbalance related to NPO state. This usually is not necessary, however.

When a person can drink but is not drinking sufficient amounts, the nursing diagnosis *Fluid Volume Deficit related to decreased desire to drink fluids secondary to fatigue and pain* may apply.

Focus Assessment Criteria

Subjective Data

History of symptoms
    The person complains of

Nausea/vomiting/anorexia	Thirst
Weight loss	Polyuria/dysuria
Diarrhea/loose stool	Fever/diaphoresis

History of contributing and causative factors
    Diabetes mellitus (diagnosed, family history)/diabetes insipidus
    Cardiac disease
    Renal disease
    Blood loss
    Gastrointestinal disorders or surgery
    Alcohol use
    Medications

Laxatives/enemas	Side effects that are GI irritants
Diuretics	(antibiotics)

    Allergies (food, milk)
    Extreme heat/humidity
    Extreme exercise effort accompanied by sweating
    Depression
    Pain
Current antihypertensive or diuretic therapy
    Type, dosage   Frequency (last dose taken when?)

Objective Data

Assess for presence of contributing factors
    Abnormal or excessive fluid loss

Liquid stools	Abnormal or excessive drainage
Vomiting or gastric suction	(*e.g.,* fistulas, drains)
Diuresis or polyuria	Loss of skin surfaces (*e.g.,* burns)
Diaphoresis	Fever

    Decreased fluid intake related to

Fatigue	Depression/disorientation
Decreased level of consciousness	Nausea or anorexia
	Physical limitations (*e.g.,* unable to hold glass)

Assess for signs of dehydration
    Skin
        Mucosa (lips, gums) (dry)
        Tongue (furrowed/dry)
        Turgor (decreased)
        Color (pale or flushed)

      Moisture (dry or diaphoretic)
      Fontanelles of infants (depressed)
      Eyeballs (sunken)
  Urine output
      Amount (varied; very large or minimal amount)
      Color (amber; very dark or very light)
      Specific gravity (increased or decreased)
      Intake vs. output (less intake than output)
  Weight (loss/gain)
  Neck veins (collapsed when lying flat)
Diagnostic studies
  Hemoglobin/hematocrit
  Electrolytes
  Blood urea nitrogen (BUN)
  Urinalysis
  Creatinine

Principles and Rationale for Nursing Care

Generic Considerations

1. Human beings constantly excrete body fluids containing electrolytes. The average amount of daily fluid loss and the major electrolytes excreted in the fluids are as follows:
   - Urine = 1500 mL (K^+ and Na^+ loss)
   - Stool = 200 mL (K^+ loss)
   - Perspiration/respiration (insensible loss) = 1000–1300 mL (Na^+, Cl^- loss)
2. A normal balance of cations (positive ions), anions (negative ions), and buffers is necessary for normal blood pH. (Normal arterial pH is 7.37–7.45.) *A very slight variation in these normals can cause death.*
3. Normal serum electrolytes are

Cations	Sodium (137–148 mEq/L)
(positive ions)	Potassium (3.5–5 mEq/L)
	Calcium (8.5–10.5 mg/dL)
	Magnesium (1.5–2.5 mEq/L)
Anions	Chloride (95–106 mEq/L)
(negative ions)	Bicarbonate (21–28 mEq/L)
	Protein (6.0–8.5 g/dL)
	Organic acids (2.4–4.5 mg/dL)
	Phosphate (2.5–4.8 mg/dL)
	Sulfate (minuscule)

4. A balance of water and sodium is necessary for normal body fluid levels. Water provides 90–93% of the volume of body fluids, while sodium provides 90–95% of the solute of extracellular fluid.
5. Vomiting or gastric suctioning results in potassium and hydrogen loss.
6. To maintain homeostasis, human beings must consume daily fluids and electrolytes to replace what has been lost; replacement comes from food and drink absorbed through the GI tract (major source) and from the cellular oxygenation of nutrients.
7. Fluid intake is primarily regulated by the sensation of thirst. Fluid output is primarily regulated by the kidneys' ability to concentrate urine.
8. The specific gravity of the urine reflects the kidney's ability to concentrate urine; the

range of urine specific gravity varies with the state of hydration and the solids to be excreted. (Specific gravity is elevated when dehydration is present, signifying concentrated urine.) Values are

Normal: 1.010–1.025
Concentrated: >1.025
Diluted: <1.010

9. Potassium is the major cation of the intracellular fluid-influencing acid-base balance and cellular hydration. High or low potassium interferes with the conduction of nerve impulses through skeletal, smooth, and cardiac muscle. *This may be manifested by cardiac and muscular irritability or flaccidity, which can cause life-threatening arrhythmias.*

10. Conditions that increase the incidence of hypokalemia (low potassium) are

Diuretic therapy (K^+ loss in urine)
Ascites (K^+ loss to accumulation of fluid in the abdomen)
Poor dietary habits (poor K^+ intake)
Extreme diaphoresis (Na^+ and K^+ loss)
Prolonged diarrhea/malabsorption syndrome (K^+ loss via stool)
Prolonged gastric suction (K^+ loss from gastric contents)
Surgery/tissue trauma (cellular loss of K^+)

11. Foods with a high potassium content include bananas, dates, raisins, oranges, tomatoes, puffed wheat cereal, potatoes, liver, Pepsi, and Gatorade.

12. Water can normally be found in three spaces of the body—within the blood vessels, within the interstitial spaces (extracellular), and within the cell itself (intracellular).

13. To correctly assess a person's potential for fluid imbalance, close examination of the previous 24–72 hours' intake and output is necessary. (In renal or cardiac disease, it may be necessary to consider intake and output for the previous 5–7 days, as well as body weight.)

14. People at high risk for fluid imbalance include:
    a. People on medication for fluid retention, high blood pressure, seizures, or "anxiety" (tranquilizers)
    b. People who suffer from diabetes, cardiac disease, excessive alcohol intake, malnourishment, obesity, or GI distress
    c. Adults over 60, and children under 6
    d. People who are confused, depressed, comatose, or lethargic (no sensation of thirst)

15. Blood is the cooling fluid of the body. Dehydration (and resulting decrease in blood volume) causes an increased body temperature, pulse, respirations.

16. Dehydration may occur within the vascular tree, while water within the interstitial spaces may be excessive (edema). Abnormal shifts between body compartments may cause fluid excess or deficit.

17. Excessive fluid loss can be expected during

Fever or increased metabolic rate
Extreme exercise or diaphoresis
Climate extremes (heat/dryness)
Excessive vomiting or diarrhea
Burns, tissue insult, fistulas

18. Large amounts of sugar, alcohol, and caffeine act as diuretics that increase urine production and may cause dehydration.

19. People receiving tube feedings are at high risk for dehydration, because the high solute concentration of the tube feeding may cause diarrhea and diuresis. *Tube feedings must be supplemented with specific amounts of water to maintain adequate hydration.*

Fluid and Nutrient Requirements

1. The average adult requires 2000 mL–3000 mL of fluid intake per day. Under normal conditions, a nonperspiring adult needs 1500 mL of fluids daily. An additional 1000 mL of fluids comes from solid foods and oxidation during metabolism.
2. In determining the 24-hour intake requirement for an infant or child, both caloric and fluid intake should be measured. The following calculations can be utilized:

   Calorie Intake

   For a child up to 10 kg of body weight: 100 cal/kg
   For a child between 11 kg and 20 kg: 1000 cal plus 50 cal/kg for each kg above 20

   Fluid Intake (for maintenance)

   Approximately 120 mL 100 cal of metabolism
   Abnormal fluid loss must be replaced in addition to the above.
3. With inadequate caloric intake, metabolism of the body's stores of fat and muscle may provide a significant increase in total body water, resulting in weight gain that may hide malnutrition (*e.g.,* the "bloating" of terminal malnutrition).
4. Adequate protein intake is necessary to maintain normal osmotic pressures. Foods that have a high protein content are meats, fish, fowl, soybeans, eggs, legumes, and cheese.

Pediatric Considerations

1. Infants are vulnerable to fluid loss due to the following factors:
   a. More water can be lost rapidly because their bodies have a higher proportionate water content. A greater proportion of fluid is in the extracellular space, from which it is lost more easily.
   b. Infants have a greater metabolic turnover of water.
   c. Homeostatic regulation, *i.e.,* renal function, is immature.
   d. Infants have a greater surface area relative to body mass (Rimar, 1989; Whaley & Wong, 1989).

Gerontologic Considerations

1. Phillips (1984) reported a general decrease in thirst with aging, which puts an elderly person at risk for not drinking sufficient fluids to maintain adequate hydration.
2. The elderly are more susceptible to fluid loss and dehydration because of:
   a. Decreased renal blood flow
   b. Decreased glomerular filtration
   c. Impaired ability to regulate temperature
   d. Decreased ability to concentrate urine
   e. Increase in physical disabilities decreases access to fluids
   f. Self-limiting of fluids for fear of incontinence
3. About 75% of the fluid intake in elderly persons typically occurs between 6 A.M. and 6 P.M. (Adams, 1988).
4. Cognitive impairments can interfere with recognition of cues of thirst.

■ Fluid Volume Deficit
Related to Decreased Oral Intake

Assessment

Subjective Data

The person reports
Nausea and vomiting/anorexia
Altered ability to drink or swallow (sore throat, dysphagia)
Upper limb limitations
Decreased motivation to obtain fluids (weakness, depression, fatigue)

Objective Data

Decreased intake (< 2000 mL/day)
Decreased urine output
Increased specific gravity of urine
Dry skin or dry mucous membranes
Decreased lacrimal secretions and decreased saliva
Poor skin turgor
Upper limb limitations
Difficulty swallowing

Outcome Criteria

The person will
- Increase intake of fluids to a minimum of 2000 mL (unless contraindicated)
- Relate the need for increased fluid intake during stress or heat
- Maintain a urine specific gravity within a normal range
- Demonstrate no signs and symptoms of dehydration

Interventions

A. Assess causative factors
  1. Inability to feed self
  2. Dislike of available liquids
  3. Sore throat/mouth
  4. Extreme fatigue or weakness
  5. Lack of knowledge (of the need for increased fluid intake)
  6. Difficulty swallowing (see *Impaired Swallowing*)

B. Reduce or eliminate causative factors
  1. Inability to feed self; see *Self-Care Deficit*
  2. Dislike of available liquids
     a. Assess likes and dislikes; provide favorite fluids within dietary restrictions.
     b. Plan an intake goal for each shift (*e.g.*, 1000 mL during day; 800 mL during evening; 300 mL at night).

    c. Make a set schedule for supplementary liquids.

    d. For children, offer
- Appealing forms of fluids (popsicles, frozen juice bars, snow cones, water, milk, Jell-O with vegetable coloring added; let child help make it)
- Unusual containers (colorful cups, straws)
- A game or activity

    e. Read a book to child and have him drink a sip when a page is turned, or have a tea party.

    f. Have child take a drink when it is his turn in a game.

    g. Make a set schedule for supplementary liquids to promote the habit of in-between meal fluids (*e.g.,* juice or Kool-Aid at 10 A.M. and 2 P.M. each day).

3. Sore throat/mouth

    a. Offer warm or cold fluids; consider frozen ices.

    b. Consider warm saline gargle or anesthetic lozenges before fluids.

4. Extreme fatigue or weakness

    a. Give smaller amounts more frequently.

    b. Provide for periods of rest prior to meals.

5. Lack of knowledge

    a. Assess the person's understanding of the reasons for maintaining adequate hydration and methods for reaching goal of fluid intake.

    b. Include significant others.

    c. Proceed with teaching.

    d. See Principles and Rationale for Nursing Care under *Health-Seeking Behaviors.*

C. Have person maintain a written record (log) of fluid intake and urinary output and daily weight (if necessary)

D. Prevent dehydration in high-risk individuals (see Principles for high-risk persons)

1. Monitor intake; ensure at least 2000 mL of oral fluids every 24 hours.
2. Monitor output; ensure at least 1000–1500 mL every 24 hours.
3. Offer fluids in large glasses, 120 or 240 mL (Adams, 1988).
4. Weigh daily in same clothes, at same time. A 2–4% weight loss indicates mild dehydration; 5–9% weight loss indicates moderate dehydration.
5. Monitor serum electrolytes, blood urea nitrogen, urine and serum, osmolality, creatinine, hematocrit, and hemoglobin.
6. For persons scheduled for fasting prior to diagnostic studies, increase their fluid intake 8 hours before fasting.
7. Review client's medications. Do they contribute to dehydration (*e.g.,* diuretics)? Do they require increased fluid intake (*e.g.,* lithium)?
8. Teach that coffee, tea, and grapefruit juice are diuretics and can contribute to fluid loss.
9. Consider the additional fluid losses associated with vomiting, diarrhea, fever.

E. Initiate health teaching as indicated

1. Give verbal and written directions for desired fluids and amounts.
2. Include the person/family in keeping a written record of fluid intake, output, daily weights.
3. Provide a list of alternative fluids (*e.g.,* ice cream, pudding).
4. Explain the need to increase fluids during exercise, fever, infection, and hot weather.

5. Teach how to observe for dehydration (especially in infants) and to intervene by increasing fluid intake (see Objective and Subjective Data for signs of dehydration).
6. Seek medical consultation for continued dehydration.

■ Fluid Volume Deficit
Related to Abnormal Fluid Loss

Abnormal fluid loss describes fluid loss by vomiting, diarrhea, excessive diaphoresis, or drains, not hemorrhage or acute burns.

Assessment

Subjective Data

The person reports
"I keep going to the bathroom all the time."
"I have to get up several times a night to urinate."
"I have loose bowels [diarrhea]."
"I've been vomiting a lot."
"I break out in a cold sweat."
"I'm thirsty all the time."

Objective Data

Extreme diaphoresis
Increased body drainage
    Vomitus/nasogastric suction
    Chest tubes/thoracentesis
    Sump drains/paracentesis
    T tubes
    Liquid or loose stools
    Polyuria
    Wound drainage (pus, serous, etc.)
Weight loss
Output exceeds intake

Outcome Criteria

The person will
- Maintain adequate intake of fluid and electrolytes as evidenced by (specify)
- Identify abnormal fluid loss, relate methods of decreasing this loss (if possible) and replace fluids as needed
- Maintain a urine specific gravity within normal range

Interventions

A. Assess causative factors
   1. Vomiting
   2. Fever
   3. Gastric suction
   4. Diarrhea/loose stools
   5. Impaired swallowing (see *Impaired Swallowing*)

B. Remove or reduce causative factors
   1. Vomiting
      a. Encourage small, frequent amounts of ice chips or clear liquids such as weak tea or flat cola or ginger ale* (adults 30 mL, children 15 mL; see *Altered Nutrition; Less Than Body Requirements*).
   2. Fever (see also *Hyperthermia*)
      a. Maintain temperature lower then 101° F (38.4° C) through tepid water sponging and medication (*e.g.,* A.S.A. or acetaminophen).*
         • Eliminate excessive clothing and bed covers.
         • Keep the room temperature cool.
         • Encourage cool, clear liquids when medication is at peak effectiveness and temperature is lowest.
         • Substitute frozen ices or popsicles if necessary (be resourceful).
         • If the temperature is extremely high, >103° F (39.5° C), apply ice packs to pulse points (groin, axilla).*
      b. Specifically for children under 5 with a sudden rise in temperature ("spiking fever"):
         • Work to attain a temperature <101° F (38.4° C) as soon as possible with medication* (A.S.A., acetaminophen) and sponging.
         • Use tepid water (85°–90° F/29.4°–37.7° C) for sponging or bathing the child.
         • Caution parents not to cover the child with blankets and to be aware of the increased risk of febrile seizures.
         • Give the child small amounts of *clear liquids only* (15 mL).
         • Teach the parents how to protect the child should a seizure occur, and *instruct them to seek immediate medical consultation.*
   3. Gastric suction (nasogastric or other)
      a. Use only normal saline for irrigation of gastric tubes to minimize electrolyte imbalance.
      b. Do not allow swallowing of water or ice chips; a "few small sips" can readily add up over a period of time.
      c. For the thirsty individual with gastric suction, *unless contraindicated by surgery or renal failure,* consult with the physician concerning ingestion of measured sips of Gatorade (1 oz/hr).
      d. Always subtract all fluid ingested (via either tube or mouth) from any total gastric drainage to attain net drainage.
      e. Keep a careful, clear record of intake and output: amount, character, color.
      f. Offer frequent mouth care.
   4. Diarrhea/loose stools, see *Diarrhea*

---

*May require a physician's order.

5. Wound drainage
   a. Keep careful records of the amount and type of drainage.
   b. Weigh dressings, if necessary, to estimate fluid loss (weigh the wet dressing; weigh a dry dressing of the same type; compare the difference).
   c. Weigh the person daily if the drainage is excessive and difficult to measure (*e.g.,* soaked sheets).
   d. Replace fluid loss (may be contraindicated in cardiac failure, renal failure, or head trauma).

C. Initiate health teaching as indicated

1. Assess the person's understanding of the type of fluid loss he is experiencing (what electrolytes are lost) and the fluids that provide replacement (see Principles and Rationale for Nursing Care).
2. Give verbal and written instructions for fluid replacement (*e.g.,* "Drink at least 3 quarts of liquid a day, including 1 quart of Gatorade").
3. Teach the person to
   a. Avoid sudden exposure and overexposure to heat, sun, and exercise.
   b. Gradually increase exposure and activity in hot weather.
   c. Eat three balanced meals a day.
   d. Increase fluid intake during hot days.
   e. Decrease activity during extreme weather.

References/Bibliography

See *Fluid Volume Excess*

Fluid Volume Excess

■ *Related to* **(Specify)**

DEFINITION

Fluid volume excess: The state in which an individual experiences or is at risk of experiencing intracellular or interstitial fluid overload.

DEFINING CHARACTERISTICS

Major (must be present)

Edema (peripheral, sacral)
Taut, shiny skin

RELATED FACTORS

Pathophysiologic

Renal failure, acute or chronic
Decreased cardiac output
    Myocardial infarction   Valvular disease
    Congestive heart failure   Tachycardia/arrhythmias
    Left ventricular failure
Varicosities of the legs
Liver disease
    Cirrhosis   Cancer
    Ascites
Tissue insult
    Injury to the cell wall   Hypoxia of the cell
Inflammatory process
Hormonal disturbances
    Pituitary   Estrogen
    Adrenal

Treatment-related

Steroid therapy
Chemotherapy

Situational (personal, environmental)

Excessive sodium intake/fluid intake
Low protein intake
    Fad diets   Malnutrition
Dependent venous pooling/venostasis
    Immobility   Standing or sitting for long
                                  periods of time

Venous pressure point
    Tight cast or bandage

Pregnancy
Inadequate lymphatic drainage

Maturational
Elderly (decreased cardiac output)

Diagnostic Considerations

Fluid Volume Excess frequently is used to describe pulmonary edema, ascites, and renal failure. This diagnosis represents a situation for which nurses can prescribe if the focus is on peripheral edema. Nursing interventions would center on teaching the client or family how to minimize edema and on protecting tissue.

Errors in Diagnostic Statements

High Risk for Fluid Volume Excess related to left-sided mastectomy

For this diagnosis, the nurse would institute strategies to reduce edema and teach the client how to manage the edema. Thus, the diagnosis should be written as: *High Risk for Fluid Volume Excess related to lack of knowledge of techniques to reduce edema secondary to compromised lympatic function.*

If edema were present, the nurse might use *High Risk for Impaired Physical Mobility related to effects of lymphedema on motion.*

Fluid Volume Excess related to portal hypertension and decreased colloid osmotic pressure secondary to cirrhosis

This diagnosis requires frequent monitoring, electrolyte replacement, diuretic therapy, dietary restrictions, and plasma expander therapy. These interventions call for three collaborative problems to describe this situation:

Potential Complication: Ascites
Potential Complication: Negative nitrogen balance
Potential Complication: Hypokalema

Because edema predisposes skin to injury and breakdown, the nurse also could use the diagnosis: *High Risk for Impaired Skin Integrity related to vulnerability of skin secondary to edema.*

Focus Assessment Criteria

Subjective Data

1. History of symptoms
   Complaints of
      Shortness of breath   Weakness/fatigue
      Weight gain   Edema
   Onset/duration
   Location
   Description
   Aggravated by?
   Precipitated by?
   Relieved by?
2. History of contributing and causative factors
   Family or personal history of diabetes
   Pregnancy

Premenses
Cardiac or renal disease
Liver disease
Alcoholism
Hyper- or hypothyroidism
Hypertension
Steroid therapy
Malnutrition
Excessive salt intake
Excessive use of tap-water enemas
Lymphatic obstruction (*e.g.,* after lymph node dissection)
Excessive parenteral fluid replacement

3. Current drug therapy
Type, dosage
Frequency
Last dose taken when?

4. Dietary intake
Estimated protein intake (adequate/inadequate)
Estimated caloric intake (adequate/inadequate/excess)
Estimated fluid intake (adequate/inadequate/excess)
Daily alcohol consumption   Type _____,   Amount _____

Objective Data

1. Assess vital signs for signs of fluid overload.
Pulse (bounding or dysrhythmic)
Respirations
Rate (tachypnea)
Quality (labored or shallow)
Lung sounds (rales or rhonchi)
Blood pressure (elevated)

2. Palpate for edema.
Press thumb for at least 5 seconds into the skin and note any remaining indentations.
Note degree and location (feet, ankles, legs, arms, sacral, generalized)

3. Assess for weight gain (weigh daily on the same scale, at the same time).

4. Assess for neck vein distention (distended neck veins at 45° elevation of the head may indicate fluid overload or decreased cardiac output).

5. Check results of diagnostic studies:
Electrolytes
Hemoglobin and hematocrit
Blood urea nitrogen (BUN)
Creatinine
Urinalysis

Principles and Rationale for Nursing Care

See *Fluid Volume Deficit* for Generic Principles

Edema

1. People with cardiac pump failure are at high risk for both vascular and tissue fluid excess (*i.e.,* pulmonary and peripheral edema). Acute pulmonary edema should be considered a medical emergency.

2. The most frequent vascular cause of tissue edema is increased venous pressure, which causes increased capillary blood pressure.
3. Edema inhibits blood flow to the tissue, resulting in poor cellular nutrition and increased susceptibility to injury.
4. Edema is often seen as a result of
   a. Venous obstruction (pressure point, such as sitting with legs crossed) and resulting venous pooling
   b. Heart failure (decreased cardiac output) resulting in backup of blood in the heart, lungs, and vessels
   c. Lymphatic obstruction (*e.g.*, after a lymph node dissection)
   d. Trauma (tissue injury that releases histamines, causing vasodilation and increased permeability and movement of fluid); examples are burns, sprains, fractures
   e. Hypoxia of the cell
   f. Vitamin C deficiency or extreme malnutrition
   g. Prolonged steroid therapy
5. A high intake of sodium causes increased retention of water. Foods with high sodium content include salted snacks, bacon, cheddar cheese, pickles, soy sauce, processed luncheon meats, MSG (monosodium glutamate), canned vegetables, catsup, and mustard. Some over-the-counter drugs such as antacids.
6. Research has suggested that edema during pregnancy may be better reduced by rest periods in water (*i.e.*, taking a bath) than by bed rest (Staff, 1990).

Gerontologic Considerations

1. The older adult is prone to stasis edema of the feet and ankles due to (Miller, 1990)
   a. Increased vein tortuosity
   b. Increased vein dilatation
   c. Decreased valve efficiency.

■ Fluid Volume Excess
Related to (Specify)

Assessment

Subjective Data

The person reports
  "I'm not supposed to eat salt."
  "I feel bloated (tired, weak)."
  Sudden or abnormal weight gain
  History of
    Fingers, feet, or ankles swelling
    "Bad heart"
    "Bad kidneys"
    Hypertension
  Cancer or lymph node dissection
  Immobility or neurologic deficit (*e.g.*, stroke or spinal cord injury)

Objective Data
  Pedal or sacral puffiness
  Puffing of extremities
  Shiny, taut skin
  Pitting edema (skin, when depressed by thumb, remains indented)
  Weight gain

Outcome Criteria

The person will
  • Relate causative factors and methods of preventing edema
  • Exhibit decreased peripheral and sacral edema

Interventions

A. Identify contributing and causative factors
  1. Improper diet (excessive sodium intake; inadequate protein intake)
  2. Dependent venous pooling/venostasis
  3. Venous pressure point (*e.g.,* tight cast or bandage)
  4. Inadequate lymphatic drainage
  5. Immobility/neurologic deficit
  6. Lack of knowledge of or compliance with medical regimen

B. Reduce or eliminate causative and contributing factors
  1. Improper diet
    a. Assess dietary intake and habits that may contribute to fluid retention.
      • Be specific; record daily and weekly intake of food and fluids.
      • Assess weekly diet for adequate protein or excessive sodium intake.
        Discuss likes and dislikes of foods that provide protein
        Teach to plan weekly menu that provides protein at a price that is
          affordable
    b. Encourage the person to decrease salt intake.
      • Teach the person to
        Read labels for sodium content
        Avoid convenience foods, canned foods, and frozen foods
        Cook without salt and use spices to add flavor (lemon, basil, tarragon,
          mint)
        Use vinegar in place of salt to flavor soups, stews, etc. (*e.g.,* 2–3
          teaspoons of vinegar to 4–6 quarts, according to taste)
      • Ascertain with physician whether salt substitute may be used (caution
        individual that he must use exactly the substitute prescribed)
  2. Dependent venous pooling
    a. Assess for evidence of dependent venous pooling or venostasis.
    b. Encourage alternating periods of horizontal rest (legs elevated) with vertical
       activity (standing) (this may be contraindicated in congestive heart failure).
    c. Keep edematous extremity elevated above the level of the heart whenever
       possible (unless contraindicated by heart failure).
      • Keep edematous arms elevated on two pillows or with IV pole sling.

- Elevate legs whenever possible, using pillows under legs (avoid pressure points, especially behind knees).
- Discourage leg and ankle crossing.
  d. Reduce constriction of vessels.
  - Assess wearing apparel for proper fit and constrictive areas.
  - Instruct person to avoid panty girdles/garters, knee highs, and leg crossing and to practice keeping legs elevated when possible.
  e. Consider using antiembolism stockings or Ace bandages; measure legs carefully for stockings/support hose.*
  - Measure from back of heel to back of knee, or top of thigh, depending on desired stocking length.
  - Measure circumference of calf and thigh.
  - Consider both measurements in choosing a stocking, matching measurements with size requirement chart that accompanies the stockings.
  - Apply stockings while lying down (*e.g.*, in the morning before arising).
  - Check extremities frequently for adequate circulation and evidence of constrictive areas.
3. Venous pressure points
  a. Assess for venous pressure points associated with casts, bandages, tight stockings.
  - Observe circulation at edges of casts, bandages, stockings.
  - For casts, insert soft material to cushion pressure points at edges.
  - Check circulation frequently.
  b. Shift body weight in cast to redistribute weight within the cast (unless contraindicated).
  - Encourage person to do this himself every 15–30 minutes during waking hours to prevent venostasis.
  - Encourage wiggling of fingers or toes and isometric exercise of unaffected muscles within the cast.*
  - If the person is unable to do this himself, assist him at least hourly to shift body weight.
  - See *Impaired Physical Mobility.*
4. Inadequate lymphatic drainage
  a. Keep extremity elevated on pillows.
  - If edema is marked, the arm should be elevated, *but not in adduction* (this position may constrict the axilla).
  - The elbow should be higher than the shoulder.
  - The hand should be higher than the elbow.
  b. Take blood pressures in unaffected arm.
  c. Do not give injections or start intravenous fluids in affected arm.
  d. Protect the affected arm from injury.
  - Teach the person to avoid strong detergents, carrying heavy bags, holding a cigarette, injuring cuticles or hangnails, reaching into a hot oven, wearing jewelry or a wristwatch, or using Ace bandages.
  - Advise the person to apply lanolin or similar cream several times a day to prevent dry, flaky skin.
  - Encourage the person to wear a "Medic Alert" tag engraved with *Caution: lymphedema arm—no tests—no needle injections.*

---

* May require a physician's order.

- Caution the person to see a physician if the arm becomes red, swollen, or unusually hard.
    e. After a mastectomy, encourage ROM exercises and use of affected arm to facilitate development of a collateral lymphatic drainage system (explain to the person that lymphedema is often decreased within a month, but that she should continue massaging, exercising, and elevating the arm for 3 or 4 months following surgery).
5. Immobility/neurologic deficit
    a. Plan passive or active ROM exercises for all extremities every 4 hours, including dorsiflexion of the foot to massage veins.
    b. Change the individual's position at least every 2 hours, using the four positions (left side, right side, back, abdomen), if not contraindicated (see *Impaired Skin Integrity*).
    c. If the person must be maintained in high Fowler's position, assess for edema of the buttocks and sacral area and help the person to shift body weight every 2 hours to prevent pressure on edematous tissue.
6. Lack of knowledge
    a. Assess the person's knowledge of
    - Medical diagnosis (*e.g.,* congestive heart failure, renal failure)
    - Diet
    - Medications (*e.g.,* diuretics, cardiotonics)
    - Activity
    - Use of Ace bandages, antiembolus stockings

C. Protect edematous skin from injury

1. Inspect skin for redness and blanching.
2. Reduce pressure on skin areas; pad chairs and footstools.
3. Prevent dry skin.
    a. Use soap sparingly.
    b. Rinse off soap completely.
    c. Use a lotion to moisten skin.
4. See *Impaired Skin Integrity* for additional information on preventing injury

D. Initiate health teaching and referrals as indicated

1. Give clear instructions verbally and in writing for all medications: what, when, how often, why, side-effects; pay special attention to drugs directly influencing fluid balance (*e.g.,* diuretics, steroids).
2. Write down instructions for diet, activity, use of Ace bandages, stockings, etc.
3. Have the person demonstrate his understanding of the instructions.
4. Have the person keep a written record of intake/output.
5. With severe fluctuations in edema, have the person weigh himself every morning and before bedtime daily; instruct the person to keep a written record of weights.
6. For less severe illness, the person may need to weigh himself daily only and record.
7. Caution the person to call physician for excessive edema/weight gain (>2 lb/day) or increased shortness of breath at night or on exertion.
8. Explain that the above may be indicative of early heart problems and may require medication to prevent them from getting worse.
9. Consider home care or visiting nurses referral to follow at home.
10. Provide literature concerning low-salt diets; consult with dietitian if necessary.

References/Bibliography

Fluid Volume Deficit and Fluid Volume Excess

Books

Aspinall, M. J., & Tanner, C. (1981). *Decision making and the nursing process.* New York: Appleton-Century-Crofts.

Bates, B. (1991). *A guide to physical examination and history taking* (5th ed.). Philadelphia: J. B. Lippincott.

Brunner, L., & Suddarth, D. (1988). *Textbook of medical surgical nursing* (6th ed.). Philadelphia: J. B. Lippincott.

Bulechek, G., & McCloskey, J. (1985). *Nursing interventions.* Philadelphia: W. B. Saunders.

Carnevali, D., & Patrick, M. (1987). *Nursing management for the elderly.* Philadelphia: J. B. Lippincott.

Carpenito, L. (1989). *Handbook of nursing diagnosis* 1989–1990. Philadelphia: J. B. Lippincott.

Fischbach, F. (1988). *A manual of laboratory diagnostic tests for nurses* (3rd ed.). Philadelphia: J. B. Lippincott.

Jacobs, M., & Geels, W. (1985). *Signs and symptoms in nursing.* Philadelphia: J. B. Lippincott.

Kintzel, K. C. (1977). *Advanced concepts in clinical nursing* (2nd ed.). Philadelphia: J. B. Lippincott.

Metheny, N. M., & Snively, W. D., Jr. (1987). *Nurses' handbook of fluid balance* (5th ed.). Philadelphia: J. B. Lippincott.

Miller, C. A. (1990). *Nursing care of older adults.* Glenview, IL: Scott, Foresman.

Porth, C. (1990). *Pathophysiology: Concepts of altered health status* (3rd ed.). Philadelphia: J. B. Lippincott.

Rimar, J. M. (1989). Principles of fluid and electrolyte maintenance. In Foster, R. L., Hunsberger, M. M., & Anderson J. J. T. (Eds.). *Family-centered nursing care of children.* Philadelphia: W. B. Saunders.

Taylor, C., Lillus, C., & LeMone, P. (1989). *Fundamentals of nursing: The art and science of nursing care.* Philadelphia: J. B. Lippincott.

Webber, J. (1988). *Nurses' handbook of health assessment.* Philadelphia: J. B. Lippincott.

Whaley, L. F., & Wong, D. L. (1989). *Essentials of pediatric nursing* (3rd ed.). St. Louis: C. V. Mosby.

Articles

Adams, F. (1988). How much do elders drink? *Geriatric Nursing, 9*(4), 218–221.

Beckett, C., et al. (1988). The venous pump of the foot. *Nursing Times, 84*(19), 45–47.

Brown, P., et al. (1989). The dying patient and dehydration. *Cancer Nurse, 85*(5), 14–16.

Carriere, G. (1988). Edema: Its development and treatment using lymph drainage massage. *Clinical Management of Physical Therapy, 8*(5), 19–21.

Chambers, J. (1981). Assessing the dialysis patient at home. *American Journal of Nursing, 81,* 750–754.

Chambers, J. (1987). Common fluid and electrolyte disorders. *Nursing Clinics of North America, 22*(4), 749–872.

Dale, R. (1980). Symposium on fluid, electrolyte, and acid-base balance. *Nursing Clinics of North America, 15*(3), 535–536.

Erkert, J. (1988). Dehydration in the elderly. *Journal of American Academy of Physicians, 1*(4), 261–269.

Felver, L. (1980). Understanding the electrolyte maze. *American Journal of Nursing, 80,* 1591–1599.

Folk-Lighty, C. (1984). Solving the puzzles of patients' fluid imbalances. *Nursing, 14*(2), 34–41.

Gershan, J., et al. (1990). Fluid volume deficit: Validating indicators. *Heart & Lung, 19*(2), 152–156.

Gray, B. (1988). Management of limb oedema in advanced cancer. *Nursing Times, 83*(4), 19–21.

Gray, G. (1987). Management of limb oedema in advanced cancer. *Physiotherapy, 73*(10), 504–506.

Hazinski, M. (1988). Understanding fluid balance in the seriously ill child. *Pediatric Nursing, 14*(3), 231–236.

Huber, M., & Calliiari, D. (1985). Hereditary angioedema—The swelling disorder. *American Journal of Nursing, 85*(10), 1090–1092.

Lane, G. (1982). When persistence pays off: Resolving the mystery of unexplained electrolyte imbalance. *Nursing, 12*(1), 44–47.

McConnell, E. (1982). Urinalysis: A common test, but never routine. *Nursing, 12*(2), 108–111.

Nardone, D., et al. (1987). Causes of peripheral edema. *Hospital Medicine, 23*(9), 162–163, 166–169, 172–175.

National Academy of Sciences, Food and Nutrition Board. (1980). *Recommended dietary allowances* (9th ed rev.). Washington DC: The Academy.

Phillips, P. A., et al. (1984). Reduced thirst after water deprivation in healthy elderly men. *New England Journal of Medicine, 311*, 753–759.

Renard, G. (1989). Edema in water intoxication. *American Journal of Nursing, 89*(12), 1635.

Smith, L. (1987). Home treatment of mild, acute diarrhea and secondary dehydration of infants and small children: An educational program for parents in a shelter for the homeless. *Journal of Professional Nursing, 4*(1), 60–63.

Staff. (1987). Facial swelling: A summary guide to some important systemic causes. *Hospital Medicine 23*(9), 180–181.

Staff. (1990). Clinical news. Watering down edema. *American Journal of Nursing, 90*(7), 18.

Stanley-Tilf, C. (1989). Recognizing psychiatric water intoxication. *American Journal of Nursing, 89*(12), 1636.

Turner, J. (1987). Problems of recognizing dehydration in hospital patients. *Nursing Times, 83*(51), 44.

Turner, J. (1988). Helping the dehydrated patient. *Nursing Times, 84*(16), 40–41.

Reedy, D. (1988). How you can prevent dehydration. *Geriatric Nursing, 9*(4), 224–226.

Twombly, M. (1978). The shift into third space. *Nursing, 8*(1), 38–46.

Urrows, S. T. (1980). Physiology of body fluids. *Nursing Clinics of North America, 15*, 603–615.

Grieving

Grieving, Anticipatory

Grieving, Dysfunctional

Grieving*

■ *Related to* **an Actual or Perceived Loss**

DEFINITION

Grieving: A state in which an individual or family experiences an actual or a perceived loss (person, object, function, status, relationship).

DEFINING CHARACTERISTICS

Major (must be present)

The person

Reports an actual or perceived loss (person, object, function, status, relationship) or
  Anticipates a loss

Minor (may be present)

Denial	Worthlessness	
Guilt	Suicidal thoughts	Delusions
Anger	Crying	Phobias
Despair	Sorrow	Anergia
Inability to concentrate		

Visual, auditory, and tactile hallucinations about the deceased

RELATED FACTORS

Many situations can contribute to feelings of loss. Some common situations are:

Pathophysiologic

Loss of function (actual or potential) related to a disorder

Neurologic	Musculoskeletal	Respiratory
Cardiovascular	Digestive	Renal
Sensory		

Loss of function or body part related to
  Trauma

*This diagnosis is not currently on the NANDA list but has been included for clarity or usefulness.

Treatment-related

Dialysis
Surgery (mastectomy, colostomy, hysterectomy)

Situational (personal, environmental)

Negation of loss by others
Secondary gains from grieving
Chronic pain
Terminal illness
Death
Changes in life-style

Childbirth   Child leaving home (*e.g.*, college
Marriage   or marriage)
Separation   Loss of career
Divorce

Expectations to "be strong"
Type of relationship (with the person who is leaving or is gone)
Multiple losses or crises
Lack of social support system
Stillbirth, abortion, miscarriage

Maturational

Loss associated with aging

Friends   Function
Occupation   Home

Diagnostic Considerations

Grieving, Anticipatory Grieving, and *Dysfunctional Grieving* represent three types of responses of individuals or families experiencing a loss. *Grieving* describes normal grieving after a loss and participation in grief work. *Anticipatory Grieving* describes someone engaged in grief work prior to an expected loss. *Dysfunctional Grieving* represents a maladaptive process occurring when grief work is suppressed or absent or when a person exhibits prolonged exaggerated responses. For all three diagnoses, the goal of nursing is to promote grief work. In addition, for *Dysfunctional Grieving,* the nurse will direct interventions to reduce excessive, prolonged, problematic responses.

In many clinical situations, the nurse expects a grief response, *e.g.,* loss of body part, death of significant other. Other situations that evoke strong grief responses are sometimes ignored or minimized, *e.g.,* abortion, newborn death, death of one twin or triplet, death of illicit lover, suicide, loss of children to foster homes, adoption (Lazare, 1979).

Errors in Diagnostic Statements

Dysfunctional Grieving related to excessive emotional reactions (crying, anger) to recent death of son

People respond to losses in highly individualized ways. Regardless of its severity, no response to acute loss should be labeled as "Dysfunctional." *Dysfunctional Grieving* is characterized by a sustained or prolonged detrimental response; validation of this diagnosis cannot be done until several months to a year after the loss. This diagnosis should be reworded as *Grieving related to recent death of son, as evidenced by emotional responses of anger and profound sadness.*

Anticipatory Grieving related to perceived effects of spinal cord injury on life goals
Using *Anticipatory Grieving* in this situation places the focus on anticipated losses rather than current actual losses. Because this individual is grieving over both actual and anticipated losses, the diagnosis should be rewritten as *Grieving related to actual or anticipated losses associated with recent spinal cord injury.*

Focus Assessment Criteria

Subjective Data

Family
>Previous coping patterns for crisis
>Quality of the relationship of the ill or deceased person with each family member
>Position or role responsibilities of the ill or deceased person
>Sociocultural expectations for bereavement
>Religious expectations for bereavement

Individual family members
>Previous experiences with loss or death (as child, adolescent, or adult)
>>Did family talk out their grief?
>>Did they practice any particular religious rituals associated with bereavement?

Present interactions between or among family members
>Adults
>Children
>>Maturational level
>>Understanding of crisis
>>Degree of participation
>Knowledge of expected grief reactions
>Relationship to ill or deceased person

Expressions of
>>Ambivalence
>>Denial
>>Fear
>>Concerns

>>Anger
>>Depression
>>Guilt

Report of
>Gastrointestinal disturbances
>>Indigestion
>>Nausea or vomiting
>>Anorexia

>>Weight gain or loss
>>Constipation or diarrhea

>Insomnia
>Preoccupation with sleep
>Fatigue (decreased or increased activity level)
>Inability to carry out self-care, social and work responsibilities
>Length of time in grief work

Objective Data

Normative
>>Shock
>>Disbelief, denial
>>Anger
>>Crying

>>Sorrow
>>Withdrawal
>>Preoccupation with lost object
>>Hopelessness

Pathologic pattern (profound; increases in intensity; continuous over 12 months)

Anger	Denial
Depression	Regression
Isolation	Obsession
Despair	Hallucinations
Worthlessness	Delusions
Guilt	Phobias
Suicidal thoughts	
Stoic	

Principles and Rationale for Nursing Care

Generic Considerations

1. American culture is devoted to youth and life. Even though death surrounds each person, it is viewed as pertaining to someone else, not oneself.
2. Loss can be viewed as consisting of four components: dying, death, grief, and mourning.
3. Loss can occur without death; when a person experiences any loss (object, relationship), grief and mourning ensue.
4. Grief is the emotional response to loss; grief work, the adaptive process of mourning. Grief work involves:
   a. Accepting the reality of the loss
   b. Experiencing the pain of grief
   c. Adjusting to an environment from which the lost person or object is missing
   d. Reinvesting in another relationships (Worden, 1982)
5. An individual's grief is affected by many factors, such as personality, previous losses, intimacy of relationship, and personal resources.
6. Staging (of grieving process) can create problems if the nurse applies the stages universally to all persons, disregarding individual differences. Staging also may encourage the nurse to focus on the symptoms as opposed to the strength of the person/family.
7. The following stages (Engle, 1964) are specific enough to assist the nurse to intervene and broad enough to prevent labeling.

I. Shock and disbelief
   Initial denial   Decreased activity
   Numbed feelings   Sporadic periods of despair
II. Developing awareness of loss
   Sadness   Guilt
   Anger   Crying
III. Restitution (usually requires at least a year)
   The work of mourning   Preoccupation with thoughts
   Painful void in life   of loss
IV. In the months to follow
   Beginning to put the lost relationship
     in perspective (its positive and neg-
     ative qualities)

---

8. "The notion that grief is a neat, orderly, linear process completed at some arbitrary point in time" has been refuted (Haylor, 1987).
9. Grief work cannot begin until the loss is acknowledged. Nurses can encourage this acknowledgment by open honest dialogue and by providing the family with an opportunity to view the dead person.
10. Life review is a process whereby a dying person reminisces about the past, especially unresolved conflicts, in an attempt to resolve them. Life review also provides the person with an opportunity to evaluate his successes and failures.
11. Terminal illness with its concurrent treatments and its progression produces a multitude of losses
    Loss of function (all systems)
    Loss of financial independence
    Change in appearance
    Loss of friends
    Loss of self-esteem
    Loss of self
12. Divorce presents many losses for the partners, children, grandparents, etc. The losses are roles, relationships, homes, possessions, finances, control, routines, and patterns.

Unresolved Grief

1. Unresolved grief is a pathologic response or prolonged denial of the loss or a profound psychotic response. Examples of such responses are
    Suppression or absence of grief process
    Progressively deeper regression, depression
    Progressively deeper isolation
    Somatic manifestations (prolonged)
    Obsessions, phobias
    Delusions, hallucinations
    Attempted suicide
2. Factors that contribute to unresolved grief are
    Quality of the individual's attachment to the loved object
    Presence of ambivalence toward the loved object
    Presence of lowered self-esteem
    Inability to grieve
3. Lazare (1979) describes the social factors that can contribute to unresolved grief as social negation of the loss (*e.g.*, abortion, newborn, death of twin, death of frail elderly parent) and socially defined as inappropriate to discuss (*e.g.*, death of lover, suicide).

Pediatric Considerations

1. The child responds to death depending on his developmental age and the response of significant others:
    a. Age <3 yrs.: Cannot comprehend death, fears separation
    b. Age 3–5: Views illness as a punishment for real or imagined wrongdoing
        Has little concept of death as final because of immature concept of time
        May view death as a kind of sleep
        May feel he caused the event to happen (magical thinking) (*e.g.*, by bad thoughts about person)
    c. Age 6–10: Begins to fear death
        Attempts to put meaning to the event (*e.g.*, devil, ghost, God)
        Associates death with mutilation and punishment
        Can feel responsibility for the event

    d. Age 10–12: Usually has an adult concept of death (inevitable, irreversible, universal)

        Attitudes greatly influenced by reactions of parent and others

        Very interested in postdeath services and rituals

    e. Adolescence: Has a mature understanding of death

        May suffer from guilt and shame

        Least likely to accept death, particularly if it is their own (Whaley & Wong, 1989)

2. Children may learn early that discussions about death are taboo (Homedes & Ahmed, 1987).
3. Children may use symbolic or nonverbal language to communicate their awareness of death and dying (McCowan, 1989).
4. Children can be encouraged to communicate symbolically through writing or telling stories or by drawing pictures (see Appendix IX for play therapy guidelines) (McCowan, 1989).
5. Children need to feel the joys and sorrows of life to begin to incorporate both in their lives appropriately (Kübler-Ross, 1983).
6. Children can feel rejected or unloved if parents or significant other is unable to offer emotional support and nurturing because of their own grief (Bourne & Meier, 1988; McCowan, 1989).

Gerontologic Considerations

1. Persons over age 60 who lose spouses to chronic illness of greater than 6 month's duration seem to experience more psychosomatic complaints, visit their doctors more frequently, and use larger amounts of drugs and alcohol (Hauser, 1983; Matteson & McConnell, 1988).
2. Three predominant factors seem to affect the grieving process in the elderly: support network, presence of concurrent losses, and individual coping skills. A greater number of resources is related to less psychosocial and/or physical dysfunction. Studies have revealed a 2.3 to 2.8-fold risk of mortality in individuals who have no social or community ties (Dimond, 1981; Kaprio & Koskenvuo, 1987; Matteson & McConnell, 1988).
3. Grief in elderly persons often can be related to losses within self, such as role changes, body image changes, or decreased body function. These losses sometimes are less easily accepted than the loss of a significant other (Matteson & McConnell, 1988).
4. In many cultures, the death of a mate is documented as the most stressful life event. Increasing longevity brings increased potential for 50 plus years of marriage to the same spouse, with a concomitantly greater impact of the loss of that spouse. The spouse possibly could be the older person's only close family member and social contact (Gallagher, Breckenridge, Thompson, & Peterson, 1983).
5. One study of persons over age 50 looked at the following factors over a period of 2 years after the loss of spouse: emotional shock, helplessness/avoidance, psychologic strength/coping, anger/guilt/confusion, and grief resolution behaviors. Statistically significant changes were seen in all areas except psychologic strength/coping. There also was no significant change in life satisfaction scores in this study (Caserta, Lund, & Dimond, 1985).
6. In another study, 12% of recently bereaved elders, compared with 8% of nonbereaved elders, were shown to be experiencing significant depression approximately 2 months after the death of their spouses. Although this is a relatively small percentage, caution should be taken in interpreting this finding; Perhaps greater depression

develops as the individual is confronted with multiple situations and limited assistance and support (Gallagher, Breckenridge, Thompson, & Peterson, 1983).

7. Some research indicates that older men have greater difficulty adapting to loss of spouse than older women. Speculation on reasons for this include unfamiliarity with household roles necessary to daily living that were performed by the spouse or possibly the role of the wife as organizer of social activities and a void created by this deficit. Other research has shown no significant differences between sexes (Gallagher, Breckinridge, Thompson, & Peterson, 1983).

8. Risk of death is greater in men than in women during the first 6 months of conjugal bereavement. Changes in health behavior patterns, such as nutrition, alcohol use, smoking, and decreased physical activity levels, may contribute to this increased mortality rate (Kaprio & Koskenvuo, 1987).

9. There seems to be some support for extending traditional bereavement periods to an expected point of at least 24 months for older individuals who have lost a spouse. More than the loss of significant other is the loss of a crucial relationship that provides meaning to the person's life. Even in young widows, the estimate of adjustment period has been extended, based on research showing movement at the 24-month mark from high distress to low distress (as measured on the Goldberg General Health Questionnaire) (Caserta, Lund, & Dimond, 1985; Ebersole & Hess, 1990; Oberfield, 1984; Vachon, Lyall, Rogers, Freedman-Letofsky, & Freeman, 1980).

10. Feelings of loneliness prevail even after widows report an increase in social activities and less feelings of depression. Loneliness has been reported to be the single greatest problem after death of a spouse (Constantino, 1981; Hogstel, 1990).

11. Bereavement is a risk factor for suicide. About 25% of all suicides are committed by older adults. Suicide attempts are less frequent in the elderly; however, the rate of attempted suicide to successful suicide increases to 4:1 after age 60, compared with 20:1 in the 40-year-old and younger group. Males aged 65 and older have the highest incidence of suicide: men aged 65–74 have 30.4 suicides per 100,000: men aged 75–84 have 42.3 suicides per 100,000; and men aged 85 + have 50.6 suicides per 100,000 (Abrams & Berkow, 1990; Hogstel, 1990).

12. The death of a pet can be a significant loss for an isolated older person and result in a grieving process (Hungelman, Kenkel-Rossi, Klassen, & Stollenwerk, 1985).

13. The elderly individual is at greater risk of experiencing multiple losses and thus has even greater weakness in adapting to losses (Ebersole & Hess, 1990; Matteson & McConnell, 1988).

14. Some losses are expected with aging as a life event and consequently are considered to be "on time"; *e.g.*, death of a 90-year-old as opposed to a 5-year-old. Sometimes this expected aspect can facilitate the grief process (Matteson & McConnell, 1988).

15. Chronic grief pattern can occur if a symbiotic relationship existed between the older individual and the deceased significant other. Helplessness becomes a prominent feeling for the grieving individual (Hauser, 1983; Oberfield, 1984).

16. Reminiscence therapy or life review can help integrate losses. Frequently, the older person uses reminiscence to move through Erikson's eighth developmental stage of Ego Integrity versus Despair (Matteson & McConnell, 1988).

17. Social supports, strong religious beliefs, good prior mental health, and a greater number of resources are related to less psychosocial and/or physical dysfunction (Matteson & McConnell, 1988).

■ Grieving
Related to an Actual or Perceived Loss

Assessment

Subjective Data

The person expresses

Sadness	Fear	Anergia; anxiety
Depression	Denial	Visual, auditory
Shock	Guilt	and/or tactile hal-
		lucinations about
		the deceased

Objective Data

Crying
Inability to cry
Withdraw behavior
Apathetic behavior
Changes in grooming, hygiene, weight, or health status

Outcome Criteria

The individual will
- Express his grief
- Describe the meaning of the death or loss to him
- Share his grief with significant others (children, spouses)

Interventions

A. Assess for causative and contributing factors that may delay the grief work

Unavailable or lack of support system	Inability to grieve (cultural, social, age-related)
Denial	History of previous emotional illness
Shock	
Anger	Personality structure
Depression	Early object loss
Guilt	Nature of the relationship with the lost person or object
Fear	
Dependency	
Multiple losses	
Uncertainty of loss (*e.g.,* MIA, missing children)	
Failure to grieve prior losses	

B. Reduce or eliminate causative or contributing factors if possible

1. Promote a trust relationship.
   a. Promote feelings of self-worth through one-on-one and/or group sessions.

b. Allow for established time to meet and discuss feelings.

c. Communicate clearly, simply, and to the point.

d. Never try and lessen the loss (*e.g.,* "She didn't suffer long"; "You can have another baby").

e. Assess what the person and the family are learning by the use of feedback.

f. Offer support and reassurance.

g. Create a therapeutic milieu.

h. Establish a safe, secure, and private environment.

i. Demonstrate respect for the person's culture, religion, race, and values.

2. Support the person and the family's grief reactions.

   a. Explain grief reactions.
      - Shock and disbelief
      - Developing awareness
      - Restitution

   b. Describe varied acceptable expressions.
      - Elated or manic behavior as a defense against depression
      - Elation and hyperactivity as a reaction of love and protection from depression
      - Various states of depression
      - Various somatic manifestations (weight loss or gain, indigestion, dizziness)

   c. Assess for past experiences with loss.
      - Loss of significant other in childhood
      - Losses in later life

3. Promote family cohesiveness.

   a. Support the family at its level of functioning.

   b. Encourage self-exploration of feelings with family members.

   c. Explain the need to discuss behaviors that interfere with relationships.

   d. Recognize and reinforce the strengths of each family member.

   e. Encourage the family to evaluate their feelings and support one another.

4. Promote grief work with each response.

   a. Denial
      - Recognize that this is a useful and necessary response.
      - Explain the use of denial by one family member to the other members.
      - Do not push client to move past denial without emotional readiness.

   b. Isolation
      - Convey a feeling of acceptance by allowing grief.
      - Create open, honest communications to promote sharing.
      - Reinforce the person's self-worth by allowing privacy.
      - Encourage client/family to gradually increase social activities (support groups, church groups, etc.).

   c. Depression
      - Reinforce the person's self-esteem.
      - Identify the level of depression and develop the approach accordingly.
      - Use empathetic sharing; acknowledge grief ("It must be very difficult").
      - Identify any indications of suicidal behavior (frequent statements of intent, revealed plan).
      - See *High Risk for Self-harm* for additional information.

   d. Anger
      - Understand that this feeling usually replaces denial.
      - Explain to family that anger serves to try to control one's environment more closely because of inability to control loss.

- Stress that the illness or death did not result from being bad or because the well child wished it.
6. Assist parents of a deceased infant (newborn, stillbirth, miscarriage) with grief work (Mina, 1985):
    a. Promote grieving.
        - Use baby's name when discussing loss.
        - Allow parents to share the hopes and dreams they had for the child.
        - Provide parents with access to hospital chaplain and/or own religious leader.
        - Encourage parents to see and hold their infant to validate the reality of the loss.
        - Design a method to communicate to auxiliary departments that the parents are in mourning (*e.g.,* rose sticker on door, chart).
        - Prepare a memory packet (wrapped in clean baby blanket) (photograph [Polaroid], ID bracelet, footprints with birth certificate, lock of hair, crib card, fetal monitor strip, infant's blanket).
        - Encourage parents to take memory packet home. If they prefer not to, keep the packet on file in case parents change their minds later.
        - Encourage parents to share the experience with siblings at home (refer to pertinent literature for consumers).
        - Provide for follow-up support and referral services after discharge (*e.g.,* social service, support group).
    b. Assist others to comfort grieving parents.
        - Stress the importance of openly acknowledging the death.
        - If the baby or fetus was named, use the name in discussions.
        - Never try to lessen the loss with discussions of future pregnancies or other healthy siblings.
        - Send sympathy cards.
        - Be sensitive of the gravity of loss for both the mother and father.
        - Create a remembrance for the infant (*e.g.,* plant a tree).
7. Identify persons who are at high risk for potential pathologic grieving reactions
    a. Absence of any emotion
    b. Previous conflict with deceased person
    c. History of ineffective coping patterns
8. Teach individual/family signs of pathologic grieving, especially persons who are at risk
    a. Prolonged hallucinations
    b. Continued searching for the deceased (frequent moves/relocations)
    c. Delusions
    d. Isolation
    e. Egocentricity
    f. Overt hostility (usually toward a family member)

C. Provide health teaching and referrals as indicated

1. Teach the person and the family signs of resolution.
    a. Griever no longer lives in the past but is future oriented and establishing new goals.
    b. Griever breaks ties with lost object/person after approximately 6–12 months of grieving.
    c. Griever begins to resocialize.

2. Identify agencies that may be helpful.
   a. Community agencies
   b. Religious groups

Grieving, Anticipatory

■ *Related to* **(Specify)**

DEFINITION

Anticipatory grieving: The state in which an individual/group experiences feelings in response to an expected significant loss.

DEFINING CHARACTERISTICS

Major (must be present)
Expressed distress at potential loss

Minor (may be present)
Denial
Guilt
Anger
Sorrow
Change in eating habits
Change in sleep patterns
Change in social patterns
Change in communication patterns
Decreased libido

RELATED FACTORS
See *Grieving*

■ Anticipatory Grieving
Related to (Specify)

Assessment

Subjective Data
The person expresses

Sadness	Fear	Anorexia
Depression	Denial	
Shock	Guilt	
Anger	Anergia	

Objective Data
Crying
Inability to cry
Withdrawn behavior
Apathetic behavior

Outcome Criteria

The person will
• Express his grief
• Participate in decision-making for the future
• Share his concerns with significant others

Interventions

A. Assess for causative and contributing factors of anticipated or potential loss

Terminal illness	Socioeconomic status
Separation, (divorce, hospitalization, marriage, relocation, job)	Alteration in body image
	Alteration in self-esteem
	Aging

B. Assess individual response

Denial	Shock
Rejection	Anger
Bargaining	Depression
Isolation	Guilt
Helplessness	Fear

1. Encourage the person to share concerns.
   a. Utilize communication techniques of open-ended questions and reflection ("What are your thoughts today?" "Are you sad?").
   b. Acknowledge the value of the person and his grief by using touch and by sitting with him and verbalizing your concern ("This must be a very difficult time for you").
   c. Recognize that some individuals may choose not to share their concerns, but convey that you are available if they desire to do so later.
2. Assist the person and the family to identify strengths.
   a. "What do you do well?"
   b. "What are you willing to do to improve your life?"
   c. "Is religion a source of strength for you?"
   d. "Do you have close friends?"
   e. "Who do you turn to in times of need?"
   f. "What does this person do for you?"
3. Promote the integrity of the person and the family by acknowledging strengths.

   a. "Your brother looks forward to your visit."

   b. "Your family is so concerned for you."

4. Support person and family with grief reactions.

   a. Prepare person and family for grief reactions.

   b. Explain grief reactions to person and family.

   c. Focus on the present life situation until the person or family indicates the desire to discuss future.

5. Promote family cohesiveness.

   a. Identify availability of a support system.

     • Meet consistently with family members.

     • Identify family member roles, strengths, weaknesses.

   b. Assess communication patterns.

     • Listen and clarify the messages being sent.

     • Identify the patterns of communication within the family unit by assessing positive and negative feedback, verbal and nonverbal communications, and body language.

   c. Provide for the concept of hope by

     • Supplying accurate information

     • Resisting the temptation to give false hope

     • Discussing concerns willingly

   d. Promote group decision-making to enhance group autonomy.

     • Establish consistent times to meet with person and family.

     • Encourage members to talk directly with each other and to listen to each other.

6. Promote grief work with each response.

   a. Denial

     • Initially support and then strive to increase the development of awareness (when individual indicates readiness for awareness).

   b. Isolation

     • Listen and spend designated time consistently with person and family.

     • Offer the person and the family opportunity to explore their emotions.

     • Reflect on past losses and acknowledge loss behavior (past and present).

   c. Depression

     • Begin with simple problem solving and move toward acceptance.

     • Enhance self-worth through positive reinforcement.

     • Identify the level of depression and indications of suicidal behavior or ideas.

     • Be consistent and establish times daily to speak with person and family.

   d. Anger

     • Allow for crying to release this energy.

     • Listen to and communicate concern.

     • Encourage concerned support from significant others as well as professional support.

   e. Guilt

     • Listen and communicate concern.

     • Allow for crying.

     • Promote more direct expression of feelings.

     • Explore methods to resolve guilt.

   f. Fear

     • Help person and family recognize the feeling.

     • Explain that this will help cope with life.

- Explore person's and family's attitudes about loss, death, etc.
- Explore person's and family's methods of coping.

   g. Rejection
- Allow for verbal expression of this feeling state to diminish the emotional strain.
- Recognize that expression of anger may create a rejection of self to significant others.

7. Provide for expression of grief.
   a. Encourage emotional expressions of grieving.
   b. Caution the use of sedatives and tranquilizers, which may prevent and/or delay emotional expressions of loss.
   c. Encourage verbalization of clients and families of all age groups.
- Support family cohesiveness.
- Promote and verbalize strengths of the family group.

   d. Encourage person and family to engage in life review.
- Focus and support the social network relationships.
- Reevaluate past life experiences and integrate them into a new meaning.
- Convey empathetic understanding.

8. Identify potential pathologic grieving reactions.

Delusions	Difficulty crying or controlling
Hallucinations	crying
Phobias	Loss of control of environment
Obsessions	leading to hopelessness,
Isolations	helplessness
Conversion hysteria	Intense reactions lasting longer
Agitated depression	than 6 months with few signs
Delay in grief work	of relief
Suicidal indications	Restrictions of pleasure

9. Refer individual with potential for pathologic grieving responses for counseling (psychiatrist, nurse therapist, counselor, psychologist)

C. Provide health teaching and referrals as indicated

1. Explain what to expect

Sadness	Fear
Feelings of aloneness	Rejection
Guilt	Anger
Emotions will be very labile initially and become more stable as grief work is accomplished	

2. Teach person and family signs of resolution.
   a. Griever no longer lives in past but is future oriented, establishing new goals.
   b. Griever breaks ties with lost object/person after approximately 6–12 months of grieving.
   c. Griever begins to resocialize.

3. Teach signs of pathologic responses and referrals needed.
   a. Defenses used in uncomplicated grief work that become exaggerated or maladaptive responses
   b. Persistent absence of any emotion
   c. Prolonged intense reactions of anxiety, anger, fear, guilt, helplessness

4. Identify agencies that may enhance grief work
   a. Self-help groups
   b. Widow-to-widow groups
   c. Parents of deceased children
   d. Single parent groups
   e. Bereavement groups

Grieving, Dysfunctional

■ *Related to* **(Specify)**

DEFINITION

Dysfunctional grieving: The state in which an individual or group experiences prolonged unresolved grief and engages in detrimental activities.

DEFINING CHARACTERISTICS

Major (must be present)

Unsuccessful adaptation to loss
Prolonged denial, depression
Delayed emotional reaction

Minor (may be present)

Social isolation or withdrawal
Failure to develop new relationships/interests
Failure to restructure life after loss

RELATED FACTORS

See *Grieving*

■ Dysfunctional Grieving
Related to (Specify)

Assessment

Subjective Data

Reported:
 History of ineffective coping
 Poor or ambivalent feelings toward the lost person/object
 Inadequate support system
 Unexpected death
 Multiple losses
 Absence of any emotion

Outcome Criteria

The individual/group will
 • Acknowledge the loss
 • Describe feelings expected with loss
 • Verbalize an intent to seek professional assistance

Interventions

A. Assess for causative and contributing factors that may contribute to dysfunctional grieving
 1. Unavailable (or lack of) support system
 2. Negation of the loss by others
 3. History of a difficult relationship with the lost person or object
 4. Multiple past losses
 5. Ineffective coping strategies
 6. Unexpected death
 7. Expectations to "be strong"

B. Promote a trust relationship
 1. Promote feelings of self-worth through one-on-one and/or group sessions.
 2. Allow for established time to meet and discuss feelings.
 3. Communicate clearly, simply, and to the point.
 4. Assess what the person and the family are learning by the use of feedback.
 5. Offer support and reassurance.
 6. Create a therapeutic milieu.
 7. Establish a safe, secure, and private environment.
 8. Demonstrate respect for the person's culture, religion, race, and values.

C. Support the person and the family's grief reactions
 1. Explain grief reactions.
  a. Shock and disbelief
  b. Developing awareness
  c. Restitution
 2. Describe varied acceptable expressions.
  a. Elated or manic behavior as a defense against depression
  b. Elation and hyperactivity as a reaction of love and protection from depression
  c. Various states of depression
  d. Various somatic manifestations (weight loss or gain, indigestion, dizziness)
 3. Assess for past experiences with loss.

       a. Loss of significant other in childhood

       b. Losses in later life

    4. Promote family cohesiveness.

       a. Support the family at its level of functioning.

       b. Encourage self-exploration of feelings with family members.

       c. Slowly and carefully identify the reality of the situation (*e.g.*, "After your husband died, who helped you most?").

       d. Explain the need to discuss behaviors that interfere with relationships.

       e. Recognize and reinforce the strengths of each family member.

       f. Encourage the family to evaluate their feelings and support one another.

D. Promote grief work with each response

    1. Denial

       a. Explain the use of denial by one family member to the other members.

       b. Do not force client to move past denial without emotional readiness.

    2. Isolation

       a. Convey a feeling of acceptance by allowing grief.

       b. Create open, honest communications to promote sharing.

       c. Reinforce the person's self-worth by allowing privacy.

       d. Encourage client/family to gradually increase social activities (support groups, church groups, etc.).

    3. Depression

       a. Reinforce the person's self-esteem.

       b. Identify the level of depression and develop the approach accordingly.

       c. Use empathetic sharing; acknowledge grief ("It must be very difficult").

       d. Identify any indications of suicidal behavior (frequent statements of intent, revealed plan).

       e. See *High Risk for Self-Harm* for additional information.

    4. Anger

       a. Understand that this feeling usually replaces denial.

       b. Explain to family that anger serves to try to control one's environment more closely because of inability to control loss.

       c. Encourage verbalization of the anger.

       d. See *Anxiety* for additional information for anger.

    5. Guilt/ambivalence

       a. Acknowledge the person's expressed self-view.

       b. Role play to allow person to "express" to the dead person what he wants to say or how he feels.

       c. Encourage client to identify positive contributions/aspects of the relationship.

       d. Avoid arguing and participating in the person's system of shoulds and should nots.

       e. Discuss the person's preoccupation with him and attempt to move verbally beyond the present.

    6. Fear

       a. Focus on the present and maintain a safe and secure environment.

       b. Help the person to explore reasons for a meaning of the behavior.

       c. Consider alternative ways of expressing his feelings.

E. Provide health teaching and referrals as indicated

    1. Teach the person and the family signs of resolution.

       a. Griever no longer lives in past but is future oriented and establishing new goals.

  b. Griever begins to break ties with lost object/person after approximately 6–12 months of grieving.
  c. Griever begins to resocialize, seeks new relationships, experiences.
 2. Teach individual/family signs of pathologic grieving, especially persons who are at risk, and to seek professional counseling.
  a. Prolonged depression
  b. Denial
  c. Lives in past
  d. Prolonged hallucinations
  e. Continued searching for the deceased (frequent moves/relocations)
  f. Delusions
  g. Isolation
  h. Egocentricity
  i. Overhostility (usually toward a family member)
 3. Identify agencies that may be helpful.
  a. Community agencies' support groups, mental health agencies
  b. Religious groups
  c. Psychotherapists, grief specialists

References/Bibliography

Books

Abrams, S., & Berkow, R. (Eds.). (1990). *The Merck manual of geriatrics*. Rahway, NJ: Merck & Co.

Backer, B. A. Hannon, N. & Russell, N. (1982). *Death and dying individuals and institutions*. New York: Wiley & Sons.

Barton, D. (Ed.). (1977). *Dying and death: A clinical guide for caregivers*. Baltimore: Williams & Wilkins.

Battin, D., Aakin, A., Gerber, I., et al. (1975). Coping and vulnerability among the aged bereaved. In Schroenber, B., Gerber, I., Wiener, A. (Eds.) (1975). *Bereavement: Its psychosocial aspects*. New York: Columbia University Press.

Beitler, R. (1968). The life review: An interpretation of reminiscence in the aged. In Neugarten, B. L. (Ed.). *Middle life and aging*. Chicago: University of Chicago Press.

Caughill, R. (Ed.). (1976). *The dying patient: A supportive approach*. Boston: Little, Brown.

dePaola, T. (1973). *Nana upstairs and nana downstairs*. New York: Putnam.

Ebersole, P., & Hess, P. (1990). *Toward healthy aging: Human needs and nursing response* (3rd ed.). St. Louis: C. V. Mosby.

Fulton, R. (Ed.). (1976). *Death and identity*. Bowie, MD: Charles Press.

Hamilton, M., Reid, H. (Eds.). *A hospice handbook: A new way to care for the dying*. Grand Rapids: W. B. Eerdmans.

Hogstel, M. O. (1990). *Geropsychiatric nursing*. St. Louis: C. V. Mosby.

Kastenbaum, R. (1977). *Death, society, and human experience*. St. Louis: C. V. Mosby.

Kastenbaum, R. (1969). Psychological death. In Pearson, L. (Ed.). *Death and dying*. Cleveland: Case Western Reserve University Press.

Kennedy, E. (1981). *Crisis counseling: The essential guide for nonprofessional counselors*. New York: Continuum.

Kyes, J. J., & Hofling, C. K. (1980). *Basic psychiatric concepts in nursing* (4th ed.). Philadelphia: J. B. Lippincott.

Kübler-Ross, E. (1975). *Death: The final stage of growth*. Englewood Cliffs, NJ: Prentice-Hall.

Kübler-Ross, E. (1983). *On children and death*. New York: Macmillan.

Lazare, A. (1979). Unresolved grief. In Lazare, A. (Ed.). *Outpatient psychiatry, diagnosis and treatment*. Baltimore: Williams & Wilkins.

Matteson, M. A., & McConnell, E.S. (1988). *Gerontological nursing: Concepts and practice*. Philadelphia: W. B. Saunders.

McCowan, D. (1989). Impact of death and dying. In Foster R. L. Hunsberger, M. M., & Anderson, J. J. T. (Eds.). *Family-centered nursing care of children*. Philadelphia: W. B. Saunders.

Packes, C. (1972). *Bereavement: Studies of grief in adult life*. New York: International Universities Press.

Rando, T. A. (1984). *Grief, dying, and death: Clinical interventions for caregivers*. Champaign, IL: Research Press.

Schiff, H. S. (1977). *The bereaved parent*. New York: Crown Publishers.

Viorst, J. (1971). *The tenth good thing about Barney*. Hartford: Atheneum.

Werner-Beland, J. A. (1980). *Grief responses to long-term illness and disability*. Reston, VA: Reston Publishing.

Whaley, L. F., & Wong, D. L. (1989). *Essentials of pediatric nursing* (3rd ed.). St. Louis: C. V. Mosby.

Worden, J. (1982). *Grief counseling and grief therapy, a handbook for the mental health practitioner*. New York: Springer Publishing.

Periodicals

Antonacci, M. (1990). Sudden death: Helping bereaved parents in the PICU. *Critical Care Nurse, 10*(4), 65–70.

Benfield, D. G., et al. (1988). Grief response of parents after referral of the critically ill newborn to a regional center. *New England Journal of Medicine, 294*(18), 975–978.

Benoliel, J. Q. (1985). Loss and adaptation: Circumstances, contingencies and consequences. *Death Studies, 9*, 217–233.

Benoliel, J. Q. (1985). Loss and terminal illness. *Nursing Clinics of North America, 20*(2), 439–448.

Bourne, V., & Meier, J. (1988). What happens now? A book to be read to children who have lost a loved one. *Oncology Nursing Forum, 15* (1), 81–85.

Butler, R. N. (1963). The life review. *Psychiatry, 26*, 65–76.

Caserta, M. S., Lund, D. A., & Dimond, M. F. (1985). Assessing interviewer effects in a longitudinal study of bereaved elderly adults. *Journal of Gerontology, 40*(5), 637–640.

Constantino, R. E. (1981). Bereavement crisis intervention in grief and mourning. *Nursing Research, 30*(6), 351–353.

Dimond, M. (1981). Bereavement and the elderly: A critical review with implications for nursing practice and research. *Journal of Advanced Nursing, 6*, 461–470.

Domming, J., Stackman, J., O'Neill, P., et al. (1973). Experiences with dying patients. *American Journal of Nursing, 73*, 1058–1064.

Engle, G. (1964) Grief and grieving. *American Journal of Nursing, 64*, 93–97.

Friedmann-Campbell, M., & Hart, C. A. (1984). Theoretical strategies and nursing interventions to promote psychosocial adaptation to spinal cord injuries and disability. *Journal of Neurosurgical Nursing, 16*(6), 335–342, 1984

Gallagher, D. E., Breckenridge, J. N., Thompson, L. W., & Peterson, J. A. (1983). Effects of bereavement on indicators of mental health in elderly widows and widowers. *Journal of Gerontology, 38*(5), 565–571.

Grogan, L. B. (1990). Grief of an adolescent when a sibling dies. *Maternal Child Nursing, 15*(1), 21–24.

Gyulag, J. (Ed.) (1989). The death of a child. *Issues in Comprehensive Pediatric Nursing, 12*(4), 1–137.

Hauser, M. J. (1983). Bereavement outcomes for widows. *Journal of Psychosocial Nursing and Mental Health Services, 21*(9), 23–31.

Haylor, M. (1987). Human response to loss. *Nurse Practitioner, 12*(5), 63.

Homedes, N., & Ahmed, S. M. (1987). In my opinion . . . death education for children. *Children's Health Care, 16*(10), 34–36.

Hungelman, J., Kenkel-Rossi, Klassen, L., & Stollenwerk, R. M. (1985). Spiritual well-being in older adults, harmonious interconnections. *Journal of Religion and Health, 24*(2), 147–153.

Hutton, L. (1981). Annie is alone: The bereaved child. *Maternal-Child Nursing Journal, 6*, 274–277.

Kaprio, J., & Koskenvuo, R. H. (1987). Mortality after bereavement: A prospective study of 95,647 widowed persons. *American Journal of Public Health, 77*(3), 283–287.

Kowalsky, E. (1978). Grief, a lost life-style. *American Journal of Nursing, 78*(3), 418–420.

Kowalski, K. (1978) Osborn, M. R. Helping mothers of stillborn infants to grieve. *Maternal-Child Nursing Journal, 2*, 29–32.

Lake, C. Marian, B., et al. (1983). The role of a grief support team following stillbirth. *American Journal of Obstetrics and Gynecology, 146*, 877–881.

Lawson, L. V. (1990). Culturally sensitive support for grieving parents. *Maternal Child Nursing, 15*(2), 76–79.

Mina, C. (1985) A program for helping grieving parents. *Maternal-Child Nursing Journal, 10*, 118–121.

Philpot, T. (1980). St. Joseph's Hospice: Death—a part of life. *Nursing Mirror, 151*(16), 20–23.

Oberfield, R. A. (1984). Terminal illness: Death and bereavement: Toward an understanding of its nature. *Perspectives in Biology and Medicine*, 287–301.

Oehler, J. (1981). The frog family books: Color pictures sad or glad. *Maternal-Child Nursing Journal 6*, 281.

Page-Liegerman, J., & Hughes, C. (1990). How fathers perceive perinatal death. *Maternal Child Nursing, 15*(5), 320–322.

Pazola, K., Gerberg, A. K. (1990). Priviledged communication—talking with a dying adolescent. *Maternal Child Nursing, 15*(1), 16–21.

Poncar, P. J. The elderly widow: Easing her role transition. *Journal of Psychosocial Nursing, 27*(2), 6–11.

Radford, C. (1980). Nursing care to the end. *Nursing Mirror, 150*(2), 30–31.

Ross-Alaolmolki, K. (1985). Supportive care for families of dying children. *Nursing Clinics of North America, 20*(2), 457–466.

Schultz, C. A. (1979). The dynamics of grief. *Journal of Emergency Nursing, 15*(5), 26–30.

Sheer, B. L. (1977). Help for parents in a difficult job: Broaching the subject of death. *Maternal-Child Nursing Journal, 5*, 320–324.

Steele, L. L. (1990). The death surround: Factors influencing the grief experience of survivors. *Oncology Nursing Forum, 17*(2), 235–241.

Vachon, M. L., Lyall, W. A., Rogers, J., Freedman-Letofsky, B., & Freeman, S. J. (1980). A controlled self-help intervention for widows. *American Journal of Psychiatry, 137*(11), 1380–1384.

Wass, H., & Corn, C. (Eds.). (1985). Childhood and death. *Issues Comprehensive Pediatric Nursing, 8*(1–6), 1–383.

Willans, J. H. (1980). Appetite in the terminally ill patient. *Nursing Times, 76*(10), 875–876.

Williams, H., Rivara, F. P., & Rothenberg, M. B. (1981). The child is dying: Who helps the family? *Maternal-Child Nursing Journal, 6*, 261–265.

Wong, D. (1980) Bereavement: The empty mother syndrome. *Maternal-Child Nursing Journal, 5*, 384–389.

Wooten, B. (1981). Death of an infant. *Maternal-Child Nursing Journal, 6* 257–260.

Resources for the Consumer

Literature

Newborn death ($2.35), *Miscarriage* ($2.35), *Where's Jess* ($3.00), Centering Corporation, Box 3367, Omaha, NE 68103-0367

Answers to a child's questions about death, by Peter Stillman, Guideline Publications, Stanford, NY 12167

Grollman, E. A. (Ed.). (1967). *Explaining death to children*. Boston: Beacon Press (See prologue; explains what *not* to tell children.)

Kushner, H. S. (1981). *When bad things happen to good people*. New York: Schocken (Offers a compassionate and humane approach to dealing with questions of suffering and life and death in a way that affirms humanity and inspires peace of mind.)

For Children

Buscaglia, L. D. (1982). *The fall of Freddie the leaf*. New York: Charles B. Slack.

Dodge, N. C. *Thumpy's story—A story of love and grief* (shared by Thumpy, the Bunny; English and Spanish editions)

Rofes, E. (Ed). (1986). *The kids book about death and dying.* New York. Little, Brown (Researched and written by 11-to-14-year-old students who also recommend other books about death and dying; covers topics such as euthanasia, organ donation, autopsy, emotions, and how children feel about the death of a friend, pet, parent, or their own life-threatening illness. However, section on brain death needs updating.)

What happens now? (single copy): St. Luke's Hospital, 2900 West Oklahoma Avenue, Milwaukee, WI 53215

Organizations

Children's Hospice International (CHI), 1101 King Street, Suite 131, Alexandria, VA 22314, (703) 684-0330 or 684-0331

The Compassionate Friends, National Headquarters, P.O. Box 3696, Oak Brook, IL 60522, (312) 323-5010

Growth and Development, Altered

■ *Related to* **(Specify)**

DEFINITION

Altered Growth and Development: The state in which an individual has, or is at risk for, impaired ability to perform tasks of his/her age group or impaired growth.

DEFINING CHARACTERISTICS

Major (must be present)

Inability or difficulty performing skills or behaviors typical of his/her age group (*e.g.,* motor, personal/social, language/cognition) (see Table II-7) and/or

Altered physical growth: weight lagging behind height by 2 standard deviations; pattern of height and weight percentiles indicate a drop in pattern

Minor (may be present)

Inability to perform self-care or self-control activities appropriate for age (see Table II-7)

Flat affect, listlessness, decreased responses, slow in social responses, shows limited signs of satisfaction to caregiver, shows limited eye contact, difficulty feeding, decreased appetite, lethargic, irritable, negative mood, regression in self-toileting, regression in self-feeding (see Focus Assessment)

Infants: watchfulness, interrupted sleep pattern

RELATED FACTORS

Pathophysiologic

Circulatory impairment: congenital heart defects, congestive heart failure

Neurologic impairment: cerebral damage, congenital defects, cerebral palsy, microencephaly

Gastrointestinal impairment: malabsorption syndrome, gastroesophageal reflux, cystic fibrosis

Endocrine or renal impairment: hormonal disturbance

Musculoskeletal impairment

Congenital anomalies of extremities   Muscular dystrophy

Acute illness

Prolonged pain

Repeated acute illness, chronic illness

Inadequate caloric, nutritional intake

Treatment-related

Prolonged, painful treatment	Repeated or prolonged hospitalization
Traction or casts	Prolonged bed rest
Isolation	Confinement

(Text continues on page 426)

Table II-7 **Age-Related Developmental Tasks**

Developmental Tasks/Needs	Parental Guidance	Implications for Nursing
Birth to 1 Year		
Personal/social		
Learns to trust and anticipate satisfaction	Encourage parent to respond to cry, meet infants need *consistently*	Encourage parent to participate in care:
Sends cues to mother/caretaker		Bathing
Begins understanding self as separate from others (body image)	Teach parent not to be afraid they will "spoil" infant with too much attention	Feeding
	Talk and sing to child; hold and cuddle often	Holding
Motor		Teach parent guidance information
Responds to sound	Provide variety of stimulation	Provide ongoing stimulation while confined
Social smile	Allow infant to feed self (cereal, etc.)	through use of toys, mirrors, mobiles, music
Reaches for objects	Do not prop bottle	Hold, speak to infant, maintain eye contact
Begins to sit, creep, pull up and stand with support	*Toys*	Investigate crying
	Brightly colored crib toys, mobiles	Do not restrain
Attempting to walk	Stuffed toys: of varied textures	
	Music boxes	
Language/cognition		
Learns to signal wants/needs with sounds, crying	*Safety*	
	Be aware of rapidly changing locomotive ability (*i.e.,* childproof kitchen, stairways; small objects within reach; tub safety)	
Begins to vocalize with meaning (two syllable words: Dada, Mama)		
Comprehends some verbal/nonverbal messages (no, yes, bye-bye)		
Learns about words through senses		
Fears		
Loud noises		
Falling		
1–3½ Years		
Personal/social		
Establishes self-control, decision-making, self-independence (autonomy)	Provide child with peer companionship	Allow child to take liquids from a cup (including medicines)
	Allow for brief periods of separation under	

(continued)

Table II-7 **Age-Related Developmental Tasks** (continued)

Developmental Tasks/Needs	Parental Guidance	Implications for Nursing
Extremely curious, prefers to do things himself	familiar surroundings	Allow child to perform some self-care tasks:
Demonstrates independence through negativism	Practice safety measures that guard against child's increased motor ability and curiosity (poisoning, falls)	Wash face and arms
		Brush teeth
Very egocentric: believes he controls the world	Tell the truth	Expect resistant behavior to treatments; reinforce treatments, not punishments
Learns about words through senses	Disciplining child for violation of safety rules:	Use firm, direct approach and provide child with choices only when possible
Motor	Running in street	Restrain child when needed
Begins to walk and run well	Touching electrical wires	Explain to parents methods for disciplining child:
Drinks from cup, feeds self	Allow child some control over fears:	
Develops fine-motor control	Favorite toy	Slap hand once (for dangerous touching, e.g., stove)
Climbs	Night light	Sit in chair for 2 minutes (if child gets up, put him back and reset timer)
Begins self-toileting	Allow exploration within safe limits	
Language/cognition	Explain as simply as possible why things happen	Explain the need for consistency
Has poor time sense		Allow expression of fear, pain, displeasure
Increasingly verbal (4–5 word sentences by age 3½)	Allow child to explain why he thinks things are happening	Assign consistent caregiver
Talks to self/others	Correct misconceptions	Let child play with simple equipment (stethoscope)
Misconceptions about cause/effect	Include child in domestic activities when possible:	
		Provide materials for play (favorite toy, night light, etc.)
Fears	Dusting	Be honest about procedure
Loss/separation from parents	Cleaning spoons	Praise child for helping you:
Darkness	Discuss differences in opinions (between parents) in front of child	Holding still
Machines/equipment	Do not threaten child with what will happen if he does not behave	Holding the Band-Aid
Intrusive procedures	Always follow through with punishment	Give child choices whenever possible
		Tell child he can cry or squeeze your hand, but you expect him to hold still
	Toys	Have parents present for procedures when at all possible
	Manipulative toys	
	Puzzles	

(continued)

Bright-colored, simple books
Large-muscle devices (gym sets, etc.)
Music (songs, records)

Explore with child his fantasies of the situation:
Use play therapy
Explain the procedure immediately before-hand if short (e.g., injection) and two hours before if longer or intrusive (e.g., x-ray, IV insertion)
Follow home routines when possible

3½–5 Years

Personal/social

Attempts to establish self as like his parents, but independent
Explores environment on his own initiative
Boasts, brags, has feelings of indestructibility
Family is primary group
Peers increasingly important
Assumes sex roles
Aggressive

Motor

Locomotion skills increase, and coordinates easier
Rides tricycle/bicycle
Throws ball, but has difficulty catching

Language/cognition

Egocentric
Language skills flourish
Generates many questions; how, why, what?
Simple problem-solving; uses fantasy to understand, problem-solve

Fears

Mutilation
Castration
Dark
Unknown

Teach parents to listen to child's fears, feelings
Encourage hugs, touch as expressions of acceptance
Provide explanations—simply
Limit stimulation from television to avoid intense material
Focus on positive behaviors
Allow child to help as much as possible
Provide child with regular contract with other children (e.g., nursery school)
Explain that television, movies are make-believe
Practice definite limit-setting on behavior
Offer child choices
Allow child to express anger verbally but limit motor aggression ("You may slam a door but you may not throw a toy")
Discipline (examples):
Sit in chair 5 minutes
Forbid a favorite pastime (no bicycle riding for 2 hours)
Be consistent and firm
Teach safety precautions about strangers

Toys and Games

Enjoys "make-believe" play (play house, toy models, etc.)

Encourage expressing of fears
Reinforce reality of body image
Encourage self-care, decision-making when possible
Involve parents in teaching
Provide peer stimulation
Limit physical restraint
Provide play opportunities for acting out fantasy, story-telling
Explain to child how he can cooperate (e.g., hold still), and expect that he will
Use play therapy to allow child free expression
Explain all procedures:
Use equipment if possible; allow therapeutic play
Encourage child to ask questions
Tell child the exact body parts that will be affected
Use models, pictures
Explain when procedure will occur in relation to daily schedule (e.g., after lunch, after bath)

(continued)

Table II-7 **Age-Related Developmental Tasks** (continued)

Developmental Tasks/Needs	Parental Guidance	Implications for Nursing
Inanimate, unfamiliar objects	Simple games with others, books, puzzles, coloring	Promote family and peer interactions (i.e., visiting, telephone, etc.)
5–11 Years Personal/social	Teach appropriate foods needed each day, provide choices	Explain all procedures and impact on body
Learns to include values and skills of school, neighborhood, peers	Encourage interaction outside home	Encourage questioning, active participation in care
Peer relationships important	Include cooking and cleaning in home activities	Be direct about explanation of procedures (i.e., body part involved, use anatomic names, pictures, etc.); explain step by step
Focuses more on reality, less on fantasy	Teach safety (bicycle, street, playground equipment, fire, water, strangers)	Be honest
Family is main base of security and identity	Maintain limit-setting and discipline	Reassure child that he is liked
Sensitive to reactions of others	Prepare child for bodily changes of pubescence and provide with concrete sex education information (late childhood)	Provide privacy
Seeks approval, recognition	Expect fluctuations between immature and mature behavior	Involve parents but make direction of care the child's decision
Enthusiastic, noisy, imaginative, desires to explore	Respect peer relationships but do not compromise your values (e.g., "But, Mom, all the other girls are wearing makeup!")	Reason and explain
Likes to complete a task	Promote responsibility, contribution to family (i.e., duties for helping, etc.)	Encourage continuance of school work, activities if condition permits (i.e., homework, contact with classmates)
Enjoys helping	Promote exploration and development of skills (i.e., joining clubs, sports, hobbies, etc.)	Encourage continuance of hobbies, interests
Motor	Toys and Games	
Moves constantly	Group games, board games, art activities, crafts, video games, reading	
Physical play prevalent (sports, swimming, skating, etc.)		
Language/cognition		
Organized, stable thought		
Concepts more complicated		
Focuses on concrete understanding		
Fears		
Rejections, failure		
Immobility		
Mutilation		
Death		

(continued)

11–15 Years

Personal/social

Family values continue to be significant influence

Peer group values have increasing significance

Early adolescence: outgoing and enthusiastic

Emotions are extreme, mood swings, introspection

Sexual identity fully mature

Wants privacy/independence

Develops interests not shared with family

Concern with physical self

Explores adult roles

Motor

Well-developed

Rapid physical growth

Secondary sex characteristics

Language/cognition

Plans for future career

Able to abstract solutions and problem-solve in future tense

Fears

Mutilation

Disruption in body image

Rejection from peers

Encourage independent problem-solving, decision-making within established values

Be available

Compliment child's achievements

Listen to interests, likes, dislikes without passing judgment

Respect privacy

Allow independence while maintaining safety limits

Provide concrete information about sexuality, function, bodily changes

Teach about:

Auto safety

Drug abuse

Alcohol abuse

Tobacco hazards

Mechanical safety

Sexual abuse

Dating

Games/interests

Intellectual games

Reading

Arts, crafts, hobbies

Video games

Problem-solving games

Computers

Respect privacy

Accept expression of feelings

Direct discussions of care and condition to child

Ask for opinions, allow input into decisions

Be flexible with routines, explain all procedures/treatments

Encourage continuance of peer relationships

Listen actively

Identify impact of illness on body image, future functioning

Correct misconceptions

Encourage continuance of school work, hobbies, interests

Situational (personal and environmental)

Parental knowledge deficit
Stress (acute, transient, or chronic)
Hospitalization or change in usual environment
Separation from significant others (parents, primary caretaker)
Inadequate, inappropriate parental support (neglect, abuse)
Inadequate sensory stimulation (neglect, isolation)
Parent-child conflict
School-related stressors
Parental anxiety
Loss of significant other
Loss of control over environment (established rituals, activities, established hours of contact with family)
Multiple caretakers

Maturational

Infant-Toddler	*Lack of Stimulation*
(birth–3 years)	Separation from parents/significant others
	Change in environment
	Restriction of activity
	Inadequate parental support
	Inability to trust significant other
	Inability to communicate (deafness)
Preschool Age	*Restriction of Activity*
(4–6 years)	Loss of ability to communicate
	Lack of stimulation
	Lack of significant other
	Loss of significant other (death, divorce)
	Loss of peer group
	Loss of independence
	Fear of mutilation, pain, abandonment
	Removal from home environment
School Age	*Loss of Individual Control*
(6–11 years)	Loss of significant others
	Loss of peer group
	Fear of immobility, mutilation, death
	Fear of intrusive procedures
	Strange environment
Adolescent	
(12–18 years)	Loss of independence and autonomy
	Disruption of peer relationships
	Disruption of body image
	Interruption of intellectual achievement
	Loss of significant others

Diagnostic Considerations

Specific developmental tasks are associated with various age groups (*e.g.*, age 18–30, to establish lasting relationships; age 1–3, to gain autonomy and self-control [*e.g.*, toileting]). An adult's failure to accomplish a developmental task may cause or contribute to altered functioning in a functional health pattern; *e.g.*, *Impaired Social Interactions, Powerlessness*. Because nursing interventions will focus on the altered functioning rather than on achievement of past developmental tasks, the diagnosis *Altered Growth and Development* has limited uses for adults. It is most useful for a child or adolescent experiencing difficulty achieving a developmental task.

Errors in Diagnostic Statements

Altered Growth and Development related to inability to perform toileting self-control appropriate for age (4 years)

Inability to perform toileting self-control is not a contributing factor, but rather a diagnostic cue. The diagnosis should be rewritten as *Altered Growth and Development related to unknown etiology, as evidenced by inability to perform toileting self-control appropriate for age (4 years)*. The use of "unknown etiology" directs nurses to collect more data on reasons for the problem.

Altered Growth and Development related to mental retardation secondary to Down syndrome

When *Altered Growth and Development* is used to describe an individual with mental or physical impairment, what is the nursing focus? What client goals would nursing interventions achieve? If physical impairments represent barriers to achieving developmental tasks, the diagnosis can be written as *High Risk for Altered Growth and Development related to impaired ability to achieve developmental tasks (specify—e.g., socialization) secondary to disability*.

For a mentally impaired child, the nurse should determine what functional health patterns are altered or at high risk for alteration and amenable to nursing interventions and address the specific problem, *e.g., Self-Care Deficit*.

Focus Assessment Criteria

See Table II-7 for descriptions of appropriate developmental milestones/behaviors for each age group, as well as information for nursing intervention and parental guidance.

Subjective Data

(Data should be verified with primary caregiver.)
1. Current nutritional patterns
   Diet recall for past 24 hours (from parent or child, type of food, amounts)
   Diet history
   Height/weight at birth
   Intake pattern
   Child's reaction to eating, feeding
   Parental/child knowledge of nutrition
2. Physiologic alterations
   Presence of nausea, vomiting, diarrhea
   Allergies
   Food intolerances
   Dysphagia
   Fatigue
   Report of other physical symptoms (*e.g.*, rash, URI)

3. Parental attitudes

What are the parents' expectations for the child?

What are the parents' feelings about being parents?

Did the parents experience poor parenting themselves?

Parenting approach to care and discipline of child?

How do the parents feel about home situation?

How do the parents feel about child's illness, treatments/hospitalization?

Assess family functioning with appropriate assessment tool.

4. Stressors in environment

Illness in family

Conflict in family

History of illness or hospitalization of child

Child's behavior/success in school

Child's peer/sibling relationships

5. Developmental level: Behaviors listed under Developmental Tasks (Table II-7) may be assessed through direct observation or report of parent/primary caregiver. The Denver Developmental Screening Tool may be used for children under 6 years of age.

Objective Data

1. General appearance

Cleanliness, grooming

Eye contact

Facial responses

Response to stimulation

Mood (*i.e.,* crying, elated, etc.)

2. Response/interaction with parent

Spontaneous, happy when comforted by parent

Reaction when separated

Response to procedures, strangers

3. Nutritional status

Height/weight (compare to norms in Principles and Rationale for Nursing Care)

Frontal/occipital circumference (also see Focus Assessment Criteria, *Nutrition, Altered: Less Than Body Requirements*)

4. Elimination patterns

Bowel and bladder

Description, frequency of stool

5. Personal/social

Language/cognition

Motor activity: Assess for achievement of developmental skills in appropriate age group (Table II-7)

6. Type of illness, treatments

7. Developmental level (see behaviors described under Developmental Tasks [Table II-7])

Principles and Rationale for Nursing Care

1. Development can be defined as the patterned, orderly, lifelong changes in structure, thought, or behavior that evolve as a result of maturation of physical and mental capacity, experiences, and learning. Development results in the person achieving a new level of maturity and integration. Growth refers to increase in body size, function, complexity of body cell content (Whaley & Wong, 1990). For the purpose of

this diagnosis, growth and development are synonymous, because any disruption that does not affect development will most likely result in a diagnosis of *Altered Nutrition*.

2. The following assumptions concerning development are relevant (Santrock, 1989; Whaley & Wong, 1990):
   a. The most rapid growth and development occurs in the early stages of life.
   b. Childhood is the foundation period of life and establishes the basis for successful or unsuccessful development throughout life.
   c. Growth and development are continuous and occur in spurts, rather than in a straight, upward direction.
   d. Development follows a definable, predictable, and sequential pattern.
   e. Critical periods exist when development is occurring rapidly and the individual's ability to respond to stressors is limited.
   f. Development proceeds in a cephalocaudal, proximodistal direction.
   g. Development proceeds from simple to complex.
   h. Development occurs in all components of a person (*i.e.*, motor, intellectual, personal, social, language).
   i. Development results from biologic, maturational, and individual learning.

3. Often development is defined in terms of stages or levels, as is illustrated in Erikson's stages of man and Piaget's stages of cognition. In addition, development may be defined in terms of tasks that must be accomplished. A developmental task is a growth responsibility that occurs at a particular time in the life of a person. Successful achievement of the task leads to success with later tasks. Development is affected through either an acceleration of the process or a slowing down of the process by a variety of influences. Physiologic disruptions, through either genetic malfunction or insult from illness, may potentially alter development, temporarily or permanently. Psychologic and social influences may also alter development positively or negatively. The alteration of development in a child is particularly critical because the alteration may establish a basic foundation that then remains faulty for the life of the child. Because of the rapid acceleration of development in childhood, several critical periods exist when influences can easily modify development (Whaley & Wong, 1989).

4. Of the range of possible physiologic, psychological, and social influences that may affect development, many exist within the context of illness and wellness care and are often encountered by nurses as they provide care to children. As a result, nursing interventions should be designed with particular developmental tasks and developmental information as a basis for intervention. As part of the care of the child, the nurse must also consider the impact of the primary caregiver or parent figure on the development of the child. The parent essentially controls most of the psychologic and social influences present in the early years of childhood. By virtue of the child's dependence on the parent, these influences can modify development (Hunsberger, 1989; Whaley & Wong 1989).

5. Illness, hospitalization, separation from parents, conflict, or inadequate support from parents, as well as specific pathophysiologic processes that interfere with growth, may ultimately affect development in a child. The nurse must support the family as well as the child in ensuring continuance of the child's developmental processes throughout the course of his illness if optimal recovery is to be achieved. In addition, the nurse must seek to stimulate as well as maintain the child's unique developmental level to promote optimal recovery. Stimulation of the developmental process may occur through parental support, parental teaching, referral, or direct intervention (see also *Altered Parenting*) (Farkas, 1983).

■ Altered Growth and Development
Related to (Specify)

Assessment
See Defining Characteristics

Outcome Criteria

The child will
- Demonstrate an increase in behaviors in personal/social, language, cognition, motor activities appropriate to age group (specify the behaviors)

Interventions

A. Assess causative or contributing factors
 1. Lack of knowledge—parental (caregiver)
 2. Acute or chronic illness
 3. Stress
 4. Inadequate stimulation
 5. Parent–child conflict
 6. Change in environment

B. Teach parents the age-related developmental tasks and parental guidance information (see Table II-7)

C. Carefully assess child's level of development in all areas of functioning by utilizing specific assessment tools (*e.g.,* Brazelton Assessment Table, Denver Developmental Screening Tool)

D. Provide opportunities for an ill child to meet age-related developmental tasks
(See Implications for Nursing [Table II-7] to assist with designing interventions)

- Birth to 1 year
 1. Provide increased stimulation using variety of colored toys in crib (*e.g.,* mobiles, musical toys, stuffed toys of varied textures, frequent periods of holding and speaking to infant).
 2. Hold while feeding; feed slowly and in relaxed environment.
 3. Provide periods of rest prior to feeding.
 4. Observe mother and child during interaction, especially during feeding.
 5. Investigate crying promptly and consistently.
 6. Assign consistent caregiver.
 7. Encourage parental visits/calls and involvement in care, if possible.
 8. Provide buccal experience if infant desires (*i.e.,* thumb, pacifier).
 9. Allow hands and feet to be free, if possible.

- 1–3½ years
1. Assign consistent caregiver.
2. Encourage self-care activities (*e.g.*, self-feeding, self-dressing, bathing).
3. Reinforce word development by repeating words child uses, naming objects by saying words, and speaking to child often.
4. Provide frequent periods of play with peers present and with a variety of toys (puzzles, books with pictures, manipulative toys, trucks, cars, blocks, bright colors).
5. Explain all procedures as you do them.
6. Provide safe area where the child can locomote, use walker, creeping area, hold hand while taking steps.
7. Encourage parental visits/calls and involvement in care, if possible.
8. Provide comfort measures after painful procedures.

- 3½–5 years
1. Encourage self care: self-grooming, self-dressing, mouth care, hair care.
2. Provide frequent play time with others and with variety of toys (*e.g.*, models, musical toys, dolls, puppets, books, mini-slide, wagon, tricycle, etc.).
3. Read stories aloud.
4. Ask for verbal responses and requests.
5. Say words for equipment, objects, and people and ask the child to repeat.
6. Allow time for individual play and exploration of play environment.
7. Encourage parental visits/calls and involvement in care, if possible.
8. Monitor television and utilize television as means to help child understand time ("After Sesame Street, your mother will come.").

- 5–11 years
1. Talk with child about care provided.
2. Request input from child (*e.g.*, diet, clothes, routine, etc.).
3. Allow child to dress in clothes instead of pajamas.
4. Provide periods of interaction with other children on unit.
5. Provide craft project that can be completed each day or week.
6. Continue school work at intervals each day.
7. Praise positive behaviors.
8. Read stories, and provide variety of independent games, puzzles, books, video games, painting, etc.
9. Introduce child by name to persons on unit.
10. Encourage visits with and/or telephone calls from parents, sibling, and peers.

- 11–15 years
1. Speak frequently with child about feelings, ideas, concerns over condition or care.
2. Provide opportunity for interaction with others of the same age on unit.
3. Identify interest or hobby that can be supported on unit in some manner and support it daily.
4. Allow hospital routine to be altered to suit child's schedule.
5. Dress in his own clothes if possible.
6. Involve in decisions about his care.
7. Provide opportunity for involvement in variety of activities (*i.e.*, reading, video games, movies, board games, art, trips outside or to other areas).
8. Encourage visits and/or telephone calls from parents, siblings, and peers.

E. Initiate health teaching and referrals when indicated

1. Provide anticipatory guidance for parents regarding constructive handling of developmental problems and support of developmental process (Table II-7) (see *Altered Parenting*).
2. Refer to appropriate agency for counseling or follow-up treatment of abuse, parent-child conflict, chemical dependency, etc. (see *Disabled Family Coping*).
3. Refer to appropriate agency for structured, ongoing stimulation program when functioning is likely to be impaired permanently (*e.g.*, schooling).
4. Refer to community programs specific to contributing factors (*e.g.*, WIC, social services, family services, counseling).
5. Provide list of parent support groups (*i.e.*, ARC, Down Syndrome Awareness, Muscular Dystrophy Association, National Epilepsy).

References/Bibliography

Briggs, D C. (1979). *Your child's self esteem.* New York: Doubleday.

Chase, R A., & Rubin, R. R. (1979). *The first wondrous year.* New York: Macmillan.

Damon, W. (1983). *Social and personality development, essays on the growth of the child.* New York: W. W. Norton.

Erikson, E. (1963). *Childhood and society* (2nd ed.). New York: W. W. Norton.

Farkas, S. C. (1983). *Hospitalized children: The family's role in care and treatment.* Washington, DC: The Catholic University of America.

Garmezy, N., & Rutter, M. (Eds.). (1983). *Stress, coping, and development in children.* St. Louis: McGraw-Hill.

Hagnes, U. (1983). *Holistic health care for children with developmental disabilities.* Baltimore: University Park Press.

Hunsberger, M. (1989). Nursing care during hospitalization. In Foster, R. L., Hunsberger, M. M., & Anderson, J. J. T. (Eds.). *Family-centered nursing care of children.* Philadelphia: W. B. Saunders.

Petrillo, M., & Sanger, S. (1980). *Emotional care of hospitalized children* (2nd ed.). Philadelphia: J. B. Lippincott.

Piaget, J. (1969). *The theory of stages in cognitive development.* New York: McGraw-Hill.

Poster, E. C. (1983). Stress immunization: Techniques to help children cope with hospitalization. *Maternal-Child Nursing Journal, 12*(2), 21–24.

Samuels, M., & Samuels, N. (1979). *The well baby book.* New York: Summit Books.

Santrock, J. W. (1989). *Lifespan development.* Dubuque, IA: William C. Brown.

Whaley, L. F., & Wong, D. L. (1989). *Essentials of pediatric nursing* (3rd ed.). St. Louis: C. V. Mosby.

Wong, D. L., & Whaley, L. F. (1990). *Clinical manual of pediatric nursing* (3rd ed.). St. Louis: C. V. Mosby.

Yoos, L. (1987). Chronic childhood illness: Developmental issues. *Pediatric Nursing, 13*(1), 25–28.

Health Maintenance, Altered

■ *Related to* **Insufficient Knowledge of Effects of Tobacco Use and Self-Help Resources Available**

■ *Related to* **Increased Food Consumption in Response to Stressors and Insufficient Energy Expenditure for Intake**

■ *Related to* **Insufficient Knowledge (Specify): High Risk for**

■ *Related to* **Insufficient Knowledge of Ostomy Care: High Risk for**

DEFINITION

Altered Health Maintenance: The state in which an individual or group experiences or is at risk of experiencing a disruption in health because of an unhealthy life-style or lack of knowledge to manage a condition.

DEFINING CHARACTERISTICS (IN THE ABSENCE OF DISEASE)

Major (must be present)

Reports or demonstrates an unhealthy practice or life-style, *e.g.:*
    Reckless driving of vehicle
    Substance abuse
    Participation in high-risk activities (*e.g.*, recreational: sky/scuba diving, hang-gliding, occupational: police, firefighter, mining, etc.)
    Presence of obvious behavior disorders (compulsiveness, belligerence)
    Overeating

Minor (may be present)

Reports or demonstrates:
    Skin and nails
        Malodorous   Unusual color, pallor
        Skin lesions (pustules, rashes,   Unexplained scars
           dry or scaly skin)
    Respiratory system
        Frequent infections   Chronic cough   Dyspnea with exertion
    Oral cavity
        Frequent sores (on tongue,   Lesions associated with lack of
           buccal mucosa)   oral care or substance abuse
        Loss of teeth at early age   (leukoplakia, fistulas)
    Gastrointestinal system and nutrition
        Obesity   Chronic bowel irregularity
        Chronic anemia   Chronic dyspepsia
    Musculoskeletal system
        Frequent muscle strain, backaches, neck pain
        Diminished flexibility and muscle strength
    Genitourinary system
        Frequent venereal lesions and infections

Frequent use of potentially unhealthful over-the-counter products (chemical douches, perfumed vaginal products, nasal sprays, etc.)
Constitutional
Chronic fatigue, malaise, apathy
Neurosensory
Presence of facial tics (nonconvulsant)
Headaches
Psychoemotional
Emotional fragility
Behavior disorders (compulsiveness, belligerence)
Frequent feelings of being overwhelmed

RELATED FACTORS

A variety of factors can produce *Altered Health Maintenance*. Some common causes are listed below.

Pathophysiologic
New medical condition

Treatment-related
Lack of previous exposure
New or complex treatment

Situational (personal, environmental)
Lack of exposure to the experience
Language differences
Information misinterpretation
Personal characteristics

Lack of motivation
Lack of education or
readiness

Ineffective coping patterns (*e.g.,* anxiety, depression, nonproductive denial of situation, avoidance coping)

Changes in finances
Lack of access to adequate health care services
Inadequate health practice
External locus of control
Religious beliefs
Cultural beliefs

Maturational
Lack of education of age-related factors. Examples include
Children

Sexuality and sexual
development
Safety hazards

Substance abuse
Nutrition

Adolescents

Same as children
Automobile safety
practices

Substance abuse
(alcohol, other
drugs, tobacco)
Health maintenance practices

Adults

Parenthood
Sexual function

Safety practices
Health maintenance practices

Elderly
Effects of aging   Sensory deficits
See Table II-8 for age-related conditions.

Diagnostic Considerations

The nursing diagnosis *Altered Health Maintenance* is applicable to both well and ill populations. Health is a dynamic, ever-changing state defined by the individual based on the perception of his or her highest level of functioning, *e.g.*, a marathon runner's definition of health will differ from a paraplegic person's. Because individuals are responsible for their own health, *Altered Health Maintenance* represents a diagnosis that the individual is motivated to treat. An important nursing responsibility associated with health maintenance involves raising the person's consciousness that better health is possible.

This diagnosis is appropriate for a person expressing a desire to change an unhealthy life-style. Examples of an unhealthy life-style are excessive dissatisfaction with occupation; lack of exercise; failure to be refreshed after rest; diet high in fat, salt, simple carbohydrates; tobacco use; obesity; excessive alcohol use; and insufficient social support.

The nursing diagnosis *High Risk for Altered Health Maintenance* is useful to describe an individual who needs teaching or referrals prior to discharge from an acute care center to prevent problems with health maintenance after discharge.

Health-Seeking Behaviors is used to describe an individual or a group desiring health teaching related to the promotion and maintenance of high-level wellness (*e.g.*, preventive behavior, age-related screening, optimal nutrition) or, according to the NANDA definition, "seeking ways to alter personal health habits in order to move to a higher level of health." In most cases, this diagnosis describes an asymptomatic person. However, it also can be used for a person with a chronic disease to help that person attain a higher level of wellness in a particular area. Different from good health, high-level wellness can be defined as an integrated method of functioning oriented toward maximizing the potential of which the individual is capable (Dunn, 1959). For example, a woman with multiple sclerosis with many physical problems could be taught self-breast examination or relaxation exercises using the diagnosis *Health-Seeking Behaviors: Self-breast exam.*

Health Seeking-Behaviors is best written as a one-part diagnostic statement with the sought-out health practice specified, *e.g.*, *Health-Seeking Behaviors: Self-breast exam.* Using "related to" for *Health-Seeking Behaviors* is unnecessary; it is understood that all persons with the diagnosis are motivated to achieve a higher level of health. Related factors could not represent causative or contributing factors, unless the nurse wants to repeat the same factors for each client, *e.g.*, *Health-Seeking Behaviors: Self-breast exam related to desire to maximize health.*

As focus shifts from an illness/treatment-oriented health care system to a health-oriented one, *Altered Health Maintenance* and *Health-Seeking Behaviors* are becoming increasingly significant nursing diagnoses. The increasingly high acuity and shortened lengths of stay in hospitals require that nurses be creative in addressing health promotion—for example, by using printed materials, TV instruction, and community-based programs.

(Text continues on page 441)

Table II-8 **Primary and Secondary Prevention for Age-Related Conditions**

Developmental Level	Primary Prevention	Secondary Prevention

Infancy (0–1 year)	Parent education
	  Infant safety
	  Nutrition
	  Breast feeding
	Sensory stimulation
	  Infant massage and touch
	  Visual stimulation
	    Activity
	    Colors
	  Auditory stimulation
	    Verbal
	    Music
	Immunizations
	  DPT ⎱ at 2, 4, and 6 months
	  TOPV ⎰
	Oral hygiene
	  Teething biscuits
	  Fluoride
	  Avoid sugared food and drink
		Complete physical exam every 2–3 months
		Screening at birth
		  Congenital hip
		  PKU
		  G-6-PD deficiency in blacks, Mediterranean and Far Eastern origin children
		  Sickle cell
		  Hemoglobin or hematocrit (for anemia)
		  Cystic fibrosis
		  Vision (startle reflex)
		  Hearing (response to and localization of sounds)
		  TB test at 12 months
		Developmental assessments
		Screen and intervene for high risk
		  Low birth weight
		  Maternal substance abuse during pregnancy
		    Alcohol: fetal alcohol syndrome
		    Cigarettes: SIDS
		    Drugs: addicted neonate, AIDS
		  Maternal infections during pregnancy

Preschool (1–5 years)	Parent education
	  Teething
	  Discipline
	  Nutrition
	  Accident prevention
	  Normal growth and development
	Child education
	  Dental self-care
		Complete physical exam between 2 and 3 years and preschool (U/A, CBC)
		TB test at 3 years
		Development assessments (annual)
		  Speech development
		  Hearing
		  Vision
		Screen and intervene
		  Lead poisoning

(continued)

Dressing
Bathing with assistance
Feeding self-care
Immunizations
DPT } at 18 months
TOPV }
MMR at 15 months
Hib at 24 mos.
Dental/oral hygiene
Fluoride treatments
Fluoridated water
Dietary counsel

Developmental lag
Neglect or abuse
Strong family history of arteriosclerotic diseases (e.g., MI, CVA, peripheral vascular disease), diabetes, hypertension, gout or hyperlipidemia—fasting serum cholesterol at age 2 years, then every 3–5 years if normal
Strabismus
Hearing deficit
Vision deficit

School age
(6–11 years)

Health education of child
"Basic 4" nutrition
Accident prevention
Outdoor safety
Substance abuse counsel
Anticipatory guidance for physical changes at puberty
Immunizations
Tetanus age 10
DPT } boosters between 4 and 6 years
TOPV }
Dental hygiene every 6–12 months
Continue fluoridation
Complete physical exam

Complete physical exam
TB test every 3 years (at ages 6 and 9)
Developmental assessments
Language
Vision: Snellen charts at school
  6–8 years, use "E" chart
  Over 8 years, use alphabet chart
Hearing: audiogram
Cholesterol profile, if high risk, every 3–5 years
Serum cholesterol one time (not high risk)

Adolescence
(12–19 years)

Health education
Proper nutrition and healthful diets
Sex education
"Safe Sex"
  Use of condoms

Complete physical exam (prepuberty or age 13)
Blood pressure
Cholesterol profile
TB test at 12 years
VDRL, CBC, U/A

(continued)

Table II-8 **Primary and Secondary Prevention for Age-Related Conditions** (continued)

Developmental Level	Primary Prevention	Secondary Prevention
	Sexually transmitted diseases	Female: breast self-exam (BSE)
	Safe driving skills	Male: testicular self-exam (TSE)
	Adult challenges	Female, if sexually active: Pap and pelvic exam twice, 1 year apart (cervical gonorrhea culture with pelvic); then every 3 years if both are negative
	Seeking employment and career choices	Screening and interventions if high risk
	Dating and marriage	Depression
	Confrontation with substance abuse	Suicide
	Safety in athletics	Substance abuse
	Skin care	Pregnancy
	Dental hygiene every 6–12 months	Family history of alcoholism or domestic violence
	Immunizations	
	Tetanus without trauma	
	TOPV booster at 12–14 years	
Young adult (20–39 years)	Health education	Complete physical exam at about 20 years, then every 5–6 years
	Weight management with good nutrition as BMR changes	Cancer checkup every 3 years
	Low cholesterol diet	Female: BSE monthly
	Life-style counseling	Male: TSE monthly
	Stress management skills	All females: baseline mammography between ages 35 and 40
	Safe driving	Parents-to-be: high-risk screening for Down syndrome, Tay-Sachs
	Family planning	Female pregnant: screen for VD, rubella titer, Rh factor, amniocentesis for women 35 years or older (if desired)
	Divorce	Screening and interventions if high risk
	Step-parenting	Female with previous breast cancer: annual mammography at 35 years and after
	Single-parenting	Female with mother or sister who has had breast cancer, same as above
	"Safe sex"	Family history colorectal cancer or high risk: annual stool guaiac, digital rectal, and sigmoidoscopy
	Parenting skills	PPD if exposed to TB
	Regular exercise	
	Environmental health choices	

(continued)

Dental hygiene every 6–12 months
Immunizations
  Tetanus at 20 years and every 10 years
  Female: rubella, if serum negative for antibodies
  Hepatitis-B for high-risk persons (male homosexuals with multiple partners; occupations at risk—dentist, nurse in dialysis unit, lab technician)

Glaucoma screening at 35 years and along with routine physical exams
Cholesterol profile every 5 years, if normal
Cholesterol profile every 1–2 years if borderline

Middle-aged adult (40–59 years)

Health education: continue with young adult
Midlife changes, male and female counseling
"Empty nest syndrome"
Anticipatory guidance for retirement
Grandparenting
Dental hygiene every 6–12 months
Immunizations
  Tetanus every 10 years
  Influenza—annual if high risk (i.e., major chronic disease [COPD, CAD])
  Pneumococcal—single dose

Complete physical exam every 5–6 years with complete laboratory evaluation (serum/urine tests, x-ray, ECG)
Cancer checkup every year
Female: BSE monthly
Male: TSE monthly
All females: mammogram every 1–2 years (40–49 years) then annual mammography 50 years and over
Schiotz's tonometry (glaucoma) every 3–5 years
Sigmoidoscopy at 50 and 51, then every 4 years if negative
Stool guaiac annually at 50 and thereafter
Screening and intervention if high risk
Endometrial cancer: have endometrial sampling at menopause
Oral cancer: screen more often if substance abuser

Elderly adult (60–74 years)

Health education: continue with previous counseling
Home safety
Retirement
Loss of spouse
Special health needs
  Nutritional changes
  Changes in hearing or vision
  Alterations in bowel or bladder habits
Dental/oral hygiene every 6–12 months

Complete physical exam every 2 years with laboratory assessments
Annual cancer checkup
Blood pressure annually
Female: BSE monthly
Male: TSE monthly
Female: annual mammogram
Annual stool guaiac
Sigmoidoscopy every 4 years
Schiotz's tonometry every 3–5 years
Podiatric evaluation with foot care PRN

(continued)

Table II-8 **Primary and Secondary Prevention for Age-Related Conditions** (continued)

Developmental Level	Primary Prevention	Secondary Prevention
	Immunizations Tetanus every 10 years Influenza—annual if high risk Pneumococcal—(one time only)	Screen for high risk Depression Suicide Alcohol/drug abuse "Elder abuse"
Old-age adult (75 years and over)	Health education: continue counsel Anticipatory guidance Dying and death Loss of spouse Increasing dependency upon others Dental/oral hygiene every 6–12 months Immunizations Tetanus every 10 years Influenza—annual Pneumococcal—if not already received	Complete physical exam annually Laboratory assessments Cancer checkup Blood pressure Stool guaiac Female: annual mammogram, sigmoidoscopy every 4 years Schiotz's tonometry every 3–5 years Podiatrist PRN

Errors in Diagnostic Statements

Altered Health Maintenance related to refusal to quit smoking

Refusal to quit smoking represents significant data that require further clarification, *e.g.,* is the person making an informed decision? Does the person know the effects of smoking on respiratory and cardiovascular functioning? Does the person know where assistance can be acquired to stop smoking? If the answers to these questions are yes, then the diagnosis *Altered Health Maintenance* is incorrect. On the other hand, if the person is not fully aware of the deleterious effects of smoking and/or the availability of self-help resources, the diagnosis *Altered Health Maintenance related to insufficient knowledge of effects of tobacco use and self-help resources available* may be appropriate.

Note: The nurse should be cautioned about timing attempts to encourage a person to quit smoking or control eating after an acute episode, such as myocardial infarction. In such a situation, denying the person his or her usual coping mechanism, no matter how unhealthy it is, may be more problematic to the person's overall health. The nurse should emphasize teaching so the person can make informed choices, not merely prohibit certain choices.

Health-Seeking Behaviors related to increased alcohol and tobacco use in response to marital break-up and heavy family demands

This represents an inappropriate diagnosis for this person, who wants to alter personal habits but is not in good or excellent health. A more appropriate focus would be to promote constructive stress management without tobacco or alcohol, through the nursing diagnosis *Ineffective Individual Coping related to inability to constructively manage the stressors associated with marital break-up and family demands.*

Focus Assessment Criteria

This assessment is structured primarily to collect data to determine the person's learning capabilities, limitations, and health habits.

Subjective Data

1. Does the individual/family report or demonstrate an unhealthy life-style?
2. Does the individual/family report frequent colds, infections, flus, etc.?
3. Determine present knowledge of
   Illness
   Severity   Susceptibility to complications
   Prognosis   Ability to cure it or control its
                                          progression
   Treatment/diagnostic studies
   Preventive measures
4. What is the pattern of adhering to prescribed health behaviors?
   Complete   Not adhering
   Modified
5. Does anything interfere with adherence to the prescribed health behavior?
6. History of disease
   Onset
   Symptoms
   Effects on life-style (relationships, work, leisure activities, finances)
7. Stage of adaptation to disease
   Disbelief   Anger
   Denial   Awareness
   Depression   Acceptance

8. Learning needs (perceived by client, family)
9. Learning ability (client, family)
   Level of education   Language spoken
   Ability to read   Language understood
10. Sociocultural factors
    Traditions   Health care beliefs and practices
    Life-style   Values

Objective Data

1. Ability to perform prescribed procedures
   Competency   Accuracy
2. Level of cognitive and psychomotor development
   Age   Ability to read and write
3. Presence of sensory deficits
   Vision
       Problems in focusing   Partial or total blindness
       Inability to distinguish colors
   Hearing
       Partial or total deafness   Tinnitus
   Sense of smell (altered or lost)
   Sense of taste (altered or lost)
   Sense of touch
       Anesthesia   Paresthesia
4. Physical stability
   Circulation/tissue perfusion
       General appearance
       Arterial blood pressure
       Pulse rate and regularity
       Pulse volume (weak, thready, full, bounding)
       Skin (color, temperature, moisture)
       Urine output
       Level of consciousness
   Respiratory status
       Rate
       Pattern
       Presence of abnormal breath sounds
       Altered blood gases
       Restlessness
       Irritability
   Nutritional/hydration status
       Fluid and electrolyte balance (Na, K, urine specific gravity, skin turgor)
       Intake and output
       Weight change
   Activity tolerance (good, fair, poor; see *Activity Intolerance* for additional assessment criteria)

Principles and Rationale for Nursing Care

Generic Considerations

1. Many members of the population view health as absence of disease. Rather, health can be viewed as a return (or recovery) to a previous state or to a heightened awareness of the individual's full potential and life meaning (Flynn, 1980).

2. The control of major health problems in the U.S. depends directly on modification of individual behavior and habits of living (Flynn, 1980).
3. Belloc and Breslow (1972) correlated well-being and increased life span to the following seven practices:
   a. Sleeping 7–8 hours nightly
   b. Eating three meals at regular times
   c. Eating breakfast daily
   d. Maintaining desirable body weight
   e. Avoiding excessive alcohol consumption
   f. Participating in regular exercise
   g. Abstaining from smoking
4. In addition to addressing life-styles to promote wellness, total health depends on (Flynn, 1980):
   a. Eradication of poverty and ignorance
   b. Availability of jobs
   c. Adequate housing, transportation, and recreation
   d. Public safety
   e. Aesthetically pleasing and beneficial environment

Weight Reduction

1. Intake must be reduced to 500 cal/day less than requirement to obtain a 1 lb/wk weight loss.
2. The desirable weight loss rate is 1–2 lb/wk.
3. Overeating is a complex multidimensional problem with physical, social, and psychologic components.
4. Overweight persons are usually nutritionally deprived.
5. Internal motivation is essential for a successful weight loss program.
6. An individual's body image and coping patterns influence the weight loss program's success or failure.
7. An American's diet currently consists of 42% fat, 12% protein, 22% complex carbohydrates (CHO), and 24% simple carbohydrates. Recommended U.S. dietary goals are 30% fat, 12% protein, 48% complex carbohydrates (CHO), and 10% simple carbohydrates (Brody, 1981).
8. Any increase in activity will increase energy output and increase caloric deficits of a person following a dietary regimen.
9. Often, obesity is facilitated/aggravated by inappropriate response to external cues, including, most often, stressors. This response sets off an ineffective pattern whereby the individual eats in response to stress cues rather than physiologic hunger.
10. The body uses a higher percent of energy (calories) to convert CHO to body fat than it does to convert fat to body fat. The body only needs 135–225 fatty calories to supply daily essential fatty acids.
11. The safest activities for the unconditioned obese person are walking, water aerobics, swimming, and cycling.
12. Fluctuations in body weight are common, especially in females. Daily weights can be misleading and disheartening. Body measurements are a better measurement of losses. Regular exercise will cause lean muscle mass to increase. Since muscle weighs more than fat, this may be reflected on the scale as a weight gain.

Prevention of Disease, Injuries

1. The goals of prevention are
   a. Avoidance of disease by choosing a healthy life-style

  b. Decrease in mortality due to disease by early detection and intervention
  c. Improvement of quality of life
2. The three levels of prevention are primary, secondary, and tertiary.
3. The primary level of prevention involves actions that prevent disease and accidents and promote well-being. Key concepts are as follows:

Concept	Examples
Wellness	Diet low in salt, sugar, and fat
A life-style that incoroprates the principles of health promotion and is directed by self-responsibility	Regular exercise and stress management
	Elimination of smoking
	Minimal alcohol intake
Self-help	
Mutual sharing with others who have similar needs	LaLeche League
	Childbirth education
	Assertiveness training
	Specific written resources (books, pamphlets, magazines)
	Public media (radio, television)
Safety	Adherence to speed limits
	Use of seat belts and car seats
	Proper storage of household poisons
Immunizations	Children: DPT
	Nonpregnant women of childbearing age: Rubella vaccine if antibody titer is negative
	Elderly: influenza, pneumonia

4. The secondary level of prevention concerns actions that promote early detection of disease and subsequent intervention, both routine physical examination by a health professional at regular intervals and self-examination.
5. The tasks of screening are to
  a. Identify major disabling conditions
  b. Investigate the personal and social benefits of early detection and intervention for asymptomatic persons with the condition (*e.g.,* facilitate family coping, minimize disability and cost, prevent premature death, improve productivity of affected persons, decrease overall morbidity and mortality)
  c. Identify persons at high risk for specific conditions through *personal medical history (e.g.,* concurrent disease such as diabetes mellitus involves greater risk for hypertension), *family medical history (e.g.,* breast cancer, diabetes, hypertension), and *social history (e.g.,* substance abuse—cancer, heart disease; sexual patterns—venereal disease; domestic violence—person abuse)
  d. Identify tests and procedures that accurately detect the condition (who will do them? how often are they done? who bears the cost?)
  e. Plan a strategy for disseminating screening information to health care professionals and the public
  f. Plan evaluation of screening effectiveness
6. Types of screening measures include
  a. Physical findings (periodic exams by health care professionals and self-exams of breast, testicles, and skin)
  b. Survey of risk factors (smoking, alcohol abuse)
  c. Laboratory tests (serum—*e.g.,* sickle-cell in blacks, PKU in newborns; urine—*e.g.,* renal disease in the elderly; x-ray—*e.g.,* dental caries, chest TB)
7. The tertiary level of prevention involves actions that restore and rehabilitate in the presence of illness. For example, for a person with coronary artery disease, these would be

    a. Restorative (surgery, such as coronary artery bypass, angioplasty and medications)

    b. Rehabilitative (stress management, exercise program, stop smoking, "zipper club" [self-help group])

8. Potential barriers to prevention are found both in the health care system and in the individual.

    a. The system may be

- Disease-oriented rather than health-oriented
- Composed of health care professionals who are taught to focus on fragment systems of the human body rather than to take a holistic approach
- Functioning on a financial system that rewards treatment of illness, not prevention
- Difficult to reach or may have previously proved unsatisfactory

    b. The client may:

- Believe that the health/illness state is determined by forces (fate, luck) outside himself (external locus of control)
- Perceive the behavior needed as unacceptable or uncomfortable
- Practice sociocultural behaviors that are not healthful (*e.g.*, obesity is considered desirable, salt is prevalent in diet)
- Experience psychologic disturbances that impede incentive to practice healthy behaviors
- Lack financial resources

Teaching/Learning Process

1. Patient/health education is the teaching-learning process of influencing client and family behavior through changes in knowledge, attitudes, and beliefs and through the acquisition of psychomotor skills. The goal of patient teaching is to help the client assume responsibility for self-care.

    The teaching-learning process consists of "steps," which are actually the components of the nursing process: assessment, planning, implementing, and evaluating. Patient education is a constellation of interventions, including self-modification (Pender, 1985), patient contracting (Jensen, 1985), values clarification (Wilberding, 1985), and preparatory sensory information (Christman & Kirchoff, 1985). It may be appropriate to use one of these interventions in the assessment phase (*i.e.*, values clarification) to determine the optimal combination of educational interventions for a particular client.

2. Each person should be assessed for the knowledge and skill needed to monitor health status (*e.g.*, home blood glucose monitoring in diabetes), control or cure disease, or prevent disease (*e.g.*, diet, medication therapy, life-style changes), and prevent recurrence or complications (*e.g.*, postoperative leg exercises).

3. Inaccurate perceptions of health status usually involve misunderstanding of the nature and seriousness of the illness, susceptibility to complications, and the need for procedures for cure or control of illness.

4. Psychologic manifestations of anxiety and denial may have resulted from misconceptions, not knowing what to do, or not knowing how to carry out prescribed behaviors.

5. Teaching should be routinely incorporated as an integral part of nursing care whenever a new diagnosis or change in regimen is made or when the client faces an unfamiliar situation.

6. An assessment prior to teaching will facilitate the meaningfulness, efficacy, and overall success of the teaching-learning process by defining *what* content should be present, *how* the content should be given, *when* the client is ready to learn, and *who* should be included in the process.

7. Learning depends on physical and emotional readiness. The client needs to be relatively free of pain and extreme anxiety in order to learn.
8. High anxiety decreases learning, while slight anxiety may increase learning.
9. Client motivation is one of the most important variables affecting the amount of learning that takes place.
10. Factors affecting learning/factors affecting the learner
   a. Physical factors that affect learning include
      • Presence of acute illness
      • Fluid and electrolyte imbalance
      • Nutritional status
      • Illness or treatments that interfere with mental alertness (pain, medications)
      • Illness or treatments that interfere with motor abilities (fatigue, equipment)
      • Activity tolerance (endurance)
   b. Personal factors that affect learning include

Age	Stage of adaptation to illness
Intelligence	Past experiences or knowledge
Level of motivation	Locus of control
Level of anxiety	Perception of
Denial of disease process	Seriousness of condition
Depression	Susceptibility to complications
	Prognosis
	Ability to control progression or to cure condition

   c. Socioeconomic factors that affect learning include

Language	Past experiences with health care
Life-style	Cultural background
Support system	Transportation
Financial status	Health care facility
	Drugstore

11. Factors resulting in ineffective teaching
   Inadequate or no assessment prior to teaching
   Assessment data were not communicated or not considered when teaching (the most influential assessment factors are psychologic status, physical stability, educational level, cultural background, socioeconomic status)
   Teaching was not individualized
   Information not presented at a level consistent with the client's ability
   Tendency to talk down to client
   Use of misunderstood terms
   Fragmented presentation of information
   Too much information given, with important information hidden or lost among irrelevant information
   No repetition of information
   No feedback given in relation to process (or client is punished for not learning)
   No evaluation of client learning made

Smoking

1. Smoking has immediate and long-term effects on the respiratory system.
2. Immediate effects are paralysis of the ciliary cleansing mechanism of the lungs (which should keep breathing passages free of inhaled irritants and bacteria); irritation of the lining of the lungs, causing an inflammatory response; increased production of mucus; and decreased oxygenation.
3. Long-term effects are *permanent* disabling of the ciliary cleansing mechanism;

reduction of the number of macrophages in the airways; a *permanent* decrease in the lung's ability to fight infection; increased production of mucus cells; a significant increase in the risk of developing pulmonary disease (a history of 15–20 "pack years" indicates a high risk); possible enlargement of the distal air passages; and chronic CO_2 retention, which results in hypoxia's becoming the drive to breathe, rather than hypercarbia (increased CO_2).

4. Smoking has immediate and long-term effects on the cardiovascular system.
5. Immediate effects are vasoconstriction and decreased oxygenation of the blood, elevated blood pressure, increased heart rate and possible dysrhythmias, and an increase in the work of the heart.
6. Long-term effects include an increased risk for coronary artery disease and myocardial infarction. Smoking also contributes to hypertension, peripheral vascular disease (*e.g.*, leg ulcers), and chronically abnormal arterial blood gases (low oxygen, or PO_2, and high carbon dioxide, or pCO_2).
7. The use of smokeless tobacco (snuff, chewing tobacco) is associated with oral leukoplakia (premalignant lesions), oral cancer, and nicotine addiction. At least 12 million Americans are at risk, mostly male teens and male adults (Young, Koch, & Mauger, 1988).
8. Tobacco use is a significant risk factor for the following cancer sites: tongue and oral mucosa, larnyx, lungs, bladder, and cervix. Combined with other carcinogens (*e.g.*, alcohol, asbestos, coal dust, radon), the health risk intensifies. The rate of cancer recurrence increases in clients who continue tobacco use during and after treatment.
9. Nicotine is the primary addicting substance in tobacco smoke and juice. Tobacco use is an addiction; these clients need special assistance with short-term withdrawal and long-term maintenance of a tobacco-free life.
10. Passive smoking, the inhalation of tobacco smoke by nonsmokers, has been shown to have negative health effects.
    a. Persons with angina experience more discomfort in a smoke-filled room.
    b. Bronchospasm is increased when an asthmatic is exposed to tobacco smoke.
    c. Children living with smoking parents have more upper respiratory infections than those living with nonsmokers.
    d. Preliminary studies suggest that nonsmokers living with smokers are at increased risk for lung cancer; children may be at greater risk for childhood malignancies (Kuller et al., 1986).
11. Smoking during pregnancy has been associated with small-for-gestational-age newborns, miscarriage, stillbirths, and sudden infant death syndrome (Institute of Medicine, 1985).
12. In the last 25 years, most health professions have seen a significant decline in the smoking behavior of its members—*but not nursing*. Estimates show that 25–29% of nurses still smoke. Studies of nurses link occupational stress and social influences with tobacco use (Cinelli & Glover, 1988). A nurse who smokes sends the wrong signals to clients. According to Ash (1987), "a role model does not smoke, thus exemplifying behavior which is desired, and behaves in a way that provides guidance and that others will want to imitate."

Nutrition

See Principles and Rationale for Nursing Care for *Altered Nutrition*

Exercise

1. A regular exercise program should
   Be enjoyable
   Utilize a minimum of 400 calories in each session

> Sustain a heart rate of approximately 120–150 beats/minute
>
> Involve rhythmical alternate contracting and relaxing of muscles
>
> Be integrated into the person's life-style 4–5 days/week (at least 30–60 minutes)

2. Regular exercise can provide the person with increased

> Cardiovascular-respiratory endurance
>
> Muscle strength
>
> Muscle endurance
>
> Flexibility
>
> Ability to deliver nutrients to tissue
>
> Ability to tolerate psychologic stress
>
> Ability to reduce body fat content

3. An exercise program should include

> A warm-up session (10 minutes of stretching exercises)
>
> Endurance exercises
>
> A cool-down session (5–10 minutes)

4. Before beginning an exercise program, the person must consider

> Physical limitations (consult nurse or physician)
>
> Personal preferences
>
> Life-style
>
> Community resources
>
> What clothing is needed (shoes)
>
> How to monitor pulse before, during, and after exercise

5. The person is taught to monitor his pulse before, during, and after exercise to assist him to achieve his target heart rate and not to exceed his maximum advisable heart rate for his age.

Age	Maximum Heart Rate	Target Heart Rate
30	190	133–162
40	180	126–153
50	170	119–145
60	160	112–136

Osteoporosis

1. Age-related changes beginning around age 40 decrease cortical bone by 3%/decade for men and women (Riggs & Melton, 1986).

2. Postmenopause, women experience an increase in cortical bone loss to 9–10%/decade (Riggs & Melton, 1986).

3. Loss of trabecular bone begins in the 30s and progresses at a rate of 6–8%/decade. The rate is accelerated in women postmenopause (Riggs & Melton, 1986).

4. Osteoporosis is classified as primary (associated with age and menopause-related changes) or secondary (caused by medications or diseases) (Miller, 1990).

5. Factors that contribute to a woman's risk of osteoporosis include loss of female hormones after menopause, low calcium intake, insufficient exercise, small stature, fair skin, family history, cigarette smoking, excessive alcohol consumption, excessive caffeine intake and excessive protein consumption, excessive use of aluminum-type antacids, and long-term use of corticosteroids (Chestnut, 1984).

6. Estrogen replacement therapy is effective in preventing bone loss and in decreasing the incidence of fractures in women postmenopause (Lindsay, 1989).

7. Estrogen in low doses and in cyclic administration with progesterone can substantially reduce the risk of uterine cancer (Bellantoni & Blackman, 1988).

Pediatric Considerations

1. The child depends on a parent/adult caregiver to provide a safe environment and promote health, *e.g.,* immunizations, well-child check-ups, and chronic disease management (Whaley & Wong, 1989).
2. The risk of altered health maintenance varies with the child's age and health status. For example, the toddler is at risk for accidental poisoning, while the adolescent is more likely to engage in high-risk behavior (Whaley & Wong, 1989).
3. Malnutrition, lack of immunizations, or an unsafe environment may be related to parental knowledge deficit, alteration in parenting, or barriers to health care (Whaley and Wong, 1989).
4. Many factors can influence a child's nutritional needs, including periods of rapid growth, stress, illness, metabolic errors, some medications, and socioeconomic factors such as inadequate income, poor housing, and lack of food (Scipien, Chard, Howe & Barnard, 1990).
5. It can be difficult to establish criteria for a definition of obesity in children due to great variations in height and weight among normal children (Williams, 1985).
6. An increase in the use and abuse of drugs (including alcohol and tobacco) has been reported among school-agers and adolescents (Scipien, Chard, Howe & Barnard, 1990; Whaley & Wong, 1989).
7. Health maintenance begins with the prenatal visit and continues with comprehensive health supervision during the child's developmental years. (Whaley and Wong, 1989).
8. Anticipatory health promotion, or anticipatory guidance, is an essential component of comprehensive health care and varies in content with the age of the child. It involves teaching parents and older children what is likely to occur in the child's development in the upcoming weeks or months (Scipien, Chard, Howe & Barnard, 1990).
9. Current trends in the care of chronically ill or disabled children focus on the developmental vs. chronological age of the child, and on normalization (Whaley & Wong, 1989).
10. Children with chronic illness or disability can achieve wellness when they function at their optimal level (Hunsberger, 1989).

Gerontologic Considerations

1. According to Miller (1990), health is "the ability of older adults to function at their highest capacity, despite the presence of age-related changes and risk factors.
2. Miller (1990) also states "Of all the age-related changes . . . osteoporosis is the one that is most likely to cause serious negative functional consequences, even in the absence of additional risk factors."
3. About 70% of people over age 65 rate their health as excellent (US Department of Health & Human Services, 1987).
4. It is important to differentiate between age-related changes and risk factors that affect functioning of older persons. Such risk factors as inadequate nutrition, fluid intake, exercise, and socialization can have a greater effect on functioning than can most age-related changes.
5. The mortality rate from pneumonia or influenza for persons over 65 years is 9/100,000. For persons who smoke, have kyphosis, or have chronic diseases, this rate increases to 979/100,000 (Schneider, 1983).
6. Older adults should be immunized yearly against influenza in late fall (Miller, 1990).
7. Oxygen consumption at anaerobic threshold varies inversely with age. Therefore, in

the older individual there is a lower anaerobic threshold, with earlier rise in lactic acid accumulation and earlier onset of muscle fatigue (Posner, Gorman, Klein, & Woldow, 1986).

8. Maximal aerobic capacity and maximal heart rate decline with age. For aerobic conditioning, an older individual must exercise to reach target heart rate for at least 20–30 minutes three times a week. The following formula will obtain target heart rate: 220 − Individual's age = × 60–70% = Target Training Heart Rate. Older adults must be taught to monitor carotid pulse for rate and rhythm. There is a greater time threshold for older individuals to return to baseline heart rates, blood pressure, and respiratory rate after exercise (Harris, 1982).

9. Elderly persons have decreased thermoregulation with diminished ability to cool the body via perspiration after physical exertion, affecting their tolerance of physical activity (Matteson & McConnell, 1988).

10. There is an age-related increase in systolic blood pressure at rest and at submaximal workloads. The cardiovascular system has a diminished sensitivity to the chronotropic, inotropic and vasodilatory effects of catecholamines. Studies have shown that catecholamines or β-adrenergic stimulation when administered during exercise had greater effects on young individuals as opposed to those of advanced age (Abrams & Berkow, 1990; Fleg, 1986).

11. Because the current generation of elderly persons has not typically been involved in structured exercise programs and fitness clubs, many individuals have not developed endurance for sustained physical activity. In their culture, exercise and perspiration resulted in a completed task such as a plowed field or a painted house.

12. A regular exercise program has been shown to positively correlate with increased self-esteem. Adult learning principles support encouraging an exercise program or regular activity that has meaning to the older individual if compliance is expected. When exercising, the older individual should be encouraged to exercise to the point of mild symptoms of intolerance and then cut back by 25% (Matteson & McConnell, 1988).

■ Altered Health Maintenance
Related to Insufficient Knowledge of Effects of Tobacco Use and Self-Help Resources Available*

Assessment

Subjective Data

Individual reports
    History of smoking and/or
    History of chewing smokeless tobacco

---

* This nursing diagnosis can be used in two different situations—for the individual who does not know the hazards of tobacco use and for the individual who desires to quit.

Objective Data

Tobacco use behavior (smoking, chewing)
Odor of tobacco on breath if smoked
Spitting behavior if chewed
Staining of teeth, fingernails, and fingertips
Cough unrelated to infectious process
Frequent respiratory infections (upper and lower tracts)
Increased sputum production
Presence of oral lesions on mucosal and/or periodontal tissues

---

Outcome Criteria

The individual will
- Identify short-term and long-term health effects of tobacco use
- Identify benefits of abstinence from tobacco use
- Verbalize commitment to personal health and desire to eliminate tobacco use*
- Devise strategies to assist in smoking/chewing cessation*
- Significantly decrease amount of tobacco used or stop altogether*

Interventions

A. Assessment

1. Define tobacco use behavior.
   a. Type and quantity
      - Cigarettes
         Filter/nonfilter
         Regular/reduced tar and nicotine
         Pack years
      - Cigars
         Inhaled/not inhaled
         Number/day, number of years
      - Pipe
         Inhaled/not inhaled
         Number of bowls/day
      - Smokeless tobacco (chewing)
         Number of minutes/day
         Number of years
   b. Associated activities
      - Job (note exposure to carcinogens in work place, *e.g.,* asbestos, arsenic, coal-tar fumes)

---

*These outcome criteria are established only *if* the client desires to quit tobacco use. For the client who does not wish to change tobacco use behaviors, provide information regarding health risks and benefits so that an *informed* choice is made. Avoid being judgmental. Always "keep the door open" should the client later change his mind.

- Home
- Relaxation
- Stressful events
- Recreation
- Use of alcohol/drugs
  c. Previous attempts to abstain from tobacco use
  - What strategies were used?
  - Why were they not successful?
2. Promote understanding of personal tobacco use behavior.
   a. Identify negative aspects of tobacco use with client.
   - Physical: exercise intolerance, cough, sputum, frequent respiratory infections, dental disease
   - Environmental: burned clothing/furniture, discolored interiors of home/workplace, malodorous clothing/furniture, dirty ashtrays, house and occupational fires
   - Social: inability to smoke in public places; offensive nature of tobacco use behaviors to family members, friends, coworkers
   - Financial: calculate monetary cost of client's habit with client
   - Psychological: unpleasant withdrawal symptoms that occur when tobacco is not available (*e.g.*, midnight "nicotine fits"), decreased self-esteem due to dependency
   b. Identify positive aspects of tobacco use with client (use client's own words).
3. Provide information.
   a. Health risks of tobacco use to self
   - Cancer (oral, lung, bladder)
   - COPD and respiratory infections
   - Arteriosclerosis (coronary and peripheral)
   - Hypertension and CVA
   - Periodontal disease
   b. Health risks of tobacco use to others
   - Unborn child
   - Infants
   - Asthmatics
   - Persons with angina
   - Persons with allergies
   - Persons sharing living/working space
   c. Benefits of quitting
   - Decreased pulse and blood pressure
   - Decreased sputum production
   - Pulmonary mucosa regenerates
   - Decreased risk of cancer, stroke, MI, COPD
   - Improved dental hygiene
   - Improved senses of taste/smell
   - Increased social acceptance
   d. Strategies available
   - Individual methods: self-help books and tapes, "cold turkey"
   - Group methods: contact local chapters of American Cancer Society, American Lung Association, and private businesses
   - Hypnosis
   - Acupuncture

- Over-the-counter products: filters, tablet regimens, nontobacco cigarettes*
- Nicotine-containing chewing gum (prescription only)

e. Discuss strategies to minimize weight gain and increase exercise.

f. Discuss symptoms of nicotine withdrawal and assist client to prepare for them.

- Craving for tobacco
- Irritability
- Anxiety
- Difficulty concentrating
- Restlessness
- Headache
- Drowsiness
- Gastrointestinal upsets: diarrhea, cramps
- If client has experienced these symptoms before, suggest he choose a time to quit in which he is experiencing relatively low stress.

4. Provide support and encouragement to promote success.

a. Identify with client significant others who will provide ongoing support of client's abstinence from tobacco use.

b. Identify with client persons who may sabotage efforts and devise strategies to minimize their impact.

c. Reinforce with client his personal reasons for tobacco use cessation; encourage client to make visible reminders.

■ Altered Health Maintenance
Related to Increased Food Consumption in Response to Stressors and Insufficient Energy Expenditure for Intake

Assessment

Subjective Data

Client states

"I like to eat,"

"Eating calms my nerves,"

"I don't have time for exercise,"

"I don't like sports or exercise,"

"I can't exercise,"

Objective Data

Weight >10% over ideal for height and frame

Triceps skin fold greater than 15 mm in men and 25 mm in women

---

*Caution: risks of the combustion of these products when inhaled are yet undetermined.

Outcome Criteria

The individual will
- Identify detrimental patterns of eating
- Identify stressors and effective response patterns
- Describe the relationship among metabolism, intake, and exercise
- Commit to exercise (specify type, amount)

Interventions

A. Assess for causative and contributing factors
   1. Lack of knowledge
      a. Balanced nutritional intake
      b. Exercise requirements
   2. Inappropriate response to external stressors
   3. Lack of initiative, motivation
   4. Imbalance in composition of foods (*e.g.,* excess fat or simple carbohydrate intake)
   5. Cultural, familial factors
   6. Poor eating habits (*e.g.,* eating out, eating on the run, skipping meals)
   7. Sedentary life-style, occupation
   8. Sabotage by family and significant others

B. Increase awareness of components of intake/activity balance
   1. Multiply female weight by 11 and male weight by 12 to determine calorie intake/day needed to maintain current weight.
   2. One pound of fat is roughly equivalent to 3500 cal. To lose 2 lb/wk, one must cut 7000 cal from weekly intake.
   3. Exercise caloric expenditure charts may be used to determine amount of calories burned per duration increment of activity.
   4. Weight-loss goals may be achieved through a combination of caloric intake reduction and energy expenditure (via exercise) in calories.
   5. Successful weight reduction/maintenance is contingent upon a balance reduced caloric intake and caloric expenditure via exercise.

C. Assist client to identify realistic weight-loss program to fit his or her needs
   1. Decide on amount of loss desired
   2. Time and duration of program
   3. Cost of various programs
   4. Nutritional soundness
   5. Compatibility with life-style

D. Assist client to anticipate environmental considerations
   1. Friends, family, coworkers—what are their habits? Would they be supportive?
   2. What types of foods are found in the home? At parties? At work? In the lunch room?
   3. What types of leisure/recreational activities are engaged in? Is person sedentary?
   4. What routes are taken to work? Does client pass by fast-food establishments?
   5. Who does the housework? Gardening? Yard? Errands?

6. How much television is watched? Do commercials trigger eating?
7. Has person responded to gimmick advertisements for rapid weight loss (*e.g.,* "sleep away," belts, garments, wraps, lotions, etc.)?

E. Assist client to self-assess present eating/exercise habits by keeping a diary for a week, including usual
1. Food intake/exercise
2. Location/time of meals
3. Emotions around meal time
4. Whom client eats with
5. Skipped meals
6. Snacks

F. Familiarize client with cues that often trigger eating
1. Eating while doing another activity, *e.g.,* watching TV
2. Eating standing up, *e.g.,* can give illusion of not eating
3. Eating out of boredom or stress because you need a break
4. Eat because everyone else is eating

G. Teach client basics of balanced nutritional intake, including supportive measures
1. Choose a diet plan that encourages high intake of complex carbohydrates (CHO) and limited fat intake.
2. Know what you are eating. The "basic four" label is misleading, *e.g.,* a chicken-fried steak is a protein converted to high fat content through its preparation (frying).
3. Attempt to obtain fat calories from fruits and vegetables instead of meat and dairy products.
4. Eat more chicken and fish because they contain less fat and fewer total calories than beef. Remove fat and skin.
5. Be aware of salad toppings and especially dressings with mayonnaise (216–308 calories per 2-oz serving).
6. Completely avoid fast foods, because they have high fat and total caloric content.
7. Dine in or make special requests in restaurants for food selection/preparations, *e.g.,* salad dressing on side, omit sauce from entree.
8. Plan meals in advance.
9. If attending a party or restaurants, decide what you will eat ahead of time and stick to it.
10. Adhere to grocery list.
11. Involve family in meal planning for better nutrition.
12. Buy the highest quality beef. Ground round = 10% fat and hamburger = 25% fat.
13. Choose a variety of foods.
14. Avoid serving family-style.
15. Drink 8–10 8-oz glasses of water daily.
16. Measure foods and count calories; keep records.
17. Read labels on foods and note food composition and calories per serving.
18. Eat slowly.
19. Experiment with spices, substitutes, and low-calories recipes.

H. Discuss benefits of exercise
   1. Reduces caloric absorption
   2. Is an appetite suppressant
   3. Increases metabolic rate
   4. Preserves lean muscle mass
   5. Increases oxygen uptake
   6. Improves self-esteem
   7. Decreases depression, anxiety, and stress
   8. Increases caloric expenditure
   9. Increases the odds for weight-loss maintenance
   10. Increases restful sleep
   11. Improves body posture
   12. Provides fun, recreation, and diversion
   13. Increases resistance to degenerative diseases of middle/later years (*e.g.,* heart, blood vessels)

I. Assist client to identify realistic exercise program to fit his or her needs, considering
   1. Personality, life-style
   2. Time factor, time of day
   3. Season—anticipate and plan
   4. Sedentary/active occupation
   5. Safety, *e.g.,* sports injuries, environmental hazards
   6. Costs—club membership, equipment
   7. Age, physical size, physical condition

J. Monitor or discuss getting started on the exercise program
   1. Start slow and easy.
   2. Choose activities using many parts of the body.
   3. Choose an activity that is vigorous enough to cause "healthful fatigue."
   4. Read, consult experts, talk with friends/coworkers who exercise.
   5. Plan a daily walking program and gradually increase rate and length of walk.
      a. Start out at 5–10 blocks for 0.5–1.0 mile/day; increase 1 block or 0.1 mile/wk.
      b. Remember, progress slowly.
      c. Avoid straining or pushing too hard and becoming overly fatigued.
      d. Stop immediately if any of the following signs occur:

Lightness or pain in chest	Dizziness
Severe breathlessness	Loss of muscle control
Lightheadedness	Nausea

      e. If pulse is 120 beats/minute (BPM) 5 minutes after stopping exercise, 100 BPM 10 minutes after stopping exercise, or if short of breath 10 minutes after exercise, slow down either the rate of walking or the distance.
      f. If unable to walk 5 blocks or 0.5 mile without signs of overexertion appearing, decrease length of walking for 1 week to point before signs appear and then start to add 1 block/0.1 mile each week.
      g. Walk at same rate; time self with stopwatch or second hand on watch; after reaching 10 blocks (1 mile) try to increase speed.
      h. Remember, increase only the rate or the length of walk at one time.
      i. Establish a regular time of day to exercise, with the goal of 3–5 times/week for a duration of 15–45 minutes and with a heart rate of 80% of stress test or

gross calculation (170 BPM for 20–29 age group; decrease 10 BPM for each additional decade of life, *e.g.,* 160 BPM for ages 30–39, 150 BPM for ages 40–49, etc.).

6. Encourage significant others also to engage in walking program.
7. Add supplemental activity, *e.g.,* park far away, work on garden, walk up stairs, spend weekends at leisure activities, such as festivals or art fairs, that require walking.
8. Work up to 1 hour of exercise per day at least 4 days per week.
9. Avoid lapses of more than 2 days between exercise days.

K. Teach client about the risks of obesity
   1. Vascular insufficiency
   2. Arteriosclerosis, heart disease, hypertension
   3. Left ventricular hypertrophy
   4. Diabetes mellitus, gallbladder disease
   5. Increased risk of complications of surgery
   6. Respiratory disease
   7. Joint degeneration
   8. Increased risk of cancer, *e.g.,* breast
   9. Increased risk of accident/injury

L. Assist client to increase interest and motivation in weight reduction/exercise program
   1. Contract re: realistic short- and long-term goals.
   2. Keep intake/activity records.
   3. Hang an admired photograph on the refrigerator.
   4. Get family involved in project.
   5. Record body measurements and limit weighing to once per week.
   6. Increase knowledge by reading and talking with health-conscious friends and coworkers.
   7. Make new friends who are health-conscious.
   8. Get a friend to go on program too or to be a central support.
   9. Avoid persons who may sabotage attempts.
   10. Reward self on a regular basis.
   11. Remind self that self-image and behavior are learned and can be unlearned.
   12. Build a support system of people who value growth and value you as an individual.
   13. Be aware of rationalization, *e.g.,* a lack of time may be a lack of prioritization.
   14. Keep a list of positive outcomes.

M. Reduce inappropriate responses to stressors
   1. Teach to distinguish between urge and hunger.
   2. Use distraction, relaxation, imagery.
   3. Use alternative response training.
      a. Make a list of external cues/situations that lead to off-target behavior.
      b. List what you can do constructively instead of indulging in off-target behavior when this occurs (*e.g.,* take a walk).
      c. Post the list of alternate behaviors on the refrigerator.
      d. Reevaluate whether plan is realistic and effective every 1–2 weeks.

N. Assist client to plan for life-long weight maintenance
1. Understand issues of dependency, control, and esteem.
2. Decide on *your* plan for *your* control.
3. Set realistic short- and long-term goals: revise as necessary.
4. Think positively, start slowly.
5. Give self credit for each achievement; avoid perfectionism.
6. Build healthy support system.

O. Initiate health teaching and referrals as indicated
1. Refer to support groups (*e.g.,* Weight Watchers, Overeater Anonymous, TOPS, trim clubs, The Diet Workshop, Inc.).
2. Dietitian for meal planning
3. Physician for morbid obesity and evaluation of other health problems

---

■ High Risk for Altered Health Maintenance
Related to Insufficient Knowledge of (Specify)

Example: Lack of Knowledge of Dietary Management of Diabetes Mellitus or Lack of Knowledge of Newborn Care

Assessment

Subjective Data
The person states that he
Is aware of a knowledge deficit
Is anxious and fearful of unfamiliar situations
Needs instruction

Objective Data
The person
Does not participate in his care (when other reasons for noncompliance have been ruled out)
Exhibits anxious behavior, such as
Increased verbalization
Inability to concentrate
and retain information
Restlessness
Sweating palms
Tremulousness
Delays seeking medical assistance when it is needed
Misuses health care system (seeks assistance when he himself could have solved the problem or used a more appropriate resource)

Outcome Criteria

The person will

- Actively participate in the health behaviors prescribed or desired (such as those behaviors required in preparation for a diagnostic test, surgery, or physical examination, or those behaviors related to recovery from illness and prevention of recurrence of complications)
- Relate less anxiety, related to fear of the unknown, fear of loss of control, misconceptions, or previously given misinformation
- Describe disease process, causes, and factors contributing to symptoms, and the procedure(s) for disease or symptom control

Interventions

The following interventions represent the teaching/learning activities to deal with a new diagnosis or treatment or the anticipation of an unfamiliar test, procedure, or surgery.

A. Assess the causative and contributing factors (in situations requiring a planned teaching/learning intervention)

1. New diagnosis
2. Change in existing medical condition/health status
3. New or altered treatment regimen

B. Reduce or eliminate barriers to learning

1. Assist person in meeting basic physiologic needs, if necessary.
2. Support person in progressing through stages of psychosocial adaptation to illness
   a. Stage of disbelief (denial)
      - Orient person to hospital setting, routines affecting him.
      - Teach with a focus on the present.
      - Provide simple explanations of procedures as they are carried out.
      - Help person feel safe, secure.
      - Concentrate on one-to-one teaching, rather than group teaching.
      - Teach family about the denial that person is having.
   b. State of developing awareness (guilt, anger)
      - Listen carefully to person.
      - Continue teaching with a present-tense focus.
      - Allow hostility to be safely vented.
      - Avoid arguing with person.
3. Delay teaching until person is ready.
4. Adapt teaching to person's physical and psychologic status.
5. Allow person to work through and express intense emotions prior to teaching.
6. Examine person's health beliefs and past experiences related to his illness and assess their impact on his desire to learn.

C. Promote person/family learning

1. Individualize the teaching approach after a thorough assessment.
2. Plan and share necessity of learning outcomes with person/family.
3. Follow the principles of teaching/learning previously listed.

4. Evaluate person/family behaviors as evidence that learning outcomes have been achieved.

D. Promote a positive attitude and active participation of the person and his family

1. Solicit expressions of feelings, concerns, and questions from person and family.
2. Encourage person/family to seek information and make informed decisions.
3. Explain person/family responsibilities and how these can be assumed.

E. Reduce anxiety

1. Encourage verbalization.
2. Listen attentively.
3. Meet person's expressed needs prior to giving other information.
4. Develop trust with frequent, consistent interactions.
5. Give correct, relevant information.
6. Give nonthreatening information before more anxiety-producing information.
7. Explain reason for and intended effect of treatment; emphasize the positive.
8. Explore with person the effects of a new diagnosis, treatment, or surgery on his significant others.
9. Do not overwhelm person with too much information if anxiety is high or physical condition is unstable.
10. Allow person to maintain some control over himself and his routines by involving person in care.
11. Prepare person and family for what to expect concerning his environment, routines, the personnel giving care, sensations experienced, etc.

F. Proceed with health teaching and referrals as indicated

■ High Risk for Altered Health Maintenance
Related to Insufficient Knowledge of Ostomy Care*

Assessment

Subjective Data

The person states that he

Has a lack of knowledge of ostomy care

Is anxious and fearful because he does not know about ostomy care

Needs instruction in ostomy care

*Persons undergoing ostomy surgery frequently question whether or not they will be able to lead normal lives. The most commonly expressed fear is that of being offensive to themselves and others. Multiple factors contribute to this fear. During the perioperative period, patients consistently ask the same questions about how the ostomy will effect their life-style: "How will I go to the bathroom? Can I really contain the drainage? Will I have an offensive odor? Will the pouch show through my clothing? How do you empty the pouch? How will I know when to change/empty the pouch? Can I work, travel, swim, play, make love? Can I eat regular food? Can I drink beer? Will my partner still love me? What can I do with the pouch during lovemaking? Can I exercise?"

Satisfactory answers to these questions provide knowledge that will decrease the person's fear and facilitate ostomy self-care. If a person can be taught how to contain the ostomy output in a discreet manner, it may provide the confidence that is necessary to begin working through the emotional issues related to having an ostomy. Because control over elimination is a primary concern, teaching the stoma pouching procedure is used as an example of a nursing intervention to reduce the lack of knowledge of ostomy care (Maklebust, 1985).

Objective Data

The person does not participate in ostomy care.

The person is:

Unable to state own disease/indications for surgery

Unable to identify own type of ostomy

Unable to describe routine ostomy care

Unable to identify stoma pouching equipment

Unable to apply, change, or empty stoma pouch

Unable to maintain peristomal skin integrity

Outcome Criteria

The person will

• Actively participate in the health behaviors prescribed or desired (such as those behaviors required in preparation for surgery or those behaviors needed to care for own ostomy

• Relate less anxiety related to fear of the unknown, fear of loss of control, misconceptions, or previously given misinformation

• Verbalize methods of incorporating ostomy care into own life-style

---

Interventions

A. Assess knowledge regarding ostomy and effects on life-style

1. Level of understanding of disease
2. Knowledge of structure and function of affected organs
3. Surgical procedure/stoma location
4. Type of ostomy effluent
5. Knowledge of ostomy care (*e.g.,* diet, activity, hygiene, clothing, sexual function, community resources, employment, travel, odor, skin care, appliances, and irrigation, if applicable)
6. Prior exposure to person with ostomy
7. Familiarity with stoma pouching equipment
8. Emotional status, cognitive ability, and physical limitations (*e.g.,* anxiety, memory, vision, manual dexterity)
9. Life-style/strengths/coping mechanisms
10. Available support systems

B. See other possible nursing diagnoses for additional interventions, for example:

1. *Anticipatory grief related to perceived loss of adult toileting behavior*
2. *Powerlessness related to loss of control over elimination following removal of anal sphincter or urethra*
3. *Self-concept disturbance related to sudden change in body structure following ostomy surgery or*
4. *Social isolation related to fear of rejection by others*

C. Instruct person on stoma and related information
1. Dispel misinformation/misconceptions regarding ostomy.
2. Explain normal anatomic structure and function of GI or GU tract.
3. Explain effects of disease on affected organs.
4. Use diagram/model to show altered route of elimination.
5. Describe appearance and anticipated location of stoma:
   a. Stoma will be same color and have same degree of moistness as oral mucous membrane.
   b. Stoma has no nerve endings for pain and will not hurt when touched.
   c. Stoma will become smaller as the surgical area heals—color will remain the same.
   d. Stoma size may change depending on illness, hormone levels, weight gain, or loss.
6. Discuss need for wearing pouch as a prosthesis or substitute for the removed colon or bladder.
7. Encourage handling of stoma pouching equipment.
8. Teach basic stoma pouching principles:
   a. Peristomal skin should be clean and dry so that appliance will adhere to skin.
   b. A well-fitting appliance should protect all the surrounding skin surface from drainage.
   c. Pouch should be changed when the least amount of drainage is anticipated, usually upon rising.
   d. Pouch should be emptied when one-third to one-half full.
   e. Pouch should be changed routinely before a leak occurs.
   f. Pouch should be changed if burning or itching occurs under the appliance.
   g. Condition of stoma and peristomal skin should be observed during pouch changes.
9. Proceed with teaching necessary procedures. Consistently use same sequence while teaching.
   a. Teach procedure for preparing stoma pouch.
      - Measure stoma.
      - Use appliance manufacturer's stoma-measuring card if possible.
      - Select pouch with a precut hole to accommodate stoma size. Allow about a $1/8$-inch margin of skin around stoma. If peristomal skin is uneven or stoma is flush with skin, use stoma paste to surround stoma.
      - If appliance manufacturer's stoma-measuring card does not accommodate stoma size or shape, teach person to make individual pattern of stoma. Place clear plastic wrap from skin barrier wafer over stoma. Trace stoma with a marking pen. Cut hole in plastic to accommodate stoma.
      - Use pattern to trace opening onto the reverse side of a skin barrier wafer.
      - Cut opening in center of skin barrier wafer that is slightly larger (approximately $1/8$ inch) than stoma
      - Secure appropriate odor-proof pouch onto skin barrier wafer (if using two-piece appliance system)
      - Remove white paper backing from skin barrier wafer.
      - Set pouch aside.
   b. Teach procedure for changing disposable stoma pouch.
      - Remove old pouch by gently pushing skin away from paper tape and skin barrier wafer.
      - Fold old pouch over on itself and discard in plastic bag.
      - Clean peristomal skin with wash cloth and warm tap water.

- Blot or pat skin dry.
- Apply new pouch to abdomen carefully, centering the hole in the skin barrier wafer over the stoma.
- Press on wafer for a few minutes so that heat and pressure of hand will help wafer adhere to skin.
- Secure pouch by "picture framing" wafer with four strips of hypo-allergenic paper tape (if wafer does not already have tape attached).

c. Teach procedure for emptying stoma pouch.
- Sit on toilet.
- Float some toilet tissue in toilet bowel so that water does not splash when contents are emptied.
- Remove pouch clamp from tail of pouch.
- Empty contents of pouch into toilet by leaning forward and letting ostomy appliance hang between legs.
- Flush toilet.
- Clean inside and outside of pouch tail with toilet paper.
- Insert ostomy appliance deodorant into end of pouch.
- Reapply clamp to tail of pouch.
- Apply stoma paste to even out dips or uneven skin surfaces. Use it only if necessary, as it is expensive and often makes it more difficult to learn needed care. If necessary to use stoma paste, wet the finger first so that it does not stick to the skin in unwanted places.
- When applying the wafer, push down well around the stoma. This is the area where stool leakages occur.
- Itching or burning under an appliance means that stool is getting under the wafer and the pouch needs changing. Do not tape the edges to try to secure a leaking appliance. Instead, change the pouch immediately. A good washing and a new appliance are usually all that is necessary. If the skin is irritated, it will almost always heal itself under a new appliance.

D. Incorporate emotional support into technical self-ostomy care sessions

1. This allows resolution of emotional issues during acquisition of technical skills. Derricks (1974) identified four stages of psychologic adjustment that ostomy patients experience.
   a. Narration—Each person recounts his illness experience and reveals his understanding of how and why he finds himself in his current situation.
   b. Visualization and verbalization—The person looks at and expresses feelings about his stoma.
   c. Participation—The person progresses from observer to assistant and then to independent performer of the mechanical aspects of ostomy care.
   d. Exploration—The person begins to explore methods of incorporating the ostomy into his life-style.
2. Using this adjustment framework helps to establish guidelines for arranging patient experiences in an organized manner.

E. Encourage person to become active in care by gradually increasing his responsibility; have the person:

1. Look at and touch stoma. Assumptions cannot be made about a person's reaction to a situation. The reality of the altered body function may overwhelm the person.
2. Verbalize feelings about stoma. Assure person that his responses are normal and appropriate. Person's perceptions must be validated by the nurse.

3. Practice using pouch clamp on empty pouch. Beginning with a necessary skill that is apart from the body is less threatening.
4. Assist with emptying pouch. During ostomy care, person watches health care professionals for signs of revulsion. The nurse's attitude and support are of primary importance.
5. Participate in pouch removal. Give feedback on progress. Reinforce positive behavior, proper techniques.
6. Participate in pouch application. Point out degrees of success achieved toward self-care.
7. Demonstrate stoma pouching procedure independently in presence of resource person. Evaluate need for further teaching.
8. Involve significant other in learning ostomy care principles. Assess interactions with significant other.
9. Explain that with a sigmoid colostomy, it may be possible to wash out the colon for up to 24 hours with a colostomy enema; this allows the choice of bowel evacuation time. However, the person should NEVER irrigate an ileostomy. Absence of output from an ileostomy accompanied by abdominal cramping may signal a small bowel blockage and necessitates prompt medical evaluation.
10. Discuss plans to incorporate ostomy into own life-style. Suggest a visitor from the United Ostomy Association who can share similar experiences.

F. Initiate health teaching and referrals as indicated

1. Review follow-up care and signs/symptoms to report to enterostomal (ET) nurse or physician.
2. Teach tips for daily living (Maklebust, 1990):
   a. Wardrobe
   - Wear two pairs of underpants. The inside pair should be low-rise or bikini-height cotton knit worn *under* the ostomy appliance to absorb perspiration and keep the pouch away from the skin. The outside pair can be cotton or nylon, should be waist-high, and is worn *over* the ostomy appliance.
   - The ostomy pouch can be tucked between the two pairs of underwear like a kangaroo pouch. Special pouch covers are expensive, soil rapidly, and are not necessary.
   - Avoid too-tight clothing, which can restrict the appliance and can cause leakage. A boxer-type bathing suit is preferable for men. For women, a patterned bathing suit with shirring can camouflage the appliance well.
   b. Diet
   - Chew all food well.
   - Postoperatively, with progression to a regular diet, the noise from passing flatus will decrease.
   - Eat on a regular schedule to help decrease the noise from an empty gut.
   - Avoid mushrooms, Chinese vegetables, popcorn, and other foods that may cause blockage. (Note: Pillsbury microwave popcorn is specially made to be tolerated because the kernels can be finely ground by adequate chewing.)
   - Keep in mind that fish, eggs, and onions cause odor in the stool.
   - Drink at least several 8-oz. glasses of water a day to prevent dehydration in an ileostomate and constipation in a colostomate. Concentrated urine or decreased urinary output is a good indicator of dehydration.
   c. Odor Control
   - Explain that odor is caused from bacteria in the stool.
   - Because most ostomy appliances are made to be odorproof, do not poke a

hole in the ostomy appliance to allow flatus to escape; constant odor will result.

- Control offensive odors with good hygiene and ostomy pouch deodorants. (Super Banish appliance deodorant works best because it contains silver nitrate, which kills the bacteria.) Hydrogen peroxide and mouthwashes such as Binaca can be placed in the ostomy pouch as inexpensive appliance deodorants.
- Do not use aspirin tablets as a deodorant in the ostomy pouch; aspirin tablets coming in contact with the stoma may cause stomal irritation and bleeding.
- Eating yogurt and cranberry juice may help reduce fecal odor. Certain oral medications reduce fecal odor, but these should be used only with the advice of a physician.

d. Hygiene
- Use a hand-held shower spray to wash the skin around the stoma and irrigate perineal wounds.
- Showers can be taken with the ostomy appliance on or off. On days when the appliance is changed, a shower can be taken when the old pouch is removed but before the new pouch is applied.
- The new pouch should be readied before getting in the shower. On days between appliance changes, showering with the appliance on only requires that the paper tape around the wafer be covered with a liquid sealant in order to waterproof the tape.

e. Exercise
- Normal activities (even strenuous sports, in most cases) can be resumed after recovery from surgery.
- Be aware that increased incidence of peristomal herniation is associated with heavy lifting.
- Also keep in mind that increased perspiration from strenuous exercise may require more frequent ostomy appliance changes due to increased melting of the appliance skin barrier.

f. Travel
- Take all ostomy supplies along when traveling.
- Do not leave ostomy appliances in automobiles parked in the sun, as the heat will melt the skin barrier.
- When flying, always keep appliances in carry-on luggage to avoid loss.

g. Sexual Activity
- Remember that an ostomy does not automatically make you undesirable; as in any sexual encounter, you may have to indicate sexual interest to your partner, who may be afraid of hurting you.
- Wearing a stretch tube top around the midriff will cover the ostomy appliance while leaving the genitals and breasts exposed.
- If male impotence is a problem, the man can be referred to a urologist for discussion or investigation of a penile prosthesis.
- Keep in mind that in many cases, sexual problems following ostomy surgery are manifestations of problems that existed prior to surgery. If the ostomate had a strong supportive relationship prior to surgery, there usually are no problems after surgery.

3. Discuss community resources/self-help groups.
  a. Visiting nurse
  b. United Ostomy Association
  c. Foundation for Ileitis and Colitis

    d. Recovery of male potency—help for the impotent male

    e. American Cancer Foundation

    f. Community suppliers of ostomy equipment

    g. Financial reimbursement for ostomy equipment

References/Bibliography

Albert, M. (1987). Health screening to promote health for the elderly. *Nurse Practitioner, 12*(5), 42.

Belloc, N. & Breslow, L. (1972). The relation of physical health status and health practice. *Preventive Medicine, 1,* 409–421.

Bille, D. (Ed.). (1981). *Practical approaches to patient teaching.* Boston: Little, Brown.

Christman, N. J., & Kirchhoff, K. T. (1985). Preparatory sensory information. In Bulechek, G., McCloskey, J. (Eds.). *Nursing interventions: Treatments for nursing diagnoses.* Philadelphia: W. B. Saunders.

Cohen, N. (1980). *Three steps to better patient teaching. Nursing, 10*(2), 72–74.

Doak, C. C., Doak, L. G., & Root, J. H. (1985). *Teaching patients with low literacy skills.* Philadelphia: J. B. Lippincott.

Dunn, H. L. (1959). What high-level wellness means. *Canadian Journal of Public Health, 50*(11), 447–457.

Duvall, E. M. (1977). *Marriage and family development* (5th ed.). Philadelphia: J. B. Lippincott.

Eisenberg A., & Eisenberg, H. (1979). *Alive and well: Decision in health.* New York: McGraw-Hill.

Falvo, D. R. (1985). *Effective patient education.* Rockville, MD: Aspen Systems.

Flynn, P. A. (1980). *Holistic health: The art and science of care.* Bowie MD: Robert J. Brady.

Hill L., & Smith, N. (1985). *Self-care nursing.* Englewood Cliffs, NJ: Prentice-Hall.

Hymovich, D. P., & Barnard, M. V. (1979). *Family health care* (2nd ed.). New York: McGraw-Hill.

Jensen, D. P. (1985). Patient contracting. In Bulechek, G., & McCloskey, J. (Eds.). *Nursing interventions: Treatments for nursing diagnoses.* Philadelphia: W. B. Saunders.

Kandzari, J., & Howard, J. (1981). *The well family: A developmental approach to assessment.* Boston: Little, Brown.

Ouslander, J. C., & Beck, J. C. (1982). Defining the health problems of the elderly. *Annual Review of Public Health, 3,* 55–83.

Pender, N. J. (1985). Self-modification. In Bulechek, G., & McCloskey, J. (Eds.). *Nursing interventions: Treatments for nursing diagnoses.* Philadelphia: W. B. Saunders.

Periodic health exam: A guide for designing individualized preventive health care in the asymptomatic adult. (1981). *Annals of Internal Medicine, 95,* 729–732.

Redman, B. K., & Thomas, S. A. (1985). Patient teaching. In Bulechek, G., & McCloskey, J. (Eds.). *Nursing interventions: Treatments for nursing diagnoses.* Philadelphia: W. B. Saunders.

Rimar, J. M. (1986). *Haemophilus influenzae* type b polysaccharide vaccine. *Maternal-Child Nursing, 11,* 57.

Todd, B. (1984). Preventing influenza and pneumonia. *Geriatric Nursing,* Nov—Dec, 399–401.

Wilberding, J. Z. (1985). Values clarification. In Bulechek, G., & McCloskey, J. (Eds.). *Nursing interventions: Treatments for nursing diagnoses.* Philadelphia: W. B. Saunders.

Woldum, K. M., Ryan-Morrell, V., & Towson, M. C. (1985). *Patient education: Foundations of practice.* Rockville, MD: Aspen Systems.

Gerontologic

Abrams, W. B., & Berkow, R. (Eds.). (1990). *The Merck manual of geriatrics.* Rahway, NJ: Merck & Co.

Fleg, J. L. (1986). Alterations in cardiovascular structure and function with advancing age. *American Journal of Cardiology, 5*(7), 33C–44C.

Harris, R. (1982). Exercise and sex in the aging patient. *Medical Aspects of Human Sexuality,* 152–157.

Matteson, M. A., & McConnell, E. S. (1988). *Gerontological nursing: Concepts and practices.* Philadelphia: W. B. Saunders.

Miller, C. A. (1990). *Nursing care of older adults.* Glenview, IL: Scott Foresman.

Posner, J. D., Gorman, K. M., Klein, H. S., & Woldow, A. (1986). *American Journal of Cardiology, 57,* 52C–58C.

Schneider, E. L. (1983). Infectious diseases in the elderly. *Annals of Internal Medicine, 98,* 395–400.

US Dept of Health & Human Services. (1987). *Current estimates for the national health survey.* Hyattsville, MD: USDHHS.

Tobacco Use

Ash, C. R. (1987). Smoking and lung cancer, *Cancer Nursing, 10*(4), 171.

Cinelli, B., & Glover, E. (1988). Nurses' smoking in the work-place: Causes and solutions. *Journal of Community Health Nursing, 5*(4), 255–261.

Hughes, J. R., & Miller, S. A. (1984). Nicotine gum to help stop smoking. *Journal of the American Medical Association, 252*(20), 2855–2858.

Institute of Medicine. (1985). *Preventing low birthweight.* Committee to Study the Prevention of Low Birthweight, Division of Health Promotion and Disease Prevention. Washington, DC: National Academy Press.

Kuller, L., Garfinkel, L., Corren, P., Haley, N., Hoffmann, D., Preston-Martin, S., & Sandler, D. (1986). Contribution of passive smoking to respiratory cancer. *Environmental Health Perspectives, 70,* 57–69.

Lefcoe, N. M., Ashley, M. J., Pederson, L. L., & Keays, J. J. (1983). The health risks of passive smoking. *Chest, 84*(1), 90–95.

McMahon, A., & Maibusch, R. (1988). How to send quit-smoking signals. *American Journal of Nursing, 88*(11), 1498–1499.

Mennies, J. H. (1983). Smoking: The physiologic effects. *American Journal of Nursing, 83*(8), 1143–1146.

Young, E. W., Koch, P. B., & Mauger, J. L. (1988). Smokeless tobacco: Substituting the spittoon for the ashtray. *Journal of Community Health Nursing, 5*(3), 167–76.

Ostomy Care

Alterescu, V. (1985). The ostomy: What do you teach the patient? *American Journal of Nursing, 85*(11), 1250–1253.

Boarini, J. (1985). The ostomy, what can go wrong? *American Journal of Nursing, 85*(12), 1361.

Bollinger, B. *A teenager's ostomy guide.* Available from Hollister, Inc., 2000 Hollister Drive, Libertyville, IL 60048

Borgland, E. (1990). Care of peristomal skin: A dermatologist's view. In *Proceedings of the seventh biennial congress of the World Council of Enterostomal Therapists.* Barcelona: Palex International SA.

Broadwell, D. C., Sorrells, S. L.
Summary of Your Ileostomy Care
Summary of Your Colostomy Care
Summary of Your Urinary Diversion Care
Ostomy Care for Children
Available from Bard Home Health Division, C. R. Bard, Inc., P. O. Box 18, Berkeley Heights, NJ 07922

Brogna, L. (1985). Self-concept and rehabilitation of the person with an ostomy. *Journal of Enterostomal Therapy, 12*(6), 205–209.

Derricks, V. (1974). Nursing practices that affect the dynamics of rehabilitation for patients with an ostomy (ANA Clinical Sessions). Kansas City: ANA.

Felice, P. (1988). Teaching the child and family how to manage a urinary diversion. *Ostomy/Wound Management, 19,* 20–22.

Fleming, L. B. (1988). Using Orem's theory: A self-care program for the ostomy client. *Ostomy/Wound Management, 18,* 14–20, 63.

Gillen, P. B. (1988). Health care practitioner interventions to help the pediatric ostomate. *Ostomy/Wound Management, 19,* 14–20.

Hedrick, J. K., (1987). Effects of ET nursing intervention on adjustment following ostomy surgery. *Journal of Enterostomal Therapy, 14*(6), 229–239.

IAET. (1989). *Standards of care: Patient with a colostomy.* Irving, CA: International Association of Enterostomal Therapy.

Jacobs, M., & Geels, W. (1985). *Signs and symptoms in nursing: Interpretation and management.* Philadelphia: J. B. Lippincott.

Jeter, K. F. "Help For Incontinent People" Report. Available from HIP, P. O. Box 544, Union, SC 29373

Maklebust, J. (1990). Assisting with adjustment to home care following ostomy surgery. *Hospital Home Health, 7*(7), 91–94.

Maklebust, J. (1985). United Ostomy Association visits and adjustment following ostomy surgery. *Journal of Enterostomal Therapy, 12*(3), 84–92.

Moss, R. C. (1986). Overcoming fear, a review of research on patient, family instruction. *AORN Journal, 43*(5), 1107–1114.

Mullen, B. D., & McGinn, K. *The ostomy book.* Available from Bull Publishing Co., P. O. Box 208, Palo Alto, CA 94302

Nortridge, J. A., (1987). Teaching the concept of body image: Use of the affective and cognitive domains. *Journal of Enterostomal Therapy, 14*(6), 255–258.

Petillo, M. H., (1987). The patient with a urinary stoma: Nursing management and patient education. *Nursing Clinics of North America, 22*(2), 263–279.

Price, A., Allen, L., & Atwood, T. (1989). Healthcare practitioners help ostomy patients adjust nutritionally. *Ostomy/Wound Management, 24,* 30–41.

Rideout, B. W., (1987). The patient with an ileostomy: Nursing management and patient education. *Nursing Clinics of North America, 22*(2), 253–262.

Ritter, M. (1987). Assessing the educational needs of ostomy patients. *Ostomy/Wound Management, 16,* 14–15.

Shettle, P. E. (1989). The impact of isolation on an ostomy patient with AIDS. *Ostomy/Wound Management, 25,* 58–61.

Shipes, E., (1987). Psychosocial issues: The person with an ostomy. *Nursing Clinics of North America, 22*(2), 291–302.

Smith, D. B. (1986). Patient teaching. In Smith, D. B., & Johnson, D. E. (Eds.). *Ostomy care and the cancer patient: Surgical and clinical considerations.* Orlando: Grune & Stratton.

Smith, D. B., & Johnson, D. E. (1986). Preoperative preparation. In Smith, D. B., & Johnson, D. E. (Eds.). *Ostomy care and the cancer patient: Surgical and clinical considerations.* Orlando: Grune & Stratton.

Watson, P. G. (1985). Meeting the needs of patients undergoing ostomy surgery. *Journal of Enterostomal Therapy, 12*(4), 121–124.

Watt, R. C. (1985). The ostomy, why is it created? *American Journal of Nursing, 85*(1), 1242–1245.

Obesity

See *Altered Nutrition: Less Than Body Requirements* for additional sources of information.

Brody, J. (1981). *Jane Brody's nutrition book.* New York: W. W. Norton.

Brownell, K. D., & Stunkard, A. J. (1980). Exercise in the development and control of obesity. In Stunkard, A. J. (Ed.). *Obesity.* Philadelphia: W. B. Saunders.

Danforth, E. (1985). Diet and obesity. *American Journal of Clinical Nutrition, 41,* 1132–1145.

Fernstein, A. R. (1960). The treatment of obesity: An analysis of methods, results, and factors that influence success. *Journal of Chronic Diseases, 11,* 349–393.

Holmes, N., Ardito, E. A., Stevenson, D., & Lucas, C. P. (1984). In Storlie, J., & Jordan, H. A. (Eds.). *Behavioral management of obesity.* New York: Spectrum Publications.

Jacobson, P. (1979). Help for fat teenagers. *Pediatric Nursing, 5*(2), 49–50.

Overeaters Anonymous. (1981). A self-help group. *American Journal of Nursing, 81,* 560–563.

Pavlou, K. N., Steffee, N. P., Lerman, R. H. & Burrows, B. A. (1985). Effects of dieting and exercise on lean body mass, oxygen uptake and strength. *Medicine and Science in Sports and Exercise, 17,* 466–469.

Pitta, P., Alpert, M., & Perelle, A. (1980). Cognitive stimulus-control program for obesity with emphasis on anxiety and depression reduction. *International Journal of Obesity, 4,* 227–233.

Wadden, T. A., Stunkard, A. J., & Brownell, K. D. (1983). Very low calorie diets: Their efficacy, safety and future. *Annals of Internal Medicine, 99,* 675–684.

Stress Management

Alberti, R. E., & Emmons, M. L. (1974). *Your perfect right: A guide to assertive behavior.* San Luis Obispo, CA: Impact Publishers.

Bloom, L., Coburn, K., & Pearlman, J. (1976). *The new assertive woman.* New York: Dell Publishers.

Girdano, D. D., & Everly, G. S. (19). *Controlling stress and tension.* Englewood Cliffs, NJ: Prentice-Hall.

Girdano, D. D., & Everly, G. S. (1980). *The stress-mess solution.* Bowie, MD: Robert J. Brady.

Martin, R. A., & Poland, E. Y. (1980). *Learning to change: A self-management approach to adjustment.* New York: McGraw-Hill.

Thomas, D., Shoffner, D., & Groer, M. (1988). Adolescent stress factors: Implications for the nurse practitioner. *Nurse Practitioner, 13*(6), 20–29.

Osteoporosis

Bellantoni, M. F., & Blackman, M. R. (1988). Osteoporosis: Diagnostic screening and its place in current care. *Geriatrics, 43*(2), 63–70.

Chestnut, C. H. (1984). Treatment of postmenopausal osteoporosis. *Comprehensive Therapy, 10*(7), 41–47.

Coralli, C., (19). Osteoporosis: Significance, risk factors and treatment. *Nurse Practitioner, 11*(9), 25.

Lindsay, R. (1989). Osteoporosis: An updated approach to prevention and management. *Geriatrics, 44*(1), 45–54.

Miller, C. A. (1990). *Nursing care of older adults.* Glenview IL: Scott, Foresman.

Riggs, L. B., & Melton, L. J. (1986). Involutional osteoporosis. *New England Journal of Medicine, 314*(26), 1676–1685.

Pediatric

Hunsberger, M. (1989). Impact of acute illness. In Foster, R. L., Hunsberger, M. M. & Anderson, J. J. T. (Eds.). *Family-centered nursing care of children.* Philadelphia: W. B. Saunders.

Scipien, G. M., Chard, M. A., Howe, J., & Barnard, M. U. (1990). *Pediatric nursing care.* St. Louis: C. V. Mosby.

Whaley, L. F., & Wong, D. L. (1989). *Essentials of pediatric nursing* (3rd ed.). St. Louis: C. V. Mosby.

Williams, S. R. (1985). *Nutrition and diet therapy* (5th ed.). St. Louis: Times Mirror/Mosby.

Wong, D. L., & Whaley, L. F. (1990). *Clinical manual of pediatric nursing* (3rd ed.). St. Louis: C. V. Mosby.

Resources for the Consumer

Osteoporosis: The silent thief, AARP BOOKS/Scott, Foresman and Co., 1865 Miner Street, Des Plaines, IL 60018, (800) 238-2300

The health consequences of smoking, PHS, US Dept. of Health and Human Services, Office on Smoking and Health, Rockville, MD 1989

The health consequences of involuntary smoking, PHS, US Dept. of Health and Human Services, Office on Smoking and Health, Rockville, MD 1989

National Self-Health Clearinghouse, Graduate School and University Center of the City University of New York (CUNY), 33 West 42nd Street, Room 1227, New York, NY 10036, (212)840-7606. Publishers of *Self-Help Reporter.*

Community Wellness Resource Centers

The Center for Health Promotion, 601 Brookdale Towers, 2810 Fifty-seventh Avenue N, Minneapolis, MN 55430

Good Health Program, Skokie Valley Community Hospital, 9600 Gross Point Road, Skokie, IL 60076

Organizations

American Cancer Society, American Dental Association, American Heart Association

Health-Seeking Behaviors

■ *Related to* **(Specify)**

DEFINITION

Health-Seeking Behaviors: The state in which an individual in stable health actively seeks ways to alter personal health habits and/or the environment in order to move toward a higher level of wellness.*

DEFINING CHARACTERISTICS

Major (must be present)

> Expressed or observed desire to seek information for health promotion

Minor (may be present)

> Expressed or observed desire for increased control of health practice
> Expression of concern about current environmental conditions on health status
> Stated or observed unfamiliarity with wellness community resources
> Demonstrated or observed lack of knowledge in health-promotion behaviors

RELATED FACTORS

Situational (personal, environmental)

> Role changes
> > Marriage
> > Parenthood
> Lack of knowledge of need for:
> > Preventive behavior (disease)
> > Screening practices for age and risk
> > Optimal nutrition and weight
> > > control

> "Empty-nest" syndrome
> Retirement

> Regular exercise program
> Constructive stress management
> Supportive social networks
> Responsible role participation

Maturational

See Table II-8 for age-related situations.

Diagnostic Considerations

See *Altered Health Maintenance*

Focus Assessment Criteria

Subjective

> Does the individual/family report good or excellent health?
> Does the person/family desire to adopt a behavior to maximize health?

---

* Stable health status is defined as age-appropriate illness prevention measures achieved, client reports good or excellent health, and signs and symptoms of disease, if present, are controlled.

Principles and Rationale for Nursing Care

Generic Considerations

1. A major focus of nursing care is to promote effective health-seeking behaviors in clients.
2. According to Nyamathi (1989), "The health goals of the client and desired goals of the nurse are mutually concerned with enhancing the individual's motivation to attain and maintain health and function, to avoid disease and disability, and to attain or retain the highest possible level of health, function or productivity."
3. Nursing activities that promote health-seeking behaviors include nurturing, encouraging, teaching, communicating, and providing (Nyamathi, 1989).
4. Health-seeking and coping behaviors are closely intertwined; nurses assist clients to maximize their abilities to handle stress throughout life (Nyamathi, 1989).
5. Many situational, maturational, and demographic factors influence the client's ability to pursue health-seeking behaviors (see Related Factors).

Health-Seeking Diet

1. Adequate dietary intake of complex carbohydrates, found in grains, fruits, legumes and vegetables, improves human health in many ways, *e.g.,* decreasing the incidence of obesity, cardiovascular disease, cancer, malnutrition, diabetes, and dental caries. Current recommendations advise an increase in total dietary carbohydrates to 55% of daily calories and a reduction of total simple sugars (concentrated nonnutritive sweets) to only 10% of daily calories.
2. Recent studies prove that the risk of heart disease can be reduced by decreasing serum cholesterol via diet and drugs, if necessary (American Heart Association, 1989).
   a. Recommended dietary changes (to reduce serum cholesterol) include:
      - A decrease in total fats, saturated fats, and cholesterol
      - In overweight persons, reduced daily caloric intake to attain desired body weight (Ernst & Cleeman, 1989).
      - Increased intake of nutrients that may help decrease the risk of cardiovascular disease (*e.g.,* oat bran and other water-soluble fibers, fruit gums, vegetables, garlic, polyunsaturated fats, olive oil, legumes and fatty fish)
   b. Many people find it difficult to maintain health-seeking diets even when they have been successful. Examples of helpful approaches include behavioral contracts (Neale, Singleton, Dupins, & Hess, 1989), positive self-talk (Kayman, 1989), and strengthening family supports (Torisky, Hertzler, Johnson, Keller, Hodges, & Mifflin, 1989).
   c. Risk factors for cardiovascular disease include (Ernst & Cleeman, 1989).
      - Male gender
      - Family history of MI or sudden death in parent or sibling less then 55 years of age
      - Smokes more than 10 cigarettes/day
      - Hypertension
      - HDL-cholesterol level less than 35 mg/dL
      - History of definite occlusive vascular disease (peripheral or cerebral)
      - Morbid obesity (greater than 30% overweight).
   d. Guidelines for cholesterol screening are (Ernst & Cleeman, 1989):
      - Less than 200 mg/dL: Desirable
      - 200–239 mg/dL: Borderline high

- 240 mg/dL and over: High blood cholesterol
        For all readings over 200 mg/dL, the test should be repeated within 8
        weeks, along with lipoprotein analysis and medical follow-up.
  e. Dietary recommendations for children over age 2 include (American Heart
     Association, 1990):
     - Provide a variety of foods daily
     - Maintain desirable body weight
     - Limit total dietary fat to 30% of calories
     - Limit total daily cholesterol to 100 mg/1000 calories and not more than 300
       mg/day
     - Limit daily protein intake to 15% of calories
     - Limit daily carbohydrate intake to 55% of calories
     - Limit sodium intake by reducing processed foods and keeping salt shaker off
       the table
3. There has been much research on both animals and human beings that suggests a
   link between nutrition and cancer; some nutrients act as promoters of carcinogens,
   others are protectors against cancer (Whitney, Cataldo, & Rolfes, 1987).
   a. Dietary behaviors associated with cancer include high consumption of fats (all
      types), vitamin A deficiency, excessive use of nitrite-containing foods, consump-
      tion of cancer-producing chemicals via food chain (*e.g.*, pesticides, herbicides,
      radiation, toxic waste in water source), high intake of alcohol.
   b. Dietary nutrients that protect against cancer include vegetable and grain fibers,
      vitamins A and C, cruciferous vegetables, and vegetables and fruits rich in
      carotene.
4. The exact relationship between dietary sodium and essential hypertension has yet to
   be unequivocally described. Studies show, however, that blood pressure in many (not
   all) clients with hypertension will decrease when dietary sodium is restricted. All
   hypertensive persons should be given a trial of a reduced sodium diet (2 g sodium/
   day.) If successful, continued dietary support is needed.

■ Health-Seeking Behaviors:
(Specify)

Assessment
Refer to Related Factors

Outcome Criteria

The person will
- Describe screening that is appropriate for age and risk factors
- Perform self-screening for cancer
- Participate in a regular physical exercise program
- State an intent to use positive coping mechanisms and constructive stress
  management
- Agree with self-responsibility for wellness (physical, dental, safety, nutri-
  tional, family)

Interventions

A. Assess for factors that contribute to the promotion and the maintenance of health
   1. Knowledge of disease and preventive behavior
   2. Appropriate screening practices for age and risk
   3. Good nutrition and weight control
   4. Regular exercise program
   5. Constructive stress management
   6. Supportive social networks

B. Promote health behaviors in the person and the family
   1. Determine the person's or family's knowledge or perception of
      a. Specific diseases (*e.g.,* heart disease, cancer, respiratory disease, childhood diseases, infections, dental disease)
      b. Susceptibility (*e.g.,* presence of risk factors, family history)
      c. Seriousness
      d. Value of early detection
   2. Determine the person's or family's past patterns of health care.
      a. Expectations
      b. Interactions with health care system or providers
      c. Influences of family, cultural group, peer group, mass media
   3. Provide specific information concerning screening for age-related conditions (refer to Table II-8).
   4. Discuss the role of nutrition in health maintenance and the prevention of illness (see Principles and Rationale for Nursing Care for *Altered Nutrition* for specific explanations).
      a. Basic four food groups
      b. Nutrient needs related to age, level of physical activity, pregnancy, and lactation
      c. The prudent use of
         • Salt (see *Fluid Volume Excess* for foods high in sodium)
         • Canned vegetables
         • Fried foods
         • Red meats
         • Fats (butter, margarines)
         • High-calorie desserts
         • Snack foods (potato chips, candy, soda)
         • Refined sugar
         • Foods containing nitrosamines (smoked meats, preservatives)
      d. The generous use of health-promoting foods
         • Cruciferous vegetables (broccoli, cabbage, cauliflower, Brussels sprouts)—protect against colorectal cancer
         • High-fiber foods—protect against colorectal cancer
         • Calcium-containing foods (dairy, dark leafy vegetables, etc.)—protect against osteoporosis
      e. See *Altered Health Maintenance* for specific information concerning weight control.
   5. Discuss the benefits of a regular exercise program.
      a. See Principles and Rationale for Nursing Care for the positive effects of a regular exercise program.

    b. Determine the optimal exercise for the individual, considering physical limitations, preferences, and life-style.
- Walking briskly
- Jogging
- Running
- Aerobic exercises
- Aerobic dancing
- Swimming
- Bicycling
- Skipping rope

    c. Stress the importance of beginning any physical activity slowly.

6. Discuss the elements of constructive stress management.
    a. Assertiveness training
    b. Problem-solving
    c. Relaxation techniques
    d. See Appendix X for relaxation techniques and Appendix VII for guidelines for problem-solving.
    e. See Pertinent Literature for the Consumer on assertiveness and problem-solving self-help books.

7. Discuss strategies for developing positive social networks.
    a. Relate the functions of a support system:
- Provide love and affection
- Share common social concerns
- Serve as buffers for life's stressors
- Prevent isolation
- Respect mutual pursuits of members
- Cooperate for the common purpose
- Provide dependable assistance (emotional and economic, if appropriate)

    b. Suggest methods for strengthening this system:
- Be supportive of others
- Practice active listening by allowing yourself to listen attentively to the other person, such as:
  Don't interrupt the person
  Allow a few seconds to lapse between dialogue to provide time to gather thoughts and to reduce the "rush to speak"

    c. Provide others with opportunities to share their concerns without judgment. Refrain from giving solutions to problems of others; rather, a discussion of options may be indicated (*e.g.,* "You have several options: You can quit your job, request a transfer, discuss the problem with your boss, or do nothing")

    d. When confronted with a relationship problem, review the situation.
- What is the problem?
- Who/what is responsible for the problem?
- What are the options?
- What are the advantages and disadvantages of each option?
  (See Appendix VII for guidelines for problem-solving.)

    e. Provide warmth and affection to significant others.
- Praise a child's accomplishments.
- Praise all attempts at accomplishments.
- Practice open shows of affection (*e.g.,* with children [boys and girls], with spouse, and with others).

    f. Practice mutual goal setting to direct common efforts and reevaluate them periodically.

    g. Offer sincere assistance to individuals to promote trust.

    h. Build relationships with individuals and families who share common interests and values.

    i. Recognize when additional assistance is needed.
- Marital counseling
- Self-help groups
- Health professional
- Religious affiliation

    j. Allow oneself and each member of the family—children, spouse, parents—to enhance personal identity by pursuing individual interests (refer to *Altered Growth and Development* for age-related needs of children).

C. Initiate health teaching and referrals as indicated

1. Review the daily health practices of the individual (adults, children).

    a. Dental care

    b. Food intake

    c. Fluid intake

    d. Exercise regimen

    e. Leisure activities

    f. Responsibilities in the family

    g. Use of
- Tobacco
- Salt, sugar, fat products
- Alcohol
- Drugs (over-the-counter, prescribed)

    h. Knowledge of safety practices
- Fire prevention
- Water safety
- Automobile (maintenance, seat belts)
- Bicycle
- Poison control

2. Suggest selective disease-preventing behaviors when appropriate.

    a. Skin cancers
- Avoid frequent sun exposure
- Avoid tanning salons
- Wear effective sunscreens and protective clothing
- Plan outdoors activities for before 10 A.M. and after 2 P.M. During these hours, wear a hat and sunscreen.

    b. Venereal diseases
- Use barrier contraceptive methods.

    c. AIDS
- Use condoms.
- Avoid high-risk sexual practices.

    d. Hepatitis B
- Hepatitis vaccine, if high risk

    e. Hearing loss
- Use ear protection routinely (*e.g.,* mowing lawn, around machinery).
- Avoid loud music (headphones, etc.).
- Avoid prolonged exposure to loud noises.

    f. Congenital deformities
- Avoid the use of alcohol and drugs during pregnancy.

    g. Oral cancers
- Avoid tobacco chewing.
- Avoid concurrent heavy use of alcohol and tobacco.

    h. Lung cancers, COPD
- Avoid tobacco smoking.
- Avoid chronic exposure to known inhalable carcinogens (*e.g.,* asbestos).
- Include carotene-rich foods in diet (*e.g.,* yellow vegetables and fruits).
- Avoid smoke-filled rooms; discourage smoking in your living and work spaces.

    i. Coronary artery disease
- Avoid obesity.
- Avoid cholesterol.
- Avoid tobacco use.
- Practice stress management.
- Exercise regularly.
- Avoid dietary cholesterol and saturated fats, and reduce total dietary fats.
- Maintain normal blood pressure.
- Increase daily intake of water-soluble fibers in diet (*e.g.,* oat bran, fruit pectins, psyllium).

    j. Stroke
- Avoid tobacco use, especially if taking oral contraceptives.
- Maintain normal blood pressure.
- Avoid dietary cholesterol and saturated fats, and reduce total dietary fats.

    k. Reye syndrome
- Avoid aspirin products in children with viruses.

    l. Osteoarthritis
- Avoid obesity.
- Avoid repeated trauma to joints.

    m. Osteoporosis for high-risk women (refer to Principles for high-risk characteristics)
- Vitamin D supplement
- Calcium supplement
- Regular exercise
- Reduction of or abstinence from caffeine, alcohol

    n. Colorectal cancer
- Avoid chronic constipation.
- Avoid foods containing nitrites (cured and smoked meats) and consume orange juice or other vitamin C–rich product with same meal when nitrites are included in diet.
- Include generous amounts of cruciferous vegetables (*e.g.,* cabbage, broccoli, brussel sprouts, cauliflower) and other sources of fiber in diet.

    o. Breast cancer
- Avoid high-fat diet.

3. Refer to selected nursing diagnoses for additional information on and assessment of
    a. Safety needs: see *High Risk for Injury*
    b. Activity needs: see *Diversional Activity Deficit*
    c. Affiliative needs: see *Social Isolation*
    d. Parenting needs: see *Altered Parenting*
    e. Family needs: see *Altered Family Processes*
    f. Spiritual needs: see *Spiritual Distress*

g. Sexual needs: see *Altered Sexuality Patterns*
h. Self-care needs: see *Impaired Home Maintenance Management*
i. Emotional needs: see *Ineffective Individual Coping; Anxiety; Fear; Grieving; Disturbance in Self-Concept; and Powerlessness*

References/Bibliography

See also References/Bibliography for *Altered Health Maintenance*

American Heart Association. (1990). *Help your heart: Children and cholesterol.* Philadelphia.

American Heart Association. (1989). *Cholesterol and your heart.* Dallas: National Center.

Australian National Health and Medical Research Council Dietary Salt Study Management Committee. (1989). Fall in blood pressure with modest reduction in dietary salt intake in mild hypertension. *Lancet, 1,* 399–402.

Block, G. Clifford, C., Naughton, M., Henderson, M., & McAdams, M. (1989). A brief dietary screen for high fat intake. *Journal of Nutrition Education, 21*(5), 199–205.

Bruhn, J. G., Cordova, F. G., William, J. A., & Fuentes, R. G., Jr. (1977). The wellness process. *Journal of Community Health, 2*(3), 209–221.

Dunn, H. L. (1977). *High level wellness.* Thorofare, NJ: Charles B. Slack.

Ernst, N. & Cleeman, J. (1989). Reducing high blood cholesterol levels: Recommendations from the National Cholesterol Education Program. *Journal of Nutrition Education, 20*(1), 23–29.

Hall, B. A., Allan, J. D. (1986). Sharpening nursing's focus by focusing on health. *Nursing Health Care, 7*(6), 315–320.

Hill, M. (1979. Helping the hypertensive patient control sodium intake. *American Journal of Nursing, 79*(5), 906–909.

Kayman, S. (1989). Applying theory from social psychology and cognitive behavioral psychology to dietary behavior change and assessment. *Journal of the American Dietetic Association, 89*(2), 191–193.

Laffrey, S. C., Loveland-Cherry, C. J., & Winkler, S. J. (1986). Health behavior: Evolution of two paradigms. *Public Health Nursing, 3*(2), 92–100.

Neale, A., Singleton, S., Dupius, M., & Hess, J. Correlates of adherence to behavioral contracts for cholesterol reduction. *Journal of Nutrition Education, 21*(5), 221–225.

Nyamathi, A. (1989). Comprehensive health seeking and coping paradigm. *Journal of Advanced Nursing, 14*(4), 281–290.

Pender, N. J. (1982). *Health promotion in nursing practice.* Norwalk, CT: Appleton-Century-Crofts.

Rakowski, W. (1986). Personal health practices, health status and expected control over future health. *Journal of Community Health, 11*(3), 189–203.

Shah, M., Jeffrey R. W., Laing, B., Saure, S. G., Van Natta, M., & Strickland, D. (1990). Hypertension prevention trial (HPT): Food pattern changes resulting from intervention on sodium, potassium, and energy intake. *Journal of the American Dietetic Association, 90,* 69–76.

Subcommittee on Nonpharmacologic Therapy of the 1984 Joint National Committee on Detection, Evaluation, and Treatment of High Blood Pressure. *Nonpharmacologic approaches to the control of high blood pressure.* US Department of Health and Human Services, PHS, NIH, US Government Printing Office: 1986-491-292-41147.

Torisky, C., Hertzler, A., Johnson, J., Keller, J., Hodges, P., & Mifflin, B. (1990). Virginia EFNEP homemakers' dietary improvement and relation to selected family factors. *Journal of Nutrition Education, 21*(6), 249–257.

Travis, J. W. (1981). *Wellness workbook for helping professionals.* Mill Valley, CA: Wellness Associates.

Whitney, E., Cataldo, C., & Rolfes, S. (1987). *Understanding normal and clinical nutrition.* St. Paul: West Publishing.

Home Maintenance Management, Impaired

■ *Related to* **(Specify)**

DEFINITION

Impaired home maintenance management: The state in which an individual or family experiences or is at risk to experience a difficulty in maintaining self or family in a home environment.

DEFINING CHARACTERISTICS

Major (must be present)

Outward expressions of difficulty by individual or family
In maintaining the home (cleaning, repairs, financial needs) or
In caring for self or family member at home

Minor (may be present)

Poor hygienic practices
Infections
Infestations
Accumulated wastes
Impaired caregiver
Overtaxed
Anxious
Unavailable support system

Unwashed cooking and eating equipment
Offensive odors

Lack of knowledge
Negative response to ill member

RELATED FACTORS

Pathophysiologic

Chronic debilitating disease
Diabetes mellitus
Chronic obstructive pulmonary disease
Congestive heart failure

Cerebral vascular accident
Cancer
Arthritis

Multiple sclerosis
Muscular dystrophy
Parkinson's disease

Situational (personal, environmental)

Injury to individual or family member (fractured limb, spinal cord injury)
Surgery (amputation, ostomy)
Impaired mental status (memory lapses, depression, anxiety–severe panic)
Substance abuse (alcohol, drugs)
Unavailable support system
Loss of family member
Addition of family member (newborn, aged parent)
Lack of knowledge
Insufficient finances

Maturational

Infant: Newborn care, high risk for sudden infant death syndrome

Elderly: Family member with deficits (cognitive, motor, sensory)

Diagnostic Considerations

In the last 20 years, the health care system has undergone dramatic changes. Costcontainment has reduced hospital lengths of stay, resulting in discharge of many functionally comprised individuals to their homes. At the same time, individuals and family members have assumed an increasingly active role in health care decisions and activities.

According to Miller (1990), "eighty to ninety percent of care given to dependent older adults in the community is provided by family and friends, most often middle-aged women." But although the home is the primary site of care, less than 1% of Medicare expenditures go to home care.

Impaired Home Maintenance Management describes situations in which a person or family needs teaching, supervision, and/or assistance to manage home care of a household member or to manage the household. For the most part, assessment of the home environment and the person's functioning at home is best accomplished by a community health nurse. The nurse in the acute setting can make a referral for a home visit for assessment.

A nurse who diagnoses the need for teaching to prevent home care problems may use the diagnosis *High Risk for Impaired Home Maintenance Management related to insufficient knowledge of (specify)* to describe this situation.

Errors in Diagnostic Statements

Impaired Home Maintenance Management related to caregiver burnout

The nurse would have insufficient data for the above diagnosis. Although caregiver burnout is a possible sign of *Impaired Home Maintenance Management,* the related factors are not validated. Instead, the diagnosis should be written as *Impaired Home Maintenance Management related to unknown etiology, as evidenced by reports of caregiver burnout.*

After focus assessment, the nurse may validate factors such as inadequate finances, caregiver health problems, or failure to delegate some responsibilities to other household members. Caregiver burnout also could be a sign of *Ineffective Individual Coping.*

Focus Assessment Criteria

Owing to the variability and complexity of this diagnosis, the nurse must determine whether the entire assessment must be performed or just selected areas. For example, if an elderly man lives alone, delete the assessment of the family. If a family is in crisis (financial or emotional), delete assessment of the functional status of the individual.

If a member is ill or disabled, the entire assessment may be indicated.

Subjective Data

Assessment of Individual Function

Vision

Adequate

Corrected (date of last prescription)

Complaints of
    Blurriness   Difficulty in focusing
    Loss of side vision   Inability to adjust to darkness

Hearing
    Adequate
    Use of hearing aid (condition, batteries)
    Need to lip-read

Thermal/tactile
    Adequate
    Altered sense of cold/hot

Mental status
    Alert
    Drowsy
    Confused
    Oriented to time, place, events
    Complaints of
        Vertigo   Orthostatic hypotension
        Altered sense of balance

Mobility
    Ability to ambulate
        Around room   Around house
        Up and down stairs   Outside house
    Ability to travel
        Drive car (date of last   Use public transportation
          reevaluation)   Get in and out of vehicles
    Devices
        Cane   Prosthesis
        Wheelchair   Condition of devices
        Walker   Competence in their use
    Shoes/slippers
        Proper fit   Nonskid soles
        Condition

Self-care activities: ability to
    Dress and undress   Use the toilet
    Groom self   Eat
    Bathe

Housekeeping activities: ability to
    Clean   Shop
    Launder clothes   Prepare food

Miscellaneous
    Drug therapy
        Type, dosage   Storage
        Labeling   Ability to self-medicate safely
    Communication: ability to
        Write   Contact emergency assistance
        Use phone
    Support system
        Help available from relatives,   Club or religious contacts
          friends, neighbors   Emergency help available
    Community resources (*e.g.,* public health nurses, homemaker service, Meals on
        Wheels)
    Public transportation

Objective Data

Assessment of Individual Function
Physical appearance (groomed, unkempt)
Gait (steady, unsteady, use of aids)
Cognitive processes
    Ability to communicate needs
    Ability to interact
    History of wandering (witnessed, reported by others)
    Assess for presence of

Anger	Withdrawal
Depression	Faulty judgment

Treatment-related activities
    Presence of barriers to performance

Lack of knowledge	Sensory deficits (visual, tactile)
Lack of resources (support system, equipment, financial)	Cognitive deficits
	Emotional deficits
Motor deficits (weakness, paralysis, amputation)	Environmental (bathroom/water not accessible)

Assessment of Family Function. (The following focuses on the assessment of the ability of the family to care for family member at home. For an assessment of the family unit, refer to assessment criteria for *Altered Family Processes*.)
Knowledge and skills
    Assess the family or caretaker for ability to perform the following safely and correctly

Treatments	Emergency treatment if appropriate
Bathing	(*e.g.,* cardiac arrest, seizures)
Medication administration	

Emotional response
    Assess the family or caretaker for the presence of

Overprotecting the person	Inability to ask for or accept relief from responsibilities
Neglect of other family members	
Neglect of other responsibilities	Unrealistic expectations of future recovery
Resentment of responsibilities	

    Assess the disabled or ill individual for the presence of

Impossible demands on time of caretaker	Lack of diversional activities
	Lack of vocational or educational pursuits
Resentment when caretaker is away	

Resources
    Assess knowledge of family or caretaker of resources available for

Emergency care	Relief from caretaking responsibilities
Equipment	
Purchase	Close relative or neighbor
Maintenance	Church group
Repair	Community agency
Financial support	Medical follow-up care

Assessment of Home Environment of Children
Presence of/Report of
    Provisions for play
        Appropriate play materials
        Safe play area (indoors, outdoors)

Special place designated for child's possessions
Stimulating environment
Selected use of television (amount, type)
Activities for age-related development (see *Altered Growth and Development*)
Family time (meal, joint activities)
Family outings
Affectionate environment
Touching, holding
Speaks with pride about child
Conversations convey positive feelings

Assessment of Housing
Type (rent, own)

Apartment	Duplex	Single family house

Appearance: presence of

Insects (flies, roaches)	Unwashed cooking equipment
Rodents/vermin	Accumulation of dirt, food
Offensive odors	wastes, or hygiene wastes

Physical facilities

Number of rooms for family members	Lighting
	Water supply
Toilet facilities (accessibility)	Sewage disposal
Heating	Garbage disposal
Ventilation	Screens
Handrails (stairs)	

Safety
Are there any adaptations that need to be made in the home for the individual?
Better communication (telephone)
Access (in and out of home, to rooms)
Bathroom (*e.g.*, grab bar, bath bench, nonskid floors)
Refer to Focus Assessment Criteria for *High Risk for Injury* for an assessment of hazards in the home.

Principles and Rationale for Nursing Care

Generic Considerations

1. Home care by professionals should be preventive, supportive, and therapeutic.
   a. *Preventive* measures include health education, home safety, and stress management.
   b. *Supportive* care can be legal, financial, nutritional, social, religious, and home-making.
   c. *Therapeutic* care involves nursing care, therapists (occupational, speech), dental, and medical.
2. Discharge planning begins at admission, with the nurse determining the anticipated needs of the person and family after discharge: the individual's self-care ability, the availability of support, homemaker services, equipment needs, community nursing services, and therapy (physical, speech, occupational).
3. The home environment must be assessed for safety prior to discharge: location of bathroom, access to water, cooking facilities, and environmental barriers (stairs, narrow doorways).
4. Community agencies can provide the opportunity for home care and allow for the person to remain at home.

5. In determining an individual's ability to care for himself at home, assess his ability to function and protect self. Consider such things as: motor deficits, sensory deficits, and mental status.

6. To assess, teach, and evaluate the individual or the family's ability to perform learned skills after discharge, use on-unit situations, whereby the person(s) takes responsibility for care, and day, overnight, or weekend leave to home. A home visit may be indicated by a nurse or a community health nurse.

7. Some families are unable to meet the home needs of ill members and require assistance. Families who are able to meet the needs of ill members should also be provided with periodic assistance or relief.

8. The effects on the life of a caretaker of a chronically ill person depend on (Goldstein, 1981):
   a. The ill person's level of disability and dependence
   b. The health and functional mobility of the caretaker
   c. The availability of assistance (type and frequency)
   d. The other responsibilities the caretaker has

9. The time and energy demands of caretaking may compete with other role responsibilities (*e.g.,* spouse, mothering, occupational).

10. Role fatigue describes the situation in which the caregiver must devote the majority of time to caregiving, thus requiring that all other roles and responsibilities be subordinated to the demands of caretaking.

11. Persons and families with cancer have certain ongoing needs that may necessitate interventions at home:
    a. Teaching needs (disease, treatment, diagnostic studies)
    b. Surgery (recovery, wound care)
    c. Coping with the diagnosis
    d. Fear of the future
    e. Treatment effects and side-effects (radiotherapy, chemotherapy)
    f. Inability to perform role responsibilities
    g. Biologic needs (disease- or treatment-related, *e.g.,* nutrition, elimination, comfort)

12. Stetz (1987) reported that spouse caregivers of individuals with cancer described the following caregiving demands (in priority):
    a. Physical care treatment regimen coping with the changes
    b. Household responsibilities, finances
    c. Witnessing the experience
    d. Fatigue, illness, change in pattern of living (*e.g.,* social life)
    e. Constant vigilance
    f. Unsatisfactory information exchange with health care provider or institution
    g. The meaning of cancer
    h. Unknown future
    i. Changes in relationship with ill spouse

13. Male caregivers experienced greater difficulty in managing the household, while female caregivers experienced greater difficulty with observing their ill mate's suffering (Stetz, 1987).

14. The following negative functional consequences of caregiving have been identified (Miller, 1990):
    a. Infringement of privacy
    b. Diminished social contact
    c. Decrease in income
    d. Increased family conflict
    e. Life void of personal activities

    f. Increased use of alcohol and/or psychotropic drugs

    g. Loss of job

    h. Chronic fatigue, anger, anxiety, depression

    i. Poorer physical health

15. Ory, Williams, and Emr (1985) identified positive functional consequences of caregiving as:

    a. Drawing family closer

    b. Financial assistance

    c. Companionship

    d. Feelings of increased self-worth

    e. Improved relationships

    f. Broader perspective on life

Pediatric Considerations

1. Children are dependent on family members for managing home care (Foster, 1989).
2. Trends in the treatment of children with chronic illness or disability include home care, early discharge, focus on the developmental age of the child, and assessment of the strengths and uniqueness of the child (Whaley & Wong, 1989).
3. Interventions are geared toward the family as a whole rather than merely toward the ill child (Foster, 1989).
4. High-risk graduates of neonatal intensive care units require technically complex home care. Discharge is planned as early as possible for cost containment and to help reduce the adverse effects of hospitalization on the infant and the family system (Baker, Kuhlmann, & Magliaro, 1989).

Gerontologic Considerations

1. Older persons have a greater incidence of chronic disease, impaired function, diminished economic resources, and a smaller social network than do younger persons (Arling, 1987; Matteson & McConnell, 1988).
2. After age 75, most elderly persons living in the community live alone. Of older people living alone, 60% own a home (Matteson & McConnell, 1988).
3. Functional ability includes activities of daily living (ADLs) and also instrumental activities of daily living (IADLs)—those skills needed to live independently, *e.g.*, procuring food, cooking, using the telephone, housekeeping, and handling finances. IADLs are integrally connected to physical and cognitive abilities (Kane & Kane, 1981; Kane, Orslander, & Abrass, 1984; Matteson & McConnell, 1988). The elderly person who lives alone is at great risk of being institutionalized if he cannot perform IADLs. There is a great possibility that there is no social network to meet these deficits (Hogstel, 1990).
4. Approximately 9 of 10 older persons have one or more chronic health problems with differing affects on function (Hogstel, 1990).
5. Chronic conditions cause approximately 6 of 10 persons over age 75 to limit their ADLs (Hogstel, 1990).
6. Along with diminished cognitive and/or physical ability, the older individual frequently has diminished financial resources, sporadic kin, or neighborhood social supports. The person also may live in substandard housing or housing that does not allow simple adaptation to meet individual physical or cognitive deficits (Matteson & McConnell, 1988; Schank & Lough, 1990).
7. About 30% of older persons living alone or with unrelated individuals have incomes below the poverty level ($4979 per year). This limits ability to hire others to assist with even minimal deficits (Matteson & McConnell, 1988; US Senate, 1987–1988).

8. In some cultures and some family structures, older adults can seek assistance in some areas of home management and still retain a feeling of independence. These individuals have determined that by choosing selective resources to meet their needs, they will be able to maintain independent living for a longer period of time (Arling, 1987; Schank & Lough, 1990).

◼ Impaired Home Maintenance Management
Related to (Specify)

Statement Examples: **Inability to Perform Household Activities Secondary to Postmyocardial Infarction**
Inability to Perform Home Activities Secondary to Impaired Vision

Assessment
Refer to Defining Characteristics

Outcome Criteria

The person or caretaker will
• Identify factors that restrict self-care and home management
• Demonstrate the ability to perform skills necessary for the care of the individual or home
• Express satisfaction with home situation

Interventions
The following interventions apply to many individuals with impaired home management, regardless of etiology.

A. Assess for causative or contributing factors
   1. Lack of knowledge
   2. Insufficient funds
   3. Lack of necessary equipment or aids
   4. Inability to perform household activities (illness, sensory deficits, motor deficits)
   5. Impaired cognitive functioning
   6. Impaired emotional functioning

B. Reduce or eliminate causative or contributing factors if possible
   1. Lack of knowledge for home care
      a. Determine with the person and family the information needed to be taught and learned.

- Monitoring skills needed (pulse, circulation, urine)
- Medication administration (procedure, side-effects, precautions)
- Treatment/procedures
- Equipment use/maintenance
- Safety issues (*e.g.,* environmental)
- Community resources
- Follow-up care
- Anticipatory guidance (*e.g.,* emotional and social needs of family, alternatives to home care)

  b. Initiate the teaching and give detailed written instruction.
  c. Refer to a community nursing agency for follow-up.
2. Lack of necessary equipment or aids
  a. Determine the type of equipment needed, considering availability, cost, and durability.
  b. Seek assistance from agencies that rent or loan supplies.
    - Teach the care and maintenance of supplies that increase length of use.
    - Consider adapting equipment to reduce cost.
3. Insufficient funds
  a. Consult with social service department for assistance.
  b. Consult with service organizations for assistance.
    - American Heart Association
    - The Lung Association
    - American Cancer Society
4. Inability to perform household activities
  a. Determine the type of assistance needed (*e.g.,* meals, housework, transportation) and assist the individual to obtain them.
    - Meals
        Discuss with relatives the possibility of freezing complete meals that require only heating (*e.g.,* small containers of soup, stew, casseroles).
        Determine the availability of meal services for ill persons (Meals on Wheels, church groups).
        Teach persons about foods that are easily prepared and nutritious (*e.g.,* hardboiled eggs).
    - Housework
        Contract with an adolescent for light housekeeping.
        Refer to community agency for assistance.
    - Transportation
        Determine the availability of transportation for shopping and health care.
        Request rides with neighbors to places they drive routinely.
5. Impaired mental processes
  a. Assess the ability of the individual to safely maintain a household.
  b. Refer to *High Risk for Injury* related to lack of awareness of hazards.
  c. Initiate appropriate referrals.
6. Impaired emotional functioning
  a. Assess the severity of the dysfunction.
  b. Refer to *Ineffective Individual Coping* for additional assessment and interventions.

C. Provide anticipatory guidance

1. Discuss the implications of caring for a chronically ill family member.
  a. Amount of time

      b. Effects on other role responsibilities (spouse, children, job)

      c. Physical requirements (lifting)

  2. Share alternatives to reduce strain and fatigue of caretaking responsibilities.

      a. Acquire relief from responsibilities at least twice a week for at least 3 hours (sitter, neighbors, relatives).

      b. Enlist the aid of others to meet some of the needs of the ill person (hairdresser, transporting to physician's office).

      c. Plan to utilize at least 1 hour a day as leisure time (*e.g.*, after ill person is asleep).

      d. Maintain contacts with friends and relatives even if only by phone; let friends know that you do use sitters so they can include you in some social activities.

      e. Allow the caretaker opportunities to share problems and feelings.

  3. Commend caregivers for their concern, diligence, and perseverance in caring for the loved one at home.

D. Initiate health teaching and referrals as indicated

  1. Refer to support groups (*e.g.*, stroke club, local Alzheimer's Association, American Cancer Society).

  2. Refer to community nursing agency.

  3. Refer to community agencies (*e.g.*, volunteer visitors, meal programs, homemakers, adult day care).

References/Bibliography

Archbold, P. (1980). Impact of parent caring on middle-aged offspring. *Gerontology Nursing, 6,* 60.

Arling, G. (1987). Strain, social support and distress in old age. *Journal of Gerontology, 42*(1), 107–113.

Baker, K., Kuhlmann, T., & Magliaro, B. (1989). Homebound. *Nursing Clinics of North America, 24*(3), 655–664.

Coyle, N. (1985). A cancer centers outreach . . . maintain these patients at home, Sloan-Kettering. *American Journal of Nursing, 85*(5), 590, 594.

Davis, A. J. (1980). Disability, home care, and the caretaking role in family life. *Journal of Advanced Nursing, 5,* 475–484.

Dewis, M. E. (1990). The older dyadic family unit and chronic illness. *Home Healthcare Nurse, 8*(2), 42–48.

Edstrom, S., & Miller, M. W. (1981). Preparing the family to care for the cancer patient at home: A home care course. *Cancer Nursing, 4,* 49–52.

Fitting, M., Rabins, P., Lucas, M. J., & Eastham, J. (1986). Caregivers for dementia patients: A comparison of husbands and wives. *Gerontologist, 26,* 248–252.

Fortinsky, R., Granger, C. V., & Seltzer, G. B. (1981). The use of functional assessment in understanding home care needs. *Medical Care, 19,* 489–497.

Foster, R. L. (1989). Principles and strategies of home care. In Foster, R. L., Hunsberger, M. M., & Anderson, J. J. T. (Eds.). *Family-centered nursing care of children.* Philadelphia: W. B. Saunders.

Goldstein, V. (1981). Caretaker role fatigue. *Nursing Outlook, 29,* 23–30.

Googe, M., & Varricchio, C. (1981). A pilot investigation of home health care needs of cancer patients and their families. *Oncology Nursing Forum, 8*(3), 24–28.

Harrell, J. S., McConnell, E. S., Wildman, D. S., & Samsa, G. P. (1989). Do nursing diagnoses affect functional status? *Journal of Gerontological Nursing, 15*(10), 13–19.

Heller, B. R., Walsh, F. J., & Wilson, K. M. (1981). Seniors helping seniors: Training older adults as new personnel resources in home health care. *Journal of Gerontological Nursing, 7,* 552–555.

Hogstel, M. O. (1990). *Geropsychiatric nursing.* St. Louis: C. V. Mosby.

Jelneck, L. J. (1977). The special needs of the adolescent with chronic illness. *Maternal-Child Nursing Journal, 2,* 57–61.

Kane, R. A., & Kane, R. L. (1981). *Assessing the elderly: A practical guide to measurement.* Lexington MA: Lexington Books.

Kane, R. L., Orslander, J. G., & Abrass, I. B. (1984). *Essentials of clinical geriatrics.* New York: McGraw-Hill.

Klopovich, P., Suenram, D., & Cairns, N. (1980). A common sense approach to caring for children with cancer: The community health care nurse. *Cancer Nursing, 3,* 201–208.

Mailick, M. (1979). The impact of severe illness of the individual and family: An overview. *Social Work Health Care, 5,* 117–128.

Matteson, M. A., & McConnell, E. S. (1988). *Gerontological nursing.* Philadelphia: W. B. Saunders.

Miller, C. A. (1990). *Nursing care of older adults.* Glenview, IL: Scott, Foresman.

Ory, M. G., Williams, T. F., & Emr, M. (1985). Families, informal supports and Alzheimer Disease. *Research on Aging, 7*(4), 623–644.

Pappas, J. P. (1983). Strategic planning for home health care. *Caring, 4*(10), 24–25, 27–29.

Schank, M. J., & Lough, M. A. (1990). Profile: Frail elderly women, maintaining independence. *Journal of Advanced Nursing, 15,* 674–682.

Schmidt, M. D. (1983). Meet the health care needs of older adults by using a chronic care model in the home setting. *Journal of Gerontological Nursing, 11*(9).

Stetz, K. M. (1987). Caregiving demands during advanced cancer—The spouse's needs. *Cancer Nursing, 10*(5), 260–268.

Symposium on community health/home care. (1988). *Nursing Clinics of North America, 23*(1).

US Senate Special Committee on Aging: *Aging America: Trends and projections 1987–1988.* Washington DC: Department of Health and Human Services.

Walsh, J., Persons, C. B., & Wieck, L. (1987). *Manual of home health care.* Philadelphia: J. B. Lippincott.

Whaley, L. F., & Wong, D. L. (1989). *Essentials of pediatric nursing* (3rd ed.). St. Louis: C. V. Mosby.

White, H. A., & Briggs, A. M. (1980). Home care of persons with respiratory problems. *Topics in Clinical Nursing, 2*(4), 69–77.

Resources for the Consumer

Literature

Aronson, M. K. (1988). *Understanding Alzheimer's disease.* New York: Charles Scribner's Sons.

Cohen, D., & Eisdorfer, C. (1986). *The loss of self.* New York: NAL Penguin.

Mace, N. L., & Rabins, P. V. (1981). *The 36-hour day.* New York: Warner.

Organizations

Alzheimer's Disease and Related Disorders Association, 70 East Lake Street, Chicago, IL 60601-5997

American Cancer Society, 90 Park Avenue, New York, NY 10016

American Parkinson Disease Association, 116 John Street, New York, NY 10038

National Multiple Sclerosis Society, 205 East 42nd Street, New York, NY 10017

National Parkinson Foundation, 1591 N.A. Ninth Avenue, Miami, FL 31316

National Spinal Cord Injury Association, 369 Elliot Street, Newton Upper Falls, MA 02164

Hopelessness

DEFINITION
Hopelessness: A sustained subjective emotional state in which an individual sees no alternatives or personal choices available to solve problems or to achieve what is desired and cannot mobilize energy on own behalf to establish goals.

DEFINING CHARACTERISTICS

Major (must be present)
Expresses profound, overwhelming, sustained apathy in response to a situation perceived as impossible with no solutions (overt or covert).
Examples of expressions are:
"I might as well give up because I can't make things better."
"My future seems awful to me."
"I can't imagine what my life will be like in 10 years."
"I've never been given a break, so why should I in the future?"
"Life looks unpleasant when I think ahead."
"I know I'll never get what I really want."
"Things never work out how I want them to."
"It's foolish to want or get anything because I never do."
"It's unlikely I'll get satisfaction in the future."
"The future seems vague and uncertain."
Physiologic
Slowed responses to stimuli
Lack of energy
Increased sleep
Emotional
The hopeless person often has difficulty experiencing feelings, but may feel:
Unable to seek good fortune, luck, or God's favor
A lack of meaning or purpose in life
"Empty or drained"
A sense of loss and deprivation
Helpless
Incompetent
Person exhibits
Passiveness
Decreased verbalization
Lack of ambition, initiative, and interest
"Giving up–given up complex"
Inability to accomplish anything
Pessimism
Impaired interpersonal relationship
Slowed thought processes
Does not take responsibility for own decisions and life

Cognitive

    Decreased problem-solving and decision-making capabilities

    Deals with past and future, not here and now

    Decreased flexibility in thought processes

    Rigid (*e.g.,* all or none thinking)

    Lacks imagination and wishing capabilities

    Unable to identify and/or accomplish desired objectives and goals

    Unable to plan, organize, or make decisions

    Unable to recognize sources of hope

    Suicidal thoughts

Minor (may be present)

Physiologic

    Anorexia

    Weight loss

Emotional

    Person feels:

        "A lump in his throat"

        Discouraged with self and others

        "At the end of his rope"

        Tense

        Helpless

        Overwhelmed (feels he just "can't . . . ")

        Loss of gratification from roles and relationships

        Vulnerable

    Person exhibits

        Poor eye contact; turns away from speaker; shrugs in response to speaker

        Apathy (decreased response to internal and external stimuli)

        Decreased motivation

        Despondency

        Sighing

        Social withdrawal

        Lack of involvement in self-care (may be cooperative in nursing care but offers little help to self)

        Regression

        Resignation

        Depression

Cognitive

    Decreased ability to integrate information received

    Loss of time perception for past, present, and future

    Decreased ability to recall from the past

    Confusion

    Decreased ability to communicate effectively

    Distorted thought perceptions and associations

    Unreasonable judgment

RELATED FACTORS

Pathophysiologic

Any chronic and/or terminal illness can cause or contribute to hopelessness (*e.g.,* heart disease, kidney disease, cancer, AIDS).

Associated factors include:
    Failing or deteriorating physiologic condition
    Impaired body image
    New and unexpected signs or symptoms of previous disease process
    Prolonged pain, discomfort, weakness
    Impaired functional abilities (walking, elimination, eating)

Treatment-related

Prolonged treatments (*e.g.*, chemotherapy, radiation) that cause discomfort
Prolonged treatments with no positive results
Treatments that alter body image (*e.g.*, surgery, chemotherapy)
Prolonged diagnostic studies that yield no significant results
Prolonged dependence on equipment for life support (*e.g.*, dialysis, respirator)
Prolonged dependence on equipment for monitoring bodily functions (*e.g.*, telemetry)

Situational

Prolonged activity restriction (*e.g.*, fractures, spinal cord injury)
Prolonged isolation due to disease processes (*e.g.*, infectious diseases, reverse isolation for suppressed immune system)
Separation from significant others (parents, spouse, children, others)
Inability to achieve goals in life that one values (marriage, education, children)
Inability to participate in activities one desires (walking, sports, work)
Loss of something or someone valued (spouse, children, friend, financial resources)
Prolonged caretaking responsibilities (spouse, child, parent)
Exposure to long-term physiologic or psychologic stress
Loss of belief in transcendent values/God

Maturational

Child
Loss of caregiver
Loss of trust in significant other (parents, sibling)
Abandonment by caregivers
Loss of autonomy related to illness (*e.g.*, fracture)
Loss of bodily functions
Inability to achieve developmental tasks (trust, autonomy, initiative, industry)

Adolescent
Loss of significant other (peer, family)
Loss of bodily functions
Change in body image
Inability to achieve developmental task (role identity)

Adult
Impaired bodily functions, loss of body part
Impaired relationships (separation, divorce)
Loss of job, career
Loss of significant others (death of children, spouse)
Inability to achieve developmental tasks (intimacy, commitment, productiveness)

Elderly
Sensory deficits
Motor deficits
Loss of independence

Loss of significant others, things
Inability to achieve developmental tasks (integrity)

Diagnostic Considerations

Hopelessness describes a person who sees no possibility that his or her life will improve and maintains that no one can do anything to help. *Hopelessness* differs from *Powerlessness*, in that a hopeless person sees no solution to his problem and/or no way to achieve what is desired, even if he feels in control of his life. In contrast, a powerless person may see an alternative or answer to the problem, yet be unable to do anything about it due to lack of control and/or resources. Sustained feelings of powerlessness may lead to hopelessness. Hopelessness is commonly related to grief, depression, and suicide. For a person at risk for suicide, the nurse also should use the diagnosis *High Risk for Self-Harm.*

Errors In Diagnostic Statements

Hopelessness related to AIDS

This diagnostic statement does not describe a situation that the nurse can treat. The statement should include specific factors that the person has identified as overwhelming, as in the following diagnostic statement: *Hopelessness related to recent diagnosis of AIDS and rejection by parents.*

Focus Assessment Criteria

Hopelessness is a subjective emotional state in which the nurse must validate with the individual. Emotional and cognitive areas must be assessed carefully by the nurse to make the inference that the person is experiencing hopelessness. Some of these same cues may be seen in persons with diagnoses of *Social Isolation, Powerlessness, Self-Concept Disturbance,* and/or *Spiritual Distress.*

Subjective Data

1. Presence of illness and/or treatment
   a. Chronic, prolonged, deteriorating, exhausting
2. Activities of daily living
   a. Exercise: amount, type
   b. Sleep: time, amount, quality
   c. Hobbies: self-interest activities
   d. Self-care participation
   e. Appetite: eating habits
3. Energy and motivation
   a. Does the person feel exhausted, tired?
   b. Does the person have any goals or desires?
   c. What are these goals and desires? Are they realistic?
   d. Does this person feel he can achieve them?
   e. Does this person feel overwhelmed?
   f. What does he feel he can achieve?
   g. Does he express an interest in self-care?
   h. Does he express an interest in social activities?
   i. Does he express an interest in any activities?

4. Meaning and purpose in life
   a. What does this person value most in life? Why?
   b. Is he able to achieve this value?
   c. What does this person describe as his purpose and/or role in life?
   d. Is this purpose/role fulfilled?
   e. What in life has the most meaning to this person?
   f. Is this available to this person at this time?
   g. Are his perceptions of his meaning and purpose realistic and/or achievable?
   h. What kind of relationship does he have with God or a higher being?
   i. Does this relationship give meaning or purpose to his life?
5. Choice and/or control in situations
   a. What does he perceive as his most difficult problem? Why?
   b. What does he feel the solution to the problem is? Is this solution realistic?
   c. What kind of problem-solving and/or decision-making skills does this person have? Planning skills? Organizing skills?
   d. Is his perception of the problem distorted? If so, how?
   e. Have other alternatives to his problem been considered and/or tried?
   f. Does this person feel he has any controlling influence in the situation?
   g. How flexible or rigid are this person's thought processes?
6. Future options
   a. What does the person believe the future will bring? Negative or positive things?
   b. Does this person look forward to the future? What does he say about his past?
   c. What does he see as worth living for?
   d. How does the future look to this person?
   e. How does this person perceive his present illness? Its effect on his life? Its effect on his relationships?
   f. How does this person perceive his current treatments for his illness? Promising, or stressful and useless?
   g. Does this person recognize any sources of hope?
   h. Does this person have any wishes or dreams?
   i. What does he want most in life?
   j. Does this person have suicidal thoughts? If so, explore why.
7. Significant relationships
   a. Who does this person perceive as the most significant other in his life?
   b. What is this person's current relationship with this significant other person?
   c. What are this person's feelings toward this significant other now?
   d. Is this relationship currently pleasing and/or helpful to this person?
   e. Does this person have contact with this significant other now?
   f. Has divorce or death of spouse, or death of child, sibling, friend, pet, occurred recently?
   g. Has this person moved away from significant others recently?

Objective Data
General appearance
- Grooming
- Posture
- Eye contact
- Speed of activities

Principles and Rationale for Nursing Care

Generic Considerations

Hope

1. Hope is a multidimensional dynamic human attribute (Notwotny, 1989).
2. Hope is an unconscious cognitive behavior that energizes and allows one to act, achieve, and use crisis as an opportunity for growth. It activates the motivation system and defends against despair (Korner, 1970).
3. Hope is closely related to confidence, wishing, faith, inspiration, determination, choice, and autonomy.
4. Although wishing and hoping are related, a person may not be committed to his wishes but may be committed to his hoped-for events. Therefore, giving up hope is more harmful than giving up a wish. Hope is more rational and logical than wishing (Korner, 1970).
5. A hopeful person has realistic desires that he feels will in some way improve his life when they occur.
6. Hope is future- and reality-oriented. A hopeful person wants a desired change in his current life. He feels that change is possible and that there is a way out of his difficulties.
7. Early childhood experiences influence a person's ability to hope. A person learns to hope if a trusting environment is promoted.
8. Hope is related to faith because many people experience hope by recognizing their reliance on higher powers to restore meaning and purpose in their lives.
9. Hope is related to help from others, in that a person feels his external resources may be supportive to him when his internal resources and strengths seem insufficient to cope with a situation (*e.g.*, a family and/or significant other is often a source of hope).
10. Watson (1979) has identified hope as both a curative and a "carative" factor in nursing. Hope, along with faith and trust, provides psychic energy to draw upon to aid in the curative process.
11. It has been observed that hope prolongs life in critical survival conditions, while a loss of hope often results in death (Korner, 1970).
12. A hoping person feels autonomous in making decisions about choices open to him.
13. Hope can be shared, but this involves close human relationships, trust, and understanding.
14. Kübler-Ross (1975) observed that those who expressed hope coped more effectively during their difficult dying periods. She also noted that death occurred soon after these individuals stopped expressing hope.
15. Hope helps a person to feel whole.
16. Maintaining family role responsibilities is essential for hope and coping (Herth, 1989). In addition, the hope concept is essential for families of the critically ill to facilitate coping and adjustment (Coulter, 1989).
17. A person's level of hope is directly related to his level of coping and vice versa (Herth, 1989).
18. Hope directly influences survival, response to therapy, and the quality of life (Engel, 1989).
19. According to Hickey (1986), "hope enables the living to continue on and the dying to die better."
20. Nurses are in a unique position to encourage hope within the patient and family (Hickey, 1986).

21. Nowotny (1989) identified six dimensions of hope: confidence in outcome, possibility of a future, relating to others, spiritual beliefs, emergence from within, and active involvement.
22. Owen (1989) found hopeful cancer patients able to set goals, be optimistic, redefine the future, find meaning in life, feel peaceful, and give out or use energy.
23. Miller (1989) studied sixty critical ill patients to determine hope-inspiring strategies; findings included:
    a. Thinking to buffer threatening perceptions
    b. Positive thinking
    c. Feelings that life has meaning and growth results from crises
    d. Beliefs and practices enabling transcendence of suffering
    e. Receiving from caregivers a constructive view of patient, expectations of patient's ability to manage difficulty, and confidence in therapy
    f. Sustaining relationships with loved ones
    g. Perception that one's knowledge and actions can affect an outcome
    h. Having desired activities and outcomes to attain
    i. Other specific coping behaviors that thwarted feelings of despair, including distraction and humor

Hopelessness

1. Hopelessness is an emotional state in which a person feels that life is too much to handle—that it is impossible. A person who lacks hope sees no possibility that his life will improve and no solution to problems. He believes that neither he nor others can do anything to help.
2. Hopelessness is related to despair, helplessness, doubt, grief, apathy, sadness, depression, and suicide.
3. A hospitalized person is often depressed but not necessarily hopeless.
4. It has been observed that hope reflected in clients' drawings has a direct relationship to the clients' improvement, whereas a lack of hope is related to recurrence of disease. Therefore, a nurse can be helpful to clients in finding their resources of hope. The presence of cancer has been significantly predicted in individuals on the basis of identifying the presence of hopelessness in the person's life prior to the diagnosis of cancer. Therefore, terminal illness may result in hopelessness, and a life state of hopelessness may result in terminal illness (Schmale & Iher, 1966).
5. Hopelessness results in three basic categories of feelings:
    a. Sense of the impossible; what the person feels he must do, he cannot; he feels trapped
    b. Overwhelmed; tasks and others are perceived as too big and difficult to handle and the self is perceived as small
    c. Apathy; the person has no goals; no sense of purpose
6. A person experiencing hopelessness cannot imagine anything that can be done or is worth doing, nor can he imagine beyond what is currently occurring.
7. Hopeless persons lack internal resources or strengths (*e.g.*, autonomy, self-esteem, integrity) to draw upon. Regardless of age, they reach outside themselves for help because their internal resources may be depleted.
8. Some degree of hopelessness is involved in everyone's life. It occurs in various forms and is a more common and usual feeling than reported (*e.g.*, we all must die; it is hopeless to hope for anything else).
9. Hopelessness is most often observed in those who are rigid and inflexible in their thoughts, feelings, and actions.

10. Often people have ideals that are hopeless in reality (*e.g.,* not to die, we can trust everyone, all people should always act appropriately).
11. If hopelessness is recognized and dealt with imaginatively, it can result in movement, growth, and resourcefulness. Rigidity never overcomes hopelessness.
12. A person can cope with a part of his life he views as hopeless if he is able to realize that there are other factors in his life that are hopeful. For example, a person may realize he may never walk again, yet he will be able to go home and be in the company of his grandchildren and move around. Therefore, hopelessness can lead to the discovery of alternatives that provide meaning and purpose in life. It is essential to keep hopelessness out of the way of hope.
13. Motivation is essential in the recovery process of hopelessness. The client must determine a goal even if he has low expectations of achieving it. The nurse is the catalyst to encourage the client to take the first step to identify a goal. After this is accomplished, another goal must be created.
14. The health care team must be hopeful if the client is to be hopeful; otherwise, the client views all efforts of the team as a waste of time.
15. The more the client believes he can attain a goal, the more important that goal becomes in providing hope for the client.
16. The nurse mobilizes the client's internal and external resources to strengthen his hope, motivation, and will to live.
17. Engel (1989) identified the "giving up–given up" complex as having five characteristics:
    a. Feeling of giving up experienced as helplessness or hopelessness
    b. Depreciated image of the self
    c. Sense of loss of gratification from relationships or roles
    d. Feeling of disruption
    e. Reactivation of memories of earlier periods of giving up
    Engel proposed that this state of coping activates neurally regulated biologic emergency patterns, which may decrease one's capacity to fight off pathogenic processes. Therefore, this "giving up–given up" complex" is a contributing factor for development of disease.
18. Often when a person's internal and external resources are exhausted, he relies on his relationship with God for hope. He may feel more secure in placing hope in God than in other people or himself. Hoping in God may not mean an abrupt end to crisis, but gives the person a sense of God's control of circumstances and ability to support a person during this time. Meaning and purpose for life and suffering may be found in a client's relationship with God and the knowledge of His control. Hope for a client's future may depend on his perception of a promise of eternal fellowship with God that continues after this present life on earth ends. With this eternal relationship with God comes the belief in God's promise to end all suffering and restore harmonious relationships—man with God, himself, and others.

Pediatric Considerations

1. Hope may be fostered in children by conveying a sense of friendliness, trust, warmth, loyalty, and committment (Ranking, 1987).
2. Families of children with life-threatening diseases may feel hopeless and become dysfunctional. The nurse may need to identify dysfunctional family interactions, use strategies from family therapy, and/or make appropriate referrals (Heiney, 1988).
3. Hinds (1984) introduced a definition of hope for adolescents through the use of

grounded theory methodology. Hope was defined as the degree to which an adolescent believes that a personal tomorrow exists.

4. To achieve adulthood, an adolescent must first achieve hopefulness. Hinds and Martin (1988) found that adolescents with cancer progress through four sequential self-sustaining phases to cope and achieve hopefulness:
   a. Cognitive discomfort
   b. Distraction
   c. Cognitive comfort
   d. Personal competence
   These phases have implications for nurses in planning appropriate strategies to assist the adolescent achieve hopefulness.
5. Hinds (1988) identified that adolescent hopefulness differs from adult's hopefulness in that adolescents experience a wider range or greater intensity of hopefulness. In addition, adolescents generally focus on hope for others and believe in the value of forced effort; that is, identifying an area of hope and fostering it.
6. Nursing interventions that have been found to influence hopefulness in adolescents include truthful explanations, doing something with them, nursing knowledge of survivors, caring behaviors, focusing on future, competency, and conversing about less sensitive areas. In addition, humor has been identified as promoting cognitive distraction and facilitating hope. Nursing interventions that inhibit cognitive distraction, such as focusing on nursing tasks and on negative adolescent behaviors, promote hopelessness (Hinds, Martin, & Vogel, 1987).

Gerontologic Considerations

1. The elderly are at risk for hopelessness due to the numerous psychosocial and physiologic changes that are part of the normal aging process. These changes often are perceived as losses. The elderly also have decreased energy, which is necessary for hopefulness (Busse & Pfeiffer, 1969).
2. Healthy coping in the elderly is related to the acquisition of developmental resources in later adulthood. The elderly must learn to give up less useful operations and acquire more effective resources to deal with life changes, which is part of the aging process (Reed, 1986).
3. Stressors for elderly persons are unique and differ from those of other age groups. These include changes in personal care, longing for missing children or grandchildren, fear of being a victim of crime, and fear of being taken advantage of by the system (Stokes & Gordon, 1988). The nurse may be able to assist the elderly client with identifying these stressors and locating resources to assist the elderly and prevent hopelessness.

■ Hopelessness
Related to (Specify)

Assessment
See Defining Characteristics

Outcome Criteria

Short Term
The person will
- Share suffering openly and constructively with others
- Reminisce and review his life positively
- Consider his values and the meaning of life
- Express feelings of optimism about the present
- Express confidence in a desired outcome and goals
- Express confidence in self and others
- Practice energy conservation

Long Term
- The person will demonstrate an increase in energy level as evidenced by activities (*i.e.,* self-care, exercise, hobbies, etc.)
- Express positive expectations about the future
- Demonstrate initiative, self-direction, and autonomy in decision-making and problem-solving
- Make statements similar to the following:
   "I am looking forward to ..."
   "When things are not so good, it helps me to think of ..."
   "I have enough time to do what I want."
   "There are more good times ahead."
   "I expect to succeed in ..."
   "I expect to get more out of the good things in life."
   "My past experiences have helped me be prepared for my future."
   "In the future, I'll be happier."
   "I have faith in the future."
- Develop, improve, and maintain positive relationships with others
- Participate in a significant role
- Expresses spiritual beliefs
- Redefine the future and set realistic goals
- Exhibits peace and comfort with situation

Interventions

A. Assist the person to identify and express feelings

1. Listen actively and treat the person as an individual.
2. Convey empathy to promote verbalization of doubts, fears, and concerns.
3. Validate and reflect impressions with the person.
4. Accept the person's feelings (*i.e.,* trust his will to live if it exists, accept his anger).
5. Encourage the person to verbalize why and how hope is significant in his life.
6. Encourage expressions of how hope is uncertain in his life and areas in which hope has failed him.
7. Assist the person to recognize that hopelessness is a part of everyone's life that demands recognition. It can be utilized as a source of energy, imagination, and freedom that encourages a person to consider alternate choices. It leads to self-discovery.

8. Assist the person to understand that he can deal with the hopeless aspects of his life by separating them from the hopeful aspects. Help the person identify areas of hopelessness in his life and acknowledge them. Help him to distinguish between the possible and the impossible. The nurse mobilizes a client's internal and external resources in order to promote hope as follows. Assist clients to identify their own personal reasons for living.

B. Assess and mobilize the person's internal resources (autonomy, independence, rationale, cognitive thinking, flexibility, spirituality)

1. Emphasize the client's strengths, not weaknesses.
2. Compliment the client on appearance and/or efforts when appropriate.
3. Promote motivation by:
   a. Identifying client's values and interests
   b. Identifying client's areas of success and usefulness; emphasize his past accomplishments. Use this information to develop goals with the client
   c. Assist clients to identify things they have fun doing and things they perceive as humorous. This can serve as a distraction to discomfort and allow the client to move on to cognitive comfort (Hinds & Martin, 1988).
   d. Assist the client to identify sources of hope (*i.e.*, relationships, faith, things to accomplish).
   e. Assist the client to develop realistic short-term and long-term goals (progress from simple to more complex; may use a "goals poster" to indicate type and time for achieving specific goals).
   f. Teach the client to monitor specific signs of progress to use as self-reinforcement.
   g. Encourage "means–end" thinking in positive terms (*i.e.*, If I do this and . . . , then I'll be able to . . .).
4. Assist the client with problem-solving and decision-making (See Appendix VII).
   a. Respect the client as a competent decision-maker; treat his decisions and desires with respect.
   b. Encourage verbalization to determine the client's perception of choices.
   c. Clarify and modify the client's perceptions of reality.
   d. Correct misinformation.
   e. Assist the client to identify those problems he cannot resolve to advance to problems he can resolve. In other words, assist the client to move away from dwelling on the impossible and hopeless and to begin to deal with matters that are realistic and hopeful.
   f. Assess the client's perceptions of self and others in relation to size. (This person often perceives others in the world as large and difficult to deal with and perceives himself as small.) If his perceptions are unrealistic, assist him to reassess them in order to restore proper size to his world.
   g. Promote flexibility. Encourage the client to try alternatives and take risks.
   h. Teach and support the client to use rational inquiry (to seek more information).
5. Assist the client to learn effective coping skills.
   a. Assist the client with setting realistic attainable goals.
   b. Teach the client the importance of mutuality in sharing concerns.
   c. Explain the benefits of distraction from negative events.
   d. Teach the client the value of confronting issues.

   e. Teach and assist patient relaxation techniques (see Appendix X) prior to anticipated stressful events.
   f. Encourage mental imagery to promote positive thought processes (see Appendix X).
   g. Allow the client time to reminisce to gain insight into past experiences.
   h. Teach the client to "hope to be" the best person possible today and to appreciate the fullness of each moment.
   i. Teach the client to maximize esthetic experiences (*e.g.*, smell of coffee, back rub, or feeling the warmth of the sun or a breeze).
   j. Teach the client to anticipate experiences he takes delight in each day (*e.g.*, walking, reading favorite book, writing letter).
   k. Assist client in expressing spiritual beliefs.
   l. Teach the client ways to conserve and generate energy.

C. Assess and mobilize person's external resources (significant others, health care team, support groups, God and/or higher powers)
   1. Family and/or significant others
      a. Involve family and/or significant others in plan of care.
      b. Encourage family to express their love and need for the person.
      c. Emphasize the importance of sustaining and supportive positive relationships.
      d. Foster and encourage the client to spend increased time and/or thoughts with loved ones in healthy relationships.
      e. Teach the family their role in sustaining hope.
      f. Convey hope, information, and confidence to family as their feelings will be conveyed to the client.
      g. Discuss the client's meaningful goals with family.
      h. Utilize touch and closeness with the client to demonstrate to the family that this is acceptable (provide privacy).
      i. Help the client to recognize that he is loved, cared about, and important to the lives of others regardless of his failing health.
      j. Use and emphasize family strengths of endurance, courage, and patience.
   2. Health care team
      a. Develop positive-trusting nurse-client relationship by:
         • Answering questions
         • Respecting client's feelings
         • Providing consistent care
         • Following through on requests
         • Touch
         • Providing comfort
         • Honesty
      b. Convey attitude of "We care too much about you to let you just give up" and/or "I can help you."
      c. Hold conferences and share client's goals with staff.
      d. Provide staff support groups, use team care conferences.
      e. Encourage the client to use and work with the health care team to cope with problems.
      f. Share advances in technology and research for treatment of diseases.
   3. Support groups
      a. Encourage person to share concerns with others who have had similar

problem and/or disease and have had positive experiences from coping effectively with it.

    b. Provide information on self-help groups (*i.e.,* "Make today count"—40 chapters in US and Canada; "I can cope"—series for cancer patients; "We Can Weekend"—for families of cancer patients).

    c. Initiate referrals when indicated.

  4. God and/or higher powers

    a. Assess belief support system (value, past experiences with, religious activities, relationship with God, meaning and purpose of prayer; refer to *Spiritual Distress*).

    b. Create environment in which client feels free to express self spiritually.

    c. Acknowledge the client's belief system.

    d. Allow the client time and opportunities to reflect on the meaning of suffering, death, and dying.

    e. Accept, respect, and support the patient's hope in God.

D. Identify the individual at risk for self-harm (Refer to *High Risk for Self-harm*)

E. Initiate referrals as indicated

  1. Counseling

    a. Spiritual

    b. Family

  2. Crisis hot line

References/Bibliography

Beck, A. T., & Weissman, A. (1972). The measurement of pessimism: The hopelessness scale. *Journal of Consulting and Clinical Psychology, 42*(6), 861–865.

Beck, M. B., Rawlins, R. P., & Williams S. R. (1984). *Mental health psychiatric nursing, a holistic life-cycle approach.* St Louis: C. V. Mosby.

Buehler, J. A. (1975). What contributes to hope in the cancer patient? *American Journal of Nursing, 75,* 1353–1356.

Busse, E., & Pfeiffer, E. (1969). *Behavior and adaptation in later life.* Boston: Little, Brown.

Bruss, C. R. (1988). Nursing diagnoses of hopelessness. *Journal of Psychosocial Nursing, 26*(3), 28–31.

Coulter, M. A. (1989). The needs of family members of patients in intensive care units. *Intensive Care Nursing, 5,* 4–10.

Dubree, M., & Vogelpohl, R. (1980). When hope dies—so might the patient. *American Journal of Nursing, 80,* 2046–2049.

Ellerhurst, A. & Ryan, B. (1987). Oncology nurses: Enablers of hope. *Ohio Nurses Review, 9*(3), 10–12.

Engel, G. (1989). A life setting conducive to illness: The giving up-given up complex. *Annals of Internal Medicine, 69,* 293–300.

Fish, S., & Shelly, J. A. (1983). *Spiritual care: The nurse's role* (2nd ed.). Downers Grove, IL: Intervarsity Press.

Gottschalk, L. A. (1974). A hope scale applicable to verbal samples. *Archives of General Psychiatry, 30,* 779–787.

Herth, K. A. (1989). The relationship between level of hope and level of coping response and other variables in patients with cancer. *Oncology Nursing Forum, 16*(1), 67–72.

Heiney, S. P. (1988). Assessing and interviewing with dysfunctual families. *Oncology Nursing Forum, 15,* 585–590.

Hickey, S. S. (1986). Enabling hope. *Cancer Nursing, 9*(3), 133–137.

Hinds, P. (1988). Adolescent hopefulness in illness and health. *Advances in Nursing Science, 10*(3), 79–88.

Hinds, P. S. (1984). Inducing a definition of "hope" through the use of grounded theory methodology. *Journal of Advanced Nursing, 9,* 357–362.

Hinds, P. S., & Martin, J. (1988). Hopefulness and the self-sustaining process in adolescents with cancer., *Nursing Research, 37*(6), 336–340.

Hinds, P., Martin, J., & Vogel, R. (1987). Nursing strategies to influence adolescent hopefulness during oncologic illness. *Journal of the Association of Pediatric Oncology Nurses, 4*(1/2), 14–23.

Korner, I. N. (1970). Hope as a method of coping. *Journal of Consultation and Clinical Psychology, 34*(2), 134–139.

Kübler-Ross, E. (1975). *Death: The final stage of growth.* Englewood Cliffs, NJ: Prentice-Hall.

Lynch, W. F. (1965). *Image of hope: Imagination as a healer of the hopeless.* Baltimore: Helicon.

Limandri, B. J., & Boyle, D. W. (1978). Instilling hope. *American Journal of Nursing, 78,* 79–80.

Martocchio, B. C., & Dufault, K. (1985). In hospice compassionate care and the dying experience. *Nursing Clinics of North America, 20*(2), 380–391.

Miller, J. F. (1985). Inspiring hope. *American Journal of Nursing, 85,* 22–25.

Miller, J. F., & Powers, M. J. (1988). Development of an instrument to measure hope. *Nursing Research, 37*(1), 6–9.

Miller, J. F. (1989). Hope inspiring strategies of the critically ill. *Applied Nursing Research, 2*(1), 23–29.

Notwotny, M. L. (1989). Assessment of hope in patients with cancer: Development of an instrument. *Oncology Nursing Forum, 16*(1), 57–61.

Owen, D. C. (1989). Nurses' perspective as the meaning of hope in patient's with cancer: A qualitative study. *Oncology Nursing Forum, 16*(1), 75–79.

Peck, M. L. (1981). The therapeutic effect of faith. *Nursing Forum, 20*(2), 154–167.

Ranking, W. W. (1987). More deeply human. *Journal of Pediatric Nursing, 2*(6), 432–433.

Reed, P. G. (1986). Developmental resources and depression in the elderly. *Nursing Research, 35*(6), 368–373.

Schmale, A. H., & Iher, H. P. (1966). The affect of hopelessness and the development of cancer. *Psychosomatic Medicine, 28*(5), 714–721.

Schnieder, J. S. (1980). Hopelessness and helplessness. *Journal of Practical Nursing and Mental Health Services, 6*(2), 12–16.

Stokes, S. A., & Gordon, S. E. (1988). Development of an instrument to measure stress in the older adult. *Nursing Research, 37*(2), 16–19.

Taylor, P. B., & Gideon, M. D. (1982). Holding out hope to your dying patient; paradoxical but possible. *Nursing, 12,* 45–55.

Watson, J. (1979). *Nursing: The philosophy and science of caring.* Boston: Little, Brown.

Infection, High Risk for

■ *Related to* **(Specify Risk Factors)**

DEFINITION

High Risk for Infection: The state in which an individual is at risk to be invaded by an opportunistic or pathogenic agent (virus, fungus, bacteria, protozoa, or other parasite) from external sources.

RISK FACTORS

Evidence of risk factors such as:
   Altered production of leukocytes
   Altered immune response
   Altered circulation (lymph, blood)
   Presence of favorable conditions for infection (see Etiologic, Contributing, Risk Factors)
   History of infection

RELATED FACTORS

A variety of health problems and situations can create favorable conditions that would encourage the development of infections.* Some common factors are:

Pathophysiologic
   Chronic diseases
      Cancer
      Renal failure
      Arthritis
      AIDS
   Alcoholism
   Immunosuppression
   Immunodeficiency
   Altered or insufficient leukocytes
   Blood dyscrasias
   Impaired circulation
   Altered integumentary system
   Periodontal disease
   Obesity
   Altered mental status
   Hormonal factors
   Dysphagia
   Splenectomy
   Anatomic abnormality

Hematologic
   disorders
Diabetes mellitus
Hepatic disorders

Respiratory disorders
Collagen disorder
Heritable disorders
Renal disorder

*See *High Risk for Infection Transmission:* Principles and Rationale for Nursing Care

Treatment-related

Medications

Antibiotics	Insulin	Immunosuppressants
Steroids	Antifungal agents	Antacids
Antiviral agents	Tranquilizers	

Surgery
Radiation therapy
Dialysis
Total parenteral nutrition
Chemotherapy
Presence of invasive lines (circulatory, gastrointestinal, respiratory, urinary)
Intubation
Enteral feedings

Situational (personal, environmental)

Prolonged immobility
Trauma (accidental, intentional)
Postpartum
Exposure to contagious agents (nosocomial or community acquired)
Postoperative period
Prolonged length of hospital stay
Malnutrition
Stress
Bites (animal, insect, human)
Thermal injuries
Moist skin areas
Inadequate personal hygiene
Lack of immunizations
Smoking

Maturational

Newborns
   Lack of maternal antibodies (dependent on maternal exposures)
   Lack of normal flora
   Open wounds (umbilical, circumcision)
   Immature immune system
Infant/childhood
   Lack of immunization
Elderly
   Debilitated
   Diminished immune response
   Chronic diseases

Diagnostic Considerations

All individuals are at risk for infection; secretion control, environmental control, and handwashing before and after client care reduce the risk of transmission of organisms. Included in the population at risk for infection is a smaller group at high risk for infection. *High Risk for Infection* describes an individual whose host defenses are compromised, thus increasing susceptibility to environmental pathogens, *e.g.,* a person with chronic liver dysfunction or with an invasive line. Nursing interventions for such a person focus on minimizing introduction of organisms and on increasing resistance to infection, *e.g.,* by improving nutritional status. For an individual with an infection, the situation is best described with the collaborative problem *Potential Complication: Sepsis.*

High Risk for Infection Transmission describes an individual at high risk for transferring an infectious agent to others. Some persons are at high risk both for acquiring opportunistic agents and for transmitting infecting organisms, warranting the use of both *High Risk for Infection* and *High Risk for Infection Transmission.*

Errors in Diagnostic Statements

High Risk for Infection related to progression of sepsis secondary to failure to treat infection

Sepsis is a collaborative problem, not a nursing diagnosis. This person is not at risk for infection but rather requires medical and nursing interventions to treat the sepsis and prevent septic shock.

High Risk for Infection related to direct access to bladder mucosa secondary to Foley catheter and lack of staff knowledge of aseptic technique

If the staff's lack of knowledge of aseptic technique is valid, the nurse should proceed with reporting the situation to nursing management via an incident report. Adding this to a nursing diagnosis statement would be legally and professionally inadvisable. Nursing diagnostic statements should never be used to criticize a client, group, or a member of the health team or to expose unsafe or unprofessional practices or behavior. Other organizational channels of communication must be used for this latter purpose.

Focus Assessment Criteria

Subjective Data

1. Does the person complain of:
   a. Fever, continuous or intermittent
   b. Previous infections
      - Urinary tract
      - Pneumonia
      - Surgical wound
      - Skin and soft tissue
      - Reproductive tract
      - Lower respiratory tract
      - Bloodstream
      - Bone and joint
      - Cardiovascular system
      - Central nervous system
      - Eye, ear, nose, throat, mouth
      - Systemic
      - GI system
   c. Pain or swelling
      - Generalized
      - Localized

2. History of recent travel
   a. Within US
   b. Outside US
3. History of exposure to infectious diseases*
   a. Airborne (most childhood infections communicable diseases, *e.g.*, chickenpox, tuberculosis)
   b. Vector-borne and other vector-associated infections (malaria, plague)
   c. Vehicle-borne and other food- and water-borne infections (hepatitis A, Salmonellas)
   d. Contact-spread (most common type of exposure)
      • Direct (person to person)
      • Indirect (instruments, clothing, etc., to person)
      • Contact droplet (pneumonias, colds, etc.)
4. History of risk factors associated with infections (see Related Factors)

Objective Data

1. Presence of wounds
   a. Surgical
   b. Burns
   c. Invasive devices (trach, IV, drains)
   d. Self-induced
2. White blood cell count (WBC)
3. Temperature
4. Cultures and other laboratory diagnostic tests for infection

Principles and Rationale for Nursing Care

Generic Considerations

1. There are two parameters that can assist in identifying individuals at risk for infection—predictive factors and confounding factors (Owen & Grier, 1987).
2. Predictors are controllable factors that have been identified as increasing the risk of infection by interfering or compromising the host defenses. Intervention can be implemented to control or influence the degree of risk associated with these factors (Owen & Grier, 1987).
3. Confounding factors augment the risk of infection. They are not singularly controllable during hospitalization but can enhance one's predictive risk for infection significantly (Owen & Grier, 1987).
4. Confounding factors are
   a. Age
   b. Anatomic determinants
   c. Metabolic determinants
   d. Decreased numbers of neutrophils
   e. Diminished or defective immunoglobulin synthesis or rapid loss of immunoglobulin
   f. Defective cell-mediated immune mechanisms
   g. Antimicrobial therapy
5. Resistance to infection depends on the host's immune response (susceptibility), the dose of the infecting agent, and the virulence of the organism. Factors influencing the host's immune response include:
   a. Anatomic barriers—each system has specific lines of defenses.
   b. Therapies—pose a threat to normal lines of defense by either invasiveness or alteration of body function.

c. Developmental and heritable factors—factors that have negative impact on the individual's immune system function (*e.g.*, newborn status); agammaglobulinemia.

d. Hormonal factors—the male is more vulnerable to infection than the female; pregnancy increases the female's vulnerability; steroid therapy increases vulnerability in both sexes.

e. Age—includes both extremes of age (immaturity or degeneration of the immune system).

f. Nutrition influences protein synthesis and phagocytosis, decreasing the body's vulnerability to infection.

g. Fever—hyperthermia may inhibit the growth of organisms; hypothermia may decrease the effects of the fever.

h. Secretions such as mucus, saliva, and skin secretions contain substances that are bactericidal, decreasing the risk of infection and colonization.

i. Endotoxins, a product of some gram-negative bacteria, have a limited ability to kill other bacteria or increase an individual's resistance to some infections.

j. Interference—the interaction between two distinct organisms that are parasitizing the host leads to interference, in which one remains dominant and the other is suppressed.

k. The inflammatory response consists of the following: (1) activation of leukocytes, (2) plasma proteins, which localize and phagocytize the infectious process, and (3) increased blood and lymph flow that dilutes and flushes out toxic materials; this process causes a local increase in temperature.

l. Phagocytosis is the process by which parasites are removed by means of engulfment and digestion.

6. Nurses must use precautions with blood and body fluids from all patients to protect themselves from exposure to all infectious organisms.

a. Wash hands before and after all patient or specimen contact.

b. Handle the blood of all patients as potentially infectious.

c. Wear gloves for potential contact with blood and body fluids.

d. Place used syringes immediately in nearby impermeable container; do not recap or manipulate needle in any way!

e. Wear protective eyewear and mask if splatter with blood or body fluids is possible (*e.g.*, bronchoscopy, oral surgery).

f. Wear gowns when splash with blood or body fluids is anticipated

g. Handle all linen soiled with blood and/or body secretions as potentially infectious.

h. Process all laboratory specimens as potentially infectious.

i. Wear mask for TB and other respiratory organisms (HIV is not airborne).

j. Place resuscitation equipment where respiratory arrest is predictable (California Nurses Association, 1988).

Host Defenses

Specific host defenses of each system that influence the immune response include:

Central Nervous System
Because the most common route for both bacterial and viral infections of the central nervous system is the hematogenous route, blood host defenses play an important primary role.

Cutaneous

1. Skin provides a first line of defense against organisms, both anatomically and chemically.

2. Sweat glands and sebaceous glands do not allow overgrowth of bacteria.
3. The acid *p*H of the skin does not allow pathogenic organisms to grow or survive on the skin for any length of time.
4. Eye infections are controlled by the flushing and lysozyme action of tears. Organisms are flushed through the lacrimal duct and deposited in the nasopharynx.

Blood

1. The circulating blood is the major vehicle for transporting internal defense mechanisms.
2. The febrile response is associated with circulating pyrogens to the hypothalamus.

Genitourinary Tract

1. Anatomic structure eliminates easy ascent of perineal microorganisms into the bladder.
2. Mucous layer allows entrapment of organisms and engulfment by bladder cells.
3. The *p*H and osmolality of urine prevent bacterial multiplication.
4. The ability to empty the bladder completely eliminates stasis of invading organisms and allows for continual flushing.

Respiratory Tract

1. The nares entrap the majority of foreign matter on the mucus membranes as a result of turbulence caused by the turbinates and hairs.
2. The mucociliary transport system consists of cilia and mucus, which remove additional matter passing to the upper and lower bronchi.
3. Lysozymes and Ig-A, a secretion of phagocytes, are found in nasal secretions and assist in the prevention of colonization.
4. Particles reaching as far as the alveoli can be removed through the expulsive action of sneezing and coughing, and the gag reflex.
5. Phagocytosis occurs in the alveoli, with the macrophages used as a major defense mechanism.

GI Tract

1. A mucous layer traps ingested microbes in the epithelium of the GI tract.
2. Gastric acids kill most organisms.
3. Peristalsis aids in the removal of organisms.
4. Intestinal secretions contain antibody (IgA), bile salts, lysozyme, glycolipids, and glycoproteins that prevent proliferation and adherence.
5. Normal gut flora interact to restrict overproliferation.

Wounds

1. Skin provides a first line of defense; the opening of the skin, either surgically or traumatically, potentiates infection.
2. A wound essentially closes within 24 hours, eliminating the risk of direct inoculations of organisms.
3. Wound infections rely on the capabilities of other host defenses to assist in the healing process.
4. Risk factors associated with wound infections depend on (1) endogenous factors such as presence of confounding factors, skin preparation, and the use of prophylactic antibiotics, and (2) exogenous factors such as the preoperative scrub, barrier techniques, airborne contamination, environmental disinfection, wound care, and the condition of the wound at the time of closure.

Pediatric Considerations

1. Approximately 80% of all childhood illnesses are due to infections, with respiratory infections occurring two to three times as often as other illnesses combined (Whaley & Wong, 1989).
2. Generally, acute illness is less frequent in children under age 6 months, increases from then on until age 3 or 4 years, and then gradually decreases throughout middle and older childhood (Whaley & Wong, 1989).
3. According to Kliegman (1990), "the neonate is at higher risk for infections." By the time a child is a toddler, the production of antibodies is well established. Phagocytosis is much more efficient in toddlers than in infants (Whaley & Wong, 1989).
4. Children who attend day care centers are at increased risk for infections caused by such organisms as shigella, rotavirus, *Haemophilus influenzae* type b, and hepatitis A (Whaley & Wong, 1989).
5. Good hygiene, optimal nutrition, immunizations, and strict sanitary practices can reduce the incidence of infectious disease during childhood.

Gerontologic Considerations

1. A slower rate of epidermal proliferation causes injured skin to take twice as long to heal in older adults (Grove, 1982).
2. Older adults also have compromised dermal immunologic responses due to a reduced number of Langerhan's cells and reduced microcirculation (Miller, 1990).
3. Older adults have diminished efficiency of the gag reflex (Close & Woodson, 1989).
4. In elderly persons, the lung's alveolar surface and elastic recoil are slightly decreased, and gas exchange in lower lung regions is decreased (Sparrow & Weiss, 1988).
5. Age-related changes in respiratory function do not significantly increase elderly persons' for infection. Rather, the presence of non–age-related risk factors, such as smoking and exposure to occupational toxins, increase risk.

■ High Risk for Infection
Related to (Specify Risk Factors)

Assessment
See Related Factors

Outcome Criteria

The person will:
- Demonstrate meticulous handwashing technique by the time of discharge.
- Demonstrate knowledge of risk factors associated with potential for infection and will practice appropriate precautions to prevent infection.

Interventions

A. Identify individuals at high risk for nosocomial infections
   1. Assess for predictors.
      a. Remote site of infection
      b. Abdominal or thoracic surgery
      c. Surgery longer than 2 hours
      d. GU procedure
      e. Instrumentation (ventilator, suction, catheters, nebulizers, tracheostomy, invasive monitoring)
      f. Anesthesia
   2. Assess for confounding factors.
      a. Age less than 1 year or greater than 65 years
      b. Obesity
      c. Underlying disease conditions (COPD, diabetes, cardiovascular blood dyscrasias)
      d. Substance abuse
      e. Medications (steroids, chemotherapy, antibiotic therapy) that modify immune response
      f. Nutritional status (intake less than minimum daily requirements)
      g. Smoker
   3. Consider a person who has one or more confounding factors and one or more predictors to be at *High Risk for Infection.*

B. Reduce the entry of organisms into individuals (Owen & Grier, 1987; used with permission):

Surgical Wound

   1. Prior to surgery, assess client for risk of remote site of infection.
   2. If abdominal surgery, teach client (preop) importance and correct coughing, turning, and deep breathing technique.
   3. If surgery is greater than 2 hours, assess client every shift for signs/symptoms of infection at surgical site.
   4. Monitor temperature every 4 hours; notify physician if greater than 100.8° F.
   5. Assess nutritional status to provide adequate protein and calorie intake for healing.
   6. Assess wound site every 24 hours and during dressing changes, documenting any abnormal findings.
   7. Evaluate all abnormal lab findings, especially culture/sensitivities, CBC.
   8. Notify epidemiologist of any abnormal findings related to the development of infection.
   9. Administer all prophylactic antibiotics within 15 minutes of scheduled administration time to ensure adequate therapeutic levels at surgery.
   10. Instruct client and family on appropriate aseptic practice.
   11. Use aseptic technique during dressing changes, changing every _____ hour as ordered to maintain dry and intact dressing.
   12. Use body substance precautions with all body fluids from client.

Urinary Tract

   1. Evaluate all abnormal lab findings, especially cultures/sensitivities, CBC.
   2. Assess client for abnormal signs/symptoms following any urologic procedure, including frequency, urgency, burning, abnormal color, odor.

3. Monitor client temperature at least every 24 hours for elevation and notify physician if greater than 100.8° F.
4. Encourage fluids when appropriate.
5. Notify epidemiologist of any abnormal findings related to the development of infection.
6. Assess other wounds and systems to evaluate client's increased risk for development of infections at other sites.
7. Instruct client and family as to risk for development of urinary tract infections.
8. Use body substance precautions with all fluids from client.
9. Use aseptic technique when emptying any urinary drainage device; keep bag off the floor, but below bladder or clamped during transport.
10. Administer all antibiotics within 15 minutes of scheduled administration time to ensure adequate therapeutic levels are maintained.
11. Reassess need for indwelling urinary catheter daily.

Circulatory

1. Assess all invasive lines every 24 hours for signs of redness, inflammation, drainage, tenderness.
2. Monitor client temperature at least every 24 hours and notify physician if greater than 100.8° F.
3. Maintain aseptic technique for all invasive devices, changing sites, dressings, tubing, and solutions per policy schedule.
4. Evaluate all abnormal lab finding especially cultures/sensitivities, CBC.
5. Notify epidemiologist of any abnormal findings related to the development of infection.
6. Administer all antibiotics within 15 minutes of scheduled administration time to ensure adequate therapeutic levels are maintained.
7. Instruct client and family on appropriate aseptic practices to prevent infection.
8. Use body substance precautions with all body fluids from client.
9. Assess nutritional status of client to provide adequate protein and calorie intake for healing.
10. Evaluate client for secondary sites of infection, either to bloodstream from another site or from bloodstream to other high risk sites on patient.

Respiratory Tract

1. Evaluate client risk for infection following any instrumentation of the respiratory tract for at least 48 hours following procedure.
2. Notify epidemiologist of any abnormal findings related to the development of infection.
   a. Monitor temperature at least every 8 hours and notify physician if greater than 100.8° F.
   b. Evaluate sputum characteristics for frequency, purulence, blood, odor.
   c. Evaluate sputum and blood cultures if done, for significant findings.
   d. Evaluate CBC for significant shift in WBC counts.
   e. Assessment of lung sounds every 8 hours or PRN.
3. If client has abdominal/thoracic surgery, instruct client on importance of coughing, turning, and deep breathing prior to surgery.
4. If client has had anesthesia, monitor for appropriate clearing of secretions in lung fields.
5. Cardiopulmonary treatments as ordered, with assessment of response to treatment documented.
6. Evaluate need for suctioning if patient unable to adequately clear secretions.

7. Use body substance precautions with all body fluids from patient.
8. Use aseptic technique with all invasive procedures of the respiratory tract.
9. Assess client for risk of aspiration, keeping head of bed elevated 30° unless otherwise contraindicated.
10. Assess nutritional status of patient to provide adequate protein and calorie intake for healing.
11. If oral feedings not tolerated without aspiration, contact physician for further action.
12. Instruct client on principles of cough and deep breathing and prevention of infection.

C. Protect the immune-deficient individual from infection

1. Place in private room.
2. Instruct client to ask all visitors and personnel to wash their hands before approaching.
3. Limit visitors when appropriate.
4. Screen all visitors for known infections or exposure to infections.
5. Limit invasive devices to those that are absolutely necessary.
6. Teach client and family members signs and symptoms of infection.
7. Evaluate client's personal hygiene habits.
8. Provide immune globulin to those exposed to specific diseases that might be life-threatening (*i.e.,* chickenpox, hepatitis, measles).

D. Reduce client's susceptibility to infection

1. Encourage and maintain caloric and protein intake in diet (see *Altered Nutrition*).
2. Assess the client for adequate immunizations against childhood diseases, bacterial infections (*e.g.,* pneumococcal and *Haemophilus influenzae* vaccines), and other viral infections (flu virus vaccines).
3. Monitor use or overuse of antimicrobial therapy.
4. Administer prescribed antimicrobial therapy within 15 minutes of scheduled time to ensure adequate maintenance of therapeutic levels (prevention of resistant strains or organisms).
5. Observe for clinical manifestations of infection in individuals at high risk.
6. Minimize length of stay in hospital to prevent colonization with nosocomial organisms.
7. Observe for superinfection development in clients currently receiving antimicrobial therapy.

E. Initiate health teaching and referrals as indicated

1. Instruct client and family regarding the causes, risks, and communicability of the infection.
2. Report communicable diseases as appropriate to public health department.
3. Collaborate with nurse epidemiologist on needs of client and family.

References/Bibliography

Axnick, K., & Yardbrough, M. (1984). *Infection control: An integrated approach.* St Louis: C. V. Mosby.
Bennett, J. V., & Brachman, P. S. (1986). *Hospital infections* (2nd ed.). Boston: Little, Brown.
Brunner, L. S., & Suddarth D. S. (1986). *The Lippincott manual of nursing practice* (4th ed.). Philadelphia: J. B. Lippincott.

California Nurses Association. (1988). *AIDS education and training*. San Francisco: CNA.

Close, L. G., & Woodson, G. E. (1989). Common upper airway disorders in elderly and their management. *Geriatrics, 44*(1), 67–72.

Garner, J. S., & Jarvis, W. R. (1988). CDC definitions for nosocomial infections 1988. *AJIC, 16*(3), 128–140.

Grove, G. L. (1982). Age related differences in healing of superficial skin wounds in humans. *Archives of Dermalogical Research, 272*(5), 381–385.

Haley, R. W. (1986). *Managing hospital infection control for cost-effectiveness: A strategy for reducing infectious complications*. Chicago: American Hospital Association.

Hoeprich, P. D. (1983). *Infectious diseases*. Philadelphia: Harper & Row.

Kliegman, R. M. (1990). Fetal and neonatal medicine. In Behrman, R. E., & Kliegman, R. (Eds.). *Nelson essentials of pediatrics*. Philadelphia: W. B. Saunders.

Larson, E. (1984). *Clinical microbiology and infection control*. Boston: Blackwell Scientific Publications.

Miller, C. A. (1990). *Nursing care of older adults*. Glenview, IL: Scott, Foresman.

Owen, M., & Grier, M. (1987). *Infection risk assessment guide*. Unpublished.

Sparrow, D., & Weiss, S. T. (1988). Pulmonary systems. In Rowe, J. W., & Besdive, C. (Eds.): *Geriatric medicine*. Boston: Little, Brown.

Thompson, J. M., McFarland, G. K., Hirsch, J. E., Tucker, S. M., & Bowers, A. C. (1989). *Mosby's manual of clinical nursing* (2nd ed.). St. Louis, C. V. Mosby.

Wenzel, R. P. (1981). *CRC handbook of hospital acquired infections*. Boca Raton, FL: CRC Press.

Whaley, L. F., & Wong, D. L. (1989). *Essentials of pediatric nursing* (3rd ed.). St. Louis: C. V. Mosby.

Infection Transmission, High Risk for*

■ *Related to* **(Specify Risk Factors)**
■ *Related to* **Lack of Knowledge of Reducing the Risk of Transmitting the AIDS Virus**

DEFINITION
High Risk for Infection Transmission: The state in which an individual is at risk for transferring an opportunistic or pathogenic agent to others.

RISK FACTORS
Presence of risk factors (See Related Factors)

RELATED FACTORS
Pathophysiologic
Colonization with highly antibiotic-resistant organism
Airborne transmission exposure
Contact transmission exposure (direct, indirect, contact droplet)
Vehicle transmission exposure
Vector-borne transmission exposure

Treatment-related
Contaminated or dirty surgeries (I&D, traumatic wound)
Drainage devices (urinary, chest tubes)
Suction equipment
Invasive devices

Situational (personal, environmental)
Disaster with hazardous infectious material
Unsanitary living conditions (sewage, personal hygiene)
Areas considered high risk for vector-borne diseases (malaria, rabies, bubonic plague)
Areas considered high risk for vehicle-borne disease (hepatitis A, *Shigella, Salmonella*)
Lack of knowledge
Intravenous drug use
Multiple sex partners

Maturational
Newborn
Birth outside hospital setting in uncontrolled environment
Exposure during prenatal or perinatal period to communicable disease via maternal source.

*This diagnostic category is not currently on the NANDA list but has been included for clarity or usefulness.

Focus Assessment Criteria

(Refer also to *High Risk for Infection*)

Subjective Data

History of infection
Onset of symptoms
Exposure to communicable disease
Sexual practices
Life-style practices

Objective Data

Extent of infection—amount of coughing, bleeding, drainage
Hygienic practices of patient
Mode of transmission
Infectivity of disease
  • Virulence of organism
  • Dose in blood/body fluids

Principles and Rationale for Nursing Care

General

1. To spread an infection, three elements are required (refer to Figure II-2):
   a. A source of infecting organisms
   b. A susceptible host
   c. A means of transmission for the organism
2. Sources of infecting organisms include:
   a. Clients, personnel, and visitors with acute disease, incubating infection, or colonized organisms without apparent disease
   b. Person's own endogenous flora (autogenous infection)
   c. Inanimate environment, including equipment and medications
3. Susceptibility of the host varies according to
   a. Immune status of the host
   b. Ability to develop a commensal relationship with the infecting organism and become an asymptomatic carrier
   c. Preexisting diseases affecting the client
4. Means of transmission for the organism include one or more of the following:
   a. Contact transmission, the most frequent method of transferring organisms. It can be divided into three subgroups:
      • Direct contact—involves direct physical transfer between a susceptible host and an infected or colonized person
      • Indirect contact—involves the exchange of organisms between a host and contaminated objects, usually inanimate
      • Droplet contact—involves the transfer of organisms from coughing, sneezing, or talking by an infected person into the conjunctivae, nose, or mouth of a susceptible host. Droplets travel no more than 3 feet.
   b. Vehicle route transmission infections are spread through a means such as:
      • Food (*e.g.*, hepatitis A, *Salmonella*)
      • Water (*e.g.*, *Legionella*)
      • Drugs (*e.g.*, IV-contaminated products)
      • Blood (*e.g.*, hepatitis B, AIDS)

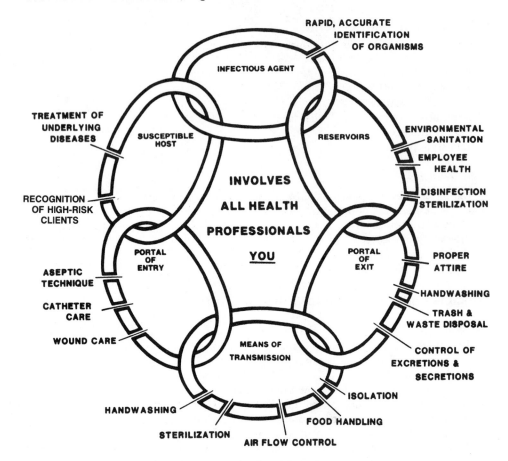

Fig. II-2 Breaking the chain of infection. (Adapted from the APIC Starter Kit with permission from the Association for Practitioners in Infection Control, Mundelein, Illinois, copyright APIC, 1978)

    c. Airborne transmission infections are disseminated via droplet nuclei (residue of evaporated droplets that may remain suspended in the air for long periods of time) or dust particles in the air containing the infectious agent.

    d. Vector-borne transmission infections are spread through vectors such as animals or insects.

5. The practice of universal body substance precautions requires that precautions be taken with all blood and body fluids. However, those clients with suspected or confirmed medical diagnosis indicative of an infectious disease process need to be documented with a comprehensive plan of care for that infection or potential infection. That can be done most expeditiously through the nursing diagnosis *High Risk for Infection Transmission.*

6. Nurses must use precautions with blood and body fluids from all clients to protect themselves from exposure to HIV and hepatitis B virus.

Acquired Immunodeficiency Syndrome (AIDS)

1. AIDS is caused by a retrovirus labeled human immunodeficiency virus (HIV). Transmission is by exposure to contaminated semen, vaginal fluids, or blood.

2. Routes of transmission
   a. Sexual: homosexual or heterosexual
   b. Exposure to blood through drug use needle sharing, transfusions, or occupational exposure (needle stick or splash)
   c. Perinatal: during pregnancy, intrapartum and postpartum (via breastfeeding) (HHS/PHS, CDC)
3. AIDS has a latency or incubation period of 18 months to 5 years. During this period the individual is transmitting disease through sexual activity or contaminated blood.
4. HIV destroys the body's T and B lymphocytes, thus making the host susceptible to a select group of diseases (refer to Table II-9).
5. AIDS is a terminal disease with a mortality rate of greater than 95% at 2 years.

Pediatric Considerations

1. Infections in the newborn can be acquired transplacentally or transcervically. These can occur before, during, or after birth (Kliegman, 1990).
2. Children are at greater risk for transmission of disease because of the following factors:
   a. Close contact with other children
   b. Frequency of infectious disease in children
   c. Lack of hygienic habits, *i.e.*, not washing hands after toileting or before eating
   d. Frequent hand-to-mouth activity, increasing risk for infection and reinfection, *e.g.*, pinworms (Whaley & Wong, 1989)

◼ Potential for Infection Transmission
Related to (Specify Risk Factors)

Assessment
See Related Factors

Outcome Criteria

The person will
- Relate the need to be isolated until noninfectious
- Describe the mode of transmission of disease by the time of discharge
- Demonstrate meticulous hand washing during hospitalization

Interventions

A. Identify susceptible host individuals based on focus assessment for high risk for infection and history of exposure

Table II-9 **List of Most Frequent Infections and Neoplasms in Acquired Immunodeficiency Syndrome (AIDS)**

Problem	Site
AIDS-Related Complex	
Candida albicans	Mouth (thrush)
Herpes simplex	Mucocutaneous; may be severe
Herpes zoster	Disseminated; may be severe
Lymphadenopathy	Generalized (always more than one lymph node)
Fevers	Usually greater than 100° F; persistent over months
Diarrhea	No organisms recovered, or conventional organisms recovered
Weight loss	Progressive and sustained
Night sweats	Characteristically severe and drenching; persistent and sustained over months
Thrombocytopenia	Often accompanied by petechia; may be severe and life-threatening
HIV encephalopathy	Clinical findings of disabling cognitive and/or motor dysfunction in absence of concurrent illness or condition other than HIV infection
HIV wasting syndrome	Profound, in the absence of concurrent illness or condition other than HIV infection
Infections	
Candida albicans	Mouth (thrush); throat
Cryptococcus neoformans	Central nervous system (CNS); pulmonary; disseminated
Pneumocystis carinii	Pneumonia
Toxoplasma gondii	CNS
Histoplasma gondii	CNS
Cryptosporidium	Intestine; diarrhea
Cytomegalovirus (CMV)	Retinas; intestine; pulmonary; disseminated
Herpes simplex	Mucocutaneous; severe
Herpes zoster	Disseminated; severe
Human immunodeficiency virus (HIV)	CNS, disseminated
Progressive multifocal leukoencephalopathy	CNS
Mycobacterium avium-intracellulare (MAI)	Disseminated
Mycobacterium tuberculosis	Pulmonary (TB)
Neoplasms	
Kaposi's sarcoma	Skin; disseminated
Burkitt's lymphoma	Lymphatic system
Non-Hodgkin's lymphoma	Lymphatic system
Mycosis fungoides	Skin (dermal lymphoma)

(Source: Keating, S. B., & Kelman, G. B. (1988). *Home health care nursing concepts and practice*, p 251. Philadelphia: J. B. Lippincott, with amendment)

B. Identify the mode of transmission based on infecting agent
   1. Airborne
   2. Contact
      a. Direct
      b. Indirect
      c. Contact droplet
   3. Vehicle-borne
   4. Vector-borne

C. Reduce the transfer of pathogens
   1. Isolate clients with airborne communicable infections (see Table II-10).
   2. Secure appropriate room assignment dependent on the type of infection and hygienic practices of the infected person.

■ Potential for Infection Transmission
Related to Lack of Knowledge of Reducing the Risk of Transmitting the AIDS Virus

Focus Assessment Criteria

Subjective Data
Individual states that he is fearful of contracting AIDS

Objective Data
   The person reports
   • Not using preventive methods
   • High-risk sexual behaviors
   The person practices high-risk behaviors

Outcome Criteria

The person will
• Describe the causes of AIDS and situations/factors contributing to its transmission
• Relate practices that reduce the transmission of the AIDS virus sexually
• Describe how to disinfect equipment

Interventions

A. Identify susceptible host individual
   1. Homosexual practices
   2. Bisexual practices
   3. Intravenous drug users

Table II-10 **Airborne Communicable Diseases**

Disease	Apply Airborne Precautions for How Long	Comments
Anthrax, inhalation	Duration of illness	Promptly report to infection control office
Chickenpox (Varicella)	Until all lesions are crusted	Immune person does not need to wear a mask. Exposed susceptible clients should be placed in a private special airflow room on STOP SIGN alert status beginning 10 days after initial exposure until 21 days after last exposure. Report to epidemiology.
Diphtheria, pharyngeal	Until 2 cultures from both nose and throat taken at least 24 hr after cessation of antimicrobial therapy are negative for *Corynebacterium diphtheriae*	Promptly report to epidemiology
Epiglottitis, due to *Haemophilus influenzae*	For 24 hr after cessation of antimicrobial therapy	Report to epidemiology
Erythema infectiosum	For 7 days after onset	Report to epidemiology
Hemorrhagic fevers	Duration of illness	Call epidemiology office immediately. Physician may call the State Health Department and Centers for Disease Control for advice about management of a suspected case.
Herpes zoster (varicella zoster), disseminated	Duration of illness	Localized does not require STOP SIGN
Lassa fever Marburg virus disease	Duration of illness	Call epidemiology office immediately. Physician may call the State Health Department and Centers for Disease Control for advice about management of a suspected case.
Measles (rubeola)	For 4 days after start of rash, except in immunocompromised patients with whom precautions should be maintained for duration of illness	Immune persons do not need to wear a mask. Exposed susceptible clients should be placed in a private special air flow room on STOP SIGN alert status beginning the 5th day after exposure until 21 days after last exposure.
Meningitis *Hemophilus influenza* known or suspect	For 24 hr after start of effective antibiotic therapy	Call epidemiology to report
Neisseria meningitidis (meningococci) known or suspect	For 24 hr after start of effective antibiotic therapy	Promptly report to epidemiology

(continued)

Table II-10   **Airborne Communicable Diseases** (*continued*)

Disease	Apply Airborne Precautions for How Long	Comments
Meningococcal pneumonia	For 24 hr after start of effective antibiotic therapy	Promptly report to epidemiology
Meningococcemia	For 24 hr after start of effective therapy	Consult with epidemiology
Multiply resistant organisms	Until culture negative or as determined by epidemiology	Consult with epidemiology
Mumps (infectious parotitis)	For 9 days after onset of swelling	Persons with history do not need to wear a mask. Call epidemiology office to report.
Pertussis (whooping cough)	For 7 days after start of effective therapy	Call epidemiology to report
Plague, pneumonic	For 3 days after start of effective therapy	Promptly report to epidemiology
Pneumonia, hemophilus in infants and children any age	For 24 hr after start of effective antibiotic therapy	Call epidemiology
Pneumonia, meningococcal	For 24 hr after start of effective antibiotic therapy	Promptly report to epidemiology
Rubella (German measles)	For 7 days after onset of rash	Immune persons do not need to wear a mask. Promptly report to epidemiology
Tuberculosis, bronchial, laryngeal, pulmonary, confirmed or suspect	In most instances, duration can be guided by clinical response and a reduction in numbers of TB organisms on sputum smear. Usually this occurs within 2–3 weeks after chemotherapy is begun. When the patient is likely to be infected with INH-resistant organisms, apply precautions until patient is improving and sputum smear is negative for TB organisms.	Call epidemiology to report; prompt use of effective anti-tuberculosis drugs is the most effective means of limiting transmission.
Varicella (Chickenpox)	Until all lesions crusted over	See chickenpox

4. Multiple blood transfusions (prior to March 1985)
5. Human immunodeficiency virus (HIV)–positive persons
6. Multiple sexual partners
7. High-risk behaviors

B. Counsel susceptible host individuals to be tested for AIDS

C. Discuss the mode of transmission of the virus in semen or vaginal fluids and blood (Source: *Understanding AIDS*)

1. Vaginal, anal, or oral sex with susceptible host persons
2. Unprotected sex with infected person
3. Sharing drug needles and syringes

4. Use appropriate universal body substance precautions for all body fluids:
   a. Wash hands before and after all patient or specimen contact.
   b. Handle the blood of all patients as potentially infectious.
   c. Wear gloves for potential contact with blood and body fluids.
   d. Place used syringes immediately in nearby impermeable container; do not recap or manipulate needle in any way!
   e. Wear protective eyewear and mask if splatter with blood or body fluids is possible (*e.g.,* bronchoscopy, oral surgery).
   f. Wear gowns when splash with blood or body fluids is anticipated (*e.g.,* L & D)
   g. Handle all linen soiled with blood and/or body secretions as potentially infectious.
   h. Process all laboratory specimens as potentially infectious.
   i. Wear mask for TB and other respiratory organisms (HIV is not airborne).
   j. Place resuscitation equipment where respiratory arrest is predictable (California Nurses Association, 1988).
5. Administer all antibiotics within 15 minutes of scheduled administration time to ensure adequate maintenance of therapeutic levels.
6. Monitor temperature at least every 4 hours during infectious process.
7. Evaluate all abnormal lab findings and report to physician, including culture with sensitivities to antibiotic administration.
8. Assess for contributing risk factors to infection if etiology is unknown.
9. Discontinue airborne communicable isolation when appropriate.
10. Evaluate client for secondary sites of infection related to the spread of infection from a primary site.

D. Initiate health teaching and referrals as indicated
1. Referral to infection control practitioner for follow-up with the Health Department regarding family exposure and cause of exposure and to assist in appropriate plan of care for client
2. Patient education regarding hand-washing as the single most important measure to prevent the spread of infection
3. Patient education regarding the chain of infection and patient responsibility in both the hospital and at home
4. Assess nutritional status of client to encourage healing.

E. Prevent the transfer of virus
1. Abstain from sexual activity.
2. Engage in sexual activity with one mutually, faithful, uninfected partner.
3. Avoid intravenous drug (street) use.

F. Reduce the risk of transmission of AIDS with susceptible host persons
1. Explain low-risk sexual behaviors.
   a. Mutual masturbation
   b. Massage
   c. Vaginal intercourse with condom
2. Explain the risk of ejaculate contact with broken skin or mucous membranes (oral, anal).
3. Teach to use condoms of latex rubber, not "natural membrane" condoms; teach appropriate storage to preserve latex.
4. Explain the need to use water-based lubricants to reduce prophylactic breaks. Avoid petroleum-based lubricants, which dissolve latex.

5. Explain that a condom with a spermicide may provide additional protection by decreasing the number of viable HIV particles.

G. Teach how to disinfect equipment possibly contaminated with the AIDS virus at home (needles, syringes, sex aids)

1. Wash under running water.
2. Fill or wash with household bleach.
3. Rinse well with water.

H. Provide facts to dispel the myths regarding AIDS transmission

1. The AIDS virus is not transmitted by mosquitoes, swimming pools, clothes, eating utensils, telephones, toilet seats, or close contact (at work, school, etc.).
2. Saliva, sweat, tears, urine, and feces do not transmit the AIDS virus.
3. Donating blood cannot transmit the AIDS virus.
4. Blood for transfusions is tested to substantially reduce the risk of contracting the AIDS virus.

I. Initiate health teaching and referrals as indicated

1. Refer to infection control practitioners.
2. Provide with AIDS hot line (1-800-342-AIDS) for more information.
3. Emphasize the need to be careful about the person you become sexually involved with (past sexual partners, experimented with drugs).
4. Provide the community and schools with the facts regarding the transmission of AIDS and dispel myths.

References/Bibliography

Books and Articles

AIDS symposium. (1988). *Nursing Clinics of North America, 23*(4), 683–862.

Becker, C. E., Cone, J. E., & Gerberding, J. (1989). Occupational infection with human immunodeficiency virus: Risks and risk reduction. *Annals of Internal Medicine, 110*(8), 653–656.

Bennett, J. V., & Brachman, P. S. (Eds.). (1986). *Hospital infections* (2nd ed.). Boston, Little, Brown & Co.

Centers for Disease Control. (1987). Human immunodeficiency virus infection in the United States: A review of current knowledge. *MMWR, 36*(Suppl. 5–6).

Centers for Disease Control. Health worker's needle-stick survey: A federal study of health workers who have possible exposure to AIDS via needle stick or other work-related incidents. The project is interested in hearing from hospital infection control coordinators who want to enroll employees in the project. Call: (404) 639-1644.

Centers for Disease Control. (1987). Revision of the CDC surveillance case definition for acquired immune deficiency syndrome. *MMWR, 36*(Suppl. 1S).

Centers for Disease Control. (1987). Recommendations for prevention of HIV transmission in health care settings. *MMWR, 36*(Suppl. 2S).

Centers for Disease Control. (1988). Update: Universal precautions for prevention of transmission of human immunodeficiency virus, hepatitis B virus and other bloodborne pathogens in health-care settings. *MMWR, 37*(24), 377–388.

Department of Health and Human Services. (1987). Advisory notice: Protection against occupational exposure to hepatitis B virus (HBV) and human immunodeficiency virus (HIV). *Federal Register, 52*(210), 41818–41823.

Garner, J. S., & Favero, M. S. (1985). *Guideline for handwashing and hospital environmental control* (Publication no. 99-1117). Atlanta: Centers for Disease Control.

Garner, J. S., & Hughes, J. M. (1987). Options for isolation precautions [editorial]. *Annals of Internal Medicine, 107*, 248–250.

Garner, J. S., & Simmons, B. P. (1983). Guideline for isolation precautions in hospitals. *Infection Control, 4,* 245–325.

Gerberding, J. L., Bryant-LeBlanc, C. E., Nelson, K., et al. (1987). Risk of transmitting the human immunodeficiency virus, cytomegalovirus, and hepatitis B virus to health care workers exposed to patients with AIDS and AIDS-related conditions. *Journal of Infectious Diseases, 156,* 1–8.

Jackson, M. M., Lynch, P., McPerson, D., et al. (1987). Why not treat all body substances as infectious? *American Journal of Nursing, 87,* 1137–1139.

Kliegman, R. M. (1990). Fetal and neonatal medicine. In Behrman, R. E., & Kliegman R. (Eds.). *Nelson essentials of pediatrics.* Philadelphia: W. B. Saunders.

Lynch, P., Jackson, M. M., Cummings, M. F., & Stamm, W. E. (1987). Rethinking the role of isolation precautions in the prevention of nosocomial infections. *Annals of Internal Medicine, 107,* 243–246.

Whaley, L. F., & Wong, D. L. (1989). *Essentials of pediatric nursing* (3rd ed.). St. Louis: C. V. Mosby.

Williams, W. W. (1983). Guidelines for infection control in hospital personnel. *Infection Control, 4,* 326–349.

Resources for the Consumer

Literature
Available through county health departments (all major communicable diseases)
Understanding AIDS. HHS Publication No. (CDC) HHS-88-8404
Surgeon General

Organizations
American Lung Association
Association for Practitioners in Infection Control (APIC, Mundelein, Illinois)

Injury, High Risk for

Aspiration, High Risk for

Poisoning, High Risk for

Suffocation, High Risk for

Trauma, High Risk for

Injury, High Risk for

- *Related to* **Lack of Knowledge of Precautions Needed Secondary to Sensory or Motor Deficits**
- *Related to* **Lack of Awareness of Environmental Hazards**
- *Related to* **Lack of Awareness of Environmental Hazards Secondary to Maturational Age of Hospitalized Child**
- *Related to* **Vertigo Secondary to Orthostatic Hypotension**

DEFINITION

High Risk for Injury: The state in which an individual is at risk for harm because of a perceptual or physiologic deficit, a lack of awareness of hazards, or maturational age.

RISK FACTORS

Presence of risk factor (*e.g.*)

Evidence of environmental hazards*
Lack of knowledge of environmental hazards
Lack of knowledge of safety precautions

History of accidents
Impaired mobility
Sensory deficits

RELATED FACTORS

Pathophysiologic

Altered cerebral function

Tissue hypoxia
Post trauma
Vertigo

Syncope
Confusion

*See Related Factors and Focus Assessment Criteria for specific hazards.

525

Altered mobility
   Unsteady gait   Loss of limb
Impaired sensory function
   Vision   Thermal/touch
   Hearing   Smell
Pain
Fatigue
Orthostatic hypotension
Vertebrobasilar insufficiency
Cervical spondylosis
Subclavian steal
Vestibular disorders
Carotid sinus syncope
Seizures
Hypoglycemia
Electrolyte imbalance
Amputation
Arthritis
Cerebrovascular accident
Parkinsonism
Congestive heart failure
Dysrhythmias
Depression

Treatment-related

Medications
   Sedatives   Hypoglycemics
   Vasodilators   Diuretics
   Antihypertensives   Phenothiazines
Casts/crutches, canes, walkers

Situational (personal, environmental)

Lack of knowledge
Dehydration (*e.g.,* in summer)
Prolonged bed rest
Stress
Vasovagal reflex
Faulty judgment
Alcohol
Poisons (plants, toxic chemicals)
Household hazards
   Unsafe walkways   Faulty electric wires
   Unsafe toys   Improperly stored poisons
Automotive hazards
   Lack of use of seat belts   Mechanically unsafe vehicle
      or child seats
Fire hazards
   Smoking in bed   Improperly stored petroleum
   Gas leaks   products
Unfamiliar setting (hospital, nursing home)
Improper footwear

Inattentive caretaker
Improper use of aids (crutches, canes, walkers, wheelchairs)
Environmental hazards (home, school, hospital)
History of accidents

Maturational

Infant/child
High risk for maturational age
Suffocation hazards (improper crib, pillow in crib, plastic bags, unattended in water—bath, pool, choking on toys, food)
Improper use of bicycles, kitchen utensils/appliances, sports equipment, lawn equipment
Poison (plants, cleaning agents, medications)
Fire (matches, fireplace, stove)
Falls
Adolescent: Automobile, bicycle, alcohol, drugs
Adult: Drugs, automobile, alcohol
Elderly: Motor and sensory deficits, medication (accidental overdose), cognitive deficits

Diagnostic Considerations

This diagnostic category has four subcategories—*High Risk for Aspiration, Poisoning, Suffocation,* and *Trauma.* The interventions to prevent poisoning, suffocation, and trauma are included under the general category *High Risk for Injury.* Should the nurse choose to isolate interventions only for prevention of poisoning, suffocation, or trauma, then the diagnostic category *High Risk for Poisoning, High Risk for Suffocation,* or *High Risk for Trauma* would be useful.

Nursing interventions related to *High Risk for Injury* focus on protecting a person from injury and teaching precautions to reduce the risk of injury. When the nurse is teaching a client or family safety measures to prevent injury but is not providing on-site protection (as in the community or out-patient department, or for discharge planning), the diagnosis *High Risk Altered Health Maintenance related to insufficient knowledge of safety precautions* may be more appropriate than *High Risk for Injury.*

Errors in Diagnostic Statements

High Risk for Injury: Hemorrhage related to abnormal blood profile secondary to cirrhosis

This diagnosis does not represent a situation that a nurse can prevent, but rather one that the nurse monitors and co-manages as the collaborative problem *Potential Complication: Hemorrhage related to altered clotting factors.* For this same person, the nursing diagnosis *High Risk for Injury related to lack of knowledge of precautions needed to protect soft tissue* also could apply.

Focus Assessment Criteria

This entire assessment is indicated only when the client is at high risk for injury because of personal deficits, alterations (*e.g.,* mobility problems), or maturational age. In households without such a family member, the functional assessment of the individual can be deleted.

Subjective Data

Physical Capabilities of the Person (as reported by person or caretaker)

1. Vision
    Adequate
    Corrected (date of last prescription)
    Complaints of
        Blurriness   Difficulty in focusing
        Loss of side vision   Inability to adjust to darkness
2. Hearing
    Adequate   Need to read lips
    Use of hearing aid (condition,   Inadequate
        batteries)
3. Thermal/tactile
    Adequate   Altered sense of hot/cold
4. Mental status
    Alert   Complaints of
    Drowsy   Vertigo
    Confused   Altered sense of balance
    Oriented to time, place, events   Orthostatic hypotension
    Cognitive stage (immature reason
        ing/judgment)
5. Mobility
    Reports of
        Feeling lightheaded, dizzy   Losing balance
        Difficulty standing, sitting   Wandering
        Falling or almost falling
    Ability to ambulate
        Around room   Around house
        Up and down stairs   Outside house
    Ability to travel
        Drive car (date of last   Use public transportation
            reevaluation)
    Devices
        Cane   Prosthesis
        Wheelchair   Condition of devices
        Walker   Competence in their use
    Shoes/slippers
        Condition   Nonskid soles
        Fit
    Abilities related to developmental milestones
        Turning over   Climbing
        Sitting   Crawling
        Standing   Walking
6. Self-care activities: ability to
    Dress and undress   Bathe self
    Groom self   Eat
    Reach the toilet
7. Housekeeping activities: ability to
    Clean   Shop
    Launder clothes   Prepare food

8. Miscellaneous
  Drug therapy
    Type, dosage
    Labeling
  Communication
    Can write
    Use phone
  Support system/primary caregiver
    Help available from relatives,
      friends, neighbors
    History of "blackouts"

    Storage
    Ability to self-medicate safely

    Contact emergency assistance
    Can make needs known

    Club and church contacts

    Urinary frequency or
      incontinence

Objective Data

Physical Capabilities of the Person
  Blood pressure (left, right, sitting/lying > 5 minutes, 1 minute after standing)
  Gait/mobility
    Steady   Unsteady   Requires aids
  Cognitive processes
    Ability to communicate needs
    Ability to interact
    History of wandering (witnessed and reported by others)
    Ability to understand cause and effect
  Assess for presence of
    Anger   Withdrawal
    Depression   Faulty judgment
  Self-care activities: ability to
    Dress and undress   Bathe
    Groom self   Eat
    Reach toilet
Housing Assessment
  Rent or own
  Type (apartment, duplex, single family house)
  Physical amenities
    Number of rooms for family   Lighting
      members   Water supply
    Toilet facilities   Sewage
    Heating   Garbage disposal
    Ventilation
  Safety
  Adaptations that may need to be made
    Replace nonsturdy furniture
    Gates for stairs
    Better communication facilities (telephone)
    Easier passage from room to room and into and out of house
    Bathroom safety (grab bar, bath bench, nonskid floors)
  Walkways (inside and outside)
    Sidewalks (uneven, broken)
    Stairs (inside and outside)
      Broken steps   Lighting
      No hand rails   Protection for children

Halls
    Cluttered   Poor lighting
Electrical considerations
    Absence of outlet covers
    Cords frayed and unanchored
    Outlets overloaded; accessible to children; near water
    Switches too far from bedside
Lighting
    Adequate or inadequate
    At night; and outdoors
    To bathroom at night
Floors
    Even or uneven
    Highly polished
    Rugs not anchored
Kitchen
    Pot handles not turned inward
    Stove (grease or flammable objects on stove)
    Refrigerator (improperly stored food; inadequate temperatures)
Toxic substances
    Stored in food containers, not properly labeled and accessible to children
    Medications kept beyond date of expiration
    Poisonous household plants
Fire protection
    Matches/lighters accessible to children
    No fire extinguishers
    Improper storage of corrosives, combustibles
    Lack of furnace maintenance
    No fire escape plan, no fire extinguishers
    Emergency telephone numbers not accessible (firehouse, police)
Hazards for children in nursery
    Cribs near drapery cords
    Cribs with wide slat openings
    Plastic bags
    Pillows in crib
    Space between mattress and crib rails
    Unattended without crib rails up
    Unattended on changing table
    Pacifier hung around infant's neck
    A propped bottle placed in infant's crib
    Toys with pointed edges, removable parts
Hazards for children in household
    Accessible purses with medications, lighters, matches
    Objects with lead paint
    Poisonous plants (see Table II-11 for specific plants)
    Open windows without screens or loose screens
    Plastic bags
    Furniture with glass or sharp corners
    Open doorways, stairways
Outdoor hazards for children
    Porches without rails

Table II-11 **Poisonous Substances Around the House**

Drugs

Aspirin	Cough medicines	Laxatives
Tranquilizers	Vitamins	Oral contraceptives
Barbiturates	Acetaminophen	

Petroleum Products

Cleaning Agents

| Soaps and polishes | Disinfectants | Drain cleaners |

Poisonous Plants

Amaryllis	Holly	Oleander
Azalea	Iris	Poinsettia
Baneberry	Jack-in-the-pulpit	Poison hemlock
Belladonna	Jerusalem cherry	Poison ivy
Bittersweet	Jimsonweed	Pokeweed
Bloodroot	Lily of the valley	Potato leaves
Castor-bean plant	Marijuana	Rhododendron
Climbing nightshade	Mistletoe	Rhubarb leaves
Daffodil	Morning glory	Tomato leaves
Dieffenbachia	Mountain laurel	Wisteria
Foxglove	Mushrooms	Yew

Miscellaneous

| Baby powder | Cosmetics | Lead paint |

Play area without fence
Backyard pools
Domestic/wild animals
Poisonous plants
Fall assessment
See Figure II-3.

Principles and Rationale for Nursing Care

Generic Considerations

1. Injury is the fourth leading cause of death in the general population (40.1 deaths/100,000), and the leading cause of death for children and young adults (National Center for Health Statistics, 1985).
2. The differentiation between accidents and injuries is a useful distinction for nurses to understand. The term accident implies lack of control of external forces. Nursing focuses on identifying variables (host, agent, environment) that can be controlled to prevent injuries (Green, 1989).
3. The nurse can reduce host variables that increase risk for injury, such as lack of knowledge; agent variables, such as shear forces in bed; and environmental variables, such as spills and other hazards.
4. Accidents occur more frequently
   During the initial period of hospitalization and between the hours of 6 and 9 P.M.
   During peak activity periods (mealtime, playtime)
   In unfamiliar surroundings

1. Name: 2. D.O.B.:   3. Sex:
4. Date: 5. Day of week: 6. Time of day:
7. Diagnoses:
8. Witnessed by staff: ( ) yes   ( ) no
9. Location of fall: ( ) Room   ( ) BR   ( ) DR   ( ) Lounge
              ( ) outdoors   ( ) shower   ( ) hallway   ( ) other
10. Vital signs: BP _____   P _____   R _____   T _____
              Orthostatic BP: lying _____,   standing _____
11. Description of fall (if applicable):
     ( ) from bed, side rails ( ) up, ( ) down
     ( ) getting in and out of bed
     ( ) from wheelchair
     ( ) ambulatory: ( ) assisted, ( ) unassisted
     ( ) tub, shower
     ( ) found on floor, wet floor ( ) yes, ( ) no
     ( ) restraints ordered: ( ) yes, ( ) no
           In place? ( ) yes, ( ) no
     ( ) from stretcher
     ( ) assistive devices: ( ) yes, ( ) no
           ( ) wheelchair, ( ) walker, ( ) cane
     ( ) environmental hazard identified? Describe:
12. Patient's account of fall:
13. Nurse's account of fall:
14. Patient's mental status prior to fall (baseline):
15. Patient's mental status at time of fall: ( ) alert, ( ) disoriented, ( ) confused,
           ( ) sedated, ( ) other _____
16. Type of injury: ( ) laceration, ( ) hematoma, ( ) burn, ( ) abrasion, ( ) sprain,
           ( ) fracture, ( ) other _____
17. Was the patient experiencing any of the following at the time of the fall:
     ( ) acute confusion
     ( ) difficulty with ambulation
     ( ) bowel or bladder urgency
     ( ) emotional upset, anger, or agitation
     ( ) medically unstable at time of fall
     ( ) lightheadedness
     ( ) palpitations
     ( ) chest pain
     ( ) shortness of breath
     ( ) one-side weakness
18. After the fall, did the patient:
     Lose consciousness ( ) yes, ( ) no
     Lose bladder/bowel control ( ) yes, ( ) no
19. Previous falls: ( ) yes, ( ) no
     No. during past 6 months _____
     No. resulting in injury _____
20. Number of different medications patient has taken during the last 24 hours, including
     prns: _____.
21. Medication categories:
     ( ) cardiac meds
     ( ) diuretic or antihypertensive
     ( ) neuroleptic (sedative, hypnotic, antidepressant, psychotropic, antianxiety)
     ( ) analgesic
     ( ) laxative or stool softener
22. What measures can be taken to prevent recurrence:
23. Postinjury care given:
24. Treatment plan:

Fig. II-3 Fall assessment. (Data from Hernandez and Miller, 1986; Barbieri, 1983; Tideiksaar, 1984; Schulman and Acquaviva, 1987)

With inadequate lighting
At holidays
On vacations
During home repairs

5. Color contrast between the object and the background increases visualization (*e.g.*, white against black).
6. Fasting for diagnostic tests causes dehydration and weakness that contribute to accidents.
7. Falls can result when urinary urgency and frequency cause a person to rush to the bathroom.
8. Table II-11 lists common sources of poisoning in the home.

Postural Hypotension

1. Postural hypotension refers to a sudden drop in blood pressure of 20 mm Hg or greater for at least 1 minute when standing.
2. Studies have shown that postprandial hypotension occurs in about one-third of healthy adults 1 hour after eating breakfast and lunch (Lipsitz & Fullerton, 1986).
3. Postural hypotension can seriously affect a person's quality of life if it contributes to falls or fear of falling.
4. Postural hypotension also can precipitate stroke and myocardial infarctions (Cunha, 1987).
5. Prolonged bed rest causes skeletal muscle weakness and decreased venous tone, predisposing to postural hypotension.
6. The blood pressure drop may be greater in the morning, because blood volume tends to decrease during the night.
7. Some common drugs contributing to postural hypotension are:

Diuretics	Antihistamines
Pheothiazines	Alcohol
Antidepressants	Levodopa
Barbiturates	Diazepam

Pediatric Considerations

1. Injuries rank as the number one cause of death in persons between age 1 and 19 years (Whaley & Wong, 1989).
2. Five leading risk areas include traffic accidents, drownings, burns and scalds, choking, poisoning, and falls (Children's National Medical Center, 1989).
3. Each year, car crashes injure and kill more children than any disease. Used properly, child safety seats and safety belts protect children in a crash and help save lives (Children's National Medical Center, 1989).
4. School-age children are at greatest risk for bicycle accidents. Every day, more than 1000 children are injured, and one dies, in bicycle accidents. One-third of children treated in emergency rooms for bicycle accidents have head injuries. The use of bicycle helmets could reduce the incidence of these injuries by 85% (*American Journal of Nursing,* 1990).
5. Drowning is the second leading cause of death from injury during childhood. Children under 4 are at especially high risk (Children's National Medical Center, 1989).
6. Children should be taught early (when 2 years old) and constantly reminded about rules regarding streets, playground equipment, fires, water (pools, bathtubs), animals, strangers.
7. In 1982 in the US, 738 children drowned and 3000 children experienced near-

drowning, with one-third left with neurologic deficits; 68,000 persons had nonsubmersion accidents in and around swimming pools (Baxter, 1987).

8. Sixty-eight percent of the near-drowning accidents take place while a parent is supervising the child, resulting from a momentary lapse of attention (Baxter, 1987).

9. Effective swimming depends on intellectual as well as physical maturity. Organized swimming lessons may give parents a false sense of security that their child "can swim" (Baxter, 1987).

10. Swimming programs that use total submersion put an infant at risk for water intoxication, hypothermia, and bacterial infections. In addition, infants may learn to fear the water (Brill, 1987).

11. Children age 1–3 years are at greatest risk for scalds. More than one-third of children aged 3–8 years are burned while playing with matches. When a fire strikes, young children need help to escape (Children's National Medical Center, 1989).

12. For children under age 3 years, choking is the fourth leading cause of accidental death (Children's National Medical Center, 1989).

13. Toddlers are at highest risk for poisoning. Children are poisoned by medications as well as by common household items, e.g., plants, make-up, and cleaning products (Children's National Medical Center, 1989).

14. For children age 1–4 years, the leading cause of accidental death and serious injury is falls in the home (Children's National Medical Center, 1989).

15. The nurse should assess each child's unique risk of potential for injury. This includes the child with sensory or motor deficits and developmental delay. Environmental changes, such as hospitalization, visiting relatives' homes, and celebrating holidays pose special hazards for children.

Gerontologic Considerations

1. Falls occur with greater frequency in the elderly, and the mortality, dysfunction, disability, and need for medical services that result are greater than in younger age groups. Unintentional injury, a category including falls, motor vehicle accidents, and burns, is the seventh leading cause of death in the elderly, and the incidence of falls represents over 60% of that category.

2. Approximately 25% of hospital admissions for older adults are directly related to falling; 47% of these people are admitted to long-term care facilities (Tideiksaar, 1989).

3. Goals for prevention and management of falls focus on reducing the likelihood of falls by reducing environmental hazards, strengthening individual competence to resist falls and fall-related injury, and providing postfall injury care.

4. "Fallaphobia" refers to fears related to a person's loss of confidence to perform activities without falling. These fears actually increase the risk for falling, and the person eventually becomes house-bound (Tideiksaar, 1989).

5. A fall-free existence is not always possible for some individuals. Increased independence and mobility may be an important and valuable trade-off for an increased risk of falling. Collaboration among the client, family, and team members helps arrive at the decision of a less restricted environment.

6. The following factors increase the risk for falls in older adults:
   a. History of falls
   b. Sensory–motor deficits (e.g., vision, hearing, hemianopsia, paresis, aphasia)
   c. Gait instability
   d. Improper footwear or foot problems (corns, bunions, calluses)
   e. Postural hypotension, especially with complaints of dizziness
   f. Confusion (persistent or acute)

g. Incontinence, urinary urgency
h. Cardiovascular disease affecting cerebral perfusion and oxygenation: dysrhythmias syncopal episodes, congestive heart failure, fibrillation
i. Neurologic disease affecting movement or judgment: cerebrovascular accident with impulsivity; parkinsonism; moderate Alzheimer's disease; seizure disorder, vertigo
j. Orthopedic disorders or devices affecting movement or balance: casts, splints, stings, prostheses, recent surgery, severe arthritis
k. Medications affecting blood pressure or level of consciousness: psychotropics, sedatives, analgesics, diuretics, antihypertensives, medication change, more than five drugs
l. Agitation, increased anxiety, emotional lability
m. Willfulness, uncooperativeness
n. Situational factors: new admission, room change, roommate change
7. Osteoporosis is the age-related change most likely to cause serious negative functional results (Miller, 1990). Refer to *Health-Seeking Behaviors* for additional information on prevention of osteoporosis.
8. Older adults cannot compensate to hypertensive or hypotensive stimuli as efficiently as younger adults and thus are more sensitive to these states. (See also Postural Hypotension.)
9. Visual difficulty because of glare is often responsible for falls in the aged, who have an increased susceptibility to glare. Incandescent (nonfluorescent) lighting produces less glare and therefore provides better illumination for the aged.

■ High Risk for Injury
Related to Lack of Knowledge of Precautions Needed Secondary to Sensory or Motor Deficits

---

Assessment

Subjective Data

The person reports
Past history of falls and injuries
Decreased or absent vision
Decreased or absent hearing
Decreased or absent thermal
    perception

Limited movement
Pain
Vertigo

Objective Data

Inflamed joints
Contractures
Skeletal deformities
Unsteady gait
Paralysis
Weakness

Muscle spasms
Crutches
Walker, cane
Prosthesis
Evidence of past injuries
    (bruises, burn marks)

Outcome Criteria

The person will
- Identify factors that increase the risk for injury
- Relate an intent to use safety measures to prevent injury (*e.g.*, remove throw rugs or anchor them)
- Relate an intent to practice selected prevention measures (*e.g.*, wear sunglasses to reduce glare)
- Increase his daily activity, if feasible

Interventions

A. Assess for the presence of causative or contributing factors
1. Unfamiliar surroundings
2. Impaired vision
   a. Altered spatial judgment
   b. Blurred vision
   c. Diplopia
   d. Blind spots
   e. Cataracts
   f. Altered peripheral vision
   g. Hemianopia (loss of half the visual field)
   h. Increased susceptibility to visual glare
   i. Decreased ability to distinguish object from background
3. Decreased hearing acuity
4. Decreased tactile sensitivity (touch)
5. Orthostatic hypotension
6. Hypoglycemia
7. Unstable gait
8. Pain
9. Fatigue
10. Improper shoes or slippers
11. Improper use of crutches, canes, walkers
12. Joint immobility
13. Side-effects of medication (*e.g.*, tranquilizers, diuretics)
14. Hazardous environmental factors

B. Reduce or eliminate causative or contributing factors if possible
1. Unfamiliar surroundings
   a. Orient each new admission to surroundings, explain the call system, and assess the person's ability to use it.
   b. Closely supervise the person during the first few nights to assess safety.
   c. Use night light.
   d. Encourage the person to request assistance during the night.
   e. Teach the person about side-effects of certain drugs (*e.g.*, dizziness, fatigue).
   f. Keep bed at lowest level during the night.
   g. Consider use of soft restraints or a movement-detection monitor, if needed.

2. Impaired vision
   a. Provide safe illumination or teach person to
      - Provide adequate lighting in all rooms, with soft light at night
      - Have light switch easily accessible, next to bed.
      - Provide background light that is soft.
   b. Teach person to reduce glare.
      - Avoid all glossy surfaces (*e.g.,* glass, highly polished floors).
      - Use diffuse light rather than direct light; use shades that darken the room.
      - Turn head away when switching on a bright light.
      - Wear sunglasses or hats with brims, or carry umbrellas, to reduce glare outside.
      - Avoid looking directly at bright lights (*e.g.,* headlights).
   c. Teach person or family to provide sufficient color contrast for visual discrimination and to avoid green and blue.
      - Color-code edges of steps (*e.g.,* with colored tape).
      - Avoid white walls, dishes, counters.
      - Avoid clear glasses (*i.e.,* use smoked glass).
      - Choose objects colored black on white (*e.g.,* black phone).
      - Avoid colors that merge (*e.g.,* beige switches on beige walls).
      - Paint doorknobs bright colors.
3. Decreased tactile sensitivity
   a. Teach preventive measures.
      - Assess temperature of bath water and heating pads prior to use.
      - Use bath thermometers.
      - Assess extremities daily for undetected injuries.
      - Keep feet warm and dry and skin softened with emollient lotion (lanolin, mineral oil).
   b. See *Altered Tissue Perfusion: Peripheral* for additional interventions.
4. Decreased hearing acuity
   a. Determine if the person has had his hearing evaluated professionally.
   b. Assist him in making a decision regarding the use or type of hearing aid if indicated.
   c. Teach him, when driving, to leave car window partially open to allow warning signals to be heard (*e.g.,* sirens) and set air conditioner, heater, or radio low so that outside noises can be heard.
5. Orthostatic hypotension
   a. See *High Risk for Injury Related to Vertigo Secondary to Orthostatic Hypotension* for additional interventions.
6. Unstable gait
   a. Crutches
      - Teach exercises to strengthen arm and shoulder muscles to facilitate use of crutches; use weights and parallel bars.
      - Measure and fit crutches to each person (2–3 inches between top of crutch and armpit); improper length of crutches may cause nerve damage or falls.
      - Instruct person to wear shoes that fit properly and have nonskid soles.
      - Assess ability to walk and climb up and down stairs.
      - Consult with physical therapist for proper gait training.

      b. Canes
- Teach person to hold cane in hand opposite affected leg and move cane and impaired limb together.
- Cane should be proper length to allow person to extend elbow and bear weight on hand.
- Cane should be fitted with rubber tip.
- Consult with physical therapist for proper gait training.

      c. Walkers
- Teach person exercises to strengthen triceps muscles used in proper crutch walking.
- See that floors are clean and dry and free of obstacles and that rugs are anchored.
- Instruct person to wear properly fitted shoes with nonslip soles.
- Consult with physical therapist for proper gait training.

      d. Prosthesis
- Teach person to bathe and inspect stump daily.
- Instruct person to put on prosthesis soon after rising to minimize stump swelling.
- Prepare person for crutch walking with triceps exercises using weights and parallel bars.
- Consult with physical therapist for proper gait training.

7. Side-effects of medications

      a. Assess for the presence of side-effects of drugs that may cause vertigo.
- Hypotension
- Sedation
- Hypokalemia
- Vasodilation
- Vasoconstriction

8. Hazardous environmental factors

      a. Teach person to
- Eliminate throw rugs, litter, and highly polished floors
- Provide nonslip surfaces in bathtub or shower by applying commercially available traction tapes
- Provide hand grips in bathroom
- Provide railings in hallways and on stairs
- Remove protruding objects (*e.g.,* coat hooks, shelves, light fixtures) from stairway walls

      b. Instruct staff to
- Keep side rails on bed in place and bed at the lowest position when person is left unattended
- Keep bed at lowest position with wheels locked when stationary
- Teach person in wheelchair to lock and unlock wheels
- Ensure that person's shoes or slippers have nonskid soles

C. Describe and document falls

1. Refer to Focus Assessment (Fig. II-3) for fall assessment.
2. Document the results of the assessment.

D. Initiate health teaching and referrals as indicated

1. Teach measures to prevent auto accidents.
      a. Frequently reevaluate ability to drive vehicles.

b. Wear good-quality sunglasses (gray or green) to reduce glare.

c. Keep windshields clean and wipers in good condition.

d. Place mirrors on both sides of car.

e. Stop periodically to stretch and rest eyes.

f. Know the effects of medications on driving ability.

g. Do not smoke while driving or drive after drinking.

2. Teach measures to prevent pedestrian accidents.

a. Allow enough time to cross streets.

b. Wear garments that reflect light (beige, white) at night.

c. Wait to cross on the sidewalk, not the street.

d. Look both ways.

e. Do not rely solely on green traffic lights to provide safe crossing (right turn on red light may be legal, or driver may disobey traffic regulations).

3. Teach measures to prevent burns.

a. Equip home with smoke alarm system and check its function each month.

b. Have a hand fire extinguisher.

c. Set thermostats for water heater to provide warm but not scalding water.

d. Use baking soda or a lid cover to smother a kitchen grease fire.

e. Do not wear loose-fitting clothing (*e.g.,* robes, nightgowns) when cooking.

f. Do not smoke when sleepy.

g. Ensure that portable heaters are safely used.

h. See *High Risk for Injury Related to Lack of Awareness of Environmental Hazards* for additional safety measures.

4. Refer individuals with motor or sensory deficits for assistance in identifying environmental hazards.

a. Local fire company

b. Community nursing agency

c. Accident-prevention information (see References/Bibliography)

5. Discuss the benefits of a walking program to increase circulation if permissible; instruct to

a. Rest 10–15 minutes before walking

b. Start slowly (10 minutes)

c. Increase time gradually

d. Refrain from drinking caffeine products (coffee, tea, chocolate, cola) 2–3 hours before walking

e. Wait 2 hours after meals to walk

f. Expect some muscle soreness; reduce activity if pain or breathlessness occur

6. Assist person and family to evaluate environmental hazards and the effects of restrictions on quality of life.

7. Refer person to public health or visiting nurse for home visit.

8. Refer person to physical therapist for evaluation of gait.

■ High Risk for Injury
Related to Lack of Awareness of Environmental Hazards

Assessment

Subjective Data
The person reports
Past history of accidents

Objective Data
Presence of hazards (see Focus Assessment Criteria)

Outcome Criteria

The person or family will
- Identify potentially hazardous factors in the environment
- Report safe practices in the home
- Teach children safety habits

Interventions

A. Identify situations that contribute to accidents

Unfamiliar setting (homes of others, hotels)
Children
Peak activity periods (during meal preparation, holidays)
New equipment (bicycle, chain saw, lawn mower, snow blower)
Lack of awareness of or disregard for environmental hazards

1. Unfamiliar setting
   a. Instruct to leave a light on for access to bathroom during night.
   b. With small children, instruct parents to
      - Inspect the area (inside and outside) for hazards before allowing child to play
      - Expect the child to explore hidden areas
      - Have infants sleep on floor on padding rather than in beds without rails

2. Children
   a. Teach parents to expect frequent changes in infants' and children's ability and to take precautions (*e.g.,* infant who suddenly rolls over for the first time might be on a changing table unattended).
   b. Discuss with parents the necessity of constant monitoring of small children.
   c. Provide parents with information to assist them in selecting a babysitter.
      - Determine previous experiences and knowledge of emergency measures.
      - Observe the interaction of the sitter with the child (*e.g.,* pick up the sitter one-half hour before you are ready to leave).

d. Teach parents to expect children to mimic them and to teach children what they can do with or without supervision.
  - Tell the child to ask you before attempting a new task.
  - Don't take pills in front of children.
e. Explain and expect compliance with certain rules (depending on age) regarding

Streets	Fire
Playground equipment	Animals
Water (pools, bathtubs)	Strangers
Bicycles	

f. Role-play with children to assess understanding of the problem
  "You are walking home from school and a strange man pulls up in a car near you. What do you do?"
  "While walking past a barbecue, your dress catches on fire. What do you do?"

3. Peak activity periods
  a. Provide the child with a special distraction (*e.g.,* clay) while preparing meal.
  b. Place the child in a playpen to provide a safe place that does not require close supervision.
  c. Assess the safety of holiday decorations prior to use.

Christmas trees	
Fire or electrical hazard	Lighted candles
Poorly anchored	Ceramic pieces

4. New equipment
  a. Teach to read directions completely before using a new appliance or a piece of equipment.
  b. Determine the limitations of the equipment.
  c. Unplug and turn off any appliance that is not functioning before examining (*e.g.,* lawn mower, snow blower, electric mixer).
  d. Determine that a new bicycle is the correct size for the child before allowing unrestricted riding.
  e. Examine new toys for removable parts and chemical and electrical hazards before allowing child to play.

5. Lack of awareness of environmental hazards
  a. Teach to avoid unsafe practices and prevent injury
    - Automobiles
        Driving a mechanically unsafe vehicle
        Not using or misusing seat restraints
        Driving after partaking of alcohol or drugs
        Driving with unrestrained babies and children in the car
        Driving at excessive speeds
        Driving without necessary visual aids
        Driving with unsafe road or road crossing conditions
        Nonuse or misuse of necessary headgear for motorcyclist
        Children riding in front seat of car
        Backing up without checking location of small children
        Warming a car in a closed garage
    - Bicycles, wagons, skateboards, and skates carrying passengers
        No reflectors or lights
        Not in single file
        Riding a too-large bicycle
        Lack of knowledge of rules of the road
        Use of skateboards or skates in heavily traveled areas

- Flammables
    - Igniting gas leaks
    - Delayed lighting of gas burner or oven
    - Experimenting with chemicals or gasoline
        - Unscreened fires, fireplaces, heaters
        - Inadequately stored combustibles, matches, or oily rags
        - Smoking in bed or near oxygen
        - Highly flammable children's toys or clothing
        - Playing with fireworks or gunpowder
        - Playing with matches, candles, cigarettes, lighters
        - Wearing of plastic aprons or flowing clothing around open flame
- Household
    - Kitchen
        - Grease waste collected on stoves
        - Wearing of plastic aprons or flowing clothing around open flame
        - Use of cracked glasses or dishware
        - Use of improper canning, freezing, or preserving methods
        - Knives stored in an uncovered fashion
        - Pot handles facing front of stove
        - Use of thin or worn potholders or oven mitts
        - Stove controls on front
    - Bathroom
        - Unlocked medicine cabinet
        - Lack of grab rails in bathtub
        - Lack of nonskid mats or emory strips in bathtub
        - Poor lighting in bathroom and hallways
        - Improper placement of electrical outlets
    - Chemicals and irritants
        - Improperly labeled medication containers
        - Medications kept in containers other than original ones
        - Poor illumination at the medicine cabinet
        - Improperly labeled containers of poisons and corrosive substances
        - Expired medications that dangerously decompose
        - Toxic substances stored in accessible areas (*e.g.,* under sink)
        - Inadequately stored corrosives (*e.g.,* lye)
        - Contact with intense cold
        - Overexposure to sun, sunlamps, heating pads
    - Lighting and electrical
        - Uncovered outlets
        - Unanchored electrical wires
        - Overloaded electrical outlets
        - Overloaded fuse boxes
        - Faulty electrical plugs, frayed wires, or defective electrical appliances
        - Inadequate lighting over landings and stairs
        - Inaccessible light switches (*e.g.,* bedside)
        - Use of machinery or appliances without prior instruction
    - Water and pools
        - Discourage use of flotation or swim aids (water wings, tubs) with children who can't swim.

Teach safe water behavior
  No running, pushing
  No jumping on others
  No swimming alone
  No playful screaming for help
  No diving in water less than 8 feet deep
  No swimming after meals
  No swimming during electrical storms
  Avoid excessive alcohol use
Enclose pool
  Use a 5–5½ foot fence
  Use a fence that children can't climb
  Use self-locking gates
Remove pool cover completely
Avoid free-floating pool covers
Teach safe diving and sliding techniques
  Allow diving only from diving boards
  Discourage running dives
  Teach to steer upward with hands and head
  Descend pool slide sitting with feet first
Have life-saving equipment at pool side (life preserver, rope, or
  hook)
Learn CPR and how to respond to accidental submersion.
  Remove from water
  If spinal injury is suspected, immobilize on a board and apply a
    cervical collar
  Clear airway of debris
  If person is unresponsive, place on side if vomiting occurs
  Remove wet clothes, dry, and cover with blankets (including
    head)
  Begin CPR and continue until help arrives
Miscellaneous
  Unsupervised contact with animals and poisons in environment
    (plants, pool chemicals, pills)
  Obstructed passageways
  Unsafe window protection in home with young children
  Guns or ammunition stored in unlocked fashion
  Large icicles hanging from roof
  Icy walkways
  Glass sliding doors that look open when closed
  Low-strung clothesline
  Discarded or unused refrigerators or freezers without removed
    doors
• Infants and children
  Household
    Pillows in crib
    Staircases without stair gates
    Crib mattresses that do not fit snugly
    Cribs with slat opening to allow child's body to fall through,
      catching the head

> Glass or sharp-edged tables
> Porches and decks without railings
> Poisonous plants (see Table II-11)
> Furniture painted with lead paint
> Unsupervised bathing
> Open windows
> Propped bottle in crib
>
> Toys
> > Sharp edges
> > Easily breakable parts
> > Removable small pieces
> > Balloons
> > Lollipops
> > Pacifier around neck
>
> Miscellaneous
> > Unattended in shopping cart
> > Unattended in car
> > Cribs, walkers, high chairs with movable parts that trap child (*e.g.*, springs)

B. Initiate health teaching and referrals as indicated

1. Instruct parents how to "child proof" the home.
2. Instruct parents to keep poisons and corrosive substances in tightly closed, carefully marked containers in locked closets.
3. Parents should discard unused supplies of medications and keep needed medications in locked, inaccessible medicine closet.
4. Parents should be taught how to administer antidotes for specific toxic substances.
5. Parents should also have the phone number of the Poison Control Center in a convenient place.
6. Refer individuals to local poison control center for "Mr. Yuk" poison warning stickers and advice on emergency procedures; teach the child what a Mr. Yuk sticker means.
7. Instruct parents on the use of ipecac and its availability.
8. Assist family to evaluate environmental hazards in home; consult public health agency.
9. Install specially designed locks to prevent children from opening closets where combustible, corrosive, or flammable materials or medications are stored.
10. Instruct parents to use socket covers to prevent accidental electrical shocks to children.
11. Teach parents about hazards of lead paint ingestion and how to identify "pica" in a child.
12. Refer parents to public health department if lead paint screening is necessary.
13. Encourage use of child-proof caps.
14. Advise parents to avoid storing dangerous substances in containers ordinarily used for foods.
15. Refer parents to automobile club for information regarding safety car seats for children.
16. Refer parents to local fire department for assistance in staging home fire drills.

■ High Risk for Injury
Related to Lack of Awareness of Environmental Hazards Secondary to Maturational Age of Hospitalized Child

Assessment

Subjective Data

The parent (primary caregiver) reports child's unique cognitive and motor abilities
Developmental milestones the child has achieved

Objective Data

Presence of hazards (see Focus Assessment Criteria)
Evidence that child/adolescent's abilities are changing (*e.g.*, the infant may turn over for the first time in the hospital)

Outcome Criteria

The child/adolescent will be
- Free from injury from potentially hazardous factors that are identified in the hospital environment

The family will
- Reinforce and demonstrate safe practices in the hospital

Interventions

A. Protect the infant/child from injury in the hospital by controlling hazards that are age-related

Infant (1–12 months)
Ensure that the infant can be identified by an identification band and a tag on his crib.
Do not shake powder directly on infant; rather, place powder in hand and then on infant's skin. Keep powder out of infant's reach.
Keep unsafe toys out of reach (*e.g.*, buttons, beads, balloons, broken toys, sharp-edged toys, other small toys).
Use restraints to prevent infant from removing catheters, eye patches, IV infusions, dressings, and feeding tubes, as needed.
Keep siderails up in locked position when child is in crib.
Pad siderails if infant is able to move out of bed or is at risk for seizures.
Do not use foam cushions for holding/feeding infant. (This type of pillow is filled with foam pellets.)
Use a cool-mist vaporizer.
Do not use an infant walker.
Ascertain identity of all visitors.

Use a firm mattress that fits crib snugly.

Do not feed honey to infants under age 6 months due to danger of botulism.

Fasten safety straps on infant seats, swings, highchairs, and strollers.

Do not allow bottles to be propped. The infant should be held with his head in an upright position.

Do not place pillows in crib.

Place one hand over the child while weighing, changing diapers, etc., to keep infant safe.

Do not allow infant to wear pacifier on a string around the neck.

Check bath water to make sure that the temperature is appropriate. Never leave infant alone while bathing! Support the small infant's head out of the water.

Check the temperature of formula, especially if it is heated in the microwave.

Position crib away from bedside stand, infusion pumps, etc., to prevent child from reaching unsafe objects (e.g., dials on infusion pump, suction machine, electrical outlets, flowers).

Do not allow parents to smoke or drink hot beverages in infant's room.

Foods that must be chewed or are small enough to occlude the airway should not be offered (i.e., nuts, popcorn, hard candy, whole hot dogs). Forks and knives are not appropriate utensils for infants.

Discard syringes, needles, med packets, plastic bags safely.

Protect with shoes or slippers the feet of the infant who is able to walk.

Transport the infant safely to other areas of the hospital (i.e., x-ray, laboratory).

Remind parents to have approved car seat in their automobile to transport the child home.

Assess each unique situation for high risk for injury to the infant. Inform parents of the infant's high risk for injury.

Early Childhood (13 months–5 years)

Ensure that the young child is identifiable by name band and name tag on crib.

Keep siderails up in locked position when child is in crib—top and bottom compartments; use siderails on youth beds.

Monitor child at all times when eating, bathing, playing, and toileting.

Keep cleaning agents, sharp items, and plastic bags out of reach.

Secure thermometer while taking temperature (use rectal or axillary method with toddler and oral method when child is old enough not to bite down on thermometer).

Assess for loose teeth, and document on records.

Check the temperature of bath water before immersing child.

Use electric beds with extreme caution. For example, children may get their fingers caught or get under the bed and be at risk for a crushing injury.

Position crib/bed away from bedside stand, infusion pumps, flowers, etc., to prevent child from reaching unsafe objects.

Keep child safe when mobile:

Protect child's feet with shoes or slippers when ambulating.

Keep bathroom and closet doors firmly shut.

Check any tubing attached to child to prevent kinking or dislodgment.

Apply safety straps when child is in highchair, stroller or on a cart.

Transport safely to other areas of the hospital (i.e., x-ray).

Use restraints to prevent child from removing catheters, eye patches, IV infusion, dressings, and feeding tubes, as needed.

Place one hand over child when weighing, changing diapers, etc., to prevent falls.

Do not call medications "candy."

Do not permit the child to chew gum, eat hard candy, nuts, whole hot dogs, or fish with bones.

Set limits. Enforce and repeat to child what he can do in the hospital and to which areas he may go.

Provide with age-appropriate, safe toys (see manufacturer's guidelines.)

Do not allow parents to smoke or drink hot beverages in the child's room.

Feed the child in a quiet environment; ensure that the child is seated while eating to prevent choking.

Remind parents to have approved car seat in automobile to transport child home.

Ascertain identity of all visitors.

Assess each unique situation for high risk for injury to the young child. Inform parents of the young child's high risk for injury.

School-ager/adolescent (6–12 years/13–18 years)

Ensure that the school-ager/adolescent can be identified by a name band and a tag on his bed. School-agers may claim to be someone else to joke with the nurse, not realizing the danger of this.

Assess for loose teeth and document on records.

Assess for self-care deficits and activity intolerance because the school-ager/adolescent may not ask for help when ambulating, bathing, toileting, and so forth.

Apply safety straps when transporting via cart or wheelchair.

Set limits: Enforce and reiterate to the child what he can do and to what areas he may go in the hospital.

Provide with age-appropriate activities. Supervise therapeutic play closely and do not allow child to use syringes as squirt guns.

Do not allow parents to smoke or drink hot beverages in the child's room.

Encourage child/adolescent to wear Medic Alert necklace or bracelet, if appropriate. Encourage to carry I.D. in wallet/purse.

Remind to wear seat belt in auto when discharged.

Discourage smoking and use of illicit drugs, including alcohol.

Assess each unique situation for high risk for injury to the school-ager/adolescent. Inform parents of child's/adolescent's high risk for injury.

■ High Risk for Injury Related to Vertigo
Secondary to Orthostatic Hypotension

Assessment

Subjective Data

Individual reports
  Dizziness
  Blurred vision
  Vertigo
  History of "blackouts"

Objective Data
Brachial systolic blood pressure decreases 20 mm Hg when standing

---

Outcome Criteria

The individual will
• Relate methods of preventing sudden decreases in cerebral blood flow due to orthostatism
• Demonstrate maneuvers to change position and avoid sudden drop in cerebral pressure
• Relate fewer episodes of dizziness or vertigo

Interventions

A. Identify contributing factors, which may include:
1. Cardiovascular disorders (hypertension, cerebral infarct, anemia, dysrhythmias)
2. Fluid and/or electrolyte imbalances
3. Peripheral neuropathy, Parkinson's disease
4. Diabetes
5. Certain medications (antihypertensives, anticholinergics, barbiturates, vasodilators, tricyclic antidepressants, levodopa, nitrates, monoamine oxidase inhibitors, phenothiazines)
6. Alcohol
7. Age 75 years or older
8. Prolonged bed rest
9. Surgical sympathectomy
10. Valsalva maneuver during voiding (Miller, 1990)

B. Assess for orthostatic hypotension
1. Take bilateral brachial pressures with the person supine.
2. If the brachial pressures are different, use the arm with the higher reading and take the blood pressure immediately after the client stands up quickly; report differences to the physician.
3. Ask the client to describe sensations.

C. Discuss physiology of orthostatic hypotension with client
1. Age-related changes in vessel
2. Volume of blood in lower extremities
3. Sympathetic nervous system response
4. Effects of prolonged bed rest
5. Postprandial effects

D. Teach techniques to reduce orthostatic hypotension
1. Change positions slowly.
2. Move from lying to an upright position in stages.
   a. Sit up in bed.
      • Dangle first one leg, then the other over the side of the bed.
   b. Allow a few minutes before going on to each step.

     c. Gradually pull oneself from a sitting to a standing position.

     d. Place a chair, walker, cane, or other assistive device nearby to use to steady oneself when getting out of bed.

  3. During day, rest in a recliner rather than in bed.

  4. Avoid prolonged standing.

  5. Avoid stooping to pick something from the floor; use an assistive device available from an orthotics department or a self-help store to pick up items from the floor.

  6. Use waist-high elastic stockings.

     a. Place stockings on in A.M. before getting out of bed

     b. Avoid sitting for long periods of time

     c. Remove stockings when supine

E. Encourage person to increase daily activity if permissible

1. Discuss the value of daily exercise (increases circulation, decreases the process of osteoporosis, increases energy levels, reduces stress, and contributes to an overall state of well-being).
2. Establish an exercise program.

F. Teach to avoid dehydration and vasodilation

1. Replace fluids during periods of excess fluid loss (*e.g.,* in hot weather).
2. Avoid diuretic fluids (*e.g.,* coffee, tea, cola).
3. Avoid alcohol consumption.
4. Avoid sources of intense heat, *e.g.,* direct sun, hot showers, baths, electric blankets.
5. Avoid taking nitroglycerin while standing.

G. Teach to reduce postprandial hypotension (Miller, 1990)

1. Take antihypertensive medications after meals rather than before.
2. Eat small, frequent meals.
3. Remain seated or lie down after meals.

H. Institute environmental safety measures

(Refer to *High Risk for Injury Related to Lack of Awareness of Environmental Hazards.*)

High Risk for Aspiration

■ *Related to* **(Specify)**

DEFINITION

High Risk for Aspiration: The state in which a person is at risk for entry of secretions, solids, or fluids into the tracheobronchial passages.

RISK FACTORS

Presence of favorable conditions for aspiration (see Etiologic, Contributing, and Risk Factors)

RELATED FACTORS

Pathophysiologic

Reduced level of consciousness/unconsciousness
Dementias
Seizures
Alcohol/drug-induced
Depressed cough/gag reflexes
Cerebral vascular accident
Parkinsonism
Head injury
Debilitating conditions
Paralysis
Increased intragastric pressure (decreased gastrointestinal motility, delayed gastric emptying)
  Autonomic dysfunction
  Pregnancy
  Obesity
  Electrolyte imbalance
  Ileus
  Intestinal obstruction
  Gastrointestinal outlet syndrome
Impaired swallowing (refer to *Impaired Swallowing*)
  Achalasia   Myasthenia gravis
  Scleraderma   Guillain-Barré syndrome
  Hiatal hernia   Multiple sclerosis
  Esophageal strictures   Muscular dystrophy
Tracheoesophageal fistula
Catatonic

Treatment-related

Facial/oral surgery/trauma
Neck surgery/trauma
Wired jaws
Gastrointestinal tubes
Tracheostomy or endotracheal tubes
Enteral feedings
Anesthesia

Situational

Inability/impaired ability to elevate upper body
Alcohol use during meals

Maturational

Newborns
  Premature
  Cleft palate

Children (high-risk age 1–3)
Elderly
    Poor dentition

Diagnostic Considerations

High Risk for Aspiration is a clinically useful diagnosis for persons at high risk for aspiration due to reduced level of consciousness, structural deficits, mechanical devices, and neurologic and gastrointestinal disorders. Although persons with swallowing difficulties often are at risk for aspiration, the nursing diagnosis *Impaired Swallowing* should be used to describe a client who has difficulty swallowing who also is at risk for aspiration. *High Risk for Aspiration* should be used to describe persons who require nursing interventions to prevent aspiration but not to improve swallowing for nutritional purposes.

Errors in Diagnostic Statements

High Risk for Aspiration related to bronchopneumonia

    This diagnostic statement does not direct the nurse to the risk factors that could be reduced. If the nurse were monitoring and comanaging bronchopneumonia, the correct statement would be the collaborative problem *Potential Complication: Bronchopneumonia.*

High Risk for Aspiration related to anesthesia

    Anesthesia is not specific enough; thus, the correct statement would be *High Risk for Aspiration related to impaired gag reflex and somnolence secondary to anesthesia.*

Focus Assessment Criteria

Subjective Data

History of a problem with swallowing or aspiration
Presence or history of: (see pathophysiologic etiologies)

Objective Data

Height and weight
Ability to swallow, chew, feed self
Neuromuscular impairment
    Decreased/absent gag reflex
    Decreased strength on excursion of muscles involved in mastication
    Perceptual impairment
    Facial paralysis
Mechanical obstruction
    Edema
    Tracheostomy tube
    Tumor
Perceptual patterns/awareness
Level of consciousness
Condition of oropharyngeal cavity
Nasal regurgitation
Hoarseness
Aspiration

Coughing a second or two after swallowing
Dehydration
Apraxia

Principles and Rationale for Nursing Care

Generic Considerations

1. Swallowing is a complicated mechanism with three stages: voluntary, pharyngeal and esophageal.
2. The voluntary stage is the moving of the food from the palate to the pharynx.
3. The pharyngeal stage is automatic.
   a. Soft palate is pulled up to close the posterior nares.
   b. Palatopharyngeal folds on the sides of the pharynx constrict to permit passage of properly masticated food.
   c. Epiglottis swings backward over larynx opening to prevent aspiration into the trachea.
   d. Relaxation of hypopharyngeal sphincter stretches the opening of the esophagus.
   e. Rapid peristaltic wave forces food into the upper esophagus.
4. The esophageal stage moves the food from the pharynx to the stomach by peristaltic movements controlled by vagal reflexes.
5. Central nervous system depression interferes with the protective mechanism of the sphincters.
6. Nasogastric and endotracheal tubes cause incomplete closure of the esophageal sphincters and depress gag and cough reflex.
7. Verifying correct placement of feeding tubes is done most reliably via radiography. Aspiration of green-colored fluid or gastric aspirant with a pH of 6.5 or lower is also reliable. Verifying placement by instilling air and simultaneously auscultating or by aspirating non-green fluid have proved inaccurate.
8. After radiographic verification of correct feeding tube placement and knowledge that the position of the tube has not changed, routine testing of placement before feeding is not needed.
9. Clients with debilitating conditions who aspirate are at high risk for aspiration pneumonia.
10. The volume and characteristics of the aspirated contents influence morbidity and mortality. Food particles can cause mechanical blockage. Gastric juice erodes alveoli and capillaries and causes chemical pneumonitis.
11. Regurgitation is often silent in persons with decreased sensorium or depressed mental states.
12. Tracheostomy tubes interfere with the synchrony of the glottic closure. Inadequate cuff inflation provides a path for aspirate.
13. Increased intragastric pressure can contribute to regurgitation and aspiration. Situations that increase intragastric pressure are bolus tube feedings, obstructions, obesity, pregnancy, and autonomic dysfunction.

Pediatric Considerations

1. A proportionately oversized airway diameter in infants and small children increases the risk of aspiration of foreign objects (Hunsberger, 1989).
2. Common household objects and food items that are aspirated include:
   a. Baby powder
   b. Hot dogs, candy, nuts, grapes
   c. Balloons
   d. Small batteries (Whaley & Wong, 1989)

3. Children with certain congenital anomalies (*e.g.,* tracheoesophageal fistula, cleft palate, and gastroesophageal reflux) are at greater risk for aspiration.
4. To prevent aspiration, infants should be held upright for feedings, and young children should be fed while sitting (Hunsberger, 1989).

■ High Risk for Aspiration
Related to (Specify)

Assessment
See Defining Characteristics

Outcome Criteria

The person will
- Not experience aspiration
- Relate measures to prevent aspiration

Interventions

A. Assess causative or contributing factors ·
1. Susceptible individual
   a. Reduced level of consciousness
   b. Autonomic disorders
   c. Debilitated
   d. Newborns
2. Tracheostomy/endotracheal tubes
3. Gastrointestinal tubes/feedings

B. Reduces the risk of aspiration in:
1. Individuals with decreased strength, decreased sensorium, or autonomic disorders
   a. Maintain a side-lying position if not contraindicated by injury.
   b. If the person cannot be positioned on his side, open oropharyngeal airway by lifting the mandible up and forward, with the head tilted backward (for a small infant, hyperextension of the neck may not be effective).
   c. Assess for position of the tongue, assuring that it has not dropped backward, occluding the airway.
   d. Keep the head of the bed elevated, if not contraindicated by hypertension or injury.
   e. Maintain good oral hygiene: Clean teeth and use mouthwash on cotton swab; apply petroleum jelly to lips, removing encrustations gently.
   f. Clear secretions from mouth and throat with a tissue or gentle suction.
   g. Reassess frequently for presence of obstructive material in mouth and throat.
   h. Reevaluate frequently for good anatomic positioning.
   i. Maintain side-lying position after feedings.

2. With tracheostomies or endotracheal tubes:
   a. Inflate cuff:
      • During continuous mechanical ventilation
      • During and after eating
      • During and 1 hour after tube feedings
      • During IPPB treatments
   b. Suction every 1–2 hours and p.r.n.
3. With gastrointestinal tubes and feedings:
   a. Confirm that the placement of the tube has been verified by radiography or aspiration of greenish fluid.
   b. Confirm that tube position has not changed since it was inserted and verified.
   c. Elevate head of bed 30–45 minutes during feeding periods, and 1 hour after to prevent reflux by use of reverse gravity.
   d. Aspirate for residual contents before each feeding for tubes positioned gastrically.
   e. Administer feeding if residual contents are less than 150 mL (intermittent) or administer feeding if residual is not greater than 150 mL at 10–20% of hourly rate (continuous).
   f. Regulate gastric feedings using an intermittent schedule allowing periods for stomach emptying between feeding intervals.
4. With newborns and premature infants with cleft lip and/or palate:
   a. Position infant's head in an upright position.
   b. Use a large soft nipple with large hole or Lamb's nipple (long, soft).
   c. The nipple hole should be large enough for the feeding to be under 30 minutes.
   d. Do not position the nipple through the cleft.
   e. Apply gentle counter pressure on the base of the bottle to assist the infant with tongue and palate control of the milk flow.
   f. Burp frequently because of excessive air swallowing.
   g. If nipple feeding is unsuccessful, use a rubber-tipped syringe to deposit the formula on the back of the tongue.
5. With an elderly person with difficulties chewing and swallowing (see *Impaired Swallowing*)

C. Initiate health teaching and referrals as indicated

1. Instruct person and/or family on causes and prevention of aspiration.
2. Have family demonstrate tube feeding technique.
3. Refer to community nursing agency for assistance at home.
4. Teach about the danger of eating when under the influence of alcohol.
5. Teach the Heimlich or abdominal thrust maneuver to remove aspirated foreign bodies.

High Risk for Poisoning

DEFINITION

High Risk for Poisoning: The state in which a person is at high risk of accidental exposure to or ingestion of drugs or dangerous substances.

RISK FACTORS

Presence of risk factors (see Related Factors for *High Risk for Injury*)

High Risk for Suffocation

DEFINITION

High Risk for Suffocation: The state in which a person is at high risk for smothering and asphyxiation.

RISK FACTORS

Presence of risk factors (see Related Factors for *High Risk for Injury*)

High Risk for Trauma

DEFINITION

High Risk for Trauma: The state in which a person is at high risk of accidental tissue injury (*e.g.,* wound, burns, fracture).

RISK FACTORS

Presence of risk factors (see Related Factors for *High Risk for Injury*)

References/Bibliography

Barbiere, E. (1983). Patient falls are not patient accidents. *Journal of Gerontological Nursing, 9*(3), 164–173.

Cooper, S. (1981). Accidents and older adults. *Geriatric Nursing, 2,* 287–290.

Green, P. M. (1989). Potential for injury. In McFarland, G., & McFarlane, E. (1989). *Nursing diagnosis and interventions.* St. Louis: C. V. Mosby.

Hernandes, M., & Miller, J. (1986). How to reduce falls. *Geriatric Nursing, 7*(2), 97–102.

Lipsitz, L. A., & Fullerton, K. J. (1986). Postprandial blood pressure reduction in health elderly. *Journal of the American Geriatrics Society, 34,* 267–270.

Lynn, F. H. (1980). Incidents—need they be accidents? *American Journal of Nursing, 80,* 1098–1101.

Masters, R., & Marks, S. (1990). The use of restraints. *Rehabilitation Nursing, 15*(1), 22–25.

Miller, C. A. (1990). *Nursing care of older adults: Theory and practice.* Glenview, IL: Scott, Foresman.

National Center for Health Statistics. (1985). Monthly vital statistics report, 1984. Hyattsville, MD: US Public Health Service Publications.

Rauckhorst, L. M. (1980). Community and home assessment. *Journal of Gerontological Nursing, 6,* 319–327.

Riffle, K. (1982). Falls: Kinds, causes, and prevention. *Geriatric Nursing, 3,* 165–169.

Schulman, B., & Acquaviva, T. (1987). Falls in the elderly. *Nurse Practitioner, 12*(11), 30.

Simons, R. S. (1980). The occupational health nurse: Safety's overlooked resource. *Occupational Health Nurse, 28*(2), 7–12.

Spellbring, A., et al. (1988). Improving safety for hospitalized elderly. *Journal of Gerontological Nursing, 14*(2), 31–37.

Symposium on injuries and injury prevention. *Pediatric Clinics of North America, 32*(1).

Tideiksaar, R. (Ed.). (1989). *Falling in old age: Its prevention and treatment.* New York: Springer Publishing.

Tideiksaar, R. (1984). Fall assessment record. *Journal of American Geriatric Society, 32*(7), 539.

Witte, N. (1979). Why the elderly fall. *American Journal of Nursing, 79,* 1154–1160.

Child Safety

Baxter, L. (1987). Report on 1986–1987 CPSC study on immersion accidents. Presented at Conference on Childhood Drowning: Current Issues and Strategies on Prevention, Newport Beach, CA, May 4, 1987.

Brill, J. (1987). Dispelling the myth of the drown proof child. *Contemporary Pediatrics, 4*(6), 30.

Children's National Medical Center. (1989). *Safe kids are no accident.* Washington, D.C.: Author.

Hayman, L. L., Weill, V. A., Tobias, N. E., Stashinko, E. E., & Meininger, J. C. (1988). Reducing risk for heart disease in children. *Maternal-Child Nursing, 13,* 442–448.

Hunsberger, M. (1989). Nursing strategies: Altered respiratory function. In Foster, R. L., Hunsberger, M. M., & Anderson, J. J. T. (Eds.). *Family-centered nursing care of children.* Philadelphia: W. B. Saunders.

Karp, S. (1987). A 10 point program for bicycle safety. *Contemporary Pediatrics, 4*(6), 16.

McIntire, M., & Angle, C. R. (1976). Poison control: A model for childhood safety. *Pediatrician, 5,* 180–184.

Newest guidelines on pediatric CPR and first aid. (1987). *Contemporary Pediatrics, 4*(6), 47.

Small doses. Bike helmet activism. (1990). *American Journal of Nursing, 90,* 41.

Whaley, L. F., & Wong, D. L. (1989). *Essentials of pediatric nursing* (3rd ed.). St. Louis: C. V. Mosby.

Wheatley, G. (1977). Introduction: Childhood accidents. *Pediatrics Annals, 6*(11), 12–26.

Orthostatic Hypotension

Adelman, E. M. (1980). When the patient's blood pressure falls: What does it mean? What do you do? *Nursing, 10*(2), 26.

Alfaro, R. (1982). Pneumatic antishock trousers, how and when to use them. *Dimensions of Critical Care Nursing, 1*(1), 7–16.

Berne, R. M., & Levy, M.N. (1981). *Cardiovascular physiology.* St Louis: C. V. Mosby.

Cunha, U. V. (1987). Management of orthostatic hypotension in the elderly. *Geriatrics, 42*(9), 61–68.

Rubenstein, L. Z., & Robbins, A. S. (1984). Falls in the elderly: A clinical perspective. *Geriatrics, 39*(4), 67–78.

Wade, D. W. (1982). Teaching patients to live with chronic orthostatic hypotension. *Nursing, 12*(7), 64–65.

West, C. M. (1986). Ischemia in pathophysiological phenomena. In Carrieri, V. K., Lindsey, A. M., & West, C. M. (Eds.). *Nursing: Human responses to illness.* Philadelphia: W. B. Saunders.

Resources for the Consumer

Literature

Making products safer (Pamphlet no. 524)

What should parents expect from children? (Pamphlet no. 357)

Request the above and a list of other publications from Public Affairs Pamphlets, 381 Park Avenue South, New York, NY 10016 (50 cents for each pamphlet)

Fontana, V.J. (1973). *A parent's guide to child safety.* New York: T.Y. Crowell.

Poison Prevention Packaging available free from the Consumer Product Safety Commission, Washington, DC 20207

Kids aren't drownproof, The kids aren't drownproof coloring book, Is your pool safe? and *What every parent should know about water safety.* The Community Association for the Retarded, 3864 Middlefield Road, Palo Alto, CA 94303

Never leave a child alone. Accident Prevention Committee, American Academy of Pediatrics, PO Box 2134, Inglewood, CA 90305

Safe swimming for your boy or girl. The Injury Prevention Program (TIPP), American Academy of Pediatrics, Publications Department, 141 Northwest Point, PO Box 927, Elk Grove Village, IL 60007

Knowledge Deficit

DEFINITION

Knowledge Deficit: The state in which an individual or group experiences a deficiency in cognitive knowledge or psychomotor skills regarding the condition or treatment plan.

DEFINING CHARACTERISTICS

Major (must be present)

Verbalizes a deficiency in knowledge or skill/request for information

Expresses "inaccurate" perception of health status

Does not perform correctly a desired or prescribed health behavior

Minor (may be present)

Lack of integration of treatment plan into daily activities

Exhibits or expresses psychologic alteration (*e.g.,* anxiety, depression) resulting from misinformation or lack of information

---

Diagnostic Considerations

Knowledge deficit does not represent a human response, alteration, or a pattern of dysfunction but rather a related factor.* Lack of knowledge can contribute to a variety of responses, *e.g.,* anxiety, self-care deficits, noncompliance. All nursing diagnostic categories have related patient/family teaching as a part of nursing interventions, *e.g., Altered Bowel Elimination, Impaired Verbal Communication.* When the teaching directly relates to a specific nursing diagnosis, incorporate the teaching in the plan. When lack of or insufficient knowledge is the primary cause of a diagnosis or a risk factor for a potential diagnosis, list lack of knowledge as a "Related to." For example, when specific teaching is indicated prior to a procedure, *Anxiety related to unfamiliar environment and procedures* can be used. When information giving is directed to assist a person or family with a decision, *Decisional Conflict* may be indicated. Other examples of diagnostic statements with lack of knowledge as the "Related to" are *High Risk for Altered Health Maintenance related to lack of knowledge of diabetes mellitus, management, and signs/symptoms of complications; High Risk Impaired Home Maintenance Management related to lack of knowledge of home care and community resources;* and *High Risk for Injury related to lack of knowledge of bicycle safety.*

---

*Jenny, J. (1987). Knowledge Deficit: Not a nursing diagnosis. *Image, 19*(4), 184–185.

Mobility, Impaired Physical

- *Related to* **Insufficient Knowledge of Techniques to Increase Lower Limb Function**
- *Related to* **Insufficient Knowledge of Techniques to Increase Upper Limb Function**

DEFINITION

Impaired Physical Mobility: A state in which the individual experiences or is at risk of experiencing limitation of physical movement.

DEFINING CHARACTERISTICS

Major (must be present)

Inability to move purposefully within the environment, including bed mobility, transfers, ambulation

Minor (may be present)

Range-of-motion (ROM) limitations
Limited muscle strength or control
Impaired coordination

RELATED FACTORS

Pathophysiologic

Neuromuscular impairment
Autoimmune alterations (multiple sclerosis, arthritis)
Nervous system diseases (parkinsonism, myasthenia gravis)
Muscular dystrophy
Partial or total paralysis (spinal cord injury, stroke)
Central nervous system (CNS) tumor
Increased intracranial pressure
Sensory deficits
Musculoskeletal impairment
Spasms
Flaccidity, atrophy, weakness
Connective tissue disease (systemic lupus erythematosus)
Edema (increased synovial fluid)

Treatment-related

External devices (casts or splints, braces, IV tubing)
Surgical procedures (amputation)

Situational (personal, environmental)
    Trauma
    Depression
    Pain

Maturational
    Elderly: Decreased motor agility, muscle weakness

Diagnostic Considerations

Impaired Physical Mobility describes an individual with limited use of arm(s) or leg(s) and/or limited muscle strength. This diagnosis should not be used to describe complete immobility, in this case, *High Risk for Disuse Syndrome* would be more applicable. Limitation of physical movement also can be the etiology of other nursing diagnoses, such as *Self-Care Deficit* and *High Risk for Injury.*

Nursing interventions for *Impaired Physical Mobility* focus on strengthening and restoring function and preventing deterioration.

Errors in Diagnostic Statements

Impaired Physical Mobility related to traumatic amputation of left arm

Listing traumatic amputation of the left arm as a related factor does not describe the problem. Rather, the diagnostic statement should reflect how the loss of a left arm has affected functioning. A more appropriate diagnosis might be *Self-Care Deficit: Feeding related to insufficient knowledge of adaptations needed secondary to loss of left arm.*

Impaired Physical Mobility related to limited muscle strength secondary to cerebrovascular accident (CVA)

Limited muscle strength is a sign of *Impaired Physical Mobility,* not a related factor. The related factors should represent direction for nursing intervention, as reflected in the diagnosis *Impaired Physical Mobility related to insufficient knowledge of techniques needed to increase motor function secondary to upper motor neuron damage.*

Focus Assessment Criteria

Subjective Data

1. History of systemic disorders
    Neurologic
        CVA, head trauma, increased intracranial pressure
        Multiple sclerosis, polio, Guillain-Barré, myasthenia gravis
        Spinal cord injury, tumor, birth defect
    Cardiovascular
        Myocardial infarction   Congenital heart anomaly
        Congestive heart failure
    Musculoskeletal
        Osteoporosis   Fractures
        Arthritis
    Respiratory
        Chronic obstructive pulmonary   Orthopnea
            disease (COPD)   Pneumonia
        Dyspnea on exertion

Debilitating diseases

Cancer   Endocrine disease

Renal disease

2. History of symptoms that interfere with mobility

Onset	Frequency
Duration	Precipitated by what?
Location	Relieved by what?
Description	Aggravated by what?

3. History of symptoms (complaints of)

Pain

Muscle weakness

Fatigue

Attributed to?	Amount of time out of bed
Induced by?	Amount of time sleeping or resting

4. History of recent trauma or surgery

Fractures	Head injury	Abdominal surgery or injury

5. Current drug therapy

Sedatives, hypnotics,

CNS depressants	Laxatives	Other

Objective Data

1. Dominant hand

Right	Left	Ambidextrous

2. Motor function

Right arm	Strong	Weak	Absent	Spastic
Left arm	Strong	Weak	Absent	Spastic
Right leg	Strong	Weak	Absent	Spastic
Left leg	Strong	Weak	Absent	Spastic

3. Mobility

Ability to turn self	Yes	No	Assistance needed (specify)
Ability to sit	Yes	No	Assistance needed (specify)
Ability to stand	Yes	No	Assistance needed (specify)
Ability to transfer	Yes	No	Assistance needed (specify)
Ability to ambulate	Yes	No	Assistance needed (specify)

Weight-bearing (assess both right and left sides)

Full	As tolerated
Partial	Non–weight-bearing

Gait

Stable	Unstable

Assistive devices

Crutches	Walker	Prosthesis
Cane	Wheelchair	Other
Braces		

Restrictive devices

Cast or splint	Ventilator	IV
Traction	Drain	Monitor
Braces	Foley	Dialysis

Range of motion (shoulders, elbows, arms, hips, legs)

Full	Limited (specify)	None

4. Endurance (see *Activity Intolerance* for additional information)
   Assess
   > Resting pulse, blood pressure, respirations
   > Blood pressure, respirations, and pulse immediately after activity
   > Pulse every 2 minutes until pulse returns to within 10 beats of resting pulse
   > After activity, assess for presence of indicators of hypoxia (showing intensity, frequency, or duration of activity must be decreased or discontinued) as follows

   Blood pressure

Failure of systolic rate to increase	Increase in diastolic of 155 mm Hg

   Respirations

Excessive rate increases	Dyspnea
Decrease in rate	Irregular rhythm

   Cerebral and other changes

Confusion	Weakness
Uncoordination	Pallor
Change in equilibrium	Cyanosis

5. Peripheral circulation
   > Capillary refill time (normal <3 sec)
   > Skin color, temperature, and turgor
   > Peripheral pulses (rate, quality)

Brachial	Popliteal
Radial	Posterior tibial
Femoral	Pedal

6. Motivation (as perceived by nurse and stated by person)

Excellent	Satisfactory	Poor

Principles and Rationale for Nursing Care

Generic Considerations

1. According to Miller (1990), "mobility is one of the most important aspects of physiological functioning because it is essential for the maintenance of independence."
2. Activity, mobility, and flexibility are integral to one's life-style. Compromised mobility has a serious impact on self-concept and life-style (Christian, 1982).
3. There are three ROM categories—passive, active, and functional.
   a. *Passive ROM* keeps muscles and joints limber. One person passively moves another person's muscles (*e.g.,* the helper lifts and moves the person's legs).
   b. *Active ROM* exercise limbers and strengthens muscles and joints. The person actively uses his muscles (*e.g.,* while lying down, the person moves his legs).
   c. *Functional ROM* strengthens muscles and joints while performing necessary activity (*e.g.,* walking). Performed by individual himself.
4. Exercise enhances independence. Incorporating ROM exercises into a person's daily routine encourages regular performance.
5. Active ROM increases muscle mass, tone, and strength and improves cardiac and respiratory functioning. Passive ROM improves joint mobility and circulation.
6. Prolonged immobility and impaired neurosensory function can cause permanent contractures.
7. Prolonged bed rest or decreased blood volume can cause a sudden drop in blood pressure (orthostatic hypotension) as blood returns to peripheral circulation. Gradual progression to increased activity reduces fatigue and increases endurance.

Pediatric Considerations

See *Potential for Disuse Syndrome.*

Gerontologic Considerations

1. About one-tenth of noninstitutionalized elderly persons report some limitation in mobility, and of the institutionalized elderly, over 90% are dependent in at least one activity of daily living (Brody & Foley, 1985). Problems with mobility are often the reason for nursing home admission or extensive in-home care. Assessment of mobility determines the extent of functional impairment as a result of disease or disability.
2. The effects of immobility in the elderly are particularly dangerous. Muscle weakness, atrophy, and decreased endurance are quick to occur, and the biochemical and physiologic effects such as nitrogen loss and hypercalciuria are important to consider (Hogue, 1985). Permanent functional loss is more likely with prolonged immobility, and in addition, elderly persons are vulnerable to new morbidity such as pneumonia, pressure sores, falls and fracture, osteoporosis, incontinence, confusion, and depression. Every effort toward prevention and mobilization should be made.
3. Pain and depression are linked in the elderly; effective management of both is sometimes necessary. Inadequate pain relief may be a primary factor leading to depression in some individuals, but depression should not be discounted as a secondary feature of pain. Depression may require aggressive management including drugs and other therapies (Kwentus, Harkins, & Lignon, 1985).
4. The age-related changes in joint and connective tissue cause impaired flexion and extension movements, decrease flexibility, and reduce cushioning protection for joints (Whitbourne, 1985).

■ Impaired Physical Mobility
Related to Insufficient Knowledge of Techniques to Increase Lower Limb Function

Assessment

Subjective Data

Pain

Fatigue

Numbness and tingling

Weakness

Objective Data

Inability to move or coordinate one or both lower limbs

Limitations in ROM of lower limbs

Mechanical devices restricting mobility (*e.g.,* cast, traction)

Refusal to acknowledge existence of limbs (*e.g.,* post-CVA)

Impaired ability to transfer with or without adaptive devices (bed-chair, chair-commode)

Impaired ability to perform activities of daily living

Impaired sitting or standing balance

Impaired ability to ambulate with or without assistive devices
Alterations in gait patterns
Partial or total loss of one or both lower limbs
Impaired ability to move within physical environment (*e.g.,* curbs, stairs)

Outcome Criteria

The person will
• Demonstrate the use of adaptive devices to increase mobility
• Utilize safety measures to minimize potential for injury
• Describe rationale for interventions
• Demonstrate measures to increase mobility
• Report an increase in strength and endurance of upper limbs

---

Interventions

A. Assess causative factors
1. Trauma (*e.g.,* cartilage tears, fractures, amputations)
2. Surgical procedure (*e.g.,* joint replacement, reduction of fractures, vascular surgery)
3. Debilitating disease (*e.g.,* diabetes, cancer, rheumatoid arthritis, multiple sclerosis, stroke)

B. Reduce or eliminate contributing factors
1. Increase limb mobility
   a. Perform ROM exercises (frequency to be determined by condition of the individual):
      • Teach the client to perform active ROM exercises on unaffected limbs at least 4 times a day, if possible.
      • Perform passive ROM on affected limbs. Do the exercises slowly to allow the muscles time to relax, and support the extremity above and below the joint to prevent strain on joints and tissues.
      • During ROM, the client's legs and arms should be moved gently to within his pain tolerance; perform ROM slowly to allow the muscles time to relax.
      • For passive ROM, the supine position is the most effective. The individual who performs ROM himself can use a supine or sitting position.
      • Do ROM daily with bed bath, 3 to 4 times daily if there are specific problem areas. Try to incorporate into activities of daily living.
   b. Support extremity with pillows to prevent or reduce swelling.
   c. Medicate for pain as needed, especially before activity* (see *Altered Comfort*).
   d. Apply heat or cold to reduce pain, inflammation, and hematoma.*
   e. Apply cold to reduce swelling postinjury (usually first 48 hr).*
   f. Encourage the person to perform exercise regimens for specific joints as prescribed by physician or physical therapist.
2. Position the person in alignment to prevent complications;
   a. Use a foot board.

*May require a physician's order.

b. Avoid prolonged periods of sitting or lying in the same position.

c. Change position of the shoulder joints every 2 to 4 hours.

d. Use a small pillow or no pillow when in Fowler's position.

e. Support the hand and wrist in natural alignment.

f. If the client is supine or prone, place a rolled towel or small pillow under the lumbar curvature or under the end of the rib cage.

g. Place a trochanter roll or sand bags alongside the hips and upper thighs.

h. If the client is in the lateral position, place pillow(s) to support the leg from groin to foot, and a pillow to flex the shoulder and elbow slightly; if needed, support the lower foot in dorsal flexion with a sandbag.

i. Use hand-wrist splints.

3. Maintain good body alignment when mechanical devices are used.

a. Traction devices
   - Assess for correct position of traction and alignment of bones.
   - Observe for correct amount and position of weights.
   - Allow weights to hang freely, with no blankets or sheets on ropes.
   - Assess for changes in circulation; check pulse quality, skin temperature, color of extremities, and capillary refill (should be < 2 sec).
   - Assess for changes in circulation (numbness, tingling, pain).
   - Assess for changes in mobility (ability to flex/extend unaffected joints).
   - Assess for signs of skin irritation (redness, ulceration, blanching).
   - Assess skeletal traction pin sites for loosening, inflammation, ulceration, and drainage; clean pin insertion sites (procedure may vary with type of pin and physician's order).
   - Encourage isometrics* and prescribed exercise program.

b. Casts
   - Assess for proper fit of casts (they should not be too loose or too tight).
   - Assess circulation to the encasted area every 2 hr (color and temperature of skin, pulse quality, capillary refill < 2 sec).
   - Assess for changes in sensation of extremities every 2 hr (numbness, tingling, pain).
   - Assess motion of uninvolved joints (ability to flex and extend).
   - Assess for skin irritation (redness, ulceration, or complaints of pain under the cast).
   - Keep cast clean and dry; do not allow sharp objects to be inserted under cast; petal rough edges with adhesive tape; place soft cotton under edges that seem to be causing pressure points.
   - Allow cast to air dry while resting on pillows to prevent dents.
   - Observe cast for areas of softening or indentation.
   - Exercise joints above and below cast if allowed (*e.g.,* wiggle fingers and toes every 2 hr).
   - Assist with prescribed exercise regimens and isometrics of muscles enclosed in casts.*
   - Keep extremities elevated after cast application to reduce swelling.

c. Braces
   - Assess for correct positioning of braces.
   - Observe for signs of skin irritation (redness, ulceration, blanching, itching, pain).

---

*May require a physician's order.

- Assist with exercises as prescribed for specific joints.
- Have the client demonstrate correct application of the brace.

d. Prosthetic devices
- Observe for signs of skin irritation of the stump before applying prosthetic device (stump should be clean and dry; Ace bandage should be rewrapped and securely in place).
- Have the client demonstrate the correct application of the prosthesis.
- Assess the client for gait alterations or improper walking technique.
- Proceed with health teaching, if indicated.

e. Ace bandages
- Assess for correct position of Ace bandage.
- Apply Ace bandage with even pressure, wrapping from distal to proximal portions, and making sure that the bandage is not too tight or too loose.
- Observe for "bunching" of the bandage.
- Observe for signs of irritation of skin (redness, ulceration, excessive tightness).
- Rewrap Ace bandage twice daily or as needed, unless contraindicated (*e.g.*, if the bandage is a postoperative compression dressing, it should be left in place).
- When wrapping lower extremity, leave the heel exposed, using figure-8 technique.

Note: Some mechanical devices may be removed for exercises, depending on nature of injury or type and purpose of device. Consult with the physician to ascertain when the person may remove the device.

4. Provide progressive mobilization.
   a. Assist the person slowly to sitting position.
   b. Allow the person to dangle his legs over the side of the bed for a few minutes before he stands up.
   c. Limit time to 15 minutes, three times a day, the first few times out of bed.
   d. Increase the person's time out of bed, as tolerated by 15-minute increments.
   e. Progress to ambulation with or without assistive devices.
   f. If unable to walk, assist the person out of bed to a wheelchair or chair.
   g. Encourage ambulating for short frequent walks (at least 3 times daily), with assistance if unsteady.
   h. Increase lengths of walks progressively each day.

C. Provide health teaching as indicated

1. Teach the person methods of transfer from bed to chair or commode and to standing position.
   a. Before transferring anyone, assess the number of personnel needed for assistance.
   b. The individual should be positioned on the side of the bed. His feet should be touching the floor, and he should be wearing stable shoes or slippers with nonskid soles.
   c. For getting in and out of bed, weight-bearing on the uninvolved or stronger side should be encouraged.
   d. Wheelchair should be locked before transfer. If using a regular chair, be sure it will not move.
   e. The person should be instructed to use the arm of the chair closer to him for support while standing.

f. Place arm around the person's rib cage and keep back straight, with knees slightly bent.

g. The person should be told to place his arms around the nurse's waist or rib cage, *not her neck.*

h. Support the person's legs by bracing his with hers. (While facing the person, she should lock his knees with her knees.)

i. Hemiplegic individuals should be instructed to pivot on the uninvolved foot.

j. For individuals with lower limb weakness or paralysis, a sliding board transfer may be used.
  • The person should wear pajamas so he will not stick to the board.
  • The person needs good upper extremity strength to be able to slide his buttocks from the bed to the chair or wheelchair. (Wheelchairs should have removable arms.)

k. When the person's arms are strong enough, he should progress to a sitting transfer without the board, if he can lift buttocks enough to clear bed and chair seat.

l. If the person's legs give out, the nurse should guide him gently to the floor and *seek additional assistance.*

2. Teach how to ambulate with adaptive equipment (*e.g.,* crutches, walkers, canes).

  a. Instruct the individual in weight-bearing status.

  b. Observe and teach the use of
    • Crutches
      No pressure should be exerted on axilla; hand strength should be used.
      Type of gait varies with individual's diagnosis.
      Measure crutches 2 to 3 inches below axilla and tips 6 inches away from feet.
    • Walkers
      Use arm strength to support weakness in lower limbs.
      Gait varies with individual's problems.
    • Wheelchairs
      Practice transfers.
      Practice maneuvering around barriers.
    • Prostheses (teach about the following)
      Stump wrapping prior to application of the prosthesis
      Application of the prosthesis
      Principles of stump care
      Importance of cleaning the stump, keeping it dry, and applying the prosthesis only when the stump is dry

  c. Teach the individual safety precautions.
    • Protect areas of decreased sensation from extremes of heat and cold.
    • Practice falling and how to recover from falls while transferring or ambulating.
    • For decreased perception of lower extremity (post-CVA "neglect"), instruct the individual to check where limb is placed when changing positions or going through doorways; and check to make sure both shoes are tied, that affected leg is dressed with trousers, and that pants are not dragging.
    • Instruct individuals who are confined to wheelchair to shift position and lift up buttocks every 15 minutes to relieve pressure; maneuver curbs, ramps, inclines, and around obstacles; and lock wheelchairs prior to transferring.

    d. Practice proper positioning, ROM (active or passive), and prescribed exercises.
    e. Practice stair-climbing if individual's condition permits.
    f. Observe for complications of immobility.
- Phlebitis (*i.e.*, redness, tenderness, swelling of calves)
- Pressure ulcer (*i.e.*, blanching of skin, redness, itching, pain)
- Infection after limb surgery (*i.e.*, pain, swelling, redness)
- Neurovascular compromise (*i.e.*, numbness, tingling, pain, blanching, decreased pulse quality, coolness of skin)

■ Impaired Physical Mobility
Related to Insufficient Knowledge of Techniques to Increase Upper Limb Function

Assessment

Subjective Data

The person reports

Pain	Fatigue
Loss of sensation (numbness, tingling)	Weakness

Objective Data

Inability to move one or both upper extremities
Impaired grasp
Limited ROM of one or more upper limbs
Mechanical devices preventing full ROM (*e.g.*, traction, cast)
Inability to perform self-care activities
Neglect of one or both upper limbs
Partial or total loss of upper limb(s)
Impaired coordination of upper limb(s)

Outcome Criteria

The person will
- Demonstrate modes of adaptation to disability (*e.g.*, use of adaptive equipment such as universal cuff)
- Relate rationale for interventions
- Report on increase in strength and endurance of upper limbs

---

Interventions

A. Assess causative factors
    1. Trauma (*e.g.*, fractures, crushing injuries, lacerations, amputations)
    2. Surgical procedure (*e.g.*, joint replacement, reduction of fractures, removal of tumors, mastectomy)

3. Systemic disease (*e.g.,* multiple sclerosis, CVA, Guillain-Barré, rheumatoid arthritis, Parkinson's, lupus)

B. Reduce or eliminate contributing factors

1. Increase limb mobility if possible.
   a. Assist with ROM exercises.*
   b. Elevate extremity with pillows or sling above level of the heart to prevent or reduce swelling (may be contraindicated in congestive heart failure).
   c. Medicate for pain as needed, especially before activity* (see *Altered Comfort*).
   d. Apply cold to reduce swelling postinjury (usually first 48 hr).*
   e. Assist with exercise regimens for specific joints as prescribed by physician or physical therapist (*e.g.,* for joint replacements).*
2. Position the person in alignment to prevent complications.
   a. Arms abducted from the body with pillows
   b. Elbows in slight flexion
   c. Wrist in a neutral position, with fingers slightly flexed, and thumb abducted and slightly flexed
   d. Position of shoulder joints changed during the day (*e.g.,* adduction, abduction, range of circular motion)
3. Prevent injury when mechanical devices are used.
   a. Traction devices
      • Assess for correct alignment of bones and position of weights.
      • Allow weights to hang freely with no blankets or sheets on ropes.
      • Assess for changes in circulation; check pulse quality, skin temperature, color of extremities, and capillary refill (should be < 2 sec).
      • Assess for changes in sensation (numbness, tingling, pain).
      • Assess for changes in mobility (ability to flex/extend unaffected joints).
      • Assess for signs of skin irritation (redness, ulceration, flaking).
      • Assess skeletal traction, pin sites for loosening, inflammation, or skin ulceration; clean pin insertion sites twice daily (procedure may vary with type of pin and physician's order).
      • Encourage isometrics and prescribed exercise program.*
   b. Casts
      • Assess for tightness of cast.
         Circulation: temperature, color, check pulses, capillary refill should be < 2 seconds
         Sensation: numbness, tingling, increased pain
         Motion: ability to flex, extend
      • Assess for skin irritation: redness ulceration, complaints of pain under cast.
      • Keep cast clean and dry; petal edges with adhesive tape if necessary; no sharp objects down into cast.
      • Allow cast to air dry; observe for areas of softening.
      • Exercise joints above and below cast; prescribed exercise regimens and isometrics of muscles enclosed in casts.
      • After application, elevate extremity on pillows to prevent or reduce swelling.
   c. Slings
      • Assess for correct application; sling should be loose around neck and

* May require a physician's order.

should support elbow and wrist above level of the heart.
- Remove slings for ROM.*

d. Ace bandages (care as for lower limbs' bandages)
- Observe for correct position.
- Apply with even pressure, wrapping distally to proximally.
- Observe for "bunching."
- Observe for signs of skin irritation (redness, ulceration) or tightness (compression).
- Rewrap Ace bandages twice daily or as needed, unless contraindicated (*e.g.,* if bandage is postoperative compression dressing, check physician's orders).

4. Encourage use of affected arm when possible.
  a. Encourage the person to use affected arm for self-care activities (*e.g.,* feeding himself, dressing, brushing hair).
  b. For post-CVA neglect of upper limb (see also *Unilateral Neglect*):
  - Place objects to affected side to encourage him to use "forgotten" limb.
  - Stand to the person's side and encourage him to use all fields of vision.
    Note: Some mechanical devices may be removed for exercises, depending on nature of injury or type and purpose of device. Physician's orders should be consulted.
  c. Instruct the person to utilize unaffected arm to exercise the affected arm.
  d. Use appropriate adaptive equipment to enhance the use of arms.
  - Universal cuff for feeding in individuals who have poor control in both arms, hands
  - Large-handled or padded silverware to assist individuals with poor fine motor skills
  - Dishware with high edges to prevent food from slipping
  - Suction-cup aids to hold dishes in place to prevent sliding of plate
  e. Use a warm bath to alleviate early morning stiffness and improve mobility.
  f. Encourage the individual to practice handwriting skills, if able.
  g. Allow time for the individual to practice using affected limb.

C. Proceed with health teaching as indicated

1. Have the person demonstrate ROM and prescribed exercises.
2. Have the person demonstrate the care of adaptive and mechanical devices.
3. Teach the person safety precautions.
4. Practice difficult maneuvers (*e.g.,* cooking with one hand).
5. For areas of decreased sensation, instruct the person to take precautions with heat, cold, and sharp objects.
6. For neglect of upper extremity, instruct the person to observe and check for positioning, exposure to irritants, or sharp objects.
7. Teach person methods of performing self-care activities (see *Self-Care Deficits*).
8. Teach individual when to alternate rest and activity of joints.

References/Bibliography

Banwell, B. F. (1984). Exercise and mobility in arthritis. *Nursing Clinics of North America, 19*(4), 605–616.
Brody, J., & Foley, E. (1985). Epidemiologic considerations. In Schneider, E. (ed.): *The teaching*

*May require a physician's order.

nursing home: A new approach to geriatric research, education, and clinical practice. New York: Raven Press, pp. 9–25.

Christian, B. J. (1982). Immobilization: Psychosocial aspects. In Normis, C. (Ed.). *Concept clarification in nursing.* Rockville, MD: Aspen Publications.

Farell, J. (1982). *Illustrated guide to orthopedic nursing* (2nd ed.). Philadelphia: J. B. Lippincott.

Gartland, J. (1965). *Fundamentals of orthopedics.* Philadelphia: W. B. Saunders.

Hogue, C. (1985). Mobility. In Schneider, E. (Ed.): *The teaching nursing home: A new approach to geriatric research, education, and clinical care.* New York: Raven Press, pp. 231–244.

Krusen, F. H., Kottke, F. J., & Elwood, P., Jr. (Eds.). (1971). *Handbook of physical medicine and rehabilitation.* Philadelphia: W. B. Saunders.

Kwentus, J., Harkins, S., & Lignon, N. (1985). Current concepts of geriatric pain and its treatment. *Geriatrics, 40*(4), 48–57.

Lieberson, S., & Mendes, D. G. (1979). Walking in bed: Strength and mobility of the lower extremities of bedridden patients. *Physical Therapy, 59,* 1112–1115.

Meissner, J. E. (1980). Elevate your patient's level of independence. *Nursing, 10*(9), 72–73.

Milazzo, V. (1981). Exercise class for patients in traction. *American Journal of Nursing, 81,* 1843–1844.

Miller, C. A. (1990). *Nursing care of older adults.* Glenview, IL: Scott, Foresman.

Olson, E. V. (Ed.). (1967). The hazards of immobility. *American Journal of Nursing, 67,* 780–797.

Sine, R. (Ed.). (1981). *Basic rehabilitation techniques* (2nd ed.). Rockville, MD: Aspen Systems.

Whitbourne, S. K. (1985). Appearance and movement. In Whitbourne, S. K. *The aging body.* New York: Springer-Verlag.

Noncompliance

- *Related to* **Anxiety**
- *Related to* **Negative Side-Effects of Prescribed Treatment**
- *Related to* **Reported Unsatisfactory Experiences in Health Care Environment**

DEFINITION

Noncompliance: The state in which an individual or group desires to comply but is prevented from doing so by factors that deter adherence to health-related advice given by health professionals.

DEFINING CHARACTERISTICS

Major (must be present)

Verbalization of noncompliance or nonparticipation or confusion about therapy and/or

Direct observation of behavior indicating noncompliance

Minor (may be present)

Missed appointments
Partially used or unused medications
Persistence of symptoms*
Progression of disease process*
Occurence of undesired outcomes* (postoperative morbidity, pregnancy, obesity, addiction, regression during rehabilitation)

RELATED FACTORS

Pathophysiologic

Impaired ability to perform tasks because of disability (*e.g.,* poor memory, motor and sensory deficits)
Chronic nature of illness
Increasing amount of disease-related symptoms despite adherence to advised regimen.

Treatment-related

Side-effects of therapy
Previous unsuccessful experiences with advised regimen
Impersonal aspects of referral process
Nontherapeutic environment
Complex, unsupervised, or prolonged therapy
Financial cost of therapy
Nontherapeutic relationship between client and nurse

* When these characteristics are considered to be the result of noncompliance, one is assuming that the therapy prescribed has been proved to be effective and is appropriate.

Situational (personal, environmental)

Concurrent illness of family member
Inclement weather preventing client from keeping appointment
Nonsupportive family, peers, community
Knowledge deficit
Lack of autonomy in health-seeking behavior
Health beliefs run counter to professional advice
Poor self-esteem
Disturbance in body image
Homelessness

Maturational

Developmental maturity of client is incompatible with his/her age

Diagnostic Considerations

Compliance depends on various factors, including the person's motivation, perception of vulnerability, and beliefs about controlling or preventing illness; environmental variables; quality of health instruction; and ability to access resources (cost, accessibility).

The diagnosis *Noncompliance* describes a person desiring to comply but is prevented from doing so by certain factors, *e.g.*, lack of understanding, inadequate finances, too-complex instructions. The nurse must attempt to reduce or eliminate these factors to ensure that interventions are successful.

The widespread view that compliance "is the extent to which a person's behavior coincides with medical advice" (Haynes,) is problematic for nurses.

A person's right to self-determination is protected through the process of informed consent. Informed consent has three conditions: the person must be capable of giving consent, must understand the advantages and disadvantages of consenting, and must not be coerced (Cassells & Redman, 1989). When a person refuses to comply with advice or instructions, it is important that the nurse assess for and validate that all required elements for an informed consent are present. The nurse is cautioned against using *Noncompliance* to describe a person who has made an informed autonomous decision not to comply. As Cassells and Redman (1989) state, "human dignity is respected by granting individuals the freedom to make choices in accordance with their own values."

Errors in Diagnostic Statements

Noncompliance related to reports of not following low-salt diet and resulting increased edema

The factors above would not have caused or contributed to noncompliance, but instead represent evidence of noncompliance. If the reason for the noncompliance is not known, the diagnosis *Noncompliance related to unknown etiology, as evidenced by reports of (specify)* would be appropriate.

When the reasons are identified, the nurse must determine whether these factors can be reduced or eliminated. If the person has made an informed decision not to follow the prescribed diet, *Noncompliance* may not be the correct nursing diagnosis. Perhaps the nurse and client could examine the prescribed diet. Is it realistic? What is the probability that compliant behavior will improve quality of life?

Focus Assessment Criteria

Subjective Data

What is the person's general health motivation?
  Does client seek help when needed?
  Does client accept the diagnosis as valid?
  Does client intend to make the advised life-style alterations?
What is the person's perception of his present state of health?
  Does client consider himself to be generally well?
  Is there fear of a specific illness?
  Does client believe his illness is severe?
How does the person view the advised treatment regimen?
Does the person report
  Unacceptable side-effects of therapy?

Unpleasant taste	Pain	Time-consuming or
Difficulty swal-		
lowing	Heavy expenses	inconvenient

  Inability to repeat or demonstrate the prescribed behavior?

Exercise program	Drug names and	Treatment procedure
Next appointment		
date	schedule	

  Situations that interfere with prescribed behavior?

Family demands	Occupations	Travel (hotels, restau-
Stress	Lack of transportation	rants)

  Does family member report any of the above problems?

Objective Data

  Assess for the presence of
    Missed appointments
    Obstacles to self-care

Inability to read	Musculoskeletal deficits
Immaturity	Cognitive deficits
Memory lags	Pain

    Evidence of obstacles in caregiving environment

Long waiting period	Hurried atmosphere

    Evidence of noncompliance

Persistence of symptoms	With medications (pill count, serum
Progression of disease	drug levels)

Principles and Rationale for Nursing Care

Generic Considerations

1. Compliance is a "positive behavior that patients exhibit when moving toward mutually defined therapeutic goals" (Conway-Rutkowski, 1982).
2. Compliance involves a behavioral change, which is positively influenced by (Hussey & Gilliland, 1989):
   a. Usual pattern of compliance
   b. Family influence, stability
   c. Perception of own susceptibility to the disease
   d. Perception that the disease is serious
   e. Efficacy of treatment

3. Compliance is negatively influenced by (Hussey & Gilliland, 1989):
   a. Duration of therapy
   b. Number of concurrent drugs or treatments
   c. Presence of side-effects
4. Since the diagnosis of noncompliance has a high subjective component, the nurse is cautioned not to utilize the diagnosis as a reflection of the nurse's value judgment but, rather, to seek to identify causative and contributing factors.
5. Both clients and health care professionals share the responsibility for noncompliance and must work together to correct it.
6. There is a gray area between noncompliance and making an informed decision not to adhere to health-related advice. For example, the individual who does not take his medication because he is unable to swallow pills is different from the person who refuses chemotherapy because he is exhausted from previous treatments and is ready to die. In both cases, the nurse intervenes to elicit reasons for this behavior.
7. The nurse–client relationship is the tool that facilitates compliance. According to Hildegard Peplau, the nurse "stimulates the patient to use and thereby to develop further his own competencies to understand situations and problems" (O'Toole & Welt, 1989).

Medication Regimens

1. When evaluating noncompliance related to medication, the nurse must consider the following factors that may affect drug absorption, metabolism, effectiveness, side-effects, and excretion: body weight, age, time of administration, route of administration, genetic factors, basal metabolic rate, interactions with other drugs and foods, presence of organ disease (*e.g.,* liver and kidneys), altered body chemistry (*e.g.,* hypokalemia), and infection. For example, serum theophylline levels will be diminished in a person who smokes cigarettes.
2. When a client reports symptomatic side-effects from a new drug, consider the many manifestations of the human allergic response: hives and the entire spectrum of rashes, respiratory discomfort and distress, pruritus, watery eyes, swelling of mucous membranes, and gastrointestinal discomforts.
3. Other adverse reactions to drugs include:
   a. Drug toxicity: dose-related effects that can occur in anyone taking the drug and result from expected pharmacologic action of the drug
   b. Drug idiosyncrasy: not related to allergy or toxicity, these reactions result from the client's tissue sensitivity to the drug and are not generally predictable. May be due to genetic factors in some people.

Pediatric Considerations

1. Following a particular treatment regimen can be difficult and trying for an ill child and family. For example, certain drugs may affect behavior, alertness, or school performance (Scipien, Chard, Howe, & Barnard, 1990).
2. Disturbances in body image may occur in older school-age children and adolescents as a result of treatment with drugs such as certain chemotherapeutic agents (Scipien, Chard, Howe, & Barnard, 1990).
3. The adolescent is particularly vulnerable to problems with compliance. A young child may accept the prolonged and regular use of drugs such as insulin or Dilantin but may rebel against the regimen in adolescence (Scipien, Chard, Howe, & Barnard, 1990).
4. Compliance or acceptance of the treatment regimen may interfere with the adolescent's desire for independence (Stevens, 1989).

Gerontologic Considerations

1. It is assumed that there is a high incidence of noncompliance in elderly persons. However, studies have shown that about 50% of *all* adults, not just the elderly, on long-term medications are noncompliant (O'Hanrahan & O'Malley, 1981; Vestal & Dawson, 1985).
2. Simonson (1984) has identified the following factors that contribute to noncompliance in older adults: living alone, adverse medication effects, financial impact, type of disease, poor client–physician relationship, complexity of regimen, cognitive and sensory impairments, and poor understanding.

■ Noncompliance
Related to Anxiety

Assessment

Subjective Data
The person states
    He is anxious or fearful
    He has not followed advice of health care professional

Objective Data
The person exhibits nonverbal signs of anxiety

Tachycardia	Chest pain
Perspiration	Dyspnea
Headache	Cold extremities
GI discomfort	Tachypnea
Insomnia	

Outcome Criteria

The person will
- Verbalize fears related to health needs
- Identify factors that are contributing to anxiety
- Identify alternatives to present coping patterns

Interventions

A. Assess causative or contributing factors

1. Negative experiences with disease or with health care system (either personally or through others)
2. Stressors

B. Reduce or eliminate causative or contributing factors if possible

1. Negative experiences with health care system

a. Using open-ended questions, encourage person to talk about previous experiences with health care (*e.g.,* hospitalizations, family deaths, diagnostic tests, blood tests, x-rays).

b. Ask client directly, "What are your concerns about

. . . taking this drug?"

. . . following this diet?"

. . . having a blood test?"

. . . going through the cystoscopy?"

. . . having your gallbladder removed?"

. . . using a diaphragm?"

. . . paying for the operation?"

c. Encourage client to talk about how the diagnosis and treatment might affect him and/or significant others.

d. Acknowledge appropriateness of being fearful.

e. Correct any misconceptions.

f. Give appropriate instructions.

g. Discuss the effects of anxiety on pain, breathing, healing, and general comfort (see also *Anxiety; Fear*).

2. Stressors

a. Assess person for recent changes in life-style (personal, work, family, health, financial).

b. Facilitate recognition by person of how those factors are affecting his health.

c. Assist person to manage his stressors; see the appropriate diagnosis that reflects the stressor:

Fear	*Spiritual Distress*
Anxiety	*Altered Thought Processes*
Grieving	*Ineffective Individual Coping*
Altered Nutrition	*Altered Family Processes*
Self-Care Deficit	

C. Initiate referrals if indicated

1. Dietitian
2. Nutrition support
3. Home health
4. Social service
5. Other community agencies

■ Noncompliance
Related to Negative Side-Effects of Prescribed Treatment

Assessment

Subjective Data

The person states that he has altered the prescribed health behavior because of discomforts related to treatment(s)

"Medications make me sick."

"Medications make me tired."

The person describes symptoms such as

Dizziness	Indigestion
Headache	Drowsiness
Dry mouth	Sexual difficulties
Pain	Depression
Diarrhea	

The person states that treatments are inconvenient

Family member describes changes in person, such as:

"He is not himself."

Decreased ability to care for himself

Change in appetite

Change in sleep pattern

Constipation/diarrhea

Incontinence of urine/stool

Objective Data

Any lab test indicative of treatment effects (*e.g.,* toxic drug levels, hypokalemia due to diuretics)

Physical findings

Rashes	Hyperpigmentation
Hives	Dehydration
Loss or growth of hair	Drowsiness
Fat deposits	Altered vital signs
Weight changes	Tarry stools
Edema	Ataxia/tremors
Wheezing	

Outcome Criteria

The person will
- Describe experiences that cause him to alter prescribed behavior
- Describe appropriate treatment of side-effects, if necessary
- Demonstrate appropriate alternatives to the previous plan

Interventions

A. Assess causative or contributing factors of prescribed therapy
   1. Requires prolonged period of time
   2. Is unsupervised
   3. Is complex, with numerous medications, or special equipment is needed
   4. Is very costly
   5. Involves changes in lifelong habits
   6. Is inconvenient in terms of time, place, or side-effects
   7. Is culturally unacceptable

B. Assess the person's complaints
   1. Onset and duration?
   2. Associated with activity? food? stress?
   3. Effects on activities of daily living (may need to consult family member/caretaker)

C. Review present medication therapy (prescribed and over-the-counter)
   1. Identify present therapy (names, dosages, time taken).
   2. Identify possible adverse interactions among drugs (consult pharmacist).
   3. Establish whether toxicity is present (blood level of drug).*

D. Assist person to reduce causative factors
   1. For gastric irritation, suggest that drug be taken with milk or food; may be advisable to eat yogurt (unless contraindicated).
   2. For drowsiness, take medication at bedtime or late in afternoon; consult physician for dose reduction.
   3. For leg cramps (hypokalemia), increase intake of foods high in potassium (oranges, raisins, tomatoes, bananas).
   4. For other side-effects, consult pertinent references.
   5. Use long-acting intramuscular preparations whenever possible; this includes some antibiotics and antipsychotic medications.
   6. Suggest that physicians use combination pills if available (Maxzide [hydrochlorothiazide and triamterene] and Triavil [perphenazine and amitriptyline]).
   7. When appropriate, be sure client is taking the fewest number of pills possible (check dosages to provide the largest dose available in the fewest number of pills).*
   8. Instruct client to take pills twice rather than four times a day whenever appropriate.*
   9. Encourage prescription of generic drugs for persons with financial concerns.
   10. When treatments require more than one set of hands, evaluate home help situation (see *Impaired Home Maintenance Management*).
   11. When expensive equipment is involved for treatments at home, make appropriate referrals to social workers and local agencies.

E. Initiate health teaching and referrals as indicated
   1. Teach importance of adhering to prescribed regime.
   2. Teach what to expect (effects of drug or treatment, side-effects).

---

*May require a physician's order.

3. Offer praise for honesty about noncompliance and for sharing reasons. For example,

"I'm glad you told me that you stopped Motrin because it made your stomach hurt. Now I understand why your hands still ache. Let's talk to the doctor about ways we can get you some comfort." Or "It's a good thing that you told me about your stopping the blood pressure pills. That explains your headaches and higher pressure today. Let's discuss how those pills made you feel."

4. At discharge from hospital or outpatient setting, provide written name and phone number of professional to call with questions or concerns about prescribed drug regimen.

■ Noncompliance
Related to Reported Unsatisfactory Experiences in Health Care Environment

Assessment

Subjective Data

Verbalizes dissatisfaction with setting, caregivers, or treatment regime
Client states lack of motivation
"I'm too busy to remember those pills."
"I enjoy junk food too much to give it up."

Objective Data

Clients seen in waiting areas for long periods of time
Schedules overbooked
Shortage of caregiving personnel
Clients and caregivers culturally unrelated
Client seen by a different caregiver at each visit
Physical setting lacks privacy
Setting located in dangerous or inaccessible area
Prescribed therapies not provided by caregiving setting
Treatments prescribed are complex or costly
Therapeutic plan lacks incentives or motivators

Outcome Criteria

The person will
- Express anger, frustrations, confusion related to aspects of the clinical setting to nurse
- Identify sources of dissatisfaction
- Offer suggestions of what would be more satisfactory

Interventions

A. Assess causative or contributing factors

1. Referral process
   a. Prolonged period between referral and scheduled appointment
   b. Referral to a clinic rather than to a specific caregiver
   c. Referral by person other than self
2. Method of scheduling
   a. Block scheduling, or "first come, first serve," rather than individual appointments
   b. Overbooked schedule preventing reasonable amount of time for visit
3. Communication barriers
   a. Presence of language barrier
   b. Teaching center in which a variety of students see clients and disturb continuity
   c. Goals of personnel and clients differ.
   d. Personnel use chatty, social communication style rather than teaching-focused techniques.
   e. Personnel are apathetic and "burned-out" (Rorer, Tucker, & Blake, 1988).
   f. Personnel lack interest or expertise necessary to develop trust of clients.
   g. Personnel make decisions *for* client, rather than *with* him.
   h. Conflicting messages from variety of health professionals to client.
4. Physical setting
   a. Crowded, impersonal seating in waiting areas
   b. Clients seen in curtained booths rather than individual rooms
   c. Location is not on public transportation lines.
   d. Location is in a neighborhood different from client's.

B. Eliminate or reduce contributing factors if possible

1. Referral process
   a. Whenever possible, allow client to make own appointments.
   b. Shorten referral waiting time.
   c. Personnel handling referral appointments should inquire about transportation and child care, suggesting help available if needed.
   d. Send reminder postcard to client before appointment.
   e. Personnel initiating referral should give client adequate explanations as to why it is indicated and what is expected from the visit.
2. Method of scheduling
   a. If possible, give individual appointments.
   b. Do not schedule unreasonable number of clients for a given time period.
3. Communication barriers
   a. Allow person an opportunity to make the decisions about his own health care; assume an advisory approach when counseling, rather than one that is dictatorial.
   b. Provide creative incentives to spark motivation, *e.g.*, free visit, t-shirts, graduation party for support groups, incentive charts using stickers when appropriate.
   c. Schedule regular follow-up appointments with nurses to reinforce teaching, answer questions, and offer praise and encouragement.
   d. Tailor written instructions to client's reading abilities.
      • Use clock faces and symbols when necessary.
      • Print instructions in all capital letters for beginning readers.

- Use large printing for a visually impaired client.
- Individualize forms based on client's needs, *e.g.,* poster for kitchen wall, small card for a wallet or bathroom mirror.

e. Provide name and phone number of accessible health professional for questions and concerns that may arise at home.

f. For nonreaders, encourage memorization whenever possible. Be nonjudgmental and caring. Include significant other during instruction.

g. For a sensory-impaired client, ensure that assistive devices (eyeglasses, hearing aids) are available and working before giving instructions.

h. Assist client to find additional resources when high cost of therapy causes noncompliance.

i. Help client set daily priorities, including desirable health behaviors.

j. Consider the use of contracting when behavior modification is indicated; include caregiver in the contract as well as the client.

k. Schedule interpreters whenever non–English speaking clients are anticipated (consult "language banks" in larger institutions).

l. For the caregiver who knows small amounts of a language (Spanish, for example), make note cards inscribed with key words appropriate to the clinical setting.

m. In teaching centers where clients may see different students at each visit, schedule primary nurses to stop in to see each patient.

n. Plan patient care conferences, including members of all involved health professions, at regular intervals to promote seeing clients as individuals.

4. Physical setting

a. Use waiting time for teaching (*e.g.,* group classes).

b. Use as many resources as possible to make waiting and caregiving areas pleasant, welcoming, and nonclinical.

c. Use blank wall space for health education materials, pictorial progress of client, holiday decorations, original artwork by clients, etc.

d. Ensure privacy during interviews, examinations, and procedures.

e. Causative factors related to the location of the clinical setting, safety, and transportation are difficult problems to correct; nurses may make proposals for

- Special buses
- Enhanced security
- Ramps for wheelchairs
- Improved lighting in parking areas and walkways
- More nearby parking facilities

f. Arrange for home visit, if appropriate.

g. Use community resources (*e.g.,* transportation for disabled or senior citizens).

C. Encourage person to verbalize frustrations with the clinical setting in the context of a therapeutic nursing relationship

References/Bibliography

Books and Articles

Becker, H. (Ed). (1974). *The health belief model and personal health behavior.* Thorofare, NJ: Charles B. Slack.

Byham, L., & Vickery, C. (1988). Compliance and health promotion. *Health Values, 12*(4), 5–12.

Cassells, J. M., & Redman, B. K. (1989). Preparing students to be moral agents in clinical nursing practice. *Nursing Clinics of North America, 24*(2), 463–473.

Conway-Rutkowski, B. (1982). The nurse, also an educator, patient advocate, and counselor. *Nursing Clinics of North America, (17),* 134–139.

Doak, C., Doak, L., & Root, J. (1985). *Teaching patients with low literacy skills.* Philadelphia: J. B. Lippincott.

Edel, M. K. (1985). Noncompliance: An appropriate nursing diagnosis? *Nursing Outlook, 33*(4), 183–185.

Hussey, L., & Gilliland, K. (1989). Compliance, low literacy and locus of control. *Nursing Clinics of North America, 24*(3), 605–611.

Jay, M. E., DuRant, R., & Litt, I. (1989). Female adolescents' compliance with contraceptive regimens. *Pediatric Clinics of North America, 38*(3), 731–746.

Kinnaird, L.S., Yoham, M. A., & Kieval, Y. M. (1982). Patient compliance in rehabilitating programs. *Nursing Clinics of North America, 17*(3), 523–532.

Komaroff, L. (1976). The practitioner and the compliant patient. *American Journal of Public Health, 66*(9), 833–835.

Marston, M. V. (1970). Compliance with medical regimes: A review of the literature. *Nursing Research, 19*(4), 312–323.

Neale, A. V., et al. (1989). Correlates to adherence to behavioral contracts for cholesterol reduction. *Journal of Nutrition Education, 6*(2), 221–225.

Nyamathi, A., & Shuler, P. (1989). Factors affecting prescribed medication compliance of the urban homeless adult. *The Nurse Practitioner, 14*(8), 47–54.

O'Hanrahan, M., & O'Malley, K. (1981). Compliance with drug treatment. *British Medical Journal, 283,* 298–300.

O'Toole, A., & Welt, S. (Eds.). (1989). *Interpersonal theory in nursing practice: Selected works of Hildegard Peplau.* New York: Springer.

Rorer, B., Tucker, C., & Blake, H. (1988). Long-term nurse–patient interactions: Factors in patient compliance to the dietary regimen. *Health Psychology, 7*(1), 35–46.

Ryan, P., & Falco, S. M. (1985). A pilot study to validate the etiologies and defining characteristics of the nursing diagnosis of noncompliance. *Nursing Clinics of North America, 20*(4), 685–695.

Scherwitz, L., & Leventhal, H. (1978). Strategies for increasing patient compliance. *Health Values, 2*(6), 301–306.

Scipien, G. M., Chard, M. A., Howe, J., & Barnard, M. U. (1990). *Pediatric nursing care.* St. Louis: C. V. Mosby.

Simonson, W. (1984). *Medication and the elderly.* Rockville, MD: Aspen Systems.

Steckel, S. B. (1982). Predicting, measuring, implementing and follow-up on patient compliance. *Nursing Clinics of North America, 17*(3), 491–497.

Stevens, B. (1989). Impact of chronic illness. In Foster, R. L., Hunsberger, M. M., & Anderson, J. J. T. (Eds.). *Family-centered nursing care of children.* Philadelphia: W. B. Saunders, pp. 746–747.

Vestal, R. E., & Dawson, G. W. (1985). Pharmacology and aging. In Finch, C. E., & Schneider, E. L. (Eds.). *Handbook of the biology of aging* (2nd ed.). New York: Van Nostrand Reinhold, pp. 744–819.

Resources for the Consumer

Literature

Center for Medical Consumers and Health Care Information
237 Thompson St
New York, NY 10012
(212) 674–7105

Food-drug interactions: Can what you eat affect your medication? Elizabeth, NJ: Wakefern Food Corporation.

National Council on Patient Information and Education
666 11th St NW
Suite 810
Washington, DC 20001
(202) 347–6711

Nutrition, Altered:
Less than Body Requirements

Impaired Swallowing

Altered Nutrition:
Less than Body Requirements

- ■ *Related to* **Chewing or Swallowing Difficulties**
- ■ *Related to* **Anorexia Secondary to (Specify)**
- ■ *Related to* **Difficulty or Inability to Procure Food**

DEFINITIONS

Altered Nutrition: Less Than Body Requirements: The state in which an individual who is not NPO experiences or is at risk experiencing reduced weight related to inadequate intake or metabolism of nutrients.

DEFINING CHARACTERISTICS

Major (must be present)

> One who is not NPO reports or has: inadequate food intake less than recommended daily allowance (RDA) with weight loss and/or
> Actual or potential metabolic needs in excess of intake with weight loss

Minor (may be present)

> Weight 10% to 20%+ below ideal for height and frame
> Triceps skin fold, mid-arm circumference, and mid-arm muscle circumference less than 60% standard measurement
> Muscle weakness and tenderness
> Decreased serum albumin
> Decreased serum transferrin or iron-binding capacity

RELATED FACTORS

Pathophysiologic

> Hyperanabolic/catabolic states
> > Burns (postacute phase) Cancer
> > Infection Trauma
> Chemical dependence
> Faulty metabolism
> > Cirrhosis Gastric resection

Dysphagia
    Cerebrovascular accident (CVA)   Muscular dystrophy
    Amyotrophic lateral sclerosis   Parkinson's disease
    Cerebral palsy   Neuromuscular disorders
Absorptive disorders
    Crohn's disease
    Cystic fibrosis
    Diverticulosis
Stomatitis
Trauma
Altered level of consciousness

Treatment-related
Surgery
Medications (chemotherapy)
Surgical reconstruction of mouth
Wired jaw
Radiation therapy
Inadequate absorption as a side effect
    Colchicine   Neomycin
    Pyrimethamine   Para-aminosalicyclic acid
    Antacid

Situational (personal, environmental)
Fear of choking
Anorexia
Depression
Stress
Social isolation
Nausea and vomiting
Allergy
Parasites
Inability to procure food (physical limitations, financial or transportation problems)
Crash or fad diet
Inability to chew (wired jaw, damaged or missing teeth, ill-fitting dentures)
Diarrhea
Lactose intolerance
Ethnic/religious eating patterns

Maturational
Infants/children/premature neonates: Congenital anomalies, growth spurts, develop-
    mental eating disorders, malabsorption, metabolism disorders, chronic illness
Adolescent: Anorexia nervosa (postacute phase)
Elderly: Altered sense of taste

Diagnostic Considerations
Nurses usually are the primary diagnosticians and prescribers for improving patients' nutritional status. Although *Altered Nutrition* is not a difficult diagnosis to
validate, it can challenge the nurse in the area of interventions.

Food habits and nutritional status are influenced by many factors: personal, family, cultural, financial, functional ability, nutritional knowledge, disease and injury, and treatment regimens. *Altered Nutrition: Less Than Body Requirements* describes persons who can ingest food but eat an inadequate or imbalanced quality or quantity. For instance, the diet may have insufficient protein or excessive fat content. Quantity of intake may be insufficient due to increased metabolic requirements (*e.g.,* resulting from cancer or pregnancy) or to interference with nutrient utilization (*e.g.,* impaired storage of vitamins in cirrhosis).

The nursing focus for *Altered Nutrition* is on assisting the person or family improving nutritional intake. This should not be used to describe individuals who are NPO or cannot ingest food. Those situations should be described by the collaborative problem of:

Potential Complication: Electrolyte imbalances
                          Negative nitrogen balance

Errors in Diagnostic Statements

Altered Nutrition: Less Than Body Requirements related to insulin deficiency, altered consciousness and hypermetabolic state

This diagnosis represents a diabetic patient experiencing diabetic ketoacidosis. In such a situation, nursing responsibility focuses on two major problems, managing the ketoacidosis with the physician and teaching the person and family how to prevent future episodes. Neither of these problems involves altered nutrition. The first problem described by the collaborative problem. *Potential Complication: Ketoacidosis,* for which the nurse would be responsible for monitoring for physiologic instability, initiating timely interventions, and evaluating the client's response. For the second problem, described by the nursing diagnosis *Possible Noncompliance related to adherence to diabetic diet and insufficient knowledge of adaptation needed when sick,* would be investigated after the client was stable.

Altered Nutrition: Less Than Body Requirements related to parenteral therapy and NPO status

This diagnosis represents a situation with which nurses are intricately involved (parenteral therapy). However, from a nutritional perspective, what interventions do nurses prescribe to improve the nutritional status of an NPO client? Parenteral nutrition in a client who is NPO influences several actual or potential responses that nurses treat, representing both nursing diagnoses, such as *High Risk for Infection* and *Altered Comfort,* and the collaborative problems *PC: Hypo/hyperglycemia* and *PC: Negative Nitrogen Balance.*

Impaired Swallowing related to tracheotomy tube

A tracheotomy represents a risk factor for the diagnosis *High Risk for Aspiration;* a more specific diagnosis for the focus of nursing care would be *High Risk for Aspiration related to increased secretions and loss of epiglottis protection secondary to tracheotomy.*

Focus Assessment Criteria

Subjective

General
  Weight 3 months ago
  Current weight

Ideal weight
Height
Usual intake
Diet recall for 24 hours
Is this the usual intake pattern?
Is there sufficient intake of basic four food groups?
Is there sufficient fluid intake?
Appetite (usual, changes)
Dietary patterns
Food/fluid dislikes, preferences
Religious dietary practices
Activity level
Occupation, exercise (type, frequency)
Food procurement/preparation
Functional ability
Transportation
Kitchen facilities
Income adequate for food needs
Knowledge of nutrition
Basic four food groups
Recommended intake of carbohydrates, fats, salt
Relationship of activity and metabolism
Physiologic risk factors
Medical conditions
Surgical history
Medications (prescribed, over-the-counter)
Reports of

Allergies	Dysphagia
Nausea	Indigestion
Vomiting	Chewing problems
Anorexia	Constipation
Fatigue	Diarrhea
Sore mouth	Pain

Objective Data

General
Appearance (muscle mass, fat distribution)
Height and weight
Hair, skin, nails
Mouth, teeth
Anthropometric measurements
Mid-arm circumference
Mid-arm muscle circumference
Triceps skin fold
Ability to chew, swallow, feed self

Diagnostic Studies

Hemoglobin	Iron
Serum albumin	Vitamin B_{12}
Serum transferrin or iron-binding capacity	Folic acid

Total lymphocyte count   Urinary creatinine level
Thyroid function   Lipoproteins
Triglycerides   Potassium
Cholesterol   Serum uric acid
Calcium

Principles and Rationale for Nursing Care

Generic Considerations

1. For proper metabolic functioning the body requires adequate carbohydrates, protein, fat, vitamins, minerals, electrolytes, and trace elements. Table II–12 describes the functions of these nutrients.
2. Factors influencing nutrient requirements include age, activity, gender, health status (presence of disease, injuries), and nutrient metabolism (storage, absorption, use, excretion).
3. Factors influencing nutrient intake include personal (appetite, chewing and swallowing ability, functional ability, psychologic status, culture) and structural (socialization, finances, ability to obtain food, kitchen facilities, transportation) (Miller, 1990).
4. The body requires a minimum level of nutrients for health and growth. During the life span, the nutritional needs of individuals vary, as indicated in Table II–13.
5. Inability to meet metabolic requirements results in loss of weight, poor health, and decreased ability of the body to grow or repair itself. Metabolic needs are increased in the presence of trauma, sepsis, infection, and cancer.
6. Tables II–14 and II–15 can be used to compare the individual's weight for height and anthropometric measurements.
7. Most Americans and Canadians consume insufficient amounts of complex carbohydrates and excessive amounts of animal protein and fat. For adults age 25 to 50,

---

Table II-12 **Functions of Nutrients**

Carbohydrates
Preferred source of energy for cellular activity; needed for:
- Transport of substrates, ensurance of cellular functions
- Secretion of specific hormones
- Muscular contraction
- Protein-sparing for other uses

Protein
Structural basis of body (e.g., bones, blood, muscles, hair, nails, tendons, skin); needed for:
- Initiation of chemical reactions
- Transportation of apoproteins
- Preservation of antibodies
- Maintenance of osmotic pressure
- Maintenance of buffer system (blood)
- Tissue growth and repair
- Detoxification of harmful substances

Fat
Maintains body functions, provides a stored source of energy; needed for:
- Alternate source of energy (lipolysis)
- Body insulation
- Cushioning of internal organs
- Absorption of fat-soluble vitamins

Table II-13 **Age-Related Daily Nutritional Requirements**

Age	Daily Nutritional Requirements
Infants	
Newborn	12–18 oz milk
2–3 months	20–30 oz milk
4–5 months	25–35 oz milk; strained vegetables and fruits; egg yolks
6–7 months	28–40 oz milk; above solids, plus meat
8–11 months	24 oz milk; 3 regular meals
1–2 years	24 oz milk; 1000 calories
Children	

Preschool (3–5 years)	1500 calories; 40 g protein
	Basic 4 food groups
	    4–6 servings fruits and vegetables
	    2 or more servings meat/protein (2 oz portions)
	    4 servings bread or cereal
	    4 servings dairy

School (6–12 years)	80 calories/kg; 1.2 (g/kg) protein
	Basic 4 food groups (as preschool)
	    1.5–2 g calcium
	    400 units vitamin D
	    1.5–3 liters water

Adolescent (13–17 years)	2200–2400 calories for females
	3000 calories for males
	Basic 4 food groups (as preschool)
	    50–60 g protein
	    3 g calcium
	    400 units vitamin D

Adults	

	1600–3000 calorie range (based on physical activity, emotional state, body size, age, and individual metabolism)
	Basic 4 food groups
	    2 servings dairy (low fat)
	    At least 2 servings protein
	    4–6 servings fruits/vegetables
	    4 servings bread or cereal/pasta
	Males need increased protein, ascorbic acid, riboflavin, and vitamins E and B_6
	Females need the above and also increased iron and vitamins A and B_{12}

Pregnant women (2nd and 3d trimesters)	Daily calorie requirement
	    11–15 years, 2500
	    16–22 years, 2400
	    23–50 years, 2300

(continued)

Table II-13 **Age-Related Daily Nutritional Requirements** (continued)

Age	Daily Nutritional Requirements
	Increase protein 10 g or 1 serving meat 1.2–3.5 g calcium Increase vitamins A, B, and C 30–60 mg iron

Lactating women	2500–3000 calories (500 over regular diet)
	Basic 4 food groups
	    4 servings protein
	    5 servings dairy
	    4+ servings grain
	    5+ servings vegetables
	        2+ servings vitamin C-rich
	        1+ green leafy
	        2+ others
	Fluids 2–3 quarts (1 qt milk)
	Increase in vitamin A, C, niacin

Over 65	Basic 4 food groups (same as adult) Caloric requirements decrease with age (1600–1800 for women, 2000–2400 for men) but dependent on activity, climate, and metabolic needs Ensure intake of essential amino acids, fatty acids, vitamins, elements, fiber, and water 60 mg ascorbic acid 40–60 mg protein 800 mg calcium (1500 mg for women) 10 mg iron

   recommended percentages of total caloric intake are 60% carbohydrates, 10% protein, and 30% fat (National Research Council, 1980).

8. For most people, meals are social events. Loneliness at mealtime can reduce the incentive to prepare nutritious meals (Weinburg, 1969).
9. Anorexia is a complex multidimensional problem involving physical, social, and psychologic components.
10. The person with cancer experiences disease- and treatment-related nutritional problems, as indicated below.

Disease-Related	*Treatment-Related*
Malabsorption	Stomatitis
Diarrhea	Diarrhea
Constipation	Nausea and vomiting
Anemia	Anorexia
Protein deficits	Fatigue
Fatigue	

Pregnancy Considerations

1. Nutritional needs change during pregnancy (refer to Table II–13).
2. Recommendations for total weight gain during pregnancy vary; the most common recommendation is 25–30 lb.

Table II-14 **Weight for Height and Body Frame***

Men

Height Feet	Inches	Small Frame	Medium Frame	Large Frame
5	2	128–134	131–141	138–150
5	3	130–136	133–143	140–153
5	4	132–138	135–145	142–156
5	5	134–140	137–148	144–160
5	6	136–142	139–151	146–164
5	7	138–145	142–154	149–168
5	8	140–148	145–157	152–172
5	9	142–151	148–160	155–176
5	10	144–154	151–163	158–180
5	11	146–157	154–166	161–184
6	0	149–160	157–170	164–188
6	1	152–164	160–174	168–192
6	2	155–168	164–178	172–197
6	3	158–172	167–182	176–202
6	4	162–176	171–187	181–207

Women

Height Feet	Inches	Small Frame	Medium Frame	Large Frame
4	10	102–111	109–121	118–131
4	11	103–113	111–123	120–134
5	0	104–115	113–126	122–137
5	1	106–118	115–129	125–140
5	2	108–121	118–132	128–143
5	3	111–124	121–135	131–147
5	4	114–127	124–138	134–151
5	5	117–130	127–141	137–155
5	6	120–133	130–144	140–159
5	7	123–136	133–147	143–163
5	8	126–139	136–150	146–167
5	9	129–142	139–153	149–170
5	10	132–145	142–156	152–173
5	11	135–148	145–159	155–176
6	0	138–151	148–162	158–179

To Make an Approximation of Your Frame Size . . . .

Extend your arm and bend the forearm upward at a 90-degree angle. Keep fingers straight and turn the inside of your wrist toward your body. If you have a caliper, use it to measure the space between the two prominent bones on *either side* of your elbow. Without a caliper, place thumb and index finger of your other hand on these two bones. Measure the space between your fingers against a ruler or tape measure. Compare it with these tables that list elbow measurements for *medium-framed* men and women. Measurements lower than those listed indicate you have a small frame. Higher measurements indicate a large frame.

Men

Height in 1" Heels	Elbow Breadth
5'2"–5'3"	2½"–2⅞"
5'4"–5'7"	2⅝"–2⅞"
5'8"–5'11"	2¾"–3"
6'0"–6'3"	2¾"–3⅛"
6'4"	2⅞"–3¼"

Women

Height in 1" Heels	Elbow Breadth
4'10"–4'11"	2¼"–2½"
5'0"–5'3"	2¼"–2½"
5'4"–5'7"	2⅜"–2⅝"
5'8"–5'11"	2⅜"–2⅝"
6'0"	2½"–2¾"

*Weights at ages 25–59 based on lowest mortality. Weight in pounds according to frame (in indoor clothing weighing 5 lb for men and 3 lb for women; shoes with 1" heels). (Revised Height–Weight Tables derived from life-insurance statistics prepared by the Metropolitan Life Insurance Company men and women. Copyright 1983, Metropolitan Life Insurance Company)

Table II-15   **Anthropometric Measurements (adult)***

Test	Sex	Reference	>90% Reference	90%–60% Reference	<60% Reference
Mid-Arm Circumference (MAC)(in cm)					
	Male	29.3	>26.3	26.3–17.6	<17.6
	Female	28.5	>25.7	25.7–17.1	<17.1
Mid-Arm Muscle Circumference (MAMC)(in cm)					
	Male	25.3	>22.8	22.8–15.2	<15.2
	Female	23.2	>20.9	20.9–13.9	<13.9
Triceps Skin Fold (TSF)(in mm)					
	Male	12.5	>11.3	11.3–7.5	< 7.5
	Female	16.5	>14.9	14.9–9.9	< 9.9

*If measurements are below 90% reference, nutritional support program may be indicated. (Jelliffe, D. B. [1986]. *The assessment of the nutritional status of the community.* World Health Organization Monograph No. 53. Geneva: WHO)

3. Naeye (1985) reported that the weight gain during pregnancy should be related to prepregnancy weight, *i.e.,* a mother of average weight can gain 20 lb, while a thin mother should gain 30 lb.
4. Dieting during pregnancy may result in insufficient maternal intake to provide the fetus with the necessary energy for growth. The fetus depends on the mother's dietary intake for growth and development, taking only iron and folate from maternal stores (Neelson & May, 1986).

Pediatric Considerations

1. Each growth period is characterized by changes in nutritional needs:
   a. Infant: Immaturity of digestive system and limited ability to absorb and excrete metabolites; period of rapid growth
   b. Toddler: Calcium and phosphorus needs rise. Lower energy needs are related to a slower growth rate.
   c. Preschooler: Food jags are related to erratic growth rates and activity levels.
   d. School-ager: Food habits are influenced by peers.
   e. Adolescent: Increased caloric and nutrient needs are related to this period of rapid physical growth and sexual maturation. Social and peer pressure put the adolescent girl at risk to restrict food intake for weight control. This may lead to anorexia nervosa or other eating disorders (Williams, 1985).
2. Children at special risk for inadequate nutritional intake include those with:
   a. Congenital anomalies (*e.g.,* TEF, cardiac or neuroanomalies)
   b. Prematurity, intrauterine growth retardation
   c. Inborn errors of metabolism (*e.g.,* phenylketonuria)
   d. Malabsorption disorders
   e. Developmental disorders (*e.g.,* cerebral palsy)
   f. Chronic illness (*e.g.,* cystic fibrosis, chronic infections, diabetes)
   g. Accelerated growth rates (*e.g.,* prematurity, infancy, adolescence)
   h. Parents who have inadequate attachment

3. Parents must follow sound feeding practices to prevent nutritional deficits in infancy (Anderson, 1989). Such practices include:
   a. Feeding the infant breast milk or iron-fortified formula for the first year of life (Whaley and Wong, 1989)
   b. Adding solid foods by age 5 to 6 months (Whaley & Wong, 1989)
   c. Assessing the infant's cues for burping or satiation (Whaley & Wong, 1989)
   d. Holding the infant during the feeding versus propping the bottle
   e. Selecting foods appropriate to the infant's physiologic and motor development
   f. Preparing formula correctly (Whaley & Wong, 1989)

Gerontologic Considerations

1. In general, the elderly need the same kind of balanced diet as any other group but with fewer calories. However, diets of elderly clients tend to be insufficient in iron, calcium, and vitamins (Drugay, 1986). The combination of long-established eating patterns, income, transportation, housing, social interaction, and the effects of chronic or acute disease influence the person's nutritional intake and health.
2. The decreased energy needs of many older adults require a change in nutrient intake, as shown below:

	Age *25 to 50 years*	*Age* *over 50 years*
Carbohydrates	60%	55%
Protein	10%	20%
Fat	30%	25%
kcal/day		
Female	2200	1900
Male	2900	2300

3. Several situations that affect the elderly client's ability to procure or ingest food are:
   a. Anorexia due to medications, grief, depression, illness
   b. Impaired mental status leading to inattention to hunger or selecting insufficient kinds/amounts of food
   c. Impaired mobility or manual dexterity (paresis, tremors, weakness, joint pain, or deformity)
   d. Voluntary fluid restriction for fear of urinary incontinence
   e. Small frame or history of undernutrition
   f. Inadequate income to purchase food
   g. Lack of transportation to buy food or facility to cook
   h. New dentures or poor dentition
   i. Dislike of cooking and eating alone
   j. Refusal to eat related to death wish or depression
4. Constipation, a frequent geriatric complaint, has been shown to be well managed without laxatives when fluids and fiber (*e.g.,* bran) are increased in the diet and activity is increased or abdominal exercises are initiated. Clients with diverticulosis also benefit from a high-fiber diet.
5. Adequate intake of calcium and vitamin D can maintain bone strength and calcium stores, a most important consideration in osteoporosis.
6. Persons receiving diuretics must be closely observed for adequate hydration (intake and output) and electrolyte balance, especially sodium and potassium. Potassium-rich foods should be regularly included in the diet.
7. Anorexia or dry mouth due to medication can be attenuated by altering the time of medication administration or offering fluids shortly before mealtime to stimulate the appetite and moisten the oral mucosa.

8. Persons who are impaired either physically or cognitively should receive the necessary support and supervision in selecting foods and in self-feeding.
9. Persons with lactose intolerance should try foods such as yogurt and ice cream, which seem to cause less flatulence and cramping, to meet their calcium needs.
10. Anemia due to iron deficiency usually occurs over a period of time and may be affected by chronic diseases and insufficient dietary iron intake. Increasing the intake of foods rich in vitamin C, folic acid, and dietary iron can improve the conditions necessary for optimal absorption of iron. Iron supplementation is often necessary.

■ Altered Nutrition: Less Than Body Requirements
Related to Chewing or Swallowing Difficulties

Assessment

Subjective Data
The person reports
  Dry mouth
  Sores in mouth
  "Can't chew (swallow)"

Objective Data
  Wired jaw
  Paresis involving muscles required for chewing or swallowing
  Impaired or broken teeth, missing teeth, ill-fitting dentures
  Stomatitis
  Decreased/absent gag reflex

Outcome Criteria

The person will
  • Describe causative factors when known
  • Describe rationale and procedure for treatment
  • Experience adequate nutrition through oral intake
  • Increase oral intake as evidenced by (specify)

Interventions

A. Assess causative factors
  1. Mechanical obstruction (wired jaw)
  2. Neurologic condition causing muscle weakness, slowness, uncoordination, paralysis, or a combination of these (CVA, amyotrophic lateral sclerosis, parkinsonian syndrome) (see *Impaired Swallowing*)

3. Decreased salivation (radiation therapy)
4. Dental disorders
5. Stomatitis (see *Altered Oral Mucous Membrane*)

B. Reduce or eliminate causative and contributing factors if possible
1. Mechanical obstruction
   a. Instruct or assist person to
      • Keep a record of intake.
      • Perform oral hygiene immediately after eating (*e.g.,* Water Pik-type cleansing [preferred]).
         Swishing low-calorie carbonated beverage around mouth
         Swishing solution of $1/2$ or $1/4$ hydrogen peroxide and $1/2$ or $3/4$ water around mouth (solution can be flavored with mouthwash)
   b. Teach techniques to maintain adequate nutritional intake and stimulate appetite.
      • Vary liquids to allow for different textures and tastes (*e.g.,* juices, cream soups).
      • Use commercially prepared or home-made high-protein/calorie supplements (*e.g.,* enrich milk [mix 1 qt fresh milk with 1 cup instant nonfat milk] and blenderize with various flavorings—ripe banana, ice cream, syrups, fresh or frozen fruit).
2. Decreased salivation
   a. Instruct or assist person to
      • Increase liquid intake with meals.
      • "Wet" food to make up for lack of saliva.
      • Use artificial saliva.
      • Use papain tablets, 10 minutes before eating.
      • Use meat tenderizer made from papaya enzyme applied to oral cavity with lemon glycerin swab 10 minutes before eating.
      • Suck on lemon immediately before eating to stimulate salivation (overuse can damage tooth enamel).
      • Avoid consuming only milk and milk products because they tend to form a tenacious mucus.
   b. Check medications person is on for side-effects of dry mouth/decreased salivation.
   c. Teach person to rinse mouth whenever needed to remove debris, stimulate gums, or lubricate and refresh mouth.
3. Swallowing difficulties
   a. Before beginning feeding, assess that person is adequately alert and responsive, is able to control mouth, has cough/gag reflex, and can swallow own saliva.
   b. Have suction equipment available and functioning properly.
   c. Position person correctly.
      • Have individual sit upright (60°–90°) in chair or dangle feet at side of bed if possible (prop pillows if necessary).
      • Have individual assume position 10 to 15 minutes before and after eating.
      • Have individual flex head forward on the midline about 45° to keep esophagus patent.
   d. Start with small amounts and progress slowly as person learns to handle each step.
      • Part of eyedropper filled with water

- Whole eyedropper
- Use juice in place of water
- ¼ teaspoon semi-solid (applesauce)
- ½ teaspoon semi-solid
- 1 teaspoon semi-solid pureed food or commercially prepared baby foods
- ½ cracker
- Soft diet
- Regular diet
- For person who has had a CVA, place food at back of tongue and on side of face he can control
- Feed slowly, making certain previous bite has been swallowed

e. Reduce noxious stimuli.
- Minimize distractions by turning off television or radio and secluding individual for the feeding session.
- Keep patient focused on task by giving directions until he has finished swallowing each mouthful.
    "Move food to middle of tongue."
    "Raise tongue to roof of mouth."
    "Think about swallowing."
    "Swallow."
    "Cough to clear airway."

f. Check that mouth is empty before continuing.
- Make sure food has not collected in the cheek pouches.

g. Instruct or assist person to
- Administer good oral hygiene before and after feedings.
- Avoid spicy, acid, or salty foods.
- Avoid rough foods (raw vegetables, bran).
- Soak "dry" foods (toast) to soften.
- If cold foods are soothing to individual, add ice or ice cream to gain extra coldness.
- Avoid smoking and alcohol (they may irritate mouth or throat).

C. Initiate health teaching and referrals as indicated

1. Consult with speech pathologist for assistance with persons with swallowing difficulties.
2. Consult with dietitian for assistance with diet plan.
3. Explain to individual and significant others rationale of treatment and how to proceed with it.
4. See *Altered Oral Mucous Membrane,* if indicated.
5. See *Impaired Swallowing,* if indicated.

■ Altered Nutrition: Less Than Body Requirements
Related to Anorexia Secondary to (Specify)

Anorexia is a diminishment or lack of appetite for food or fluids.

Assessment

Subjective Data

The person reports
  He is not hungry
  Nausea
  Cannot concentrate on food

Objective Data

  Weight loss
  Intake less than RDA

Outcome Criteria

The person will
  • Increase oral intake as evidenced by (specify)
  • Describe causative factors when known
  • Describe rationale and procedure for treatments

Interventions

A. Assess causative factors
   1. Alteration in sense of taste or smell
   2. Social isolation
   3. Radiation therapy or chemotherapy
   4. Alteration in body image or self-concept
   5. Early satiety
   6. Noxious stimuli (pain or painful or unpleasant procedures, fatigue, odors, nausea and vomiting)

B. Reduce or eliminate contributing factors if possible
   1. Altered sense of taste or smell
      a. Explain to person the importance of consuming adequate amounts of nutrients.
      b. Teach person to use spices to help improve the taste and aroma of food (lemon juice, mint, cloves, basil, thyme, cinnamon, rosemary, bacon bits).
      c. Teach protein sources he may find more acceptable than red meat.
         • Eggs and dairy products
         • Chicken and turkey
         • Fish (if not strong-smelling)
         • Marinated meat (in wine, vinegar)
         • Soy products (tofu)

      d. Chopped or ground meats/protein sources may be more acceptable.

      e. Mixing protein and vegetables may be more acceptable.

      f. Refer to meals as "snacks" to make them sound smaller.

  2. Social isolation

      a. Encourage individual to eat with others (meals served in dining room or group area, at local meeting place such as community center, by church groups).

      b. Provide daily contact through phone calls by support system.

      c. See *Social Isolation* for additional interventions.

  3. Noxious stimuli (pain, fatigue, odors, nausea, and vomiting)

      a. Pain

- Plan care so that unpleasant or painful procedures do not take place before meals.
- Medicate individual for pain 1/2 hour before meals according to physician's orders.
- Provide pleasant, relaxed atmosphere for eating (no bedpans in sight; don't rush); try a "surprise" (*e.g.,* flowers with meal).
- Arrange plan of care to decrease or eliminate nauseating odors or procedures near mealtimes.

      b. Fatigue

- Teach or assist individual to rest before meals.
- Teach individual to spend minimal energy in food preparation (cook large quantities and freeze several meals at a time; request assistance from others).

      c. Odor of food

- Teach him to avoid cooking odors—frying foods, brewing coffee—if possible (take a walk; select foods that can be eaten cold).
- Suggest using foods that require little cooking during periods of anorexia.

      d. Nausea and vomiting

- Encourage frequent small amounts of ice chips or cool clear liquids (dilute tea, Jell-O water, flat ginger ale or cola) unless vomiting continues (adults 30–60 mL every 1/2–1 hr; children 15–30 mL every 1/2–1 hr).
- Consider giving medications by suppository rather than by mouth.
- Decrease the stimulation of the vomiting center.

          Reduce unpleasant sights and odors.

          Provide good mouth care after vomiting.

          Teach person to practice deep breathing and voluntary swallowing to suppress the vomiting reflex.

          Instruct him to sit down after eating but not to lie down.

          Encourage him to eat smaller meals and eat slowly.

- Restrict liquids with meals to avoid overdistending the stomach; also avoid fluids 1 hour before and after meals.
- If possible, avoid the smell of food preparation.
- Try eating cold foods, which have less odor.
- Loosen clothing.
- Sit in fresh air.
- Avoid lying down flat for at least 2 hours after eating (an individual who must rest should sit or recline so head is at least 4 inches higher than feet).

  4. See *Impaired Swallowing* for additional interventions.

C. Promote foods that stimulate eating and increase protein consumption
  1. Maintain good oral hygiene (brush teeth, rinse mouth) before and after ingestion of food.
  2. Offer frequent small feedings (6/day plus snacks) to reduce the feeling of a distended stomach.
  3. Allow individual to choose food items as close to actual eating time as possible.
  4. Arrange to have highest protein/calorie nutrients served at the time individual feels most like eating (*e.g.,* if chemotherapy is in early morning, serve in late afternoon).
  5. Encourage significant others to bring in favorite home foods.
  6. Instruct person to
      a. Eat dry foods (toast, crackers) upon arising.
      b. Eat salty foods if permissible.
      c. Avoid overly sweet, rich, greasy, or fried foods.
      d. Try clear cool beverages.
      e. Sip slowly through straw.
      f. Take whatever he feels he can tolerate.
      g. Eat small portions low in fat and eat more frequently.
  7. Try commercial supplements available in many forms (liquids, powder, pudding); keep switching brands until some are found that are acceptable to individual in taste and consistency.
  8. Teach techniques to individual and family for home food preparation.
      a. Add powdered milk or egg to milkshakes, gravies, sauces, puddings, cereals, meatballs, or milk to increase protein calorie content.
      b. Add blenderized or baby foods to meat juices or soups.
      c. Use fortified milk (*i.e.,* 1 c instant nonfat milk to 1 qt fresh milk).
      d. Use milk or half-and-half instead of water when making soups and sauces; soy formulas can also be used.
      e. Add cheese or diced meat whenever able.
      f. Add cream cheese or peanut butter to toast, crackers, celery sticks.
      g. Add extra butter or margarine to soups, sauces, vegetables.
      h. Spread toast while hot.
      i. Use mayonnaise (100 cal/T) instead of salad dressing.
      j. Add sour cream or yogurt to vegetables or as dip.
      k. Use whipped cream (60 cal/T).
      l. Add raisins, dates, nuts, and brown sugar to hot or cold cereals.
      m. Have extra food (snacks) easily available.
  9. Review high-calorie versus low-calorie foods.
  10. If lactose-intolerant, explore alternate dairy source to drinking milk (*i.e.,* cheese, yogurt, acidophilus milk).

D. Initiate health teaching and referrals as indicated
  1. Dietitian for meal planning
  2. Psychiatric therapy when indicated
  3. Community meal centers
  4. Support groups for anorexics

■ Altered Nutrition: Less Than Body Requirements
Related to Difficulty or Inability to Procure Food

Altered ability to procure food is the inability to acquire food because of physical, economic, or sociocultural barriers.

Assessment

Subjective Data
The person reports
"Can't afford to buy food."
"Don't know how to fix food."
"Too much bother to fix meals for one person."

Objective Data
Inability to speak or understand English
Activity restriction

Outcome Criteria

The person will
• Describe causative factors when known
• Identify a method to acquire food on a regular schedule

Interventions

A. Assess causative factors
   1. Inadequate economic resources to obtain adequate nutrition
   2. Sociocultural barrier
   3. Physical inability to procure food, related to health problem such as chronic obstructive pulmonary disease, condition, CVA, or quadriplegia

B. Eliminate or reduce contributing factors if possible
   1. Inadequate economic resources
      a. Assess eligibility for food stamps or other government-funded programs for low-income groups; consult with social service.
      b. Suggest cooperatives or local farmers' markets for shopping.
      c. Buy foods and meats on sale and freeze; utilize cheaper cuts and tenderize.
      d. Suggest foods that are low in cost and nutritionally high; decrease use of prepackaged or prepared items.
         • Beans and legumes as protein source
         • Powdered milk (alone or mixed half-and-half with whole milk)
         • Seasonal foods when plentiful

  e. Encourage growing a small garden or participating in a community plot.

  f. Freeze or can fruits and vegetables in season (refer to county agricultural agent for information on canning and freezing).

2. Sociocultural barrier

  a. Introduce individual to locally available foodstuffs and instruct in their preparation.

  b. Suggest substitutions of locally available foodstuffs for those to which individual is accustomed.

  c. Refer to adult education home economics classes for food preparation.

  d. Assist individual in recognizing and using additional outlets and sources of food (grocery stores, meat and fruit markets).

  e. Encourage peer group meetings among people of similar backgrounds to allow learning and exchange of ideas.

  f. Acquaint with ethnic food store locations, if available.

3. Physical deficits

  a. Promote alternate methods of food procurement and preparation.

   • Assess support systems for someone willing to purchase or prepare food for individual or take him to store.

     Supermarkets that deliver

     Meals on Wheels or similar service

     Homemaker

     Group housing

     Door-to-store bus service

   • Teach the individual or others to cook enough for six meals at one time and freeze; make own complete "frozen dinners."

  b. Aid person in planning daily activities to account for energy need in shopping for food and preparing meals.

   • Rest periods before and after activity

   • Rest periods during activity, if needed

C. Teach techniques for meal planning and preparation for one

1. Buy small cans of food (it may be more expensive, but spoiled food is costly).

2. When buying fruit, select three stages of ripeness (ripe, medium ripe, green).

3. Ask the grocer to break open family-sized packages of meat or fresh vegetables.

4. When you must buy in large quantity, make soups and stews with the extra.

5. Use powdered milk instead of fresh milk in recipes.

6. Buy fresh milk in pints or quarts.

7. Store large-quantity items, (rice, flour, corn meal, dry milk, cereal) in glass jars. Place tightly-sealed jars in the freezer for one night to kill any organisms and their eggs.

8. Experiment with stir-frying vegetables (e.g., Chinese cabbage, celery) in a little chicken broth.

9. If freezer space is available, prepare four to six times as much as you need and freeze in individual portions, dating the packages.

10. Store half a loaf of bread well-wrapped in freezer. (It will become stale in the refrigerator.)

11. Buy large bags of frozen vegetables, use small amounts, and close with twist ties.

12. Finely chop and freeze fresh herbs (parsely, dill, basil) in small zip-loc type bags. Flatten so that small portions can be broken off after freezing.

13. Buy large quantities of meat and freeze in foil wrap (not freezer paper).

D. Initiate health teaching and referrals as indicated
1. Refer to social worker, occupational therapist, or visiting nurse, as needed.
2. Refer to local extension office for information on vegetable gardening, community gardens, and techniques of freezing and canning foods.
3. Refer to dietitian for meal planning.

References/Bibliography

Books and Articles

Anderson, J. J. (1989). Families with infants. In Foster, R. L., Hunsberger, M. M., & Anderson J. J. T. (Eds.). *Family-centered nursing care of care of children.* Philadelphia: W. B. Saunders, p. 239.

Cockram, D., & Kaminski, M. (1986). Current concepts in nutritional assessment. *Nutritional Support Services, 6*(5), 14–15.

Drugay, M. (1986). Nutritional evaluation: Who needs it. *Journal of Gerontological Nursing, 12*(4), 14–18.

Ewald, E. B. (1973). *Recipes for a small planet.* New York: Ballantine Books.

Forlaw, L., & Bayu, L. (Eds.). (1983). Symposium on nutrition. *Nursing Clinics of North America, 18*(1).

Grant, M., Rhiner, M., & Padilla, G. V. (1989). Nutritional management in the head and neck cancer patient. *Seminars in Oncology Nursing, 5*(3), 195–204.

Hess, L. V. (1989). Nutritional care of the geriatric patient. *Journal of Home Health Care Practice, 2*(1), 29–38.

Kaminsky, M. V., Jr., & Jeejeebhoy, K. N. (1979). Modern clinical nutritional assessment—diagnosis of malnutrition and selection of therapy. *American Journal of Intravenous Therapy and Clinical Nutrition, 6*(3), 31–50.

Light, I., & Contento, I. R. (1989). Changing the course; a school nutrition and cancer education curriculum developed by the American Cancer Society and the National Cancer Institute. *Journal of School Health, 59*(5), 205–209.

Miller, C. A. (1990). *Nursing care of older adults.* Glenview, IL: Scott, Foresman.

Naeye, R. L. (1985). Weight gain and outcome of pregnancy. *American Journal of Obstetrics and Gynecology, 153*(1), 3–9.

National Research Council. (1980). *Recommended dietary allowances* (9th ed.). Washington, D.C.: National Academy of Science.

Neeson, J., & May, K. (1986). *Comprehensive maternity nursing.* Philadelphia: J. B. Lippincott.

Prendergast, J. M. (1989). Clinical validation of nutritional risk index. *Journal of Community Health, 14,*(3), 125–135.

Ralfes, S. R., DeBruyne, L. K., & Whitney, E. N. (Eds.). (1990). *Life span nutrition.* St. Paul: West Publishing.

Rang, M. L. (1980) Bibliography for nutrition in pregnancy. *Journal of Obstetric, Gynecologic and Neonatal Nursing, 9,* 55–58.

Recommended nutrient intakes for Canadians. (1983). Ottawa, Canada: Bureau of Nutritional Sciences, Department of National Health and Welfare.

Roudeu, J. R. (1980). *Dysphagia: An assessment and management program for the adult.* Minneapolis: Sister Kenny Institute-Abbott-Northwestern Hospital.

Tait, N., & Aisner, J. (1989). Nutritional concerns in cancer patients. *Seminars in Oncology Nursing, 5*(2 [suppl.]), 58–62.

Thelan, L., Davie, J., & Urden, L. (1990). *Textbook of critical care nursing.* St. Louis: C. V. Mosby.

Weinburg, J. (1969). Psychlogical implications of the nutritional needs of the elderly. *Journal of the American Dietetic Association, 60*(3), 293–296.

Whaley, L. F., & Wong, D. L. (1989). *Essentials of pediatric nursing* (3 ed.). St. Louis: C. V. Mosby.

Williams, S. R. (1985). *Nutrition and diet therapy* (5th ed.). St. Louis: Times Mirror/Mosby.

Resources for the Consumer

Literature

Chamberlain, A. S. *The soft foods cookbook.* Garden City, NY: Doubleday.

Chemotherapy and you (N.I.H. Pub. No. 81-1136). These three pamphlets available from U.S. Department of Health, Office of Cancer Communications, National Cancer Institute, Building 31, Room 108A18, Bethesda, MD 20205.

Diet and nutrition (N.I.H. Pub. No. 81-2038). A resource for parents of children with cancer.

Eating hints (N.I.H. Pub. No. 81-2079). Recipes and tips for better nutrition during cancer treatment.

Goldbeck, N. *As you eat so your baby grows: A guide to nutrition in pregnancy.* Available from Ceres Press, Box 87, Dept D, Woodstock, NY 12498 ($1.75)

McGill, M., & Pye, O. (1982). *The no-nonsense guide to food and nutrition.* Piscataway, NJ: New Century.

List of publications. Society for Nutrition Education, 2140 Shattuck Avenue, Suite 1110, Berkeley, CA 94704.

Impaired Swallowing

■ *Related to* **(Specify)**

DEFINITION

Impaired Swallowing: The state in which an individual has decreased ability to voluntarily pass fluids and/or solid foods from the mouth to the stomach.

DEFINING CHARACTERISTICS

Major (must be present)

Observed evidence of difficulty in swallowing and/or
Evidence of aspiration
Stasis of food in oral cavity

Minor (may be present)

Coughing
Choking
Apraxia (ideational, constructional, or visual)

RELATED FACTORS

Pathophysiologic

Cleft lip/palate
Neuromuscular disorders (*e.g.,* cerebral palsy, muscular dystrophy, myasthenia gravis, Guillain-Barré, botulism, poliomyelitis, Parkinson's disease)

Neoplastic disease (disease affecting brain and/or brain stem)
CVA
Right or left hemispheric damage to brain
Damage to 5th, 7th, 9th, 10th, or 11th cranial nerve
Tracheoesophageal fistula
Tracheoesophageal tumors, edema

Treatment-related

Surgical reconstruction of the mouth and/or throat
Anesthesia
Mechanical obstruction (tracheostomy tube)

Situational (personal, environmental)

Altered level of consciousness
Fatigue
Limited awareness
Altered sense of taste
Irritated oropharyngeal cavity

Maturational

Infant/children: congenital anomalies, developmental disorders

Diagnostic Considerations

See *Altered Nutrition: Less Than Body Requirements*

Errors in Diagnostic Statements

See *Altered Nutrition: Less Than Body Requirements*

Focus Assessment Criteria

Subjective Data

History of problem with swallowing
Diet recall for past 24 hours
    Is that the usual intake pattern?
History of problem foods
Diet history
Weight change
Present dietary pattern
    Diet diary
    Food source and preparation
    Living arrangements
    Financial status
Coping pattern
    Perception of problem
    Perception of causation
Knowledge of nutrition
    Basic food groups
    Foods high and low in calories

Physiologic alterations
    Medical history
    Presence of
        Allergies
        Vomiting
        Fatigue
        Dysphagia
        Pain
        Stomatitis

Objective Data

Height and weight
Ability to swallow, chew, feed self
Neuromuscular impairment
    Decreased/absent gag reflex
    Decreased strength on excursion of muscles involved in mastication
    Perceptual impairment
    Facial paralysis
Mechanical obstruction
    Edema
    Tracheostomy tube
    Tumor
Perceptual patterns/awareness
Level of consciousness
Condition of oropharyngeal cavity
Nasal regurgitation
Hoarseness
Aspiration
Cough a second or two after swallowing
Dehydration
Apraxia

Principles and Rationale for Nursing Care

1. Swallowing has an intellectual component as well as a physical one.
2. Swallowing (deglutition) can be divided into three phases:
   - Voluntary
   - Pharyngeal
   - Esophageal
3. The 5th, 7th, 9th, 10th, and 11th cranial nerves are involved in deglutition.
4. Swallowing is a complex activity.
5. A cough reflex is essential for rehabilitation, but a gag reflex is not.
6. Do not confuse the ability to chew with the ability to swallow. See also *Altered Nutrition: Less Than Body Requirements*.
7. An individual may have more than one type of swallowing impairment.

■ Swallowing, Impaired
Related to (Specify)

Some statement examples are:
- Related to mechanical impairment of mouth
- Related to muscle paralysis or paresis
- Related to inability to participate in automatic eating behavior secondary to decreased cognition

Assessment

See Defining Characteristics

Outcome Criteria

The person will
- Report improved ability to swallow

The person and/or family will
- Describe causative factors when known
- Describe rationale and procedures for treatment

Interventions

A. Assess for causative or contributing factors
  1. Mechanical impairment of oropharyngeal structures
     a. Congenital anomalies
     b. Cleft lip/palate
     c. Cranial nerve damage (5th, 7th, 9th, 10th, and/or 11th)
     d. Surgical reconstruction of mouth
     e. CVA
     f. Altered level of consciousness
     g. Fatigue
     h. Reddened, irritated oropharyngeal cavity
     i. Decreased/absent gag reflex
  2. Muscle paralysis or paresis
     a. Post-CVA
     b. Cranial nerve damage
     c. Decreased/absent gag reflex (*e.g.*, postradiation)
  3. Impaired cognition or awareness
     a. Cortical damage
     b. Apraxia
     c. Aphasia

B. Reduce or eliminate causative/contributing factors in individuals with
  1. Mechanical impairment of mouth—assist the individual with moving the bolus of food from the anterior to the posterior of mouth.
     a. Place food in the posterior mouth where swallowing can be assured, using
        - A syringe with a short piece of tubing attached

- A glossectomy spoon
- Soft food of a consistency that can be manipulated by the tongue against the pharynx, such as gelatin, custard, or mashed potatoes

   b. Prevent/decrease thick secretions.

- Artifical saliva
- Papain tablets dissolved in mouth 10 minutes before eating
- Meat tenderizer made from papaya enzyme applied to oral cavity 10 minutes before eating
- Frequent mouth care
- Increase fluid intake
- Check medications for potential side-effects of dry mouth/decreased salivation

2. Muscle paralysis or paresis

   a. Strengthen muscles by the following measures:

- Pass a #14 or #16 feeding tube several times a day while verbally encouraging person to swallow.
- Talk the person through the process of swallowing a feeding tube.
- Instruct/guide person through swallowing tube himself.
- Increase size of feeding tube to #18 tube if further strengthening is required.
- Encourage person to think about swallowing while doing it.
- Progress to ice chips, water, and then food when danger of aspiration is decreased.

3. Impaired cognition or awareness

   a. General

- Remove feeding tube during training if increased gag reflex is present.
- Concentrate on solids rather than liquids, since liquids are generally less well tolerated.
- Keep extraneous stimuli at minimum while eating (*e.g.*, no television or radio, no verbal stimuli unless directed at task).
- Have person concentrate on task of swallowing.
- Have person sit up in chair with neck slightly flexed.
- Instruct person to hold breath while swallowing.
- Observe for swallowing and check mouth for emptying.
- Avoid overloading mouth, because this decreases swallowing effectiveness.
- Give solids and liquids separately.

   b. Person with aphasia, or left hemispheric damage

- Demonstrate expected behavior.
- Reinforce behaviors with simple one-word commands.

   c. Person with apraxia, or right hemispheric damage

- Divide task into smallest units possible.
- Assist person through each task with verbal commands.
- Allow person to complete one unit fully before giving next command.
- Continue verbal assistance at each eating session until no longer needed.
- Incorporate written checklist as a reminder to person.

Note: Person may have both left and right hemispheric damage and require a combination of the above techniques.

C. Reduce the possibility of aspiration

1. Before beginning feeding, assess that person is adequately alert and responsive, is able to control mouth, has cough/gag reflex, and can swallow own saliva.

2. Have suction equipment available and functioning properly.
3. Position person correctly
   a. Have individual sit upright (60°–90°) in chair or dangle feet at side of bed if possible (prop pillows if necessary)
   b. Have individual assume position 10 to 15 minutes before eating and maintain position for 10 to 15 minutes after finishing eating.
   c. Have individual flex head forward on the midline about 45° to keep esophagus patent.
4. Keep individual focused on task by giving directions until he has finished swallowing each mouthful.
   a. "Take a breath"
   b. "Move food to middle of tongue"
   c. "Raise tongue to roof of mouth"
   d. "Think about swallowing"
   e. "Swallow"
   f. "Cough to clear airway"
   g. Reinforce voluntary action
5. Start with small amounts and progress slowly as person learns to handle each step
   a. Ice chips
   b. Part of eyedropper filled with water
   c. Whole eyedropper
   d. Use juice in place of water
   e. ¼ teaspoon semisolid
   f. ½ teaspoon semisolid
   g. 1 teaspoon semisolid
   h. Pureed food or commercial baby foods
   i. One-half cracker
   j. Soft diet
   k. Regular diet
   l. For person who has had a CVA, place food at back of tongue and on side of face he can control.
   m. Feed slowly, making certain previous bite has been swallowed.
   n. Some individuals do better with foods that hold together, such as soft-boiled eggs or ground meat and gravy.

D. Initiate health teaching and referrals as indicated
   1. Consult with speech pathologist.
   2. Consult with dietitian for meal planning.
   3. Explain to individual and significant others rationale of treatment and how to proceed with it.
   4. See *Altered Oral Mucous Membrane,* if indicated.
   5. See *Nutrition, Altered: Less Than Body Requirements.*

Note: If the above strategies are unsuccessful, consultation with physician may be necessary for alternative feeding techniques such as tube feedings or parenteral nutrition.

References/Bibliography

DiIorio, C., Price, M. (1990). Swallowing: An assessment guide. *American Journal of Nursing, 90* (7), 38–48.

Emick-Herring, B., & Wood, P. (1990). A team approach to neurologically based swallowing disorders. *Rehabilitation Nursing, 15*(3), 126–132.

Forlaw, L. (1983). The critically ill patient: Nutritional implications. *Nursing Clinics of North America, 18,* 111–117.

Iverson, T., Carpenter, M., Haskin, D., Mass M., et al. (1988). Fulfilling nutritional requirements. *Journal of Gerontological Nursing, 14* (4), 16–24.

Lang, C., Cooning, S., & Newman, S. (1982). Nutritional support: A foundation for critical care. *Critical Care Quarterly, 5* (2), 45–47.

Larsen, G L. (1981). Chewing and swallowing. In Martin, N., Holt, N. B., & Hicks, D. B. (Eds.). *Comprehensive rehabilitation nursing.* New York: McGraw-Hill, pp. 173–185.

McNally, J., Stair, J., & Somerville, E. (Eds.). (1985). *Guidelines for cancer nursing practice.* Orlando: Grune & Stratton.

Salmond, S. (1980). How to assess the nutritional status of acutely ill patients. *American Journal of Nursing, 80,* 922–924.

Tilton, C. N., & Maloof, M. (1982). Diagnosing the problem in stroke. *American Journal of Nursing, 82,* 596–601.

Welnetz, K. (1983). Maintaining adequate nutrition and hydration in the dysphagic ALS patient. *Canadian Nurse, 79*(3), 30–34.

Worthington-Roberts, B., & Karkeck, J. M. (1986). Nutrition. In Carnevali, D. & Patrick, M. (Eds.). *Nursing management for the elderly* (2nd ed.). Philadelphia: J. B. Lippincott, pp. 189–218.

Nutrition, Altered: More Than Body Requirements

■ *Related to* **Increased Intake Secondary to Chemical or Metabolic Changes, High Risk for**

DEFINITION

Altered Nutrition: More Than Body Requirements: The state in which the individual experiences or is at risk of experiencing weight gain related to an intake in excess of metabolic requirements.

DEFINING CHARACTERISTICS

Major (must be present)

Overweight (weight 10% over ideal for height and frame), or
Obese (weight 20% or more over ideal for height and frame)
Triceps skin fold greater than 15 mm in men and 25 mm in women

Minor (may be present)

Reported undesirable eating patterns
Intake in excess of metabolic requirements
Sedentary activity patterns

RELATED FACTORS

Pathophysiologic

Altered satiety patterns
Decreased sense of taste and smell

Treatment-related

Medications (corticosteroids)
Radiation (decreased sense of taste and smell)

Situational (personal, environmental)

Pregnancy (at risk to gain more than 25–30 lb)

Maturational

Adult/elderly: Decreased activity patterns; decreased metabolic needs

---

Diagnostic Considerations

Using this diagnosis to describe persons who are overweight or obese places the focus of interventions on nutrition. Obesity is a complex condition with sociocultural, psychologic, and metabolic implications. When the focus is primarily on limiting food intake, as with many weight loss programs, the chance of permanent weight loss is slim. To be successful, a weight loss program must focus on behavior modification and life-style changes.

The nursing diagnosis *Altered Nutrition: More Than Body Requirements* does not describe this focus. Rather, *Altered Health Maintenance related to intake in excess of metabolic requirements* better reflects the need to increase metabolic requirements through exercise and decrease intake. For some persons who desire weight loss, *Ineffective Individual Coping related to increase in eating in response to stressors* could be a useful diagnosis in addition to *Altered Health Maintenance*.

The nurse should be cautioned against applying nursing diagnosis for an overweight or obese person who does not want to participate in a weight loss program. A person's motivation for weight loss usually must come from within. Nurses can gently and expertly teach the hazards of obesity, but must respect a person's right to choose, the right of self-determination.

Altered Nutrition: More Than Body Requirements does have clinical usefulness in persons at risk for or who have experienced abnormal weight gain because of family eating patterns, pregnancy, taste or smell changes, or medications (*e.g.,* corticosteroids).

Errors in Diagnostic Statements

Altered Nutrition: More Than Body Requirements related to excessive calorie intake and sedentary life-style

As discussed in Diagnostic Considerations, *Altered Nutrition* does not describe the complex nature of obesity or overweight conditions. Obesity is not a nutritional problem, but rather a problem with coping and life-style choices. *Altered Health Maintenance* and *Ineffective Individual Coping* are more useful diagnoses for the focus of nursing interventions.

Altered Nutrition: More Than Body Requirements related to reports of gaining 50 lb with first pregnancy

A report of gaining 50 lb during first pregnancy should prompt the nurse to initiate a focus assessment to explore other variables. For example, the nurse could ask "What do you think contributed to your weight gain during your first pregnancy?" "What was the pattern of weight gain during each trimester?" The nurse also should discuss the difference between dieting during pregnancy versus a diet not excessive in simple CHO or fat. After additional data collection, the following diagnosis possibly could prove valid: *High Risk for Altered Nutrition: More Than Body Requirements related to lack of knowledge of nutritional needs during pregnancy and exercise needed and history of 50-lb weight gain during previous pregnancy.*

Focus Assessment Criteria

See *Altered Nutrition: Less Than Body Requirements*

Pediatric Considerations

1. Obesity is the most common nutritional disturbance of children (Whaley & Wong, 1989). Up to 25% of children and adolescents are obese (Anderson, Scott, & Boggs, 1989).
2. Overeating frequently begins in infancy and continues throughout childhood (Whaley & Wong, 1989).

Assessment

Presence of risk factors (see Related Factors)

Outcome Criteria

The person will
- Describe reasons why he is at risk for weight gain
- Describe reasons for increase intake with taste or olfactory deficits
- Discuss the nutritional needs during pregnancy
- Discuss the effects of exercise on weight control

Interventions

A. Assess for causative or contributing factors, such as
   1. Decreased sense of smell or taste
   2. Effects of medications
   3. History of weight gain over 30 lb during pregnancy.

B. Explain the effects of decreased sense of taste and smell on perception of satiety after eating. Encourage the person to
   1. Evaluate intake by calorie counting, not feelings of satiety.
   2. If not contraindicated, spice foods heavily to satisfy decreased sense of taste. Experiment with seasonings (*e.g.,* dill, basil).
   3. When taste is diminished, concentrate on food smells.

C. Explain the rationale for increased appetite due to use of certain medications (*e.g.,* steroids, androgens).

D. Discuss nutritional intake and weight gain during pregnancy (refer to Principles and Rationale for Nursing Care under *Altered Nutrition: Less Than Body Requirements*).

E. Assist to decrease unnecessary calorie intake and to increase metabolic activity.
   1. Increase the client's awareness of actions that contribute to excessive food intake.
      a. Request that he write down all the food he ate in the past 24 hours.
      b. Instruct client to keep a diet diary for 1 week that specifies the following:
         - What, when, where, and why eaten
         - Whether he was doing anything else (*e.g.,* watching TV, cooking) while eating
         - Emotions before eating
         - Others present (*e.g.,* snacking with spouse, children)
      c. Review the diet diary to point out patterns (*e.g.,* time, place, emotions, foods, persons) that affect food intake.
      d. Review high- and low-calorie food items.
   2. Teach behavior modification techniques to decrease caloric intake, such as:
      a. Eat only at a specific spot at home (*e.g.,* the kitchen table).
      b. Do not eat while performing other activities.

    c. Drink an 8-oz glass of water immediately before a meal.
    d. Decrease second helpings, fatty foods, sweets, and alcohol.
    e. Prepare small portions, just enough for one meal and discard leftovers.
    f. Use small plates to make portions look bigger.
    g. Never eat from another person's plate.
    h. Eat slowly and chew food thoroughly.
    i. Put down utensils and wait 15 seconds between bites.
    j. Eat low-calorie snacks that must be chewed to satisfy oral needs (*e.g.*, carrots, celery, apples).
3. Instruct to increase activity level to burn calories; encourage the following:
    a. Use the stairs instead of elevators.
    b. Park at the farthest point in parking lots and walk to buildings.
    c. Plan a daily walking program with a progressive increase in distance and pace.

Note: Urge the person to consult with a physician before beginning any exercise program.

F. Initiate referral to a community weight loss program, if indicated (*e.g.*, Weight Watchers)

References/Bibliography

Anderson, J. J., Scott, P. N., & Boggs, K. (1989). Nursing strategies: Behavioral and psychiatric alterations. In Foster, R. L., Hunsberger, M. M., & Anderson, J. J. T. (Eds.). *Family-centered nursing care of children*. Philadelphia: W. B. Saunders.

Whaley, L. F., & Wong, D. L. (1989). *Essentials of pediatric nursing* (3rd ed.). St. Louis: C. V. Mosby.

Nutrition, Altered: Potential For More Than Body Requirements

DEFINITION

Altered Nutrition: Potential for More Than Body Requirements: The state in which an individual is at risk of experiencing an intake of nutrients that exceeds metabolic needs.

RISK FACTORS

Reported or observed obesity in one or both parents
Rapid transition across growth percentiles in infants or children
Reported use of solid food as major food source before 5 months of age
Observed use of food as reward or comfort measure
Report of observed higher baseline weight at beginning of each pregnancy
Dysfunctional eating patterns

Diagnostic Considerations

This nursing diagnosis is similar to *High Risk for Altered Nutritions: More Than Body Requirements*. It describes an individual who has a family history of obesity, is demonstrating a pattern of higher weight, and/or has had a history of excessive weight gain (*e.g.,* previous pregnancy). Until clinical research differentiates this diagnosis from other presently accepted diagnoses, use *Altered Health Maintenance (Actual* or *High Risk for)* or *High Risk for Altered Nutrition: More Than Body Requirements* to direct teaching to assist families and individuals to identify unhealthy dietary patterns.

Parenting, Altered

Parental Role Conflict

Parenting, Altered

■ *Related to* **(Specify) as evidenced by Impaired Parental–Infant Attachment (Bonding)**

DEFINITION

Altered Parenting: The state in which one or more caregivers experiences a real or potential inability to provide a constructive environment that nurtures the growth and development of his/her/their child (children).

DEFINING CHARACTERISTICS

Major (must be present)

> Inappropriate parenting behaviors
> Lack of parental attachment behavior

Minor (may be present)

> Frequent verbalization of dissatisfaction or disappointment with infant/child
> Verbalization of frustration of role
> Verbalization of perceived or actual inadequacy
> Diminished or inappropriate visual, tactile, or auditory stimulation of infant
> Evidence of abuse or neglect of child
> Growth and development lag in infant/child

RELATED FACTORS

Individuals or families who may be at high risk for developing or experiencing parenting difficulties

Parent(s)

Single	Emotionally disturbed	Terminally ill
Adolescent	Alcoholic	Acutely disabled
Abusive	Addicted to drugs	Accident victim

Child

Of unwanted pregnancy	Physically handicapped	Terminally ill
Of undesired sex	Mentally handicapped	Rebellious
With undesired characteristics	Hyperactive characteristics	

Situational (personal, environmental)
Separation from nuclear family
Lack of extended family
Lack of knowledge
Economic problems
    Inflation   Unemployment
Relationship problems
    Marital discord   Step-parents
    Divorce   Live-in boy/girl friend
    Separation   Relocation
Change in family unit
    New child   Relative moves in

Other
History of ineffective relationships with own parents
Parental history of abusive relationship with parents
Unrealistic expectations of child by parent
Unrealistic expectations of self by parent
Unrealistic expectations of parent by child
Unmet psychosocial needs of child by parent
Unmet psychosocial needs of parent by child

Diagnostic Considerations

The family environment should provide the basic needs for a child's physical growth and development: stimulation of the child's emotional, social, and cognitive potential; consistent, stable reinforcement to learn impulse control; reality testing; freedom to share emotions; and moral stability (Pfeffer, 1981). This environment nurtures a child to develop, as Pfeffer (1981) states, "the ability to disengage from the family constellation as part of a process of life-long individuation." It is the role of parent(s) to provide such an environment. Most parenting difficulties stem from lack of knowledge or inability to manage stressors constructively. The ability to parent effectively is at high risk when the child or parent has a condition that increases stress on the family unit, *e.g.*, illness, financial problems.

    Altered Parenting describes a parent experiencing difficulty creating or continuing a nurturing environment for a child. *Parental Role Conflict* describes a parent or parents whose previously effective functioning ability is challenged by external factors. In certain situations, such as illness, divorce, or remarriage, role confusion and conflict are expected. If parents do not receive assistance in adapting their role to external factors, *Parental Role Conflict* can lead to *Altered Parenting*.

Errors In Diagnostic Statements

Altered Parenting related to child abuse
    Child abuse is a sign of family dysfunction. Usually, each child abuse situation involves an abusing adult and a knowing nonabusing adult; the treatment plan must include both. Thus, the diagnosis *Ineffective Family Coping* would be more descriptive of this problem. *Altered Parenting* is most appropriate when an external factor challenges the parents. External factors do not cause child abuse; rather emotional disturbances and ineffective coping do.

Focus Assessment Criteria

Applies to each individual (mother and father) and to family unit

1. Attachment behavior

Pregnancy

Planned?	Was an abortion considered?
Desired?	If yes, why was decision changed?

Prenatal

Verbalizes anticipation	Seeks prenatal care
Selects name	Follows the regimen
Plans layette	Decides about infant feeding (breast or bottle)

Intrapartum

Participates in the decision and the birthing process

Verbalizes positive feelings

Attempts to see infant as soon as delivered

Responds positively (happy) or negatively (sad, apathetic, disappointed, angry, ambivalent)

Holds and talks to infant

Uses baby's name

Talks to baby's father

Postpartum

Verbalizes positive feelings

Seeks proximity by holding infant closely; touches and hugs

Smiles and gazes at infant; seeks eye-to-eye contact

Seeks family resemblance (*i.e.*, "has my eyes," "sleeps like his father")

Refers to infant by name and sex

Expresses interest in learning infant care

Performs nurturing behavior (*i.e.*, feeding, changing)

2. Family structure/roles

Characteristics of the family: age and sex of family members, cultural and religious backgrounds, occupations of parent(s).

Roles of parent(s) within and outside of family structure; identify potential for role conflicts

Demands of daily living (employment, financial)

Social support systems of parent(s)

Location of most relatives

Frequency of visits with relatives

Length of time lived at present residence

Patterns of parental socialization with friends and relatives

Interrelationship between parents

3. Parenting knowledge/experience

Parents' recall of their relationship with their parent or caretakers and types of discipline and punishment used

Experiences with previous pregnancies

Knowledge of developmental needs and demands

Parental expectations of child

4. Parent/child relationship

Subjective

Parental level of satisfaction with child

Amount of play activities between mother and child

          Amount of play activities between father and child
          Amount of caretaking activities between mother and child
          Amount of caretaking activities between father and child
          Provisions for child development (toys, verbal stimulation)
          Reasons for disciplining
          Methods of discipline or punishment

5. Individuals (parent, child) at high risk for parenting problems
          Assess for presence of at-risk factors in parent and child (see Related Factors)
          Objective
              Child's affect (animated, warm, apathetic, cold, withdrawn)
              Presence of touching/holding behavior
              Presence of injuries
                    Explanation by child and parent
                    Correlation of explanation to injury
                    History of injuries (type, causes)
          Observe
              Parent-child interactions
              Parental participation in caretaking activities
              Parental comforting of child
              Parental gathering and assimilation of information related to their child
                and themselves
              Family communication patterns
              Visiting patterns and changes in visiting patterns

Principles and Rationale for Nursing Care

In the past, because of living in extended families, young children observed and frequently assisted in the birth and care of infants. Today in the United States, because of our mobile society and the more isolated nuclear family life-style, young men and women often approach parenthood with only a vague recollection of their own childhood, little knowledge of the birthing process, and limited, if any, experience in infant and child care.

Generic Considerations

1. Parenting is a learned behavior, and in general, people parent as they were parented.
2. Support groups partially replacing the extended family have become very popular and useful in providing knowledge regarding the birth process and in developing parenting skills.
3. Parents need confidence, as well as skill, in order to be comfortable in their new role. The nurse is in the enviable position of being able to assist families by providing them with information on parenting (Gaffney, 1988; McKay & Phillips, 1984).
4. Situations that contribute to potential or actual alteration in parenting are often related to ineffective individual or family coping. (See *Ineffective Family Coping: Disabling, as evidenced by child abuse.*)
5. See *Altered Growth and Development* for age-related developmental tasks with related interventions.
6. Observations of parent–child interactions should be guided by attention to the reciprocal aspect to the interaction. Parenting behaviors may be hampered by an interactive "mismatch," evidenced when the infant is demanding and the parent lacks resilience or when the child's behavior is normal and the parents' expectations of the child are unrealistic (Barnes, 1986).

7. In 1990, an estimated 375,000 drug-addicted infants will be born; 11% of these infants will suffer chronic mental and physical disorders beyond their initial recovery period. In addition, 8000 alcohol-damaged babies will be born (Statistics at a Glance, 1990). These children will pose special difficulties for their parents and will require specialized parenting skills that will challenge the already at-risk parents. Nurses will have to develop strategies to promote attachment, bonding, and healthy parenting practices (Adams, 1990).
8. Parenting behaviors are affected by perception of their child's vulnerability. Early life-threatening events (*e.g.*, illness, accident, prematurity) may lead to disturbed parent-child relationships, which may result in problematic psychosocial development. This phenomenon, termed the "vulnerable child syndrome," has important implications for nurses working with parents during the recovery phase of an illness (Culley, 1989).

Bonding/Attachment

1. Research indicates that there is a "sensitive period" during the newborn's first minutes and hours of life during which the child is beautifully equipped to meet and interact with the parents. Close contact at this time and in the days to follow is most beneficial to the bonding process (Klaus & Kennell, 1976).
2. The process of bonding begins before conception by planning the pregnancy and its conception as described by the following steps (Josten, 1981): planning the pregnancy, confirming the pregnancy, accepting the pregnancy, feeling fetal movement, accepting the fetus as an individual, giving birth, hearing and seeing the baby, touching and holding the baby, and caring for the baby.
3. The period from birth to 3 days is an important period for father-child bonding (Greenberg & Morris, 1974).
4. Bonding is promoted by seeing, touching, and caring for the infant (Klaus & Kennell, 1976).
5. Participation of the father in caregiving activities in American society has increased. Fathers who choose the traditional role (allowing the mother to be totally responsible for caretaking activities) must be assessed in their sociocultural context.
6. Attachment during the postpartum period is influenced by three factors: the characteristics of the baby—its appearance (attractive) and behavior (alert); the characteristics of each parent (satisfaction with baby, beliefs about ability to care for baby, ability to console and comfort baby, frequency of interactions with baby); and support—the availability of a positive resource person (relative, neighbor) and the availability of follow-up for high-risk families.
7. The bonding process is impeded when the parent(s) and child are separated because of the condition of the infant or a parent (Klaus & Kennell, 1976).
8. Parents are reluctant to form attachments to a sick infant because of their fear of loss. This reluctance creates tremendous guilt.
9. Parents of a premature infant or an infant with malformations may feel a sense of failure, leading to low self-esteem and subsequent difficulties with attachment (Klaus & Kennell, 1976).
10. Parents must be given the opportunity for grief work in the case of an ill or defective infant before attachment can begin.
11. No single behavior during pregnancy or in the postpartum period can be a conclusive sign of attachment difficulty. The presence of several characteristic signs should direct the nurse to gather more data.
12. The use of birthing rooms enhances the bonding process because of the decrease in interruptions.

13. Disorders of attachment may lead to manifestation of non-organic failure to thrive—failure of a child to grow without an organic cause (Barnes, 1986).
14. In multiple births, attachment takes longer because a mother can only attach optimally to one infant at a time. Mothers may feel differently about each infant of a multiple birth based on characteristics of the infants, such as health status or birth weight (Theroux, 1989).

General Guidelines for Nurses and Parents in Interactions with Children

1. Practice open, honest dialogues. Never threaten (*e.g.,* "If you are bad I will not take you to the movies").
2. Do not lecture. Tell the child he was wrong and let it go. Spend time talking about pleasant experiences.
3. Compliment children on their achievements. Make each child feel important and special. Especially tell a child when he has been good; try not to focus on negative behavior.
4. Do not be afraid to hold and hug (boys as well as girls).
5. Set limits and keep them. Expect cooperation. Encourage the child to participate in activities that conform to your values. Do not be trapped by, "But everybody else can."
6. Let the child help you as much as possible.
7. Discipline the child by restricting his activity. For a younger child, sit him in a chair for 3 to 5 minutes. If the child gets up, spank him once and put him back. Continue until the child sits for the prescribed time. For an older child, restrict bicycle riding or movie-going (pick an activity that is important to him).
8. Make sure the discipline corresponds to the unacceptable behavior. Children should be allowed opportunities to make mistakes and to verbally express anger.
9. Spank only once (the first spank is for the child, the rest are for you). Stay in control. Try not to discipline when you are irritated.
10. Remember to examine what you are doing when you are not disciplining your child (*e.g.,* enjoying each other, loving each other).
11. Never reprimand a child in front of another person (child or adult). Take the child aside and talk.
12. Never decide you cannot control a child's destructive behavior. Examine your present response. Are you threatening? Do you follow through with the punishment or do you give in? Has the child learned you do not mean what you say?
13. Be a good model (the child learns from you whether you intend it or not). Never lie to a child even when you think it is better; the child must learn that you will not lie to him, no matter what.
14. Children learn to be responsible adults by having responsibilities as children. Give each child a responsibility suited to his age, such as picking up toys, making beds, or drying dishes. Expect the child to complete the task.
15. Share your feelings with children (happiness, sadness, anger). Respect and be considerate of the child's feelings and of his right to be human.

■ Altered Parenting
Related to (Specify) as evidenced by Impaired Parental–Infant Attachment (Bonding)

Bonding is the strong attachment formed between parent and child.

Assessment

Subjective Data
The parent verbalizes
  Feelings of inadequacy
  Disgust at infant's bodily functions
  Resentment toward infant
  Disappointment in sex or physical characteristics of infant

Objective Data
  Does not hold infant close
  Does not seek eye-to-eye contact
  Does not talk to infant or call infant by name
  Inattentive to infant's needs
  Asks no questions about care
  Cries, appears sad
  Is hostile to father

Outcome Criteria

The parent will
  • Demonstrate increased attachment behaviors, such as holding infant close, smiling and talking to infant, and seeking eye contact with infant
  • Request to be involved in infant's care
  • Begin to verbalize positive feelings regarding the infant

---

Interventions

A. Assess causative or contributing factors
  1. Maternal
    a. Unwanted pregnancy
    b. Prolonged or difficult labor and delivery
    c. Postpartum pain or fatigue
    d. Lack of positive support system (mother, spouse, friends)
    e. Lack of positive role model (mother, relative, neighbor)
  2. Parental inadequate coping patterns (one or both parents)
    a. Alcoholic
    b. Drug addict
    c. Marital difficulties (separation, divorce, violence)

      d. Change in life-style related to new role

      e. Adolescent parent

      f. Career change (*e.g.,* working woman to mother)

      g. Illness in family

   3. Infant

      a. Premature, defective, ill

      b. Multiple birth

B. Eliminate or reduce contributing factors if possible

   1. Illness, pain, fatigue

      a. Establish with mother what infant-care activities are feasible.

      b. Provide mother with uninterrupted sleep periods of at least 2 hours during the day and 4 hours during the night.

      c. Provide relief for discomforts.

        • Episiotomy

          Evaluate degree of pain.

          Assess for hematomas and abscesses.

          Provide with comfort measures (ice, warm compresses, analgesics*).

        • Hemorrhoids

          Prevent and treat constipation.

          Provide comfort measures (compresses with witch hazel, suppositories,* analgesics*).

        • Breast engorgement of nursing mother

          Nurse as frequently as possible.

          Apply warm compresses (shower) before nursing.

          Apply cold compresses following nursing.

          Try hand massage, hand expressing, or breast pump between nursing.

          Offer mild analgesics.

          See *Ineffective Breast-feeding.*

        • Breast engorgement of non-nursing mother

          Offer analgesics as ordered.

          Apply ice packs.

          Encourage use of a good supporting brassiere that covers the entire breast.

   2. Lack of experience or lack of positive mothering role model

      a. Explore with mother her feelings and attitudes concerning her own mother.

      b. Assist her to identify someone who is a positive mother and encourage her to seek that person's aid.

      c. Outline the teaching program available to her during hospitalization.

      d. Determine who will assist her at home initially.

      e. Identify community programs and reference material that can increase her learning about child care after discharge (see References/Bibliography).

   3. Lack of positive support system

      a. Identify mother's support system and assess its strengths and weaknesses.

      b. Assess the need for counseling.

        • Encourage the parent(s) to express feelings about the experience and about the future.

        • Be an active listener to the parent(s).

        • Observe the parent(s) interacting with the infant.

* May require a physician's order.

- Assess for resources (financial, emotional) already available to the family.
- Be aware of resources available both within the hospital and in the community.
- Counsel the parent(s) on assessed needs.
- Refer to hospital or community services.

C. Provide opportunities for the bonding process

1. Promote bonding in the immediate postdelivery phase.
   a. Encourage mother to hold infant following birth (may need a short recovery period).
   b. Provide skin-to-skin contact if desired; keep room warm (72°–76° F°) or use a heat panel over the infant.
   c. Provide mother with an opportunity to breast-feed if desired.
   d. Delay the administration of silver nitrate to allow for eye contact.
   e. Give family as much time as they need together with minimum interruption from the staff (the "sensitive period" lasts from 30–90 min).
   f. Encourage father to hold infant.
2. Facilitate the bonding process during the postpartum phase.
   a. Check mother regularly for signs of fatigue, especially if she had anesthesia.
   b. Offer flexible rooming-in to the mother; establish with her the amount of care she will assume initially and support her requests for assistance.
   c. Discuss the future involvement of the father in the infant's care (if desired, plan opportunities for father to participate in his child's care during visits).
3. Provide support to the parent(s).
   a. Listen to the mother's replay of her labor and delivery experience.
   b. Allow for verbalization of feelings.
   c. Indicate acceptance of feelings.
   d. Point out the infant's strengths and individual characteristics to the parent(s).
   e. Demonstrate the infant's responses to the parents.
   f. Have a system of follow-up following discharge, especially for families considered at risk (*e.g.*, phone call or a home visit by the community health nurse).
   g. Be aware of resources and support groups available within the hospital and the community and refer the family as needed.
4. Assess the need for teaching.
   a. Observe the parent(s) interacting with the infant.
   b. Support each parent's strengths.
   c. Assist each parent in those areas in which they are uncomfortable (role modeling).
   d. Offer classes in infant care.
   e. Have handouts and audiovisual aids available for parent(s) to view at odd hours.
   f. Assess for level of knowledge in the area of growth and development and provide information as needed.
   g. See References/Bibliography for recommended printed material on parenting and child care.
5. When immediate separation of the child from the parents is necessary due to prematurity or illness, provide for bonding/attachment experiences, as possible.
   a. Allow parents to see and touch infant prior to transport.
   b. Encourage father to visit NICU and bring back verbal reports of infant and pictures if possible (Brazelton, 1981).

    c. Encourage earliest visiting for mother as feasible, with frequent phone contact with infant's caregivers if visiting not possible.

    d. When both parents are able to visit infant, continue with family-centered interventions per parental role conflict due to hospitalization of a child.

D. Initiate referrals as needed

    1. Consult with community agencies for follow-up visits if indicated.

    2. Refer parents to pertinent organizations (see References/Bibliography).

Parental Role Conflict

■ *Related to* **Illness and/or Hospitalization of a Child**

DEFINITION

Parental Role Conflict: The state in which a parent or primary caregiver experiences or perceives a change in role in response to external factors (*e.g.*, illness, hospitalization, divorce, separation).

DEFINING CHARACTERISTICS

Major (must be present)

Parent(s) express(es) concerns about changes in parental role

Demonstrated disruption in care and/or taking routines

Minor (may be present)

Parent(s) express(es) concerns/feelings of inadequacy to provide for child's physical and emotional needs during hospitalization or in the home

Parent(s) express(es) concerns about effect of child's illness on family

Parent(s) express(es) concerns about care of siblings at home

Parent(s) express(es) guilt about contributing to the child's illness through lack of knowledge, judgment, etc.

Parent(s) express(es) concern about perceived loss of control over decisions relating to the child

Parent(s) is (are) reluctant, unable, or unwilling to participate in normal caretaking activities, even with encouragement and support

Parent(s) verbalize(s), demonstrate(s) feelings of guilt, anger, fear, anxiety, and/or frustration

RELATED FACTORS

Situational (personal, environmental)

Illness of child

Birth of a child with a congenital defect and/or chronic illness

Hospitalization of a child with an acute or chronic illness

Change in acuity, prognosis, or environment of care (*e.g.,* transfer to or from an ICU)

Invasive or restrictive treatment modalities (*e.g.,* isolation, intubation, etc.)

Home care of a child with special needs (*e.g.,* apnea monitoring, postural drainage, hyperalimentation)

Interruptions of family life due to treatment regimen

Separation

Divorce	Death
Remarriage	Illness of caretaker

Change in family membership

Birth, adoption

Addition of relatives (*e.g.,* grandparent, siblings)

Diagnostic Considerations

See *Altered Parenting*

Focus Assessment Criteria

Subjective Data

1. Family structures/roles
   a. Characteristics of the family unit (as defined by the family) members, relationships, ages, sex, cultural and religious backgrounds
   b. Living accommodations, distance from hospital, transportation
   c. Roles of parent(s)
   d. Employment, means of support
   e. Change (relocation, addition, deletion, economic)
2. Family social support systems
   a. Presence of extended family
   b. Support from neighbors, church group, parent support group
3. Recent changes, events
   a. Change in household members
   b. Occupation
   c. Marital status
4. Child illness or hospitalization
   a. History of illness
      • Acute or chronic
      • Congenital or acquired
      • Resulting from an accident
      • When diagnosis first made
      • Knowledge of parent(s) about diagnosis, prognosis, treatment
      • Knowledge of child about diagnosis, prognosis, treatment

b. Parent's knowledge/experiences
- Experience with own hospitalizations
- Experiences with previous hospitalizations of this child or other children
- Involvement with medical/nursing care in the home
- Knowledge of hospital systems
- Assertiveness
- Communication style and level
- Knowledge of child development and understanding of effect of hospitalization of child
- Understanding of need for this hospitalization
- Desired outcomes from current hospitalization
- Involvement in case management for child, if any

c. Plans for dealing with this hospitalization
- Visiting plans and travel arrangements
- Desired involvement in care
- Plans for acquiring information about child
- Plans for self-care
- Plans for payment of medical and hospital bills
- Plans for meeting other roles while child is hospitalized, *i.e.,* working, care of home and other children
- Other emergent family situations that will impact upon time and energy needed for parenting the ill child

Objective Data

Parent(s)–child interaction (observe each parent/caretaker)

Involvement in caretaking

Comforting of child

Discipline of child

Interpreting hospitalization/illness related events to child

Support of child's development

Principles and Rationale for Nursing Care

1. The parental role is one of the most complex in our society due to the great number of role expectations and skills required for effective parenting.
2. Parenting behaviors are learned through role modeling, role rehearsal, and reference group interaction. External factors, both developmental (birth of a child) and situational (illness and/or hospitalization of a child) require the acquisition of new behaviors or the modification of existing parenting behaviors (Hymovich & Barnard, 1979). Difficulty in mastering the behaviors required for the role transition will lead to role strain; uncertainty about what behaviors are required in the new role will lead to lack of role clarity; and experiencing incompatibility between the new role expectations and already existing expectations will lead to role conflict (Burr, 1972).
3. Parents experiencing their child's illness in an acute or a chronic situation are faced with the challenge of role transition in order to continue effective parenting on either a temporary or permanent basis. The parent must give up the role of parenting a well child and acquire the role of parenting a sick child (Jay, 1977). Parents may be hampered in their acquisition of new effective parenting behaviors by feelings of anxiety, guilt, powerlessness, and diminished competence; and lack of information and/or unfamiliarity with hospital surroundings, personnel, and systems (Chan & Leff, 1982; Freiberg, 1972; Lewandowski, 1980; Ogden-Burke, 1989; Smith, 1987). Parents also may have self-reported factors that interfere with parenting a hospi-

talized child, including: not being used as a source of information about their child and receiving conflicting information about their child (Ogden-Burke, 1989), waiting for information (Saveora, 1987), separation from the child for long periods of time, not knowing how to comfort the child, and not being able to provide physical care for the child (Miles & Carter, 1982).

4. Nurses are in an exceptional position to use interventions to assist parents in acquiring effective parenting skills for their ill child by providing role cues (Algren, 1985; Roy, 1967) and role supplementation strategies such as role rehearsal and role modeling (Meleis, 1975). Nursing interventions that are instrumental in alleviating the environmental, situational, and personal stressors experienced by parents of a hospitalized child and that maximize the personal and environmental resources available to parents will enhance role transition (Miles & Carter, 1982).

5. Support and enhancement of role transition for parents of an ill child can best be achieved in a setting that is guided by principles of family-centered care (Shelton, 1987) and by a nursing process that also is guided by this family-focused philosophy (Arango, 1990; Mott, 1990; Rushton, 1990). The basic tenets of the family-centered philosophy include (Shelton, 1987):

    a. Recognition that the family is the constant in the child's life while the service systems and personnel within those systems fluctuate
    b. Facilitation of parent/professional collaboration at all levels of health care
    c. Sharing of unbiased and complete information with parents about their child's care on an ongoing basis in an appropriate and supportive manner
    d. Implementation of appropriate policies and programs that are comprehensive and provide emotional and financial support to meet the needs of families
    e. Recognition of family strengths and individuality and respect for different methods of coping
    f. Understanding and incorporating the developmental needs of children and families into the health care delevery system
    g. Encouragement and facilitation of parent-to-parent support
    h. Assurance that the design of the health care delivery system is flexible, accessible, and responsive to family needs

6. Nursing strategies based on an empowerment model will be the most effective in helping parents resolve role conflict and move through role transition. These strategies can help parents acquire parenting behaviors that will be effective in the caring for their ill child in the hospital or the home on a temporary or long-term basis. Based on the promotion of self-determination, decision-making capabilities, and self-efficacy, the family-centered empowerment model requires three beliefs: 1) parents are competent in or have the capacity to become competent in the care of their ill child; 2) parents must be given opportunities to display competencies in the care of their ill children; and 3) parents need the necessary information to make informed decisions, to obtain resources to meet needs and thus acquire control over their child's care (Dunst, 1988). Dunst's enablement model of helping specifies caretaker behaviors that support parental empowerment, including:

    a. Emphasis on parental responsibility for meeting needs and solving problems
    b. Emphasis on building on parental strengths
    c. Active and reflective listening
    d. Offer of normative help that is congruent with parental appraisal of need
    e. Promotion of acquisition of competencies
    f. Use of parent-professional collaboration as the mechanism for meeting needs
    g. Allowing locus of control to reside with the parent
    h. Acceptance and support of parental decisions.

7. Role conflicts can develop easily when a child receives home care from a parent or from a combination of parents and health care professionals. Role diffusion caused by the intrusion of treatments and/or providers into the home is a source of stress for the entire family and requires careful role negotiation on the part of parents and professionals (Hochstadt & Yost, 1989).

8. With the passage of federal legislation (PL 99–457) that mandates early intervention services for handicapped infants and toddlers and their families through statewide programs, the issue has been raised about the potential for parents to serve in the role of official "service coordinator" (case manager) for their own child.

9. Clements (1990) reports in a study of 30 families with chronically ill children that parenting is more difficult at certain critical times: initial diagnosis; increase in physical symptoms; relocation of the child, such as rehospitalization; developmental changes for the child, such as the entrance into school; and the physical or emotional absence of one parent (*e.g.*, illness, pregnancy).

■ Parental Role Conflict
Related to Effects of Illness and/or Hospitalization of a Child

Assessment

Subjective Data

Parent(s) reports unwillingness or fear of inadequacy in providing physical care for the child

Parent(s) reports frustration in comforting child and/or in helping child cope with pain

Parent(s) reports inability to help child understand the events of hospitalization

Parent(s) expresses anger at hospital staff for not sharing information about the child

Parent(s) expresses confusion and lack of understanding of diagnosis, prognosis, and treatment

Parent(s) expresses frustration/anger at not understanding the complex hospital system

Parent verbalizes prognosis or treatment plan that is incongruent with documented information

Child verbalizes concerns about parent(s)'s ability to perform usual parenting behaviors

Objective Data

Parent(s)'s visiting pattern decreases in frequency with no plausible explanation from personal situation

Parent(s) visits constantly while expressing concern about home or work responsibilities

Parent(s) visits but does not interact with child or participate in normal caretaking activities

Parent(s) makes no attempts to gather information about the child from nursing or medical staff

Communication among family members does not happen or is strained

Parent(s) appears to be tired, lacking hygiene, adequate nutrition

Parent(s) have no visits from other family members or friends; do not interact with parents of other patients

Parent(s) encourages inappropriate coping behaviors for the child

---

Outcome Criteria

Parent(s) will

- Demonstrate control over decision-making regarding the child, collaborate with health professionals in making decisions about the health/illness care of the child
- Relate information about the child's health status and treatment plan
- Participate in caring for the child in the home/hospital setting to the degree he/she/they desire
- Verbalize feelings about the child's illness and the hospitalization
- Identify and use available support systems that will allow parent time and energy to cope with ill child's needs

---

Interventions

A. Help parent(s) adapt parenting behaviors to allow for continuation of parenting role during hospitalization and/or illness (Meleis, 1975) and role cues (Roy, 1967)

1. Use role-supplementation strategies to help parents adapt parenting role to meet the needs of the child.
2. Use role model parenting behaviors appropriate to child's developmental stage and medical condition.
   a. Instruct parents to continue limit-setting strategies and demonstrations of caring behaviors (*e.g.*, touching, hugging despite hospitalization and equipment).
3. Provide information to empower parent(s) to adapt parenting role to the situation of hospitalization and/or the event of chronic illness of the child (Dunst, 1988).
4. Provide information about hospital routines and policies such as visiting hours, mealtimes, division routines, medical and nursing routines, rooming-in, etc. (Flint & Walsh, 1988; Miles & Carter, 1983).
5. Introduce self and other health care workers involved in the child's care and explain the role of each member of the team.
6. Explain procedures and tests to parent(s); help them interpret these activities to the child; discuss child's age-appropriate range of responses.
7. Assess usual parenting role or interpretation of real or perceived parental role.
8. Assess parental knowledge about child's normal growth and development, safety issues, etc., and offer supplemental information as appropriate (see *Altered Growth and Development*).
9. Teach parent(s) special skills needed to provide for the physical and health care needs of the child.

B. Facilitate parent(s) receiving information about the child's health status and treatment plan
   1. Foster open communication between self and parent(s), allowing time for questions, frequent repetition of information; provide direct and honest answers.
   2. Facilitate open communication between parent(s) and other members of the health care team.
   3. Approach parent(s) with new information, do not make them assume the responsibility for seeking out the information (Rushton, 1990).
   4. When parent(s) cannot be with their child, facilitate information-sharing through telephone calls; allow parents to call primary nurse or nurse caring for child.
   5. Facilitate interdisciplinary communication so that all members of the health care team will have congruent and consistent information to share with the family.
   6. Minimize waiting time for parents whenever possible (Savedra, 1987).
   7. Assess parental understanding of the child's illness.
   8. Explain and intepret medical terminology to parent(s) to aid in their understanding of the child's condition. Pass and Pass (1987) suggest providing parents with a list of questions they should be asking about their child's hospitalization. The list includes:
      a. What is the reason for the child's hospitalization?
      b. What is going to be done to the child during hospitalization?
      c. Will the child be awake for the procedures?
      d. Will the child feel pain or discomfort?
         • Where will it hurt?
         • What will be done for the discomfort?
      e. Will the child be changed in any way after the procedure? Is the change temporary or permanent?
      f. Who may visit the child? When?
      g. What may be brought to the hospital from home?
      h. How long will the child be in the hospital?
      i. Will there be any restrictions for the child at home?
   9. Interpret hospital environment and events to parent(s).
   10. Use role model interpretations of events to child, help parents interpret to child and other family members.
   11. Respect confidentiality of information, share information about child with parent(s) only, instruct other family members to obtain information from parent(s).

C. Support continued decision-making of parent(s) regarding the child's care
   1. Provide parent(s) opportunity to help formulate plan of care for their child.
   2. Use parent(s) as source of information about the child, his/her usual behaviors, reactions, and preferences (Ogden-Burke, 1989).
   3. Recognize parent(s) as "expert(s)" about their child (Rushton, 1990).
   4. Allow parent(s) the choice to be present during treatments and procedures.
   5. Involve parent(s) in decisions about the child's care, giving them choices whenever possible (Scharer & Dixon, 1989).
   6. Encourage both parents to share responsibility in decision-making as appropriate to their usual pattern.

D. Allow parents to participate in caring for their child to the degree they desire (Rushton, 1990)

1. Provide for 24-hour rooming-in for at least one parent and extended visiting for other family members. Alexander (1988) found significantly higher anxiety levels in nonrooming-in parents of hospitalized children, especially as the duration of hospitalization increased.
2. Collaborate and negotiate with parent(s) about parental tasks they wish to continue to do, tasks they wish others to assume, tasks they wish to share, and task they want to learn to do; continually assess changes in their desired involvement in care. Knafl and Dixon (1984) reported that 24% of the fathers in their study reported role expansion as a result of the hospitalization of their child. Expansion included the responsibility for monitoring the child's care.
3. Assess parental ability to comfort the child, use comfort strategies that parent(s) have indicated for the child (Miles & Carter, 1983).
4. Allow parent(s) to have uninterrupted time with the child (Scharer & Dixon, 1989).
5. Provide consistent caregivers for the family through primary nursing; explain the primary nurse's role, responsibilities, and commitment to the parent and child (Miles & Carter, 1983; Ruston, 1990).
6. Explore with parent(s) their personal responsibilities (i.e., work schedule, sibling care, household responsibilities, responsibilities to extended family); assist them in establishing a schedule that allows for sufficient caretaking time for the child and/or visiting time with the hospitalized child without frustration in meeting other role responsibilities (*e.g.,* if visiting is not possible until evening hours, delay child's bath time and allow parent to bathe child then). Alexander (1988) found a significant level of high anxiety in nonrooming-in fathers with greater members of children at home, suggesting a shift in home responsibilities.

E. Support parental ability to normalize the hospital/home environment for themselves and the child (Scharer & Dixon, 1989)

1. Orient parent(s) and child to hospital setting prior to admission, if possible, through prehospitalization or pretransfer tour (Miles & Carter, 1983).
2. Orient parent(s) to the hospital environment: kitchen, playroom, tub room, treatment room, parent's lounge.
3. Orient parent(s) on how to obtain needed supplies for self and child.
4. Orient parent(s) to other hospital area: cafeteria, chapel, gift shop, library, Ronald McDonald house.
5. Encourage parent(s) to bring clothing and toys from home.
6. Allow parent(s) to prepare home-cooked food or bring food from home if desired.
7. Encourage opportunities for families to eat meals together.
8. Provide for sibling visitation. Help parents prepare siblings for the visit (Flint & Walsh, 1988).
9. Construct daily routine around home routine as indicated by parent(s).
10. Provide privacy for parent-child interactions (*i.e.,* privacy for breast-feeding of infants, family time for teens and parents).
11. Provide parent(s) with comfortable visiting and sleeping accommodations at the bedside, if possible, for easy access to the child.
12. Attempt to minimize stressors of the unit/division (*i.e.,* noise level, overaccess by hospital personnel, unplanned patient care) that disrupt quiet/rest periods.

13. Provide age-appropriate developmental (school) and diversional activities for the child to provide for parenting opportunities.
14. Encourage opportunities for parent(s) to take the child on leaves from the hospital, including visits home, as possible.
15. Use an interdisciplinary approach to care planning to minimize the length of hospitalization.

F. Help parent(s) verbalize feelings about the child's illness and/or hospitalization and adaptation of the parenting role to the situation (Miles, 1979)

1. Encourage parent(s) to express feelings and concerns about the child's illness and/or hospitalization and about the perceived need for parental role change (Meyer, 1988; Rushton, 1990).
2. Provide opportunities for parent(s) to be alone, not in the presence of the child, so they may feel free to express feelings, frustrations, fears.
3. Indicate acceptance of parental feelings.
4. Provide supportive climate in which parents feel comfortable sharing their concerns.
5. Identify members of the staff who have established a therapeutic relationship with the parent(s).
6. Provide opportunities for parent(s) to talk about themselves, events related to hospitalization/illness, and real/perceived conflicts and changes in their role, whether temporary or permanent.
7. Facilitate process of adjustment to the diagnosis/prognosis and planning for future care.

G. Provide for physical and emotional needs of parent(s) so that they have the energy and support to continue parenting during illness/hospitalization

1. Assess and facilitate parental ability to meet self-care needs (i.e., rest, nutrition, activity, privacy, etc.) (Miles, 1979).
2. Allow parent(s) an opportunity to determine the caregiving schedule to correspond with a schedule to meet their own needs.
3. Assess support systems: parent to parent, family, friends, minister, etc.
4. Assess, acknowledge, and facilitate family strengths.
5. Facilitate and reinforce effective coping strategies used by parent(s).
6. Continue to listen to parental concerns regarding the child and parental role.
7. Continue to assess additional stressors in the family setting.

H. Initiate referrals if indicated

1. Chaplain, social service, community agencies (respite care), parent self-help groups.
2. Provide information to parent(s) for self-referral (Austin, 1990; Meyer, 1988).

References/Bibliography

General

Admire, G., & Byer, L. (1981). Counseling the pregnant teenager. *Nursing, 11*(14), 62–63.

Aguilera, D. C., & Messick, J. M. (1974). *Crisis intervention: Theory and methodology.* St. Louis: C. V. Mosby.

Ayer, A. (1978). Is partnership with parents really possible? *American Journal of Maternal Child Nursing, 3*(2), 107.

Bishop, B. (1975). A guide to assessing parenting capabilities. *American Journal of Nursing, 75,* 1784–1787.

Brink, R. (1982). How serious is the child's behavioral problem? *Maternal-Child Nursing Journal, 7*(1),33–36.

Cameron, J. (1979). Year-long classes for couples becoming parents. *Maternal-Child Nursing Journal, 4*(5), 358–362.

Dressen, S. (1976). The young adult: Adjusting to single parenting. *American Journal of Nursing, 76,* 1286–1289.

Dunst, C. J., Trivette, C. M., & Deal, A. G. (1988). *Enabling and empowering families: Principles and guidelines for practice.* Cambridge, MA: Brookline Books.

Ferraro, A., & Longo, D. (1985). Nursing care of the family with a chronically ill, hospitalized child: An alternative approach. *Image, 16*(3), 77–81.

Fife, B., Huhman, M., & Keck, J. (1986). Development of a clinical assessment scale: Evaluation of the psychosocial impact of childhood illness on the family. *Issues in Comprehensive Pediatric Nursing, 9*(1), 11–31.

Hawkins-Walsh, E. (1980). Diminishing anxiety in parents of sick newborns. *Maternal-Child Nursing Journal, 5*(1), 30–34.

Hayes, V., & Knox, J. (1984). The experience of stress in parents of children hospitalized with long term disabilities. *Journal of Advanced Nursing, 9,* 333–341.

Hill, R. (1966). Generic features of families under stress. In Paral, H. J. (Ed.). *Crisis intervention: Selected readings.* New York: Family Service Association of America.

Hobbs, N., & Perrin, J. (1985). *Issues in the care of children with chronic illness.* San Francisco: Jossey-Bass.

Hymovich, D. (1976). Parents of sick children, their needs and tasks. *Pediatric Nursing, 2*(6), 9–13.

Hymovich, D. (1981). Assessing the impact of chronic childhood illness on the family and parent coping. *Image, 13,* 71–74.

Jackson, P., Braadham, R. & Burwel, H. (1978). Child care in the hospital: A parent/staff partnership. *American Journal of Maternal Child Nursing, 3*(2), 104–107.

Johnson, S. H. (1986). *Nursing Assessment and strategies for the family at risk: High-risk parenting* (2nd ed.). Phildelphia: J. B. Lippincott.

Johnston, M. (1980). Cultural variations in professional and parenting patterns. *Journal of Obstetric, Gynecologic and Neonatal Nursing, 8*(4), 9–15.

Malinowski, J. S. (1979). Answering a child's questions about sex and a new baby. *American Journal of Nursing, 79,* 1956–1968.

McKeever, P. (1981). Fathering the chronically ill child. *Maternal-Child Nursing Journal, 6*(2), 124–128.

Melichar, M. (1980). Using crisis theory to help parents cope with a child's temper tantrums. *Maternal-Child Nursing Journal, 5*(3), 181–185.

Mercer, R. T. (1980). Teenage motherhood: The first year. *Journal of Obstetric Gynecologic and Neonatal Nursing, 9*(1), 16–29.

Miezio, P. (1983). *Parenting children with disabilities: A professional source for physicians and a guide for parents.* New York: Dekker.

Mishel, M. (1983). Parents' perception of uncertainty concerning their hospitalized child. *Nursing Research, 32*(6), 324–330.

Moore, M. L. (1981). *Newborn, family, and nurse.* Philadelphia: W. B. Saunders.

Morrow, N., Johnson, R. (1985). Coping strategies used by parents during their child's hospitalization in an intensive care unit. *Children's Health Care, 14,*(1), 14–21.

Nelms, B. (1981). What is a normal adolescent? *Maternal-Child Nursing Journal, 6*(6), 402–406.

Petrillo, M., & Sangay, S. (1980). *Emotional care of the hospitalized child.* Philadelphia: J. B. Lippincott.

Pfeffer, C. R. (1981). Development issues among children of separation and divorce. In Stuart, I. R. & Abt, L. E. (Eds.). *Children of separation and divorce: management and treatment.* New York: Van Nostrand Reinhold.

Rapoff, M. (1986). Helping parents to help their children comply with treatment regimens for chronic disease. *Issues in Comprehensive Pediatric Nursing, 9*(3), 147–156.

Shelton, T., Geppson, E., & Johnson, B. (1987). *Family-centered care for children with special health care needs.* Washington, D.C.: Association for Care of Children's Health.

Stranik, J. K., & Hogberg, B. L. (1979). Transition into parenthood. *American Journal of Nursing, 79,* 90–93.

Trahd, G. E. (1986). Siblings of chronically ill children: Helping them cope. *Pediatric Nursing, 12*(3), 191–193.

Whaley, L. & Wong, D. (1979). *Nursing care of infants and children.* St. Louis: C. V. Mosby.

Woolery, L., & Barkley, N. (1981). Enhancing couple's relationship during prenatal and postnatal classes. *Maternal-Child Nursing Journal, 6*(3), 184–188.

Abuse

Helfer, R. E., & Kempe, C. H. (1972). *Helping the battered child and his family.* Philadelphia: J. B. Lippincott.

Olson, R. J. (1976). Index of suspicion: Screening for child abusers. *American Journal of Nursing, 76,* 108–110.

Symposium on child abuse and neglect. (1981). *Nursing Clinics of North America, 16*(2).

Tagg, P. I. (1976). Nursing interventions for the abused child and his family. *Pediatric Nursing, 2*(5), 36–39.

Wegmann, M., & Lancaster, J. (1981). Child neglect and abuse. *Family and Community Health, 11*(2), 11–17.

Bonding

Dean, P., Morgan, P., Towle, J. M., et al. (1982). Making baby's acquaintance a unique attachment. *Strategy, 7*(1), 37–41.

Jenkins, R., & Westhus, N. K. (1981). The nurse role in parent-infant bonding: Overview, assessment, intervention. *Journal of Obstetric, Gynecologic, and Neonatal Nursing, 10*(2), 114–118.

Josten, L. (1981). Prenatal assessment guide for illuminating possible problems with parenting. *Maternal-Child Nursing Journal, 6*(2), 113–117.

Klaus, M. H., & Kennell, J. H. (1976). *Maternal/infant bonding.* St. Louis: C. V. Mosby.

Mercer, R. (1977). *Nursing care for parents at risk.* Thorofare, NJ: Charles B. Slack.

Parenting, Altered

Adams, C., Eyler, F.D., & Behnke, M. (1990). Nursing interventions with mothers who are substance abusers. *Journal of Perinatal and Neonatal Nursing, 3*(4), 43–51.

Barnes, C., Beardslee, C. I., Schafer, P., & Shannon, R. (1986). The child with failure to thrive, *Pediatric Nursing Forum, 1*(1), 3–11.

Brazelton, T. B. (1981). *On becoming a family—the growth of attachment.* New York: Delta/Seymour Laurence.

Culley, B., Perrin, E.C., & Jordan-Chaberski, M. (1989). Parental perceptions of vulnerability of formerly premature infants. *Journal of Pediatric Health Care, 3*(5), 237–243.

Gaffney, K. (1988). New directions in maternal attachment research. *Journal of Pediatric Health Care, 2*(4), 81–87.

Greenberg, M., & Morris, N. (1974). Engrossment: The newborn's impact upon the father. *American Journal of Orthopsychiatry, 44,* 520–531.

Klaus, M., & Kennell, J. (1976). *Maternal-infant bonding.* St. Louis: C. V. Mosby.

McKay, S., & Phillips, C. (1984). *Family centered maternity care: Implementation strategies.* Rockville, MD: Aspen Systems.

Office of Public Information, Ohio Department of Human Services. (1990). *Statistics at a glance.* Columbus, Oh.

Theroux, R. (1989). Multiple birth: A unique parenting experience. *Journal of Perinatal and Neonatal Nursing, 3* (1), 35–45.

Parental Role Conflict

Alexander, D., Powell, G.M., Williams, P., White, M., & Conlon, M. (1988). Anxiety levels of rooming-in and non-rooming-in parents of young hospitalized children. *Maternal-Child Nursing Journal, 17*(2), 79–98.

Algren, C. (1985). Role perceptions of mothers who have hospitalized children. *Children's Health Care, 14*(1), 6–9.

Arango, P. (1990). Family-centered care: Making it a reality. *Children's Health Care, 19*(1), 57–62.

Austin, J. (1990). Assessment of coping mechanisms used by parents and children with chronic illness. *America Journal of Maternal Child Nursing, 15*(2), 98–102.

Burr, W. (1972). Role transitions: A reformation of theory. *Journal of Marriage and the Family, 17*(3), 407–415.

Chan, J. M., & Leff, P. T. (1982). Parenting the chronically ill child in the hospital: Issues and concerns. *Children's Health Care, 11*(1), 9–16.

Clements, D., Copeland, L., & Loftus, M. (1990). Critical times for families with a chronically ill child. *Pediatric Nursing, 16*(2), 157–161.

Dunst, C. J., Trizette, C. M., Davis, M., & Wheeldreyer, J.C. (1988). Enabling and empowering families of children with health empairments. *Children's Health Care, 17*(2), 71–81.

Flint, N., & Walsh, M. (1988). Visiting policies in pediatrics: Parents' perceptions and preferences. *Journal of Pediatric Nursing, 3*(4), 237–245.

Freiberg, K. (1972). How parents react when their child is hospitalized. *American Journal of Nursing, 72*(7), 1270–1272.

Hochstadt, N., & Yost, D. (1989). The health care-child welfare partnership: Transitioning medically complex children to the community. *Children's Health Care, 18*(1), 4–11.

Hymovich, D., & Barnard, M. (1979). *Family health care, Volume two: Developmental and situational crises* (2nd ed.). New York: McGraw-Hill.

Jay, S. (1977). Pediatric intensive care: Involving parents in the care of their child. *Maternal-Child Nursing Journal, 6*, 195–204.

Knafl, K., & Dixon, D. (1984). The participation of fathers in their children's hospitalization. *Issues in Comprehensive Pediatric Nursing, 7*, 269–281.

Lewandowski, L. (1980). Stress and coping styles of children undergoing open-heart surgery. *Critical Care Quarterly, 3*(1), 75–84.

Meleis, A. (1975). Role insufficiency and role supplementation: A conceptual framework. *Nursing Research, 24*(4), 264–271.

Miles, M. (1979). Impact of the intensive care unit on parents. *Issues in Comprehensive Pediatric Nursing, 3*, 72–90.

Miles, M. S., & Carter, M. (1983). Assessing parental stress in intensive care units. *American Journal of Maternal Child Nursing, 8*(5), 354–359.

Miles, M. S., & Carter, M. (1982). Sources of parental stress in pediatric intensive care units. *Children's Health Care, 11*(2), 65–68.

Mott, S., et al. (1990). *Nursing care of children and families: A holistic approach* (2nd ed.). Redwood City, CA: Addison-Wesley.

Myer, P. (1988). Parental adaptation to cystic fibrosis. *Journal of Pediatric Nursing, 2*(1), 20–28.

Opden-Burke, S., Castello, E.A., & Handley-Derry, M. H. (1989). Maternal stress and repeated hospitalizations of children who are physically disabled. *Children's Health Care, 18*(2), 82–90.

Pass, M., & Pass, C. (1987). Anticipatory guidance for parents of hospitalized children. *Journal of Pediatric Nursing, 2*(4), 250–258.

Roy, M. C. (1967). Role cues and mothers of hospitalized children. *Nursing Research, 16*(2), 178–182.

Rushton, C. H. (1990). Strategies for family-centered care in the critical care setting. *Pediatric Nursing, 16*(2), 195–199.

Savedra, M. (1987). Parent's waiting: Is it an inevitable part of the hospital experience? *Journal of Pediatric Nursing, 2*(5), 328–332.

Scharer, K., & Dixon, D. (1989). Managing chronic illness: Parents with a ventilator-dependent child. *Journal of Pediatric Nursing, 4*(4), 236–246.

Shelton, T., Jeppson, E.S., & Johnson, B.H. (1987). *Family-centered care for children with special health care needs.* Washington, D.C.: Association for the Care of Children's Health.

Smith, M., & Goodman, J. (1987). *Child and family: Concepts of nursing practice* (2nd ed.). New York: McGraw-Hill.

Resources for Parents

Literature

Adams, D.W., & DeVeau, E. J. (1984). *Coping with childhood cancer.* Reston, VA: Reston.

Child care manual. ROCOM Press, P.O. Box 1577, Newark, NJ 07101

Christophersen, E.R. (1977). *Little people: Guidelines for common sense childrearing.* Lawrence, KS: H & H Enterprises.

Mash, E.J. (1976). *Behavior modification approaches to parenting.* New York: Brunner/Mazel Publishers.

Parent resource directory. Washington, D.C.: Association for the Care of Children's Health.

Salk, L., & Kramer, R. (1973). *How to raise a human being.* New York: Warner Books.

Your child from 1 to 6. U.S. Department of Health, Education, and Welfare, Children's Bureau, Publication No. 30, Washington, D.C. 20014

Organizations

Parents Without Partners, 7910 Woodmount Avenue, 1000 Washington, D.C. 20014; also local chapters

LaLeche League International, 9616 Minneapolis Avenue, Franklin Park, IL 60131; also local chapters

Parent Effectiveness Training, 531 Stevens Avenue, Solana Beach, CA 92075

Parents for Parents, Inc., 125 Northmore Drive, Yorktown Heights, NY 10598

Federation for Children with Special Needs, 312 Stuart Street, Boston, MA 02116

Parent Training and Information Centers (PTI's), U.S. Department of Education, 400 Maryland Ave S.W., Washington DC 20202, (202) 732–1032

Parents Helping Parents (PHP), 535 Race St, Suite 220, San Jose, CA 95126, (408) 288–5010

Sick Kids (Need) Involved People (SKIP), 216 Newport Drive, Severna Park, MD 21146, (301) 261–2602

Local Counseling Services

Catholic Charities, Jewish Family Services, Christian Family Services, community agencies, and mental health centers

Post-Trauma Response

Rape Trauma Syndrome

Post-Trauma Response

■ *Related to* **(Specify The Traumatic Event[s])**

DEFINITION

Post-Trauma Response: A state in which the individual experiences a sustained painful response to (an) overwhelming traumatic event(s), which has not been assimilated.

DEFINING CHARACTERISTICS

Major (must be present)

Re-experience of the traumatic event, which may be identified in cognitive, affective, and/or sensory motor activities such as:

Flashbacks, intrusive thoughts
Repetitive dreams/nightmares
Excessive verbalization of the traumatic event(s)
Survival guilt or guilt about behavior required for survival
Painful emotion, self-blame, shame, or sadness
Vulnerability or helplessness, anxiety, or panic
Fear of repetition, death, or loss of bodily control
Angry outbursts/rage, startle reaction
Hyperalertness or hypervigilance

Minor (may be present)

Psychic/emotional numbness
Impaired interpretation of reality, impaired memory
Confusion, dissociation, or amnesia
Vagueness about the traumatic event(s)
Narrowed attention or inattention/daze
Feeling of numbness, constricted affect
Feeling detached/alienated
Reduced interest in significant activities
Rigid role-adherence or stereotyped behavior
Altered life-style
Submissiveness, passiveness, or dependency
Self-destructiveness (alcohol/drug abuse, suicide attempts, reckless driving, illegal activities, etc.)

Thrill-seeking activities
Difficulty with interpersonal relationships
Development of phobia regarding trauma
Avoidance of situations or activities that arouse recollection of the trauma
Social isolation/withdrawal, negative self-concept
Sleep disturbances, emotional disturbances
Irritability, poor impulse control, or explosiveness
Loss of faith in people or the world feeling of meaninglessness in life
Feeling of not achieving normally expected life goals
Sense of foreshortened future or disturbance in orientation of the future
Chronic anxiety and/or chronic depression
Somatic preoccupational/multiple physiologic symptoms

RELATED FACTORS

Situational (personal, environmental)

Natural-origin traumatic events, including floods, earthquakes, volcanic eruptions, storms, avalanches, epidemics (may be of human origin), or other natural disasters that are overwhelming to most people

Human-origin traumatic events, such as wars, airplane crashes, serious car accidents, large fires, bombing, concentration camps, torture, assault, rape, industrial disasters (nuclear, chemical, or other life-threatening accidents), or other human-origin traumatic events that involve death and destruction or threat of such

Other influential factors such as personal vulnerability, severity of trauma, and post-trauma context, including social support

Diagnostic Considerations

The diagnosis *Post-Trauma Response* represents a group of emotional responses to a traumatic event of either natural origin (*e.g.,* floods, epidemics, earthquakes) or human origin (*e.g.,* war, rape, torture). The emotional responses (*e.g.,* guilt, nightmares, fear, anger) interfere with interpersonal relationships and can precipitate self-destructive behavior (*e.g.,* alcohol/drug abuse, suicide attempts). The nurse may find it necessary to use additional diagnoses when specific interventions are indicated, *e.g., Ineffective Family Coping, High Risk for Self-Harm.*

The diagnosis *Rape-Trauma Syndrome* was described in 1975 as encompassing an acute phase of disorganization and a long-term phase of reorganization. Based on the most recent definition of syndrome nursing diagnoses as a cluster of associated nursing diagnoses, this diagnosis does not represent a syndrome and would be more accurately labeled *Rape Trauma Response.* The inclusion of causative or contributing factors with this category is unneccessary, because the etiology is always rape. Thus, the second part of the diagnostic statement is omitted; however, the individual's report of the rape can be added to the statement. For example, *Rape Trauma Syndrome as evidenced by the report of a sexual assault and sodomy on June 22 and multiple facial bruises* (refer to ER record for description).

Errors in Diagnostic Statements

Post-Trauma Response related to expressions of survival guilt and recovering nightmares of auto accident

Survival guilt and nightmares of a traumatic event represent possible manifestations of post-trauma response, not related factors. The diagnosis should be restated as *Post-Trauma Response related to auto accident, as evidenced by recurring nightmares and expressions of survival guilt.*

Focus Assessment Criteria

Subjective Data

1. History of the trauma*
   a. Ask if person was exposed to very stressful, disturbing situations like major earthquakes or floods, very serious accidents or fires, physical assault or rape, seeing other people killed or dead, being in war or heavy combat, or some other type of disaster during his/her life.
   b. List all traumas, including dates and duration.
2. The person's responses to the traumatic event(s)
   a. Ask about person's thoughts, feelings, or actions that he/she feels have been different since the traumatic experience to assess signs and symptoms of re-experiencing or numbing responses.
   b. Ask if person's general life-style/pattern has changed since the traumatic event(s) to assess any readjustment difficulties.

Objective Data

1. Make observations and collect information from family members or other appropriate persons as possible.
   a. Excessive verbalization of the traumatic events
   b. Preoccupation with trauma-reminders, such as sorting through pictures or other trauma-related objects
   c. Use of denial, distortion, minimization, exaggeration, disavowal, fantasy, or avoidance
   d. Evidence of indifference or dissociation to stimuli (questions, noise, activities around him/her)
   e. Sudden or significant behavioral/personality changes since the traumatic event

Principles and Rationale for Nursing Care

Generic Considerations

1. Trauma victims are identified as having specific health-related problems that need nursing care.
2. Trauma is defined in terms of the subjective experience of (an) overwhelming event(s) that cannot be dealt with or assimilated in the usual way.
3. Traumatic situations differ from ordinary experience in that they involve realistic danger of physiologic or psychologic destruction that could mobilize fear of death.
4. A traumatic event may affect only a single person or many people at once, and it may be of human origin (*e.g.,* rape or wars) or natural origin (*e.g.,* avalanches or volcanic eruptions).
5. In general, traumatic events of natural origins are less severe or long-lasting when compared with those of human origin (Green, 1985), because those of human origin are often characterized by indifference, negligence, or malice.

---

*The purpose of securing a history is to substantiate evidence of trauma and not to explore details of trauma. This should be done in an appropriate therapy session.

6. Despite different types of traumatic events, there are commonly shared human responses: re-experiencing the trauma, reduced psychic and emotional functioning, and altered adaptation pattern and life-style.
7. Horowitz (1986a, b) conceptualized these phenomena and postulated a phasic tendency in human responses to traumatic events.
    a. The initial response to trauma is to survive and function in the immediate life-threatening situation by using all resources.
    b. The powerful coping method of "numbing" is used to reduce psychologic and emotional impact.
    c. However, in an attempt to master the traumatic experience, intrusive recollection or re-enactment of the trauma erupts into conscious awareness.
    d. There is a pattern of oscillation between "numbing" and intrusive reactions peculiar to each individual.
    e. Gradually, the individual works through the trauma by using a broader perception and rationale for the event and the aftermath.
    f. Finally, such an experience is assimilated into a meaningful whole that is congruent with basic beliefs and values.
8. Severity of trauma is associated with intensity, duration, and frequency of the traumatic experience.
9. It involves a complex interaction of environmental conditions (Lindy, 1984) and the person's subjective experiences such as degree of warning, threat to life, exposure to the grotesque, bereavement, displacement, and moral conflict about the role of the survivor.
10. Individual characteristics, such as early childhood experience, developmental phase, and character strength, may affect the outcome of responses to trauma.
    a. Unresolved childhood conflicts may be reactivated by the current trauma.
    b. Age can be a crucial factor because trauma can interrupt a stage of human development.
    c. Individual coping resources are important when one is confronted by a traumatic situation, and they will influence the effectiveness of adaptation.
11. The process of working through the trauma may be interrupted when there is a lack of support or additional stresses.
12. Cultural background also plays an important role in defining how a survivor deals with trauma (Kroll, 1989).
13. Nurses need to explore their own feelings about traumas they encounter before attempting to intervene effectively with trauma victims.
14. The nurse may not see every symptom of trauma response, particularly when a victim is coping with "numbing."
15. Short-term trauma crisis intervention should begin as soon as victims are identified.
16. Follow-up counseling and long-term support therapy in the community should be arranged.
17. Victims need to work through trauma at their own pace; for some, it may take a lifetime.

Pediatric Considerations

1. A child's response to trauma depends on the nature and the extensiveness of the trauma, developmental age, and the response of significant others (Whaley & Wong, 1989).
2. Nursing assessment should include the child's symbolic or nonverbal language communication (Whaley & Wong, 1989).
3. Play therapy, such as writing, drawing, telling stories, or playing with dolls, should

be offered so that the children can act out, express feelings, and/or communicate their experience safely (see Appendix IX) (Kelley, 1985; Wright, 1989).

■ Post-Trauma Response
Related to (Specify the Traumatic Event[s])

Assessment
See Defining Characteristics

Outcome Criteria

Short-term goals

The person will
- Report a lessening of re-experiencing the trauma or numbing symptoms
- Acknowledge the traumatic event and begin to work with the trauma by talking over the experience and expressing feelings such as fear, anger, and guilt
- Identify and make connection with support persons/resources

Long-term goals

The person will
- Assimilate the experience into a meaningful whole and go on to pursue his/her life as evidenced by goal setting

---

Interventions

A. Determine if the person has experienced (a) traumatic event(s)
   1. When interviewing the person, secure a quiet room where there will be no interruptions but easy access to other staff in case of management problems.
   2. Be aware that talking about a traumatic experience may cause significant discomfort to the person.
   3. If the person becomes too anxious, the assessment should be discontinued and the person helped to regain control of the distress or provided with other appropriate intervention

B. Evaluate the severity of the responses and the effects on current functioning level

C. Assist person to decrease extremes of re-experiencing or numbing symptoms
   1. Provide a safe, therapeutic environment where the person can regain control.
   2. Stay with the person and offer support during an episode of high anxiety (see *Anxiety* for additional information).

3. Assist the person to control impulsive acting-out behavior by setting limits, promoting ventilation, and redirecting excess energy into physical exercise activity (gym, walking, jogging, etc.). (See *High Risk for Self-harm* and *High-Risk for Violence* for additional information.)
4. Reassure the person that these feelings/symptoms are often experienced by the individuals who underwent such traumatic events.
5. Recognize that psychic/emotional numbness cushions the person's emotional impact.

D. **Assist person to acknowledge the traumatic event and begin to work through the trauma by talking over the experience and expressing feelings such as fear, anger, and guilt**
1. Provide a safe, structured setting for the person to describe the traumatic experience and to express feelings.
2. Explain to the person that talking about the traumatic event may intensify the symptoms (nightmares, flashbacks, painful emotions, feeling of numbness, etc.).
3. Assist the person to proceed at an individual pace.
4. Listen attentively with empathy and unhurried manner.
5. Assist the person to talk about trauma, to understand what has occurred, and to validate the reality of personal involvement.
6. Help the person to ventilate feelings associated with the traumatic event and to become aware of the link between the experience and anger, depression, or anxiety.
7. Assist the person to differentiate reality from fantasy and to look back and talk about the areas of his/her life that have been changed.
8. Recognize and support cultural and religious values in dealing with the traumatic event.

E. **Assist person to identify and make connections with support persons and resources**
1. Help person to identify his/her strength and resources.
2. Explore available support system.
3. Assist person to make connections with support and resources according to his/her needs.
4. Assist person to resume old activities and begin some new ones.

F. **Assist children to understand and to integrate the experience in accordance with their developmental stage**
1. Assist child to describe the experience and to express feelings (fear, guilt, rage, etc.) in safe, supportive places, such as play therapy sessions (Zimmerman, 1987).
2. Provide accurate information and explanations to the child in terms child can understand.
3. Provide family counseling to promote family members' understanding of the child's needs.

G. **Assist family/significant others**
1. Assist them to understand what is happening to the victim.
2. Encourage ventilation of their feelings.
3. Provide counseling sessions and/or link them with appropriate community resources, as necessary.

H. Provide nursing care appropriate to each individual's traumatic experience and needs (see *Rape Trauma Syndrome* for additional information, if relevant)

I. Provide or arrange follow-up treatment where person can continue to work through the trauma and to integrate the experience into a new self-concept

References/Bibliography

American Psychiatric Association. (1987). *Quick reference to the diagnostic criteria from DSM-III-R*. Washington, D.C.: APA

Alexander, M. C. (1988). The longitudinal course of posttraumatic morbidity: The range of outcomes and their predictors. *Journal of Nervous and Mental Disease, 176*(1), 30–39.

Benner, P. (1982). Stress and coping under extreme conditions. In Dimsdale, J. E. (Ed.). *Survivors, victims, and perpetrators, essays on the Nazi holocaust.* New York: Hemisphere Publishing Co.

Card, J. (1987). Epidemiology of PTSD in a national cohort of Vietnam veterans. *Journal of Clinical Psychology, 43*(1), 6–17.

Catherall, D. R. (1986). The support system and amelioration of PTSD in Vietnam veterans. *Psychotherapy, 23*(3), 472–482.

Chodoff, P. (1970). The German concentration camp as a psychological stress. *Archives of General Psychiatry, 22,* January, 78–87.

Eth, S., & Pynoos, R. S. (1985). Developmental perspective on psychic trauma in childhood. In Figley, C. R. (Ed.). *Trauma and its wake.* New York: Brunner/Mazel.

Fischman, Y., & Ross, J. (1990). Group treatment of exiled survivors of torture. *American Journal of Orthopsychiatry, 60*(1), 135–142.

Frederick, C. J. (1984). Children traumatized by catastrophic situations. In Pynoos, R. S. (Ed.). *Posttraumatic stress disorder in children.* Washington, D.C.: American Psychiatric Press.

Goldberg, J. (1990). A twin study of the effects of the Vietnam War on posttraumatic stress disorder. *Journal of the American Medical Association, 263*(9), 1227–1232.

Goodwin, J. (1987). The etiology of combat-related post-traumatic disorders. In Williams, T. (Ed.). *Post-traumatic stress disorders: A handbook for clinicians.* Cincinnati, OH: The Disabled American Veterans.

Green, B. (1985). A conceptual framework for post-traumatic stress syndromes among survivor groups. In Figley, C. R. (Ed.). *Trauma and its wake.* New York: Brunner/Mazel.

Green, B. (1986). Posttraumatic stress disorder: Toward DSM-IV. *Journal of Nervous and Mental Disease, 173,* 406–411.

Green, B. (1990). Buffalo Creek survivors in the second decade: Stability of stress symptoms. *American Journal of Orthopsychiatry, 60*(1), 43–54.

Holmstrom, L. L., & Burgess, A. W. (1975). Development of diagnostic categories: Sexual trauma. *American Journal of Nursing, 75*(8), 1288–1291.

Horowitz, M. J. (1986a). *Stress response syndromes* (2nd ed.). New York: Aronson.

Horowitz, M. J. (1986b). Stress response syndromes: A review of posttraumatic and adjustment disorders. *Hospital and Community Psychiatry, 37*(3), 241–248.

Kelley, S. J. (1985). Drawings: Critical communications for sexually abused children. *Pediatric Nursing, 11*(6), 421–426.

Kluznik, J. C. (1986). Forty-year follow-up of United States prisoners of war. *American Journal of Psychiatry, 143*(11), 1443–1445.

Kroll, J. (1989). Depression and posttraumatic stress disorder in Southeast Asian refugees. *American Journal of Psychiatry, 146*(12), 1592–1597.

Lenehan, G. P. (1986). Emotional impact of trauma. *Nursing Clinics of North America, 21*(4), 729–740.

Lifton, R. J. (1969). *Death in life: Survivors of Hiroshima.* New York: Vintage Books.

Lifton, R. J., & Olson, E. (1976). The human meaning of total disaster: The Buffalo Creek experience. *Psychiatry, 39,* 1–18.

Lindy, J. D. (1984). Building a conceptual bridge between civilian trauma and war trauma: Preliminary psychological findings from a clinical sample of Vietnam veterans. In *Posttraumatic stress disorder.* Washington, D.C.: American Psychiatric Association.

Madakasira, S., & O'Brien, K. (1987). Acute posttraumatic stress disorder in victims of a natural disaster. *Journal of Nervous and Mental Disease, 175*(5), 286–290.

Paul, E. A., & O'Neill, J. (1986). American nurses in Vietnam: Stressors and aftereffects. *American Journal of Nursing, 86*(5), 526.

Powell, B. J., & Penick, E. C. (1983). Psychological distress following a natural disaster: A one-year follow-up of 98 flood victims. *Journal of Community Psychology, 11,* 269–276.

Pynoos, R. S. (1987). Life threat and posttraumatic stress in school-age children. *Archives of General Psychiatry, 44,* 1057–1063.

Rahe, R. (1990). Psychological and physiological assessments on American hostages freed from captivity in Iran. *Psychosomatic Medicine, 52,* 1–16.

Scurfield, R. M. (1985). Post-trauma stress assessment and treatment: Overview and formulations. In Figley, C. R. (Ed.). *Trauma and its wake.* New York: Brunner/Mazel.

Shore, J. H. (1986). The Mount St. Helen's stress response syndrome. In Shore, J. H. (Ed.). *Disaster stress studies: New methods and findings.* Washington, D.C.: American Psychiatric Press.

Solursh, D. (1990). The family of the trauma victim. *Nursing Clinics of North America, 25*(1), 155–162.

Tanaka, K. (1988). Development of a tool for assessing posttrauma response. *Archives of Psychiatric Nursing, II*(6), 350–356.

Tanaka, K. (1990). Post-trauma response. In McFarland, G., & Thomas, M. (Eds.). *Psychiatric mental health nursing.* Philadelphia: J. B. Lippincott.

Terr, L. C. (1985). Psychic trauma in children and adolescents. *Psychiatric Clinics of North America, 8*(4), 815–835.

Whaley, L. F., & Wong, D. L. (1989). *Essentials of pediatric nursing* (3rd ed.). St. Louis: C. V. Mosby.

Wright, S. (1989). Nursing strategies: Altered musculoskeletal function. In Foster, R. L., Hunsberger, M. M. & Anderson, J. J. T. (Eds.). *Family-centered nursing care of children.* Philadelphia: W. B. Saunders.

Zimmerman, M. L. (1987). Art and group work: Interventions for multiple victims of child molestation. *Archives of Psychiatric Nursing, 1*(1), 40–46.

Rape Trauma Syndrome

DEFINITION

Rape Trauma Syndrome: A state in which the individual experiences a forced, violent sexual assault (vaginal or anal penetration) against his or her will and without his or her consent. The trauma syndrome that develops from this attack or attempted attack includes an acute phase of disorganization of the victim and family's life-style and a long-term process of reorganization of life-style.*

*Holmstrom, L., & Burgess, A. W. (1975). Development of diagnostic categories: Sexual traumas. *American Journal of Nursing, 75,* 1288–1291.

DEFINING CHARACTERISTICS

Major (must be present)
Reports or evidence of sexual assault

Minor (may be present)
If the victim is a child, parent(s) may experience similar responses

Acute Phase
Somatic responses
  Gastrointestinal irritability (nausea, vomiting, anorexia)
  Genitourinary discomfort (pain, pruritus)
  Skeletal muscle tension (spasms, pain)
Psychologic responses
  Denial
  Emotional shock
  Anger
  Fear—of being alone or that the rapist will return (a child victim will fear
    punishment, repercussions, abandonment, rejection)
  Guilt
  Panic on seeing assailant or scene of the attack
Sexual responses
  Mistrust of men (if victim is a woman)
  Change in sexual behavior

Long-term Phase
Any response of the acute phase may continue if resolution does not occur.
Psychologic responses
  Phobias   Anxiety
  Nightmares or sleep disturbances Depression
  Suicidal ideation

Diagnostic Considerations
See *Post-Trauma Response*

Errors in Diagnostic Statements
See *Post-Trauma Response*

Focus Assessment Criteria

Subjective Data (must be recorded)
History of the assault
  Time and place of rape
  Identity or description of assailant
  Sexual contact (type, amount, coercion, weapon)
  Witnesses, if any
  Activities that may alter evidence (changing clothes, bathing, urinating,
    douching)

Sexual history
Date of last menses
Menstrual history
History of venereal disease
Contraceptive use
Date of last sexual contact
Response to the assault during acute phase
Assess person and family for
Somatic symptoms
Psychologic symptoms
Sexual reactions
Assess child for
Understanding of the event
Knowledge of the identity of the molester
Possibility of previous assaults
Assess parent(s), spouse, others for
Understanding of the event
Ability to help the victim cope
Ability to cope
Response to the assault during long-term phase
Assess person and family for psychologic symptoms and sexual reactions

Objective Data

Observe for injury (ecchymoses, lacerations, abrasions)
Gastrointestinal system
(mouth, anus, abdomen)
Genitourinary system
Skeletal muscle system
Assess the emotional responses
Crying
Hysteria
Withdrawal
Detachment
Composure

Principles and Rationale for Nursing Care

Generic Considerations

1. In 1987, an estimated 91,111 cases of forcible rape occurred in the United States. National trends show a 21% increase in forcible rapes over the past 10 years (U.S. Department of Justice, 1987).
2. Rape is a crime using sexual expression to humiliate or degrade the victim (Foley & Darvies, 1987). The victim's right of privacy, sense of security, safety, and well-being are always violated (McCombie, 1980).
3. Rape is a crime that must be reported by health care providers (Brozan, 1985).
4. Our past culture (and some subcultures today) supported that (Heinrich, 1987):
   a. "A woman's rightful place in society is to fulfill man's destiny."
   b. "Women are property of men and are responsible for retaining value" (therefore, women who allow themselves to get raped are bad).
   c. "Women are important to men, as symbols of their power and status and prizes of prowess."
5. Some myths about rape include (Heinrich, 1987):
   a. The rapist is a sexually unsatisfied man unable to control his urges.
   b. Committing rape is a one-time incident, representing a momentary lapse in judgment.
   c. Rapists are strangers.
   d. Rape is provoked by the victim.
   e. Only promiscuous women get raped.

f. Rapes happen to women out alone at night. If a woman stays home, she will be safe.

g. Women cannot be raped against their will—the rape can be avoided by resistance.

h. Most rapes involve black men and white women.

i. Women respect men for overpowering them; they may even enjoy the rape.

j. Rapists are mentally ill or retarded, and therefore not responsible for their acts.

6. Victims, families, society, and caregivers who subscribe to these myths may not view themselves as victims or recognize the criminality of rape, may not seek help, or may be denied supportive interventions (Heinrich, 1987).

7. Russell (1982) reported, in a random sample of 930 families, that 44% admitted experiencing rape or attempted rape. Only 8% reported it to the police.

8. Burgess and Holmstrom (1974) categorize three main types of rape:

a. *Rape:* Sex without consent in which the assailant uses confidence rape (date rape or acquaintance rape) or blitz rape (no previous interaction).

b. *Accessory to sex:* Survivors collaborate in a secondary manner to the sexual activity and consent, or lack of consent is due to cognitive or personality development. (Mentally retarded people and children are susceptible.)

c. *Sex-stress situation:* Sex is agreed on initially but then one party decides not to go through with it, usually because of exploitation, but this change of heart is not heeded.

9. Rape occurs in all age groups, all races, and all educational and economic groups (Davis & Brody, 1981; Hughes, 1987; Longo, 1981).

10. Male rape victims (including homosexuals) are unlikely to report the rape but are most likely to experience symptoms of *Rape Trauma Syndrome* (Anderson, 1981–82; Kaufman, 1980).

11. The medicolegal examination serves to assess the condition of the victim and to gather documentary evidence. It consists of a general examination; oral, pelvic, and rectal exams; a culture for sperm and veneral diseases; serum pregnancy test; blood typing; and a drug and alcohol screen. Obvious debris is placed in separate envelopes. Dried sperm is collected. The victim's pubic hair and head hair is combed, and samples are placed in separate envelopes. Fingernail scrapings are placed in separate envelopes for each hand (Heinrich, 1987).

12. Rape crisis centers provide rape victims and significant others with information regarding the medical examination, police interrogation, and court procedures; with escort service to hospital, police department, and courts; and with counseling.

13. Rape crisis centers work in the community to educate the public on rape and rape prevention, improve the response of hospitals and the police to rape victims, and improve rape-related legislation.

14. Nurses need to explore their own feelings about rape before attempting to intervene effectively with rape trauma victims. The nurse's responses to rape victims can be anxiety and overcompensation, denial of the event, condescending, anger, coercing, blaming, helplessness, and/or overinvolvement.

15. The nurse may not see every symptom of rape trauma syndrome with each rape victim.

16. Short-term rape crisis intervention should begin during the acute phase.

17. During the acute phase, hospital emergency rooms and crisis intervention centers are two places where the nurse may encounter the rape victim.

18. Nurses should consider preexisting conditions of the rape trauma (*i.e.,* physical or psychiatric illnesses, substance abuse) that may lead to compound reactions.

19. Acute symptoms overlap with long-term symptoms of rape trauma syndrome.

20. Follow-up intervention is usually counselor-initiated.

21. Nurses in community settings can teach primary prevention concepts by reviewing with clients measures to take to reduce the possibility of rape.
22. The rape victim will resolve the rape trauma event at her/his own readiness.

Pediatric Considerations

1. An estimated 75% of sexual abuse victims are girls (Kauffman, Neill, & Thomas, 1986). The adolescent female is particularly at risk for sexual assault; it is estimated that more than 50% of rape victims are between 10 and 19 years of age (Whaley & Wong, 1989).
2. When working with young rape trauma victims, nurses should be cognizant of individual developmental levels, because the impact of the event will vary according to the child's developmental stage (Whaley & Wong, 1989).
3. The child's reaction depends on age, degree of physical trauma, relationship to assailant, and parental (caretaker) reaction (Whaley & Wong, 1989).
4. The assailant of a child is most likely someone the child knows, and the assaults usually have occurred for a period of time within the child's own home or neighborhood (Pownall, 1985).
5. Play therapy should be an integral part of the treatment regimen. (Guidelines for play therapy are presented in Appendix IX.) For rape victims, provide dolls that have genitalia for play therapy; rag dolls can have genitalia attached. The child can then act out the assault with dolls of appropriate sex (a boy victim can use two male dolls). Puppets are also beneficial for play therapy (Whaley & Wong, 1989).
6. Adolescents, particularly boys, are more prone to commit suicide in the aftermath of rape (Collins, 1982).

Gerontologic Considerations

1. Incidences of rape frequently go unreported among the elderly (U.S. Department of Justice, 1985).
2. The elderly experience similar reactions to rape as other adult victims, but may have increased degrees of dependency, powerlessness, and depression. (Davis & Brody, 1981; Fielo, 1987).

Outcome Criteria

Short-term goals

The person will
- Share feelings
- Describe rationale and treatment procedures
- Identify members of support system and utilize them appropriately

Long-term goals

The person will
- Return to precrisis level of functioning

The child will
- Discuss the assault
- Express feelings concerning the assault and the treatment

The parent(s), spouse, or significant other will
- Discuss their response to the assault
- Return to precrisis level of functioning

Interventions

The interventions for rape trauma syndrome are listed for usefulness under the three types of responses: psychologic, sexual, and somatic. The nurse must assess and intervene with each response for each victim (DiVasto, 1985).

Psychologic Responses

A. Assess for psychologic responses (Jaloweic & Powers, 1981)
   1. General
      a. Phobias, nightmares
      b. Enuresis
      c. Denial, emotional shock
      d. Anger, fear, anxiety
      e. Depression, guilt
   2. Subjective
      a. Expressions of numbness, shame, self-blame
      b. Suicidal ideation
   3. Objective
      a. Crying
      b. Silence
      c. Trembling hands
      d. Excessive bathing (seen particularly with child or adolescent)
      e. Avoiding interaction with others (staff, family)
      f. Wearing excessive clothing (two or three pairs of pants or panties)

B. Assist to identify major concerns (psychologic, medical, legal) and her/his perception of the help she/he needs
   1. Explain the care and examination she/he will experience (refer to principles for specifics) (D'Epiro, 1986).
      a. Conduct the exams in an unhurried manner.
      b. Explain every detail prior to action.
      c. If this is the person's first pelvic exam, explain the position and the instruments.
      d. Discuss the possibility of pregnancy and a sexually transmitted disease and treatments available.
   2. Explain the legal issues and police investigation (Heinrich, 1987).
      a. Explain the need to collect specimens for future possible court use (Kobernick, Seiffert, & Sanders, 1985).
      b. Explain that the choice to report the rape is the victim's (Lenehan, 1983).
      c. If the police interview is permitted
         • Negotiate with victim and police for an advantageous time.
         • Explain to victim what kind of questions will be asked.
         • Remain with the victim during the interview; do not ask questions or offer answers.
         • "If the officer is insensitive, intimidating, offensive in manner or asks improper questions, discuss this with the officer in private. If the behavior continues, use proper channels and make a complaint."

C. Eliminate or reduce psychologic responses when possible
   1. Promote trusting relationship (Aguilera & Messick, 1982).
      a. Stay with person during acute stage or arrange for other support (McCombie, 1980).

    b. Brief person on police and hospital procedures during acute stage.

    c. Assist person during medical examination and explain all procedures in advance.

    d. Help person to meet personal needs (bathing *after* examination and evidence has been acquired).

    e. Listen attentively to person's requests.

    f. Maintain unhurried attitude toward person and family.

    g. Avoid rescue feelings toward person.

    h. Maintain nonjudgmental attitude.

    i. Support person's beliefs and value system and avoid labeling.

    j. Initiate play therapy with a child to explain treatments and allow child to express feelings.

2. Whenever possible, provide crisis counseling within 1 hour of rape trauma event (Kilpatrick, 1983).

    a. Ask permission to contact the rape crisis counselor.

    b. Be flexible and individualize approach according to person's needs.

    c. Observe person's behavior carefully and record objective data.

    d. Encourage victim to verbalize thoughts/feelings/perceptions of the event.

    e. Discuss her/his treatment as victim; express empathy.

    f. Assess person's verbal style (expressive, controlled).

    g. Discuss with person previous coping mechanism.

    h. Explore available support system; involve significant others if appropriate.

    i. Assess stress tolerance.

    j. Reassure person about manner in which she/he reacted.

    k. Explore with person her/his strengths and resources.

    l. Convey to person confidence in her/his ability to return to prior level of functioning.

    m. Assist person in decision-making and problem-solving; involve person in own treatment plan.

    n. Help restore person's dignity by calmly exploring basis for feelings together.

    o. Reassure person that these feelings/symptoms—fear of rapist, fear of death, guilt, loss of control, shame, short attention span, anger, anxiety, phobias, depression, flashbacks, embarrassment, and eating/sleeping pattern disturbances—are often experienced by rape trauma victims.

    p. Respect victim's right; honor wishes to restrict unwanted visitors and offer privacy when appropriate.

    q. Explain to person that this experience will disrupt his/her life and feelings that occurred during acute phase may recur; encourage person to proceed at his/her own pace.

    r. Offer explanation of any papers that need to be signed.

    s. Briefly counsel family and friends at their level.

        • Share with them the immediate needs of the victim for love and support.

        • Encourage them to express their feelings and ask questions.

3. Support person's efforts to overcome feelings (Grossman & Sutherland, 1983; Hicks, 1985).

    a. Change residence and/or telephone number.

    b. Use objects that symbolize safety (nightlight).

    c. Take a trip.

    d. Turn to support system.

    e. Plan a day at a time.

    f. Avoid highly stressful situations.

g. Engage in diversional activities.

h. Use previous coping mechanisms that proved effective.

D. Fulfill medical-legal responsibilities by documentation (Heinrich, 1987)

1. History of rape (date, time, place)
2. Nature of injuries, use of force, weapons used, threats of violence or retribution, restraints used
3. Nature of assault (fondling, oral, anal, vaginal penetration, ejaculation, use of condom)
4. Post-assault activities (douching, bathing/showering, gargling, urinating, defecating, changing clothes, eating or drinking)
5. Present state (use of drugs, alcohol)
6. Medical history, tetanus immunization status, gynecologic history (last menstrual period), last voluntary intercourse
7. Emotional state, mental status
8. Examination findings, smears/cultures taken, blood tests, evidence collected, and photographs (if appropriate)
9. Document to whom, when, and what evidence is delivered

E. Proceed with follow-up until victim is in control of reactions and feelings (Pownall, 1985)

1. Before person leaves hospital, provide card with information about follow-up appointments and names and telephone numbers of local crisis and counseling centers.
2. Plan home visit or telephone call.
3. Arrange for legal or pastoral counseling, if appropriate.
4. Recommend and make referrals to psychotherapist, mental health clinic, citizen action and community group advocacy-related services.

Sexual Responses

A. Assess for sexual responses (Furniss, 1983)

1. General
   a. Fear of intercourse
   b. Parents' fear that assault will affect child's future sexual health
2. Subjective
   a. Mistrust of men
3. Objective
   a. Change in sexual behavior
   b. Lack of sexual desire (especially if victim never had intercourse before)

B. Promote helping relationship (Ledray, 1982)

1. Encourage person to express feelings openly.
2. Provide accepting atmosphere.
3. Reassure person that her/his symptoms are frequently experienced by rape trauma victims.
4. Offer feedback to person on feelings verbalized.
5. Encourage person to recognize positive responses or support from sexual partner or members of opposite sex.
6. Discuss with person possible fear of rejection by significant others.

7. Discuss potential anxiety about resuming sexual relations with partner.
8. Explore sexual concerns with patient.

C. Proceed with referrals (McGarthy, 1986)

1. Recommend couple therapy.
2. Recommend sexual counseling.

Somatic Responses

A. Assess for somatic responses (Foley & Darvies, 1983)

1. Gastrointestinal irritability
2. Genitourinary discomfort
3. Rectal discomfort
4. Skeletal muscle tension
5. Vaginal discharge
6. Bruising and edema
7. Reports of:
   - Headaches
   - Fatigue
   - Itching
   - Anorexia
   - Nausea
   - Pain
   - Burning on urination

B. Eliminate or reduce somatic symptomatology

1. Gastrointestinal irritability
   a. Anorexia
      - Offer small, frequent feedings.
      - Provide appealing foods.
      - Record intake.
      - Refer to *Altered Nutrition* if anorexia is prolonged.
   b. Nausea
      - Avoid gas-forming foods.
      - Restrict carbonated beverages.
      - Observe for abdominal distention.
      - Offer antiemetic as per physician's order.
2. Genitourinary discomfort
   a. Pain
      - Assess pain for quality and duration.
      - Monitor intake and output.
      - Inspect urine and external genitalia for bleeding.
      - Listen attentively to person's description of pain.
      - Give pain medication as per physician's order (see *Altered Comfort*).
   b. Discharge
      - Assess amount, color, and odor of discharge.
      - Allow person time to wash and change garments after initial examination has been completed.
   c. Itching
      - Encourage bathing in cool water.
      - Avoid use of detergent soaps.
      - Avoid touching area causing discomfort.

3. Skeletal muscle tension
   a. Headaches
      - Avoid any sudden change of person's position.
      - Approach person in calm manner.
      - Slightly elevate bed (unless contraindicated).
      - Discuss with person pain-reducing measures that have been effective in the past.
   b. Fatigue
      - Assess present sleeping patterns if altered (see *Sleep Pattern Disturbance*).
      - Discuss with person precipitating factors for sleep disturbance and try to eliminate these factors if possible.
      - Provide frequent rest periods throughout the day.
      - Avoid interruptions during sleep.
      - Avoid stress-producing situations.
   c. Labile emotional responses
      - Provide person with emotionally secure environment.
      - Discuss person's daily routines and adhere to them as much as possible.
      - Avoid any sudden movements and approach in calm manner.
      - Provide frequent quiet periods throughout the day.
4. Generalized bruising and edema
   a. Avoid constrictive garments.
   b. Handle affected body parts gently.
   c. Elevate affected body part if edema is present.
   d. Apply cool, moist compress to edematous area the first 24 hours, then warm compress after 24 hours.
   e. Encourage person to verbalize discomfort.
   f. Record presence and location of bruises, lacerations, edema, or abrasions.

C. Proceed with health teaching with person and family

1. Gastrointestinal irritability: Explain to person side-effects of DES (diethylstilbestrol): nausea and vomiting; vaginal spotting when discontinued
2. Genitourinary discomfort: Advise person against scratching area causing discomfort
3. Skeletal muscle tension
   a. Explain to person potential causes of discomfort.
   b. Explain to person measures that may help release tension.
   c. Teach person relaxation methods (see Appendix X).
   d. Explain to person that these symptoms are often experienced by rape trauma victims.

References/Bibliography

Aguilera, D. C., & Messick, J. M. (1982). *Crisis intervention: Theory and methodology* (4th ed.). St. Louis, C. V. Mosby.

Anderson, C. (1981–82). Males as sexual assault victims: Multiple levels of trauma. *Journal of Homosexuality, 7,* 145–159.

Brownmiller, S. (1975). *Against our will: Men, women and rape.* New York: Simon & Schuster.

Brozan, N. (1985, August 10). Rape trauma: Seeking court acceptance. *The New York Times,* p. 43.

Burgess, A. W. (1985). Rape trauma syndrome: A nursing diagnosis. *Occupational Health Nursing, 33*(8), 405–406.

Burgess, A. W., & Holmstrom, L. L. (1974). Rape trauma syndrome. *American Journal of Psychiatry, 131*(9), 981–986.

Colao, F., et al. (1983). Therapists coping with sexual assault. *Women and Therapy, 2*(2–3), 205–214.

Collins, G. (1982, January 18). Counseling male rape victims. *The New York Times,* p. 27.

Davis, L., & Brody, E. (1981). *Rape and older women: A guide to prevention and protection.* Rockville, MD: U.S. Department of Health Education and Welfare, Public Health Service, Alcohol, Drug Abuse, and Mental Health Administration, National Institute of Mental Health.

D'Epiro, P. (1986). Examining the rape victim. *Patient Care, 20*(8), 98–123.

DiVasto, P. (1985). Measuring the aftermath of rape. *Journal of Psychosocial Nursing Mental Health Services, 23*(2), 33–35.

Donaldson, S. (1985). Male rape survivors: A checklist of consequences. Unpublished manuscript.

Fielo, S. (1987). How does crime affect the elderly? *Geriatric Nursing, 8*(2), 80–83.

Foley, T., & Darvies, M. (1983). *Rape: Nursing care of victims.* St. Louis: C. V. Mosby.

Grossman, R., & Sutherland, J. (1983). *Surviving sexual assault.* New York: Congdon & Held.

Groth, N., & Burgess, A. W. (1980). Male rape: Offenders and victims. *American Journal of Psychiatry, 136*(7), 806–810.

Heinrich, L. (1987). Care of the female rape victim. *Nursing Practice, 12*(11), 9.

Hicks, C. (1985). Survivors advocate . . . Dealing with rape victims . . . The potential role of nurses. *Nursing Times, 81*(19), 26.

Hilberman, E. (1976). *The rape victim.* New York: Basic Books.

Hughes, J. D. (1987, April). Friends raping friends: Could it happen to you? Project on the status and education of women. Association of American Colleges, pp. 1–8.

Jalowic, A., & Powers, M. (1981). Stress and coping in hypertensive and emergency room patients. *Nursing Research, 30*(1), 10–15.

Kaufman, A. (1980). Male rape victims: Non-institutionalized assault. *American Journal of Medicine, 137*(2), 221–223.

Kilpatrick, D. (1983). Rape victims: Detection, assessment and treatment. *The Clinical Psychologist, 36*(4), 92–95.

Kobernick, M., Seiffert, S., & Sanders, A. (1985). Emergency department management of sexual assault victims. *Journal of Emergency Medicine, 2,* 205–214.

Ledray, L. E. (1982). Home accommodation to self-determination: Nursing role in the development of health care policy: A nursing developed model for the treatment of rape victims . . . A nursing research demonstration project. ANA Publications, American Academy of Nursing, No. 6–153:68–76.

Lenehan, G. (1983). Rape victim protocol and chart for use in the emergency department. *Journal of Emergency Nursing, 9*(2), 83–90.

Longo, R. E. (1981). Sexual assault of handicapped individuals. *Journal of Rehabilitation, 47,* 24–25.

McCombie, S. (1980). *The rape crisis intervention handbook.* New York: Plenum Press.

McGarthy, B. (1986). A cognitive-behavioral approach to understanding and treating sexual trauma. *Journal of Sex and Marital Therapy, 12*(4), 322–324.

Moore, J. (1985). Rape: The double victim. *Nursing Times, 81*(19), 24–25.

Moyniham, B., & Duncan, J. (1981). The role of the nurse in the care of sexual assault victims. *Nursing Clinics of North America, 16*(1), 95–100.

Notman, M., & Nadelson, C. (1976). The rape victim: Psychodynamic consideration. *American Journal of Psychiatry, 133,* 408–413.

The problem of rape on campus. (1978). Project on the status and education of women. Washington, D.C.: Association of American Colleges.

Russell, D. (1982). The prevalence and incidence of forcible rape and attempted rape of females. *Victimology, 7*(1–4), 81–93.

Smith, L. (1987). Sexual assault, the nurse's role. *A D Nurse, 2*(2), 24–28.

Sutherland, S., & Scherl, S. J. (1970). Patterns of response among victims of rape. *American Journal of Orthopsychiatry, 40*(3), 503–511.

U.S. Department of Justice. (1985, March). *The crime of rape.* Bureau Of Justice Statistics Bulletin, NCJ-96777.

U.S. Department of Justice. (1987). Federal Bureau of Investigation: *Uniform crime reports for the United States.* Washington, D.C.: U.S. Government Printing Office.

Wertheimer, A. (1982). Examination of the rape victim. *Postgraduate Medicine, 71*(3), 173–180.

Children and Adolescents

Benedict, M. I. (1985). Selected perinatal factors and child abuse. *American Journal of Public Health, 75*(7), 780–781.

Burgess, A. W., & Holmstrom, L. L. (1975). Sexual trauma of children and adolescents: Pressure, sex and secrecy. *Nursing Clinics of North America, 10,* 551–563.

Committee on Adolescence. (1983). Rape and the adolescent. *Pediatrics, 72*(5), 738–740.

Dodd, K. Z. (1982). Looking for empathy . . . mother of a six year old boy. *Nursing, 12*(122), 112.

Furniss, T. (1983). Mutual influence and interlocking professional-family process in the treatment of child sexual abuse and incest. *Child Abuse and Neglect, 7*(2), 207–223.

Hamilton, J. (1986). Working with adolescent girls, new findings and clinical applications. Unpublished manuscript.

Hunka, C. D. (1985). Self-help therapy in parents anonymous. *Journal of Psychosocial Nursing and Mental Health Services, 23*(7), 24–32.

Kauffman, C. K., Neill, M. K. & Thomas, J. N. (1986). The abusive parent. In Johnson, S. H. *High-risk parenting: Assessment and nursing strategies for families at risk.* Philadelphia: J. B. Lippincott.

Kelly, S. J. (1985). Drawings: Critical communications for sexually abused children. *Pediatric Nursing, 11*(6), 421–426.

Kempe, R. S., & Kempe, C. T. (1984). *The common secret: Sexual abuse of children and adolescents.* New York: H. H. Freeman.

Lahiff, M. E. (1983). Family stress. *Nursing (Oxford), 2*(20), 580–581.

Pownall, M. (1985). Health visiting: A family affair? . . . Sexual abuse of children. *Nursing Times, 81*(43), 58, 60–61.

Schmidt, A. (1981). Adolescent female rape victims: Special considerations. *Journal of Psychosocial Nursing and Mental Health Services, 19,* 17.

Whaley, L. F., & Wong, D. L. (1989). *Essentials of pediatric nursing* (3rd ed.). St. Louis: C. V. Mosby.

Powerlessness

■ *Related to* **(Specify)**

DEFINITION

Powerlessness: The state in which an individual or group perceives a lack of personal control over certain events or situations which impacts outlook, goals, and life-style.

DEFINING CHARACTERISTICS

Major (must be present)

Overt or covert (anger, apathy) expressions of dissatisfaction over inability to control a situation (*e.g.,* work, illness, prognosis, care, recovery rate) that is negatively impacting outlook, goals, and life-style

Minor (may be present)

Refuses or is reluctant to participate in decision-making

Anxiety	Acting-out behavior
Aggressive behavior	Uneasiness
Violent behavior	Resignation
Depression	

RELATED FACTORS

Pathophysiologic

Any disease process, acute or chronic, can cause or contribute to powerlessness. Some common sources are

Inability to communicate (cerebrovascular accident [CVA], Guillain-Barré, intubation)

Inability to perform activities of daily living (CVA, cervical trauma, myocardial infarction, pain)

Inability to perform role responsibilities (surgery, trauma, arthritis)

Progressive debilitating disease (multiple sclerosis, terminal cancer)

Mental illness

Substance abuse

Obesity

Disfigurement

Situational (personal, environmental)

Lack of knowledge

Personal characteristics that highly value control (*e.g.,* internal locus of control)

Hospital or institutional limitations

Some control relinquished to others	Not consulted regarding decisions
No privacy	Social displacement
Altered personal territory	Relocation

Social isolation   Insufficient finances
Lack of explanations from   Sexual harassment
    caregivers

Maturational

Adolescent: Dependence on peer group, independence from family
Young adult: Marriage, pregnancy, parenthood
Adult: Adolescent children, physical signs of aging, career pressures, divorce
Elderly: Retirement, sensory deficits, motor deficits, losses (money, significant others)

Diagnostic Considerations

Powerlessness is a feeling that all persons experience to varying degrees in various situations. Stephenson (1979) has described two types of powerlessness. *Situational powerlessness* occurs in a specific event and is probably short-lived. *Trait powerlessness* is more pervasive, affecting general outlook, goals, life-style, and relationships. The nursing diagnosis *Powerlessness* may be more clinically useful when used to describe a person experiencing trait powerlessness rather than situational powerlessness.

Hopelessness differs from powerlessness in that a hopeless person sees no solution to his problem or no way to achieve what is desired, even if he feels in control of his life. A powerless person may see an alternative or answer to the problem, yet be unable to do anything about it because of perception of control and resources. Prolonged powerlessness may lead to hopelessness.

Errors in Diagnostic Statements

Powerlessness related to hospitalization

Hospitalization evokes varied responses in persons and families, including anxiety, fear, and powerlessness. If the hospitalization is expected to be short, the diagnosis of *Anxiety related to unfamiliar environment, loss of usual routines, and invasion of privacy* may be useful to describe situational powerlessness. If the hospitalization is a readmission for a continuing problem, the use of *Powerlessness* may be more appropriate to describe trait powerlessness. The diagnosis should be restated as *Powerlessness related to readmission for pulmonary infection and effects of illness on career and marriage.*

Focus Assessment Criteria

Because powerlessness is a subjective state, all inferences made regarding a person's feelings of powerlessness must be validated. The nurse will assess each individual to determine his usual level of control and decision-making and the effects that losing elements of control have had on him.

Subjective Data

Decision-making patterns
    "How would you describe your usual method of making decisions (career, financial, health care)?"
    Make them alone
    Consult with others for advice (who?)
    Allow others to make them for me (spouse? children? others?)

Individual and role responsibilities

"What responsibilities did you have

. . . as a school child and adolescent?"

. . . at home?"

. . . at work?"

. . . in community and religious organizations?"

Perception of control

"How would you describe your ability—high, moderate, fair, or poor—to control or cure your present health problem?" (*e.g.,* diabetes mellitus, aphasia, activity intolerance, obesity)

"To what do you attribute your (high, moderate, fair, poor) ability to control?"

Preventive measures

Good nutrition	Stress management
Weight control	Exercise program

Others

Physician	Significant others
Nurses	Peer group

No control

Fate	Luck

Objective Data

Participation in grooming and hygiene care (when indicated)

Actively seeks involvement	Reluctant to participate
Requires encouragement	Refuses to participate

Information-seeking behaviors

Actively seeks information and literature from others concerning condition	Requires encouragement to ask questions
	Expresses lack of interest

Refuses to receive information

Response to limits placed on decision-making and self-control behaviors

Acceptance	Depression
Apathy	Anger
	Withdrawal

Attempts to circumvent limits

Ignores limits

Increases attempts to exercise control

Principles and Rationale for Nursing Care

Generic Considerations

1. An individual's response to loss of control depends on the meaning of the loss, individual patterns of coping, personal characteristics (psychologic, sociologic, cultural, spiritual), and the response of others.
2. Each individual, whether well or ill, has a desire for control. Feelings of powerlessness are sometimes appropriate.
3. When an individual does not expect to be able to control outcomes, attention to and retention of information is poor (Seeman, 1967).
4. Powerlessness is very closely related to but not synonymous with the concept of external versus internal locus of control.
5. A person with internal locus of control believes he can affect his outcome by actively

manipulating himself or the environment. Examples of internal behavior are participating in a regular exercise program, acquiring printed literature about a new diagnosis, or learning assertive skills.

6. A person with external locus of control believes that affecting his outcome is outside his control and attributes what happens to him to others or to fate. Examples of external behavior are losing weight because of fear of physician's response and blaming others for his present position (*e.g.*, depression, anger).

7. Internally controlled persons motivate themselves, while externally controlled persons usually need others to motivate them. Young children are usually externally controlled but can be taught to be internally controlled. For example, a child can be taught to keep a daily chart record of the nutrients needed daily and his intake of them to assist him to understand the concept of good nutrition and to encourage him to take responsibility for his eating patterns.

8. Individuals possessing internal locus of control may experience the loss of decision-making ability more profoundly than individuals possessing external locus of control.

9. Loss of or decrease in power in one area may be counterbalanced by the introduction of a new source of power or support by an increase in a present one.

10. Powerlessness is part of a continuum with hopelessness and helplessness.

11. Simmons and West (1984–85) reported that older adults with high self-efficacy and occupational status had more difficulty with uncontrollable situations than their counterparts with lower self-efficacy. Younger adults were found to cope more effectively with uncontrollable situations if high efficacy, high income, and occupational status were present.

Pediatric Considerations

1. Hospitalized children commonly experience powerlessness. The goals of nursing interventions to treat powerlessness include modifying the hospital environment to resemble the child's home and providing opportunities for acceptable control (Wong & Whaley, 1990).

2. Children can gain mastery over stressful situations by participating in play activities while ill or hospitalized (Whaley & Wong, 1989). (See Appendix IX: Guidelines for Play Therapy.)

3. It may be difficult to differentiate the diagnosis *Powerlessness* from the diagnoses *Anxiety* and *Fear*, especially in children. Refer to the Pediatric Considerations under the diagnostic categories *Anxiety* and *Fear*.

Gerontologic Considerations

1. The elderly are at high risk for powerlessness. Miller describes seven sources of power: physical strength and reserve, psychologic stamina and support network, positive self-concept, energy, knowledge, motivation, and belief system (Miller, 1983; Spielman, 1986).

2. Internal locus of control and desired amount of control correlate with health status and high morale and life satisfaction (Chang, 1978; Fuller, 1978; Ziegler & Reid, 1979).

3. Personality traits, various effects of diseases, and environmental conditions affect powerlessness. For the elderly, disease states might place restrictions on mobility. Changes in environment (*e.g.*, relocating to an extended care facility) can remove opportunities for decision-making and autonomy. Institutional policy may require physical or chemical restraints for certain agitated behaviors (Matteson & McConnell, 1988).

4. Late life changes in role, resources, and responsibility can contribute to feelings of loss of control (Richmond & Metcalf, 1986).

5. Extensive interactions with caregivers rather than peers can lead to a sense of powerlessness. This has implications for the older individual who, with an increased chance of multiple chronic illnesses, might be in the sick role for an extended period of time (Lambert & Lambert, 1981; Matteson & McConnell, 1988).

6. Older persons often demonstrate learned compliance and dependence. This might present as a perception of powerlessness earlier than in a younger person (Farkas, 1981).

7. Alienation and boredom, which are not unknown to the elderly, have a high correlation with powerlessness (Hall, 1985).

■ Powerlessness
Related to (Specify)

Assessment

See Defining Characteristics

Outcome Criteria

The person will
- Identify factors that can be controlled by him
- Make decisions regarding his care, treatment, and future when possible

---

Interventions

A. Assess for causative and contributing factors

　1. Lack of knowledge
　2. Previous inadequate coping patterns (*e.g.,* depression; for discussion, see *Ineffective Individual Coping Related to Depression*)
　3. Insufficient decision-making opportunities

B. Eliminate or reduce contributing factors if possible

　1. Lack of knowledge
　　a. Increase effective communication between person and health care provider.
　　b. Explain all procedures, rules, and options to person; avoid medical jargon.
　　c. Allow time to answer questions; ask him to write questions down so as not to forget them.
　　d. Provide children with
　　　• Opportunities to make decisions (*e.g.,* setting time for bath, holding still for injection)
　　　• Specific play therapy (see Appendix IX) before and after a traumatic situation (refer to *Altered Growth and Development* for specific interventions for age-related development needs)

e. Provide a specific time (10–15 min) each shift that person knows can be used to ask questions or discuss subjects as desired.

f. Keep person informed about schedule condition, treatments, and results.

g. Anticipate questions/interest and offer information.

h. While being realistic, point out positive changes in person's condition, such as serum enzymes decreasing after myocardial infarction or surgical incision healing well.

i. Be an active listener by allowing person to verbalize concerns and feelings; assess for areas of concern.

j. Provide consistent staffing.

k. Single out one nurse to be responsible for 24-hour plan of care, and provide opportunities for person and family to identify with this nurse.

l. Contact self-help support groups if available (*e.g.,* mastectomy, ostomy clubs, paraplegics).

2. Provide opportunities for individual to control decisions.

a. Allow person to manipulate surroundings, such as deciding what is to be kept where (shoes under bed, picture on window).

b. Keep needed items within reach (call bell, urinal, tissues).

c. Do not offer options if none exist (*e.g.,* a deep IM Z-track injection must be rotated).

d. Discuss daily plan of activities and allow person to make as many decisions as possible about it.

e. Increase decision-making opportunities as person progresses.

f. Respect and follow individual's decision if you have given him options.

g. Record person's specific choices on care plan to ensure that others on staff acknowledge preferences ("dislikes orange juice," "take showers," "plan dressing change at 7:30 prior to shower").

h. Keep promises.

i. Provide opportunity for person and family to express feelings.

j. Provide opportunities for person and family to participate in care.

k. Be alert for signs of paternalism/maternalism in health care providers (*e.g.,* making decisions for clients).

l. Plan a care conference to allow staff to discuss methods of individualizing care; encourage each nurse to share at least one action that she discovered a particular individual liked.

m. Shift emphasis from what one cannot do to what one can do.

n. Set goals that are short-term, behavioral, practical, and realistic (walk 5 more feet every day; then in 1 week, client can walk to television room).

o. Provide daily recognition of progress.

p. Praise gains/achievements.

3. Assess the person's usual response to problems (see Focus Assessment Criteria).

a. Internal control (seeks to change own behaviors or environment to control problems)

b. External control (expects others or other factors—fate, luck—to control problems)

4. Provide person with internal locus of control the needed information to alter behavior or environment.

a. Explain the problem as explicitly as the individual requests.

b. Explain the relationship of prescribed behavior and outcome (*e.g.,* need for salt restriction, the physiologic effects of exercise, the effects of bed rest on impaired cardiac function).

    5. Monitor a person with external locus of control to encourage participation.
      a. Have him keep a record for you (*e.g.,* his food intake for 1 week; weight loss chart; exercise program—type and frequency; medications taken).
      b. Use telephone contact to monitor if feasible.
      c. Provide explicit written directions to follow (*e.g.,* meal plans; exercise regimen—type, frequency, duration; speech practice lessons—for aphasia).
      d. Teach significant others methods to manipulate behaviors, if appropriate.
      e. Provide reward for each goal/step reached.
    6. Assist client in deriving power from other sources.
      a. Give permission to use other power sources to both client and significant others (*e.g.,* prayer, stress reduction techniques).
      b. Self-help groups
      c. Support groups
      d. Offer referral to religious leader.
      e. Provide privacy and support for other measures client may request (*e.g.,* meditation, imagery, special rituals).

C. Initiate health teaching and referrals as indicated (social worker, psychiatric nurse/physician, visiting nurse, religious leader, self-help groups)

References/Bibliography

Booth, R. L. (1985). Power: A negative or positive force in relationships. *Nursing Administration Quarterly, 7*(4), 10–20.

Bulechek, G. & McCloskey, J. (1985). *Nursing interventions: Treatments for nursing diagnosis.* Philadelphia: W. B. Saunders.

Burckhardt, C. (1987). Coping strategies of the chronically ill. *Nursing Clinics of North America, 22*(3), 543–550.

Carlson, C., & Blackwell, B. (1978). *Behavioral concepts and nursing interventions* (2nd ed.). Philadelphia: J. B. Lippincott.

Chang, B. (1978). Generalized expectancy, situational perception and morale among the institutionalized aged. *Nursing Research, 27*(5), 316–324.

Farkas, L. (1981). Adaptation problems with nursing home application for elderly persons: An application of the Roy adaptation nursing model. *Journal of Advanced Nursing, 6*(5), 363–368.

Feather, N. T. (1969). Attribution of responsibility and valence of success and failure in relation to initial confidence and task performance. *Journal of Personality and Social Psychology, 13,* 129–144.

Fuller, S. (1978). Inhibiting helplessness in elderly people. *Journal of Gerontological Nursing, 4,* 18–21.

Hall, C. M. Religion and aging. *Journal of Religion and Health, 24*(1), 70–78. 1985.

Hickey, T. (1979). Powerlessness. In Carnevali, D. L., & Patrick, M. (Eds.). *Nursing management for the elderly.* Philadelphia: J. B. Lippincott.

Johnson, D. E. (1967). Powerlessness: A significant determinant in patient behavior. *Journal of Nursing Education, 6*(2), 39–44.

Kleinke, C. L. (1978). *Self-perception, the psychology of personal awareness.* San Francisco: W. H. Freeman.

Kritek, P. B. (1981). Patient power and powerlessness. *Supervisor Nurse, 12*(6), 26–34.

Lamare, E. K. (1985). Communicating personal power through nonverbal behavior. *Journal of Nursing Administration, 15*(4), 38–41.

Lambert, V. A., & Lambert, C. E. (1981). Role theory and the concept of powerlessness. *Journal of Psychosocial Nursing and Mental Health Services, 19*(9), 11–14.

Lowerly, B., & DuCutte, J. (1976). Disease-related learning and disease control in diabetes as a function of locus of control. *Nursing Research, 25*(5), 358–362.

Matteson, A. M., & McConnell, E. S. (1988). *Gerontological nursing: Concepts and practice.* Philadelphia: W. B. Saunders.

Miller, J. (1983). *Powerlessness: Coping with chronic illness.* Philadelphia: F. A. Davis.

Richmond, T. S., & Metcalf, J. A. (1986). Psychosocial responses to spinal cord injury. *Journal of Neuroscience Nursing, 18*(4), 183–187.

Roberto, S. L. (1978). *Behavioral concepts and nursing throughout the life span.* Englewood Cliffs, NJ: Prentice-Hall.

Rotter, J. B. (1966). Generalized expectancy for internal vs. external control of reinforcement. *Psychology Monograph, 80*(609), 1–28.

Seeman, M. (1967). Powerlessness and knowledge: A comparative study of alienation and learning. *Sociometry, 30*(1), 105–123.

Simmons, R., & West, G. (1984–85). Life changes, coping resources and health among the elderly. *International Journal of Aging and Human Development, 20*(3), 173–189.

Smith, F. B. (1985) Patient power. *American Journal of Nursing, 85*(11), 1260–1262.

Spielman, B. J. (1986). Rethinking paradigms in geriatric ethics. *Journal of Religion and Health, 25*(2).

Stephenson, C. A. (1979). Powerlessness and chronic illness: Implications for nursing. *Baylor Nursing Educator, 1*(1), 17–28.

Whaley, L. F. & Wong, D. L. (1989). *Essentials of pediatric nursing* (3rd ed.). St. Louis: C. V. Mosby.

Wilkinson, M. B. (1979). Power and the identified patient. *Perspectives on Psychiatric Care, 17*(6), 248–253.

Wong, D. L., & Whaley, L. F. (1990). *Clinical manual of pediatric nursing* (3rd ed.). St. Louis: C. V. Mosby.

Ziegler, M., & Reid, D. (1979). Correlates of locus of desired control in two samples of elderly persons: Community residents and hospitalized elderly patients. *Journal of Consultative Clinical Psychology, 47,* 977.

Respiratory Function, High Risk for Altered*

Ineffective Airway Clearance

Ineffective Breathing Patterns

Impaired Gas Exchange

Respiratory Function, High Risk for Altered

■ *Related to* **Immobility**
■ *Related to* **Environmental Allergen**

DEFINITION

High Risk for Altered Respiratory Function (ARF): The state in which the individual is at risk of experiencing a threat to the passage of air through the respiratory tract and to the exchange of gases (O_2–CO_2) between the lungs and the vascular system.

RISK FACTORS

Risk factors that can change respiratory function (see Related Factors).

RELATED FACTORS

The codes IAC (Ineffective Airway Clearance) and IBP (Ineffective Breathing Patterns) are used to indicate factors specific to those diagnoses. Factors without a code relate to all the diagnoses.

Pathophysiologic
    Excessive or thick secretions (IAC)
        Infection (IAC)
    Neuromuscular impairment
        Diseases of the nervous system   CNS depression
           (*e.g.,* Guillain-Barré syndrome,   Cerebrovascular accident (stroke)
           multiple sclerosis, myasthenia
           gravis)
    Allergic response
    Hypertrophy or edema of upper airway structures—tonsils, adenoids, sinuses (IAC)

*This diagnosis is not currently on the NANDA list but has been included for clarity or usefulness.

Treatment-related

Medications (narcotics, sedatives, analgesics)
Anesthesia, general or spinal (IAC, IBP)
Suppressed cough reflex (IAC)
Decreased oxygen in the inspired air
Bed rest or immobility

Situational (personal, environmental)

Surgery or trauma
Pain, fear, anxiety
Fatigue
Mechanical obstruction (IAC)
Improper positioning (IAC)
Altered anatomic structure (IAC)
    Tracheostomy
Aspiration
Extreme high or low humidity (IAC)
Smoking
Mouth breathing (IAC, IBP)
Perception/cognitive impairment (IAC)
Severe nonrelieved cough (IAC, IBP)
Exercise intolerance

Maturational

Neonate: Complicated delivery, prematurity, cesarean birth, low birth weight
Infant/child: Asthma or allergies, increased emesis (potential for aspiration), croup,
    cystic fibrosis, small airway
Elderly: Decreased surfactant in the lungs, decreased elasticity of the lungs, immo-
    bility, slowing of reflexes

Diagnostic Considerations

Nursing's many responsibilities associated with problems of respiratory function include preventing problems, reducing risk factors, reducing or eliminating contributing factors to respiratory problems, monitoring respiratory status, and managing acute respiratory dysfunction.

High Risk for Altered Respiratory Function has been added to the NANDA list to describe a state in which the entire respiratory system may be affected, not just isolated areas such as airway clearance or gas exchange. Allergy and immobility are examples of factors that affect the entire system and thus make it incorrect to say *Impaired Gas Exchange Related to Immobility,* since immobility also affects airway clearance and breathing patterns. The diagnoses *Ineffective Airway Clearance* and *Ineffective Breathing Patterns* can be used when the nurse can definitely alter the contributing factors that are influencing respiratory function, such as ineffective cough, immobility, or stress.

The nurse is cautioned not to use this diagnosis to describe acute respiratory disorders, which are the primary responsibility of medicine and nursing together (*i.e.,* collaborative problems). Such problems can be labeled *Potential Complication: Acute hypoxia* or *Potential Complication: Pulmonary edema.* When an individual's immobility is prolonged and threatens multiple systems, integumentary, musculoskeletal, vascular, as well as respiratory, the nurse should use *High Risk for Disuse Syndrome* to describe the entire situation.

Errors In Diagnostic Statements

Ineffective Breathing Patterns related to respiratory compensation for metabolic acidosis

This diagnosis represents the respiratory pattern associated with diabetic ketoacidosis. Nursing responsibilities for this situation include monitoring, early detection of changes, and rapid initiation of nursing and medical interventions. This situation does not represent a situation for which nurses diagnose and are accountable to prescribe treatment for. Rather, the collaborative problem *Potential Complication: Ketoacidosis* would represent the nursing accountability for the situation, not *Ineffective Breathing Patterns.*

Ineffective Airway Clearance related to mucosal edema and loss of ciliary action secondary to thermal injury

After sustaining burns of the upper airway, a person is at risk for pulmonary edema and respiratory distress. This potentially life-threatening situation requires both nurse- and physician-prescribed interventions. The collaborative problem *Potential Complication: Respiratory related to thermal injury* would alert nurses that close monitoring for respiratory complications, and management if they occur, are indicated.

Ineffective Airway Clearance related to decreased cough and gag reflexes secondary to anesthesia

The nursing focus for this client is on preventing aspiration through proper positioning and good oral hygiene, not on teaching effective coughing. Thus, the diagnosis should be restated as *High Risk for Aspiration related to decreased cough and gag reflexes secondary to anesthesia.*

Focus Assessment Criteria

Subjective Data

1. History of symptoms (*e.g.,* pain, dyspnea, cough)
     Onset? Precipitated by what?
     Description? Relieved by what?
     Effects on other body functions
          Gastrointestinal (nausea, vomiting, anorexia, constipation)?
          Genitourinary (impotence, kidney function)?
          Circulatory (angina, tachycardia/bradycardia, fluid retention)?
          Neurosensory (thought processes, headache)?
          Musculoskeletal (muscle fatigue, atrophy, use of accessory muscles?)
     Effects on life-style
          Occupation   Social/sexual functions
          Role functions   Financial status
2. Presence of contributing or causative factors
     Smoking ("pack years": number of packs per day times number of smoking years)
     Allergy (medication, food, environmental factors—dust, pollen, other)
     Trauma, blunt or overt (chest, abdomen, upper airway, head)
     Surgery/pain
          Healing incision of chest/neck/head/abdomen
          Recent intubation

Environmental factors
Toxic fumes (cleaning agents, smoke)
Extreme heat or cold
Daily inspired air, work and home (humid, dry, level of pollution, level of pollens)
Infection
3. Current drug therapy
What? How often? When was last dose taken?
Effect on symptoms?
4. Medical/surgical history
Cardiac disease
Pulmonary disease
5. For infants only, history of:
Immaturity? Low birth weight?
Cesarean birth? Complicated delivery?
Family history of sudden infant death syndrome (SIDS)?

Objective Data
Respiratory
1. Airway
Type
Spontaneous nasal
Spontaneous mouth breather
Oral airway
Nasal airway
Nasal endotracheal tube
Oral endotracheal tube
Tracheostomy
Condition
Clear
Nasal flaring
Loose secretions present
Bleeding (specify where, how much)
Thick secretions/encrustations present
Swelling (specify where)
Mechanical obstruction (packing/NG tube) present
2. Description
Spontaneous
Controlled mechanical ventilation (CMV)
Spontaneous intermittant mechanical ventilations (SIMV)
Rate (per minute)

Slowed	Increased

Rhythm

Regular	Smooth
Irregular	Uneven

Depth

Decreased	Symmetric
Increased	Variable
Asymmetric	Even

Type

Regular	Hyperpnea
Tachypnea	Splinted/guarded

      Bradypnea   Kussmaul

      Apnea   Cheyne-Stokes

3. Cough

    Raspy   Productive

    Barking   Dry

    Painful   None

                        Absent cough reflex

4. Sputum

Color	Character	Amount	Odor
Clear	Frothy	Small	None
Yellow	Watery	Moderate	Foul
White	Tenacious	Copious	Yeastlike
Greenish	Hemoptysic		
Reddish	(bloody)		
(bloody)			
Brown specks			

5. Breath sounds (detected by auscultation: compare right upper and lower lobes to left upper and lower lobes; listen to all four quadrants of the chest)

    Diminished   Rales (crackles)

    Absent   Rhonchi (wheezes)

    Abnormal   Rubs (squeaks)

Circulatory

Pulse

Rate	Rhythm	Quality	Baseline

Blood pressure

Usual	Present	Pulse pressure	Baseline

Skin color

    Within normal limits   Ruddy

    Pale   Cyanotic (central/peripheral)

    Ashen

Diagnostic studies

Chest x-ray

Arterial blood gas analysis

Oxygen saturation

Principles and Rationale for Nursing Care

Generic Considerations

1. Ventilation requires synchronous movement of the walls of the chest and abdomen. (Coordination and conscious control of breathing are key elements in teaching a person to breathe efficiently.) With *inspiration* the diaphragm moves downward, the intercostal muscles contract, the chest wall lifts up and out, the pressure inside the thorax lowers, and air is drawn in. *Expiration* occurs as air is forced out of the lungs by the elastic recoil of the lungs and the relaxation of the chest and diaphragm. Expiration is diminished in the elderly and with chronic pulmonary disease.

2. There are two phases of respiration. *External respiration* occurs in the lungs at the alveolar level (outside air to bloodstream). *Internal respiration* occurs between the systemic capillaries and the interstitial fluid (bloodstream to tissues; optimum perfusion needed).

3. A cough ("the guardian of the lungs") is accomplished by closure of the glottis and the explosive expulsion of air from the lungs by the work of the abdominal and chest muscles.

4. Lying flat causes the abdominal organs to shift toward the chest, thus crowding the lungs and making it more difficult to breathe.

5. Breath-holding can result in a "Valsalva" maneuver: a marked increase in intra-thoracic and intra-abdominal pressure, with profound circulatory changes (decreased heart rate, cardiac output, and blood pressure).

6. Hyperventilation (blowing off of CO_2) causes an acid-base imbalance and may result in temporary loss of consciousness (fainting).

7. The terms tachypnea, hyperpnea, hyperventilation, bradypnea, and hypoventilation are frequently confused. For our purposes, these terms will be defined as follows:

   Tachypnea: rapid, shallow respiratory rate

   Hyperpnea: rapid respiratory rate with increased depth

   Hyperventilation: increased rate or depth or respirations causing an alveolar ventilation that is above the body's normal metabolic requirements

   Bradypnea: slow respiratory rate

   Hypoventilation: decreased rate or depth of respiration, causing a minute alveolar ventilation that is less than the body's requirements

8. An insufficient supply of oxygen reaching the tissue is called *hypoxia.* The effects of hypoxia upon vital signs are:

Vital Sign	Early Hypoxia	Late Hypoxia
Blood pressures	Rising systolic/falling diastolics	Falling
Pulse	Rising, bounding, arrhythmic	Falling, shallow, arrhythmic

Vital Sign	Early Hypoxia	Late Hypoxia
Pulse pressure	Widening	Widened/narrowed
Respirations	Rapid	Slowed/rapid

9. The clinical manifestations of hypoxia are:

Early Hypoxia	Late Hypoxia
Irritability	Seizures
Headache	Coma or brain tissue swelling
Confusion	Decreased cardiac output
Agitation	Oliguria or anuria
Pain	
Oliguria	

10. Hypoxia contributes to coma and shock. Oxygen demand is greater during febrile illness, exercise, pain, and physical and emotional stress.

11. Oxygen should be administered carefully (< 3/min) to people with a history of chronic CO_2 retention, for their drive to breathe is hypoxia.

12. Oxygenation depends on the ability of the lungs to deliver oxygen to the blood and on the ability of the heart to pump enough blood to deliver the oxygen to the microcirculation of the cells.

13. Renfroe (1988) suggests that the use of progressive muscle relaxation (PMR) to control breathing produces immediate reduction in dyspnea and anxiety in patients with chronic obstructive pulmonary disease (COPD).

Pediatric Considerations

1. The characteristics of normal respiration in the newborn differ from those of older infants and children.
   a. Respirations are irregular and abdominal; to be accurate, count respirations for 1 full minute (Whaley & Wong, 1989).
   b. The rate is between 30 and 50 breaths/min (Whaley & Wong, 1989).
   c. Periods of apnea, less than 15 seconds, may occur (Whaley & Wong, 1989).
   d. Obligate nasal breathing occurs through the first 3 weeks of life (Hunsberger, 1989).
2. Characteristics of the respiratory system of the infant and young child include:
   a. Abdominal breathing continues until the child is about age 5 (Hunsberger, 1989).
   b. Retractions are more often observed with respiratory illness because of increased chest wall compliance. Children may quickly develop respiratory insufficiency (Hunsberger, 1989).
   c. Smaller airway diameter increases the risk of obstruction (Hunsberger, 1989).
   d. Infants and small children swallow sputum when it is produced (Whaley & Wong, 1989).
3. Janson-Bjerklie (1987) found that younger asthmatic patients appear to experience more intense dyspnea than older persons at a given level of airway obstruction.
4. Huckabay and Daderian (1989) noted that pediatric patients who were given a choice in the selection of color of water in blow bottles performed significantly more breathing exercises than those who were not given a choice.

Gerontologic Considerations

1. The age-related changes in the respiratory system have little effect on function in healthy adults unless they interact with risk factors such as smoking, immobility, or compromised immune system (Miller, 1990).
2. The following age-related changes in the respiratory system typically occur (Staab & Lyles, 1990; Miller, 1990).
   a. No change in total volume
   b. 50% increase in residual volume
   c. Compromised gas exchange in lower lung regions
   d. Reduced compliance of bony thorax
   e. Decreased strength of respiratory muscles and diaphragm
3. Age-related kyphosis and diminished immune response compromises respiratory function and increases the risk of pneumonia and other respiratory infections.
4. Adults age 65 and older have a yearly death rate from pneumonia or influenza of 9/100,000. When smoking, exposure to air pollutants, or occupational exposure to toxic substances is present, the rate increases to 217/100,000. If two or more risk factors are present, the rate rises to 979/100,000 (Schneider, 1978).

■ High Risk for Altered Respiratory Function
Related to Immobility

Assessment

Subjective Data
> Report of pain or discomfort with movement
> Report of being too tired to move, not wanting to move

Objective Data
> Inability to turn self
> Inability to ambulate
> Presence of respiratory rales and diminished respiratory depth

---

Outcome Criteria

The person will
- Perform hourly deep breathing exercises (sigh) and cough sessions as needed
- Demonstrate satisfactory pulmonary function (adequate tidal volume, vital capacity, forced end-expiratory volume [FEV])
- Relate importance of daily pulmonary exercises

Interventions

A. Assess causative factors
  1. Pain, lethargy
  2. Medical order of bed rest
  3. Neuromuscular impairment
  4. Lack of motivation (to ambulate; to cough and deep-breathe)
  5. Decreased level of consciousness
  6. Lack of knowledge

B. Eliminate or reduce causative factors if possible
  1. Assess for optimal pain relief with minimal period of fatigue or respiratory depression.
  2. Encourage ambulation as soon as consistent with medical plan of care.
     a. If unable to walk, establish a regime for being out of bed in a chair several times a day (*i.e.*, 1 hr after meals and 1 hr before bedtime).
     b. Increase activity gradually, explaining that respiratory function will improve and dyspnea will decrease with practice.
  3. For neuromuscular impairment
     a. Vary the position of the bed, thus gradually changing the horizontal and vertical position of the thorax, unless contraindicated.
     b. Assist to reposition, turning frequently from side to side (hourly if possible).
     c. Encourage deep breathing and controlled coughing exercises five times every hour.

  d. Teach individual to use blow bottle or incentive spirometer every hour while awake (with severe neuromuscular impairment, the person may have to be awakened during the night as well).
  e. For child, use colored water in blow bottle; have him blow up balloons.
  f. Auscultate lung field every 8 hours; increase frequency if altered breath sounds are present.
4. For the person with a decreased level of consciousness
  a. Position from *side to side* with set schedule (*e.g,* left side even hours, right side odd hours); do not leave person lying flat on back.
  b. Position on right side after feedings (nasogastric tube feeding, gastrostomy) to prevent regurgitation and aspiration.
  c. Keep head of bed elevated 30° unless contraindicated.

C. Prevent the complications of immobility

See specific diagnoses for interventions to prevent or treat the complications of immobility:

High Risk for Disuse Syndrome
Sensory–Perceptual Alterations
Activity Intolerance
Diversional Activity Deficit

■ High Risk for Altered Respiratory Function
Related to Environmental Allergens

Assessment

Subjective Data

The person states
"I'm allergic to . . . "
" . . . gives me a rash"
"I can't eat . . . "
"I have trouble breathing."
"I feel short of breath."
"I feel itchy."
"Something bit (stung) me."
"I have asthma."
History of ingestion of new food or drugs
Frequent ear infections

Objective Data

Hoarseness, wheezing/dyspnea
Coughing and sneezing, watery eyes and nose
Hives/rashes
Presence of stinger (bee)
Erythema
Edema

Outcome Criteria

The person will
- State causative allergens (if known) and describe methods of avoiding allergens
- Relate the emotional aspects of the allergic response
- Demonstrate and report decreased episodes of wheezing
- State the need to seek immediate medical attention for severe allergic response and demonstrate the use of hypodermic injection (for administration of epinephrine) if applicable

---

Interventions

A. Assess causative factors
1. Chronic allergy (known allergens such as molds, dust, pollen, food, others)
2. Stinging insect
3. Nonspecific (unknown) allergen

B. Provide the following health teaching
1. For chronic allergy to molds
   a. Avoid barns, cut grass, leaves, weeds, decaying or rotting vegetation, firewood, house plants, damp basements, attics, and crawl spaces.
   b. Avoid eating marinated or aged foods (bread, flour, cheese, fruits, vegetables).
   c. Maintain household walls clean and dry.
      - Be sure that there is adequate house drainage to keep walls dry.
      - Check walls for black or grayish blue mold spots.
      - Wash walls with chlorine bleach solution to remove mold.
   d. Maintain a dust-free environment, especially in the bedroom.*
      - Empty room to the bare walls, including closets (store contents elsewhere if possible).
      - Scrub woodwork and floors.
      - Thereafter, dust and vacuum well daily and clean thoroughly once a week.
      - Keep bedroom furniture to a minimum (preferably wood, rather than stuffed furniture).
      - Choose waxed, hardwood floors (no carpets).
      - Use pull shades rather than venetian blinds at windows; do not use curtains or draperies.
      - Use closet to a minimum; keep it as dust free as the bedroom, and keep the door closed.
      - Use bedroom for sleeping only; if it is a child's bedroom, encourage play elsewhere.
      - Do not use stuffed toys.
      - Keep animals of fur or feathers out of the area.
      - Do not use fuzzy blankets or feather comforters; cotton bedspreads are preferred.
      - Launder bed linens frequently.

---

* It is difficult to keep one's home and work environment dust free, but special efforts can readily be made to keep the area where one sleeps free of dust.

     e. Keep dust down throughout the entire house.
- Use steam or hot-water heat if available.
- Maintain a clean filter in furnace; use air conditioning if possible.
- Cover hot-air furnace outlets with cheesecloth or have a filter installed; change filter frequently.
- Avoid any room while it is being cleaned and do not handle any objects that may be dust collectors (such as books).
- Wear a mask while cleaning.

2. For chronic allergy to pollen
   a. Reduce exposure as much as possible to trees (April–May), grass (May–July), weeds (mid-May to first frost).
   b. Use air conditioning with electrostatic filters.
   c. Stay inside on windy days, avoiding drafts and cross-ventilation.
   d. Use air conditioning in cars and avoid extended rides.
   e. Wear a dampened mask while cutting lawn.
   f. Avoid strong odors (scents and perfumes).
   g. Do not drink ice-cold beverages or food (can cause spasms).
   h. Avoid granaries, barns, decaying materials, cut grass, weeds, dry leaves, firewood.
   i. Try to arrange vacations during high pollen season in a low-pollen area such as the eastern seashore.
   j. Be sure over-the-counter drugs such as antihistamines are approved by physician, for some may give the opposite intended effect.

3. To avoid stinging insects (bees, wasps, yellow jackets, hornets)
   a. Do not wear brightly colored clothing (choose lighter colors such as white, light green, khaki).
   b. Keep hair short or tied back; avoid hair sprays, perfumes, and flappy clothing.
   c. Wear shoes and socks.
   d. Avoid riding horses or bicycles in areas where bees or wasps are plentiful (*e.g.,* fields of clover, flowers).
   e. Avoid mowing lawns, trimming hedges, or pruning trees during the insect season.
   f. Carry an insect spray in the glove compartment of the car and keep one handy at home (attempts to swat or kill bees must be well planned, for a missed blow may infuriate the insect and make it more dangerous).
   g. If approached by a bee or wasp in the open, stay still or move back very slowly.
   h. Each spring, have home and garden searched for new hornets' or bees' nests and obtain professional assistance from an exterminator or fire department in eliminating them.

4. For a severe allergic reaction where hives or any respiratory symptoms appear, or *if one has had a previous severe reaction to any kind of sting,* carry out the following procedure
   a. Remove stinger if possible.
   b. Keep as quiet as possible (avoid panic).
   c. Apply ice immediately.
   d. Use emergency bee-sting kit injection if available.
   e. Call emergency medical services.

5. General instructions for unknown or nonspecific allergies
   a. Assess for introduction of new food or medication.
   b. Eliminate
- Fish and fish oils (cod-liver oil products)
- All kinds of nuts

- All fresh fruits and fresh vegetables (this elimination does not apply to cooked fruits and vegetables)
- Chocolate
- Eggs and food containing eggs
- Milk and foods containing milk
- Wheat and foods containing wheat

Ineffective Airway Clearance

■ *Related to* **(Specify)**

DEFINITION

Ineffective Airway Clearance: The state in which the individual experiences a threat to respiratory status related to inability to cough effectively.

DEFINING CHARACTERISTICS

Major (must be present)
Ineffective cough or
Inability to remove airway secretions

Minor (may be present)
Abnormal breath sounds
Abnormal respiratory rate, rhythm, depth
Absent cough reflex
Pain with coughing

RELATED FACTORS
See *High Risk for Altered Respiratory Function*

Principles and Rationale for Nursing Care
See *High Risk for Altered Respiratory Function*

■ Ineffective Airway Clearance
Related to (Specify)

Outcome Criteria

The person will
- Not experience aspiration
- Demonstrate effective coughing and increased air exchange in his lungs

---

Interventions

The nursing interventions for the diagnosis *Ineffective Airway Clearance* represent interventions for any individual with this nursing diagnosis, regardless of the related factors.

A. Assess for causative or contributing factors

1. Inability to maintain proper position
2. Ineffective cough
3. Pain or fear of pain
4. Viscous secretions (dehydration)
5. Fatigue, weakness, drowsiness
6. Lack of knowledge (of how to cough, and why it is important)
7. Chronic, nonrelieved cough

B. Reduce or eliminate factors if possible

1. Inability to maintain proper position
   a. Refer to *High Risk for Aspiration*
2. Ineffective cough
   a. Instruct person on the proper method of controlled coughing
      - Breathe deeply and slowly while sitting up as high as possible
      - Use diaphragmatic breathing
      - Hold the breath for 3 to 5 seconds and then slowly exhale as much of this breath as possible through the mouth (lower rib cage and abdomen should sink down)
      - Take a second breath, hold, and cough forcefully from the chest (not from the back of the mouth or throat), using two short forceful coughs
3. Pain or fear of pain
   a. Assess present analgesic regime.
      - Administer pain medications as needed.
      - Assess its effectiveness: Is the individual too lethargic? Is the individual still in pain?
      - Note time when person appears to have best pain relief with optimal level of alertness and physical performance: *This is the time for active breathing and coughing exercises.*
   b. Provide emotional support.
      - Stay with person for the entire coughing session.
      - Explain the importance of coughing after pain relief.

- Reassure person that suture lines are secure and that splinting by hand or pillow will minimize pain of movement.
  c. Use appropriate comfort measures for site of pain.
- Splint abdominal or chest incisions with hand, pillow, or both.
  d. For sore throat
- Assess for adequate humidity in the inspired air.
- Consider warm saline gargle every 2 to 4 hours.
- Consider use of anesthetic lozenge or gargle, especially before coughing sessions.*
- Examine throat for exudate, redness, and swelling and note if it is associated with fever.
- Explain that a sore throat is common after anesthesia and should be a short-term problem.
  e. Maintain good body alignment to prevent muscular pain and strain.
- Acquire and use extra pillows on both sides of person, especially the affected side, for support.
- Position person to prevent slouching and cramping positions of the thorax and abdomen; reassess positioning frequently.
  f. Assess person's understanding of the use of analgesia to enhance breathing and coughing effort.
- Teach person during periods of optimal level of consciousness.
- Continually reinforce rationale for plan of nursing care. ("I will be back to help you cough when the pain medicine is working and you can be most effective.")
4. Viscous (thick) secretions
   a. Maintain adequate hydration (increase fluid intake to 2–3 q a day if not contraindicated by decreased cardiac output or renal disease).
   b. Maintain adequate humidity of inspired air.
5. Fatigue, weakness, drowsiness
   a. Plan and bargain for rest periods. ("Work to cough well now; then I can let you rest.").
   b. Vigorously coach and encourage coughing, using positive reinforcement. ("You worked hard; I know it's not easy, but it is important.").
   c. Be sure coughing session occurs at peak comfort period after analgesics, but not peak level of sleepiness.
   d. Allow for rest after coughing and before meals.
   e. For lethargy or decreased level of consciousness, stimulate person to breathe. ("Take a deep breath.")
6. Lack of understanding or motivation (of how and why to cough)
   a. Assess knowledge of reasons and method for coughing.
   b. Proceed with health teaching with constant reinforcement in principles of care.
   c. Acknowledge and encourage good individual effort and progress.
7. For chronic, nonrelieved coughing
   a. Minimize irritants in the inspired air (*e.g.,* dust, allergens).
   b. Provide periods of uninterrupted rest.
   c. Administer Rx—cough suppressant, expectorant—as ordered by physician (withhold food and drink immediately after administration of medications for best results).

* May require a physician's order.

d. Relieve mucous membrane irritation through humidity (inhaling steam from shower, or sitting over pot of steaming water with a towel over the head, will loosen thick secretions and soothe the membranes).

C. Initiate health teaching and referrals as indicated
1. Instruct parents on the need for child to cough, even if painful.
2. Allow adult and older child to listen to lungs; describe if clear or if rales are present.
3. Consult with respiratory therapist for assistance, if needed.

Ineffective Breathing Patterns

■ *Related to* **(Specify) as Manifested by Hyperventilation Episodes**

DEFINITION
Ineffective breathing patterns: The state in which the individual experiences an actual or potential loss of adequate ventilation related to an altered breathing pattern

RELATED FACTORS
See *High Risk for Altered Respiratory Function*

DEFINING CHARACTERISTICS

Major (must be present)
Changes in respiratory rate or pattern (from baseline)
Changes in pulse (rate, rhythm, quality)

Minor (must be present)
Orthopnea
Tachypnea, hyperpnea, hyperventilation
Arrhythmic respirations
Splinted/guarded respirations

Principles and Rationale for Nursing Care
See *High Risk for Altered Respiratory Function*

■ Ineffective Breathing Patterns
Related to (Specify) as Manifested by Hyperventilation Episodes

Hyperpnea or hyperventilation is rapid breathing pattern that results in lowered arterial pCO_2.

Assessment

Subjective Data

The person states
"I can't catch my breath."
"My fingers tingle and my heart beats fast."
"I feel dizzy (faint)."
History of existing emotional or physical stress
Fear of anxiety

Objective Data

Tachypnea (forceful)   Rising blood pressure
Tachycardia   Anxious facial expression
Bounding pulse

Outcome Criteria

The person will
- Demonstrate an effective respiratory rate and experience improved gas exchange in the lungs
- Relate the causative factors, if known, and relate adaptive ways of coping with them

---

Interventions

A. Assess causative factors
1. Fear
2. Pain
3. Exercise/activity

B. Remove or reduce causative factors
1. Fear
   a. Remove cause of fear, if possible.
   b. Reassure that measures are being taken to ensure safety.
   c. Distract person from thinking about his anxious state by having him maintain eye contact with you (or perhaps with someone else he trusts); say, "Now look at me and breathe slowly with me like this."

     d. Consider use of paper bag as means of rebreathing expired air (expired CO_2 will be reinspired, thereby slowing respiratory rate).

     e. See *Fear*.

  2. Pain

     a. Determine location of discomfort.

     b. Use appropriate comfort measures (see *Altered Comfort*).

     c. Encourage displacement of pain perception through concentration on more efficient breathing (*e.g.*, concentrating completely on air going in and out of lungs, giving plentiful oxygen to the body).

     d. Stay with person and coach in taking slower, more effective breaths.

  3. Exercise/activity

     a. Encourage slow deep breaths, pausing when ambulating for the first time after immobility or surgery.

     b. Encourage conscious control of breathing during exercise (slower, deeper, abdominal breathing).

     c. See *Activity Intolerance* for additional interventions.

C. Proceed with health teaching

  1. Explain that one can learn to overcome hyperventilation through conscious control of breathing even when the cause is unknown.

  2. Discuss possible causes, physical and emotional, and methods of coping effectively (see *Anxiety*).

Impaired Gas Exchange

DEFINITION

Impaired Gas Exchange: The state in which the individual experiences an actual or potential decreased passage of gases (oxygen and carbon dioxide) between the alveoli of the lungs and the vascular system.

DEFINING CHARACTERISTICS

Major (must be present)

Dyspnea on exertion

Minor (may be present)

Tendency to assume three-point position (sitting, one hand on each knee, bending forward)

Pursed-lip breathing with prolonged expiratory phase

Increased anteroposterior chest diameter, if chronic

Lethargy and fatigue

Increased pulmonary vascular resistance (increased pulmonary artery/right ventricular pressure)

Decreased gastric motility, prolonged gastric emptying

Decreased oxygen content, decreased oxygen saturation, increased pCO_2, as measured by blood gas analysis

Cyanosis

Diagnostic Considerations

Impaired Gas Exchange is used clinically to describe persons with acute respiratory insufficiency. However, *Impaired Gas Exchange* does not represent a situation for which nurses prescribe definitive treatments. Nursing responsibilities in acute respiratory distress include managing physiologic changes through early detection and initiation of nurse- and physician-prescribed interventions, thus this situation is best described as the collaborative problem *Potential Complication: Respiratory Insufficiency.* The nurse also can treat the functional health patterns that decrease oxygenation and possibly affect sleep, activity, and psychologic comfort, *e.g., Anxiety related to episodes of breathlessness and fear of outcome.*

The nursing responsibilities for a person with chronic respiratory insufficiency (such as COPD) also would include the collaborative problem *Potential Complication: Respiratory insufficiency.* In addition, certain nursing diagnoses also may apply, such as *Activity Intolerance related to lack of knowledge of adaptive techniques required secondary to respiratory insufficiency.*

References/Bibliography

Books and Articles

Acosta, F. (1988). Biofeedback and progressive relaxation in wearning the anxious patient from the ventilator: A brief report. *Heart and Lung, 17*(3), 300–301.

Bates, B. (1991). *A guide to physical examination* (5th ed.). Philadelphia: J. B. Lippincott.

Burton, G., Hodgkin J. & Ward, J. (1991). *Respiratory care: A guide to clinical* practice (3rd ed.). Philadelphia: J. B. Lippincott.

Carroll, P. (1990). Safe suctioning. *Nursing, 19*(9), 48–51.

D'Agostino, J. Teaching tips for living with COPD at home. *Nursing, 14*(2), 12–57.

Erhardt, B., & Graham, M. (1990). Pulse oxymetry, an easy way to check O_2 saturation. *Nursing, 20*(3), 50–54.

Gift, A. (1989). Clinical measurement of dyspnea. *DCCN, 8*(4) 42–45.

Harimon, A. (1980). Anaphylaxis can mean sudden death. *Nursing, 10*(10), 40–43.

Harper, R. W. (1981). *A guide to respiratory care.* Philadelphia: J. B. Lippincott.

Huckabay, L., & Daderian, A. (1989). Effect of choices on breathing exercises post open heart surgery. *DCCN, 9*(4), 190–201.

Hoffman, L., Mazzocco, M., & Roth, J. (1987). Fine tuning your chest PT. *American Journal of Nursing, 87*(12), 1566–1572.

Hunsberger, M. (1989). Nursing strategies: Altered respiratory function. In Foster, R. L., Hunsberger, M. M., & Anderson, J. J. T. (Eds.). *Family-centered nursing care of children.* Philadelphia: W. B. Saunders, pp. 1166–1167.

Janson-Bjerklie, S., Ruma, S., Stulbarg, M., & Carrieri, V. (1987). Predictors of dyspnea intensity in asthma. *Nursing Research, 36*(3), 179–183.

Jecklin, J. (1979). Positioning, percussion and vibrating patients for effective bronchial drainage. *Nursing, 9*(3), 64–70.

Kaufman, J., & Woody, J. (1981). C.O.P.D.—better living through teaching. *Nursing, 10*(3), 57–61.

Largerson, J. (1982). The cough: Its effectiveness depends on you. *Respiratory Care, 27*(4), 418–434.

Larter, N. (1981). Cystic fibrosis. *American Journal of Nursing, 81*(3), 527–532.

McCaully, E. (1979). Breathing exercises as play for asthmatic children. *Maternal-Child Nursing Journal, 5*(5), 340–345.

McCreary, C., & Watson, J. (1981). Pickwickian syndrome. *American Journal of Nursing, 81*(3), 555.

McMahon, A., & Mailbusch, R. (1988). How to send quit smoking signals. *American Journal of Nursing, 88*(11), 1498–1499.

Miller, C. A. (1990). *Nursing care of older adults.* Glenview, IL: Scott, Foresman.

Pinney, M. (1981). Foreign body aspiration. *American Journal of Nursing, 81*(3), 521–522.

Porth, C. (1990). *Pathophysiology* (3rd ed.). Philadelphia: J. B. Lippincott.

Renfroe, K. (1988). Effect of progressive relaxation on dyspnea and state anxiety in patients with chronic obstructive pulmonary disease. *Heart and Lung, 17*(4), 408–413.

Rice, V. (1980) Clinical hypoxia. *Critical Care Nurse, 1*(6), 21–29.

Richard, E., & Shephard, A. (1981). Giving up smoking: A lesson in loss theory. *American Journal of Nursing, 81*(4), 755–757.

Rifas, E. (1980). How you and your patient can manage dyspnea. *Nursing, 10*(6), 34–41.

Schneider, E. L. (1978). Infectious diseases in the elderly. *Annals of Internal Medicine, 98*(4), 395–400.

Simkins, R. (1981). Asthma: Reactive airway disease. *American Journal of Nursing, 81*(3), 523–526.

Simkins, R. (1981). Croup and epiglottitis. *American Journal of Nursing, 81*(3), 519–520.

Sjoberg, E. (1983). Nursing diagnosis and the COPD patient. *American Journal of Nursing, 83*(2), 244–248.

Staab, A., & Lyles, M. (1990). *Manual of geriatric nursing.* Glenview, IL: Scott, Foresman.

Taylor, C., Lillis, C., & LeMone, P. (1989). *Fundamentals of nursing: The art and science of nursing care.* Philadelphia: J. B. Lippincott.

Taylor, D. (1985). Clinical applications. Assessing breath sounds. *Nursing, 3,* 60–63.

Webber, J. (1988). *Nurses' handbook of health assessment.* Philadelphia: J. B. Lippincott.

Westra, B. (1984). Assessment under pressure: When your patient says "I can't breathe." *Nursing, 14*(5), 34–39.

Whaley, L. F., & Wong, D. L. (1989). *Essentials of pediatric nursing* (3rd ed.). St. Louis: C. V. Mosby, pp. 194, 656.

Resources for the Consumer

Organizations

American Cancer Society, 777 3rd Avenue, New York, NY 10017

American Heart Association, 7320 Greenville Avenue, Dallas, TX 75231

American Lung Association, 1740 Broadway, New York, NY 10019

Cystic Fibrosis Foundation, 3091 Mayfield Road, Cleveland, OH 44118

SIDS Clearing House, Suite 600, 1555 Wilson Boulevard, Rosslyn, VA 22209

Literature

Tuby, J., & Bither, S. (1977). *Breathing easy: Living with emphysema and chronic bronchitis. A manual for patients with chronic obstructive disease.* Portland: Oregon Lung Association, 1977. Write for a copy: 830 Medical Arts Building, 1020 Southwest Taylor Street, Portland, OR 97205

Sources of Information on Allergy Control

Dickey Enterprise (environmentalists), 635 Gregory Road, Fort Collins, CO 80524; (303) 482–6001

Meridian, Bio-Medical (for pollen guide), 3278 Wadsworth Boulevard South, Denver, CO 80227; (303) 986–5555

Hollister-Stier Laboratories, Division of Cutter Laboratories, Inc., Box 3145, Terminal Annex, Spokane, WA 99220

Role Performance, Altered

DEFINITION

Altered Role Performance: The state in which an individual experiences or is at risk for experiencing a disruption in the way one perceives one's role performance.

DEFINING CHARACTERISTICS

Major (must be present)

Conflict related to role perception or performance

Minor (may be present)

Change in self-perception of role
Denial of role
Change in others' perception of role
Change in physical capacity to resume role
Lack of knowledge of role
Change in usual patterns of responsibility

Diagnostic Considerations

The nursing diagnosis *Altered Role Performance* has a defining characteristic of conflict related to role perception or performance. All individuals have multiple roles. Some of these roles are prescribed, such as gender and age; some acquired, such as parent and occupation; and some transitional, such as elected office or team member.

Various factors affect a person's roles, including developmental stage, societal norms, cultural beliefs, values, life events, illness, and disabilities. When a person has difficulty with role performance, it may be more useful to describe the impact of the difficulty on functioning rather than to describe the problem as *Altered Role Performance*. For example, a person who has experienced a cerebrovascular accident (CVA) may undergo a change from being the primary breadwinner to becoming unemployed. In this situation, the nursing diagnosis *Grieving related to loss of role as financial provider secondary to effects of CVA* would be appropriate. Take another example: If a woman became unable to continue her household responsibilities due to illness and these responsibilities were assumed by the other family members, the situations that may arise would better be described as *High Risk for Self-Concept Disturbance related to recent loss of role responsibility secondary to illness* and *High Risk for Impaired Home Maintenance Management related to lack of knowledge of family members*.

A conflict in a family regarding others meeting role obligations or expectations can represent related factors for the diagnosis *Altered Family Processes related to conflict regarding expectations of members meeting role obligations*.

Until clinical research defines this diagnosis and the associated nursing interventions, use "altered role performance" as a related factor for another nursing diagnosis, e.g., *Anxiety, Grieving,* or *Self-Concept Disturbance*.

Self-Care Deficit Syndrome*

Feeding Self-Care Deficit

Bathing/Hygiene Self-Care Deficit

Dressing/Grooming Self-Care Deficit

Toileting Self-Care Deficit

Instrumental Self-Care Deficit*

Self-Care Deficit Syndrome

DEFINITION

Self-Care Deficit Syndrome: The state in which the individual experiences an impaired motor function or cognitive function, causing a decreased ability in performing each of the four self-care activities.

DEFINING CHARACTERISTICS

Major (One deficit must be present in each activity)
1. Self-feeding deficits
   Unable to cut food or open packages
   Unable to bring food to mouth
2. Self-bathing deficits (includes washing entire body, combing hair, brushing teeth, attending to skin and nail care, and applying makeup)
   Unable or unwilling to wash body or body parts
   Unable to obtain a water source
   Unable to regulate temperature or water flow
3. Self-dressing deficits (including donning regular or special clothing, not night-clothes)
   Impaired ability to put on or take off clothing
   Unable to fasten clothing
   Unable to groom self satisfactorily
   Unable to obtain or replace articles of clothing

---

*These diagnoses are not currently on the NANDA list but have been included for clarity or usefulness.

4. Self-toileting deficits

    Unable or unwilling to get to toilet or commode

    Unable or unwilling to carry out proper hygiene

    Unable to transfer to and from toilet or commode

    Unable to handle clothing to accommodate toileting

    Unable to flush toilet or empty commode

RELATED FACTORS

Pathophysiologic

Neuromuscular impairment

    Autoimmune alterations (arthritis, multiple sclerosis)

    Metabolic and endocrine alterations (diabetes mellitus, hypothyroidism)

    Nervous system disorders (parkinsonism, myasthenia gravis, muscular dystrophy, Guillain-Barré)

    Lack of coordination

    Spasticity or flaccidity

    Muscular weakness

    Partial or total paralysis (spinal cord injury, stroke)

    CNS tumors

    Increased intracranial pressure

Musculoskeletal disorders

    Atrophy

    Muscle contractures

    Connective tissue diseases (systemic lupus erythematosus)

    Edema (increased synovial fluid)

Visual disorders

    Glaucoma

    Cataracts

    Diabetic/hypertensive retinopathy

    Ocular histoplasmosis

    Cranial nerve neuropathy

    Visual field deficits

    Depression

Treatment-related

External devices (casts, splints, braces, IV equipment)

Surgical procedures

Fractures

Tracheostomy

Gastrostomy

Jejunostomy

Ileostomy

Colostomy

Situational (personal, environmental)

Immobility

Trauma

Nonfunctioning or missing limbs

Coma

Maturational

Elderly: Decreased visual and motor ability, muscle weakness, dementia

Diagnostic Considerations

Self-care encompasses the activities needed to meet daily needs, commonly known as activities of daily living (ADLs), which are learned over time and become life-long habits. Involved in self-care activities is not only what is to be done (hygiene, bathing, dressing, toileting, feeding) but also how, when, where, with whom and how it is done (Hoskins, 1989).

In every person, the threat or reality of a self-care deficit evokes panic. Many persons report that they fear loss of independence more than death. A self-care deficit impacts the core of one's self-concept and self-determination. For this reason, the nursing focus for self-care deficit should not be on providing the care measure but rather on identifying adaptive techniques to allow the person the maximum degree of participation and independence possible.

The diagnosis *Total Self-Care Deficit* once was used to describe a person's inability to complete feeding, bathing, toileting, dressing, and grooming (Gordon, 1982; Carpenito, 1983). The intent of specifying "Total" was to describe a person with deficits in these ADLs. Unfortunately, sometimes its use invites, according to Magnan (1989), "preconceived judgments about the state of an individual and the nursing interventions required." The person may be viewed as in a vegetative state requiring only minimal custodial care. *Total Self-Care Deficit* has been eliminated because its language does not denote potential for growth or rehabilitation.

Currently not on the NANDA list, the diagnosis *Self-Care Deficit Syndrome* has been added here to describe a person with compromised ability in all four self-care activities. For this person, the nurse will assess functioning in each of the four areas and identify the level of participation of which the person is capable. The goal is to maintain the current level of functioning and/or to increase participation and independence. The syndrome distinction clusters all four self-care deficits together to enable grouping of interventions when indicated while also permitting specialized interventions for a specific deficit.

The danger of applying a *Self-Care Deficit* diagnosis lies in the possibility of prematurely labeling a person as unable to participate at any level, eliminating a rehabilitation focus. It is important that the nurse classify the person's functional level to promote independence. (Refer to the functional level classification scale in Focus Assessment Criteria.) Continuous reevaluation also is necessary to identify changes in the person's ability to participate in self-care.

Errors in Diagnostic Considerations

Toileting Self-Care Deficit related to insufficient knowledge of ostomy care

The diagnostic category *Toileting Self-Care Deficit* describes a person who cannot get to, sit on, or rise up from the toilet, or perform clothing and hygiene activities related to toileting. Insufficient knowledge of ostomy care does not apply to this diagnosis. Depending on presence of risk factors or signs and symptoms, the diagnosis of either *Altered Health Maintenance* or *High Risk for Altered Health Maintenance related to insufficient knowledge of ostomy care* would apply to this situation.

Dressing Self-Care Deficit related to inability to fasten clothing

Inability to fasten clothing represents a sign or symptom of *Dressing Self-Care Deficit*, not a related factor. Using a focus assessment the nurse needs to determine the contributing factors (*e.g*, insufficient knowledge of adaptive techniques needed).

Self-Care Deficit Syndrome related to cognitive deficits

As a syndrome diagnosis, no related factors are indicated and in fact are not very useful for treatment. Instead, the nurse should write the diagnosis as *Self-Care*

Deficit Syndrome: Feeding (1), Bathing (4), Dressing/Grooming (4), Toileting (5). The number code indicates the present level of functioning needed. The outcome criteria should represent improved or increased functioning.

Focus Assessment Criteria

Subjective/Objective
Evaluate each ADL using the following scale:
- 0 = Completely independent
- 1 = Requires use of assistive device
- 2 = Needs minimal help
- 3 = Needs assistance and/or some supervision
- 4 = Needs total supervision
- 5 = Needs total assistance or unable to assist

Mental Status
- Ability to remember
- Judgment
- Ability to follow directions
- Ability to identify/express needs
- Ability to anticipate needs (food, laundry)
- Self-feeding abilities
  - Swallowing
  - Chewing
  - Using utensils and cutting food
  - Selecting foods
  - Seeing
- Self-bathing abilities
  - Undressing to bathe
  - Reaching water source
  - Differentiating water temperatures
  - Obtaining equipment (water, soap, towels)
  - Washing body parts
  - Performing oral care
- Self-dressing/grooming abilities
  - Putting on or taking off necessary clothing
  - Selecting appropriate clothing
  - Retrieving appropriate clothing
  - Fastening clothing
  - Washing hair
  - Styling hair
- Self-toileting abilities
  - Getting to toilet and undressing
  - Sitting on toilet
  - Rising from toilet
  - Cleaning self/flushing toilet
  - Redressing
  - Performing proper hygiene (washing hands)

Principles and Rationale for Nursing Care

Generic Considerations
1. The concept of self-care emphasizes each person's right to maintain individual control over his own pattern of living. (This applies to both the ill individual and the well individual.)
2. Regardless of handicap, people should be given privacy and treated with dignity while performing self-care activities.
3. Self-care does not imply allowing the person to do things for himself as planned by the nurse but, rather, encouraging and teaching the person to make his own plans for optimal daily living.

4. Mobility is necessary to meet one's self-care needs and to maintain good health and self-esteem.
5. Cleanliness is important for comfort, for positive self-esteem, and for social interactions with others.
6. Inability to care for oneself produces feelings of dependency and poor self-concept. With increased ability for self-care, self-esteem increases.
7. Disability often causes denial, anger, and frustration. These are valid emotions that must be recognized and addressed.
8. It is acceptable for a limited period of time to be dependent on others to provide basic physiologic and psychologic needs.
9. Regression in ability to perform self-care activities may be a defense mechanism to threatening situations.
10. Neglect of an extremity refers to the memory loss of the presence of an extremity (*e.g.*, a person who has had a stroke or brain injury resulting in partial paralysis may ignore the arm or leg on the affected side of the body).
11. Optimal patient education promotes self-care. To teach effectively the nurse must determine what the learner perceives as his own needs and goals, determine what the nurse feels are his needs and goals, and then work to establish mutually acceptable goals.
12. Offering the individual choices and including him in planning his own care reduces feelings of powerlessness; promotes feelings of freedom, control, and self-worth; and increases the person's willingness to comply with therapeutic regimens.
13. The following key elements promote relearning of self-care tasks:
    a. Providing a structured, consistent environment and routine
    b. Repeating instructions and tasks
    c. Teaching and practicing tasks during periods of least fatigue
    d. Maintaining a familiar environment and teacher
    e. Using patience, determination, and a positive attitude (by both learner and teacher)
    f. Practicing, practicing, practicing

Endurance

1. The endurance or ability of the individual to maintain a given level of performance is influenced by the ability to use oxygen to produce energy (related to the optimal functioning of the heart, respiratory, and circulatory systems) and the functioning of the neurologic and musculoskeletal systems. Thus, individuals with alterations in these systems have increased energy demands or a decreased ability to produce energy.
2. Stress is energy consuming; the more stressors an individual has, the more fatigue he will experience. Stressors can be personal, environmental, disease-related, and treatment-related. Examples of possible stressors follow.

Personal	*Environmental*	*Disease-Related*	*Treatment-Related*
Age	Isolation	Pain	Walker
Support system	Noise	Anemia	Medications
Life-style	Unfamiliar setting		Diagnostic studies

3. The signs and symptoms of decreased oxygen in response to an activity—*e.g.*, self-care, mobility—are:
    Sustained increased heart rate 3 to 5 minutes after ceasing the activity or a change in the pulse rhythm

Failure of systolic blood pressure reading to increase with activity, or a decrease in value

Decrease or excessive increase in respiratory rate and dyspnea

Weakness, pallor, cerebral hypoxia (confusion, incoordination)

4. Refer to Principles of Nursing Care under *Activity Intolerance* for additional information.

Pediatric Considerations

1. The infant and young child depend on a caregiver for assistance in ADLs.
2. Parents/caregivers can facilitate a child's mastery of self-care skills. The desired outcome is that the child participates in his care to the maximum of his abilities (Whaley & Wong, 1989).
3. The nurse should assess each child's unique ability to engage in self-care activities to promote control over self and environment.

Gerontologic Considerations

1. Age-related changes do not in themselves cause self-care deficits. Older adults do, however, have increased incidence of chronic diseases that can compromise functional ability, *e.g.*, arthritis, cardiac disorders, visual impairment.
2. Comparing statistics from 1961 to 1981 reveals a substantial improvement in overall functioning among older adults (Palmer & Tonis, 1980).
3. About 70% of persons age 65 years and older rate their health as excellent. Only 20% of adults age 65 to 74 and 24% over age 75 report limitations in activity due to chronic illness (U.S. Department of Health and Human Services, 1987).
4. Older adults with dementia have varying difficulty with self-care activities depending on memory deficits, ability to follow directions, and judgment (Miller, 1990).

■ Self-Care Deficit Syndrome

Assessment

Subjective/Objective Data

Observed or reported inability or difficulty in performing some activity in each of the four areas of self-care

---

Outcome Criteria

The person will
- Identify preferences in self-care activities (*e.g.*, time, products, location)
- Demonstrate optimal hygiene after assistance with care
- Will participate physically and/or verbally in feeding, dressing, toileting, bathing activities

Interventions

A. Assess for causative or contributing factors
   1. Visual deficits
   2. Impaired cognition
   3. Decrease motivation
   4. Impaired mobility
   5. Lack of knowledge
   6. Inadequate social support

B. Promote optimal participation
   1. Assess present level of participation.
   2. Determine areas for potential increase in participation in each self-care activity.
   3. Explore the person's goals.

C. Promote self-esteem and self-determination
   1. Determine preferences for
      a. Schedule
      b. Products
      c. Methods
      d. Clothing selection
      e. Hair styling
   2. During self-care activities provide choices and request preferences.

D. Evaluate ability to participate in each self-care activity (feeding, dressing, bathing, toileting)
   1. Assign a number value to each activity (refer to the coding scale under *Self-Care Deficit Syndrome*).
   2. Reassess ability frequently and revise code as appropriate.

E. Refer to interventions under each diagnoses—*Feeding, Bathing, Dressing, and Toileting Self-Care Deficit*—as indicated

---

Feeding Self-Care Deficit

■ *Related to* **(Specify)**

DEFINITION

A state in which the individual experiences an impaired ability to perform or complete feeding activities for himself or herself

DEFINING CHARACTERISTICS
Unable to cut food or open food packages
Unable to bring food to mouth

RELATED FACTORS
See *Self-Care Deficit Syndrome*

Diagnostic Considerations
See *Self-Care Deficit Syndrome*

Errors in Diagnostic Statements
See *Self-Care Deficit Syndrome*

Principles and Rationale of Nursing Care
See *Self-Care Deficit Syndrome*

■ Feeding Self-Care Deficit (Specify Code)*
Related to (Specify)

Assessment

Subjective Data
The person reports
Problems with eating "I can't feed myself"
"I'm too tired to eat."
"Could you help me with my food?"
Pain

Objective Data
Impaired visual acuity
Mental lethargy
Poor oral hygiene (lack of teeth or poorly fitting dentures; oral injury, ulcer, deformity)
Drooling or facial paralysis
Uncoordination
Inability to use hands to grip a device to move food to mouth
Absence of gag reflex

* Refer to the coding scale in *Self-Care Deficit Syndrome*, Focus Assessment.

Outcome Criteria

The person will
- Demonstrate increased ability to feed self *or*
- Report that he is unable to feed self
- Demonstrate ability to make use of adaptive devices, if indicated
- Demonstrate increased interest and desire to eat
- Describe rationale and procedure for treatment
- Describe causative factors for feeding deficit

Interventions

A. Assess causative factors
   1. Visual deficits (blindness, field cuts, poor depth perception)
   2. Affected or missing limbs (casts, amputations, paresis, paralysis)
   3. Cognitive deficits (aging, trauma, cerebrovascular accident [CVA])

B. Provide opportunities to relearn or adapt to activity
   1. Common nursing interventions for feeding
      a. Ascertain from person or family members what foods the person likes or dislikes.
      b. Have meals taken in the same setting: pleasant surroundings that are not too distracting.
      c. Maintain correct food temperatures (hot foods hot, cold foods cold).
      d. Provide pain relief, since pain can affect appetite and ability to feed self.
      e. Provide good oral hygiene before and after meals.
      f. Encourage person to wear dentures and eyeglasses.
      g. Place person in the most normal eating position suited to his physical disability (best is sitting in a chair at a table).
      h. Provide social contact during eating.
      i. See *Altered Nutrition: Less Than Body Requirements.*
   2. Specific interventions for people with sensory/perceptual deficits
      a. Encourage the person to wear prescribed corrective lenses.
      b. Describe location of utensils and food on tray or table.
      c. Describe food items to stimulate appetite.
      d. For perceptual deficits, choose different-colored dishes to help distinguish items (*e.g.,* red tray, white plates).
      e. Ascertain person's usual eating patterns and provide food items according to preference (or arrange food items in clocklike pattern); record on care plan the arrangement used (*e.g.,* meat, 6 o'clock; potatoes, 9 o'clock; vegetables, 12 o'clock).
      f. Encourage eating of "finger foods" (*e.g.,* bread, bacon, fruit, hot dogs) to promote independence.
      g. Avoid placing food to blind side of person with field cut, until visually accommodated to surroundings; then encourage him to scan entire visual field.
   3. Specific interventions for people with missing limbs
      a. Provide for eating environment that is not embarrassing to individual and allow sufficient time for the task of eating.

b. Provide only the amount of supervision and assistance necessary for relearning or adaptation.

c. To enhance maximum amount of independence, provide necessary adaptive devices.
- Plate guard to avoid pushing food off plate
- Suction device under plate or bowl for stabilization
- Padded handles on utensils for a more secure grip
- Wrist or hand splints with clamp to hold eating utensils
- Special drinking cup
- Rocker knife for cutting

d. Assist with set-up if needed, opening containers, napkins, condiment packages; cutting meat; buttering bread.

e. Arrange food so person has adequate amount of space to perform the task of eating.

4. Specific interventions for people with cognitive deficits

a. Provide isolated, quiet atmosphere until person is able to attend to eating and is not easily distracted from the task.

b. Supervise feeding program until there is no danger of choking or aspiration.

c. Orient person to location and purpose of feeding equipment.

d. Avoid external distractions and unnecessary conversation.

e. Place person in the most normal eating position he is physically able to assume.

f. Encourage person to attend to the task, but be alert for fatigue, frustration, or agitation.

g. Provide one food at a time in usual sequence of eating until person is able to eat the entire meal in normal sequence.

h. Encourage person to be tidy, to eat in small amounts, and to put food in unaffected side of mouth if paresis or paralysis is present.

i. Check for food in cheeks.

j. Refer to *Impaired Swallowing* for additional interventions.

C. Initiate health teaching and referrals as indicated

1. Assess to ensure that both person and family understand the reason and purpose of all interventions.

2. Proceed with teaching as needed.

a. Maintain safe eating methods.

b. Prevent aspiration.

c. Use appropriate eating utensils (avoid sharp instruments).

d. Test temperature of hot liquids and wear protective clothing (*e.g.,* paper bib).

e. Teach use of adaptive devices.

Bathing/Hygiene Self-Care Deficit

■ *Related to* **(Specify)**

DEFINITION
Bathing/Hygiene Self-Care Deficit: A state in which the individual experiences an impaired ability to perform or complete bathing/hygiene activities for himself or herself.

DEFINING CHARACTERISTICS
Self-bathing deficits (washing entire body, combing hair, brushing teeth, attending to skin and nail care, and applying makeup)
  Unable or unwilling to wash body or body parts
  Unable to obtain a water source
  Unable to regulate temperature or water flow

RELATED FACTORS
See *Self-Care Deficit Syndrome*

Diagnostic Considerations
See *Self-Care Deficit Syndrome*

Errors in Diagnostic Statements
See *Self-Care Deficit Syndrome*

Principles and Rationale of Nursing Care
See *Self-Care Deficit Syndrome*

■ ## Bathing/Hygiene Self-Care Deficit (Specify Code)*
Related to (Specify)

Assessment

Subjective Data
  The person states
    "I can't wash myself."

*Refer to the coding scale in *Self-Care Deficit Syndrome,* Focus Assessment.

"I don't want (need) a bath."
"I'm too tired (weak) to wash myself."
"It hurts."

Objective Data

Impaired visual acuity
Impaired hearing acuity
Impaired upper limb movement
Inability to use hands
Uncoordinated movements or spasticity
Presence of restrictive devices (splints, casts, braces, traction equipment)
Decreased mental alertness

Outcome Criteria

The person will
- Perform bathing activity at expected optimal level *or*
- Report satisfaction with accomplishments despite limitations
- Relate feeling of comfort and satisfaction with body cleanliness
- Demonstrate ability to use adaptive devices
- Describe causative factors of bathing deficit
- Relate rationale and procedures for treatment

Interventions

A. Assess causative factors

1. Visual deficits (blindness, field cuts, poor depth perception)
2. Affected or missing limbs (casts, amputations, paresis, paralysis, arthritis)
3. Cognitive deficits (aging, trauma, CVA)

B. Provide opportunities to relearn or adapt to activity

1. General nursing interventions for inability to bathe
   a. Bathing time and routine should be consistent to encourage greatest amount of independence.
   b. Encourage person to wear prescribed corrective lenses or hearing aid.
   c. Keep bathroom temperature warm; ascertain individual's preferred water temperature.
   d. Provide for privacy during bathing routine.
   e. Keep environment simple and uncluttered.
   f. Observe skin condition during bathing.
   g. Provide all bathing equipment within easy reach.
   h. Provide for safety in the bathroom (nonslip mats, grab bars).
   i. When person is physically able, encourage use of either tub or shower stall, depending on which facility is at home (the person should practice in the hospital in preparation for going home).
   j. Provide for adaptive equipment as needed.
      - Chair or stool in bathtub or shower
      - Long-handled sponge to reach back or lower extremities

- Grab bars on bathroom walls where needed to assist in mobility
- Bath board for transferring to tub chair or stool
- Safety treads or nonslip mat on floor of bathroom, tub, and shower
- Washing mitts with pocket for soap
- Adapted toothbrushes
- Shaver holders
- Hand-held shower spray

   k. Provide for relief of pain that may affect ability to bathe self.*

2. Specific interventions for bathing for people with visual deficits
   a. Place bathing equipment in location most suitable to individual.
   b. Avoid placing bathing equipment to blind side if person has a field cut and is not visually accommodated to surroundings.
   c. Keep call bell within reach if person is to bathe alone.
   d. Give the visually impaired individual the same degree of privacy and dignity as any other person.
   e. Verbally announce yourself before entering or leaving the bathing area.
   f. Observe the person's ability to locate all bathing utensils.
   g. Observe the person's ability to perform mouth care, hair combing, and shaving tasks.
   h. Provide place for clean clothing within easy reach.

3. Specific interventions for bathing for people with affected or missing limbs
   a. Bathe early in morning or before bed at night to avoid unnecessary dressing and undressing.
   b. Encourage person to use a mirror during bathing to inspect the skin of paralyzed areas.
   c. Encourage the person with amputation to inspect remaining foot or stump for good skin integrity.
   d. For limb amputations, bathe stump twice a day and be sure it is dry before wrapping it or applying prosthesis.
   e. Provide only the amount of supervision or assistance necessary for relearning the use of extremity or adaptation to the handicap.
   f. For lack of sensation, encourage use of the affected area in the bathing process (an individual tends to forget the existence of body parts in which there is no sensation).

4. Specific interventions for bathing people with cognitive deficits
   a. Provide a consistent time for the bathing routine as part of a structured program to help decrease confusion.
   b. Keep instructions simple and avoid distractions; orient to purpose of bathing equipment, put toothpaste on toothbrush.
   c. If person is unable to bathe the entire body, have him bathe one part until he does it correctly; give positive reinforcement for success.
   d. Supervise activity until person can safely perform the task unassisted.
   e. Encourage attention to the task, but be alert for fatigue that may increase confusion.
   f. Apply firm pressure to the skin when bathing; it is less likely to be misinterpreted than a gentle touch.
   g. Use a warm shower or bath to help a confused or agitated person to relax.

---

*May require a physician's order.

C. Initiate health teaching and referrals as indicated
1. Communicate to staff and family the person's ability and willingness to learn.
2. Teach use of adaptive devices.
3. Ascertain bathing facilities at home and assist in determining if there is any need to make adaptations; refer to occupational therapy or social service for help in obtaining needed home equipment.
4. Teach to use tub or shower stall, depending on type of facility at home.
5. If person is paralyzed, instruct him or his family to demonstrate complete skin check on key areas for redness (buttocks, bony prominences).
6. Teach to maintain a safe bathing environment.

Dressing/Grooming Self-Care Deficit

■ *Related to* **(Specify)**

DEFINITION
Dressing/Grooming Self-Care Deficit: A state in which the individual experiences an impaired ability to perform or complete dressing and grooming activities for himself or herself.

DEFINING CHARACTERISTICS
Self-dressing deficits (including donning regular or special clothing, not nightclothes)
Impaired ability to put on or take off clothing
Unable to fasten clothing
Unable to groom self satisfactorily
Unable to obtain or replace articles of clothing

RELATED FACTORS
See *Self-Care Deficit Syndrome*

Diagnostic Considerations
See *Self-Care Deficit Syndrome*

Errors in Diagnostic Statements
See *Self-Care Deficit Syndrome*

Principles and Rationale For Nursing Care
See *Self-Care Deficit Syndrome*

Dressing/Grooming Self-Care Deficit (Specify Code)*
Related to (Specify)

Assessment

Subjective Data

The person states
"I can't wash myself."
"I don't want (need) a bath."
"I'm too tired (weak) to wash myself."
"It hurts."

Objective Data

Impaired visual acuity
Inability to use hands
Spasticity, weakness, lack of coordination
Presence of restrictive devices (traction, cats, splints, braces)
Disheveled appearance or inappropriate dress
Decreased mental alertness
Inability to dress self

Outcome Criteria

The person will
- Demonstrate increased ability to dress self *or*
- Report the need of having someone else assist him in performing the task
- Demonstrate ability to learn how to use adaptive devices to facilitate optimal independence in the task of dressing
- Demonstrate increased interest in wearing street clothes
- Describe causative factors for dressing deficits
- Relate rationale and procedures for treatments

Interventions

A. Assess causative factors
  1. Visual deficits (blindness, field cuts, poor depth perception)
  2. Affected or missing limbs (casts, amputations, arthritis, paresis, paralysis)
  3. Cognitive deficits (aging, trauma, CVA)

B. Provide opportunities to relearn or adapt to activity
  1. Common nursing interventions for self-dressing
    a. Encourage person to wear prescribed corrective lenses or hearing aid.
    b. Promote independence in dressing through continual and unaided practice.

---

* Refer to the coding scale in *Self-Care Deficit Syndrome*, Focus Assessment.

    c. Choose clothing that is loose fitting, with wide sleeves and pant legs and front fasteners.

    d. Allow sufficient time for dressing and undressing, since the task may be tiring, painful, or difficult.

    e. Plan for person to learn and demonstrate one part of an activity before progressing further.

    f. Lay clothes out in the order in which they will be needed to dress.

    g. Provide dressing aids as necessary (some commonly used aids include dressing stick, Swedish reacher, zipper pull, buttonhook, long-handled shoehorn, and shoe fasteners adapted with elastic laces, Velcro closures, or flip-back tongues; all garments with fasteners may be adapted with Velcro closures).

    h. Encourage person to wear ordinary or special clothing rather than night-clothes.

    i. Increase participation in dressing by medicating for pain 30 minutes before it is time to dress or undress, if indicated.*

    j. Provide for privacy during dressing routine.

    k. Provide for safety by ensuring easy access to all clothing and by ascertaining individual's performance level.

2. Specific interventions for dressing people with visual deficits

    a. Allow person to ascertain the most convenient location for clothing and adapt the environment to best accomplish the task (*e.g.,* remove unnecessary barriers).

    b. Verbally announce yourself before entering or leaving the dressing area.

    c. Avoid placing clothing to the blind side if person has a field cut, until he is visually accommodated to surroundings; then encourage him to turn head to scan entire visual field.

    d. Apply adaptive devices (*e.g.,* hand splints) before dressing activity.

    e. Consult or refer to physical or occupational therapy for teaching application of prosthetics to missing limbs.

3. Specific interventions for dressing for people with cognitive deficits

    a. Make a consistent dressing routine to provide a structured program to decrease confusion.

    b. Keep instructions simple and repeat them frequently, avoid distractions.

    c. Introduce one article of clothing at a time.

    d. Encourage attention to the task; be alert for fatigue, which may increase confusion.

C. Initiate health teaching and referrals as indicated

1. Assess understanding and knowledge of individual and family for above instructions and rationale.

2. Proceed with teaching as needed.

    a. Communicate the individual's ability and willingness to learn to staff and family members.

    b. Teach use of adaptive devices and techniques that are specific to each disability.

    c. Teach to maintain a safe dressing environment.

    d. Attempt to be noncritical in correcting errors.

---

*May require a physician's order.

Toileting Self-Care Deficit

■ *Related to* **(Specify)**

DEFINITION

Toileting Self-Care Deficit: A state in which the individual experiences an impaired ability to perform complete toileting activities for himself or herself.

DEFINING CHARACTERISTICS

Unable or unwilling to get to toilet or commode
Unable or unwilling to carry out proper hygiene
Unable to transfer to and from toilet or commode
Unable to handle clothing to accommodate toileting
Unable to flush toilet or empty commode

RELATED FACTORS

See *Self-Care Deficit Syndrome*

Diagnostic Considerations

See *Self-Care Deficit Syndrome*

Errors in Diagnostic Statements

See *Self-Care Deficit Syndrome*

Principles and Rationale of Nursing Care

See *Self-Care Deficit Syndrome*

■ **Toileting Self-Care Deficit (Specify Code)***
   Related to (Specify)

Assessment

Subjective Data

The person states
"I can't go to the toilet."

---

* Refer to the coding scale in *Self-Care Deficit Syndrome*, Focus Assessment.

"It hurts."
"I can't get out of bed (walk, move)."
"I can't get to the bathroom in time."
"I wet myself."
"I can't control my bowels."

Objective Data

Impaired visual acuity
Decreased mental alertness
Weakness, lack of coordination
Spasticity
Presence of restrictive devices (traction, casts, splints, braces)
Immobility

Outcome Criteria

The person will
- Demonstrate increased ability to toilet self *or*
- Report that he is unable to toilet self
- Demonstrate ability to make use of adaptive devices to facilitate toileting
- Describe causative factors for toileting deficit
- Relate rationale and procedures for treatment.

Interventions

A. Assess causative factors

1. Visual deficits (blindness, field cuts, poor depth perception)
2. Affected or missing limbs (casts, amputations, paresis, paralysis)
3. Cognitive deficits (aging, trauma, CVA)

B. Provide opportunities to relearn or adapt to activity

1. Common nursing interventions for toileting difficulties
   a. Encourage person to wear prescribed corrective lenses or hearing aid.
   b. Obtain bladder and bowel history from individual or significant other (see *Altered Bowel Elimination* or *Altered Patterns of Urinary Elimination*).
   c. Ascertain communication system person uses to express the need to toilet.
   d. Maintain bladder and bowel record to determine toileting patterns.
   e. Provide for adequate fluid intake and balanced diet to promote adequate urinary output and normal bowel evacuation.
   f. Promote normal elimination by encouraging activity and exercise within the person's capabilities.
   g. Avoid development of "bowel fixation" by less frequent discussion and inquiries about bowel movements.
   h. Be alert to possibility of falls when toileting person (be prepared to ease him to floor without causing injury to either of you).
   i. Achieve independence in toileting by continual and unaided practice.
   j. Allow sufficient time for the task of toileting to avoid fatigue (lack of sufficient time to toilet may cause incontinence or constipation).
   k. Avoid use of indwelling catheters and condom catheters to expedite bladder continence (if possible).

2. Specific interventions for toileting for people with visual deficits
   a. Keep call bell easily accessible so person can quickly obtain help to toilet; answer call bell promptly to decrease anxiety.
   b. If bedpan or urinal is necessary for toileting, be sure it is within person's reach.
   c. Avoid placing toileting equipment to the blind side of an individual with field cut (when he is visually accommodated to surroundings, you may suggest he search entire visual field for equipment).
   d. Verbally announce yourself before entering or leaving toileting area.
   e. Observe person's ability to obtain equipment or get to the toilet unassisted.
   f. Provide for a safe and clear pathway to toilet area.
3. Specific interventions for toileting for people with affected or missing limbs
   a. Provide only the amount of supervision and assistance necessary for relearning or adapting to the prosthesis.
   b. Encourage person to look at affected area or limb and use it during toileting tasks.
   c. Encourage useful transfer techniques taught by occupational or physical therapy (the nurse should familiarize herself with planned mode of transfer).
   d. Provide the necessary adaptive devices to enhance the maximum amount of independence and safety (commode chairs, spill-proof urinals, fracture bedpans, raised toilet seats, support side rails for toilets).
   e. Provide for a safe and clear pathway to toilet area.
4. Specific interventions for toileting for people with cognitive deficits
   a. Offer toileting reminders every 2 hours, after meals, and before bedtime.
   b. When person is able to indicate the need to toilet, begin toileting at 2-hour intervals, after meals, and before bedtime.
   c. Answer call bell immediately to avoid frustration and failure to be continent.
   d. Encourage wearing ordinary clothes (many confused individuals are continent while wearing regular clothing).
   e. Avoid the use of bedpans and urinals; if physically possible, provide a normal atmosphere of elimination in bathroom (the toilet used should remain constant to promote familiarity).
   f. Give verbal cues as to what is expected of the individual, and give positive reinforcement for success.
   g. Work to achieve daytime continency before expecting nighttime continency (nighttime incontinence may continue after daytime continence has returned).
   h. See *Altered Patterns of Urinary Elimination* for additional information on incontinence.

C. Initiate health teaching and referrals as indicated
1. Assess the understanding and knowledge of the individual and significant others of foregoing interventions and rationale.
   a. Communicate person's ability and willingness to learn to staff and family.
   b. Maintain a safe toileting environment.
   c. Reinforce knowledge of transferring techniques.
   d. Teach use of adaptive devices.
   e. Ascertain home toileting needs and refer to occupational therapy or social services for help in obtaining necessary equipment.

Instrumental Self-Care Deficit

■ *Related to* **Cognitive or Physical Deficits and Insufficient Knowledge of Adaptive Techniques or Resources Available**

DEFINITION

Instrumental Self-Care Deficit: A state in which the individual experiences an impaired ability to perform certain activities or access certain services essential for managing a household.

DEFINING CHARACTERISTICS

Observed or reported difficulty in one or more of the following
Using a telephone
Accessing transportation
Laundering, ironing
Preparing meals
Shopping (food, clothes)
Managing money
Medication administration

RELATED FACTORS

See *Self-Care Deficit*

Diagnostic Considerations

Instrumental Self-Care Deficit is not currently on the NANDA list, but has been added here for clarity and usefulness. This diagnosis describes problems in performing certain activities or accessing certain services needed to live in the community, *e.g.*, phone use, shopping, money management. This diagnosis is important to consider in discharge planning and during home visits by community nurses.

Errors in Diagnostic Statements

Instrumental Self-Care Deficit related to possible inability to plan meals and manage laundry

When a nurse suspects that a client or family may have compromised ability to engage in certain activities needed to live in and run a household, the nurse should label the diagnosis *Possible Instrumental Self-Care Deficit* and add related factors representing why the nurse suspects the diagnosis, *e.g., related to difficulty remembering routine tasks* or *related to poor planning skills*. The nurse detecting evidence of memory or judgment difficulties could interpret this as a risk factors for *High Risk for Instrumental Self-Care Deficit*.

Focus Assessment

Subjective/Objective Data

Mental status
  Ability to remember
  Judgment
  Ability to anticipate needs (food, laundry)
  Ability to identify/express needs
  Ability to follow directions
Social supports
  Support person(s)
  Availability of help with transportation, shopping, money management, laundry,
    housekeeping, food preparation
  Community resources
Instrumental ADLs
  Telephone
    Ability to dial
    Ability to answer
    Ability to talk, hear
  Transportation
    Ability to drive
    Access to transportation
  Laundry
    Availability of washer
    Ability to wash, iron
    Ability to put away
  Food procurement and preparation
    Ability to cook
    Ability to select foods
    Ability to shop
  Medications
    Ability to remember
    Ability to administer
  Finances
    Ability to write checks, pay bills
    Ability to handle cash transactions (simple, complex)

Principles and Rationale For Nursing Care

Generic Considerations

1. Lawton (1980) and Brody (1985) identified that to live in the community an individual not only had to perform or have assistance with six ADLs, but also had to perform
   or have assistance with additional activities.
2. Instrumental ADLs include housekeeping, food preparation and procurement, shopping, laundry, ability to self-medicate safely, ability to manage money, and access to
   transportation (Miller, 1990).
3. Instrumental ADLs are more complex tasks than ADLs.
4. Maintaining persons in the community rather than in nursing homes has significant
   financial benefit. In 1981, 25% of all health care expenditures for older adults in the
   U.S. went to nursing homes, but only 5% of the elderly population were receiving care
   in these facilities. Medicaid covers about 90% of public spending for nursing home
   care (Miller, 1990).

5. Maintaining persons in the community rather than in a nursing home also maintains autonomy, strengthens family life, and affirms the value of older adults in our society.

Pediatric Considerations
See *Self-Care Deficit*

Gerontologic Considerations
See *Self-Care Deficit*

■ Instrumental Self-Care Deficit
Related to Cognitive or Physical Deficits and Insufficient Knowledge of Adaptive Techniques or Resources Available

Assessment
See Defining Characteristics

Objective
Impaired vision, hearing
Impaired cognition
Impaired physical mobility
Impaired coordination

Outcome Criteria

The person/family will
- Demonstrate use of adaptive devices, *e.g.,* phone, cooking aids
- Describe a method to ensure adherence to medication schedule
- Report ability to call and answer telephone
- Report regular laundering by self or others
- Report daily intake of two nutritious meals
- Identify transportation options to stores, physician, house of worship, social activities
- Demonstrate management of simple money transactions
- Identify individual(s) who will assist with money matters

Interventions

A. Assess for causative and contributing factors
 1. Visual, hearing deficits
 2. Impaired cognition
 3. Impaired mobility

4. Lack of knowledge

5. Inadequate social support

B. Assist to identify self-help devices

1. Grooming-dressing aids (see *Impaired Physical Mobility*)
2. Kitchen/eating aids
    a. One side built-up dishes
    b. Built-up handles on cutlery (use plastic foam curlers)
    c. Bulldog clip to secure a straw in glass
    d. Built-up corner of cutlery board to hold and anchor food or pot, *e.g.,* to butter toast, mashed potatoes
    e. Mounted jar opener
    f. Nonslip material applied under dishes (same strips used to prevent slipping in bath tub)
    g. Two-sided suction holder to hold dishes in place
3. Communication/security
    a. Motion-activated lights near walkway/entrance
    b. Night light for path to bathroom
    c. Light next to bed
    d. Specially adapted phones (amplified, big button)

C. Promote self-care and safety for person with cognitive deficit

1. Evaluate activities that are achievable.
2. Teach safety techniques.
    a. Turn lights on before dark.
    b. Use nightlights.
    c. Keep environment simple, uncluttered.
    d. Use clocks, calenders as cues.
    e. Mark on calender (using picture symbols) reminders for shopping, laundry, cleaning, doctor's appointments, etc.
3. For laundry, teach to:
    a. Separate dark and light clothes.
    b. Use pictures to illustrate steps for washing clothes.
    c. Mark cup with line to indicate amount of soap needed.
    d. Minimize ironing.
    e. Use an iron with automatic shut-off mechanism.
4. Evaluate ability to procure, select, and prepare nutritious food daily.
    a. Prepare a permanent shopping list with cues for essential foods, products.
    b. Teach to review list before shopping and check items needed, and, in the store, check off items selected. (Use a pencil, which can be erased to reuse list.)
    c. Teach how to shop for single-person meals (refer to *Altered Nutrition* for specific techniques).
    d. If possible, teach to use a microwave to reduce the risk of heat-related injuries or accidents.
5. Teach hints to improve adherence to medication schedule.
    a. Have someone place medications in a commercial pill holder divided into 7 days.
    b. Take out exact amount of pills for the day. Divide them in small cups each labeled with time of day.

    c. If needed, draw a picture of the pills and the quantity on each cup.

    d. Teach to take pills from cup to a small plastic bag when planning to be away from home.

6. Teach who to call for instructions if a dose is missed.

D. Determine available sources of transportation

1. Neighbors, relatives
2. Community center
3. Church group
4. Social service agency

E. Determine available sources of social support

1. Discuss the possibility of bartering for services (*e.g.,* wash neighbor's clothes in exchange for shopping help).
2. Identify a person who can provide immediate help (*e.g.,* neighbor, friend, hot-line).
3. Identify sources for help with laundry, shopping, money matters.

F. Initiate health teaching and referrals as indicated

1. Discuss the importance of identifying the need for assistance.
2. Refer to community agencies for assistance (*e.g.,* Department of Social Services, area agency on aging, senior neighbors, public health nursing).
3. Refer to the References/Bibliography for material aimed at the health care consumer.

References/Bibliography

Books

Gordon, M. (1982). *Manual of nursing diagnosis.* New York: McGraw-Hill.

Guidelines for stroke care. (1976). Public Health Service Publ. No. 76-14017. Washington, DC: U.S. Department of Health Education and Welfare.

Magnan, M. (1989). Unpublished paper.

Martin, N., Holt, N. B., & Hicks, D. (1981). *Comprehensive rehabilitation nursing.* New York: McGraw-Hill.

Miller, C. A. (1990). *Nursing care of older adults.* Glenview, IL: Scott, Foresman.

Palmer, M., & Tonis, J. (1980). *Manual for functional training.* Philadelphia: F. A. Davis.

Sine, R. D., et al: (1981). *Basic rehabilitation techniques.* Rockville, MD: Aspen Systems.

Whaley, L. F., & Wong, D. L. (1989). *Essentials of pediatric nursing* (3rd ed.). St. Louis: C. V. Mosby.

Articles

General

Allen, C., & Bennett, A. (1984). One step at a time to relearn self-help skills. *Nursing Mirror, 158*(15), Clinical Forum II–IV.

Alteri, C. A. (1984). The patient with myocardial infarction: Rest prescriptions for activities of daily living. *Heart and Lung, 14*(4), 355–360.

Ciuca, R., Bradish, J., & Trombly, S. M. (1978). Active range of motion exercises: A handbook. *Nursing, 8*(8), 45–49.

Gardiner, R. (1979). Getting the right piece in the right place: Home aids. *Community Outlook, 10*(2), 39–42.

Gould, M. T. (1983). Nursing diagnoses concurrent with multiple sclerosis. *Journal of Neurosurgical Nursing, 15*(16), 339–345.

Halper, J. (1990). The functional model in multiple sclerosis. *Rehabilitative Nursing, 15*(2), 77–79, 85.

Hoskins, L. M. (1989). Self care deficit. In McFarland, G., & McFarlane, E. (Eds.): *Nursing diagnosis and intervention*. St. Louis: C.V. Mosby.

Lerner, J. F. & Alexander, J. (1981). Activities of daily living: Reliability and validity of gross vs specific ratings. *Archives of Physical Medicine and Rehabilitation, 62*(4), 161–166.

Levin, L. S. 1978. Patient education and self-care: How do they differ? *Nursing Outlook, 26*(3), 170–175.

Meissner, S. F. (1980). Evaluate your patient's level of independence. *Nursing, 10*(9), 72–73.

Orem, D. E. (1985). A concept for self-care for the rehabilitation process. *Rehabilitation Nursing, 10*(3), 33–36.

Reeder, J. M. (1984). Help your disabled patient be more independent. *Nursing 14*(11), 43.

Ross, T. (1983). Nursing process: Activities of living. *Nursing Mirror, 156*(6), 28–29.

Sullivan, L. J. (1980). Self-care model for nursing. ANA Pub. No. G-147, 57–68.

Walter, K. M. (1980). Techniques and concepts: Independent living. Perceptions by professionals in rehabilitation. *Journal of Rehabilitation, 46*(3), 57–63.

Yep, J. O. (1977). Tools for aiding physically disabled individuals increase independence in dressing. *Journal of Rehabilitation, 43*(5), 39–41.

Aged

Barton, E. M. (1980). Etiology of dependence in older nursing home residents during morning care: The role of staff behavior. *Journal of Personality and Social Psychology, 10*(3), 423–431.

Brody, E. (1985). Parent care as a normative family stress. *The Gerontologist, 25*(1), 19–29.

Garvan, P., Lee, M., Lloyd, K., et al. (1980). Self-care applied to the aged. *New Jersey Nurse, 10*(1), 3–6.

Hirschfield, M. J. (1985). Self-care potential: Is it present? The elderly. *Journal of Gerontological Nursing, 11*(8), 28–34.

Karl, C. A., et al. (1982). The effect of an exercise program on self-care activities for the institutionalized elderly. *Journal of Gerontological Nursing, 8*(5), 282–285.

Lawton, M. P. (1980). *Environment and aging.* Belmont, CA: Wadsworth.

Leering, C. (1979). A structural model of functional capacity in the aged. *Journal of the American Geriatric Society, 27*(7), 314–316.

Lundsren-Lindquist, B., et al. (1983). Functioning studies in 79 year olds. I. Performance in hygiene activities. *Scandinavian Journal of Rehabilitation Medicines, 15*(3), 109–115

Palmore, E. B. (1987). Centenarians. In G. L. Maddox (Ed.). *The encyclopedia of aging,* pp. 107–108. New York: Springer Publishing Company.

Rameizl, P. (1983). Cadet; A self care assessment tool. *Geriatric Nursing, 4*(6), 377–378.

Rodgers, J. C., & Snow, T. (1982). An assessment of the feeding behaviors of the institutionalized elderly. *American Journal of Occupational Therapy, 36*(6), 373–380.

U.S. Department of Health and Human Services. (1987, October). *Current estimates from the National Health Interview Survey, United States, 1986.* Hyattsville, MD: U.S. Department of Health and Human Services.

Warshaw, G. A. (1982). Functional disability in the hospitalized elderly. *Journal of the American Medical Association, 248*(7), 847–850.

Amputee

Weiss-Lambrou, R. (1985). Brief or new: Toilet independence for the severe bilateral upper limb amputee. *American Journal of Occupational Therapy, 39*(6) 397–399.

Brain Injury

Panikoff, L. B. (1983). Recovery trends of functional skills in the head-injured adult. *American Journal of Occupational Therapy, 37*(11), 735–743.

Talmage, E. W., & Collins, G. A. (1983). Physical abilities after head injury: A retrospective study. *Physical Therapy, 63*(12), 2007–2010.

Spinal Cord Injury

Panchal P. D. (1980). Rehabilitation of the patient with spinal cord injury. *Current Problems in Surgery, 17*(4), 254–262.

Rogers, J. C., & Figone, J. J. (1980). Traumatic quadriplegia: Follow-up study of self-care skills. *Archives of Physical Medicine and Rehabilitation, 61*(7), 316–321.

Stroke and Brain Injury

Adler, M. K. (1980). Stroke rehabilitation: Is age a determinant? *Journal of the American Geriatric Society, 28*(11), 499–503.

Dzau, R. E., & Bochme, A. R. (1978). Stroke rehabilitation: A family-team education approach. *Archives of Physical Medicine and Rehabilitation, 59*(5), 236–239.

Rogers, E. J. (1980). Goals in hemiplegia care. *Journal of the American Geriatric Society, 28*(11), 497–498.

Stonington, H. H. (1980). Rehabilitation in cerebrovascular diseases. *Primary Care, 7*(3), 87–106.

Resources for Consumers

General

Citizens for Better Care—*For information on nursing homes/extended care facilities*
Department of Social Services—*Adult Foster Care Division*
Department of Social Service—*Chore Services Division*
Home Care or Durable Medical Equipment Companies
Private Home Care Nursing Agencies
Public Health Nursing Department
Senior Neighbors—*Home-delivered meals and in-home support services*
State Bureau of Rehabilitation—*For information/financial assistance for individuals presenting with physical or mental rehabilitation needs*
Visiting Nurse Associations—*For in-home nursing; physical, occupational, and speech therapy service; nurse aides/companions*

National Organizations

Accent on Information
P.O. Box 700; Bloomington, IL 61701
(309) 378–2961
Alzheimer's Disease and Related Disorders Association
360 N. Michigan Ave., Suite 601; Chicago, IL 60601
(312) 853–3060
Human Resources Center
I.U. Willets Rd.; Albertson, NY 11507
(516) 747–5400
Information Center for Individuals with Disabilities
20 Park Plaza, Rm. 330; Boston, MA 02116
(617) 727–5540
MAINSTREAM
1200 15th St. NW; Washington, DC 20005
(202) 833–1136
National Association for Independent Living
c/o National Rehabilitation Association
633 S. Washington St.; Alexandria, VA 22314
(703) 836–0850
National Association of the Physically Handicapped
76 Elm St.; London, OH 43140
(614) 852–1664
National Self-help Clearinghouse—*Graduate School and University Center*
33 W 42nd St.; City University of New York
New York, NY 10036
(212) 840–1259

P.R.I.D.E. FOUNDATION (Promote Real Independence for the Disabled and Elderly)
1159 Poquonnock Rd.; Groton, CT 06340
(203) 447–7433

Disease-Specific Organizations

Alzheimer's Disease and Related Disorders Association, Inc.
360 North Michigan Ave
Suite 1102
Chicago, IL 60601

Amyotrophic Lateral Sclerosis Society of America
12011 San Vincent Boulevard
Los Angeles, CA 90049

Herpes Resource Center
Box 100
Palo Alto, CA 94302

Muscular Dystrophy Associations of America, Inc.
810 Seventh Ave
New York, NY 10019

National Association for Sickle-Cell Disease, Inc.
945 S Western Ave
Suite 206
Los Angeles, CA 90006

National Epilepsy League
6 N Michigan Ave
Chicago, IL 60602

National Hemophilia Foundation
Room 903
25 W 39th Street
New York, NY 10018

National Multiple Sclerosis Society
205 East 42nd Street
New York, NY 10017

United Cerebral Palsy Associations, Inc.
66 East 34th Street
New York, NY 10016

United Ostomy Association
1111 Wilshire Blvd
Los Angeles, CA 90017

Financial Assistance

American Association of Retired Persons
1909 K Street, NW
Washington, DC 20049

Equal Employment Opportunities Commission
2401 East Street, NW
Washington, DC 20506

Health Insurance Association of America
1850 K Street, NW
Washington, DC 20006

Social Security Administration
1875 Connecticut Ave, NW
Room 1120
Washington, DC 20009

Self-Concept Disturbance*

Body Image Disturbance

Personal Identity Disturbance

Self-Esteem Disturbance

Chronic Low Self-Esteem

Situational Low Self-Esteem

Self-Concept Disturbance

■ *Related to* **(Specify)**

DEFINITION
Self-Concept Disturbance: The state in which the individual experiences or is at risk of experiencing a negative state of change about the way he feels, thinks, or views himself. It may include a change in body image, self-esteem, role performance, or personal identity.

DEFINING CHARACTERISTICS
Since a self-concept disturbance may include a change in any one or combination of its four component parts (body image, self-esteem, role performance, personal identity), and since the nature of the change causing the alteration can be so varied, there is no "typical" response to this diagnosis. Reactions may include:
Refusal to touch or look at a body part
Refusal to look into a mirror
Unwillingness to discuss a limitation, deformity, or disfigurement
Refusal to accept rehabilitation efforts
Inappropriate attempts to direct own treatment
Denial of the existence of a deformity or disfigurement
Increasing dependence on others
Signs of grieving: weeping, despair, anger
Refusal to participate in own care or take responsibility for self-care (self-neglect)
Self-destructive behavior (alcohol, drug abuse)

*This diagnosis is not currently on the NANDA list but has been included for clarity or usefulness.

Displaying hostility toward the healthy
Withdrawal from social contacts
Changing usual patterns of responsibility
Showing change in ability to estimate relationship of body to environment

RELATED FACTORS

A self-concept disturbance can occur as a response to a variety of health problems, situations, and conflicts. Some common sources follow.

Pathophysiologic

Chronic or terminal disease
Loss of body part(s)
Loss of body function(s)
Severe trauma

Treatment-related

Hospitalization: chronic or terminal illness
Surgery

Situational (personal, environmental)

Divorce, separation from, or death of a significant other
Loss of job or ability to work
Pain
Obesity
Pregnancy
Immobility or loss of function
Need for nursing home placement

Maturational

Infant and preschool: Deprivation
Young adult: Peer pressure, puberty
Middle aged: Signs of aging (graying or loss of hair), reduced hormonal levels (menopause)
Elderly: Losses (people, function, financial, retirement)

Other

Women's movement
Sexual revolution

Diagnostic Considerations

Self-Concept reflects self-view, encompassing body image, self-esteem, role performance, and personal identity. In constant evolution and change, self-concept is influenced by interactions with the environment and other persons, and by perceptions of how others view you.

Self-Concept Disturbance represents a broad diagnostic category under which fall more specific nursing diagnoses. Initially, the nurse may not have sufficient clinical data to validate a more specific diagnosis such as *Chronic Low Self-Esteem* or *Body Image Disturbance;* thus, *Self-Concept Disturbance* can be used until data can support a more specific diagnosis.

Self-Esteem is one of the four components of Self-Concept. *Self-Esteem Disturbance* is the general diagnostic category. *Chronic Low Self-Esteem* and *Situational Low Self-Esteem* represent specific types of *Self-Esteem Disturbances*, thus involving more specific interventions. Initially the nurse may not have sufficient clinical data to validate a more specific diagnosis as *Chronic Low Self-Esteem* or *Situational Low Self-Esteem*. Refer to the major defining characteristics under these categories for validation.

Situational Low Self-Esteem is an episodic event; repeated occurrence and/or the continuation of negative self-appraisals over time can lead to *Chronic Low Self-Esteem* (Willard, 1990).

Errors in Diagnostic Statements

Self-Concept Disturbance related to substance abuse

Although a relationship exists between negative self-concept and alcohol and/or drug abuse, listing substance abuse as a related factor does not describe the nursing focus. If the person acknowledged a substance abuse problem and expressed a desire for assistance, the diagnosis *Ineffective Individual Coping related to inability to constructively manage stressors without alcohol or drugs* could be appropriate. If the person denied a problem, the diagnosis *Ineffective Denial related to lack of acknowledgment of substance abuse/dependency* would apply—if the nurse will be addressing the denial. A nurse with data that suggest or confirm *Self-Concept Disturbance* should explore contributing factors; *e.g.*, guilt influenced by social stigma. The nurse can use "unknown etiology" until focus assessment identifies contributing factors.

Body Image Disturbance related to mastectomy

Mastectomy can produce various responses, including grief, anger, and negative feelings about self. A woman undergoing breast surgery for cancer is at high risk for both *Body Image Disturbance* and *Self-Esteem Disturbance*. Thus, the diagnosis *High Risk for Self-Concept Disturbance related to perceived negative effects of changed appearance and diagnosis of cancer* would be most appropriate. A nurse with data to support *Self-Concept Disturbance*, should record it as an actual diagnosis with these same related factors and including "as evidenced by" to specify signs and symptoms of or manifestations, *e.g.*, *Self-Concept Disturbance related to perceived negative effects of changed appearance and diagnosis of cancer, as evidenced by reports of negative feelings about "new self" and determination of not to let husband see her.*

Focus Assessment Criteria

Self-Concept Disturbance is manifested in a variety of ways. An individual may respond with an alteration in another life process (see *Spiritual Distress, Fear, Ineffective Individual Coping*). The nurse should be aware of this and utilize the assessment data to ascertain the dimensions affected.

It may be difficult for the nurse to identify the cues and make the inferences necessary to diagnose a self-concept disturbance. Each individual reacts differently to loss, pain, disability, and disfigurement. Therefore, the nurse should determine an individual's usual reactions to problems and feelings about himself before attempting to diagnose a change.

Subjective Data

Self views
"Describe yourself."
"What do you like most/least about yourself?"

"What do others like?"
"What do you/others want to change about you?"
"What do you enjoy?"
"Has being ill affected how you see yourself?"
Identity
    "What personal achievements have given you satisfaction?"
    "What are your future plans?"
Role responsibilities
    "What do you do for a living? Job responsibilities? Home responsibilities?"
    "Are these satisfying?"
    If the person has had a role change, how has it affected life-style and relationships?
Stress management
    "How do you manage stress?"
    "To whom do you go for help with a problem?"
    Substance abuse?
    Exercise
    Religious convictions
    Problem-solving approach
Support system
    "Any problems in current relationships?"
    "How does your family feel about your illness?" "Do they understand?"
    "Does your family regularly discuss problems?"
Somatic problems
    "Do you feel fearful, anxious or nervous?"
    "Ever have panic spells?"
    "Ever feel like you are falling apart? Dizziness? Aches and pains? Shortness of
        breath? Palpitations? Urinary frequency? Nausea/vomiting? Sleep problems?
        Fatigue? Loss of sexual interest?"
Affect and mood
    "How do you feel now?"
    "How would you describe your usual mood?"
    "What things make you happy/upset?"
    "Have you ever thought of harming yourself?"
Body image
    "What do you like most/least about your body?"
    "What parts are most important to you?"
    "Before you were sick, how did you feel about people who were sick or disabled?"
    "What do you understand to be your health problem?"
    "What limitations do you think will result?"
    "How do you feel about this illness/disability?"
    "Has it changed the way you feel about yourself or the way others respond to you?"
    Children may be able to draw self-portraits.

Objective Data

General appearance
    Facial expression
    Affect
    Hygiene (cleanliness)
    Grooming (clothes, hair, makeup)
    Dress (condition, appropriateness)

Thought processes/content
    Orientation
    Feelings of depersonalization
    Appropriate
    Rambling
    Suspicious
    Homicidal/suicidal ideation
    Sexual preoccupation
    Delusions (grandeur, persecution, reference, influence, or bodily sensations)
    Difficulty concentrating
    Slowed thought processes
Behavior
    Aggressiveness
    Hyperactivity
    Delinquency
    School problems
    Social withdrawal
    Ability for self-care
    Communication patterns
        With significant others
            Relates well
            Hostile
            Dependent
            Demanding
        Physical impairment to communication (*e.g.,* deafness, aphasia, trach)
        Cultural variations in communication (*e.g.,* use of gestures, touch, etc.)
        Decision-making ability
            Indecisive
            Procrastination
    Nutritional status
        Appetite
        Eating patterns
        Weight (gain/loss)
    Rest/sleep pattern
        Recent change
        Early wakefulness
        Insomnia

Principles and Rationale for Nursing Care

Generic Considerations

1. Both the client and the nurse have their own personal self-concept. To deal effectively with others, the nurse must be aware of her own behavior, feelings, attitudes, and responses.
2. Self-concept involves a person's feelings, attitudes, and values and affects his reactions to all experiences.
3. A person's self-concept evolves from infancy through old age. With aging, new skills and challenges emerge. Successful completion of developmental tasks will contribute to a positive self-concept (Fuller & Schaeler-Ayers, 1990).
4. A person's self-concept is influenced by interactions with others, the sociocultural milieu, and developmental task completion (Fuller & Schaeler-Ayers, 1990).

5. The concept of self includes components of body image, self-esteem, role performance, and personal identity.
6. Body image is the mental idea a person has of his body. It is based on past as well as present experience. It is composed of the interrelated phenomena of body surface and depth and the attitudes, emotions, and personality reactions of the individual to his body. It is flexible and subject to change.
7. Alterations in the components of self-concept are described as follows:

   Body image: Viewing oneself differently as a result of actual or perceived changes in body structure or function

   Self-esteem: lack of confidence in ability to accomplish that which is desired

   Role performance: Inability to perform those functions and activities expected of a particular role in a given society

   Personal identity: Disturbance in perception of self ("Who am I?")
8. A nurse's attitude can hinder or facilitate the individual's adaptation to an alteration in self-concept.
9. Intrusive procedures can threaten an individual's sense of wholeness. The nurse should provide a great deal of emotional support during procedures that increase a person's sense of vulnerability.
10. Body image changes constantly. There is often a time lag between the actual body change and the change in body image. The nurse must be aware that during this lag the individual may reject both the diagnosis and the education and treatment prescribed.
11. Body image is influenced during pregnancy in relation to biologic, psychologic, and role changes.

Loss of Body Part/Function

1. The loss of a body part of function is followed by a period of grief and mourning. The grief is similar to that following the loss of any valued object.
2. The process of mourning for the loss of a body part of function may include feelings of helplessness, loneliness, sadness, guilt, and anger. The stages of adaptation to loss include shock and disbelief, anger, depression, and eventual adaption (see *Grieving*).
3. Reorganization of an altered body image is a process of recognition, acceptance, and resolution.

Self-Esteem

1. Self-esteem evolves from a comparison between the self-concept and self-ideal. The greater the congruency, the higher the self-esteem (Stuart & Sundeen, 1987).
2. Self-esteem derives from one's own perceptions of competency and efficacy and from appraisals of others. Generally, people hold positive self-enhancing beliefs about themselves, the world, and the future. These biased perceptions are considerably more positive than objective evidence indicates (Taylor, 1989).
3. The belief that a person can exert personal control in a situation tends to foster good health practices. Conversely, a belief that one usually cannot influence outcomes can result in illness or death. Studies have demonstrated that people led to believe they have control (even when they have none) exhibit dramatic differences in neuroendocrine functioning (Taylor, 1989).
4. High self-esteem is rooted in unconditional acceptance as an innately worthy person (Stuart & Sundeen, 1987). Such persons tend to attribute failures or threatening events to external causes their control—unlike persons with low self-esteem, who tend to attribute failure or threatening events to internal causes (Tenner & Herzberger, 1987).
5. Optimism enhances social relationships and enables a person to make more effective

use of social supports to maintain self-esteem. Supportive friends and family can bolster self-esteem by reinforcing a sense of personal control through suggestions and resources and a sense of confidence (Taylor, 1989).

6. Low self-esteem may be an indicator of susceptibility to depression. Low self-esteem can be a trait in some individuals that is stable over time. For others it can be initiated by a broad range of stressful situations (Tenner & Herzberger, 1987).

7. As self-esteem declines, so does a person's belief that he can exert control over his environment. Likewise, as personal control is perceived to decrease, so does self-esteem (Taft, 1985). Attributing failure to a lack of ability (internal cause) leads to decreased expectations and motivation (Antaki & Brewin, 1982).

8. In response to a threat to a person's self-concept, self-esteem is protected through three cognitive processes:
   a. Searching for meaning in the experience
   b. Regaining mastery over the event; exerting personal control
   c. Self-enhancement ("How am I managing as compared to others?") (Taylor, 1989).

9. The following behaviors are associated with low self-esteem: rigidity; procrastination; repetitive, unnecessary apologies; minimizing one's abilities; emphasizing deficits; expecting failure; self-destructive behaviors; approval-seeking behavior; inability to accept compliments; disregard for one's own opinions; difficulty in forming close relationships; and inability to say no when appropriate (Miller, 1990).

10. Increased social interaction through involvement in groups will enable one to receive social and intellectual stimulation (Taft, 1985), which will enhance self-esteem.

Pediatric Considerations

1. Self-concept is learned. A child's concept of self, for example, emerges as a result of changes occuring during earlier developmental stages (Whiting, 1986).

2. To develop and maintain self-esteem, a child needs to feel worthwhile, different in some way, and superior and more lovable than any other child (Whaley & Wong, 1989).

3. Self-esteem increases as a child develops meaningful relationships and masters developmental tasks. Early adolescence is a time of risk to self-esteem as the adolescent strives to define an identity and sense of self within a peer group (Stuart & Sundeen, 1987).

4. A child's development of body image is based on his own body, which is influenced by present and past perceptions of his body, physiologic functioning, developmental maturation, and the response of others to him (Stuart & Sundeen, 1987).

5. Adolescence is probably the critical period of development for body image formation, as pubertal changes force alteration of the adolescent's body image (Stuart & Sundeen, 1987).

6. The development of a positive body image by age is charted below (Drapo, 1986):

Age	Developmental Task
Birth to 1 year	Learns to tolerate small frustrations
	Learns to trust
1 to 3 years	Learns to like body
	Learns mastery of
	Motor skills
	Language skills
	Bowel training
3 to 6 years	Learns initiative
	Learns sex typing
	Identifies with parent models
	Increases skills (motor, language)

6 to 12 years	Develops a sense of industry
	Has a clear sex role identification
	Learns peer interaction
	Develops academic skills
Adolescence	Establishes self-identity and sexual role
	Utilizes abstract thought
	Develops personal value system

7. A child learns to see himself in the way he is seen by his parents and or significant others (Stuart & Sundeen, 1987).
8. To develop a healthy personality, a child needs a positive and accurate body image, realistic self-ideal, positive self-concept, and high self-esteem (Stuart & Sundeen, 1987).
9. Experiences with and restrictions imposed by chronic illness or disability may interfere with development of healthy self-esteem (Scipien, Chard, Howe, & Barnard, 1990).
10. Obese children and adolescents are at particular risk for developing body image or self-esteem disturbance (Whaley & Wong, 1989).

Gerontologic Considerations

1. According to Miller (1990), self-esteem is "one of the characteristics most highly associated with both depression and happiness" in elderly persons.
2. Self-esteem depends on interactions with others and on others' opinions. In Western societies, a generally negative view of aging can contribute to an elderly person's decreased self-esteem.
3. Many variables interact to produce a decline in self-esteem in the elderly, including negative societal attitudes, decreased social interactions and decreased power and control over the environment (Taft, 1985).
4. Meisenheilder (1985) reported that the following people exert the most significant influence on self-esteem in older adults: spouse, peers (most important for males), authority figures (most important to females), people they live with, and people in the immediate social work and church environment.
5. Environmental factors in long-term care facilities that can influence self-esteem of elderly residents include decor, social roles, choices available, architectural design, space, and privacy (Miller, 1990).
6. Older adults with poor health, high degree of disability, and daily pain report the lowest self-esteem (Hunter, Linn, & Harris, 1981–82).

■ Self-Concept Disturbances
Related to (Specify)

> ### Outcome Criteria
>
> The person will
> - Discuss recent change in feelings about self
> - Identify two positive characteristics

Interventions

Nursing interventions for the variety of problems that might be associated with a diagnosis of *Self-Concept Disturbance* are very similar.

A. Establish a trusting nurse/client relationship

1. Encourage person to express his feelings, especially about the way he feels, thinks, or views himself.
2. Encourage person to ask questions about his health problem, his treatment, his progress, his prognosis.
3. Provide reliable information and reinforce information already given.
4. Clarify any misconceptions the person has about himself, his care, or his care-givers.
5. Avoid negative criticism.
6. Provide privacy and a safe environment.

B. Assess for signs and symptoms

Use the Focus Assessment Criteria to isolate signs and symptoms. Refer to the Defining Characteristics of *Self-Esteem Disturbance, Body Image Disturbance,* and *Altered Role Performance.* After confirmation, utilize Interventions under the category.

C. Initiate health teaching as indicated

1. Teach person what community resources are available, if needed (*e.g.,* mental health centers, such self-help groups as Reach for Recovery, Make Today Count).

Body Image Disturbance

■ *Related to* **(Specify)**

DEFINITION

Body Image Disturbance: The state in which an individual experiences or is at risk to experience a disruption in the way one perceives one's body image.

DEFINING CHARACTERISTICS

Major (must be present)

Verbal or nonverbal negative response to actual or perceived change in structure and/or function

Minor (may be present)

Not looking at body part
Not touching body part

Hiding or overexposing body part
Change in social involvement
Negative feelings about body feelings of helplessness, hopelessness, powerlessness
Preoccupation with change or loss
Refusal to verify actual change
Depersonalization of part or loss

RELATED FACTORS

Pathophysiologic

Chronic disease
Loss of body part
Loss of body function
Severe trauma

Treatment-related

Hospitalization
Surgery
Chemotherapy
Radiation

Situational

Pain
Obesity
Pregnancy
Infertility
Immobility
Cultural influences

Maturational

Adolescent: puberty
Middle age: signs of aging (graying, menopause)
Elderly: losses (people, function, financial)

Diagnostic Considerations

See *Self-Concept Disturbance*

Errors in Diagnostic Statements

See *Self-Concept Disturbance*

Focus Assessment Criteria

See *Self-Concept Disturbance*

Principles and Rationale for Nursing Care

See *Self-Concept Disturbance*

■ Body Image Disturbance
Related to (Specify)

Assessment
See Defining Characteristics

Outcome Criteria

The person will
- Share feelings about how he views himself
- Achieve or maintain control of his body
- Begin to assume role-related responsibilities
- Develop confidence in his ability to accomplish what is desired

---

Interventions

A. Establish a trusting nurse/client relationship
   1. Encourage person to express his feelings, especially about the way he feels, thinks, or views himself.
   2. Encourage person to ask questions about his health problem, his treatment, his progress, his prognosis.
   3. Provide reliable information and reinforce information already given.
   4. Clarify any misconceptions the person has about himself, his care, or his care-givers.
   5. Avoid negative criticism.
   6. Provide privacy and a safe environment.

B. Promote social interaction
   1. Assist person to accept help from others.
   2. Avoid overprotection, but limit the demands made on the individual.
   3. Encourage movement.
   4. Support family as they adapt.
   5. Encourage visits from peers and significant others.
   6. Encourage contact (letters, telephone) with peers and family.
   7. Encourage involvement in unit activities.
   8. Provide opportunity to share with persons going through similar experiences.

C. Provide specific interventions in selected situations
   1. Pregnancy
      a. Encourage the woman to share her concerns.
      b. Attend to each concern if possible or refer her to others for assistance.
      c. Discuss the challenges and changes that pregnancy and motherhood bring.
      d. Encourage her to share expectations: her own and those of her significant others.
      e. Assist her to identify sources for love and affection.

    f. Provide anticipatory guidance to both parents-to-be regarding
- Fatigue and irritability
- Appetite swings
- Gastric disturbances (nausea, constipation)
- Back and leg aches
- Changes in sexual desire
- Mood swings
- Fear (for self, for unborn baby, of loss of attractiveness, of inadequacy as a mother)

    g. Encourage the mutual sharing of concerns between spouses.

2. Hospitalized child

    a. Prepare child for hospitalization, if possible, with an explanation and a visit to the hospital to meet personnel and examine the environment.

    b. Provide child with opportunities to share fears, concerns, anger (see Appendix IX for play therapy guidelines).
- Acknowledge the normalcy of these fears, concerns, anger.
- Correct child's misconceptions (*e.g.,* that he's being punished; that his parents are angry).
- Encourage family to stay with or visit child, despite the child's crying when they leave; teach them to provide accurate information as to when they will return to reduce fears of abandonment.
- Allow parents to help with care.

    c. Assist child to understand his experiences.
- Provide child with an explanation ahead of time, if possible.
- Explain sensations and discomforts of condition, treatments, and medications.
- Encourage crying.

    d. Maintain sense of intactness during periods of immobility.
- Encourage movement, no matter how slight.
- During bath, ask child to identify body parts: "Where is your leg?"
- Allow child access to mirror to provide visualization of body.

3. Loss of body part of function

    a. Assess the meaning of the loss for the individual and significant others, as related to visibility of loss, function of loss, and emotional investment.

    b. Expect the individual to respond to the loss with denial, shock, anger, and depression.

    c. Be aware of the effect of the responses of others to the loss; encourage sharing of feelings between significant others.

    d. Allow individual to ventilate his feelings and to grieve.

    e. Utilize role-playing to assist with sharing; if person says, "I know my husband will not want to touch me with this colostomy," take the husband's role and discuss her colostomy, then switch roles so she can act out her feelings about her husband's response.

    f. Explore realistic alternatives and provide encouragement.

    g. Explore strengths and resources with person.

    h. Assist with the resolution of a surgically created alteration of body image.
- Replace the lost body part with prosthesis as soon as possible.
- Encourage viewing of site.
- Encourage touching of site.

    i. Teach about the health problem and how to manage.

    j. Begin to incorporate person in care of operative site.

      k. Gradually allow person to assume full self-care responsibility, if feasible.

      l. Teach person to monitor own progress (Miller, 1990).

      m. Refer to *Sexual Dysfunction* for additional information, if indicated.

4. Changes associated with chemotherapy (Cooley, 1986)

      a. Discuss the possibility of hair loss, absence of menses, temporary or permanent sterility, decreased estrogen levels, vaginal dryness, mucositis.

      b. Encourage to share concerns, fears and their perception of the impact of these changes on their life.

      c. Explain where hair loss may occur (head, eyelashes, eyebrows, auxiliary hair, pubic and leg hair).

      d. Explain that hair will grow back after treatment but may change in color and texture.

      e. Select a wig prior to hair loss, wear it before hair loss. Consult a beautician for tips on how to vary the look (*e.g.,* combs, clips, etc.).

      f. Encourage the wearing of scarves, turbans when wig is not on.

      g. Teach to minimize the amount of hair loss by
- Avoiding excessive shampooing, using a conditioner twice weekly
- Patting hair dry gently
- Avoiding electric curlers, dryers, and curling irons
- Avoiding pulling hair with bands, clips, or bobby pins
- Avoiding hair spray and hair dye
- Using wide-tooth comb, avoiding vigorous brushing

      h. Refer to American Cancer Society for information regarding new or used wigs. Inform them that the wig is a tax-deductible item.

      i. Discuss the difficulty that others (spouse, friends, coworkers) may have with visible changes.

      j. Encourage the person to initiate calls and contacts with others who may be having difficulty.

      k. Encourage the person to ask for assistance of friends, relatives. Ask person if the situation were reversed, what he or she would want to do to help a friend.

      l. Allow significant others opportunities to share their feelings and fears.

      m. Assist significant others to identify positive aspects of the client and ways this can be shared.

      n. Provide information regarding support groups for couples.

D. Initiate health teaching as indicated

1. Teach person what community resources are available, if needed (*e.g.,* mental health centers, self-help groups such as Reach for Recovery, Make Today Count).
2. Teach wellness strategies (see *Health-Seeking Behaviors*).

Personal Identity Disturbance

DEFINITION
Personal Identity Disturbance: The state in which an individual experiences or is at risk of experiencing an inability to distinguish between self and nonself.

DEFINING CHARACTERISTICS
See Defining Characteristics for *Self-Concept Disturbance* or *Altered Growth and Development*.

Diagnostic Considerations
This nursing diagnosis is a subcategory under *Self-Concept Disturbance*. Until clinical research defines and differentiates this subcategory from others, refer to *Self-Concept Disturbance* or *Altered Growth and Development* for assessment criteria and interventions.

Self-Esteem Disturbance

DEFINITION
Self-Esteem Disturbance: The state in which an individual experiences or is at risk of experiencing negative self-evaluation about self or capabilities.

DEFINING CHARACTERISTICS*
Overt or covert
Self-negating verbalization
Expressions of shame of guilt
Evaluates self as unable to deal with events
Rationalizes away/rejects positive feedback and exaggerates negative feedback about self

*Source: Norris, J., & Kunes-Connell, M. (1987). Self-esteem disturbance: A clinical validation study. In McLane, A. (Ed.). *Classification of nursing diagnoses: Proceedings of the seventh conference*. St. Louis: C. V. Mosby.

Hesitant to try new things/situations
Denial of problems obvious to others
Projection of blame/responsibility for problems
Rationalizes personal failures
Hypersensitivity to slight criticism
Grandiosity

RELATED FACTORS

Self-Esteem Disturbance can be either an episodic event or a chronic problem. Failure to resolve a problem or multiple sequential stresses can result in chronic low self-esteem (CLSE). Those factors, which occur over time and are associated with chronic low self-esteem, are indicated by chronic low self-esteem.

Pathophysiologic

Loss of body parts
Loss of body function(s)
Disfigurement (trauma, surgery, birth defects)

Situational (personal, environmental)

Hospitalization
Loss of job or ability to work
Death of significant other
Separation from significant other
Increase/decrease in weight
Pregnancy
Unemployment
Financial problems
Relationship problems

Marital discord	Step-parents
Separation	In-laws

Failure in school
History of ineffective relationship with own parents (CLSE)
History of abusive relationships (CLSE)
Unrealistic expectations of child by parent (CLSE)
Unrealistic expectations of self (CLSE)
Unrealistic expectations of parent by child (CLSE)
Parental rejection (CLSE)
Overpassiveness (CLSE)
Inconsistent punishment (CLSE)
Legal difficulties
Institutionalization

Mental health facility	Orphanage
Jail	Halfway house

Cultural influences

Ethnic group	Minority

Drug/alcohol abuse by self or family member

Maturational

Infant/toddler/preschool
Lack of stimulation (CLSE)
Separation from parents/significant others (CLSE)
Restriction of activity (CLSE)

Inadequate parental support (CLSE)
Inability to trust significant other (CLSE)
School age
Loss of significant others
Failure to achieve grade level objectives
Loss of peer group
Adolescent
Loss of independence and autonomy
Disruption of peer relationships
Disruption in body image
Interruption of intellectual achievement
Loss of significant others
Career choices
Middle age
Signs of graying
Menopause
Career pressures
Elderly
Losses (people, function, financial, retirement)

Diagnostic Considerations
See *Self-Concept Disturbance*

Errors in Diagnostic Statements
See *Self-Concept Disturbance*

Focus Assessment Criteria
See *Self-Concept Disturbance*

Principles and Rationale for Nursing Care
See *Self-Concept Disturbance*

Chronic Low Self-Esteem

■ *Related to* **(Specify)**

DEFINITION
Chronic Low Self-Esteem: The state in which an individual experiences long-standing negative self-evaluation about the self's capabilities.

DEFINING CHARACTERISTICS*

Major (80–100%)

Long-standing or chronic
  Self-negating verbalization
  Expressions of shame/guilt
  Evaluates self as unable to deal with events
  Rationalizes away/rejects positive feedback and exaggerates negative feedback about
    self
  Hesitant to try new things/situations

Minor (50–79%)
  Frequent lack of success in work or other life events
  Overly conforming, dependent on others' opinions
  Lack of eye contact
  Nonassertive/passive
  Indecisive
  Excessively seeks reassurance

RELATED FACTORS
See *Self-Esteem Disturbance*

Diagnostic Considerations
See *Self-Concept Disturbance*

Errors in Diagnostic Statements
See *Self-Concept Disturbance*

Principles and Rationale for Nursing Care
See *Self-Esteem Disturbance*

■ Chronic Low Self-Esteem
Related to (Specify)

Assessment
See Defining Characteristics

---

* Source: Norris, J., & Kunes-Connell M. (1987). Self-esteem disturbance: A clinical validation study. In McLane, A. (Ed.). *Classification of nursing diagnoses: Proceedings of the seventh conference.* St. Louis: C. V. Mosby.

> **Outcome Criteria**
>
> The individual will
> - Verbalize realistic perceptions of self
> - Identify positive aspects about self
> - Interact appropriately with others
> - Participate in activities

Interventions

A. Assist the person to reduce his present anxiety level
   1. Be supportive, nonjudgmental.
   2. Accept silence, but let him know you are there.
   3. Orient as necessary.
   4. Clarify distortions; do not use confrontation.
   5. Be aware of your own anxiety and avoid communicating it to the individual.
   6. Refer to *Anxiety* for further interventions.

B. Enhance the person's sense of self
   1. Be attentive.
   2. Respect his personal space.
   3. Validate your interpretation of what he is saying or experiencing ("Is this what you mean?").
   4. Help him to verbalize what he is expressing nonverbally.
   5. Use communication that helps to maintain his own individuality ("I" instead of "we").
   6. Pay attention to person, especially new behavior.
   7. Provide encouragement as a task or skill is attempted.
   8. Provide realistic positive feedback on accomplishments.
   9. Teach person to consensually validate with others.
   10. Respect need for privacy.
   11. Provide consistency among staff (Miller, 1990).

C. Assist person in expressing his thoughts and feelings
   1. Use open-ended statements and questions.
   2. Encourage expression of both positive and negative statements.
   3. Use movement, art, and music as means of expression.
   4. If person has impaired reality-testing ability, refer to *Altered Thought Processes* for further interventions.

D. Provide opportunities for positive socialization
   1. Encourage visits/contact with peers and significant others (letters, telephone).
   2. Be a role model in one-to-one interactions.
   3. Involve in activities, especially when strengths can be utilized.
   4. Do not allow person to isolate self (refer to *Social Isolation* for further interventions).
   5. Involve in supportive group therapy.
   6. Teach social skills as required (refer to *Impaired Social Interaction* for further interventions).
   7. Encourage participation with others sharing similar experiences.

E. Set limits on problematic behavior such as aggression, poor hygiene, ruminations and suicidal preoccupation

Refer to *High Risk for Self-Harm* and/or *High Risk for Violence* if these are assessed as problems.

F. Provide for development of social and vocational skills
   1. Reinforce confidence as person demonstrates new skills.
   2. Refer for vocational counseling.
   3. Involve in volunteer organizations.
   4. Encourage participation in senior citizens groups.
   5. Arrange for continuation of education (*e.g.*, literacy class, GEDs, vocational training, art/music classes).

G. Assist in self-exploration as anxiety and trust permit
   1. Identify positive self-evaluation.
   2. Assess self-appraisal.
   3. Refer to *Situational Low Self-Esteem* for specific interventions.

Situational Low Self-Esteem

■ *Related to* **(Specify)**

DEFINITION

Situational Low Self-Esteem: The state in which an individual who previously had positive self-esteem experiences negative feelings about self in response to an event (loss, change).

DEFINING CHARACTERISTICS*

Major (80–100%)

   Episodic occurrence of negative self-appraisal in response to life events in a person with a previous positive self-evaluation
   Verbalization of negative feelings about self (helplessness, uselessness)

Minor (50–79%)

   Self-negating verbalizations
   Expressions of shame/guilt
   Evaluates self as unable to handle situations/events
   Difficulty making decisions

---

*Source: Norris, J., & Kunes-Connell, M. (1987). Self-esteem disturbance: A clinical validation study. In McLane, A. (Ed.). *Classification of nursing diagnoses: Proceedings of the seventh conference.* St. Louis: C. V. Mosby.

RELATED FACTORS
See *Self-Esteem Disturbance*

Errors in Diagnostic Statements
See *Self-Concept Disturbance*

Principles and Rationale for Nursing Care
See *Self-Esteem Disturbance*

■ Situational Low Self-Esteem
Related to (Specify)

Assessment
See Defining Characteristics

Outcome Criteria

The person will
- Identify positive aspects of self
- Express a positive outlook for the future
- Analyze his own behavior and its consequences
- Identify ways of exerting control and influencing outcomes

Interventions

A. Assist the individual in identifying and expressing feelings
   1. Be empathetic, nonjudgmental.
   2. Listen. Do not discourage expressions of anger, crying, and so forth.
   3. What was happening when he began feeling this way?
   4. Clarify relationships between life events.

B. Assist in identifying positive self-evaluations
   1. How has he handled other crises?
   2. How does he manage anxiety, exercise, withdrawal, drinking/drugs, talking?
   3. Reinforce adaptive coping mechanisms.

4. Examine and reinforce positive abilities and traits (*e.g.*, hobbies, skills, school, relationships, appearance, loyalty, industriousness, etc.).
5. Help individual accept both positive and negative feelings.
6. Do not confront defenses.
7. Communicate confidence in person's ability.
8. Involve person in mutual goal-setting.
9. Have clients write positive true statements about themselves (for their eyes only); have them read the list daily as a part of their normal routine (Grainger, 1990).

C. Explore relationship between behavior and self-appraisals
1. Encourage examination of current behavior and its consequences (*e.g.*, dependency, procrastination, isolation).
2. Assist in mutually identifying faulty perceptions.
3. Assist in identifying unrealistic expectations.
4. Help to identify negative automatic thoughts. ("I will never be able to do this.")
5. Examine if person is overgeneralizing. ("If I can't do this, then I'm a failure at everything.")
6. Assist in identifying own responsibility and control in a situation (*e.g.*, when continually blaming others for problems).

D. Assess and mobilize current support system
1. Does he live alone? Employed?
2. Does he have available friends and relatives?
3. Is the church a support?
4. Has he previously used community resources?
5. Refer to vocational rehabilitation for retraining.
6. Support returning to school for further training.
7. Assist in involving in local volunteer organizations (senior citizens employment, Foster Grandparents, local support groups).
8. Arrange continuation of school studies for students.

E. Assist individual in learning new coping skills
1. Teach about how persons respond to a life change.
2. Let him know he is not alone.
3. Assist in identifying options (*e.g.*, saying no, time off).
4. Refer to Appendix VII, Guidelines for Problem-Solving and Crisis Intervention.
5. Refer to Appendix X, Stress Management Techniques.
6. Encourage trail of new behavior.
7. Reinforce the belief that the individual does have control over the situation.

F. Assist person in managing specific problems
1. Rape—refer to *Rape-Trauma Syndrome*.
2. Loss—refer to *Grieving*.
3. Hospitalization—refer to *Powerlessness* and *Parental Role Conflict*.
4. Ill family member—refer to *Altered Family Processes*.
5. Change or loss of body part—refer to *Body Image Disturbance*.
6. Depression—refer to *Ineffective Individual Coping* and *Hopelessness*.
7. Domestic violence—refer to *Ineffective Family Coping*.

References/Bibliography

Antaki, C., & Bruoin, C. (Eds.). (1982). *Attributions and psychological change.* London: Academic Press.

Crouch, M. A., & Straub, V. (1983). Enhancement of self-esteem in adults. *Family Community Health, 6*(2), 76–78.

Cooley, M. E., Yeomans, A., & Cobb, S. (1986). Sexual and reproductive issues for women with Hodgkins disease. *Cancer Nursing, 9,* 248–255.

Drapo, P. J. (1986). Mental retardation. In Johnson, B. S. *Adaptation and growth.* Philadelphia: J. B. Lippincott, p. 443.

Fuller, J., & Schaelar-Ayers, J. (1990). *Health assessment: A nursing approach.* Philadelphia: J. B. Lippincott.

Gilberts, R. (1983). The evaluation of self-esteem. *Family Community Health, (8),* 29–49.

Grainger, R. (1990). How to feel good about being you. *American Journal of Nursing, 90*(4), 14.

Harris, M. (1986). Helping the person with an altered self-image. *Geriatric Nursing, 7*(2), 90–92.

Hunter, K, Linn, M., & Harris, R. (1981–82). Characteristics of high and low self-esteem in the elderly. *International Journal of Aging and Human Development, 14*(2), 117–126.

Meisenhelder, J. B. (1985). Self-esteem: A closer look at clinical interventions. *International Journal of Nursing Studies, 22*(2), 127–135.

Miller, C. A. (1990). *Nursing care of older adults.* Glenview, IL: Scott, Foresman.

Miller, S. (1987). Promoting self-esteem in the hospitalized adolescents: Clinical interventions. *Issues of Comprehensive Pediatric Nursing, 10*(3), 187–194.

Murray, R. (1972). The concept of body image. *Nursing Clinics of North America, 7*(4), 593–707.

Norris, J., & Kunes-Connell, M. (1985). Self-esteem disturbance. *Nursing Clinics of North America, 20*(12), 745–761.

Reasoner, R. W. (1983). Enhancement of self-esteem in children and adolescents. *Family Community Health, 6*(2), 51–63.

Scipien, G. M., Chard, M. A., Howe, J., & Barnard, M. U. (1990). *Pediatric nursing care.* St. Louis: C. V. Mosby.

Showalter J. E. Lord, R. D. (1971). The hospitalized adolescent. *Children, 18*(4), 127–132.

Stuart, G., & Sundean, S. (1987). *Principles and practice of psychiatric nursing* (3rd ed.). St. Louis: C. V. Mosby.

Taft L. B. (1985). Self-esteem in later life: A nursing perspective. *Advances in Nursing Science, 8*(1), 77–84.

Taylor, S. (1983). Adjustment to threatening events: A theory of cognitive adaptation. *American Psychologist, 38*(8), 1161–1173.

Taylor, S. (1989). *Positive illusions.* New York: Basic Books.

Tennen, H., & Herzberger, S. (1987). Depression, self-esteem and the absence of self-protective attributional biases. *Journal of Personality and Social Psychology, 52*(2), 72–80.

Utz, S. W., Hammer, J., Whitmire, V. M., & Grass, S. (1990). Perceptions of body image and health status in persons with mitral valve prolapse. *Image, 22*(1), 18–22.

Whaley, L. F., & Wong, D. L. (1989). *Essentials of pediatric nursing* (3rd ed.). St. Louis: C. V. Mosby.

Whiting, S. M. A. (1986). Development of the person. In Johnson, B. S. *Adaptation and growth.* Philadelphia: J. B. Lippincott, p. 61.

Willard, A. (1990). Personal communication.

Self-Harm, High Risk for*

■ *Related to* **(Specify)**

DEFINITION
High Risk for Self-Harm: A state in which an individual is at risk for inflicting direct harm on himself or herself.

DEFINING CHARACTERISTICS
Suicidal ideation

Minor (may be present)

Severe stress

Depression

Hallucinations/delusions

Hostility

Substance abuse

Low self-esteem

Hopelessness

Acute agitation

Poor impulse control

Lack of a support system

Helplessness

RELATED FACTORS
High Risk for Self-Harm can occur as a response to a variety of health problems, situations, and conflicts. Some sources are listed.

Pathophysiologic

Terminal illness

Chronic illness (*e.g.,* diabetes, hypertension)

Alcoholism

Organic mental disorder

Chronic pain

Treatment-related

Dialysis

Insulin injections or any ongoing treatments

Chemotherapy/radiation

Ingestion of prescribed or nonprescribed drugs

Situational

Parental/marital conflict

Job loss

Divorce/separation

Threatened or actual financial loss

Alcoholism/drug abuse in family

Wish to reunite with loved one who has died

Inadequate coping skills

Depression

Death of significant other

Loss of status, prestige

Someone leaving home

Child abuse

Threat of abandonment by significant other

---

*This diagnosis is not currently on the NANDA list but has been included for clarity or usefulness.

Maturational

> Adolescent: Separation from family, peer pressure, role changes, identity crisis, loss of significant support person, family or romantic problems
> Adult: Marital conflict, parenting, loss of family member, role changes
> Elderly: Retirement, social isolation, loss of spouse

Diagnostic Considerations

High Risk for Self-Harm currently is not on the NANDA list but has been added here for clarity. *High Risk for Violence to Self* is included under *High Risk for Violence.* The term violence is defined as a swift and intense force or a rough or injurious physical force. As you know, suicide can be either violent or nonviolent (*e.g.*, overdose of barbiturates). Using the term violence in this diagnostic context unfortunately can lead to nondetection of a person at risk for suicide due to the perception that the person is not capable of violence.

High Risk for Self-Harm clearly denotes a person as high risk for suicide and in need for protection. Treatment of this diagnosis involves validating the risk, contracting with the person, and providing protection. Treatment of the person's underlying depression and hopelessness should be addressed with other applicable nursing diagnoses; *e.g., Ineffective Individual Coping, Hopelessness.*

Errors in Diagnostic Statements

High Risk for Self-Harm related to recent diagnosis of cancer

In this situation, the recent diagnosis of cancer in itself is not a risk factor for suicide. The person must be depressed and severely stressed and exhibit suicidal intentions. The nurse must not automatically label a person as suicidal based on a single crisis or severe physical disability. All *High Risk for Self-Harm* diagnostic statements must contain both verbal and nonverbal cues to suicidal intent, *e.g., High Risk for Self-Harm related to remarks about life being unbearable and reports of giving belongings away.*

Focus Assessment Criteria

Information must be gathered from the individual and at least one significant other. The nurse must not be reluctant to ask questions about suicide. Persons with no suicidal thoughts cannot be led to suicidal thoughts through questioning. Questions to assess a person's risk for suicide should focus on encouraging sharing of feelings and perceptions of the future. Questions such as "Have you ever thought of committing suicide?" are not useful because they usually evoke a yes or no answer with no description of the person's feelings.

Subjective Data

1. Psychologic status
   a. Present concerns
      - What are you thinking about?
      - What is on your mind?
      - What brought you here?
   b. Assess for feelings of:
      - Hopelessness
      - Isolation/abandonment

- Anger, hostility
- Helplessness
- Guilt, shame
- Suicide as a viable alternative

c. Suicidal ideation
- Do you ever think
  Life is not worth living?
  About escaping from your problems?
  About harming yourself?
  How you would harm yourself?
  Under what circumstances you would act on your plan?
- Assess for a suicide plan
  Method: Is there a specific plan (pills, wrist-slashing, shooting, etc.); plans for rescue?
  Availability: Is the method accessible? Is access easy or difficult?
  Specificity: How specific is plan?
  Lethality: How lethal is the method?

d. Recent changes in behavior

e. History of psychiatric problems
- Outpatient treatment
- Previous attempts
  Number
  Recency
  Lethality
- Hospitalization

2. Medical status
  a. Acute or chronic illness—how is it affecting life?
  b. Has person consulted physician in past 6 months?
  c. History of alcoholism/drug abuse?

3. Sources of stress in current environment
  a. Job change/loss
  b. Failure in work/school
  c. Threat of financial loss
  d. Divorce/separation
  e. Death of significant other
  f. Illness/accident
  g. Threat of criminal prosecution
  h. Alcohol/drug use in family

4. Coping strategies (past and present)
  a. Assess ability of individual and family to cope with repeated stresses
  b. Available resources
  c. Level of impulse control
  d. Taking unnecessary risks (drugs, alcohol)

5. Support system
  a. Who is relied on during periods of stress?
  - Are they available?
  - Their reaction to current situation
    Denial of problem
    Not receptive to helping now
    Anger, guilt
    Helplessness, frustration
    Concern and willingness to help

b. Personal and financial resources
   Employment   Financial problems
   Housing

Objective Data

1. General appearance
   Facial expression   Dress
   Posture
2. Behavior during interview
   Withdrawn   Quiet
   Hostile   Cooperative
   Hopeless
3. Communication pattern (subjective/objective)
   Content
      Appropriate   Tangential/allusive
      Denial of problem   Suspicions
      Delusions (grandeur,   Hopelessness ("It's hopeless; it's
         persecution)   the end of the road")
      Suicidal thoughts ("I may as Negative cognitive set
         well be dead"; "I wish I
         were dead")
   Pattern of speech
      Appropriate   Jumps from one topic to another
      Blocking of ideas   Unable to come to a decision
      Ideas loosely connected   Unable to see alternatives (tunnel
                                      vision)

   Rate of speech
      Appropriate   Reduced
      Excessive   Pressured
   Reaction of significant others
      Ignoring suicidal expressions   Anger at expressions
      Leaving or turning away
         following expression
4. Activities of daily living
   Capable of caring for self   Impaired ability to care for self
5. Nutritional status
   Weight (increased, decreased)   Appetite
6. Sleep/rest pattern
   Recent change   Early wakefulness
   Insomnia   Sleeps too much
7. Personal hygiene
   Cleanliness   Clothes (condition, appropri-
   Grooming   ateness)
8. Motor activity
   Within normal limits   Increased
   Decreased   Agitated
   Repetitive
9. Evidence of self-harm
   Wrist slashes   Eye enucleation
   Burns on body   Gunshot wound
   Broken bones   Overdose

Principles and Rationale for Nursing Care

See also *Hopelessness*

Generic Considerations

1. Self-destructive behavior ranges from indirect acts (obesity, noncompliance with medical treatment) to direct acts of self-destruction. Indirect self-destructive behavior has the potential to be harmful and result in death; however, the person is unaware of this potential. With direct self-destructive behavior, usually referred to as suicidal, the intent is death, and the individual is aware.
2. Suicidal behavior is an attempt to escape from intolerable life stressors that have accumulated over time. It is accompanied by intense feelings of hopelessness (Shneidman, 1989).
3. Both the individual and the family have exhausted their resources.
4. A suicidal crisis happens both to the individual and to the person's support system.
5. Suicide may be seen as a viable alternative both by the individual and by significant others.
6. Situations that contribute to suicidal behavior include depression, loss (significant other, job, finances), debilitating disease, and alcohol/drug abuse.
7. Persons exhibiting poor reality testing, delusions, and poor impulse control are at high risk. Alcohol and drugs tend to lower impulse control.
8. Suicidal individuals are usually ambivalent about the decision. Staff can work with the positive goals to effect a change in attitude (Shneidman, 1989).
9. Changes in behavior (*e.g.*, giving away possessions) may signal an increase in risk. Individuals may appear to be better just prior to an attempt. This may be due to feelings of relief after making a decision.
10. Older men will seldom seek help from mental health agencies. Families, senior citizen centers, clergy, and physicians are the network that can most readily identify the potential problem.
11. Demographic factors can serve the caregiver in identifying people who are at risk for suicidal behavior (Jacobs, 1989).
    a. Suicide increases with age to a peak at about 50 years for white men.
    b. Adolescents also represent a high-risk group.
    c. More women attempt suicide, but men complete suicide more often.
    d. Unemployment and frequent job changes are associated with an increased risk.
    e. Alcohol is associated with a high risk.
    f. The greater the satisfaction with social relationships, the lower the risk will be; thus, divorce, separation, and widowhood increase the risk.
    g. Previous attempts place the person in a high-risk group, since they are likely to repeat the attempt.
12. The suicide rate among psychiatric inpatients markedly exceeds the general suicide rate (Modestin & Kopp, 1988).
13. The more resources are available, the more likely the crisis can be effectively managed. This includes personal support systems, employment, physical and mental abilities, finances, and housing.
14. Some individuals use suicide attempts as a way to cope with stress. The more frequent the attempts and the more lethal, the higher is the current risk.
15. To assess more accurately the risk for suicide, the caregiver must question the person directly. Ask simple, straightforward questions. The more specific, more lethal, more available the means, the higher is the present risk. The most lethal methods in our culture are shooting and hanging. The least lethal is wrist-slashing.

16. Long-term suicide risk exists for some people. This can be assessed best by evaluating
    a. Their coping strategies when confronted with stress
    b. Their life-style—is it stable or unstable?
    c. The specificity and lethality of the plan
17. Interventions are based on the type of risk the person presents. Long-term treatment is often more difficult to institute than emergency care.
18. Caregivers can become immobilized or drained by the acutely suicidal person. Feelings of hopelessness are often communicated to the caregiver. Self-awareness and use of consultation can help prevent negative consequences.
19. Use verbal and nonverbal clues to assess risk, since seriously suicidal persons may deny suicidal thoughts.
20. Prediction of suicide risk is not an exact science. Some of the errors that can be made result from:
    a. Overreliance on mood as an indicator since not all persons who commit suicide are clinically depressed
    b. Reliance on intuition, as many persons can totally conceal their intention
    c. Failure to assess support system
    d. Counter-transference, particularly the failure of the therapist to acknowledge negative feelings that are aroused (Maltsberger, 1986)
21. Levels of risk can be assessed as low or high. Not all of the following parameters are necessarily present in any one individual (Hatton & Valente, 1977).
    a. High
       - Adolescent or over 45
       - Divorced, separated, widowed
       - Professional worker
       - Chronic or terminal illness
       - Delusions/hallucinations
       - Hopelessness/helplessness
       - Intoxicated or addicted
       - Frequent or constant suicidal thoughts
       - Means—readily available
       - Male
       - Isolated socially
       - Unemployed or lack of stable job history
       - Severe depression
       - Severe anxiety
       - Multiple attempts
       - With a specific plan, method is highly lethal
    b. Low
       - 25 to 45 years of age or under 12
       - Married
       - Blue-collar worker
       - No serious medical problems
       - No specific plan, or has a plan with low lethality
       - Female
       - Socially active
       - Employed
       - Infrequent substance abuse
       - Thoughts are fleeting (if person has a vague plan)

Pediatric Considerations

1. Suicide is the second leading cause of death during adolescence. A significant trend is the rise among persons in the younger age groups (Whaley & Wong, 1989).
2. Suicide in children and adolescents may occur because of problems coping with stress, family dysfunction, and psychosis (Whaley & Wong, 1989).
3. Depression may be masked by a wide range of somatic complaints and behaviors. This could include social withdrawal, irritability, school problems, and aggression (Whaley & Wong, 1989).

Gerontologic Considerations

1. Caucasian males over age 60 have a suicide rate twice the rate in all other age groups. They comprise 18.5% of the population but commit 23% of all suicides (U.S. Bureau of the Census, 1984).
2. The self-esteem of older men is negatively affected by retirement, loss of vigor, and loss of a meaningful role (Boxwell, 1988).
3. The elderly tend to complete suicide when attempted. The rate of attempts to completion is 4:1 while for younger persons, the ratio is approximately 200:1 (McIntosh, 1985).
4. Alcohol contributes to depression. Depression increases alcohol use. Both are significant risk factors for suicide in older adults (Blazer, 1982).
5. Depressed older adults generally talk less about suicide than younger adults, but use more violent means and are more successful (Miller, 1990).
6. Suicidal potential often is overlooked due to the prevalent view that older adults are generally passive and nonviolent. In addition, complaints about depression and hopelessness may be subtle and thus easily ignored in older adults (Miller, 1990).

■ High Risk for Self-Harm
Related to (Specify)

Assessment
See Defining Characteristics

Outcome Criteria

The person will
- Not harm self
- State the desire to live
- Verbalize feelings of anger, loneliness, hopelessness
- Identify persons to contact if suicide thoughts occur
- Identify alternative coping mechanisms

Interventions

A. Assist the person in reducing his present risk for self-destruction

1. Assess level of present risk (see Principles and Rationale for Nursing Care for specific differentiation).
   a. High   b. Moderate   c. Low
2. Assess level of long-term risk.
   a. Life-style   b. Lethality of plan   c. Usual coping mechanisms

3. Provide a safe environment based on level of risk.
   Immediate management for high-risk person
   a. Acutely suicidal persons should be admitted to a closely supervised environment.
   b. Although it is impossible to create a completely safe environment, removal of dangerous objects and close observation convey a nonverbal message of concern to the individual. Restrict glass, nail files, scissors, nail polish remover, mirrors, needles, razors, soda cans, plastic bags, lighters, electric equipment, belts, hangers, knives, tweezers, alcohol, guns.
   c. Meals should be provided in a closely supervised area, usually on the unit or in individual's own room.
      • Ensure adequate food and fluid intake.
      • Use paper/plastic plates and utensils.
      • Check to be sure all items are returned on the tray.
   d. When administering oral medications, check to ensure that all medications are swallowed.
   e. Designate a staff member to provide checks on the person as designated by institution's policy. Provide relief for the staff member.
   f. Restrict the individual to the unit unless specifically ordered by physician. When off unit, provide a staff member to accompany the person.
   g. Instruct visitors on restricted items. Ensure that they do not give the person food in a plastic bag, for example.
   h. Restricted items may be used by individual in presence of staff, depending on level of risk. Acutely suicidal persons should not be allowed access to such items.
   i. The acutely suicidal person may be required to wear a hospital gown to prevent elopement. As risk decreases, client may be allowed own clothing.
   j. Room searches should be done periodically according to institution policy.
   k. Utilize seclusion and restraint if necessary (refer to *High Risk for Violence* for discussion).
   l. Notify police if the person elopes and is at risk for suicide.
   m. When the individual is being constantly observed, he is not to be allowed out of sight even though privacy is lost.
4. Notify all staff that this person is at risk for self-harm.
   a. Use both written and oral communication.
5. Make a no-suicide contract with the individual (include family if person is at home).
   a. Use a written contract.
   b. Mutual agreement
      • "I will not kill myself" or "I will not accidentally or intentionally take medicine except according to instructions." "I will talk to a staff member about my thoughts when suicidal ideas increase."

B. Help build self-esteem
   1. Be nonjudgmental and empathetic.
   2. Be aware of own reactions to the situation.
   3. Provide genuine praise.
   4. Encourage interactions with others.
   5. Divert attention to external world (*e.g.,* odd jobs).
   6. Convey sense that he is not alone (use group or peer therapy).
   7. Seek out person for interactions.

8. Set limits by informing of rules.
9. Use firm, consistent approach.
10. Provide planned daily schedules to persons with low impulse control.

C. Assist in identifying and contacting support system

1. Inform family and significant others.
2. Enlist support.
3. Do not provide false reassurance that behavior will not recur.
4. Point out vague or unclear messages from individual or support system.
5. Encourage an increase in social activity.

D. Assist individual in developing positive coping mechanism

1. Refer to *Anxiety, Ineffective Individual Coping,* and *Hopelessness* for further interventions.
2. Encourage appropriate expression of anger and hostility.
3. Set limits on ruminations about suicide or previous attempts.
4. Assist in recognizing predisposing factors: "What was happening before you started having these thoughts?"
5. Facilitate examination of life stresses and past coping mechanisms.
6. Explore alternative behaviors.
7. Anticipate future stresses and assist in planning alternatives.
8. Use appropriate behavior modification techniques for noncompliant, resistive persons.
9. Help identify negative thinking patterns and direct person to practice altering these patterns.
10. Involve person in planning the treatment goals and evaluating progress.

E. Initiate health teaching and referrals when indicated

1. Provide teaching that will prepare person to deal with life stresses (relaxation, problem-solving skills, how to express feelings constructively).
2. Refer for peer or group therapy.
3. Refer for family therapy, especially when child or adolescent is involved.
4. Teach family limit-setting techniques.
5. Teach family constructive expression of feelings.
6. Instruct significant others in how to recognize an increase in risk: change in behavior, verbal, nonverbal communication, withdrawal, signs of depression.
7. Supply phone number of 24-hour emergency hotlines.
8. Refer to vocational training if appropriate.
9. Refer to halfway houses or other agencies, as appropriate.
10. Refer to ongoing psychiatric follow-up.
11. Refer to senior citizen centers or other agencies to increase leisure time activities.

References/Bibliography

Blazer, D. G. (1982). *Depression in late life.* St. Louis: C. V. Mosby.
Blythe, M., & Pearlmutter, D. (1983). The suicidal watch: A re-examination of maximum observation. *Perspectives on Psychiatric Care, 21*(3), 90–93.
Boxwell, A. (1988). Geriatric suicide, the preventable death. *Nurse Practitioners, 13*(6), 10–14.
Bydlon-Brown, B., & Billman, R. (1988). At risk for suicide. *American Journal of Nursing, 88*(10), 1359–1361.

Gilead, M., & Muliak, J. (1983) Adolescent suicide: A response to developmental crisis. *Perspectives on Psychiatric Care, 21*(3), 94–101.

Hatton, C., & Valente, S. (1977). Assessment of suicidal risk. In Hatton, C. (Ed.). *Suicide: Assessment and intervention.* New York: Appleton-Century-Crofts.

Hradek, E. (1988). Crisis intervention and suicide. *Journal of Psychosocial Nursing, 26*(5), 24–27.

Jacobs, D. (1989). Evaluation and care of suicidal behavior in emergency settings. In Jacobs, D., & Brown, H. (Eds.). *Suicide: Understanding and responding.* Madison, CT: International University Press.

Maltsberger, J. (1986). *Suicide risk.* New York: University Press.

McIntosh, J. L. (1985). Suicide among the elderly: Levels and trends. *American Journal of Orthopsychiatry, 55*(4), 2, 288–293.

Miller, C. A. (1990). *Nursing care of older adults.* Glenview, IL: Scott, Foresman.

Modestin, J., & Kopp, N. (1988). A study of clinical suicide. *Journal of Nervous and Mental Disease, 176,* 668–673.

Richman, J. (1986). *Family therapy for suicidal people.* New York: Springer-Verlag.

Shneidman, E. (1989). Overview: A multidimensional approach to suicide. In Jacobs, D., & Brown, H. (Eds.). *Suicide: Understanding and responding.* Madison, CT: International University Press.

U.S. Bureau of the Census. (1984). *Statistical abstracts of the United States:* 1985, 105th ed. Washington, DC, pp. 75–79.

Valente, S. (1985). The suicidal teenager. *Nursing, 15*(12), 47–50.

Whaley, L. F., & Wong, D. L. (1989). *Essentials of pediatric nursing* (3rd ed.). St. Louis: C. V. Mosby.

Whall, A. (1985) Suicide in older adults. *Journal of Gerontological Nursing, 11*(8), 40.

Sensory–Perceptual Alterations

■ *Related to* **Sensory Overload**

DEFINITION

Sensory–Perceptual Alterations: A state in which the individual/group experiences or is at risk of experiencing a change in the amount, pattern, or interpretation of incoming stimuli.

DEFINING CHARACTERISTICS

Major (must be present)

Inaccurate interpretation of environmental stimuli and/or negative change in amount or pattern of incoming stimuli

Minor (may be present)

Disoriented in time or place	Restlessness
Disoriented about people	Reports auditory or visual
Altered ability to problem-solve	hallucinations
Altered behavior or communication	Fear
pattern	Anxiety
Sleep pattern disturbances	Apathy

RELATED FACTORS

Many factors in an individual's life can contribute to sensory–perceptual alterations. Some common factors are listed below.

Pathophysiologic

Sensory organ alterations (visual, gustatory, hearing, olfactory, and tactile deficits)
Neurologic alterations

Cerebrovascular accident (CVA)	Neuropathies
Encephalitis meningitis	

Metabolic alterations

Fluid and electrolyte imbalance	Acidosis
Elevated blood urea nitrogen (BUN)	Alkalosis

Impaired oxygen transport

Cerebral	Respiratory
Cardiac	Anemia

Musculoskeletal changes

Paraplegia	Quadriplegia

Treatment-related

Amputation
Medications (sedatives, tranquilizers)
Surgery (glaucoma, cataract, detached retina)

Physical isolation (reverse isolation, communicable disease, prison)
Radiation therapy
Immobility
Mobility restrictions (bedrest, traction, casts, Stryker frame, Circoelectric bed)

Situational (personal, environmental)

Social isolation (terminal or infectious patient)
Pain
Stress
Environment (noise pollution, ICU)

Diagnostic Considerations

Sensory–Perceptual Alterations describes a person with altered perception and cognition influenced by physiologic factors; *e.g.,* pain, sleep deprivation, immobility, or excessive or decreased meaningful environmental stimuli. Keep in mind that the diagnosis *Altered Thought Processes* also can manifest with altered perception and cognition. To differentiate between the two diagnoses, remember that *Sensory–Perceptual Alterations* applies when barriers or factors interfere with a person's ability to accurately interpret stimuli; in contrast, when personality or mental disorders interfere with this ability, *Altered Thought Processes* would be a more accurate diagnosis.

The diagnosis *Sensory–Perceptual Alterations* encompasses six subcategories: *Visual, Auditory, Kinesthetic, Gustatory, Tactile,* and *Olfactory.* Use of these subcategories can pose some problems in clinical situations, for example, for a person with a visual deficit, how does the nurse intervene with a diagnosis such as *Sensory–Perceptual Alterations: Visual related to effects of glaucoma?* What would the outcome criteria be? The nurse should assess for the individual's response to the visual loss and specifically label the response, not the deficit.

Sensory–Perceptual Alterations is more clinically useful without the addition of the sensory deficit. Examples of responses to sensory deficits may be:

Visual:	*High Risk for Injury*
	Self-Care Deficit
Auditory:	*Impaired Communication*
	Social Isolation
Kinesthetic:	*High Risk for Injury*
Olfactory:	*Altered Nutrition*
Tactile:	*High Risk for Injury*
Gustatory:	*Altered Nutrition*

Errors in Diagnostic Statements

Sensory–Perceptual Alterations related to impairment of sensory tracts secondary to spinal cord injury

A person suffering spinal cord injury experiences several responses related to loss of sensation, which can be described and addressed by diagnoses such as *High Risk for Injury, Diversional Activity Deficit,* and *Sensory–Perceptual Alterations.* If the nursing focus is to increase meaningful sensory input because of loss of sensation, immobility, and position restrictions, the diagnosis should be recorded as *Sensory–Perceptual Alterations related to decreased visual field when prone and inadequate tactile stimulation.*

Sensory–Perceptual Alterations: Visual related to altered sensory reception
   Visual deficits can contribute to a variety of responses, including fear, high risk for injury, self-care deficits, and sensory deprivation. Using *Sensory–Perception Alterations* to rename a visual or hearing deficit fails to clarify a problem that the nurse can treat.

Focus Assessment Criteria

Subjective Data

History of symptoms
   The person reports
      Difficulty concentrating   Fatigue or irritability
      Anxiety   Unusual sensations
   Onset and description
      Precipitated by?   Frequency?
      Relieved by?
Assess for presence or history of
      Recent surgery   Change in biorhythm pattern
      Recent hospitalization   Mobility restrictions
      Neurologic impairment   Social isolation
      Sensory organ deficit   Substance abuse (drugs, alcohol)

Objective Data

Assess sensory acuity
   Visual
      Snellen chart
      Newspaper clippings and large lettered index cards
      Aids (contact lenses, glasses)
   Auditory
      Observation of client during normal conversation
      Use of hearing aids
   Tactile
      Thermal sensation
      Sensitivity
   Olfactory/gustatory
Assess for the presence of factors that contribute to sensory–perceptual alterations
   Sensory deprivation (isolation, lack of visitors)
   Sensory overload (noise, personnel)
   Physiologic alterations
   Medication (side-effects, toxic levels)
   Sleep deprivation
   Fluid, electrolyte, nutritional imbalances
   Crisis, fears, losses

Principles and Rationale for Nursing Care

Generic Considerations

1. Receiving (reception) and accurately interpreting (perception) incoming stimuli from the environment are essential for survival.
2. People receive information via their five senses. Deficits in one or more senses can alter perception.

3. The five senses can be organized into close (olfactory, gustatory, and tactile) and distant (auditory and visual). When an individual is deprived of a distant sense, he becomes more dependent on the close senses. A blind person will develop a keener sense of touch than a sighted person.
4. Individuals adapt to the stimuli from their internal and external environments. The capacity for this adaptation varies with individuals and also varies at times in the same individual.
5. A disruption in the quality or quantity of incoming stimuli can affect an individual's physiologic, emotional, cognitive, and affective domains.
6. Manifestations of sensory deprivation vary with an individual's adaptation ability. Some common manifestations are generalized anxiety, perceptual distortions, inability to think and reason, distortion of time sense, vivid imagery, and illusions and hallucinations.
7. The quality and quantity of sensory input are reduced by immobility or confinement.
8. The elderly are more prone to develop sensory deprivation due to loneliness, physical isolation, and the increased incidence of chronic disabilities experienced during this life stage.
9. An illness state may decrease the efficiency of the sensory organs and thus alter an organism's capacity for adequate reception and perception of information.
10. Sensory overload produces the problem of sensory bombardment and also blocks out meaningful stimuli, thus concurrently producing sensory deprivation.
11. Refer to Principles and Rationale for Nursing Care for *Altered Thought Processes* for additional information.

Pediatric Considerations

1. The newborn has well-developed sensory abilities that have an important effect on growth and development (Whaley & Wong, 1989):
   a. Newborns demonstrate discrimination between patterns, sizes, and shapes but lack accommodation to distance.
   b. Newborns respond to sound stimuli by alerting, crying, and the startle reaction.
   c. Newborns differentiate between bitter and sweet taste.
   d. Newborns perceive tactile stimulation, particularly on the face (Anderson, 1989; Whaley & Wong, 1989).
2. Piaget calls the first 2 years of life the sensorimotor period. This period is characterized by integration and organization of information derived through sensorimotor experiences (Scipien, Chard, Howe, & Barnard, 1990).
3. Children with sensory–perceptual alterations have the same basic needs as other children. However, their experiences must be adapted to promote optimal development (Hunsberger, 1989).
4. Care of a hospitalized sensory–perceptually impaired child should include:
   a. Maintaining the usual method of communication
   b. Assigning consistent caregivers
   c. Fostering normal growth and development, *e.g.,* providing play opportunities, including kinetic stimulation
   d. Encouraging independence in self-care activities
   e. Incorporating special routines used at home into the plan of care (Hunsberger, 1989).

Gerontologic Considerations

1. Older adults need more time to process visual information when in unfamiliar situations; they also need more light to identify and process the input, and take longer to respond to changes in illumination (Miller, 1990).

2. Insufficient time to process auditory and visual input can lead to sensory overload.
3. Wearing hearing aids in an excessively noisy environment (*e.g.,* clinic, ICU) also can cause sensory overload.

■ Sensory–Perceptual Alterations
Related to Sensory Overload

Assessment

Subjective Data

The person reports
Visual imagery
Nightmares
Difficulty concentrating
Color perception changes
Alteration in the size and contour of objects
Hallucinations

Objective Data

(Occurs in an environment with excessive stimuli)
Mood alterations
Sleep pattern disturbances
Poor appetite
Evidence of lack of self-care
Delusions

Outcome Criteria

The person will
• Demonstrate decreased symptoms of sensory overload as evident by (specify)
• Identify and eliminate the potential risk factors if possible
• Describe the rationale for the treatment modality

Interventions

A. Assess causative and contributing factors
1. Altered sleep and rest pattern (refer to *Sleep Pattern Disturbance*)
2. Pain (refer to *Altered Comfort*)
3. Excessive noise or light
4. Critical care unit activity
5. Health care facility routines
6. Unfamiliar environment (different culture of language)

B. Reduce or eliminate causative and contributing factors when possible

1. Excessive noise or light
   a. Cover nonessential blinking lights at bedside with tape.
   b. Dim lights at night.
   c. Encourage use of blindfolds.
   d. Decrease noise output.
      - Shut off nonessential alarms.
      - Encourage use of earplugs.
      - If possible, limit the use of flasher, etc., during sleep hours.
      - Turn off unnecessary equipment.
      - Position person away from direct source of noise, if possible.
      - Curtail nonessential personnel conversation.
      - Avoid loud noises.
      - Discourage television after 10 P.M.
   e. Share with person the source of the noise.
   f. Discuss the use of a radio with earplugs to provide soft, relaxing music.
   g. Share with personnel the need to reduce noise and provide individuals with uninterrupted sleep for at least 2 to 4 hours' duration.
2. Unfamiliar environment
   a. Attempt to reduce fears and concerns by explaining equipment, its purpose and noises.
   b. Encourage person to share his perceptions of noises.
   c. Enlist the aid of an interpreter to explain the environment to person who does not speak English.

C. Promote reorientation

1. Orient to all three spheres (person, place, time).
   a. Address person by name.
   b. Introduce yourself frequently.
   c. Identify the place.
   d. Identify the time.
      "Good morning Mr. Jones. I am Mary Smith. I will be your nurse today."
      "Where are you Mr. Jones? You are in the hospital."
      "Today is May sixth and it is eight thirty in the morning."
2. Explain all activities.
   a. Offer simple explanations of each task.
   b. Allow person to handle equipment related to the task.
   c. Allow him to participate in task, such as washing his face.
   d. Acknowledge when you leave and when you will return.

D. Promote movement

1. Encourage person to remain out of bed as much as possible (eat meals in chair).
2. Teach person to perform isometric and isotonic exercises when in bed.
3. Encourage person to change his position frequently, even if it is just lifting one side off a surface by rolling slightly.
4. To encourage walking, choose a destination to reach or give the walk a purpose (walking to the lounge for breakfast).

E. Utilize measures to prevent injury

1. Keep side rails in place and bed in lowest position.
2. Place call bell in convenient location.
3. Refer to *High Risk for Injury* for additional interventions.

F. Assist person to differentiate reality from fantasy
  1. Refer to *Altered Thought Processes Related to Inability to Evaluate Reality* for additional interventions.

References/Bibliography

Anderson, J. J. (1989). Development and adaptations of the family with an infant. In Foster R. L., Hunsberger, M. M., & Anderson, J. J. T. (Eds.). *Family-centered nursing care of children.* Philadelphia: W. B. Saunders, pp. 194–195.

Bolin, R. H. (1974). Sensory deprivation: An overview. *Nursing Forum, 13*(3), 240–258.

Burnside, I. (1981). *Nursing and the aged.* New York: McGraw-Hill.

Chodil, J., & Williams, B. (1970). The concept of sensory deprivation. *Nursing Clinics of North America, 5*(3), 453–465.

Dodd, M. J. (1978). Assessing mental states. *American Journal of Nursing, 78,* 1501–1503.

Downs, F. (1974). Bed rest and sensory deprivation. *American Journal of Nursing, 74,* 434–438.

Drummond, L. K., & Scarbrough, D. (1978). A practical guide to reality orientation: A treatment approach for confusion and disorientation. *Gerontologist, 18*(12), 568–573.

Gimbel, P. (1975). The pathology of boredom and sensory deprivation. *Psychiatric Nursing, 16*(5), 12–13.

Hunsberger, M. (1989). Nursing strategies: Sensory and communication alterations. In Foster, R. L., Hunsberger, M. M., & Anderson, J. J. T. (Eds.). *Family-centered nursing care of children.* Philadelphia: W. B. Saunders.

Kintzel, K. C. (1977). *Advanced concepts in clinical nursing* (2nd ed.). Philadelphia: J. B. Lippincott.

Miller, C. A. (1990). *Nursing care of the older adult.* Glenview, IL: Scott, Foresman.

Murray, R., Huelskoetter, M., & O'Driscoll, D. (1980). *The nursing process in later maturity.* Englewood Cliffs, NJ: Prentice-Hall.

Nowakowski, L. (1980). Disorientation—signal or diagnosis? *Journal of Gerontological Nursing, 6*(4), 197–202.

Schultz, P. (1965). *Sensory restriction: Effects on behavior.* New York: Academic Press.

Scipien, G. M., Chard, M. A., Howe, J., & Barnard, M. U. (1990). *Pediatric nursing care.* St. Louis: C. V. Mosby.

Severtsen, B. (1979). Sensory impairment: Its effects on the family. In Hymovich, D., & Barnard, M. (Eds). *Family health care.* New York: McGraw-Hill, pp. 293–304.

Shelby, S. (1978). Sensory deprivation. *Image, 10*(2), 49–55.

Solomon, L. (1961). *Sensory deprivation.* Cambridge, MA: Harvard University Press.

Trockman, G. (1978). Caring for the confused or delirious patient. *American Journal of Nursing, 78,* 1495–1499.

Whaley, L. F., & Wong, D. L. (1989). *Essentials of pediatric nursing* (3rd ed.). St. Louis: C. V. Mosby.

Wyness, M. A. (1985). Perceptual dysfunction: Nursing assessment and management. *Journal of Neuroscience Nursing, 17*(2), 105–110.

Zubek, S. (1969). *Sensory deprivation: Fifteen years of research.* New York: Appleton-Century-Crofts.

Sexuality Patterns, Altered

Sexual Dysfunction

Sexuality Patterns, Altered

■ *Related to* **Stress**
■ *Related to* **the Effects of Acute or Chronic Illness**
■ *Related to* **Change in or Loss of Body Part**
■ *Related to* **Prenatal and Postpartum Changes**
■ *Related to* **Fear of Pregnancy and/or Sexually Transmitted Diseases (STDs); High Risk for**

Definition

Altered Sexuality Patterns: The state in which an individual experiences or is at risk of experiencing a change in sexual health—the integration of somatic, emotional, intellectual and social aspects of sexual being in ways that are enriching and that enhance personality, communication, and love (WHO, 1975).

DEFINING CHARACTERISTICS

Major (must be present)

Actual or anticipated changes in sexual functioning or sexual identity

Minor (may be present)

Expression of concern about sexual functioning or sexual identity
Inappropriate sexual verbal or nonverbal behavior
Changes in primary and/or secondary sexual characteristics
Major change in physical appearance or functioning
Major change in psychosocial roles or functioning

RELATED FACTORS

An alteration in sexual patterns can occur as a response to various health problems, situations, and conflicts. Some common sources are listed below.

Pathophysiologic

Endocrine
    Diabetes mellitus   Hyperthyroidism
    Decreased hormone production   Addison's disease
    Myxedema   Acromegaly

Genitourinary
    Chronic renal failure   Vaginismus
    Retrograde ejaculation   Priapism
    Altered structures   Infections
    Sexually transmitted diseases
Neuromuscular and skeletal
    Arthritis   Spinal cord injury
    Multiple sclerosis   Cerebrovascular accident (CVA)
    Amyotrophic lateral sclerosis
    Other disturbances of nerve supply to brain, spinal cord, sensory nerves, and
        autonomic nerves
Cardiorespiratory
    Peripheral vascular disorders
    Myocardial infarction
    Chronic respiratory disorders
    Congestive heart failure
Gastrointestinal
    Ulcerative colitis   Crohn's disease
    Liver disease
Cancer

Treatment-related
    Medications
    Radiation therapy
    Surgery
        Mastectomy   AP resection
        Prostatectomy   Colostomy
        Hysterectomy   Ileostomy
        Amputation   Orchiectomy

Situational (personal, environmental)
    Partner
        Unwilling   Not available
        Uninformed   Abusive
        No partner
    Environment
        Unfamiliar   Hospital
        No privacy   Extended care facility
    Stressors
        Job problems   Value conflicts
        Financial worries   Religious conflicts
    Lack of knowledge
    Fatigue
    Obesity
    Pain
    Alcohol ingestion (acute or chronic)
    Recreational drug use (acute or chronic)
    Fear of sexual failure
    Fear of pregnancy
    Infertility
    Depression

Anxiety
Guilt
Fear of sexually transmitted diseases

Maturational

Ineffective role models	Adolescence
Negative sexual teaching	Pregnancy
Absence of sexual teaching	Aging
Adjustment to parenthood	

Diagnostic Considerations

The diagnoses *Altered Sexuality Patterns* and *Sexuality Dysfunction* are difficult to differentiate. *Altered Sexuality Patterns* represents a broad diagnosis, of which sexual dysfunction can be one part. *Sexual Dysfunction* may be used most appropriately by a nurse with advanced preparation in sex therapy. Until *Sexual Dysfunction* is well differentiated from *Altered Sexuality Patterns,* it should not be used by most nurses.

Errors in Diagnostic Statements

Altered Sexuality Patterns related to reports of absent libido

Report of absent libido represents a symptom of *Altered Sexuality Patterns,* not a "related to" statement. If further assessment revealed the person's dissatisfaction with present sexual patterns, the nurse could record the diagnosis *Altered Sexuality Patterns related to unknown etiology, as evidenced by reports of absent libido.* The use of "unknown etiology" in this diagnostic statement will prompt focus assessments to determine contributing factors, *e.g.,* stress, medication side-effects.

Sexual Dysfunction related to impotence secondary to spinal cord injury

How would the nurse treat this diagnosis? A nurse planning to explore feelings and provide information and referrals would not be treating sexual dysfunction. Instead, the nursing focus would be best described in the diagnosis *Anxiety related to effects of spinal cord injury on sexual function and insufficient knowledge of causes and community resources available.*

Focus Assessment Criteria

Guidelines for Taking a Sexual History

1. Take sexual history in a private, relaxed setting to ensure confidentiality.
2. Do not judge the individual by your own beliefs/practices.
3. Permit the individual to refuse to answer.
4. Clarify vocabulary; use slang terms if needed to convey meaning
5. Assess only those areas pertinent for this client at this time.
6. Strive to be open, warm, objective, unembarrassed, and reassuring.
7. Keep in mind that it is more appropriate to assume that the client has had some sexual experience than to assume none.
8. Several sessions may be necessary to complete the interview.

Subjective Data

1. General
    Age, sex, marital status
    Sexual orientation/preference

Quality of relationship with significant other
Number of children and siblings
Religious and cultural background
Job and financial status
Medical and surgical history
Drug and alcohol use (present and past)
2. Sexual knowledge and attitudes
Source of sexual information
Knowledge of anatomy and physiology
Childhood sexual experiences (parental influence, religious influence, masturbation)
Attitudes concerning sexual variations
Myths and taboos
Menstruation
Birth control methods
3. Sexual function
Usual pattern
Present pattern
Satisfaction (individual, partner)
Erection problems for male (attaining, sustaining)
Ejaculation problems for male (premature, retarded, retrograde)
Inhibited lubrication in females
Inhibited orgasm in females
4. Sexual problem
Description
Onset (when, gradual/sudden)
Pattern over time (increased, decreased, unchanged)
Person's concept of cause
Knowledge of problem by others (partner, physician, others)
Past diagnostic studies and treatments
Expectations
5. School-aged child
Knowledge
"What is the difference between boys and girls?"
"What do you know about having babies?"
"Who taught you? At what age?"
Body changes
"Is your body changing in any way? How? Why?"
"How do you feel about these changes?"
Masturbation
"Almost everyone touches their body; how do you feel about this?"
6. Adolescent
Knowledge and attitudes
"What were your parents' attitudes toward sex, nudity, and touching?"
"Were these subjects discussed in your home?"
"How does pregnancy occur?"
"What are some methods of birth control?"
"What do you know about sexually transmitted diseases?"
Body changes
"Is your body changing in any ways? How? Why?"
"How do you feel about these changes?"

Sexual activity

"Some young people are sexually active; how do you feel about that?"

"Are you sexually active? If so, do you use birth control? Do you practice "safe sex"?"

Objective Data

Menstrual/reproductive/sexually transmitted disease history
Fertility status
Genitourinary/gynecologic assessment
Surgical/congenital alterations
Diagnostic studies
Primary/secondary sexual characteristics
Dress, grooming
General health status

Principles and Rationale for Nursing Care

Generic Considerations

1. All people are sexual beings. Sexuality is an integral part of identity.
2. Sexuality encompasses how one feels about oneself and how one interacts with others.
3. Sexual function refers to psychologic and physiologic ability to perform in a sexually satisfying manner, with or without a partner.
4. Sexuality and sexual function are influenced by age, marital status, sexual orientation, personal value system, sexual knowledge, resources (social, economic, geographic), culture, physical health, and emotional health.
5. The characteristics of a sexually healthy person are (Lion, 1982):
   a. A positive body image despite the body's packaging
   b. Acceptance of sexual and body functions as normal and natural
   c. Accurate knowledge about human sexuality and sexual functioning
   d. Recognition and acceptance of own sexual feelings
   e. Effective interpersonal relationships
   f. Acceptance of mistakes/imperfections in self and others
6. Sexuality is not restricted solely to the young and healthy.
7. Sexual expression is not limited to sexual intercourse; it includes closeness and touch, as well as other forms of verbal and nonverbal communication.
8. Sexual orientation is an individual matter. Homosexuality is not a diagnosis unless the person sees it as a problem. In such a situation, another nursing diagnosis might be appropriate, *e.g., Self-Concept Disturbance.*
9. A person must have the opportunity to make his or her own educated decisions regarding sexuality and sexual expression. Mutually satisfying acts between consenting adults are considered normal.

The Nurse's Role in Discussing Sexuality

1. Sexuality is as important as other aspects of human health and should be incorporated into nursing assessments and other aspects of nursing care.
2. The nurse must become educated regarding sexuality and sexual health through the life span. It is important to examine one's own beliefs and feelings regarding sexuality, sexual function, and what is considered sexually normal and abnormal.
3. Many nurses have difficulty providing patients with care in the area of sexuality and do not address sexual concerns unless the patient asks specific questions. Research

indicates, however, that many patients wish nurses and other health care professionals would *initiate* discussion of sexuality (Krueger, Hassell, Goggins, Ishimatso, Pablico, & Tuttle, 1979; Wilson & Williams, 1988).

4. The PLISSIT model (Annon, 1976) is very helpful for the nurse generalist providing care in the area of sexuality:

   a. **Permission:** Convey to the person and significant others a willingness to discuss sexual thoughts and feelings (*e.g.,* "Some people with your diagnosis have concerns about how their illness will affect their sexual functioning. Is this a concern for you or your partner?").

   b. **Limited Information:** Provide the person and significant other with information regarding the effects certain situations (*e.g.,* pregnancy), conditions (*e.g.,* cancer), and treatments (*e.g.,* medications) can have on sexuality and sexual function.

   c. **Specific Suggestions:** Provide specific instructions that can facilitate positive sexual functioning (*e.g.,* changes in coital positions).

   d. **Intensive Therapy:** Refer persons who need more help to an appropriate health care professional (*e.g.,* sex therapist, surgeon).

5. Giving a person "permission" to discuss sexual concerns is by far the most important aspect of nursing care in the area of sexuality. The nurse should give permission by:

   a. Including sexuality in the initial health history, and addressing questions on sexuality in a manner similar to questions on bowel and bladder function. This helps the person to see that nurses view sexuality as a routine part of human health.

   b. Offering to discuss sexual concerns at appropriate times during the client's hospitalization/visit.

6. The nurse should assure person of the confidentiality of all data regarding sexuality and obtain permission from the person before making a referral for a sexual problem.

7. If a diagnosis of *Altered Sexuality Patterns* or *Sexual Dysfunction* is made, the diagnosis, goals, and general interventions should be marked on the care plan and the name of the nurse providing care for this diagnosis indicated. Details of the assessment and interactions should not be included on the chart, in order to ensure confidentiality.

Medications and Sexuality

1. Drugs can influence sexual functioning positively and negatively (see Table II–16).
2. The patient has the right to be educated about all medication side-effects, including those affecting sexuality.

Pregnancy and Sexuality

1. Barring complications, a pregnant woman is free to engage in sexual activity with her partner to the extent that it is comfortable and desired.
2. Pregnant women have varying degrees of sexual desire during pregnancy.

   a. Some women are very sexually excitable.

   b. Some women are not very desirous of sex.

   c. Libido changes by large degrees during different stages of pregnancy.

   d. A woman's body image affects her sexuality. (If thinness is an attribute, then many pregnant women are confused about changing size.)

   e. A woman's attitude toward her body can influence her partner's sexual attraction toward her.

3. Pregnancy is a time of stress for both man and woman; to deny physical closeness at a time when both partners are struggling can add to tension and alienation.
4. The postpartum period is a time of self-doubt. For the first 6 weeks, a new mother

Table II–16 **Drugs That Alter Sexuality**

Drug	Effect on Sexuality
Alcohol	In small amounts, may increase libido and decrease sexual inhibitions In large amounts, impairs neural reflexes involved in erection and ejaculation Chronic use causes impotence and sterility in men; decreased desire and orgasmic dysfunction in women
Amyl nitrate	Peripheral vasodilator reputed to cause intensified orgasms when inhaled at time of orgasm May cause loss of erection, hypotension, and syncope
Antidepressants	Peripheral blockage of nervous innervation to sex organs Significant percentage of impotence and ejaculatory dysfunction
Antihistamines	Block parasympathetic nervous innervation of sex organs Sedative effect may decrease desire Decrease in vaginal lubrication
Antihypertensives	Libido may be decreased in both sexes Some antihypertensives cause impotence and ejaculatory problems in up to 50% of men
Antispasmodics	Inhibit parasympathetic innervation of sex organs May cause impotence
Cocaine	Short-term use is reported to enhance sexual experience Chronic use causes loss of desire and sexual dysfunction in both sexes
Hormones	Estrogen suppresses sexual function in men Testosterone may increase libido in both sexes, but causes virilization in women Chronic use of anabolic steroids causes testicular atrophy, decreased testosterone, and decreased sperm production; may cause permanent sterility
Marijuana	May decrease sexual inhibitions Chronic use may cause decreased libido and impotence
Narcotics	Chronic use causes decreased libido in both sexes Testosterone levels and amount of semen decreased Erectile and ejaculatory dysfunction common
Oral contraceptives	Remove fear of pregnancy May cause decreased libido
Sedatives/tranquilizers	Initially and in low doses may enhance sexual pleasure due to relaxation and decrease of inhibitions Long-term use decreases libido and may cause orgasmic dysfunction and impotence

feels lost, overwhelmed, tired, depressed, ignorant, and isolated. Her self-esteem as well as her sexuality may suffer.

5. A new father may experience his own adjustments postnatally, which can be manifested by a lack of interest in sex. He may feel inadequate in regard to caring for the child and may experience jealousy of the closeness of mother and infant. He may be disturbed by the woman's postpartum body, and/or may view her as changed and no longer someone he can relate to sexually since she moved into the Mother role.

Pediatric Considerations

1. Sex role identification begins in infancy and is determined by adolescence.
   a. Infants are able to identify body parts by the end of the first year.
   b. Toddler learn gender differentiation.
   c. Preschoolers frequently engage in masturbation and sex play with peers (*e.g.,* comparing genitals).
   d. School-agers continue to gain awareness about their sex role identity. While masturbation and sex play are common in young school-agers, the older school-age child becomes involved in purposeful sexual behavior (*e.g.,* hugging, kissing members of opposite sex) (Rew, 1989; Whaley & Wong, 1989).
   e. Adolescents experience altered body image in response to the physical changes of puberty. The key developmental task of adolescence is identity formation, which is influenced by sexual maturation and assuming a sex role (Whaley & Wong, 1989).
2. Parents are the primary force in sexuality education in a child's life. This includes what is not said as well as what is said (Gordon & Gordon, 1983).
3. Formal sex education, presented from a life-span approach, is best offered during middle childhood. Topics should include information about sexual maturation and the process of reproduction (Whaley & Wong, 1989).
4. A significant number of children are victims of sexual abuse. Incest accounts for 80% of child sexual abuse cases (Scipien, Chard, Howe & Barnard, 1990).

Gerontologic Considerations

1. An elderly person is psychologically and physically capable of engaging in sexual activity regardless of age-related changes in sexual anatomy and physiology.
2. Elderly females experience and decreased breast tone, thinning, and loss of elasticity of the vaginal wall, decreased vaginal lubrication, and shortening of vaginal length due to the loss of circulating estrogen.
3. Elderly males experience decreased production of spermatozoa, decreased ejaculatory force, and smaller, less firm testicles. Direct stimulation may be required to achieve an erection; however, the erection may be maintained for a longer period of time.
4. The need for intimacy and touch is especially important for the elderly, who may be experiencing diminishing meaningful relationships.
5. Past sexual function (enjoyment, interest, frequency) are predictors of sexual activity in the elderly. To be capable of sexual activity in old age, a person must participate in sexual activity throughout life.
6. Adult children and caregivers commonly view sexual activities of older adults as "immoral, inappropriate and negative" (Convey, 1989).
7. The sexual functioning of older adults is most influenced by myths and misunderstanding. According to Miller (1990), "Because sex is so closely identified with youthfulness, the stereotype of sexless seniors is widely believed."

■ **Altered Sexuality Patterns**
Related to Stress

Any situation or event which causes stress (changes in personal relationships, changes in work situations, health problems, environmental changes, etc.) may negatively influence sexual functioning.

Assessment

Subjective Data

The individual or partner voluntarily reports concern with sexual functioning or responds positively to assessment questions regarding sexuality

The above problem is accompanied by one or more stressors, such as:

Job-related stress
Financial worries
Relocation
Divorce
Separation from partner
Death of partner or significant other
Job change
Disability of spouse
Temporary change in health status
Infertility
Severe fatigue

Objective Data

Depression
Anxiety
Anger

Outcome Criteria

The person will
- Identify stressors
- Identify impact of stressors on sexual functioning
- Resume previous sexual activity or engage in alternate satisfying sexual activity

---

Interventions

A. Assess for causative or contributing factors. (Refer to Assessment, Subjective Data.)

B. Assess the person's awareness of the relationship between sexual functioning and stressors

C. Eliminate or reduce causative or contributing factors (if possible)
   1. Clarify relationship between stressors and problem in sexual functioning.
   2. Explore options available for reducing the impact of the stressor on sexual functioning (*e.g.,* increase sleep, increase exercise, modify diet, explore stress reduction methods).

D. Provide limited information and specific suggestions
   1. Explore comfort with self-pleasuring/masturbation as alternative method for sexual release.
   2. Suggest use of nonsexual touch, massage, or other techniques to take pressure off performing sexually.
   3. Explore options to meet and socialize with others.

E. Initiate referrals as needed
   1. Sex therapist
   2. Marriage counselor
   3. Psychiatrist or psychologist
   4. Social service (for assistance with job, financial, housing, or family problems

---

■ **Altered Sexuality Patterns**
Related to the Effects of Acute or Chronic Illness

Assessment

Subjective Data

Person reports change in sexual functioning associated with symptoms of acute or chronic illness, such as
   Decrease in or loss of desire
   Decreased arousal
   Impaired orgasm
   Decreased frequency of intercourse
   Decreased vaginal lubrication
   Impaired erectile ability
Person reports change in partner's interest in sexual activity associated with onset of acute or chronic illness

Objective Data

Medical diagnosis including, but not limited to
   Diabetes mellitus
   Chronic renal failure
   Cancer
   Cerebrovascular accident
   Arthritis
   Myocardial infarction
   Spinal cord injury

Chronic obstructive pulmonary disease
Multiple sclerosis
Medical treatment
Medications (see Table II–16)
Surgery
Radiation Therapy

Outcome Criteria

The person will
- Identify factual limitations on sexual activity caused by health problem
- Identify appropriate modifications in sexual practices in response to these limitations
- Report satisfying sexual activity

Interventions

A. Assess for causative or contributing factors, which may include
1. Fatigue
2. Pain
3. Shortness of breath
4. Paralysis
5. Limited oxygen reserve
6. Immobility
7. Impaired nerve innervation
8. Neutropenia
9. Hormonal changes
10. Depression
11. Lack of appropriate information

B. Eliminate or reduce causative or contributing factors (if possible). Teach the importance of adhering to medical regimen designed to reduce or control disease symptoms.

C. Provide limited information and specific suggestions
1. Provide appropriate information to patient and partner regarding actual limitations on sexual functioning caused by the illness (limited information).
2. Teach possible modifications in sexual practices to assist in dealing with limitations caused by illness (specific suggestions).
3. See Table II–17 for more details.

D. Provide referrals as indicated, which may include
1. Enterostomal therapist
2. Physician
3. Clinical specialist

(*Text continues on page 765*)

Table II–17 **Disorders That Alter Sexuality**

Health Problem	Sexual Complication	Nursing Intervention
Diabetes mellitus	Men: Erectile difficulties due to diabetic neuropathies or microangiopathy	LI: Encourage proper metabolic control. SS: Eventually may require penile implant; refer to urologist.
	Women: Decreased desire; decreased vaginal lubrication	LI: Encourage proper metabolic control; teach signs and symptoms of vaginitis. SS: Suggest use of water-soluble lubricating jelly.
Chronic obstructive pulmonary disease	Activity intolerance due to exertional dyspnea; coughing and expectoration	LI: Teach controlled breathing; plan intercourse for time of peak effect from medications; avoid sex after large meal or physical exertion, or immediately after awakening; plan for nonhurried relaxed, low-stress encounters.
	Anxiety	SS: Suggest positions that minimize chest pressure (sitting or side-lying); explain that waterbeds also help decrease exertion during sex.
Arthritis		LI: Explain that arthritis has no effect on physiologic aspects of sexual functioning.
	Pain, joint stiffness, fatigue	SS: Suggest that the couple plan intercourse for time of peak medication effects; promote joint relaxation by taking warm bath/shower alone/with partner; perform mild range-of-motion exercises.
	Decreased libido from steroid medications	LI: Teach that decreased desire is a common side-effect of medication.
Benign prostatic hypertrophy (TUR)	Retrograde ejaculation due to damage to internal bladder sphincter	LI: Explain that erection and orgasm will still occur, but ejaculate will be decreased or absent; urine will be cloudy.
Cardiovascular disease	Anxiety, fear of performance, fear of chest pain, death, decreased desire, decreased arousal, decision of partner to stop sexual activity	LI: Explain that infarction has no direct effect on physiologic sexual functioning; activity usually is safe 5–8 weeks postinfarction, based on Index of Sexual Readiness (ability to take brisk walk, climb two flights of stairs without chest pain). Teach to avoid sexual activity after large meal, drinking alcohol, or in room with extremes in temperature. Point out that some medications may cause sexual dysfunction (see Table II–16).

(continued)

Table II–17 **Disorders That Alter Sexuality** (continued)

Health Problem	Sexual Complication	Nursing Intervention
		SS: Encourage nonsexual touching; suggest positions that conserve energy (side-to-side lying, supine lying position, or sitting in chair with partner on top); explore option of masturbation; assure that oral–genital sex does not place additional strain on heart. Warn to avoid anal sex, as anal penetration stimulates vagus nerve and decreases cardiac function.
Chronic renal failure (CRF)	Chronic/recurrent uremia can produce state of depression, decreased sexual desire and arousal	LI: Acknowledge that stress of disease and dialysis may cause decreased desire; encourage nonsexual touching without pressure to perform.
	Untreated CRF causes cessation of ovulation and menses in women and causes atrophy of testicles, decreased spermatogenesis, decreased plasma testosterone, and erectile dysfunction in men. Dialysis may restore ovulation and menses in women and return testosterone levels to normal in men; sexual desire may return to predisease levels with treatment.	Reassure that these problems are usually reversible with dialysis. Warn that birth control should be continued as fertility may return. Explain that sexual dysfunction may be a product of emotional stress and the physiologic components of the disease. SS: Explain that measurement of nocturnal penile tumescence can distinguish between organic and psychologic causes of sexual dysfunction in men.
Total abdominal hysterectomy with bilateral salpingo-oophorectomy	Loss of circulating estrogen	LI: Teach signs and symptoms of menopause, use of water-soluble vaginal lubricants. Encourage discussion with physician about estrogen replacement, creams. Explain that in most cases intercourse may be resumed after 6-week postop visit.
	Postoperative psychologic adjustment or change in sexual identity, grieving, loss of reproductive capacity	Explore the meaning of uterine and ovarian loss to the woman. Assure her that the surgery will not change her ability to respond and function sexually.
Enterostomal surgery Anterior-posterior resection	Women: Loss of uterus and ovaries; shortening of vagina	LI: See above. SS: Suggest coital positions that decrease depth of penetration (e.g., side-to-side lying, man on top with legs outside the woman's, woman on top).

(continued)

Table II–17 **Disorders That Alter Sexuality** (continued)

Health Problem	Sexual Complication	Nursing Intervention
	Men: Erectile dysfunction, decrease in amount/force of ejaculate or retrograde ejaculation due to interruption of sympathetic and parasympathetic nerve supply (**Note:** Amount of rectal tissue removed appears to determine degree of dysfunction.)	LI: Explain that erectile dysfunction may be temporary or permanent. Encourage use of touch and other noncoital means of sexual communication.
Colostomy/ ileostomy	Alteration in sexual self-concept, body image	LI: Allow person to express feelings about change in body appearance; encourage communication with partner.
	Decrease in desire, arousal, and orgasm	LI: Teach that fatigue and decreased desire are common after surgery. Discuss ways to increase sexual attractiveness; suggest wearing sexy lingerie or other clothing to hide appliance.
	Anxiety regarding spillage, odor	Teach to empty bag prior to sexual activity; encourage to maintain a sense of humor, as accidents will sometimes occur.
	Erectile dysfunction in men (varies with age and type of surgery)	Encourage alternate ways to express sexuality if intercourse is not possible.
Spinal cord injury	Sexual disability depends on level and type of cord injury: after injury, separation of genital sexual functioning and cerebral eroticism. Men with complete upper motor neuron injury may not be able to ejaculate	LI: Discuss sexual options available; depend on extent of injury; e.g., a waterbed to amplify pelvic movements. Encourage continued use of contraceptives, as appropriate. SS: Discuss alternate positions; e.g., partner on top. Encourage experimentation with vibrators, massage, and other means of sexual expression.

Note: Much information is available regarding the sexual implications of spinal cord injury. The reader is referred to available literature on this subject.

Cancer	Sexual implications depend on site of disease and treatment	LI: Encourage expression of anxiety and fear; encourage grieving.
	Possible guilt associated with desiring touch and sexual activity	Assure that sexual expression even when one has cancer is natural, and that need for intimacy often increases during this time.
	Changes in role function and sexually defined gender roles	Encourage discussion between partners about this; encourage negotiation about role changes, which may be temporary.

(continued)

Table II–17 **Disorders That Alter Sexuality** (continued)

Health Problem	Sexual Complication	Nursing Intervention
	Fear of being contagious	Assure person and partner that the disease can not be transmitted through sexual activity.
	Change in body image	Discuss purchase of wig, false eyelashes prior to hair loss; suggest sexy lingerie, other ways to pamper oneself to increase feelings of sexual desirability and attractiveness.
	Fatigue	Explain that severe fatigue may hinder sexual desire and that fatigue does not indicate rejection of partner. Encourage verbal and nonverbal communication between person and partner.
Chemotherapy	Alkylating agents, antimetabolites, and antitumor antibiotics: Amenorrhea, oligospermia, azoospermia, decreased desire, ovarian dysfunction, erectile dysfunction	LI: Encourage discussion about changes in body appearance/ function. Explore option of sperm banking. Urge to continue use of contraceptives. False-positive Pap smear possible.
	Vinca alkaloids: Retrograde ejaculation, erectile dysfunction, decreased desire, ovarian dysfunction, temporary decrease in sexual desire/arousal	Encourage nonsexual touching; rest; avoidance of alcoholic beverages, narcotics and sedatives prior to sexual activity; use of water-soluble lubricants to decrease vaginal irritation; avoidance of oral and anal sex during periods of neutropenia.
	Genetic teratogenicity and mutagenicity	Encourage the couple to seek genetic counseling prior to conception.
Radiation therapy	Most side-effects will be site-dependent; however, side-effects such as fatigue, neutropenia, anorexia will generally be present in all persons	LI: Teach to plan sexual activity after rest periods and to use positions that require less exertion for the patient. Encourage nonsexual touching and communication. Teach that patient is not radioactive during external treatment. Teach site-specific side-effects and impact on sexual functioning.

LI = limited information; SS = specific suggestion.

■ Altered Sexuality Patterns
Related to Change in or Loss of Body Part

Assessment

Subjective Data

The person reports
    Feelings of undesirability
    Unwillingness or partner's unwillingness to look at affected part
    Change in own or partner's social or sexual responses
    Negative changes in sexuality
    Partner's fear of hurting person

Objective Data

Loss of or change in body part, such as in

Amputation	Ileostomy
Mastectomy	Orchiectomy
Plastic surgery	Prostatectomy
Colostomy	Hysterectomy
Trauma	Burns

(Note: Sexuality can be affected even if the loss or change is not visible externally.)
Withdrawal
Depression
Unwillingness to acknowledge loss
Unwillingness to look at affected body part

Outcome Criteria

The person will
- Identify impact of loss or change on sexual functioning
- Identify factual limitations on sexual activity caused by loss or change
- Identify appropriate modifications in sexual practices in response to these limitations
- Report satisfying sexual activity

Interventions

A. Assess for causative or contributing factors, which can include

1. Loss of or change in organ considered important for sexual attractiveness or sexual function (breast, penis, etc.)
2. Loss of or change in reproductive capacity
3. Fear of rejection or ridicule
4. Fear of drainage or odor during sexual activity
5. Increased pain during sexual activity
6. Inability to assume usual position for sexual functioning

7. Hormonal changes
8. Change in body image
9. Lack of appropriate information

B. Eliminate or reduce causative or contributing factors, if possible

C. Facilitate adaptation to change in or loss of body part by
1. Assessing the stage of adaptation of the person and partner to the loss (denial, depression, anger, resolution; see *Grieving*).
2. Encouraging adherence to the medical regimen to promote maximum recovery
3. Encouraging the couple to discuss the strengths of their relationship and to assess the influence of the loss on these strengths
4. Clarifying the relationship between loss or change and the problem in sexual functioning

D. Provide limited information and specific suggestions
1. Provide appropriate information to patient and partner regarding any actual limitations on sexual functioning caused by the change or loss (limited information).
2. Teach possible modifications in sexual practices to assist in dealing with limitations caused by illness (specific suggestions), for example,
   a. Modifications in positions
   b. Use of pillows for comfort and/or balance
   c. Techniques to control drainage or odor
   d. Use of attractive lingerie to cover affected part

E. Provide referrals when indicated, which may include
1. Enterostomal therapist
2. Physician
3. Clinical specialist
4. Reach for Recovery
5. United Ostomy Association

■ Altered Sexuality Patterns
Related to Prenatal and Postpartum Changes

Assessment

Subjective Data
The person reports
Altered sexual function
Feelings of undesirability
Partner's change in usual sexual and social responses

Outcome Criteria

The person will
- Share concerns
- Express increased satisfaction with sexual patterns

Interventions

A. Assess the sexual patterns during and after pregnancy (Reeder, Mastroianni, & Martin, 1983)

Prenatal

1. What has your physician said about sex during pregnancy?
2. How does the pregnancy make you feel? (asked of both partners)
3. How do you feel about changes in appearance?
4. How do you feel about changes in emotions?
5. How do you feel about one another's experience of the pregnancy?
6. What are your feelings about sex during pregnancy?
7. Has the pregnancy made many changes in your life and sexual relationship?
8. What have you heard about what you should or should not do sexually during pregnancy?
9. Have you experienced any physical difficulties with intercourse during pregnancy?
10. Are there any concerns or worries about your sexual relationship during pregnancy or afterwards?
11. How do you think having a baby will change your life? How do you plan to manage these changes?
12. How do you feel physically?
13. What medications do you take?
14. Have you had any recent changes in your health?

Postpartum

1. Are you still bleeding?
2. Have you resumed sexual activity?
3. Are you concerned about conceiving again?
4. Has breast-feeding altered your sexual relationship?
5. How has the baby affected your sexuality?
6. Is your episiotomy healed and comfortable during intercourse?
7. Have you experienced a lack of lubrication since delivery?
8. Do you ever have time alone with your partner?

B. Assess contributing factors

1. Body changes
2. Change in sex drive
3. Fatigue
4. Emotional lability
   a. Anxieties about taking on parental responsibilities
   b. Grief from separating from childhood
   c. Anxiety about outcome of pregnancy
   d. Ambivalence about having a baby

    e. Guilt about desiring sex when pregnancy has been achieved (religious, social pressure)

    f. Fear of dependency

    g. Fear of loss of current status (career, freedom)

    h. Self-doubt

5. Fear of damaging fetus
6. Dyspareunia in pregnancy
7. Dyspareunia in postpartum
8. Guilt due to baby

    a. Afraid to let go and enjoy sex lest something happen to baby

9. Influence of others

    a. Relatives (mother, in-laws)

      • Attitudes related to pregnancy and child care

      • Cultural attitudes toward sex during pregnancy and toward mothers as sexual beings

    b. Partner: Intrusion on time together

    c. Baby: Intrusion on time (nursing, care)

10. Fear of pregnancy
11. Breast-feeding (see *Ineffective Breast-feeding*)

C. Reduce or eliminate contributing factors

1. Body changes

    a. Provide literature or suggested reading list for person to read to establish knowledge of normalcy of pregnancy and changes.

    b. Refer to community resources.

    c. Refer to early pregnancy classes.

    d. Refer to childbirth preparation classes.

    e. View video about sex during pregnancy (see References/Bibliography for a list of available videos.)

    f. Suggest alternative sexual positions for later pregnancy.

      • Side-lying

      • Woman kneeling

      • Woman standing

      • Woman on hands and knees

      • Woman on top

      • Woman astride man

    g. Discuss postpartum changes.

      • Provide literature.

      • Give reassurance about these changes.

        Episiotomy

        Lochia—how long it will last, how it will change

        Lubrication

        Uterine resolution

        Flabby abdominal musculature

        Breast engorgement

        Breast leakage during lovemaking

      • Reassure that this is a temporary state and will resolve in 2 to 3 months.

      • Refer to postpartum exercise class.

2. Change in sex drive

    a. Reassure that sexual attitudes change throughout pregnancy from feeling very desirous of sex to wanting only to be cuddled.

    b. Support acceptance of whatever pleasuring may be desired. Encourage flexibility and alternative sexual patterns (*e.g.,* oral sex, mutual masturbation, fondling, stroking, massage, vibrators).

    c. Encourage honest communication with partner regarding desires or changes in interest.

3. Fatigue
    a. Acknowledge this as factor especially during first trimester and again during last month.
    b. Can be a major contributor to postpartum sexual problem
    c. Encourage person to make time for her relationship, in sexual as well as other contexts.
    d. Encourage to ask for help, hire a sitter, etc.

4. Emotional lability
    a. Encourage woman and/or partner to discuss emotions.
    b. Listen—allow time for person to elaborate on feelings.
    c. Reassure that these feelings are normal.
    d. Refer to reading material.
    e. Refer to other pregnant couples for verification.
    f. Relate your own experiences, if appropriate.
    g. Refer to therapy, if indicated.

5. Fear of damaging fetus
    a. Reassure that unless problems exist (preterm labor, previous early loss, bleeding or rupture of membrane) intercourse is allowed until labor begins.
    b. Refer to physician for reassurance.
    c. Explore misinformation. Use anatomic charts to show protection of baby in uterus.
    d. Inform that orgasm causes contractions that are not harmful and will subside.

6. Dyspareunia in pregnancy
    a. Explore what pain is experienced and when.
    b. Suggest alternative positions:
        - Woman on top
        - Side-lying
        - Posterior–vaginal entry
    c. Suggest use of water-soluble lubricant.
    d. Refer to physician if pain continues.

7. Dyspareunia in postpartum
    a. Explore what pain is experienced and under what circumstances.
    b. Assess healing of episiotomy.
    c. Suggest varied positions.
    d. Suggest use of water-soluble lubricant (nursing women report reduced vaginal lubrication during entire nursing experience).
    e. Teach person to identify her pelvic floor muscles and strengthen them with exercise.
        - "For posterior pelvic floor muscles, imagine you are trying to stop the passage of stool and tighten your anus muscles without tightening your legs or your abdominal muscles."
        - "For anterior pelvic floor muscles, imagine you are trying to stop the passage of urine, tighten the muscles (back and front) for 4 seconds, and then release them; repeat ten times, four times a day" (can be increased to four times an hour if indicated).
    f. Instruct person to stop and start the urinary stream several times during voiding.
    g. Refer to physician if pain continues.

8. Guilt due to baby
   a. Encourage discussion; reassure that these feelings are normal; allow time to elaborate.
   b. Expression of these feelings will often create a release and relaxation.
   c. Include partner in discussion (both may have similar feelings they have not felt free to express to one another).
   d. Refer to postpartum support groups.
   e. Refer to psychologic or social assistance if pathology is observed.
9. Influence of others
   a. Encourage discussion of mother/woman relationship.
      • Does woman see her mother as a sexual being?
      • Does she now feel confused about her roles as mother versus sex partner?
   b. Reassure that identity confusion is common.
   c. Refer to postpartum discussion groups.
   d. Allow to express feelings concerning changes in life.
   e. Include partner in discussion (perhaps at a later time)—let both parties talk about adjustment and pressures that interfere with relating sexually and otherwise.
   f. Interview partners separately. (This may allow an opening-up that may be difficult with the other person present.)
10. Fear of pregnancy
    a. Encourage discussion.
    b. Explore contraceptive choices.
    c. Refer to nurse practitioner or gynecologist for contraception.
    d. Inform patient that breast-feeding does not provide effective contraception and that prepregnancy contraceptive devices may no longer fit.
       • Warn that oral contraceptives are contraindicated while nursing.

D. Initiate health teaching and referrals

1. Teach couples to abstain from intercourse and seek the advise of their health care provider if any of the following situations are present (Zlatnik & Burmeistey, 1982):
   a. Vaginal bleeding
   b. Premature dilation
   c. Multiple pregnancy
   d. Engaged fetal head or lightening
   e. Placenta previa
   f. Rupture of membranes
   g. History of premature delivery
   h. History of miscarriage
2. Refer to suggested references for printed material.
3. Refer to counselor if resolution is not achieved.

■ Sexuality Patterns, High Risk for Altered
Related to Fear of Pregnancy and/or Sexually Transmitted Diseases (STDs)

Assessment

Subjective Data
The person reports
Actual or potential sexual intercourse without use of contraception (unless pregnancy is desired)
Improper use of contraceptive method
Dissatisfaction with contraceptive method
Lack of knowledge about available contraceptive methods
Actual or potential sexual activity without adequate protection from sexually transmitted diseases
Lack of knowledge about sexually transmitted diseases
Dissatisfaction with sexuality due to fear of pregnancy or STDs

Objective Data
Previous unplanned pregnancy
History of therapeutic abortion
Adolescent
Newly married
Recently divorced
Postpartum
History of STD

Outcome Criteria

The person will
- Report proper use of contraception and adequate protection against STDs
- Report satisfaction with contraceptive method and sexuality patterns
- Not experience an unplanned pregnancy or acquire an STD

Interventions

A. Assess for causative or contributing factors, such as
1. Lack of exposure to or understanding of information on contraception and STDs
2. Newly sexually active
3. Change in sexual partner
4. Multiple sexual partners

B. Eliminate or reduce causative or contributing factors (if possible)
1. Stress genuine risk of pregnancy or STD with unprotected sexual activity.
2. Encourage abstinence from sexual activity or thoughtful consideration in choice and number of sexual partners.

C. Provide limited information and specific suggestions
  1. Discuss advantages and disadvantages of various contraceptive methods.
  2. Provide specific information on chosen contraceptive method, including written/graphic material and return demonstration if appropriate.
  3. Teach to abstain from sexual activity if partner has symptoms of an STD.
  4. Teach danger of infertility, morbidity, or death from contracting an STD (see *High Risk for Infection*).

D. Provide referrals, as indicated
  1. Physician
  2. Nurse practioner
  3. Family planning clinic

Sexual Dysfunction

DEFINITION
Sexual Dysfunction: The state in which an individual experiences or is at risk of experiencing a change in sexual function that is viewed as unrewarding or inadequate.

DEFINING CHARACTERISTICS

Major
> Verbalization of problem with sexual function
> Reports limitations on sexual performance imposed by disease or therapy

Minor
> Fears future limitations on sexual performance
> Misinformed about sexuality
> Lacks knowledge about sexuality and sexual function
> Value conflicts involving sexual expression (cultural, religious)
> Altered relationship with significant other
> Dissatisfaction with sex role (perceived or actual)

Diagnostic Considerations
See Altered Sexuality Patterns

References/Bibliography

Andersen, B. L., & Hacker, N. F. (1983). Treatment for gynecologic cancer: A review of the effects on female sexuality. *Health Psychology, 2,* 203–221.

Andersen, B. L. (Ed.) (1986). *Women with cancer: Psychological perspectives.* New York: Springer-Verlag.

Annon, J. S. (1976). The PLISS + Model: A proposed conceptual scheme for the behavioral treatment of sexual problems. *Journal of Sex Education and Therapy, 2,* 211–215.

Baxter, R. (1978). Sex counseling and the spinal cord injured patient. *Nursing, 8,* 46–52.

Bullard, D. G., & Knight, S. E. (Eds.) (1981). *Sexuality and physical disability: Personal perspectives.* St. Louis: C. V. Mosby.

Burgener, S., & Logan, G. (1989). Sexuality concerns of the post-stroke patient. *Rehabilitation Nursing, 14,* 178–181.

Campbell, M. L. (1987). Sexual dysfunction in the COPD patient. *Dimensions in Critical Care Nursing, 6,* 70–74.

Carey, P. (1975). Temporary sexual dysfunction in reversible health limitations. *Nursing Clinics of North America, 10,* 575–585.

Comfort, A. (1978). *Sexual consequences of disability.* Philadelphia: George F. Stickley.

Convey, H. L. (1989). Preceptions and attitudes toward sexuality of the elderly during middle ages. *The Gerontologist, 29*(1), 93–100.

Cooley, M., Yeomans, A., & Cobb, S. (1986). Sexual reproductive issues for women with Hodgkin's disease, Part II: Application of PLISSIT model. *Cancer Nursing, 9,* 248–255.

Cutler, W. B., Garcia, C. R., & McCoy, N. (1987). Perimenopausal sexuality. *Archives of Sexual Behavior, 16,* 225–234.

Derogatis, L. R. (1980). Breast and gynecologic cancers: Their unique impact on body image and sexual identity in women. *Frontiers of Radiation Therapy and Oncology, 14,* 1–11.

Evans, R., Halar, E. M., & DiFreece, A. B. (1976). Multidisciplinary approach to sex education of spinal cord injured patients. *Physical Therapy, 56,* 541–545.

Gloeckner, M. R. (1984). Perceptions of sexual attractiveness following ostomy surgery. *Research in Nursing & Health, 7,* 87–92.

Gordon, S., & Gordon, J. (1983). *Raising a child conservatively in a sexually permissive world.* New York: Simon & Schuster.

Hahn, K. (1989). Sexuality and COPD. *Rehabilitation Nursing, 14,* 191–195.

Hatcher, R. A., Guest, F., Stewart, F., Stewart, G. K., Trussell, J., Bowen, S. C., & Cates, W. (1988). *Contraceptive technology 1988–1989.* New York: Irvington Publishers.

Hawton, K. (1984). Sexual adjustment of men who have had strokes. *Journal of Psychosomatic Research, 28,* 243–249.

Katzun, L. (1990). Chronic illness and sexuality. *American Journal of Nursing, 90,* 57–59.

Kolodny, R. C., Masters, W. H., & Johnson, V. E. (1979). *Textbook of sexual medicine.* Boston: Little, Brown.

Krozy, R. (1978). Becoming comfortable with sexual assessment. *American Journal of Nursing, 78,* 1036–1038.

Krueger, J. C., Hassell, J., Goggins, D. B., Ishimatsu, T., Pablico, M. R., & Tuttle, E. J. (1979). Relationship between nurse counseling and sexual adjustment after hysterectomy. *Nursing Research, 28,* 145–150.

Lion, E. (1982). *Human sexuality in nursing process.* New York: Wiley & Sons.

Mann, S., & Sandler, I. (1984). Coping and adjustment to genital herpes. *Journal of Behavioral Medicine, 7,* 391–409.

Masters, W. H., & Johnson, V. E. (1966). *Human sexual response.* Boston: Little, Brown.

McCann, M. E. (1989). Sexual healing after heart attack. *American Journal of Nursing, 89,* 1133–1140.

Metcalfe, M. C., & Fischman, S. H. (1985). Factors affecting the sexuality of patients with head and neck cancer. *Oncology Nursing Forum, 12,* 21–25.

Miller, C. A. (1990). *Nursing care of the older adult.* Glenview, IL: Scott, Foresman.

Murray, R. L. E. (1972). Principles of nursing intervention for the adult patient with body image changes. *Nursing Clinics of North America, 7,* 697–707.

Muscari, M. (1987). Obtaining the adolescent sexual history. *Pediatric Nurse, 13,* 307–310.

Peach, E. (1980). Counseling sexually active very young adolescent girls. *Maternal-Child Nursing Journal, 5,* 191–195.

Pettyjohn, R. D. (1979). Health care of the gay individual. *Nursing Forum, 17,* 367–371.

Prather, R. C. (1988). Sexual dysfunction in the diabetes female: A review. *Archives of Sexual Behavior, 17,* 277–283.

Rew, L. (1989). Promoting healthy sexuality. In Foster, R. L., Hunsberger, M. M., & Anderson, J. J. T. (Eds.). *Family-centered nursing care of children.* Philadelphia: W. B. Saunders.

Scipien, G. M., Chard, M. A., Howe, J., & Barnard, M. U. (1990). *Pediatric nursing care.* St. Louis: C. V. Mosby.

Schain, W. S. (1980). Sexual functioning, self-esteem, and cancer care. *Frontiers of Radiation Therapy Oncology, 14,* 12–19.

Shipes, E., & Lehr, S. (1982). Sexuality and the male cancer patient. *Cancer Nursing, 5,* 375–381.

Shuman, N. A., & Bohachick, P. (1987). Nurses' attitudes towards sexual counseling. *Dimensions in Critical Care Nursing, 6,* 75–81.

Steinke, E., & Bergen, B. (1986). Sexuality and aging. *Journal of Gerontological Nursing, 12,* 6–10.

Webb, C., & Askham, J. (1987). Nurses' knowledge and attitudes about sexuality in health care: A review of the literature. *Nurse Educator Today, 7,* 75–87.

Whaley, L. F., & Wong, D. L. (1989). *Essentials of pediatric nursing* (3rd ed.). St. Louis: C. V. Mosby.

Wilson, M. E., & Williams, H. A. (1988). Oncology nurses' attitudes and behaviors related to sexuality of patients with cancer. *Oncology Nursing Forum, 15,* 49–53.

Woods, N. F. (1984). *Human sexuality in health and illness* (3rd ed.). St. Louis: C. V. Mosby.

World Health Organization. (1975) Education and treatment in human sexuality: The training of health professionals. Report of a WHO Meeting, Technical Report Series no. 572. Geneva: WHO.

Zlatnick, F. J., & Burmeistey, L. F. (1982). Reported sexual behavior in late pregnancy. *Selected Medicine, 27*(3), 627–632.

Sex in Pregnancy and Postpartum

Bing, E., & Colman, L. (1977). *Making love during pregnancy.* New York: Bantam Books.

Brenner P., Greenberg, M. (1977). The impact of pregnancy on marriage. *Medical Aspects of Human Sexuality, 2,* 15–22.

Falicov, C. J. (1973). Sexual adjustment during first pregnancy and postpartum. *American Journal of Obstetrics and Gynecology, 117*(7), 991–1000.

Friday, N. (1980). *My mother myself.* New York, Dell, 1980

Genevie, L. & Margolies, C. (1987). *The motherhood report.* New York: Macmillan.

Masters, W., & Johnson, V. (1966). *Human sexual response.* Boston: Little, Brown.

Perkins, R. P., (1982). Sexuality in pregnancy: What determines behavior? *Obstetrics and Gynecology, 59*(2), 189–198.

Reeder, S., Mastroianni, L., & Martin, L. (1983). *Maternity nursing.* Philadelphia: J. B. Lippincott, p. 197.

SIECUS (Sex Information and Education Council of the U.S.). (1974). Sexual relations during pregnancy and the post-delivery period. Study Guide No. 6.

Solberg, D. A., Butler, J., & Wagner, N. N. (1973). Sexual behavior in pregnancy. *New England Journal of Medicine, 288*(5), 1098–1103.

Tolor, A., & DiGrazia, P. V. (1976). Sexual attitudes and behavior patterns during and following pregnancy. *Archives of Sexual Behavior, 5*(6), 539–551.

Zalk, S. R. (1980). Psychosexual conflicts in expectant fathers. In Blum, B. L. (Ed.). *Psychological aspects of pregnancy, birthing and bonding.* New York: Human Sciences Press, Chap. 11.

Resources/Literature for the Consumer

"Sex Can Help Arthritis" (pamphlet), available from the Arthritis Foundation (local chapters)

Sex and Spinal Cord Injured, Superintendent of Documents, U.S. Government Printing Office, Washington, DC 20402

Sex Information and Education Council of the United States, 80 Fifth Avenue, New York, NY 10011

Bibliographies for professionals and the general public (*e.g.,* aging, disabilities, children)

Planned Parenthood, Publications Section, 810 Seventh Avenue, New York, NY 10019

American Cancer Society, 77 Third Avenue, New York, 10017

American Fertility Society, 1608 14th Avenue South, Birmingham, AL 35205

National Clearinghouse for Family Planning Information, P.O. Box 2225, Rockville, MD 20852

United Ostomy Association, 1111 Wilshire Boulevard, Los Angeles, CA 90017

"Sex Education for Adolescents," American Library Association, Order Department, 50 East Huron Street, Chicago, IL 60611

Public Affairs Pamphlets, 381 Park Avenue South, New York, NY 10016 (many inexpensive pamphlets for parents; send for free catalog)

Doyee, F. S. (1982). *Private zone.* Edmonds, WA: Chas. Franklin Press.

"Sex During Pregnancy," ICEA Review, April, 1982, International Childbirth Education Association, P.O. Box 20048, Minneapolis, MN 55420-0048

"Sex During Pregnancy" by Sheila Kitzinger, 1972, Penny Press, 1100 23rd Ave. East, Seattle, WA 98112

"Sex After The Baby Comes" by Shelia Kitzinger, 1980, Penny Press, 1100 23rd Ave. East, Seattle, WA 98112

VIDEO: "Sex and Pregnancy," Glendon Association, 2049 Century Park East, #3000, Los Angeles, CA 90067

Sleep Pattern Disturbance

■ *Related to* **(Specify)**

DEFINITION

Sleep Pattern Disturbance: The state in which the individual experiences or is at risk of experiencing a change in the quantity or quality of his rest pattern that causes discomfort or interferes with desired life-style.

DEFINING CHARACTERISTICS

Adults

Major (must be present)

Difficulty falling or remaining asleep

Minor (may be present)

Fatigue on awakening or during the day
Dozing during the day
Agitation
Mood alterations
Dark circles under eyes

Children

Sleep disturbances in children are frequently related to fear, enuresis, or inconsistent responses of parents to child's requests for changes in sleep rules, such as requests to stay up late.

Reluctance to retire
Frequent awakening during the night
Desire to sleep with parents

RELATED FACTORS

Many factors in an individual's life can contribute to sleep pattern disturbances. Some common factors are listed below.

Pathophysiologic

Impaired oxygen transport
    Angina   Respiratory disorders
    Peripheral arteriosclerosis   Circulatory disorders
Impaired elimination (bowel or bladder)
    Diarrhea   Retention
    Constipation   Dysuria
    Incontinence   Frequency

Impaired metabolism
    Hyperthyroidism   Hepatic disorders
    Gastric ulcers

Treatment-related

Immobility (imposed by casts, traction)
Medications
    Tranquilizers   Steroids
    Sedatives   Soporifics
    Hypnotics   MAO inhibitors
    Antidepressants   Anesthetics
    Antihypertensives   Barbiturates
    Amphetamines

Situational (personal, environmental)

Lack of exercise
Pain
Anxiety response
Pregnancy
Life-style disruptions
    Occupational   Sexual
    Emotional   Financial
    Social
Environmental changes
    Hospitalization (noise, disturbing   Travel
      roommate, fear)

Diagnostic Considerations

The inability to rest and sleep has been described as "one of the causes, as well as one of the accompaniments of disease" (Henderson, 1969). Sleep disturbances can result from physiologic, psychologic, social, environmental, and maturational changes or problems.

The nursing diagnosis *Sleep Pattern Disturbance* must be differentiated from sleep disorders, chronic conditions (*e.g.*, sleep apnea, narocolepsy) usually not treatable by a nurse generalist. *Sleep Pattern Disturbance* should be used to describe temporary changes in usual sleep patterns and/or those which a nurse can prevent or reduce, *e.g.*, disruptions for treatments, anxiety response.

Errors In Diagnostic Statements

Sleep Pattern Disturbance related to apnea
    This diagnosis requires monitoring and comanagement by nurses and physicians; thus it should be written as the collaborative problem *Potential Complication: Sleep apnea.*
Sleep Pattern Disturbance related to hospitalization
    This diagnosis does not reflect the treatment needed. The effects of hospitalization on sleep should be specified, such as in *Sleep Pattern Disturbance related to changes in usual sleep environment, unfamiliar noises, and interruptions for assessments.*

Focus Assessment Criteria

Subjective Data
>   History of symptoms
>   Complaints of
>   Sleeplessness   Depression
>   Anxiety   Fear (nightmares, dark,
>   Irritability   maturational situations)
>   Onset and duration
>   Location
>   Description
>   Precipitated by what?   Aggravated by what?
>   Relieved by what?
>   Sleep requirements
>   To establish the amount of sleep an individual needs, have him go to bed and sleep
>   until he wakes in the morning (without an alarm clock). This should be done
>   for a few days and the average of the total sleeping hours calculated—with the
>   subtraction of 20 to 30 minutes, which is the time most people need to fall
>   asleep.
>   Sleep patterns (present, past)
>   Rate sleep on a scale of 1 to 10
>   Usual bedtime and arising time
>   Difficulty in getting to sleep, staying asleep, awakening
>   Reasons for difficulty (*e.g.,* noise, need to urinate)
>   Use of sleep aids or rituals
>   Warm bath   Pillows
>   Drink or food (milk, wine)   Position
>   Medications   Toy, book
>   Naps (frequency, length)

Objective Data
>   Physical characteristics
>   Drawn appearance (pale, dark circles under eyes, puffy eyes)
>   Yawning
>   Dozing during the day
>   Decreased attention span
>   Irritability

Principles and Rationale for Nursing Care

Generic Considerations
1. Sleep involves two distinct stages: REM (rapid eye movement) and NREM (non-rapid eye movement). NREM sleep comprises about 75% of total sleep time; REM sleep accounts for the remaining 25%.
2. The entire sleep cycle is completed in an interval of 70 to 100 minutes; this cycle repeats itself four or five times during the course of the sleep pattern.
3. Sleep is a restorative and recuperative process that facilitates cellular growth and the repair of damaged and aging body tissues. During NREM sleep, metabolic, cardiac, and respiratory rate decreased to basal levels and blood pressure decreases. There is profound muscle relaxation, bone marrow mitotic activity, and accelerated

tissue repair and protein synthesis. During REM sleep, the sympathetic nervous system accelerates, with erratic increases in cardiac output and heart and respiratory rate. Perfusion to gray matter doubles, and cognitive and emotional information is stored, filtered, and organized (Williams & Jackson, 1982).

4. The active phase of the sleep cycle, REM sleep is characterized by increased irregular vital signs, penile erections, flaccid musculature, and the release of adrenal hormones. REM sleep occurs approximately four to five times a night and is essential to one's sense of well-being. REM sleep is instrumental in facilitating emotional adaptation; a person needs substantially more REM sleep after periods of increased stress or learning (Sebilia, 1981).

5. Perception of the quality of one's sleep is influenced by the percentage of time in bed at night actually spent asleep, or *sleep efficiency*. Studies report that younger persons typically report a sleep efficiency of 80 to 95%, while older persons report 67 to 70% (Dement, Richardson, Prinz, Carskadon, Kripke, & Czeisler, 1985; Hayashi & Endo, 1982).

6. Monroe (1967) reported a high correlation between what people report about their sleep patterns and what polysomnographic evaluation (EEG, EMG, EOG) reveals. The subjects in this study were young and healthy; it is not known if the same results could be replicated with ill adults.

7. Sleep deprivation results in impaired cognitive functioning (memory, concentration, judgment) and perception, reduced emotional control, increased suspicion, irritability, and disorientation. It also lowers the pain threshold and decreases production of catecholamines, corticosteroids, and hormones (Berger & Oswald, 1962; Fuller & Schaller-Ayres, 1990).

8. The average amount of sleep needed according to age follows (William, 1971):

Age	Hours of Sleep
Newborn	14 to 18
6 months	12 to 16
Over 6 months to 4 years	12 to 13
5 to 13 years	7 to 8.5
13 to 21 year	7 to 8.75
Adults under 60	6 to 9
Adults over 60	7 to 8

10. Depression usually influences sleep in the form of initial insomnia (difficulty getting to sleep). Depressed individuals may then increase their sleeping hours (daytime and nighttime).

11. Caffeine and nicotine are CNS stimulants that lengthen sleep latency and increase nighttime wakenings (Miller, 1990).

12. Alcohol induces drowsiness but suppresses REM sleep and increases the number of awakenings (Miller, 1990).

13. Early morning naps produce more REM sleep than do afternoon naps. Naps over 90 minutes long decrease the stimulus for longer sleep cycles in which REM sleep is obtained (Thelan, 1990).

14. Researchers have reported that the chief deterrents to sleep in critical care clients were activity, noise, pain, physical condition, nursing procedures, lights, vapor tents, and hypothermia. (Dlin, Rosen, & Dickstein, 1971).

15. Environmental noise that cannot be eliminated or reduced can be masked with "white noise," *e.g.*, fan, soft music, tape-recorded sounds (rain, ocean waves) (Miller, 1990).

16. Hypnotics contribute to sleep disturbances by:
    a. Requiring increasing dosage due to tolerance
    b. Depressing CNS function
    c. Producing paradoxic effects (nightmares, agitation)
    d. Interfering with REM and deep sleep stages
    e. Causing daytime sombulence due to a very long half-life

Pediatric Considerations

1. Children exhibit a wide variation in the amount and distribution of sleep (Whaley & Wong, 1989).
2. Sleep affects a child's growth and development as well as the family unit as a whole (Hunsberger, 1989).
3. As children mature, the number of hours spent in sleep decreases. Moreover, there is a change in the quality of sleep with maturity. Sleep is characterized as being deep and restful 50% of the time in an infant, versus 80% of the time in the older child (Whaley & Wong, 1989).
4. Sleep problems commonly are related to feeding, resistance to separation, and normal fears (Hunsberger, 1989).
5. Children need to understand nighttime and be assisted to prepare for it. Preparation for bedtime involves switching the child from activity to bedtime gradually. It is a time for calmness, reassurance, and closeness.
6. Children should be helped to learn that their beds are safe places to be in.

Gerontologic Considerations

1. Age-related changes have little effect on the quantity of sleep but a significant impact on the quality of sleep and quantity of rest. It is unclear whether these changes are due to aging or to the increased incidence of certain risks factors in the elderly, *e.g.*, respiratory disorders, sleep apnea (Miller, 1990).
2. Older adults have more difficulty falling asleep, are more easily awakened, and spend more time in the drowsiness stage and less time in the dream stages (Miller, 1990).
3. Miller (1990) reports that "approximately one-third of adults complain of some type of sleep disturbance, usually involving primary symptoms of daytime sleepiness, difficulty falling asleep, and frequent arousals during the night."
4. Older adults have increased sensitivity to hypnotics and sleeping medications and experience more adverse effects, *e.g.*, constipation, confusion, and interference with quality of sleep.

■ Sleep Pattern Disturbance
Related to (Specify)

Assessment
See Defining Characteristics

Outcome Criteria

The person will
- Describe factors that prevent or inhibit sleep
- Identify techniques to induce sleep
- Report an optimal balance of rest and activity

Interventions

Since a variety of factors can disrupt sleep patterns, the nurse should consult the index for specific interventions to reduce certain factors (*e.g.,* pain, anxiety, fear). The following suggests general interventions for promoting sleep and specific interventions for selected clinical situations.

A. Identify causative contributing factors
   1. Pain (see *Altered Comfort*)
   2. Fear (see *Fear*)
   3. Stress or anxiety (see *Anxiety*)
   4. Immobility or decreased activity
   5. Pregnancy
   6. Urinary frequency or incontinence (see *Altered Patterns of Urinary Elimination*)
   7. Unfamiliar or noisy environment
   8. Temperature (too hot/cold)

B. Reduce or eliminate environmental distractions and sleep interruptions
   1. Noise
      a. Close door to room.
      b. Pull curtains.
      c. Unplug telephone.
      d. Use "white noise" (*e.g.,* fan, quiet, music, tape of rain, waves).
      e. Eliminate 24-hour lighting.
      f. Provide night lights.
      g. Decrease the amount and kind of incoming stimuli (*e.g.,* staff conversations).
      h. Cover blinking lights with tape.
      i. Reduce the volume of alarms and televisions.
      j. Place with compatible roommate if possible.
   2. Interruptions
      a. Organize procedures to provide the fewest number of disturbances during sleep period (*e.g.,* when individual awakens for medication also administer treatments and obtain vital signs).

    b. Avoid unnecessary procedures during sleep period.

    c. Limit visitors during optimal rest periods (*e.g.,* after meals).

    d. If voiding during the night is disruptive, have person limit his nighttime fluids and void before retiring.

C. Increase daytime activities as indicated

1. Establish with person a schedule for a daytime program of activity (walking, physical therapy).
2. Discourage naps longer than 90 minutes.
3. Encourage naps in the morning.
4. Limit amount and length of daytime sleeping if excessive (*i.e.,* more than 1 hr).
5. Provide others to communicate with person and stimulate wakefulness.

D. Promote sleep in agency

1. Assess with person, family, or parents the usual bedtime routine—time, hygiene practices, rituals (reading, toy)—and adhere to it as closely as possible.
2. Encourage or provide evening care.
    a. Bathroom or bedpan
    b. Personal hygiene (mouth care, bath, shower, partial bath)
    c. Clean linen and bedclothes (freshly made bed, sufficient blankets)
3. Use sleep aids.
    a. Warm bath
    b. Desired bedtime snack (avoid highly seasoned and high-roughage foods)
    c. Reading material
    d. Back rub or massage
    e. Soft music or tape-recorded story
    f. Relaxation/breathing exercises
4. Utilize pillows for support (painful limb, pregnant or obese abdomen, back).
5. Discourage naps longer than 90 minutes.
6. Ensure that the person has at least four to five periods of at least 90 minutes each of uninterrupted sleep.
7. Document the amount of the persons uninterrupted sleep each shift.
8. Children
    a. Explain night to the child (stars and moon).
    b. Discuss how some people (nurses, factory workers) work at night.
    c. Compare the contrast that when night comes for them, day is coming for other people somewhere else.
    d. If a nightmare occurs, encourage the child to talk about it if possible. Reassure child that it is a dream, even if it seems so real. Share with child that you have dreams too.
    e. Provide child with a nightlight and/or a flashlight to use to give him control over the dark.
    f. Reassure child that you will be nearby all night.
    g. Avoid allowing child to sleep with parents or parents to sleep in child's bed. Stay with child for a while (*e.g.,* sit on bed or chair, rub child's back).

E. Reduce the potential for injury during sleep

1. Utilize side rails if needed.
2. Place bed in low position.
3. Provide adequate supervision.
4. Provide night lights.

5. Place call bell within reach.
6. Ensure that an adequate length of tubing is available for turning (IV tubing, Levin tube).

F. Provide health teaching and referrals as indicated

1. Teach an at-home sleep routine (Miller, 1990):
   a. Maintain a daily schedule for waking, sleeping, and resting.
   b. Arise at the usual time even after not sleeping well; avoid staying in bed when awake.
   c. Use bed only for activities associated with sleeping.
   d. If awaken and cannot return to sleep, get out of bed and read in another room for 30 minutes.
   e. Avoid caffeine-containing foods and beverages (*e.g.*, chocolate, tea, coffee) during afternoon and evening.
   f. Avoid alcohol.
   g. Try a bedtime snack of foods high in L-tryptophan (*e.g.*, milk, peanuts).
2. Teach the importance of regular exercise (walking, running, aerobic dance and exercise) for at least 1/2 hour three times a week (if not contraindicated) to reduce stress and promote sleep.
3. Explain that hypnotic medications are not for long-term use due to the risk of developing tolerance and interference with daytime functioning.
4. Teach a pregnant woman
   a. Not to stand when she can sit
   b. To elevate feet when sitting
   c. Not to sit when she can lie down
   d. To adjust her schedule to provide for an afternoon rest (*e.g.*, upon returning home from work)
5. Explain to person and significant others the causes of sleep/rest disturbance and possible ways to avoid or minimize these causes.
6. Refer a person with a chronic sleep problem to a sleep disorders center.

References/Bibliography

Berger R. J., Oswald, I. (1962). Effects of sleep deprivation on behavior, subsequent sleep and dreaming. *Journal of Mental Science, 108,* 457.

Beyerman, K. (1987). Etiologies of sleep pattern disturbances in hospitalized patients. In McLane, A. (Ed.). *Classification of nursing diagnosis. Proceedings of the seventh conference.* St Louis: C. V. Mosby, p 193.

Dement, W., Richardson, G., Prinz, P., Carskadon, M., Kripke, D., & Czeisler, C. (1985). Changes of sleep and wakefulness with age. In Finch, C. E., & Schneider, E. L. (Eds.). *Handbook of the biology of aging* (2nd ed.). New York: Van Nostrand Reinhold, pp. 692–717.

Dlin, B., Rosen, H., Dickstein, K. (1971). The problems of sleep and rest in the intensive care unit. *Psychosomatics, 12,* 155.

Edgil, A., Wood, K., & Smith, D. (1985). Sleep problems of older infants and preschool children. *Pediatric Nursing, 11,* 88–89.

Erman, M. K. (1985). Insomnia management. *Journal of Enterostomal Therapy, 12*(6), 210–213.

Fass, G. (1971). Sleep, drugs, and dreams. *American Journal of Nursing, 71*(12), 2316–2320.

Henderson V. (1969). *Basic principles of nursing care.* New York: Macmillan Publishing Co.

Fuller, J., & Schaller-Ayers, J. (1990). *Health assessment: A nursing approach.* Philadelphia: J. B. Lippincott.

Hayashi, Y., & Endo, S. (1982). All-night sleep polygraphic recordings of healthy aged persons: REM and slow-wave sleep. *Sleep, 5,* 277–283.

Hayter, J. (1980). The rhythm of sleep. *American Journal of Nursing, 80*(3), 457–461.

Hayter, J. (1985). To nap or not to nap. *Geriatric Nursing, 2*, 104–106.

Hilton, B. A. (1976) Quality and quantity of patient's sleep and sleep disturbing factors in a respiratory intensive care unit. *Journal of Advanced Nursing, 1*(3), 453–468.

Hunsberger, M. (1989). Promoting healthy sleep patterns. In Foster, R. L., Hunsberger, M. M., & Anderson, J. J. T. (Eds.). *Family-centered nursing care of children.* Philadelphia: W. B. Saunders, pp. 649, 656.

Kleitman, N. (1963). *Sleep and wakefulness.* Chicago: University of Chicago Press.

Lareau, S., & Bonnet, M. (1985). Sleep disorders: Insomnia. *Nurse Practitioner, 10*(8), 16–17.

Miller, C. A. (1990). *Nursing care of older adults.* Glenview, IL. Scott, Foresman.

Monroe, L. J. (1967). Psychological and physiological differences between good and poor sleepers. *Journal of Abnormal Psychology, 72*(3), 225–264.

Sebilia, A. (1981). Sleep deprivation and biological rhythms in the critical care unit. *Critical Care Nurse, 3,* 19.

Thelan, L., Davie, J., & Urden, L. (1990). *Textbook of critical care nursing.* St. Louis: C. V. Mosby.

Whaley, L. F., & Wong, D. L. (1989). *Essentials of pediatric nursing* (3rd ed.). St. Louis: C. V. Mosby.

White, M. A. (1990). Sleep onset latency and distress in hospitalized children. *Nursing Research, 39*(3), 134–139.

William, D. (1971). Sleep and disease. *American Journal of Nursing, 71*(12), 2321–2324.

Williams, R. L., & Jackson, D. (1982). Problems with sleep. *Heart and Lung, 11*(3), 262.

Woods, N. (1972). Patterns of sleep in post-cardiotomy patients. *Nursing Research, 2*(4), 437–452.

Zelechowski, G. Sleep and the critically ill. *Critical Care Update, 6*(2), 5–13.

Resources for the Consumer

Sleep and aging (GPO 885-270), National Institute of Aging, U.S. Government Printing Office, Washington, DC 20402

The sleep book. AARP Books, Dept L078, 1865 Miner St, Des Plaines, IL 60018

Association of Sleep Disorders Centers, 604 Second St. SW, Rochester, MN 55902, (507) 287–6006 (provides list of accredited sleep disorder centers)

Social Isolation

■ *Related to* **(Specify)**

DEFINITION
Social Isolation: The state in which the individual or group experiences a need or desire for contact with others but is unable to make that contact.

DEFINING CHARACTERISTICS
Since social isolation is a subjective state, all inferences made regarding a person's feelings of aloneness must be validated. Because the causes vary and people show their aloneness in different ways, there are no absolute cues to this diagnosis.

Major (must be present)
Expressed feelings of aloneness and/or
Desire for more contact with people

Minor (may be present)
Time passing slowly ("Mondays are so long for me.")
Inability to concentrate and make decisions
Feelings of uselessness
Doubts about ability to survive
Feeling of rejection
Behavior changes
    Increased irritability or restlessness
    Underactivity (physical or verbal)
    Inability to make decisions
    Increased signs and symptoms of illness (a change from previous state of good health)
    Appearing depressed, anxious, or angry
    Postponing important decision-making
    Failure to interact with others nearby
    Sleep disturbance (too much sleep or insomnia)
    Change in eating habits (overeating or anorexia)

RELATED FACTORS
A state of social isolation can result from a variety of situations and health problems that are related to a loss of established relationships or to a failure to generate these relationships. Some common sources follow.

Pathophysiologic
Obesity
Cancer (disfiguring surgery of head or neck, superstitions of others)
Physical handicaps (paraplegia, amputation, arthritis, hemiplegia)
Emotional handicaps (extreme anxiety, depression, paranoia, phobias)
Incontinence (embarrassment, odor)
Communicable diseases (acquired immunodeficiency syndrome [AIDS], hepatitis)

Situational (personal, environmental)

Death of a significant other

Divorce

Extreme poverty

Hospitalization or terminal illness
(dying process)

Moving to another culture (*e.g.,*
unfamiliar language)

Drug or alcohol addiction

Homosexuality

Loss of usual means of transportation

Maturational

Child: Child in protective isolation or with a communicable disease

Elderly: Sensory losses, motor losses, loss of significant others

Diagnostic Considerations

The nurse should view *Social Isolation* as a nursing diagnosis describing loneliness. Loneliness is a subjective state that exists whenever a person says it does and is perceived as imposed by others. Social isolation is *not* the voluntary solitude that is necessary for personal renewal, nor is it the creative aloneness of the artist or the aloneness—and possible suffering—one may experience as a result of seeking individualism and independence (*e.g.,* moving to a new city, going away to college).

Errors in Diagnostic Statements

Social Isolation related to inability to engage in satisfying personal relationships since death of wife 1 year ago

When a person fails to resume activities or to renew or initiate social relationships after the death of a spouse, the nurse should suspect *Dysfunctional Grieving*. Prolonged social isolation after a death is a cue for unresolved grief. The nurse should conduct a focus assessment to identify other cues, such as prolonged denial, depression, or other evidence of unsuccessful adaption to the loss of his wife. Until additional data is confirmed, the diagnosis *Possible Dysfunctional Grieving related to failure to resume or initiate relationships after wife's death 1 year ago* would be appropriate in this situation.

Social Isolation related to multiple sclerosis

Using multiple sclerosis as a related factor clusters all persons with multiple sclerosis as socially isolated and for the same reasons. This not only does violates the uniqueness of each individual, but also does not specify how a nurse can intervene. If mobility and incontinent problems are present but no data support social isolation, the nurse can record the diagnosis as *High Risk for Social Isolation related to mobility and incontinence problems secondary to multiple sclerosis.*

Principles and Rationale for Nursing Care

Generic Considerations

1. Loneliness is an affective statement involving an awareness of being apart from others with an accompanying vague need for other persons (Leiderman, 1969).
2. Loneliness differs from aloneness, solitude, and grief. Aloneness refers to being without company, not necessarily a negative state. Solitude involves being alone with a positive affective state. Grief is a response to the experience of a traumatic loss (Hillestad, 1984).

3. Social isolation can result in intense feelings of loneliness and suffering. The suffering associated with social isolation is not always visible. To diagnose this state, nurses must first be able to identify those persons at risk.

4. The lonely or isolated person often aggravates his condition by suffering alone. The lonely tend to shun each other. The isolated person may resign himself to his situation and never seek companionship. He may deny his own feelings.

5. Persons who feel isolated may communicate and be communicated with in only the most concrete terms. "Hello, how are you?" "Do you want to eat?"

6. Illness may be the only legitimate way a socially isolated individual can get attention.

7. A socially isolated person usually is not able to initiate or coordinate various isolation-reduction activities on his or her own behalf.

8. The functional ability of a person's senses has a strong influence on his or her perception of the world, his behavior, and the behavior of others toward him or her (Yurick, 1984). A person with visible deficits may be shunned.

9. Chronic illness can contribute to social isolation due to lack of energy, decreased mobility, discomforts, fear of exposure to pathogens, and distancing by previous friends who are uncomfortable with the ill person's disabilities (Miller, 1990).

10. Lonely persons are preoccupied with self, are hypervigilant to threats, and tend to interpret social cues as being hostile (Weiss, 1973).

Pediatric Considerations

1. Children at high risk for social isolation include the chronically ill or disabled, terminally ill, and disfigured (Johnson, 1986; Stuart & Sundeen, 1987).

2. A child in protective isolation or with a communicable disease may not understand the rationale for separation from others (Hunsberger, 1989).

Gerontologic Considerations

1. Elderly persons are at high risk for social isolation because there often are fewer natural opportunities for being among people. Retirement from work, difficulty securing transportation, health problems that restrict visiting, sensory deficits making communication laborious or frustrating, or isolation from the mainstream in institutions (hospitals or nursing homes) each can significantly limit the natural encounters an elderly client would have with people.

2. Family roles become altered and stressed when parents become dependent on their children, and children begin to assume traditional parental tasks or decision-making. To help elderly individuals meet their affiliative needs and increase satisfaction with social encounters, it is suggested that small groups be formed to promote interaction (rather than large noisy crowds) and that one or two meaningful relationships (confidante) be encouraged.

3. Factors increasing social isolation in elderly persons include: hearing impairment, limited mobility, fatigue, caregiving responsibilities, inability to drive, mental or psychosocial impairments, and separation from spouse, friends, and/or relatives by death, illness, or physical distance (Miller, 1990).

4. Impaired ability to drive due to impaired vision, musculoskeletal functioning, and/or CNS functioning can increase an elderly person's social isolation and dependency on others (Miller, 1990).

5. Sensory deficits rate highest on the list of problems in the elderly that have the potential for causing social isolation (Bernardini, 1985).

6. Longino & Karl (1982) reported that the type or quality of social interactions are more important than the quantity. Informal activities promote well-being to a greater degree than formal structured activities.

Focus Assessment Criteria

The nurse must listen attentively to hear what the patient is saying. The nurse must also make astute observations of behavior if an accurate nursing diagnosis is to be made and appropriate interventions identified.

Subjective Data

Social resources (support)

"Who lives with you?"

"About how many times did you talk to someone—friends, relatives or others—on the telephone in the past week (either you called them or they called you)?" If subject has no phone, question in the following manner.

"How many times during the past week did you spend some time with someone who does not live with you; that is, you went to see them, or they came to visit you, or you went out to do things together?"

"How many times in the past week did you visit with someone, either with people who live here or people who visited you here?"

To whom does the person turn in time of need?

Are there friends or neighbors on whom he relies for such things as meals and transportation?

"Do you see your relatives and friends as often as you want to, or are you somewhat unhappy about how little you see them?"

If institutionalized: "In the past year, about how often did you leave here to visit your family and/or friends for weekends or holidays, or to go on shopping trips or outings?"

Feelings of loneliness

Does the person feel lonesome (isolated)?

Why does he think he feels this way?

Can he describe these feelings of loneliness?

Are there times (holidays or other occasions) when this feeling is more painful?

When during a 24-hour period does he feel most alone (morning, afternoon, evening, or during the night)?

What does he do to relieve this feeling?

Desire for more human contact

Who does the person think could help relieve this feeling of isolation?

What kind of relationships would he like? (Same sex or opposite sex? Same age? Someone with same situational or maturational problem?)

Is he willing to make the effort to meet new people and go to new places?

What kind of group activities does he most enjoy? (Travel? A religious service or activity?)

Has divorce or death (of spouse, child, sibling, friend, pet) occurred recently?

Has the person moved away from vicinity of significant other? (Living alone increases the likelihood of loneliness)

Barriers to social contacts

Does the person lack knowledge of resources available, where to meet others, how to initiate conversation with strangers?

Is he housebound? (Illness or incapacity—lack of mobility on steps or curbs—and weather hazards can physically isolate the elderly, as does loss of usual transportation, living in dangerous area, and lack of access to public transportation)

Are there changes in the person's sensory ability (tactile sense, hearing, visual acuity, ability to write letters)?

Change in living arrangement
  Has the person moved recently (to nursing home or child's home, to an apartment, to a strange location)?

Objective Data

Esthetic problems
  Mutilating surgery
  Odor (*e.g.,* ulcerating tumor)
  Extreme obesity
  Incontinence

■ Social Isolation
Related to (Specify)

Assessment

See Defining Characteristics

Outcome Criteria

The person will
  • Identify the reasons for his feelings of isolation
  • Discuss ways of increasing meaningful relationships
  • Identify appropriate diversional activities

Interventions

The nursing interventions for a variety of contributing factors that might be associated with a diagnosis of *Social Isolation* are very similar.

A. Identify causative and contributing factors
(See Focus Assessment Criteria)

B. Reduce or eliminate causative and contributing factors
  1. Promote social interaction
     a. Support the individual who has experienced a loss as he works through his grief (see *Grieving*).
     b. Validate the normalcy of grieving.
     c. Encourage person to talk about his feelings of loneliness and the reasons why they exist.
     d. Mobilize person's support system of neighbors and friends.
     e. Discuss the importance of quality socialization rather than a great number of interactions.
  2. Decrease barriers to social contact.
     a. Assist with identification of transportation options.

    b. Determine available transportation in the community (public, church-related, volunteer).

    c. Determine if person must be taught how to use alternate transportation (*e.g.,* drive a car).

    d. Identify activities that help keep people busy, especially during times of high risk of loneliness (see *Diversional Activity Deficit*).

    e. Assist with the development of alternate means of communication for persons with compromised sensory ability (*e.g.,* amplifier on phone; see *Impaired Communication Related to Hearing Loss*).

    f. Assist with the management of esthetic problems (*e.g.,* consult enterostomal therapist if ostomy odor is a problem; teach those with cancer to control odor of tumors by packing area with yogurt or pouring in buttermilk, then rinsing well with saline solution).

    g. Assist person in locating stores that sell clothing especially made for those who have had disfiguring surgery (*e.g.,* mastectomy).

    h. Refer to *Altered Patterns of Urinary Elimination* for specific interventions to control incontinence.

3. Identify strategies to expand the world of the isolated.

    a. Senior centers and church groups

    b. Foster grandparent program

    c. Day care centers for the elderly

    d. Retirement communities

    e. House sharing

    f. College classes opened to older persons

    g. Pets

    h. Telephone contact

C. Initiate referrals as indicated

1. Community-based groups that contact the socially isolated
2. Self-help groups for clients isolated due to specific medical problems (Reach to Recovery, United Ostomy Association)
3. Wheelchair groups

References/Bibliography

Bernardini, L. (1985). Effective communication as an intervention for sensory deprivation in the elderly client. *Topics in Clinical Nursing, 1*(4), 72–81.

Burnside, I. M. (1976). *Nursing and the aged.* New York: McGraw-Hill.

Carnevali, D., & Patrick, M. (1979) *Nursing management for the elderly.* Philadelphia: J. B. Lippincott.

Davis, B. (1990). Loneliness in children and adolescents. *Issues in Comprehensive Pediatric Nursing, 13*(1), 59–69.

Decker, S., & Kinzel, S. (1985). Learned helplessness and decreased social interactions in elderly disabled persons. *Rehabilitation Nurse, 10*(2), 31–33.

Eliopoulos, C. (Ed). (1984). *Health assessment of the older adult.* Menlo Park, CA: Addison-Wesley.

Glassman-Feibusch, B. (1981). The socially isolated elderly. *Geriatric Nursing, 2*(1), 28–31.

Hillestad, E. A. (1984). Toward understanding of loneliness. In *Proceedings of conference on spirituality.* Milwaukee, WI: Marquette University.

Holt-Ashley, M. (1988). Loneliness as a nursing diagnosis in bone marrow transplantation patients. *Dimensions in Oncology Nursing, 2*(1), 66–71.

Hunsberger, M. (1989). Principles and skills adapted to the care of children. In Foster, R. L., Hunsberger, M. M., & Anderson, J. J. T. (Eds.). *Family-centered nursing care of children.* Philadelphia: W. B. Saunders, p. 822.

Johnson, S. H. (1986). Nursing diagnosis strategies. In Johnson, S. H. *High-risk parenting: Nursing assessment and strategies for the family at risk*. Philadelphia: J. B. Lippincott, p. 458.

Leiderman, P. H. (1969). Loneliness: A psychodynamic interpretation. In Scheidman E. S., & Ortega, M. J. (Eds.). *Aspects of depression. International Psychiatric Clinics*. Boston: Little, Brown.

Longino, C. F., & Karl, C. S. (1982). Explicating activity theory: A formal replication. *Journal of Gerontology, 37*(2), 713–722.

Lynch, J. J. (1979). *The broken heart: The medical consequences of loneliness*. New York: Basic Books.

Miller, C. A. (1990). *Nursing care of older adults*. Glenview, IL: Scott, Foresman.

Miller, J. F. (1984). Loneliness and spiritual well-being. In *Proceedings of conference on spirituality*.

Perry, G. (1990). Loneliness and coping among tertiary level adult cancer patients in the home. *Cancer Nursing, 13*(5), 293–296. Milwaukee, WI: Marquette University.

Ravish, T. (1985). Prevent social isolation before it starts. *Journal of Gerontological Nursing, 11*(10), 10–13.

Roberts, S. L. (1976). *Behavioral concepts and the critically ill patient*. Englewood Cliffs, NJ: Prentice-Hall.

Roberts, S. L. (1978). *Behavioral concepts and nursing throughout the life span*. Englewood Cliffs, NJ: Prentice-Hall.

Ryan, M., & Patterson, J. (1987). Loneliness in the elderly. *Journal of Gerontological Nursing, 11*(10), 10–13.

Stuart, G. W., & Sundeen, S. J. (1987). *Principles and practice of psychiatric nursing*. St. Louis: C. V. Mosby.

Weiss, R. S. (1973). *Loneliness: The experience of emotional and social isolation*. Cambridge, MA: MIT Press.

Yurick, A., Spier, B., Robb, S., & Ebert, N. (1989). *The aged person and the nursing process* (3rd ed.). Norwalk, CT: Appleton-Century-Crofts, p. 341.

Social Interactions, Impaired

■ *Related to* **(Specify) Secondary to Chronic Illness**

DEFINITION

Impaired Social Interaction: The state in which individual experiences or is at risk of experiencing negative, insufficient, or unsatisfactory responses from interactions.

DEFINING CHARACTERISTICS

Major (must be present)

Reports inability to establish and/or maintain stable, supportive relationships

Minor (may be present)

Lack of motivation
Severe anxiety
Dependent behavior
Hopelessness
Delusions/hallucinations
Disorganized thinking
Lack of self-care skills

Distractibility/inability to
concentrate
Social isolation
Superficial relationships
Poor impulse control
Difficulty holding a job
Lack of self-esteem

RELATED FACTORS

Impaired social interactions can result from a variety of situations and health problems that are related to the inability to establish and maintain rewarding relationships. Some common sources are listed below.

Pathophysiologic

Loss of body function
Hearing deficits
Mental retardation
Terminal illness
Loss of body part

Visual deficits
Speech impediments
Chronic illness (Crohn's disease,
renal failure, epilepsy)
Psychiatric disorders

Treatment-related

Surgical disfigurement
Dialysis
Reaction to medication

Situational (personal, environmental)

Depression
Language/cultural barriers
Social isolation
Lack of vocational skills
Substance abuse

Anxiety
Divorce/death of spouse
Institutionalization
Thought disturbances

Maturational

Child/adolescent: Altered appearance, speech impediments, separation from family
Adult: Loss of ability to practice vocation
Elderly: Death of spouse, retirement

Diagnostic Considerations

Social competence refers to a person's ability to interact effectively with others. Interpersonal relationships assist a person through life experiences, both positive and negative. Positive relationships with others requires positive self-concept, social skills, social sensitivity, and acceptance of the need for independence. To interact satisfactorily with others, one must acknowledge and accept one's limitations and strengths (Maroni, 1989).

A person without positive mental health usually does not have social sensitivity, and thus is uncomfortable with the interdependence necessary for effective social interactions. A person with poor self-concept may constantly sacrifice his or her needs for those of others or always may put personal needs before the needs of others.

The diagnosis *Impaired Social Interactions* describes a person who exhibits ineffective interactions with others. If extreme and/or prolonged, this problem can lead to a diagnosis of *Social Isolation*. The nursing focus for *Impaired Social Interactions* is on increasing the person's sensitivity to the needs of others and teaching reciprocity.

Errors In Diagnostic Statements

Impaired Social Interactions related to verbalized discomfort in social situations

In this diagnosis, the person's report of discomfort represents a diagnostic cue, not a related factor. The nurse will perform a focus assessment to determine reasons for the person's discomfort; until these reasons are known, the diagnosis *Impaired Social Interactions related to unknown etiology* can be recorded.

Focus Assessment Criteria

Subjective Data

1. Interaction patterns and skills
   a. Job-related
      - Job-seeking and interviewing skills
         Able to identify own job-related assets
         Dresses appropriately
         Asks appropriate questions
         Identifies employment sources
         Ability to complete an application
      - Employment status
         Employed
         Unemployed
      - Employment history
         Length of employment
         Reasons for leaving (problems with coworkers or supervisors)
         Frequency of job changes
      - Interactions with coworkers
         Contacts outside work

   b. Living arrangements
   - Ability to live cooperatively with others
     Ability to participate with others in group tasks; such as food preparation, cleaning
     Performs assigned tasks
     Adequacy of personal hygiene
     How does he handle conflict?
     Dependability
   - Residential patterns
     Where?—family, group home, boarding house, institution
     How long?
     Frequency of relocation
     Reasons for relocation
   - Assess social isolation (see *Social Isolation*)
   c. Leisure/recreation
   - "What do you do with your free time?"
   - "Who do you share your time with?"
   - Attendance at any structured activity?
   - What interferes with participating in recreational activities?
   - Preference for individual or group activity?
2. Recent life stress (Krauss & Slavinsky, 1982)
   - Explore each of the following:
     Emergencies (*e.g.*, police, fire)
     Health (*e.g.*, others in household)
     Financial (*e.g.*, increase or decrease in income, increased debt)
     Job (*e.g.*, change in responsibility)
     Relationships (*e.g.*, new, broken)
     Treatment (*e.g.*, change in medications, therapist)
3. Support system
   - Assess availability and responses of others
     Family and significant others
       Fearful
       Frustrated
       Guilty
       Angry
       Embarrassed
       Hopeless
     Relationships
       Does he have friends?
       Does he initiate friendship?
     Health care system
       Frequency of contact
       Frequency of admissions
       Variety of services used
       Compliance with prescribed treatment—kept appointments, medications
4. Coping skills
   a. How does he respond to stress, conflict?
   - Substance abuse
   - Aggression (verbal or physical)

- Suicide
- Withdrawal

5. Legal history
   a. Arrests and convictions

Objective Data

1. General appearance
   Facial expression (*e.g.,* sad, hostile, expressionless, posture, gait)
   Dress (*e.g.,* meticulous, disheveled, seductive, eccentric)
   Personal hygiene
       Cleanliness
       Grooming
       Clothes (appropriateness, condition)
2. Communication pattern
   During interview

Quiet	Withdrawn
Hostile	Cooperative
Apathetic	Hyperactive
Elated	

   Content

Appropriate	Sexually preoccupied
Rambling	Religiosity
Suspicious	Worthlessness
Denial of problem	Delusions
	Obsessions
	Homicidal or suicidal plans

   Pattern of speech

Appropriate	Blocking (unable to finish an idea)
Circumstantial (unable to get to the point)	Jumps from one topic to another
	Indecisive
	Neologisms
	Word salad

   Rate of speech

Appropriate	Reduced
Excessive	Pressured

3. Relationship skills
   Able to listen and respond appropriately
   Has conversational skills
   Does not seek interactions
   Withdrawn/preoccupied with self
   Shows dependency, passivity
   Demanding/pleading
   Hostile
       Barriers to satisfactory relationships
           Social isolation
           Severe depression
           Panic attacks
           Thought disturbances
           Chronic mental illness
           Preoccupation with illness

Principles and Rationale for Nursing Care

Generic Considerations

1. Social competence is the ability of the individual to interact effectively with his environment.
2. Effective reality testing, ability to problem-solve, and a variety of coping mechanisms are necessary for the individual to be socially competent.
3. Both the individual and the environment contribute to impaired functioning. A person may be able to function in one environment or situation and not in others.
4. Adequate social functioning is most often associated with conjugal living and a stable occupation.

Chronic Mental Illness

1. Chronic mental illness is characterized by recurring episodes over a long period of time. The extent to which the individual is impaired in role performance varies. The extent of impairment is related to social inadequacy.
2. Alterations in thought processes may interfere with the individual's ability to engage in appropriate social or occupational role behavior.
3. Dependency is one of the most consistent features presented. It may be seen through multiple readmissions requiring a large amount of clinician's time, resistance to discharge, resistance to any change including medication, and refusal to leave home.
4. The origins of impaired social interactions in the chronically mentally ill vary. For some, it is the result of poor reality testing. If a person is unable to perceive reality accurately, it is difficult to manage everyday problems. For others, it may be the result of social isolation or the loss of interpersonal skills due to long-term institutionalization.
5. The chronically mentally ill person usually has no friends, is socially isolated, and engages in little community activity (Test & Stein, 1976).
6. Deinstitutionalization has decreased the number of institutionalized individuals and decreased the median length of hospital stay, thus changing the character of today's chronically ill population. There is now an emerging group of individuals 18 to 35 years old who are distinctly different from the older institutionalized adults, in that their lives reflect a transient existence and multiple hospital admissions versus stable, long-term residence in a state hospital (Bachrach, 1982).
7. The young chronically ill patients exhibit problems with impulse control (*e.g.,* suicidal gestures, legal problems, alcohol/drug intoxication), disturbances in affect (*e.g.,* anger, argumentativeness, belligerence), and poor reality testing especially when under stress. The population varies from system-dependent, poorly motivated persons to system-resistant persons with low frustration tolerance and refusal to acknowledge problems (Pepper, Ryglewicz, & Kirshner, 1982).
8. Despite the variations, most have several factors in common (Pepper, Ryglewicz, & Kirshner, 1982).
   a. Difficulty in maintaining stable supportive relationships—most have transient, unstable relationships with marginally functional people.
   b. Repeated errors in judgment—seen in their inability to learn from their experiences and the inability to transfer knowledge from one situation to another.
   c. Vulnerability to stress—those experiencing stress are at greater risk for relapse.
   d. Patterns of social interaction are demanding, hostile, and manipulative, which produce negative reactions among caregivers.
9. Both the individuals and families are under stress. The individual's behaviors that strain the family include their excessively demanding behavior, social withdrawal, lack of conversation, and minimal leisure interests. The family also affects the

individual's ability to survive in the community by either supportive or nonsupportive behaviors.

10. Skills learned in one situation are not transferred to another, so that skills are best taught in the environment in which the person will be functioning (Test & Stein, 1976).

11. Passivity or lack of motivation is a part of the illness and thus should not be simply accepted by the caregivers. Caregivers must use an assertive approach in which the treatment is "taken to the person" rather than waiting for him to participate (Test & Stein, 1976).

12. Treatment approaches that do not rely on verbal skills are more successful. Examples are coaching, modeling, and reinforcements for positive behaviors (Anthony, 1980).

13. Chronically mentally ill persons often lose their jobs, not because of inability to do job tasks, but because of deficits in emotional and interpersonal functions (Anthony, 1980). Research in social skills training has shown that posthospital adjustment is improved by skill building programs (Manderino & Bzdek, 1987).

Pediatric Considerations

1. A child is significantly impacted when his or her parent(s) is emotionally disturbed. Emotionally disturbed parents may not be able to meet the physical or safety needs of their children (Krone, 1986).

2. Young children depend on their parents to interpret the world for them. Parents with impaired social interaction and/or *Altered Thought Processes* may not accurately interpret experiences for the child (Krone, 1986).

3. Impaired social interaction may result in *Social Isolation*. Also, see the nursing diagnosis, *Parenting Altered.*

Gerontologic Considerations

1. Effective social interactions depend on positive self-esteem. No data suggest that older adults have diminished self-esteem when compared with younger adults (Miller, 1990).

2. In elderly persons, common threats to self-esteem include devaluation, dependency, functional impairments, and decreased sense of control (Miller, 1990).

3. Depression-related affective disturbances of daily life occur in 27% of older adults. Major depression occurs in 2% of community-living older adults and in 12% of older persons living in nursing homes (Parmelee, Katz, & Lawton, 1989).

4. Depressed older adults lose interest in social activities and do not display positive interactions when they do interact.

■ Impaired Social Interactions
Related to (Specify) Secondary to Chronic Illness

Assessment

Subjective Data

Psychiatric history
    Hospitalized several times
    Relapse in last year
    Use of several facilities and a variety of treatments ("revolving door")

Use of other social agencies
Medication
    Recent changes
    Patient response
    Problem with compliance
Suicidal ideation or attempts
History of assaults or property destruction
Examination of symptoms associated with recent life stress
    Residence change or problem
    Employment problem
    Medication change
    Problem among family members
    Medical problem
    Financial change
    Relationship change
Obstacles to community functioning
    Poor personal hygiene
    Expects self-reliance
    Lacks leisure-time activities
    Inappropriate behavior in public
    Legal problems
    Unemployed
    Unstable, transient residences
    Social isolation

Objective Data

Thought disturbances
Inappropriate dress
Lack of conversational skills
Preoccupation with self
Noncompliant with previous treatment
Demanding, hostile, manipulative
Low motivation
Dependent

Outcome Criteria

The person will
- Identify problematic behavior that deters socialization
- Substitute constructive behavior for disruptive social behavior (specify)

The family will
- Describe strategies to promote effective socialization

Interventions

A. Provide support for the maintenance of basic social skills and reduce social isolation

(Refer to *Social Isolation* for further interventions)

1. Provide an individual, supportive relationship.
   a. Assist person in managing life stresses.
   b. Focus on present and reality.
   c. Help to identify how stress precipitates problems.
   d. Support healthy defenses.
   e. Help to identify alternative courses of action.
   f. Assist in analyzing approaches that work best.
2. Provide supportive group therapy.
   a. Focus on here and now.
   b. Establish group norms which discourage inappropriate behavior.
   c. Encourage testing of new social behavior.
   d. Use snacks or coffee to decrease anxiety during sessions.
   e. Role-model certain accepted social behaviors (*e.g.*, responding to a friendly greeting versus ignoring it).
   f. Foster development of relationships among members through self-disclosure and genuineness.
   g. Use questions and observations to encourage persons with limited interaction skills.
   h. Encourage members to validate their perception with others.
   i. Identify strengths among members and ignore selected weaknesses.
   j. Activity groups, drop-in socialization centers can be used for some individuals.
3. Monitor medication compliance.
   a. Use small groups or scheduled individual sessions.
   b. Question individual regarding side-effects and symptom exacerbation (do not expect person to self-monitor).
4. Be assertive with persons who are unmotivated or passive.
   a. Contact the person when he fails to attend a scheduled appointment, job interview, etc.
   b. Do not wait for person to want to participate.
5. Hold persons accountable for their own actions.
   a. Treat as responsible citizens.
   b. Allow decision-making, but may have to outline limits.
   c. Do not allow them to use their illness as an excuse for their behavior.
   d. Set consequences and enforce when necessary, including encounters with law.
6. Allow individual to be dependent as necessary.
7. Utilize a wide variety of agencies and services (medical, psychiatric, vocational, social, residential).
   a. Services must be coordinated by one agency (individual will not be able to coordinate for self).
   b. Case managers have been successful in providing linkage.
   c. Programs must be flexible and culturally relevant.

B. Decrease problematic behavior
   1. Impaired reality testing (refer to *Altered Thought Processes*)
   2. Lack of leisure-time activities (refer to *Diversional Activity Deficit*)
      a. Companionship program
      b. Day treatment centers
   3. Social isolation (refer to *Social Isolation*)
   4. Hostility and violent outbursts (refer to *Anxiety* and *High Risk for Violence*)

5. Suicidal threats or attempts (refer to *High Risk for Self-Harm*)
6. Manipulation
   a. Use limit-setting (refer to section on anger in *Anxiety*).
   b. Be aware of own reactions.

C. Provide for development of social skills
1. Identify the environment in which social interactions are impaired.
   a. Living
   b. Learning
   c. Working
2. Provide instruction in the environment where person is expected to function when possible (*e.g.,* accompany to job site, work with person in own residence).
3. Develop an individualized social skill program. Examples of some social skills are: grooming-personal hygiene, posture, gait, eye contact, beginning a conversation, listening, ending a conversation. Include modeling, behavior rehearsal, and homework (Manderino & Bzdek, 1987).
4. Combine verbal instructions with demonstration and practice.
5. Be firm in setting parameters of appropriate social behaviors such as punctuality, attendance, managing illnesses with employers, dress, etc.
6. Use group as a method of discussing work-related problems.
7. Use sheltered workshops and part-time employment depending on person's level where success can best be achieved.
8. Give positive feedback; make sure it is specific and detailed. Focus on no more than three behavioral connections at a time; too-lengthy feedback adds confusion and increases anxiety.
9. Convey a "can-do" attitude.

D. Assist family and community members in understanding and providing support
1. Provide factual information concerning illness, treatment, and progress to family members.
2. Validate family members' feelings of frustration in dealing with daily problems.
3. Provide guidance on overstimulating or understimulating environments.
4. Allow families to discuss their feelings of guilt and how their behavior affects the person.
5. Develop an alliance with family.
6. Arrange for periodic respite care.
7. Provide support to landlords, shopkeepers, and anyone else with whom person has contact.
   a. Provide information on mental illness.
   b. Teach them relationship skills needed to manage person (*e.g.,* direct, firm, simple directions; use of modeling).
   c. Give person name and number he can call when problems arise.
   d. Provide this education as the need arises with specific individuals.

E. Initiate health teaching and referrals as indicated
1. Teach the person (McFarland & Wasli, 1986)
   a. Responsibilities of his/her role as a client (making requests clearly known, participating in therapies)
   b. To outline activities of the day and to focus on accomplishing them
   c. How to approach others in order to communicate

    d. To identify which interactions encourage others to give him/her consideration and respect

    e. To identify how he/she can participate in formulating family roles and responsibility to comply

    f. To recognize signs of anxiety and methods to relieve them

    g. To identify his/her positive behavior and to experience satisfaction with himself in selecting constructive choices

2. Teach basic coping skills necessary to live independently (home management, personal hygiene, financial management, transportation skills).
3. Teach or refer for assertive skill training.
4. Teach basic conversational skills.
5. Teach job-seeking skills.
6. Teach parenting skills.
7. Refer to a variety of social agencies; however, coordination and continuity to be maintained by one agency.
8. Refer for supportive family therapy as indicated.
9. Refer families to local self-help groups.
10. Provide numbers for crisis intervention services.

References/Bibliography

Anthony, W. A. (1980). *The principles of psychiatric rehabilitation.* Baltimore: University Park Press.

Bachrach, L. (1982) Young adult chronic patients: An analytical review of the literature. *Hospital and Community Psychiatry, 33*(6), 189–197.

Johnson, S. H. (1986). Nursing diagnosis strategies. In Johnson, S. H. *High-risk parenting: Nursing assessment and strategies for the family at risk.* Philadelphia: J. B. Lippincott, p. 458.

Krauss, J. (1980). The chronic psychiatric patient in the community—a model of care. *Nursing Outlook, 28*(7), 308–314.

Krauss, J., & Slavinsky, A. (1982). *The chronically ill psychiatric patient and the community.* Oxford: Blackwell Scientific.

Krone, C. H. (1986). The emotionally disturbed parent. In Johnson, S. H. *High-risk parenting: Nursing assessment and strategies for the family at risk.* Philadelphia: J. B. Lippincott, pp. 308, 310.

Manderino, M., & Bzdek, V. (1987). Social skill building. *Journal of Psychosocial Nursing, 25*(9), 18–22.

Maroni, J. (1989). Impaired social interactions. In McFarland, G., & McFarlane, E. *Nursing diagnosis and interventions.* St. Louis: C. V. Mosby.

McFarland, G., & Wasli, E. (1986). Manipulation in nursing diagnoses and process. In *Psychiatric mental health nursing.* Philadelphia: J. B. Lippincott, p. 92.

Miller, C. A. (1990). *Nursing care of older adults.* Glenview, IL: Scott, Foresman.

Parmelee, P. A., Katz, I. R., & Lawton, M. P. (1989). Depression among institutionalized aged. *Journal of Gerontology: Medical Sciences, 44*(1), 22–29.

Pepper, B., Ryglewicz, H., & Kirshner M. (1982, June). The uninstitutionalized generation: A new breed of psychiatric patient. In Pepper, B., & Ryglewicz, H. (Eds). *New directions for mental health services: The young adult chronic patient No. 14.* San Francisco: Jossey-Bass.

Test, M. A., & Stein, L. (1976). Practical guidelines for the community treatment of markedly impaired patients. *Community and Mental Health Journal, 12*(31), 72–82.

Spiritual Distress

- *Related to* **(Specify) as Evidenced by Inability to Practice Spiritual Rituals**
- *Related to* **Conflict Between Religious or Spiritual Beliefs and Prescribed Health Regimen**
- *Related to* **Crisis of illness/Suffering/Death**

DEFINITION

Spiritual Distress: The state in which the individual or group experiences or is at risk of experiencing a disturbance in the belief or value system which provides strength, hope and meaning to life.

DEFINING CHARACTERISTICS

Major (must be present)

Experiences a disturbance in belief system

Minor (may be present)

Questions credibility of belief system
Demonstrates discouragement or despair
Is unable to practice usual religious rituals
Has ambivalent feelings (doubts) about beliefs
Expresses that he has no reason for living
Feels a sense of spiritual emptiness
Shows emotional detachment from self and others
Expresses concern—anger, resentment, fear—over meaning of life, suffering, death
Requests spiritual assistance for a disturbance in belief system

RELATED FACTORS

Pathophysiologic

Loss of body part or function
Terminal illness
Debilitating disease
Pain
Trauma
Miscarriage, stillbirth

Treatment-related

Abortion   Isolation
Surgery   Amputation
Blood transfusion   Medications
Dietary restrictions   Medical procedures

Situational (personal, environmental)
    Death or illness of significant other
    Embarrassment at practicing spiritual rituals
    Hospital barriers to practicing spiritual rituals
        Restrictions of intensive care
        Confinement to bed or room
        Lack of privacy
        Lack of availability of special foods/diet
    Beliefs opposed by family, peers, health care providers
    Childbirth
    Divorce, separation from loved one

Diagnostic Considerations

Wellness represents a response to a person's potential for personal growth, involving utilization of all one's resources (social, psychologic, cultural, environmental, spiritual, and physiologic) (Bruhn, Cordova, Williams, & Fuentes, 1977). Nurses profess to care for the whole client, but several studies report that nurses commonly avoid addressing the spiritual dimension of clients, families, and communities (DeYoung, 1984; Martin, Burrows, & Pomilio, 1978).

To promote positive spirituality with persons and families, the nurse must possess positive spirituality. For the nurse, self-evaluation must precede assessment regarding spiritual concerns, and assessment of spiritual health should be confined to the context of nursing. The nurse can assist persons with spiritual concerns or distress by providing resources for spiritual help, by listening nonjudgmentally, and by providing opportunities for meeting spiritual needs (Stoll, 1984). The nurse should be cautioned against establishing practice patterns that routinely result in referring all spiritual needs of clients and families to religious or spiritual leaders.

Errors in Diagnostic Statements

Spiritual Distress related to critical illness and doubts about religious beliefs

Critical illness can challenge a person's spiritual beliefs and can evoke feelings of guilt, anger, disappointment, and helplessness. However, critical illness does not represent a specific contributing factor or cue to the presence of spiritual distress. Until related factors are known, the nurse can record the diagnosis as *Spiritual Distress related to unknown etiology as evidenced by expressions of doubt about religious beliefs*. The nursing focus will be on actively listening to the person's feelings and fears.

Focus Assessment Criteria

Subjective Data

The following questions may be included as part of the psychosocial nursing assessment for individuals and families.

1. "Is religion or God important to you?"
    If answer is *yes*, "To what religion do you belong?" or "In what do you believe?"
    If *no*, "Do you find a source of strength or meaning in another area?"
2. "What effect do you expect your illness (hospitalization) to have on your spiritual practices or beliefs?"

3. "Are there any religious books (statues, medals, services, places) that are especially important to you?"
4. Do you have a special religious leader (priest, pastor, rabbi)?"
5. "How can I help you maintain your spiritual strength during this illness (hospitalization)?" (*e.g.,* contact spiritual leader, provide privacy at special times, request reading materials)

Objective Data

1. Present practices
   Assess for
   The presence of religious or spiritual articles (clothing, medals, texts)
   Visits from religious leader
   Visits to religious place of worship
   Requests for spiritual counseling or assistance
2. Response to interview on spiritual needs
   Assess for the presence of anxiety, doubt, anger, depression
3. Sudden changes in spiritual practices
   Assess for
   Rejection or neglect of previous practices
   Increased interest in spiritual matters

Principles and Rationale for Nursing Care

Generic Considerations

1. According to Ellison (1983), spirituality enables and motivates a person to "search for meaning and purpose of life, to seek the supernatural or some meaning which transcends one, to wonder about one's origins and identities, to require morality and equity." It helps provide direction and order to life.
2. Spirituality involves a "direct personal experience and realization of reality" (*e.g.,* of oneself, of a higher being, of nature) (Roche de Coppens, 1980).
3. Spirituality is not synonymous with religion, religiousness, or spiritualism. As Egan (1984) states, "To serve another spiritually is to be witness, friend, and advocate of the sacredness of the human person."
4. According to Colliton (1984), "The spiritual dimension builds on nature and is nurtured through relationships. The person who assists another in the quest for spiritual experience shares a creative moment wherein a transfer of spiritual energy takes place, spiritually enriching both. This deepest touch—spirit to spirit—is founded in the patient's and nurse's intimacy with body touch in physical care and verbal "touch" in emotional support. The nurse tries to be at the disposal of the patient as a spiritual partner to satisfy the need for relatedness in such a way that the patient will find strength to come to terms with life, gain confidence, and become more fully a person."
5. No matter how overwhelmed with illness the person, the nurse may become a spiritual partner and by peaceful silent prayerful intention offer spiritual strength and will to live to someone who has lost it or for whom it hangs in balance (Colliton, 1984).
6. Before a nurse can establish a supportive relationship with another, she or he must acknowledge her or his own vulnerability and humanity (Stoll, 1984). A nurse lending others her strength is willing to open herself for joy and praise or rejection and criticism (Fish & Shelly, 1978).
7. According to Stoll (1984), "prayer, private or with a significant other, is over-

whelmingly reported as the most meaningful spiritual coping strategy and religious practice."

8. All people have a spiritual dimension, whether or not they participate in formal religious practices (Fehring & McLane, 1986).

9. The practice of nurses should not violate their own moral, ethical, spiritual, or religious values.

10. The nature of the spiritual care an individual receives may directly affect the speed and quality of his recovery from illness. An individual is a spiritual person even when disoriented, confused, emotionally ill, delirious, or cognitively impaired.

11. Religion influences attitudes and behavior related to right and wrong, family, child-rearing, work, money, politics, and many other functional areas (Taylor, Lillis, & LeMone, 1989).

12. Research shows that persons with higher levels of spiritual well-being tend to experience lower levels of anxiety (Kaczorowski, 1989). For many persons, spiritual activities provide a direct coping action (Sodestrom & Martinson, 1987).

13. To deal effectively with a person's spiritual needs, the nurse must recognize her or his own beliefs and values, acknowledge that these values may not be applicable for others, and respect the person's beliefs when helping him meet perceived spiritual needs (Taylor, Lillis, & LeMone, 1989).

14. The value of prayers or spiritual rituals to the believer is not affected by whether or not they can be scientifically "proved" to be beneficial.

15. A person's request to see a spiritual leader or counselor should not be denied except in case of extreme emergency. (The leader or counselor could even be sent to the operating room or treatment room if necessary.)

16. The nurse should function as an advocate in recognizing and respecting the individual's spiritual needs, which may sometimes be overlooked or ignored by other health professionals.

17. Research indicates that many nurses feel inadequately prepared to provide spiritual care, and that fewer than 15% include spirituality in nursing care (Piles, 1990).

18. To assist people in spiritual distress, the nurse must know certain beliefs and practices of the various spiritual groups found in this country. Table II–18 provides information on the beliefs and practices that are most directly related to health and illness. It is intended as a quick reference only. Major religions, denominations, and spiritual groups are arranged alphabetically. Denominations with similar practices and restrictions are grouped together. No attempt is made to discuss the broad beliefs and philosophies of the selected groups; see References/Bibliography for such in-depth information.

Pediatric Considerations

1. Children's spiritual needs include love and relatedness, forgiveness, meaning, and purpose (Van Heukelem, 1982).

2. Spiritual beliefs are influenced by moral and cognitive development (Whaley & Wong, 1989).

3. Children learn faith and religion from the practices of parents/significant others (Whaley & Wong, 1989).

Gerontologic Considerations

1. The White House Council on Aging in 1971 described spiritual concerns as "the human need to deal with sociocultural deprivations, anxieties and fears, death and dying, social alienation, and philosophy of life" (Moberg, 1984; Ryan, 1985).

(Text continues on page 814)

Table II–18 **Overview of Religious Beliefs**

Agnostic
Beliefs
It is impossible to know if God exists (specific moral values may guide behavior)

Amish
Illness
Usually taken care of within family
Texts
Bible
Ausbund (16th century German hymnal)
Beliefs
Rejection of all government aid
Rejection of modernization
Legally exempt from immunizations

Armenian
See Eastern Orthodox

Atheist
Beliefs
God does not exist (specific moral values may guide behavior)

Baptist, Churches of God, Churches of Christ, and Pentecostal (Assemblies of God, Four-square Church)
Illness
Some practice layong on of hands, divine healing through prayer
May request Communion
Some prohibit medical therapy
May consider illness divine punishment or intrusion of Satan
Diet
No alcohol (mandatory for most)
No coffee, tea, tobacco, pork, or strangled animals (mandatory for some)
Some fasting
Birth
Opposes infant baptism
Text
Bible
Beliefs
Some practice glossolalia (speaking in tongues)

Buddhism
Illness
Considered trial that develops the soul
May wish counseling by priest
May refuse treatment on holy days (1/1, 1/16, 2/15, 3/21, 4/8, 5/21, 6/15, 8/1, 8/23, 12/8, 12/31)
Diet
Strict vegetarianism (mandatory for some)
Discourages use of alcohol, tobacco, and drugs
Death
Last-rite chanting by priest
Death leads to rebirth, may wish to remain alert and lucid

(*continued*)

Table II–18 **Overview of Religious Beliefs** (continued)

Texts

Buddha's sermon on the "eightfold path"

The Tripitaka, or "three baskets" of wisdom

Beliefs

Cleanliness is of great importance

Suffering is universal

Christian Science

Illness

Caused by errors in thought and mind

May oppose drugs; IV fluid; blood transfusions; psychotherapy; hypnotism; physical examinations; biopsies; eye, ear, and blood pressure screening; and other medical and nursing interventions

Accepts only legally required immunizations

May desire support from a Christian Science reader or treatment by a Christian Science nurse or practitioner (a list of these nonmedical practitioners and nurses may be found in the *Christian Science Journal*)

Healing is spiritual renewal

Death

Autopsy permitted only in cases of sudden death

Text

Bible

Science and Health With Key to the Scriptures by Mary Baker Eddy

Church of Christ
See Baptist

Church of God
See Baptist

Confucian

Illness

The body was given by one's parents and should therefore be well cared for

May be strongly motivated to maintain or regain wellness

Beliefs

Respect for family and older persons very important

Cults (variety of groups, usually with living leader)

Illness

Most practice faith healing

May reject modern medicine and condemn health personnel as enemies

Therapeutic compliance and follow-up are generally poor

Illness may represent wrong thinking or inhabitation by Satan

Beliefs

Expansion of cult through conversions important

May depend on cult environment for definition of reality

Eastern Orthodox (Greek Orthodox, Russian Orthodox, Armenian)

Illness

May desire Holy Communion, laying on of hands, anointing, or sacrament of Holy Unction

Most oppose euthanasia and favor every effort to preserve life

Russian Orthodox males should be shaved only if necessary for surgery

(continued)

Table II–18 **Overview of Religious Beliefs** *(continued)*

Diet
  May fast Wednesdays, Fridays, during Lent, before Christmas, or for 6 hr before Communion
    (seriously ill are exempted)
  May avoid meat, dairy products, and olive oil during fast (seriously ill are exempted)
Birth
  Baptism 8–40 days after birth, usually by immersion (mandatory for some)
  May be followed immediately by confirmation
    Greek Orthodox only: If death of infant is imminent, nurse should baptize infant by touching
      the forehead with a small amount of water three times
Death
  Last rites and administration of Holy Communion (mandatory for some)
  May oppose autopsy, embalming, and cremation
Texts
  Bible
  Prayer book
Religious articles
  Icons (pictures of Jesus, Mary, saints) are very important
  Holy water and lighted candles
  Russian Orthodox wears cross necklace which should be removed only if necessary
Other
  Greek Orthodox opposes abortion
  Confession at least yearly (mandatory for some)
  Holy Communion 4 times yearly; Christmas, Easter, 6/30, and 8/15 (mandatory for some)
  Dates of holy days may differ from Western Christian calendar

Episcopal
Illness
  May believe in spiritual healing
  May desire confession and Communion
Diet
  May abstain from meat on Fridays
  May fast during Lent or before Communion
Birth
  Infant baptism is mandatory (nurse may baptize infant when death is imminent by pouring water
    on forehead and saying, "I baptize you in the name of the Father, the Son, and the Holy
    Spirit")
Death
  Last rites optional
Texts
  Bible
  Prayer book

Friends (Quaker)
No minister or priests; direct, individual, inner experience of God is vital
Diet
  Most avoid alcohol and drugs and favor practice of moderation
Death
  Many do not believe in afterlife
Beliefs
  Pacifism important; many are conscientious objectors to war

(continued)

Table II–18 **Overview of Religious Beliefs** (continued)

Greek Orthodox
See Eastern Orthodox

Hinduism
Illness
   May minimize illness and emphasize its temporary nature
   Considered important only as it affects spiritual quest
   Illness or injury may represent sins committed in previous life
Diet
   Various doctrines, many vegetarian; many abstain from alcohol (mandatory for some); beef and
      pork are forbidden
Death
   Seen as rebirth; may wish to be alert
   Priest may tie thread around neck or wrist of body—do not remove
   Water is poured into mouth, and family washes body
   Cremation preferred—must be soon after death
Beliefs
   Self-control, self-discipline, and cleanliness emphasized
   Opposes artificial insemination
Texts
   Vedas
   Upanishads
   Bhagavad-Gita
Worship
   Usually in home
   May involve various images, statues, and symbols of gods
   May include use of water, fire, lights, sounds, natural objects, special postures, and gestures

Jehovah's Witness
Illness
   Opposes blood transfusions and organ transplantation (mandatory)
   May oppose other medical treatment and all modern science
   Opposes faith healing
   Opposes abortion
Diet
   Refuses foods to which blood has been added; may eat meats that have been drained
Text
   Bible

Judaism
Illness
Medical care emphasized
   Rabbinical consultation necessary for donation and transplantation of organs
   May oppose surgical procedures on the Sabbath (sundown Friday to sundown Saturday); seri-
      ously ill are exempted
   May prefer burial of removed organs or body tissues
   May oppose shaving
   May wear skull cap and socks continuously, believing head and feet should be covered
Diet
   Fasting for 24 hr on holy days of Yom Kippur (in September or October) in Tisha Bab (in August)

(continued)

Table II-18 **Overview of Religious Beliefs** (continued)

Matzo replaced leavened bread during Passover week (in March or April)

May observe strict Kosher dietary laws (mandatory for some) that prohibit pork; shellfish, and the eating of meat and dairy products at same meal or with same dishes (milk products, served first, can be followed by meat in a few minutes; reverse is not Kosher); seriously ill are exempted

Birth

Ritual circumcision 8 days after birth (mandatory for some)

Fetuses are buried

Death

Ritual burial; society members wash body

Burial as soon as possible

Opposes cremation

Many oppose autopsy and donation of body to science

Most do not believe in afterlife

Generally oppose prolongation of life after irreversible brain damage

Texts

Torah (first five books of Old Testament)

Talmud

Prayer book

Religious articles

Menorah (seven-branched candlestick)

Yarmulke (skull cap, may be worn continuously)

Tallith (prayer shawl worn for morning prayers)

Tefillin, or phylacteries (leather boxes on straps containing scripture passages)

Star of David (may be worn around neck)

Krishna

Diet

Vegetarian diet; no garlic or onions

No drugs, alcohol; herbal tea only

Death

Cremation mandatory

Texts

Vedas

Srimad-Bhagavatam

Beliefs

Continual practice of mantra (chant)

Belief in reincarnation

Lutheran, Methodist, Presbyterian

Illness

May request Communion, anointing and blessing, or visitation by minister or elder

Generally encourages utilization of medical science

Birth

Baptism by sprinkling or immersion of infants, children, or adults

Death

Optional last rites or scripture reading

Texts

Bible

Prayer book

(continued)

Table II–18 **Overview of Religious Beliefs** (continued)

Mennonite
Illness
  Opposes laying on of hands
  May oppose shock treatment and drugs
Texts
  Bible
  18 articles of the Dondecht Confession of Faith
Beliefs
  Shun modernization
  No participation in government, pensions, or health plans

Methodist
See Lutheran

Mormon (Church of Jesus Christ of Latter-Day Saints)
Illness
  May come through partaking of harmful substances such as alcohol, tobacco, drugs, etc.
  May be seen as a necessary part of the plan of salvation
  May desire Sacrament of the Lord's Supper to be administered by a Church Priesthood holder
  Divine healing through laying on of hands
  Church may provide financial support during illness
Diet
  Prohibits alcohol, tobacco, and hot drinks (tea and coffee)
  Sparing use of meats
Birth
  No infant baptism
  Infants are born innocent
Death
  Cremation is opposed
Texts
  Bible
  Book of Mormon
Religious articles
  Special undergarment may be worn by both men and women and should not be removed ex-
    cept during serious illness, childbirth, emergencies, etc.
Beliefs
  Abortion is opposed
  Vicarious baptism for deceased who were not baptized in life

Muslim (Islamic, Moslem) and Black Muslim
Illness
  Opposes faith healing
  May be noncompliant due to fatalistic view (illness is God's will)
  Group prayer may be helpful—no priests
  Favors every effort to prolong life
Diet
  Pork prohibited
  May oppose alcohol and traditional Black American foods (corn bread, collard greens)
  Fasts sunrise to sunset during Ramadan (9th month of Muslim year—falls different time each
    year on Western calendar); seriously ill are exempted

(continued)

Table II–18 **Overview of Religious Beliefs** (continued)

Birth
   Circumcision practiced with accompanying ceremony
   Aborted fetus after 30 days is treated as human being
Death
   Confession of sins before death, with family present if possible
   Family follows specific procedure for washing and preparing body, which is then turned to face Mecca
   May oppose autopsy
Texts
   Koran (scriptures)
   Hadith (traditions)
Prayer
   Five times daily—upon rising, midday, afternoon, early evening, and before bed—facing Mecca and kneeling on prayer rug
   Ritual washing after prayer
Beliefs
   All activities (including sleep) restricted to what is necessary for health
   Personal cleanliness very important
   All Muslims: gambling and idol worship prohibited

Pentecostal
See Baptist

Presbyterian
See Lutheran

Quakers
See Friends

Roman Catholic
Illness
   Allowed by God because of man's sins but not considered personal punishment
   May desire confession (penance) and Communion
   Anointing of sick for all seriously ill patients (some patients may equate this with "Last Rites" and assume they are dying)
   Donation and transplantation of organs permitted
   Burial of amputated limbs (mandatory for some)
Diet
   Fasting or abstaining from meat mandatory on Ash Wednesday and Good Friday (seriously ill are exempted); optional during Lent and on Fridays
   Fasts from solid food for 1 hr and abstains from alcohol for 3 hr before receiving Communion (mandatory) (seriously ill are exempted)
Birth
   Baptism of infants and aborted fetuses mandatory (nurse may baptize in case of imminent death by sprinkling water on the forehead and saying, "I baptize you in the name of the Father, of the Son, and of the Holy Spirit")
Death
   Anointing of sick (mandatory)
   Extraordinary artificial means of sustaining life are unnecessary
Texts
   Bible
   Prayer book

(continued)

Table II–18 **Overview of Religious Beliefs** (continued)

Religious articles
  Rosary, crucifix, saints' medals, statues, holy water, lighted candles
Other
  Attendance at mass required (seriously ill are exempted) on Sundays or late Saturday and on
    holy days (1/1, 8/15, 11/1, 12/8, 12/25, and 40 days after Easter)
  Sacrament of Penance at least yearly (mandatory)
  Opposes abortion

Russian Orthodox
See Eastern Orthodox

Seventh-Day Adventist (Advent Christian Church)
Illness
  May desire baptism or Communion
  Some believe in divine healing
  May oppose hypnosis
  May refuse treatment on the Sabbath (sundown Friday to sundown Saturday)
  Healthful diet and life-style are stressed
Diet
  No alcohol, coffee, tea, narcotics, or stimulants (mandatory)
  Some abstain from pork, other meat, and shellfish
Birth
  Opposes infant baptism
Text
  Bible, especially Ten Commandments and Old Testament

Shinto
Illness
  May believe in prayer healing
  Great concern for personal cleanliness
  Physical health may be valued due to emphasis on joy and beauty of life
  Family extremely important in giving care and providing emotional support
Beliefs
  Worships ancestors, ancient heroes, and nature
  Traditions emphasized
  Esthetically pleasing area for worship important

Taoist
Illness
  Illness is seen as part of the health/illness dualism
  May be resigned to and accepting of illness
  May consider medical treatment as interference
Death
  Seen as natural part of life
  Body is kept in house for 49 days
  Mourning follows specific ritual patterns
Text
  Tao-te-ching by Lao-tzu
Beliefs
  Esthetically pleasing area for meditation important

(continued)

Table II–18 **Overview of Religious Beliefs** (continued)

Unitarian Universalist
Illness
  Reason, knowledge, and individual responsibility are emphasized, so may prefer not to see clergy
Birth
  Most do not practice infant baptism
Death
  Prefers cremation

Zen
Meditation utilizing lotus position (many hours and years are spent in meditation and contemplation); goal is to discover simplicity
Illness
  May wish consultation with Zen master

---

2. The National Interfaith Coalition on Aging describes spiritual well-being as "the affirmation of life in a relationship with God, self, community, and environment that nurtures and celebrates wholeness" (Ryan & Patterson, 1987).
3. Factors that contribute to spiritual distress and put elderly persons at risk include questions concerning life after death as the person ages, separation from formal religious community, and a value-belief system that is continuously challenged by losses and suffering (Dickinson, 1975; Matteson & McConnell, 1988; Patterson, 1984).
4. About 75% of all elderly persons are members of religious organizations. This does not necessarily mean that they attend their formal services and meetings regularly (Matteson & McConnell, 1988).
5. Elderly persons tend to participate in formal religious groups less than younger people. Nonorganizational participation increases dramatically with age, and the desire to participate in the church activities remains constant throughout their lives. Elderly persons may find religious services difficult to attend and participate in due to physical impairments. Factors such as lack of transportation, inaccessible toileting facilities, poor acoustics and sound systems for hearing-impaired, and small-print hymn books or prayer books can diminish active involvement in formal religious activities (Ainlay & Smith, 1984; Mindel & Vaughan, 1978).
6. Elderly persons must complete Erikson's developmental stage of Ego Integrity versus Despair to achieve life satisfaction. The older person may reflect on his life, expressing that he has lived in accordance with his value system, and may express contentment with his life. These behaviors demonstrate fulfillment of the need for meaning and purpose in life (Forbis, 1988; Matteson & McConnell, 1988).
7. Those who have not sought religion early in life will not automatically become more religious in later life (Ainlay & Smith, 1984; Nelsen, 1981).
8. A common coping method for elderly persons, prayer increases feelings of self-worth and hope by reducing the sense of aloneness and abandonment. In addition to private prayer and mediation, television and radio often provide adjunct stimulus for spiritual life. Estimates indicate that 60% of viewers of religious television programs are over age 50, primarily female (Ainlay & Smith, 1984; Bearon & Koenig, 1990; Carson, 1980).
9. The elderly may rely on spiritual life more than most young people because of other limitations in their lives. The spiritual realm allows for satisfying connectedness with others (Giuri, 1980; Hall, 1985). An older individual can counterbalance some of

the negative, isolating aspects of aging by identifying with tradition and institutional values. Private religion can help to motivate and provide purpose to life.

10. Older persons commonly intertwine their religious beliefs with beliefs about health and illness. The nurse must assess these beliefs appropriately to facilitate the person's understanding of his illness in the context of his religion (Bearon & Koenig, 1990).

11. For many elderly persons, religious activities and spiritual exchanges can reduce anxiety.

12. Three phases of suffering in the frail elderly can explain spiritual distress:
    a. Mute suffering, which revolves around a feeling of abandonment, belief that prayers are not answered, and self-isolation
    b. The cry of lament, which can be explained as an interpretation that bad things are happening because of earlier mistakes in life
    c. Liberation for change, which allows the person to transcend loneliness and to approach hope through suffering (Shea, 1986; Patterson, 1984; Bearon & Koenig, 1990)

13. Older adults commonly report a sense of increased power and control from religion and spiritual resources (Stevenson, 1982).

14. Spiritual well-being can be described as harmony and interconnection of relationships. These relationships are either time or person-related, e.g., ultimate other (describes a love of God), other/nature (expresses mutual love and concern), self (values inner self), past (recognizes influence in past sociocultural and religious practices), present (finds meaning and purpose in life experiences), and future (hopes in ultimate integration). In reviewing the above, it seems likely that older adults who have achieved passage through developmental phases or tasks can use their spirituality to work through Erikson's stage of Ego Integrity versus Despair. A strong sense of satisfaction with self and life conveys an inner harmony (Hungelmann, Kenkel-Rossi, Klassen, & Stollenwerk, 1985).

15. DeYoung (1984) reported a study in which 76% of older adults in nursing homes expressed a sense of spiritual well-being. About 25% of the subjects reported that a nurse had helped them with their spiritual needs, but 79% were against nursing involvement in their spiritual lives. Reasons cited included differing beliefs and the nurse's need to focus on physical care.

■ Spiritual Distress
Related to (Specify) as Evidenced by Inability to Practice Spiritual Rituals

---

Assessment

Subjective Data

The person expresses one or more of the following feelings related to spiritual belief system

Anxiety	Embarrassment
Guilt	Sense of loss
Depression	Grief

Requests spiritual articles, reading materials, sacraments, services, etc.

Questions others about their spiritual rituals

Person requests changes in medical regimen or hospital protocols to allow practice of spiritual rituals

Objective Data

Cannot go to religious services or place of worship

Cannot maintain religious diet or fast

Is separated from religious or spiritual articles, clothing, texts, etc.

Is unable to say prayers or meditate

Is unable to maintain usual contact with spiritual leader or members of spiritual group

Cannot read religious materials

Cannot assume normal position for prayer or meditation

Outcome Criteria

The person will
- Continue spiritual practices not detrimental to health
- Express decreasing feelings of guilt and anxiety
- Express satisfaction with spiritual condition

Interventions

A. Assess for causative and contribution factors

1. Hospital or nursing home environment
2. Limitations related to disease process or treatment regimen (*e.g.,* cannot kneel to pray due to traction; prescribed diet differs from usual religious diet)
3. Fear of imposing upon or antagonizing medical and nursing staff with requests for spiritual rituals
4. Embarrassment regarding spiritual beliefs or customs (especially common in adolescents)
5. Separation from articles, texts, or environment of spiritual significance
6. Lack of transportation to spiritual place or service
7. Spiritual leader unavailable due to emergency or lack of time

B. Eliminate or reduce causative and contributing factors, if possible

1. Limitations imposed by the hospital or nursing home environment
   a. Provide privacy and quiet as needed for daily prayer, for visit of spiritual leader, and for spiritual reading and contemplation.
      - Pull curtains or close door.
      - Turn off television and radio.
      - Ask desk to hold calls if possible.
      - Note spiritual interventions on Kardex and include in care plan.
   b. Contact spiritual leader to clarify practices and perform religious rites or services if desired.
      - Communicate with spiritual leader regarding person's condition.

- Address Roman Catholic, Orthodox, and Episcopal priests as "Father," other Christian ministers as "Pastor," and Jewish rabbis as "Rabbi."
- Prevent interruption during visit, if possible.
- Offer to provide table or stand covered with clean white cloth.
- Chart visit and patient's response.
    c. Inform patient about religious services and materials available within the institution.
2. Limitations related to disease process or treatment regimen
    a. Encourage spiritual rituals not detrimental to health (see Table II–18)
        - Encourage children to maintain bedtime or before-meal prayer rituals.
        - Assist individuals with physical limitations in prayer and spiritual observances (e.g., help to hold rosary; help to kneeling position, if appropriate).
        - Assist in habits of personal cleanliness.
        - Avoid shaving if beard is of spiritual significance.
        - Allow to wear religious clothing or jewelry whenever possible.
        - Make special arrangements for burial of resected limbs or body organs.
        - Allow family or spiritual leader to perform ritual care of body.
        - Make arrangements as needed for other important spiritual rituals (e.g., circumcisions).
    b. Maintain diet with spiritual restrictions when not detrimental to health (see Table II–18)
        - Consult with dietitian.
        - Allow fasting for short periods if possible.*
        - Change therapeutic diet as necessary.*
        - Have family or friends bring in special food if possible.
        - Have members of spiritual group supply meals to the person at home.
        - Be as flexible as possible in serving methods, times of meals, etc.
3. Fear of imposing or embarrassment
    a. Communicate acceptance of various spiritual beliefs and practices.
    b. Convey nonjudgmental attitude.
    c. Acknowledge importance of spiritual needs.
    d. Express willingness of health care team to help in meeting spiritual needs.
    e. Provide privacy and ensure confidentiality.
4. Separation from articles, texts, or environment of spiritual significance
    a. Question individual about missing religious or spiritual articles or reading material (see Table II–18).
    b. Obtain missing items from clergy in hospital, spiritual leader, family, or members of spiritual group.
    c. Treat these articles and books with respect.
    d. Allow person to keep spiritual articles and books within reach as much as possible, or where they can be easily seen.
    e. Protect from loss or damage (e.g., medal pinned to patient's gown can be lost in laundry).
    f. Recognize that articles without overt religious meaning may have spiritual significance for individual (e.g., wedding band).
    g. Utilize spiritual texts in large print, in Braille, or on tape when appropriate.
    h. Provide opportunity for individual to pray with others or be read to by members of own religious group or member of the health care team who feels comfortable with these activities.

---

* May require a physician's order.

  • Jews and Seventh-Day Adventists would find Psalms 23, 34, 42, 63, 71,
    103, 121, and 127 appropriate.
  • Christians would also appreciate I Corinthians 13, Matthew 5:3–11,
    Romans 12, and the Lord's Prayer.
5. Lack of transportation
    a. Take person to chapel or quiet environment on hospital grounds.
    b. Arrange transportation to church or synagogue for individual in home.
    c. Provide access to spiritual programming on radio and television when appro-
       priate.
6. Spiritual leader unavailable due to emergency or lack of time
    a. Baptize critically ill newborn of Greek Orthodox, Episcopal, or Roman Catho-
       lic parents (see Table II–18).
    b. Perform other mandatory spiritual rituals if possible.

■ Spiritual Distress
Related to Conflict Between Religious or Spiritual Beliefs and Prescribed Health Regimen

---

Assessment

Subjective Data

The person expresses one or more feelings related to spiritual beliefs

Anxiety	Depression
Guilt	Fear of God
Grief	Fear of physician
Sense of loss	Dream about angry God or
Doubt	minister
Sense of powerlessness	Ambivalence in decisions
Trapped feeling	

Objective Data

Questions or refuses therapeutic regimen
Agrees to morally or ethically unacceptable therapy
Frantically seeks advice or support for decision-making
Questions others about their beliefs and values
Experiences insomnia or nightmares
Objects to prescribed or legally required medical procedures (autopsy, blood transfu-
    sion, immunization) that conflict with personal spiritual beliefs
Objects to prescribed diet or medication that conflicts with spiritual dietary restric-
    tions

> **Outcome Criteria**
>
> The person will
> - Express religious or spiritual satisfaction
> - Express decreased feelings of guilt and fear
> - Relate he is supported in his decision regarding his health regimen
> - State that conflict has been eliminated or reduced

Interventions

A. Assess for causative and contributing factors (see Table II–18)

1. Lack of information about or understanding of spiritual restrictions
2. Lack of information about or understanding of health regimen
3. Informed, true conflict
4. Parent conflict regarding treatment of child
5. Lack of time for deliberation before emergency treatment or surgery

B. Eliminate or reduce causative and contributing factors, if possible

1. Lack of information about spiritual restrictions
   a. Have spiritual leader discuss restrictions and exemptions as they apply to those who are seriously ill or hospitalized.
   b. Provide reading materials on religious and spiritual restrictions and exemptions.
   c. Encourage person to seek information from and discuss restrictions with others in spiritual group.
   d. Chart results of these discussions.
2. Lack of information about health regimen
   a. Provide accurate information about health regimen, treatments, medications.
   b. Explain the nature and purpose of therapy.
   c. Discuss possible outcomes without therapy; be factual and honest but do not attempt to frighten or force person to accept treatment.
3. Informed, true conflict
   a. Encourage individual and physician to consider alternate methods of therapy* (e.g., utilization of Christian Science nurses and practitioners; special surgeons and techniques for surgery without blood transfusions).
   b. Support individual making informed decision—even if decision conflicts with own values.
      - Consult own spiritual leader.
      - Change patient assignment so that person can be cared for by nurse with compatible beliefs.
      - Arrange for discussions among health care team to share feelings.
4. Parent conflict regarding treatment of child
   a. If parents refuse treatment of child, follow interventions under 3a and 3b above.
   b. If treatment is still refused, physician or hospital administrator may obtain court order appointing temporary guardian to consent to treatment.*

*May require a physician's order.

c. Call spiritual leader to support parents (and possibly child).
d. Encourage expression of negative feelings.
5. Emergency treatment
a. Provide as little treatment as possible for Christian Scientists, cult members, etc. (see Table II–18).
b. Delay treatment if possible until spiritual needs have been met (*e.g.,* receiving last rites before surgery)*; send spiritual leader to treatment room or operating room, if necessary.
c. Anticipate reaction and provide support when individual chooses to accept or is forced to accept spiritually unacceptable therapy.
   • Depression, withdrawal, anger, fear
   • Loss of will to live
   • Reduced speed and quality of recovery

■ Spiritual Distress
Related to Crisis of Illness/Suffering/Death

Assessment

Subjective Data

The person asks one or more questions similar to the following:
"What did I do to deserve this?"
"Why is this happening to me?"
"Is this God's will?"
"How can God love me and still allow me to suffer?"
"Is my faith too weak?"
"Does God exist?"
The person expresses one or more of the following feelings related to spiritual beliefs:

Doubt	Anger	Depression
Ambivalence	Alienation	Emptiness
Regret	Worthlessness	Shame
Guilt	Apathy	Fear

Objective Data

Shows symptoms of depression and withdrawal
Experiences disturbances in sleep/rest patterns
Cries frequently
Questions others about their belief systems
Refuses to see or speak to spiritual leader
Reduces participation in religious/spiritual activities

---

*May require a physician's order.

> **Outcome Criteria**
>
> The person will
> - Express his feelings related to change in beliefs
> - Describe spiritual belief system positively
> - Express desire to perform religious/spiritual practices
> - Describe satisfaction with meaning and purpose of illness/suffering/death

Interventions

A. Assess for causative and contributing factors
   1. Failure of spiritual beliefs to provide explanation/comfort during crisis of illness/ suffering/impending death
   2. Doubting quality or strength of own faith to deal with current crisis
   3. Anger toward God/spiritual beliefs for allowing/causing illness/suffering/death

B. Eliminate or reduce causative and contributing factors, if possible
   1. Failure of spiritual beliefs to provide explanation/comfort during crisis of illness/ suffering/impending death
      a. Communicate that you take spiritual concerns seriously by being available to listen to feelings, questions, etc.
      b. Give "permission" to discuss spiritual matters with nurse by bringing up subject of spiritual welfare, if necessary.
      c. Use questions about past beliefs and spiritual experiences to assist person in putting this life event into wider perspective.
      d. Assist person to begin problem-solving process and move toward new spiritual understandings if necessary.
      e. Offer to contact usual or new spiritual leader.
      f. Offer to pray/meditate/read with client if you are comfortable with this, or arrange for another member of health care team if more appropriate.
      g. Provide uninterrupted quiet time for prayer/reading/meditation on spiritual concerns.
   2. Doubting quality of own faith to deal with current illness/suffering/death
      a. Be available and willing to listen when client expresses self-doubt, guilt, or other negative feelings.
      b. Silence and/or touch may be useful in communicating the nurse's presence and support during times of doubt or despair.
      c. Suggest process of "life review" to identify past sources of strength or spiritual support.
      d. Suggest guided imagery or meditation to reinforce faith/beliefs.
      e. Offer to contact usual or new spiritual leader.
   3. Anger toward God/spiritual beliefs for allowing or causing illness/suffering/death
      a. Express to person that anger toward God is a common reaction to illness/ suffering/death.
      b. Help client recognize and discuss feelings of anger.
      c. Allow client to problem-solve to find ways to express and relieve anger.
      d. Offer to contact usual spiritual leader.

e. Offer to contact other spiritual support person (such as pastoral care, hospital chaplain, etc.) if person cannot share feelings with usual spiritual leader.

References/Bibliography

Ainlay, S. C., & Smith, D. R. (1984). Aging and religious participation. *Journal of Gerontology, 39*(3), 357–363.

Bearon, L., & Koenig, H. (1990). Religious cognitions and use of payer in health and illness. *The Gerontologist, 30*(2), 249–253.

Bruhn, J. G., Cordova, F. D., Williams, J. A., & Fuentes, R. G. (1977). The wellness process. *Journal of Community Health, 2*(3), 234–240.

Burnard, P. (1987). Spiritual distress and the nursing response: Theoretical considerations and counselling skills. *Journal of Advanced Nursing, 12*(3), 377–382.

Carson, V. (1980). Meeting the spiritual needs of hospitalized psychiatric patients. *Perspectives in Psychiatric Care, 18*(1), 17–20.

Colliton, M. (1984). The spiritual dimension. In Fehring, R. (Ed.). *Proceedings of the conference on spirituality.* Milwaukee, WI: Marquette University.

Conrad, N. L. (1985). Spiritual support for the dying. *Nursing Clinics of North America, 20*(2), 415–425.

DeYoung, S. (1984). Perceptions of the institutionalized elderly regarding the nurse's role in supporting spiritual well-being. In Fehring, R. (Ed.). *Proceedings of the conference on spirituality.* Milwaukee, WI: Marquette University.

Dickinson, C. (1975). The search for spiritual meaning. *American Journal of Nursing, 75*(10), 1789–1793.

Egan, K. (1984). Spirituality: Life to the full. In R. Fehring, R. (Ed.). *Proceedings of the conference on spirituality.* Milwaukee, WI: Marquette University.

Ellison, C. W. (1983). Spiritual well-being: Conceptualization and measurement. *Pyschological Theology, 11*(4), 330–340.

Fehring, R. J., & McLane, A. M. (1986). Value belief/spiritual distress. In Thompson, J. M., McFarland, G. K., Hirsch, J. E., Tucker, S. M., & Bowers, A. C. (Eds.). *Clinical nursing.* St. Louis: C. V. Mosby.

Fish, S., & Shelly, J. (1978). *Spiritual care: The nurse's role.* Downer's Grove, IL: Intervarsity Press.

Forbis, P. A. (1988). Meeting patient's spiritual needs. *Geriatric Nursing, 9*(3).

Giuri, A. (1980). Aging and the spiritual life. *Spiritual Life, 26,* 41–46.

Hall, C. M. (1985). Religion and aging. *Journal of Religion and Health, 24*(1), 70–78.

Highfield, M. F., & Cason, C. (1983, June). Spiritual needs of patients: Are they recognized. *Cancer Nursing,* 187–192.

Hogstel, M. O. (1990). *Geropsychiatric nursing.* St. Louis: C. V. Mosby.

Hungelmann, J., Kenkel-Rossi, E., Klassen, L., & Stollenwerk, R. M. (1985). Spiritual well-being in older adults, harmonious interconnectedness. *Journal of Religion and Health, 24*(2), 147–153.

Kennedy, R. (1984). *The international dictionary of religion.* New York: Crossroad.

Kaczorowski, J. M. (1989). Spiritual well-being and anxiety in adults diagnosed with cancer. *The Hospice Journal, 5*(3/4), 105–115.

Lippy, E. H., & Williams, P. W. (Eds.). (1988). *Encyclopedia of the American religious experience: Studies of traditions and movements.* New York: Scribners.

Martin, C., Burrows, C., & Pomilio, J. (1978). Spiritual needs of patients survey. In Fish, S., & Shelly, J. A. *Spiritual care: The nurse's role.* Downers Grove, IL: Intervarsity Press.

Matteson, A. M., & McConnell, E. S. (1988). *Gerontological nursing: Concepts and practice.* Philadelphia: W. B. Saunders.

Miller, J. F. (1985). Inspiring hope. *American Journal of Nursing, 85*(1), 22–25.

Mindel, C. H., & Vaughan, C. E. (1978). A multidimensional approach to religiosity and disengagement. *Journal of Gerontology, 33,* 103–108.

Moberg, D. O. (1984). Subjective measures of spiritual well-being. *Review of Religious Research, 25*(4), 351–364.

Nelsen, H. M. (1981). Life without afterlife: Toward a congruency of belief across generations. *Journal of Scientific Study in Religion, 20,* 109–118.

Pastoral care: Spiritual resources manual. (1988). (Available from the Grey Bruce Regional Health Centre, 1400 8th St. East, P.O. Box 1400 Owen Sound, Ontario, Canada, N4K 6M9)

Patterson, R. A. (1984). The search for meaning a pastoral response to suffering. *Hospital Progress, 65,* 46–49.

Piles, C. L. (1990). Providing spiritual care. *Nurse Educator, 15*(1), 36–41.

Pumphrey, J. B. (1977). Recognizing your patients' spiritual needs. *Nursing, 7*(12), 64–70.

Roche de Coppens, P. (1980). *The spiritual perspective: Key issues and themes interpreted from the standpoint of spiritual consciousness.* Washington, D. C.: University Press of America.

Ryan, J. (1984). The neglected crisis. *American Journal of Nursing, 84*(10), 1257–1258.

Ryan, J. E. (1985). Selecting an instrument to measure spiritual distress. *Oncology Nursing Forum, 12*(2), 93–94, 99.

Ryan, M. C., & Patterson, J. (1987). Loneliness in the elderly. *Journal of Gerontological Nursing, 13*(5), 6–12.

Shannon, M. (1980). Spiritual needs and nursing responsibility. *Imprint, 10*(12), 23.

Shea, G. (1986). Meeting the pastoral care needs of an aging population. *Health Progress, 67*(5), 36–37, 68.

Sodestrom, K. E., & Martinson, I. M. (1987). Patients' spiritual coping strategies: A study of nurse and patient perspectives. *Oncology Nursing Forum, 14*(2), 41–46.

Stevenson, J. S. (1982). Construction of a scale to measure load, power and margin in life. *Nursing Research, 31*(4), 222–225.

Stoll, R. I. (1984). Spiritual assessment: A nursing perspective. In Fehring, R. (Ed.). *Proceedings of the conference on spirituality.* Milwaukee, WI: Marquette University.

Taylor, C., Lillis, C., & LeMone, P. (1989). *Fundamentals of nursing: The art and science of nursing care.* Philadelphia: J. B. Lippincott, pp. 1099–1118.

Van Heukelem, J. (1982). Assessing the spiritual needs of children and their families. In Shelley, J. A. *The spiritual needs of children.* Downers Grove, IL: Intervarsity Press, pp. 94–95.

Whaley, L. F., & Wong, D. L. (1989). *Essentials of pediatric nursing* (3rd ed.). St. Louis: C. V. Mosby.

Thought Processes, Altered

- *Related to* **(Specify) as Evidenced by Inability to Evaluate Reality**
- *Related to* **Effects of Dementia**

DEFINITION

Altered Thought Processes: A state in which an individual experiences a disruption in such mental activities as conscious thought, reality orientation, problem solving, judgment, and comprehension.

DEFINING CHARACTERISTICS

Major (must be present)

Inaccurate interpretation of stimuli, internal and/or external

Minor (may be present)

Cognitive defects, including abstraction, memory
Suspiciousness
Delusions
Hallucinations
Phobias
Obsessions
Distractibility
Lack of consensual validation

Language disturbances, *e.g.,* echolalia, neologism
Confusion/disorientation
Ritualistic behavior
Impulsivity
Suicidal/homicidal thoughts

RELATED FACTORS

Pathophysiologic

Personality and mental disorders
    Alteration in biochemical compounds
    Genetic disorder
    Hormonal changes
    Progressive dementia

Situational (personal, environmental)

Depression or anxiety
Substance abuse (alcohol, drugs)
Fear of the unknown
Actual loss (of control, routine, income, significant others, familiar object or surroundings)
Unclear communication
Emotional trauma

Rejection or negative appraisal by others
Negative response from others
Isolation
Physical/sexual abuse
Torture

Maturational

Adolescent: Peer pressure, conflict, separation
Adult: Marital conflict, family additions or deaths
Elderly: Isolation, late-life depression, dementia

Diagnostic Considerations

Altered Thought Processes describes a person with altered perception and cognition that interferes with daily living. Causes include physiologic dysfunction (*e.g.,* dementia) and psychologic disturbances (*e.g.,* depression, personality disorders, bipolar disorders). For this diagnosis, the focus of nursing is on reducing disturbed thinking and/or promoting reality orientation.

The nurse should be cautioned against using this diagnosis as a "waste-basket" diagnosis for all clients with disturbed thinking or confusion. Frequently, confusion in an elderly person is erroneously attributed to aging. Confusion in the elderly can be caused by a single factor (*e.g.,* dementia, medication side-effects, metabolic disorder) or by depression related to multiple factors associated with aging. Depression causes impaired thinking more frequently than dementia in older adults (Miller, 1990).

Errors in Diagnostic Statements

Altered Thought Processes related to depression

When a person exhibits signs and symptoms of depression and impaired cognition, use of *Altered Thought Processes* would seem appropriate. However, the impaired cognition associated with depression should be viewed as a manifestation of depression rather than as a response to be treated. Depression is a state that represents ineffective coping; thus, the following diagnosis would be more clinically useful: *Ineffective Individual Coping related to unknown etiology, as evidenced by slowed affect, reports of constant sadness, little motivation, and memory difficulties.* Because the central issue in depression is low self-esteem, the nurse will use a focus assessment to determine factors that are causing or contributing to low self-esteem, *e.g.,* disabilities, losses, feelings of rejection.

Altered Thought Processes related to loss of memory

Loss of memory can be present in many situations; *e.g.,* depression, dementia, anxiety, sensory deprivation, psychiatric disorders, endocrine disorders. The nursing focus would vary, depending on the contributing factors. For example, loss of memory with head injuries usually is very anxiety-producing; thus, a diagnosis of *Anxiety* would be more useful. Loss of memory that poses a danger would be associated with *High Risk for Injury.* If *Altered Thought Processes* were appropriate for this person, the diagnosis should be restated as *Altered Thought Process related to* (specify, *e.g., effects of hypoxia secondary to cerebrovascular accident), as evidenced by loss of memory,* etc.

Focus Assessment Criteria

Acquire data from client and significant others

Subjective Data

1. History of the individual
    Life-style
        Interests
        Work history
        Coping patterns (past and
            present)
        Strengths and limitations
        Previous level of functioning and
            handling stress
        Use of alcohol/drugs
    Support system (availability)
    History of medical problems and treatments (medications)
    Activities of daily living (ability and desire to perform)
2. History of symptoms (onset and duration)
    Acute or chronic
    Sudden or gradual
    Continuous or intermittent?
    Time of day
3. History of unusual sensations and thought productions
    Precipitating factors
    Frequency and duration
    Routine time of occurrence
    Description in individual's own
        words
4. Assess for presence of
    Feelings of
        Extreme sadness and
            worthlessness
        Guilt for past actions
        Apprehension in various
            situations
        Being rejected or isolated
        Living in an unreal world
        Mistrust or suspiciousness of
            others
        Others making him do and say
            things
        Excessive self-importance
        Depersonalization

    Fears
        That others will harm him
        That mind is being controlled by
            external agents
        Of being unable to cope
        Of falling apart
        Of thoughts racing
        Of being held prisoner
        Body is rotting or not there
    Hallucinations (visual, auditory, gustatory, olfactory, tactile—includes an objec-
        tive component)
    Dementia
        Gradual onset of impaired memory, labile affect
        Alert level of consciousness
        Evasive
        Denial of symptoms
        Inappropriate dress
        Cognitive deficits (aphasia, apraxia, agnosia, agraphia)
        Delusions used to explain deficits (e.g., theft, spouse infidelity, fears)
    Depression (Miller, 1990)
        Difficulties with memory
        Lack of motivation
        Inability to concentrate
        Consistent sadness
        Slaved apathetic responses

Physical complaints of fatigue, anorexia, constipation, insomnia, dysphagia

Delusions of foreboding gloom, diminished self-esteem, money, death, guilt

5. Orientation

Person

"What is your name?"   "What is your occupation?"

Time

"What season is it?"   "What month is it?"

Place

"Where are you?"   "Where do you live?"

6. Problem-solving ability

"What would you do if the phone rang?"

"What is the difference between the doctor and the president?"

7. Memory: immediate, recent, remote

Objective Data (includes a subjective component)

1. General appearance

Facial expression (alert, sad, hostile, expressionless)

Dress (meticulous, disheveled, seductive, eccentric)

2. Behavior during interview

Withdrawn	Cooperative
Hostile	Quiet
Apathetic	Negativism

3. Communication pattern

Content

Appropriate	Sexual preoccupations
Rambling	Delusions (grandeur,
Suspicious	persecution, reference,
Denying problem	influence, control,
Homicidal plans	or bodily sensations)
Suicidal ideas	Religiousness
Lacking content	Worthlessness
Obsessions	

Pattern of speech

Appropriate	Loose connection of ideas
Blocking (unable to finish idea)	Jumps from one topic to another
Circumstantial (unable to get to point)	Unable to come to conclusion, be decisive
Neologisms	Clang association
Word salad	Echolalia

Rate of speech

Appropriate	Reduced
Excessive	Pressured

Nonverbal behavior

Affect appropriate to verbal content	Gestures, mannerisms, facial grimaces
Affect inappropriate to verbal content	Posture

4. Interaction skills

With nurse

Inappropriate	Shows dependency

Relates well	Demanding/pleading
Withdrawn/preoccupied	Hostile
With significant others	
Relates with all (some) family	Does not seek interaction
members	Does not have visitors
Hostile toward one (all) members	

5. Activities of daily living
   Emotionally capable of self-care   Physically capable of self-care
6. Nutritional status
   Appetite   Weight (within normal limits,
   Eating patterns   decreased, increased)
7. Sleep/rest pattern
   Recent change   Early wakefulness
   Sleeps too much or too little   Insomnia
8. Personal hygiene
   Cleanliness (body, hair, teeth)   Clothes (condition,
   Grooming (clothes, hair, makeup)   appropriateness)
9. Motor activity
   Within normal limits
   Agitated
   Decreased/stuporous
   Waxy flexibility
   Echopraxia
   stereotyped behavior

Principles and Rationale for Nursing Care

Generic Considerations

1. Thought is a functioning process of the brain that integrates every individual's daily living experiences.
2. Cognitive processes are the mental processes related to reasoning, comprehension, judgment, and memory.
3. Cognitive function is influenced by physiologic functions, stimuli from the environment, and the person's emotional state.
4. The cognitive processes of remembering and perception are influenced by the individual's current needs and interests as well as his fund of knowledge.
5. Development of cognitive abilities follows a systematic pattern of maturational experiences and requires varied perceptual stimulation.
6. A disruption in the quality and quantity of incoming stimuli can affect an individual's thought processes.
7. What a person thinks about an event influences both feelings and behavior. Any changes in thoughts, feelings, or behavior will result in changes in the other two (Potocki & Everly, 1989).
8. People attempt to gain control over a situation by assigning meaning, sometimes a rational explanation, other times irrational (Sideleau, 1987).
9. Over time, irrational beliefs lead to chronic dissatisfaction; the person's thinking patterns become characterized by "shoulds" and "musts" (Sideleau, 1987).
10. Helping the person to restructure irrational belief is based on the use of objective, reality-based data. Three basic questions are raised (Everly, 1989).
    a. What is the evidence?

b. What is another explanation?

c. So what if it happens?

11. Actual events frequently become reorganized and reinterpreted individually so that they may be substantially changed and distorted during the process of remembering.

12. The ability to conceptualize develops relatively slowly and requires contact with others; the development of concrete concepts precedes the development of abstract concepts.

Reality

1. Reality testing is the objective evaluation and judgment of the world outside the self, differentiated from one's thoughts and feelings.

2. Reality testing is determined by early life experiences and by significant people in one's life.

3. Delusions—fixed false beliefs—and hallucinations originate during extreme emotional stress; they represent attempts to decrease panic (Varcarolis, 1990).

4. Delusions include those of:

    a. Grandeur: An exaggerated sense of importance of identity or of ability

    b. Persecution: A sense that one is being harassed

    c. Reference: Belief that the behavior of others refers to oneself

    d. Influence: Exaggerated sense of power over others

    e. Control: Sense that one is being manipulated by others

    f. Bodily sensations: Belief that one's organs are diseased despite contrary evidence

    g. Infidelity: Belief, due to pathologic jealousy, that one's lover is unfaithful

5. Delusions arise when the person attempts to alter reality. First, he denies his own feelings, then projects those feelings onto the environment, and finally he must explain this to others (Dixon, 1969).

6. The fundamental feelings being projected by suspicious and grandiose clients are inadequacy and worthlessness.

7. Hallucinations are perceptions that arise from within the person's own thoughts. He actually hears, sees, feels, or tastes the phenomenon.

8. Hallucinations are meeting underlying needs (*e.g.,* loneliness, anxiety, self-worth), and until a person can substitute other activities, he may be unwilling to "give these up" (Schwartzman, 1976).

9. The person may spend much time in his fantasy world, which leads to a lack of consensual validation of language. Not only are the connections between words disturbed, but the words often have a different meaning to the person than is generally accepted.

10. Verbal assaults are expressions of fear and anxiety and should not be taken personally.

11. Disorganized thinking often leads to regression in behavior, disturbed communication, and difficulty in interactions with others.

Pediatric Considerations

1. A child who consistently displays abnormal behavior patterns (*e.g.,* disturbances in interpersonal relationships, language problems, and altered affect) should be referred for evaluation (Whaley & Wong, 1989).

2. Suicide is the second leading cause of death during the adolescent years. This high rate is related to the vulnerable adolescent's struggle with problem-solving, lack of resources, and family dysfunction (Whaley & Wong, 1989).

Gerontologic Considerations

1. Thinking ability, arithmetic ability, memory, judgment, and problem-solving are measured in the elderly to give a general index of overall cognitive ability. Short-term memory may decline somewhat, but long-term memory often remains intact.

2. Intelligence does not alter, perhaps until the very later years, but the person needs more time to process information. Reaction time increases as well. There may be some difficulty in learning new information because of increased distractibility, decrease in concrete thinking, and difficulty solving new problems. However, older persons usually compensate for these deficiencies by taking more time to process the information, screening out distractions, and using extreme care in making decisions. Marked cognitive decline is usually attributed to disease processes such as atherosclerosis, loss of neurons, and other pathologic changes.

3. Elderly persons are vulnerable to acute confusion when their ability to compensate for stressors, physiologically or psychologically, is compromised. Failure to adapt to changes in the external and internal environment results in confusion. Adaptation can be assessed in the following categories:
   a. Compromised brain function (congestive heart failure, anemia, pneumonia, hypoglycemia, fluid and electrolyte imbalance, hypotension, toxic drug reactions)
   b. Sensory-perceptual problems (decreased vision, hearing, information processing)
   c. Disruption in pattern and meaning (unable to cope with chronic stress-producing situations)
   d. Altered normal physiologic states (problems in eating, sleeping, or elimination, pain, etc.)
   e. True dementias (senile dementia of the Alzheimer type, multi-infarct dementia, etc.) (Wolanin & Phillips, 1981)

4. Most older adults exhibit no cognitive impairment. Severe cognitive impairment, a consequence of disease process, occurs in only 1% of people over age 65 and 20% of people over age 85 (Katzman, 1988).

5. Anxiety influences cognitive abilities through excessive self-focusing and worrying. Depression causes decreased concentration, attention deficits, and negative expectations (Miller, 1990).

6. Age-related changes can influence medication actions and produce negative consequences. Table II–19 illustrates the age-related changes that influence medication actions.

7. Dementia describes impairments of intellectual functioning, not behavioral functioning. Dementia refers to a group of symptoms, not a disease. (Miller, 1990). Alzheimer's disease, the fourth leading case of death in adults, is one type of dementia.

8. Postmortem examination of brain tissue has identified neurofibrillory tangles and neuritic plaques with Alzheimer's disease. These changes are thought to cause the behavioral and cognitive impairments but are not the cause of the dementia (Cohen & Eisdorder, 1986). There is a 50% or greater reduction in the production of acetylcholine in areas of the brain containing tangles and plaques (Miller, 1990). The cause of Alzheimer's disease remains unknown, however.

9. Depression and dementia both cause cognitive impairments. It is critical to differentiate the underlying cause, because depression is treatable (Miller, 1990).

10. Blazer (1986) reported depressive symptoms in 27% of community-living older adults. According to Parmelee, Katz, & Lawton (1989), 12% of older adults living in nursing homes met the criteria for major depression, while 30% were identified with minor depressive symptoms.

11. Blazer (1986) describes a multiple causation theory for late-life depression, which

Table II–19 **Effects of Age-Related Physiologic Changes on Medication Actions***

Age-Related Changes	Effects on Medication Actions
Decreased total body water	Delayed absorption of water-soluble medications.
Increase body fat	Unpredictable effect of fat-soluble medications.
Decreased serum albumin	Increase levels of protein-bound medications. (e.g., warfarin, salicyclic acid, oral hypoglycemics)
Decreased cardiac output, renal and liver function	Decreased clearance rates (barbiturates, antibiotics, digoxin, cimetidine, meperidine)
Compromised homeostatic mechanisms	Increased side-effects in medications with sensitivity to changes in temperature and fluid volume (e.g., lithium)
Altered receptor sensitivity	Change therapeutic and adverse effects

(Adapted from Miller, C. A. (1990). *Nursing care of older adults*. Glenview, IL: Scott, Foresman)

emphasizes the complex interactions between several or many causative factors. Factors identified include poor economic resources, decreased social support, and decreased physical health functioning. These factors negatively impact self-esteem and motivation, which increase feelings of guilt and anger. The resulting negative emotions depress affect and increase ruminations. The person reduces social contact or is shunned, which starts the cycle again.

■ Altered Thought Processes
Related to (Specify) as Evidenced by Inability to Evaluate Reality

The inability to evaluate reality is an inability to differentiate one's thoughts and feelings from the actualities of the outside world.

Assessment

Subjective Data

Expresses mistrust
Feels he is being controlled
Fears falling apart
Fears objects are communicating
States he sees, hears, feels, tastes something that is not there

Expresses hostility: "Everyone is against me."
Has difficulty concentrating
Accuses others of making him do things
States body parts are rotting or missing

Objective Data

Mood alterations
Poor judgment
Regression (childlike behavior)

Overreaction to stimuli
Arrogant
Seclusive

Disturbed communication
Inappropriate laughter, grinning
Delayed verbal responses
Eye movements
Increased verbal/motor activity
Sleep disturbances

Reduced fluid/food intake
Social isolation
Altered interpersonal
    interactions
Poor impulse control
Poor hygiene/grooming

Outcome Criteria

The person will
- Identify situations that occur prior to hallucinations/delusions
- Express delusional material less frequently
- Communicate clearly with others
- Describe problems in relating with others
- Identify actions that can be taken when anxiety increases
- Participate in unit activities (specify)

Interventions

A. Promote communication that enhances the person's sense of integrity
   1. Encourage open, honest dialogue.
      a. Approach in a calm, nurturing manner.
      b. Persevere, be consistent.
      c. Be open and share with the person.
      d. Discuss expectations and demands.
      e. Recognize when person is testing the trustworthiness of others.
      f. Avoid making promises that cannot be fulfilled.
      g. Initial staff contact minimal and brief with suspicious person; increase time as suspiciousness decreases.
      h. Explain if appointments cannot be kept.
      i. Verify your interpretation of what person is experiencing. ("I understand you are fearful of others.")
      j. Be an attentive listener; note both verbal and nonverbal messages.
      k. Help individual verbalize what person indicates nonverbally.
      l. Use terminology that is familiar and evokes little anxiety.
      m. Recognize the importance of body posture, facial expression, and tone of voice.
      n. Present information in a matter-of-fact way that is least likely to be misinterpreted; do not use humor or bantering with suspicious persons.
      o. Use communication that helps person maintain his own individuality (*e.g.*, "I" instead of "we").
      p. Eliminate whispered comments or incomplete explanations that encourage fantasy interpretation.
   2. Maintain client's personal space.
      a. Do not touch person until you have developed an ongoing trusting relationship.
      b. Talk to the person in open space; avoid small rooms or offices.

B. Assist person to differentiate between own thoughts and reality

1. Validate the presence of hallucinations.
   a. Observe for verbal and nonverbal cues—inappropriate laughter, delayed verbal response, eye movements, moving lips without sound, increased motor movements, grinning.
      • "Are you hearing/seeing something now?"
      • "What's happening now?"
   b. Assist person in observing thoughts and feelings as they relate to the underlying need(s) being met.
      • "Has this happened before?"
      • "What were you doing/thinking?"
      • "You were lonely?"

2. Focus on here-and-now
   a. Direct the focus from delusional expression to discussion of reality-centered situations.
   b. Encourage person to validate his thoughts by sharing them with significant others.
   c. Avoid derogation or belittling when person misinterprets stimuli or is delusional; do not laugh or make fun of him.
   d. Encourage person to identify and focus on his strengths, not his weaknesses.
   e. Encourage differentiation of stimuli arising from inner sources from those from outside (*e.g.*, in response to "I hear voices," say: Those are the voices of people on TV" or "I hear no one speaking now; they are your own thoughts").
   f. Avoid the impression that you confirm or approve reality distortions; tactfully express doubt.
   g. Focus on reality-oriented aspects of the communication (*e.g.*, if person states, "The TV is controlling my mind," the nurse can say, "How does it make you feel when others try to control you?").
   h. Set limits for discussing repetitive delusional material. ("You've already told me about that; let's talk about something realistic.")
   i. Teach person to relearn to focus attention on real things and people.
   j. Identify the underlying needs being met by the delusions/hallucinations.
   k. Help person become aware that his needs are being expressed in fantasy and teach more appropriate ways to meet these needs (*e.g.*, aggression expressed through delusion of persecution can be put into constructive activity such as hammering metal objects).
   l. Do not automatically dismiss physical complaints; however, do not express undue concern.

3. Assist in restricting irrational thoughts (refer to *Anxiety*).

C. Assist the person with disordered thinking in communicating more effectively

1. Ask for the meaning of what is said; do not assume that you understand.
2. Validate your interpretation of what is being said. ("Is this what you mean?")
3. Clarify all global pronouns—we, they. ("Who is *they?*")
4. Refocus when person changes the subject in the middle of an explanation or thought.
5. Tell the person when you are not following his train of thought.
6. Do not mimic or restate words or phrases that you do not understand.
7. Teach the person to consensually validate with others.

D. Encourage a more mature level of functioning
1. Assist person to set limits on his own behavior.
   a. Discuss alternative methods of coping (*e.g.*, taking a walk instead of crying).
   b. Confront person with the attitude that regression is not acceptable behavior.
   c. Help delay gratification (*e.g.*, "I want you to wait 5 minutes before you repeat your request for help in making your bed").
   d. Encourage person to achieve realistic expectations.
   e. Pace expectations to avoid frustration.
2. Encourage and support person in the decision-making process.
   a. Help person review options and the advantages and disadvantages of each option.
   b. Assist in structuring daily living activities (*e.g.*, help schedule bath time before activity hour).
   c. Compliment the person who assumes more responsibility.
   d. Show patience and understanding when a mistake is made.
   e. Provide opportunity for person to contribute to his own treatment plan.
   f. Help establish future goals that are realistic; examine problems in achieving a goal and suggest various alternatives.
3. Assist person to differentiate between needs and demands.
   a. Explain the difference between needs and demands (*e.g.*, food and clothing are needs; expectations that others dress and feed him, if he can do it, are demands).
   b. Assist person to examine the effects of his behavior on others; encourage a change in behavior if it evokes negative responses.
   c. Teach negotiation to achieve needs and goals.
   d. Help person ask for what he wants and tell others how he feels.
   e. Help person realize that failure of others to meet his needs and demands is not always related to their regard for him.

E. Provide person with opportunities for positive socialization
1. Help him share on a one-to-one basis.
   a. Be warm, honest, and sincere in interactions.
   b. Demonstrate that you accept him.
   c. Recognize that some people deny the need for close relationships.
   d. Be sensitive to behaviors that indicate resistance to interpersonal involvement.
   e. Help person know that you recognize his uneasiness in social situations. ("It must be difficult for you.")
   f. Use touch judiciously if person fears closeness.
2. Help person recognize behaviors that stimulate rejection.
   a. Identify activities that reduce interpersonal anxiety (*e.g.*, exercise, controlled breathing exercises; see Appendix X).
   b. Set limits firmly and kindly on destructive behavior.
   c. Allow expression of negative emotions, verbally or in constructive activity.
   d. Avoid argument or debate about delusional ideas or destructive behavior.
   e. Help person accept responsibility for responses he elicits from others.
   f. Encourage discussion of problems in relating after visits with family members.
   g. Help person test new skills in relating to others in role-playing situations.
3. Refer to impaired socialization for further interventions.

F. Promote physical well-being and prevent injury
   1. Explain and monitor medication regimen.
      a. Assess person's ability to remember to take medications.
      b. Assist person to remember to take medications by color coding each bottle with a sticker and writing out the times of the day that medications are prescribed for, with the appropriate color sticker next to the time.
      c. Teach about the purpose of medications and their side-effects.
      d. Encourage person to report all physical symptoms.
      e. Encourage person to take prescribed medication, especially antipsychotic (*e.g.*, lithium).
      f. Check to ensure that medication was swallowed. If you have doubts about patient taking oral medications (*e.g.*, failure to improve), change to concentrate.
      g. Extremely suspicious and hostile persons should begin on concentrate, so that you will not have to check mouth and increase distrust.
      h. Do not mix medications with food.
   2. Monitor nutritional intake.
      a. Observe eating habits (amount, selection, frequency, food preferences and dislikes, appetite).
      b. Note weight gain or loss.
      c. Discuss adequate nutrition in relation to activity level.
      d. Allow person to choose food he especially likes; contract with individual who eats predominantly snack foods (*e.g.*, "If you eat one egg you can order a doughnut").
      e. Note delusions regarding food or body that might interfere with nutritional intake.
      f. Encourage increased calorie intake for hyperactive person.
      g. Provide finger foods that can be eaten on-the-run (*e.g.*, sandwiches).
      h. Allow choices in foods (may prefer to eat food brought in by family, in unopened packages, fruit, etc.).
      i. Refer to *Altered Nutrition* for additional interventions.
   3. Assess ability for self-care activities.
      a. Identify areas of physical care for which person needs assistance (sleep and rest, nutrition, bathing, dressing, elimination, exercise).
      b. Note person's motivation and interest in appearance.
      c. Teach skills required to assume responsibility for self-care.
      d. Assist person in planning his daily routines to foster independence and responsibility.
      e. Monitor for sleep disturbances.
      f. Provide a single room for extremely suspicious person.
      g. Suggest leaving the light on.
      h. Give nonstimulating drinks with a snack at bedtime.
      i. Assess the need for a sleeping medication.
      j. If appropriate, arrange to give last dose of antipsychotic medication at bedtime (*e.g.*, b.i.d. medication—give AM and HS).
      k. Refer to *Self-Care Deficit* for additional interventions.

G. Reduce the potential for violence to self and others
   1. Provide a minimally stimulating environment.
      a. Reduce incidence of bright colors and loud noises.

    b. Be short, concise, and matter-of-fact.

    c. Be consistent.

    d. May need to assign staff responsible for developing trusting relationship.

    e. Avoid large groups.

2. Provide activities in which he will be successful.

    a. Avoid competitive sports.

    b. Suspicious persons are often good managers.

    c. Involve in activities for a short time period.

3. Allow ventilation of hostility (as long as it is not combative/destructive).

    a. Be nonjudgmental.

    b. Do not personalize.

4. Assess for signs indicative of aggression ("Those Russian spies are going to attack me tonight"). Refer to *High Risk for Violence* for further interventions.

5. Identify cues to suicide.

    a. Sudden changes in mood or behavior

    b. Report of plan to harm himself

    c. Report of voices directing person to harm himself or others

    d. Observe closely for changes in behavior; increase vigilance.

    e. Share with personnel the individual's potential for self-harm.

    f. Refer to *High Risk for Self-harm* for further interventions.

6. Interview family and note approaches that have been beneficial in the past in controlling aggression.

7. Reduce anxiety and develop a sense of safety through a climate of care and concern.

H. Initiate health teaching and referrals as indicated

1. Anticipate difficulties in adjusting to community living; discuss concerns about returning to community and elicit family reaction to individual's discharge.

2. Provide health teaching that will prepare person to deal with life stresses (methods of relaxation, problem-solving skills, how to negotiate with others, how to express feelings constructively).

3. Review signs and symptoms of recurrent illness that indicate impending maladjustment.

4. Refer to other professions for assistance.

    a. To occupational therapist to learn leisure-time activities

    b. To industrial therapist to improve or learn new job skills

    c. To social worker to discuss living arrangements, financial problems, or family negotiations

5. Supply telephone number and address of local mental health clinic.

6. Inform individual of social agencies that offer help in adjusting to community living.

    a. General social agencies

       • Mental health and mental retardation centers

       • Mental Health Association

       • HELP (alternative to mental health center)

       • Family Service (family counseling)

       • Drug rehabilitation centers

    b. Specific social agencies

       • Alcoholics Anonymous

       • Gray Panthers

- Suicide Crisis Intervention Center
- Synanon
- Contact

■ Altered Thought Processes
Related to Effects of Dementia

Dementia describes impaired intellectual functioning not impaired behavior. The organic cause of dementia is unknown.

Assessment

Subjective Data

The person
    Denies symptoms
    Uses delusions to explain deficits

Objective Data

Denial of reality
Impaired memory
Labile affect
Evasive
Angry
Inappropriate dress
Aphasia
Agraphia
Agnosia
Apraxia

Outcome Criteria

The person will
- Participate to maximum level of independence
- Have decreased frustration when environmental stressors are reduced

---

Interventions

A. Assess history of cognitive deficits with person and family. Refer to Focus Assessment Criteria to differentiate dementia from depression. If depression is suspected, consult with a therapist (nurse, physician).

B. Promote communication that contributes to the person's sense of integrity
   1. Examine attitudes about aging (in self, caregivers, significant others).
   2. Maintain standards of empathetic, respectful care.
      a. Be an advocate when other caregivers are insensitive to the individual's needs.
      b. Function as a role model with coworkers.
      c. Provide other caregivers with up-to-date information on aging and reality orientation.
      d. Expect empathetic, respectful care and monitor its administration.
   3. Attempt to obtain information that will provide useful and meaningful topics for conversations (likes, dislikes; interests, hobbies; work history).
   4. Encourage significant others and caregivers to speak slowly and at an average volume (unless hearing deficits are present), as one adult to another, with eye contact, and as if expecting person to understand.
   5. Provide respect and promote sharing.
      a. Pay attention to what person is saying.
      b. Pick out meaningful comments and continue talking.
      c. Call person by name and introduce yourself each time a contact is made; utilize touch if welcomed.
      d. Use name the person prefers; avoid "Pops" or "Mom," which can increase confusion and is unacceptable.
      e. Convey to person that you are concerned and friendly (through smiles, an unhurried pace, humor, and praise; do not argue).

C. Provide sensory input that is sufficient and meaningful
   1. Keep person oriented to time and place.
      a. Refer to time of day and place each morning.
      b. Provide person with a clock and calendar large enough to see.
      c. If dementia is severe, remove all visible mirrors.
      d. Use night lights or dim lights at night.
      e. Turn lights on before it gets dark.
      f. Provide person with opportunity to see daylight and dark through a window or take person outdoors.
      g. Single out holidays with cards or pins (*e.g.,* wear a red heart for Valentine's Day).
   2. Encourage family to bring in familiar objects from home (*e.g.,* photographs with nonglare glass, afghan).
      a. Ask person to tell you about the picture.
      b. Focus on familiar topics.
   3. Discuss current events, seasonal events (snow, water activities); share your interests (travel, crafts).
   4. Assess if person can perform an activity with his hands (*e.g.,* latch rugs, wood crafts).
      a. Provide reading materials, audio tapes, puzzles (manual, computer, crossword).
      b. Encourage person to keep his own records if possible (*e.g.,* intake and output).
      c. Provide tasks to perform (addressing envelopes, occupational therapy).
   5. If hallucinations and delusions persist, refer to *Altered Thought Processes* for specific interventions

6. In teaching a task or activity—for example, eating—break it into small, brief steps by giving only one instruction at a time.
   a. Remove covers from food plate and cups.
   b. Locate napkin and utensils.
   c. Add sugar and milk to coffee.
   d. Add condiments to food (sugar, salt, pepper).
   e. Cut foods.
   f. Proceed with eating.
7. Explain all activities.
   a. Offer simple explanations of tasks.
   b. Allow individuals to handle equipment related to each task.
   c. Allow individual to participate in task, such as washing his face.
   d. Acknowledge that you are leaving and say when you will return.

D. Increase person's self-esteem
1. Allow former habits (*e.g.,* reading in the bathroom).
2. Encourage the wearing of dentures.
3. Assist with removal of facial hair.
4. Ask family to provide spending money.
5. Ask person his usual grooming routine and encourage him to follow it.
6. Provide privacy at all times; when it is necessary to expose a body surface, take precautions to cover all other areas (*e.g.,* if washing a back, use towels or blankets to cover legs and front torso).
7. Provide for personal hygiene according to person's preferences (hair grooming, showers or bath, nail care, cosmetics, deodorants and fragrances).

E. Promote a well role
1. Discourage the use of nightclothes during the day; have person wear shoes, not slippers.
2. Encourage self-care and grooming activities.
3. Have person eat meals out of bed, unless contraindicated.
4. Promote socialization during meals (*e.g.,* set up lunch for four individuals in lounge).
5. Plan an activity each day to look forward to (*e.g.,* bingo, ice cream sundae gathering).

F. Do not endorse confusion
1. Do not argue with person.
2. Never agree with confused statements.
3. Direct person back to reality; do not allow him to ramble.
4. Adhere to the schedule; if changes are necessary, advise person of them.
5. Avoid talking to coworkers about other topics in person's presence.
6. Provide simple explanations that cannot be misinterpreted.
7. Remember to acknowledge your entrance with a greeting and your exit with a closure. ("I will be back in 10 minutes.")

G. Utilize various modalities to promote stimulation for the individual
1. Music therapy
   a. Provide soft, familiar music during meals.
   b. Arrange group song fests.

      c. Play music during other therapies (physical, occupational).

      d. Have person exercise to music.

      e. Encourage construction of simple instruments and have individuals play them in a rhythm band.

      f. Organize guest entertainment.

      g. Use client-developed songbooks (large print and decorative covers).

  2. Recreation therapy

      a. Encourage arts and crafts (knitting and crocheting).

      b. Suggest creative writing.

      c. Provide puzzles.

      d. Organize group games.

  3. Remotivation therapy

      a. Organize group sessions into five steps (Dennis, 1984):

         • *Step 1:* Climate of Acceptance (approx. 5 min)
          Relaxed atmosphere with introductions of leaders and participants
          Provide large-letter name tags and names on chairs
          Maintain assigned places for every session

         • *Step 2:* Creating a Bridge to Reality (approx. 15 min)
          Use a prop (visual, audio, song, picture, object, poem) to introduce theme of session

         • *Step 3:* Sharing the World We Live In (approx. 15 min)
          Group members discuss the topic
          Stimulation of senses should be promoted

         • *Step 4:* Appreciation of the Work of the World (approx. 20 min)
          Discussion of how the topic relates to their past experiences (work, leisure)

         • *Step 5:* Climate of Appreciation (approx. 5 min)
          Each member is thanked individually
          Announcement of the next session's topic and meeting date

      b. Use associations and analogies.

         • "If ice is cold, then fire is . . . ?"
         • "If day is light, then night is . . . ?"

      c. Topics for remotivation sessions are chosen based on suggestions from group leaders and the interest of the group. Examples are pets, bodies of water, canning fruits and vegetables, transportation, holidays (Janssen & Giberson, 1988).

  4. Sensory training

      a. Stimulate vision (with brightly colored items of different shape, pictures, colored decorations, kaleidoscopes).

      b. Stimulate smell (with flowers, coffee, cologne).

      c. Stimulate hearing (ring a bell, play records).

      d. Stimulate touch (sandpaper, velvet, steel wool pads, silk, stuffed animals).

      e. Stimulate taste (spices, salt, sugar, sour substances).

H. Prevent injury to the individual

  1. Discourage the use of restraints; explore other alternatives.

      a. Put person in a room with others who can help watch him.

      b. Enlist aid of family or friends to watch person during confused periods.

      c. If person is pulling out tubes, use mitts instead of wrist restraints.

  2. Refer to *High Risk for Injury* for strategies for assessing and manipulating the environment for hazards.

I. Implement techniques to lower the stress threshold in individuals in middle or later stages of dementia (Hall and Buckwalter, 1987; Miller, 1990):
   1. Reduce competing or excessive stimuli.
      a. Keep environment simple and uncluttered.
      b. Use simple written cues to clarify directions for use of radio and TV.
      c. Eliminate or minimize unnecessary noise.
   2. Plan and maintain a consistent routine.
      a. Attempt to assign same caregivers.
      b. Elicit from family members specific methods that help or hinder care.
      c. Arrange personal care items in order of use (clothes, toothbrush, mouthwash, etc.).
   3. Focus on the person's ability level.
      a. Do not request performance of function beyond ability.
      b. Express unconditional positive regard for the person.
      c. Modify environment to compensate for ability.
      d. Use simple sentences, demonstrate activity.
      e. Do not ask questions that the person cannot answer.
      f. Avoid open-ended questions (*e.g.,* "What do you want to eat?" or "When do you want to take a bath?").
      g. Offer simple choices (*e.g.,* "Do you want a cookie or crackers?").
      h. Use finger foods (*e.g.,* sandwiches) to encourage self-feeding.
   4. Reduce fatigue and anxiety.
      a. Implement regular rest periods.
      b. Maintain an unconditional positive regard for the person.
      c. Use touch to convey concern.
      d. Maintain good eye contact.
      e. Identify expressions of increasing stress or anxiety and reduce environmental stimuli quickly.

References/Bibliography

Alzheimer's disease and related disorders. (1988). In *Special care for Alzheimer's patients.* Chicago: Alzheimer's Disease and Related Disorders Association, Inc.

Arnold, H. M. (1976). Working with schizophrenic patients. Four A's: A guide to one-to-one relationships. *American Journal of Nursing, 76,* 941–943.

Bayer, M. (1980). The multipurpose room: A way-out outlet for staff and clients. *Journal of Psychiatric Nursing, 18*(10), 35–37.

Blazer, D. G. (1986). Depression: Paradoxically a cause for hope. *Generations, 10*(3), 21–23.

Cohen, D., & Eisdorder, C. (1986). *The loss of self.* New York: NAL Penguin.

Dennis, H. (1984). Remotivation therapy groups. In Burnside, I. M. (Ed). *Working with the elderly group: Process and techniques* (2nd ed.). Monterey, CA: Jones & Bartlett.

Dixon, B. (1969). Intervening when the patient is delusional. *Journal of Psychiatric Nursing, 7*(1), 25–34.

Everly, G. (1989). *A guide to the treatment of human stress response.* New York: Plenum Press.

Hall, G. R., & Buckwalter, K. C. (1987). Progressively lowered stress threshold: A conceptual model for care of adults with Alzheimer's disease. *Archives of Psychiatric Nursing, 1*(6), 399–406.

Janssen, J., & Giberson, D. (1988). Remotivation therapy. *Journal of Gerontological Nursing, 14*(6), 31–34.

Katzman, R. (1988). *Alzheimer's disease as an age dependent disorder, research and the aging population* (CIBA Foundation Symposium 1334). New York: Wiley & Sons.

Knowles, R. D. (1981). Disputing irrational thought. *American Journal of Nursing, 81,* 735.

Kreigh, H., & Perko, J. *Psychiatric and mental health nursing: A commitment to cure and concern.* Reston, VA: Reston Publishing, pp. 195–203.

Libow, L. (1981). A rapidly administered, easily remembered mental status evaluation: FROMAJE. In Libow, L., & Sherman, B. (Eds.). *The core of geriatric medicine.* St. Louis: C. V. Mosby, pp. 84–85.

Miller, C. A. (1990). *Nursing care of older adults.* Glenview, IL: Scott, Foresman.

O'Brien, J. (1979). Teaching psychiatric inpatients about their medications. *Journal of Psychiatric Nursing, 17*(10), 30–32.

Ozuna, J. (1985). Alterations in mentation: Nursing assessment and intervention. *Journal of Neurosurgical Nursing, 17*(1), 65–70.

Parmelee, P. A., Katz, I. R., & Lawton, M. P. (1989). Depression among institutionalized aged: Assessment and prevalence estimation. *Journal of Gerontology: Medical Sciences, 44*(1), M22–29.

Potocki, E., & Everly, G. (1989). Control and the human stress response. In Everly, G. *A guide to the treatment of human stress response.* New York: Plenum Press, pp. 119–123.

Pullinger, W. F. Jr. (1960). Remotivation. *American Journal of Nursing, 60*(5), 682–685.

Schroeder, P. J. (1979). Nursing interventions with patients with thought disorders. *Perspectives on Psychiatric Care, 17*(1), 32–39.

Schwartzman, S. T. (1976). The hallucinating patient and nursing intervention. *Journal of Psychiatric Nursing, 13*(6), 23–28, 33–36.

Sideleau, B. (1987). Irrational beliefs and intervention. *Journal of Psychosocial Nursing, 25*(3), 18–24.

Slater, M. C. (1983). Altered levels of consciousness: Impaired thought processes. In Snyder, M. (Ed.). *A guide to neurological and neurosurgical nursing.* New York: John Wiley & Sons, pp. 157–188.

Torrey, E. F. (1983). *Surviving schizophrenia: A family manual.* New York: Harper & Row.

Varcarolis, E. (1990). *Foundations of psychiatric mental health nursing.* Philadelphia: W. B. Saunders.

Whaley, L. F. & Wong, D. L. (1989). *Essentials of pediatric nursing* (3rd ed.). St. Louis: C. V. Mosby.

Wolanin, M., & Phillips, L. (1981). *Confusion: Prevention and care.* St. Louis: C. V. Mosby.

Resources for the Consumer

Literature

Powell, L. S., & Courtice, K. (1983). *Alzheimer's disease: A guide for families.* Menlo Park, CA: Addison-Wesley.

Altered Protection

Tissue Integrity, Impaired*

Skin Integrity, Impaired

Oral Mucous Membrane, Altered

Altered Protection

DEFINITION

Altered Protection: The state in which an individual experiences a decrease in the ability to guard against internal or external threats, such as illness or injury.

DEFINING CHARACTERISTICS

Major (must be present)

Immunodeficiency
Impaired healing
Altered clotting
Maladaptive stress response
Neurosensory alterations

Minor (may be present)

Chills
Diaphoresis
Dyspnea
Cough
Itching
Restlessness
Pressure sores

Insomnia
Fatigue
Anorexia
Weakness
Immobility
Disorientation

Diagnostic Considerations

This broad diagnosis describes a person with compromised ability to defend against microorganisms and/or bleeding due to immunosuppression, myleosuppression, and/

---

*This diagnostic category was developed and submitted to NANDA by the Clinical Nurse Specialist Group, Harper Hospital, in the Detroit Medical Center.

or abnormal clotting factors. Use of this diagnosis can entail several potential problems.

The nurse should be cautioned against substituting *Altered Protection* as a name for an immune system compromise, AIDS, disseminated intravascular coagulation, diabetes mellitus, or other disorders. Rather, the nurse should focus on diagnosis describing the person's functional abilities that are or may be compromised due to altered protection, such as *Fatigue, High Risk for Infection,* and *High Risk for Social Isolation.* The nurse also should address the physiologic complications of altered protection that require nursing and medical interventions for management, identifying appropriate collaborative problems.

For example, the nurse could use *Altered Protection* in each of these three cases: Mr. A, who has leukemia, leukopenia, and no evidence of infection; Mr. B, who is experiencing sickle cell crisis; and Mr. C, who has AIDS. The problem is that this diagnosis does not describe the specific focus of nursing, but instead describes situations in which more specific responses can be diagnosed. For Mr. A, the nursing diagnosis of *High Risk for Infection related to compromised immune system* would apply. For the collaborative problem *Potential Complication: Sickle cell crisis* best describes his situation, which the nurse will monitor and manage using physician- and nurse-prescribed interventions. The nursing diagnosis *High Risk for Infection* and the collaborative *Potential Complication: Opportunistic infections* would apply for Mr. C.

As shown by these examples, in most cases the nursing diagnosis *High Risk for Infection* and selected collaborative problems will prove more clinically useful than *Altered Protection.*

Impaired Tissue Integrity

■ *Related to* **The Effects of Mechanical Destruction**
■ *Related to* **The Effects of Chemical Destruction**

DEFINITION

Impaired Tissue Integrity: A state in which an individual experiences or is at risk for damage to the integumentary, corneal, or mucous membranous tissues of the body.

DEFINING CHARACTERISTICS

Major (must be present)

Disruptions of corneal, integumentary, or mucous membranous tissue, invasion of body structure (incision, dermal ulcer, corneal ulcer, oral lesion)

Minor (may be present)

Lesions (primary, secondary)   Dry mucous membrane

Edema   Leukoplakia

Erythema   Coated tongue

RELATED FACTORS

Pathophysiologic

Autoimmune alterations
- Lupus erythematosus
- Scleroderma

Metabolic and endocrine alterations
- Diabetes mellitus
- Hepatitis
- Cirrhosis
- Renal failure
- Jaundice
- Cancer
- Thyroid dysfunction

Nutritional alterations
- Obesity
- Dehydration
- Edema
- Emaciation
- Malnutrition

Impaired oxygen transport
- Peripheral vascular alterations
- Venous stasis
- Arteriosclerosis
- Anemia
- Cardiopulmonary disorders

Medications (steroid therapy)

Psoriasis

Eczema

Infections
- Bacterial (impetigo, folliculitis, cellulitis)
- Viral (herpes zoster [shingles], herpes simplex, gingivitis, AIDS)
- Fungal (ringworm [dermatophytosis], athlete's foot, vaginitis)

Dental caries/periodontal disease

Treatment-related

NPO status

Therapeutic extremes in body temperature

Therapeutic radiation

Surgery

Drug therapy (local and systemic)
- Steroids

Imposed immobility related to sedation

Mechanical trauma
- Therapeutic fixation devices
  - Wired jaw
  - Traction
  - Casts
  - Orthopedic devices/braces

Inflatable or foam donuts
Tourniquets
Footboards
Restraints
Dressings, tape, solutions
External urinary catheters
Nasogastric tubes
Endotracheal tubes
Oral prostheses/braces
Contact lenses

Situational (personal, environmental)

Chemical trauma
Excretions
Secretions
Noxious agents/substances
Environmental
Radiation—sunburn
Temperature
Humidity
Parasites

Bites (insect, animal)
Inhalants
Poisonous plants

Immobility
Related to pain, fatigue, motivation, cognitive, sensory, or motor deficits
Depression
Allergies
Inadequate personal habits (hygiene, dental, dietary, sleep)
Body build, weight distribution, bony prominences, muscle mass, range of motion, joint mobility
Stress
Occupation
Pregnancy

Maturational

Infants/children: Diaper rash, childhood diseases (chickenpox)
Adults: Occupational (chemicals, rubber gloves)
Elderly: Dry skin, thin skin, loss of skin elasticity, loss of subcutaneous tissue

Diagnostic Considerations

Impaired Tissue Integrity is the broad diagnosis under which the more specific diagnosis of *Impaired Skin Integrity* and *Impaired Oral Mucous Membranes* fall. Since tissue is composed of epithelium, connective tissue, muscle, and nervous tissue, *Impaired Tissue Integrity* correctly describes some pressure ulcers that are deeper than the dermis. *Impaired Skin Integrity* should be used to describe disruptions of epidermal and dermal tissue only.

When a pressure ulcer is stage IV, necrotic, or infected, it may be more appropriate to label the diagnosis a collaborative problem, such as *Potential Complication: Stage IV pressure ulcer.* This would represent a situation that a nurse manages with physician-and nurse-prescribed interventions. When a stage II or III pressure ulcer needs a dressing that requires a physician's order in an acute care setting, the nurse should continue to label the situation a nursing diagnosis, because it would be appropriate and legal for a nurse to treat the ulcer independently in other settings, *e.g.*, in the community.

If an individual is immobile and multiple systems are threatened (respiratory, circulatory, musculoskeletal as well as integumentary), the nurse can use *High Risk for Disuse Syndrome* to describe the entire situation. If an individual is at risk for damage to corneal tissue, the nurse can use a diagnosis such as *High Risk for Impaired Corneal Tissue Integrity related to corneal drying and lower lacrimal production secondary to unconscious state.*

Errors in Diagnostic Statements

Impaired Skin Integrity related to surgical removal of skin/tissues

Impaired Skin Integrity should not be used as a new label for surgical incisions, tracheostomies, or burns. Surgical incisions disrupt the skin's protective mechanism, increasing vulnerability to microorganism invasion; a more clinically useful diagnosis would be *High Risk for Infection related to surgical incision.*

Impaired Skin Integrity related to fecal diversion

Fecal diversions such as colostomy or ileostomy should not be renamed with the nursing diagnosis *Impaired Skin Integrity.* Instead, the nurse should assess the person's actual or potential responses to the surgical procedure that the nurse can treat. For example, the skin around an ostomy is at risk for erosion from effluent, calling for the diagnosis *High Risk for Impaired Skin Integrity related to chemical irritation of effluent on adjacent skin.* If the adjacent skin exhibited lesions from irritants (chemical or mechanical), the diagnosis *Impaired Skin Integrity related to exposure to ostomy effluent, as evidenced by 2 cm ulcer left midline of stoma* would be appropriate.

Focus Assessment Criteria

Subjective Data
1. History of symptoms
    Onset
    Precipitated by what?
    Relieved by what?
    Frequency?
    Effects on life-style
        Occupation
        Financial
        Role functions
        Sexual/social
2. History of exposure (if allergy is suspected)
    Carrier of contagious disease
    Chemicals, paints, cleaning agents, plants, animals
    Heat or cold
3. Medical, surgical, and dental history, use of tobacco, alcohol
4. Current drug therapy
    What drugs? How often? When was last dose taken?
    Effects on symptoms

5. Factors contributing to the development or extension of tissue destruction (assess for)
    Skin deficits
        Dryness
        Edema
        Obesity
        Thinness
        Excessive perspiration
        Aging skin (dry, thin, loss of elasticity, subcutaneous tissue)
    Mucous membrane deficits
        Mouth pain
        Bleeding gums
        Coated tongue
        Oral lesions or ulcers
        Oral plaque
        Dryness
    Corneal deficits
        Absence of blink reflex
        Corneal ulcers
        Ptosis
        Excessive tearing
        Diminished tearing
        Contact lens wear
        Sensory deficits
    Impaired oxygen transport
        Edema
        Anemia
        Peripheral vascular disorders
        Arteriosclerosis
        Venous stasis
        Cardiopulmonary disorders
    Chemical/mechanical irritants
        Radiation   Casts, splints, braces
        Incontinence (feces, urine)   Contact lenses
        Oral prostheses
    Nutritional deficits
        Protein deficiencies   Mineral and trace
        Vitamin deficiencies   element deficiencies
                                        Dehydration
    Systemic disorders
        Infection
        Diabetes mellitus
        Cancer
        Hepatic or renal disorders
    Sensory deficits
        Brain or cord injury
        Decreased level of consciousness
        Confusion
        Neuropathy
        Visual or taste alterations
    Immobility

Objective Data*

Tissue Characteristics

1. Skin

Color	Texture	Turgor	Vascularity
Pigment	Coarse	Good	Bruising
Pallor	Thick	Poor	Bleeding
Cyanosis	Thin		Angioma
Jaundice			Petechiae
Flushed			Purpura
			Telangiectasis

Moisture	Temperature
Dry	Cool, <98.6° F°
Moist	Warm, >98.6° F°
Normal	Normal

2. Lesions (primary, secondary; see Table II–20)

Type	Shape
Location	Size
Distribution	Drainage
Color	

3. Circulation

   Is erythema present?

   Does the skin blanch when pressure is applied?

   Does erythema subside within 30 minutes after pressure is removed?

4. Edema

   Note degree and location

   Palpate over bony prominences for sponginess (indicates edema)

5. Oral mucous membrane

   Refer to Focus Assessment for *Altered Oral Mucous Membrane* category

Principles and Rationale for Nursing Care

Generic Considerations

1. Tissues are groupings of specialized cells that unite to perform specific functions. The human body is composed of four basic types of tissue: epithelial, connective tissue (including skeletal tissue and blood), muscle, and nervous tissue.

2. The epithelial tissue is a continuous layer of cells that either covers an outside body surface or lines an inside lumen or cavity. Epithelial tissue is classified by numbers of layers (simple—single layer; stratified—more than one layer) and by shapes of the surface cells (squamous, or flat; cuboidal, or cubes; columnar, or tall columns). All

---

*Dark or black skin should be assessed in good light (daytime preferred). Palpation is usually more beneficial than observation. Borders of rashes can be felt and the skin surface can indicate increased warmth (inflammation) and tautness (edema) when palpated.

Table II–20 **Primary and Secondary Lesions**

Primary	Secondary
Macules Circumscribed, flat discolorations of the skin Examples: freckles, flat nevi	**Scales** Dead epidermal cells that thicken and flake off Examples: dandruff, psoriasis
Papules Circumscribed, elevated, superficial, solid lesions that are smaller than 1 cm Examples: elevated nevi, warts	**Crusts** Dried exudate on the surface of the skin produced when skin is damaged Examples: impetigo, infected dermatitis
Nodules Solid elevation, usually > 1 cm in diameter, extend deeper into dermis than papules Examples: epitheliomas	**Fissures** Linear breaks in the tissue, sharply defined with abrupt walls Example: congenital syphilis, athlete's foot
Tumors Larger than 1 cm, solid lesions with depth; they may be above, level with, or beneath the skin Example: tumor stage of *Mycosis fungoides*	**Erosion** Loss of epidermis that does not extend into the dermis Example: abrasion
Plaques Circumscribed, elevated, superficial, solid lesions that are larger than 1 cm Examples: localized *Mycosis fungoides,* neurodermatitis	**Ulcers** Localized areas of tissue destruction that may extend into the mucous membrane or through the epidermis, dermis, and underlying tissue Examples: venous ulcers of the legs, tertiary syphilis
Wheals Types of plaques; result is transient edema in dermis	**Scars** Formations of connective tissue replacing tissue lost through injury or disease Example: keloids
Vesicles Up to 1 cm, circumscribed elevations of the skin of mucous membrane containing serous fluid Examples: early chickenpox, contact dermatitis	
Bullae Larger than 1 cm, circumscribed elevations containing serous fluid Examples: pemphigus, second-degree burns	

communication between the body and the outside world is through the epithelium. Under favorable conditions, the regeneration of epithelial tissue occurs rapidly by a process called epithelialization.

3. Connective tissue is the supporting, binding, and wrapping tissue of the body. It has few living cells and contains a great deal of nonliving intercellular material. Connective tissue is classified according to intercellular material (a gelatin-type ground substance and collagen, elastin, and reticular fibers) and by types of cells (fibroblasts, macrophages, reticular cells, mast cells, plasma cells, leukocytes, fat cells, and pigment cells). Connective tissue is found throughout the body as adipose tissue, ligaments, and loose or dense connective tissue. The fibroblasts of loose connective tissue reproduce rapidly, which aids in the healing of defects in other tissue that has less power to regenerate.

4. Muscle tissue is classified into three categories: involuntary, voluntary, and cardiac.

Involuntary or smooth muscle tissue is found in muscles of internal organs, the gastrointestinal tract, the respiratory tract, the genitourinary tract, the lymphatics and blood vessels, and the pupils of the eye. Voluntary or striated muscle tissue is found in the body wall and extremities. Cardiac muscle tissue is found in the heart wall and in portions of the pulmonary vein. Regeneration of muscle tissue takes place mainly by scar tissue formation.

5. Nervous tissue is found in the brain, spinal cord, and nerves throughout the body. Nervous tissue has the ability to transmit important information by way of chemical and electrical messages. Nerve cells do not regenerate by mitosis, but they do grow axons.

6. The external covering of the body is composed of epithelial tissue called the integument. Wherever the body exposes large openings to the outside, its outer covering changes from integument to an inner lining called mucous membrane, *e.g.,* mouth. Each layer of the integument has its counterpart in a complete mucous membrane. The integument includes both the skin and the subcutaneous tissue.

7. The skin is a complex organ consisting of two layers: the outer epidermis and the deeper dermis. The epidermis is approximately 0.04 mm thick, and the dermis is about 0.5 cm thick.

8. The epidermis functions as a barrier to protect inner tissues (from injury, chemicals, organisms); as a receptor for a range of sensations (touch, pain, heat, cold); as a regulator of body temperature through radiation (giving off heat), conduction (transfer of heat), and convection (movement of warm air molecules away from the body); as a regulator of water balance by preventing water and electrolyte loss; and as a receptor for vitamin D from the sun.

9. Essentially avascular, the multiple layers of epidermal cells progressively die as they reach the surface. Homeostasis of the skin surface depends on equilibrium between cell production and renewal, and cell destruction or loss.

10. Epidermal regenerations is depressed by a water-soluble mitotic inhibitor called chalone. Chalone levels are high during daytime stress and activity and lower during sleep. Healing is therefore promoted during rest and sleep.

11. Beneath the avascular epidermis lies the highly vascularized dermis. The dermis contains epithelial tissue, connective tissue, muscle, and nervous tissue. The dermis is rich in collagen, which imparts toughness to the skin. Hair follicles extend into the dermis and serve as islands of cells for rapid reepithelization of minor wounds. Sweat glands in the dermis contribute to control of body water and temperature. Small muscles within the dermis serve to produce goose pimples. Specialized dermal nerve endings for pain, touch, heat, and cold are irreplaceable once destroyed.

12. The subcutaneous tissue, which lies beneath the dermis, stores fat for temperature regulation and contains the remainder of the sweat glands and hair follicles.

13. Complex interactions between the dermis and epidermis carry messages to one another in case of injury requiring repair.

14. The skin's responses to antigens are capillary dilation (erythema), arteriole dilation (flare), and increased capillary permeability (wheal), which all contribute to localized edema, spasms, and pruritus.

15. Application of heat causes local vasodilation, which promotes healing in healthy tissue but increases pruritus and edema.

16. Application of cold causes local vasoconstriction, which decreases edema and pruritus but retards healing.

17. Skin lesions can be described as primary or secondary. Primary lesions are the initial responses of the skin to an irritant. Secondary lesions result from changes that take place in primary lesions (see Table II–20).

18. Causes of tissue destruction can be mechanical, immunologic, bacterial, chemical, and thermal. Mechanical destruction includes physical trauma or surgical incision. Immunologic destruction occurs as an allergic response to an antigen. Bacterial destruction results from an overgrowth of organisms. Chemical destruction results when a caustic substance maintains contact with unprotected tissue. Thermal destruction occurs when tissue is exposed to temperature extremes that are incompatible with cell life.

Wound Healing of Damaged Tissue

1. Wound healing is a complex sequence of events initiated by injury to the tissues. The components of wound healing are coagulation of bleeding, inflammation, epithelialization, fibroplasia and collagen metabolism, collagen maturation and scar remodeling, and wound contraction (Hudson-Goodman, Girard, & Jones, 1990).
2. A wound must be considered in relation to the entire person. Major factors that affect wound healing are nutrition, vitamins, minerals, anemia, blood volume and tissue oxygenation, steroids and anti-inflammatory drugs, diabetes mellitus, chemotherapy, and radiation.
3. Wound healing requires the following intrinsic factors (Pinchcofsky-Devin & Kaminiski, 1986):
   a. Increased protein–carbohydrate intake sufficient to prevent negative nitrogen balance, hypoalbuminemia, and weight loss
   b. Increased daily intake of vitamins and minerals
      - Vitamin A, 10,000 IU to 50,000 IU
      - Vitamin B_1, 0.5 mg to 1.0 mg/1000 diet calories
      - Vitamin B_2, 0.25 mg/1000 diet calories
      - Vitamin B_6, 2 mg
      - Niacin, 15 mg to 20 mg
      - Vitamin B_{12}, 400 mg
      - Vitamin C, 75 mg to 300 mg
      - Vitamin D, 400 mg
      - Vitamin E, 10 IU to 15 IU
      - Traces of zinc, magnesium, calcium, copper, manganese
   C. Adequate oxygen supply and the blood volume and ability to transport it
4. Wound healing occurs most efficiently with the following extrinsic factors.
   a. Humidity has been shown to affect the rate of epithelization and the amount of scar formation. A moist environment provides the optimum conditions for rapid healing.
   b. When wounds are left uncovered, epidermal cells must migrate under the scab and over the fibrous tissue below. When wounds are semioccluded and the surface of the wound remains moist, epidermal cells migrate more rapidly over the surface.
   c. Moist wound healing may be promoted with the appropriate use of dressings. Wounds that are epidermal or dermal in depth may be mechanically protected and properly humidified by the use of semiocclusive film dressings or hydrocolloid barrier wafers. These dressings bathe the wound in serous exudate and do not adhere to the wound surface when they are removed. A physician's order may be required.
5. Principles of topical treatment (Doughty, 1990)
   a. Remove necrotic tissue. Necrotic tissue delays wound healing by prolonging the inflammatory phase.
   b. Cleanse wound bed to decrease bacteria count. Bacterial counts $> 10^5$ may produce infection by overwhelming the host.

   c. Obliterate dead space in wound, which prevents premature closure and abscess formation.

   d. Absorb excess exudate, which macerates surrounding skin and increases risk of infection in wound bed.

   e. Maintain a moist wound surface, which promotes cellular migration. Dry wound surfaces delay epithelialization secondary to difficult cellular migration.

   f. Insulate the wound surface, which enhances blood flow and increases epidermal migration.

   g. Protect the healing wound from trauma and bacterial invasion. Open wounds are vulnerable to abrasion, contamination, drying, and shear mechanisms.

Pediatric Considerations

1. Although all the skin structures are present at birth, many skin functions are immature (Whaley & Wong, 1989).
2. Many childhood illnesses are characterized by rashes (Whaley & Wong, 1989).

Gerontologic Considerations

1. Elastin, which gives the skin flexibility, elasticity, and tensile strength, decreases with age. It is found in tissues associated with body movement, such as the walls of major blood vessels, heart, lungs, and skin (Goldfarb, Ellis, & Voorhees, 1990; Matteson & McConnell, 1988; Ravito, 1984).
2. Found in all connective tissue, such as blood, lymph, and bone, collagen binds together and supports other tissues. The extracellular matrix of connecting tissue is composed primarily of collagen and elastin, and approximately 80% of the dermis consists of collagen. With aging, skin strength decreases due to age-related loss of collagen from the dermis and the degeneration of the elastic properties of the remaining collagen (Goldfarb, Ellis, & Voorhees, 1990).
3. Some elderly persons exhibit shiny, loose, thin transparent skin primarily on the backs of the hands and the forearms (Macmillan, 1985).
4. Subcutaneous fat decreases with aging, reducing the cushioning of bony prominences, putting elderly persons at increased risk for pressure ulcers (Goldfarb, Ellis, & Voorhees, 1990).
5. Age-related decrease in sebum secretion and the number of sebaceous glands causes drier, coarser skin that is more prone to fissures and cracks (Gilchrist, 1982; Matteson & McConnell, 1988).
6. In older persons, cells are larger and proliferate more slowly, fibroblasts decrease in number, and dermal vascularity decreases. All these factors contribute to a slowed rate of wound healing (Macmillan, 1985).
7. With aging, the thermal threshold for sweating is raised and the sweat output is decreased (Macmillan, 1985).
8. Asteatosis (excessive skin dryness) is the most common cause of pruritus in the elderly. Its incidence is anywhere from 40% to 80%, with this wide range accounted for by varying criteria and climate differences. With scratching, small breaks in the epidermis can increase the risk of infection due to age-related changes in the immune system (Goldfarb, Ellis, & Voorhees, 1990; Matteson & McConnell, 1988; Macmillan, 1985).
9. Aging nails become dull, brittle, and thickened due to decreased blood supply to the nailbed. Splitting of the nails can occur, increasing the risk of infection. Thickening of the toenails causes the distal portion of the nail to lift from the nailbed; debris collection creates a risk of fungal infection (Matteson & McConnell, 1988).
10. More than 90% of all elderly persons have some kind of skin disorder resulting from various causes, *e.g.,* malignancies, stress, metabolic diseases, vascular disorders, and

toxic reactions to drugs. Any epidermal invasion carries the chance of infection. Immune system suppression increases the risk of systemic infection (Goldfarb, Ellis, & Voorhees, 1990; Matteson & McConnell, 1988).

11. Sun exposure is the primary cause of age-related skin changes. The current generation of elderly might be more at risk than younger persons, who have benefitted from sunscreens that have been popularized over the last decade or so. (The induction period for sun-caused cancers is 15 to 40 years.) Repeated sun exposure causes immediate sunburn erythema, thickening of the stratum corneum, and increased melanin production by melanocytes. Incidence of certain pathologic skin conditions (*e.g.,* premalignant cancers, basal cell epitheliomas, and squamous cell carcinomas) increases with sun exposure. Elderly persons also are at risk for secondary lesions (*e.g.,* scales, crusts, fissures, and ulcers), which predispose to localized or systemic infection (Goldfarb, Ellis, & Voorhees, 1990; MacMillan, 1985; Ravits, 1984).

12. Hypothermia is more common in the elderly, particularly in those who show impaired regulation of skin blood flow. This impairment of the thermoregulatory skin vascular reflexes probably is due to degenerative neurologic changes affecting the autonomic nervous system (Ravits, 1984; Macmillan, 1985; Gilchrist, 1982).

13. Many conditions leading to malnutrition are common among the elderly. It is therefore not unusual to find protein depletion and vitamin and trace element deficiencies. Many of these deficiencies involve various cutaneous lesions and mucuous membrane disruption. Hypoalbuminemia can contribute to the development of pressure ulcers and to delayed wound healing. Vitamin C seems to be of particular significance in wound healing (Allman, 1989; Goldfarb, Ellis, & Voorhees, 1988; Roe, 1990).

14. Immobility represents the most important risk factor to the development of pressure ulcers. Many chronic diseases and conditions common to the elderly (*e.g.,* stroke, dementia, arthritis) can cause immobility and put the person at risk for skin breakdown. Other significant risk factors also contribute to the development of pressure ulcers. For example, fecal and urinary incontinence precipititate epidermal excoriation of the epidermis because of the caustic, moist substances coming in contact with the skin (Allman, 1989).

■ Impaired Tissue Integrity
Related to the Effects of Mechanical Destruction

Assessment

Subjective
The person reports discomfort from physical trauma

Objective
Tissue deficits

Drain site	Erythema
Ulcer	Edema
Abrasion	Inflammation
Erosion	Induration

Laceration
Avulsion
Mechanical factors
  Pressure
  Friction
  Shear
  Excessive moisture

Drainage
Necrosis

Outcome Criteria

The person will
• Identify cause of mechanical tissue destruction
• Identify rationale for treatment
• Participate in plan to promote wound healing
• Demonstrate progressive healing of tissue

Interventions

A. Identify causative/contributing factors
  1. Removal of adhesives
  2. Pressure dressings
  3. Nasogastric tubes
  4. Endotracheal tubes
  5. Skeletal prominences with little overlying soft tissue
  6. Hard supporting sleep or sitting surfaces
  7. Prolonged sitting or lying in same position
  8. Dragging across bed linens
  9. Sitting in Fowler's position
  10. Bladder and bowel incontinence
  11. Profuse diaphoresis
  12. Cognitive, sensory, motor deficits
  13. Fixation devices
     a. Skeletal traction
     b. Oral prostheses
  14. Contact lens wear

B. Eliminate or reduce causative factors if possible
  1. Assess for risk of mechanical tissue destruction.
  2. Encourage highest degree of mobility to avoid prolonged periods of pressure.
  3. For neuromuscular impairment
     a. Teach client/significant other appropriate measures to prevent pressure, shear, friction, maceration.
     b. Teach client to recognize early signs of tissue damage.
     c. Change position at least every 2 hours around the clock.
     d. Frequently supplement full body turns with minor shifts in body weight.
  4. Keep client clean and dry.
  5. Reduce environmental sources of pressure (drains, tubes, dressings).
  6. Avoid stripping of epidermis when removing adhesives.

7. Use pressure-dispersing devices as appropriate.
8. Limit Fowler's position in high-risk clients.
9. Avoid use of knee gatch on bed.
10. Use lift sheet to reposition client.
11. Install overhead trapeze to allow clients increased mobility.
12. Use sheepskin pad to reduce friction.

C. See *Impaired Skin Integrity* for further interventions

■ Impaired Tissue Integrity
Related to the Effects of Chemical Destruction

Assessment

Subjective Data
The person reports itching, burning pain from chemical trauma

Objective Data
Tissue deficits

Burn	Ulcer
Blister	Erythema
Excoriation	Inflammation
Erosion	Edema
Stoma	Drainage
Fistula	Exudate
Abscess	Necrosis

Chemical factors

Excretions	Body soap
Secretions	Mouth wash
Chemical irritant	Dental adhesive
Topical medication	Contact lens solution
Chemotherapy	Eye drops

Outcome Criteria

The person will
- Identify cause of chemical tissue destruction
- Identify rationale for treatment
- Participate in plan to promote wound healing
- Demonstrate progressive healing of tissue

Interventions

A. Identify causative/contributing factors
1. Uncontrolled fecal or urinary incontinence
2. Poorly fitting ostomy appliances resulting in peristomal irritation
3. Uncontained draining fistulas or ulcers
4. Use of caustic topical solutions
5. Use of harsh soaps or mouth wash
6. Ingestion of acidic foods or fluids
7. Use of ophthalmic drops or solution
8. Chemotherapy—see *Altered Oral Mucous Membrane* for specific interventions

B. Eliminate or reduce causative factors if possible
1. Assess for risk of chemical tissue destruction.
2. Devise method to contain bowel or bladder incontinence. See *Altered Patterns of Urinary Elimination* and *Altered Bowel Elimination* for specific interventions.
3. Teach correct application of stoma pouch. See *Altered Health Maintenance Related to Lack of Knowledge of Ostomy Care* for specific interventions.
4. Use stoma pouching techniques to contain drainage from fistulas/ulcers.
5. Teach safe use of topical solutions; teach to test small amount of new product on inner aspect of arm.
6. Recommend mild soaps that do not alter skin *p*H.
7. Recommend saline mouth washes.
8. Follow intake of acidic food or fluid with several glasses of water.
9. Refer drug reactions to physician; stop use immediately if untoward effects occur.
10. Teach use of protective gloves/clothing when using chemical products in occupational setting.

Skin Integrity, Impaired

■ *Related to* **Immobility: High Risk for**
■ *Related to* **The Effects of Pressure, Shear, Friction, Maceration**

DEFINITION

Impaired Skin Integrity: A state in which the individual experiences or is at risk for damage to the epidermal and dermal tissue.

DEFINING CHARACTERISTICS

Major (must be present)
Disruptions of epidermal and dermal tissue

Minor (may be present)
   Denuded skin
   Erythema
   Lesions (primary, secondary)
   Pruritus

RELATED FACTORS
See *Impaired Tissue Integrity*

Diagnostic Considerations
See *Impaired Tissue Integrity*

Errors in Diagnostic Statements
See *Impaired Tissue Integrity*

Focus Assessment Criteria
See *Impaired Tissue Integrity*

Principles and Rationale for Nursing Care
See also *Impaired Tissue Integrity*

Generic Considerations
1. Pressure is a compressing downward force on a given area. If pressure against soft tissue is greater than intracapillary blood pressure (approximately 32 mm Hg), the capilaries can be occluded, and the tissue can be damaged as a result of hypoxia.
2. Shear is a parallel force in which one layer of tissue moves in one direction and another layer moves in the opposite direction. If the skin sticks to the bed linen and the weight of the sitting body makes the skeleton slide down inside the skin, the subepidermal capillaries may become angulated and pinched resulting in decreased perfusion of the tissue.
3. Friction is the physiologic wearing away of tissue. If the skin is rubbed against the bed linens, the epidermis can be denuded by abrasion.
4. Maceration is a mechanism by which the tissue is softened by prolonged wetting or soaking. If the skin becomes waterlogged, the cells are weakened and the epidermis is easily eroded.
5. Pressure relief is the one consistent intervention that must be included in all pressure ulcer treatment plans.
6. The choice of products to relieve pressure is best made by actually measuring the tissue interface pressure between a bony prominence and an external supporting surface. A product should reduce the external pressure below the amount of pressure required to keep the capillaries open. A pressure-relieving surface must not be able to be fully compressed by the body. To be effective, a support surface must be capable of first being deformed and then redistributing the weight of the body across the surface. Comfort is not a valid criterion for determining adequate pressure relief.

Pediatric Considerations

1. A newborn commonly exhibits normal skin variations, such as mongolian spots, milia, and stork bites, which can be upsetting to parents but are clinically insignificant (Whaley & Wong, 1989).
2. Several common conditions of the skin affect children in specific age groups. These include atopic, seborrheic, and diaper dermatitis in infancy and acne in adolescence (Whaley & Wong, 1989).
3. Infants and young children have a thin epidermis and require special protection from the sun (Hunsberger & Wonnecott, 1989).

■ High Risk for Impaired Skin Integrity
Related to Immobility

Assessment

Subjective Data
The person reports fatigue, discomfort over bony prominence, inability to move or turn.

Objective Data
Imposed bed rest or immobility
Contributing factors
    Skin deficits
    Impaired oxygen transport
    Nutritional deficit
    Cognitive deficits
    Motor deficits
    Sensory deficits
    Irritants
    Bowel or bladder incontinence

Outcome Criteria

If able, the person will
- Participate in risk assessment
- Express willingness to participate in prevention of pressure ulcers
- Describe etiology and prevention measures
- Explain rationale for interventions
- Demonstrate skin integrity free of pressure ulcers

Interventions

A. Use a risk assessment scale to identify persons at risk for developing pressure ulcers (Bergstro, Braden, Laguzza, & Holman, 1987; Gosnell, 1987)

Assess for
1. Skin deficits
   a. Dryness
   b. Edema
   c. Obesity
   d. Thinness
   e. Excessive perspiration
2. Impaired oxygen transport
   a. Edema
   b. Anemia
   c. Peripheral vascular disorders
   d. Arteriosclerosis
   e. Cardiopulmonary disorders
3. Chemical/mechanical/thermal irritants
   a. Radiation
   b. Incontinence (feces, urine)
   c. Casts, splints, braces
   d. Spasms
4. Nutritional deficits
   a. Protein deficiencies
   b. Vitamin deficiencies
   c. Mineral and trace elements deficiencies
   d. Dehydration
5. Systemic disorders
   a. Infection
   b. Diabetes mellitus
   c. Cancer
   d. Hepatic or renal disorders
6. Sensory deficits
   a. Neuropathy
   b. Confusion
   c. Head injury
   d. Cord injury
7. Immobility

B. Attempt to reduce contributing factors to lessen the possibility of development of a pressure ulcer
   1. Incontinence of urine or feces
      a. Determine etiology of incontinence.
      b. Maintain sufficient fluid intake for adequate hydration (approximately 2500 mL daily, unless contraindicated); check mucous membranes in mouth for moisture and check urine specific gravity.
      c. Establish a schedule for emptying bladder (begin with every 2 hr).
      d. If person is confused, determine what his incontinence pattern is and intervene before incontinence occurs.
      e. Explain problem to individual and secure cooperation for plan.
      f. When incontinent, wash perineum with a liquid soap that will not alter skin pH.
      g. Apply a protective barrier to the perineal region (incontinence film barrier spray or wipes).
      h. Check person frequently for incontinence when indicated.
      i. For additional interventions, refer to *Altered Patterns of Urinary Elimination*.

2. Immobility
   a. Encourage range-of-motion exercise and weight-bearing mobility, when possible, to increase blood flow to all areas.
   b. Promote optimal circulation when in bed.
      - Utilize repositioning schedule that relieves vulnerable area most often (*e.g.,* if vulnerable area is the back, turning schedule would be left side to back, back to right side, right side to left side, and left side to back); post "turn clock" at bedside.
      - Turn person or instruct him to turn or shift weight every 30 minutes to 2 hours, depending on other causative factors present and the ability of the skin to recover from pressure.
      - Frequency of turning schedule should be increased if any reddened areas that appear do not disappear within 1 hour after turning.
      - Position person in normal or neutral position with body weight evenly distributed (Fig. II–4). Use 30° laterally inclined position when possible.
      - Keep bed as flat as possible to reduce shearing forces; limit Fowler's position to only 30 minutes at a time.
      - Use foam blocks or pillows to provide a bridging effect to support the body above and below the high-risk or ulcerated area so that affected area does not touch bed surface. Do not use foam donuts or inflatable rings, since this will increase the area of pressure.
      - Alternate or reduce the pressure on the skin surface with:
        Foam mattresses (comfort only)
        Triple-layered air mattresses (pressure relief)
        Air fluidized beds (pressure relief and moisture control)
        Vascular boots to suspend heels
   c. Utilize enough personnel to lift person up in bed or chair rather than pull or slide skin surfaces. Have patient wear long-sleeved top and socks to reduce friction on elbows and heels.
   d. To reduce shearing forces, support feet with footboard to prevent sliding.
   e. Promote optimum circulation when person is sitting.
      - Limit sitting time for person at high risk for ulcer development.
      - Instruct person to lift self using chair arms every 10 minutes, if possible, or assist person in rising up off the chair every 10 to 20 minutes, depending on risk factors present.
      - Do not elevate legs unless calves are supported, to reduce the pressure over the ischial tuberosities.
      - Pad chair with pressure-relieving cushion.
   f. Inspect areas at risk of developing ulcers with each position change.
      Ears
      Occiput
      Heels*
      Sacrum
      Scrotum
      Elbows
      Trochanter*
      Ischia
      Scapula
   g. Observe for erythema and blanching and palpate for warmth and tissue sponginess with each position change.

*Areas with little soft tissue over a body prominence are at greatest risk.

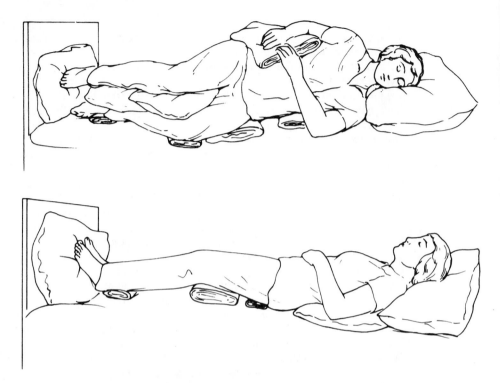

Fig. II-4 Positioning. (*Top*) Side-lying position. Pillows are used above and below the trochanter and lateral malleolus to relieve pressure. (*Bottom*) Supine position. Pillows are used above and below the sacrum and above the heels to relieve pressure. A pillow above the knees prevents hyperextension of the knees and relieves pressure on the popliteal space.

h. Use gentle massage around vulnerable areas with each position change. Do not rub reddened areas. To avoid damaging the capillaries, do not perform deep massage.

3. Malnourished state
   a. Increase protein and carbohydrate intake to maintain a positive nitrogen balance; weigh the person daily and determine serum albumin level weekly to monitor status.
   b. Ascertain that daily intake of vitamins and minerals is maintained through diet or supplements (see Principles for recommended amounts).
   c. See *Altered Nutrition: Less Than Body Requirements* for additional interventions.

4. Sensory deficit
   a. Inspect person's skin at least every 2 hours, since he will not experience discomfort.
   b. Teach person or family to inspect skin with mirror.

C. Initiate health teaching as indicated
   1. Instruct person and family in specific techniques to use at home to prevent pressure ulcers.
   2. Investigate use of long-term pressure-relieving devices for permanent disabilities.

■ Impaired Skin Integrity
Related to the Effects of Pressure, Friction, Shear, Maceration

This nursing diagnosis describes a dermal ulcer as an area of cellular necrosis (due to tissue hypoxia) resulting from pressure, friction, shear, or maceration.

Assessment

Subjective Data
The person may report no discomfort or may report pain or numbness.

Objective Data
The following signs may be noted over a bony prominence (sacrum, heel) or under a cast or brace
Erythema
Elevated skin temperature
Reactive hyperemia
Blanching on pressure
Ulcer
Blister
Drainage
Tissue erosion
Tissue sponginess

Outcome Criteria

The person will
- Identify causative factors for pressure ulcers
- Identify rationale for prevention and treatment
- Participate in the prescribed treatment plan to promote wound healing
- Demonstrate progressive healing of dermal ulcer

Interventions

A. Identify the stage of pressure ulcer development (National Pressure Advisory Panel, 1989)
1. Stage I: Nonblanchable erythema of intact skin
2. Stage II: Ulceration of epidermis and/or dermis
3. Stage III: Ulceration involving subcutaneous fat
4. Stage IV: Extensive ulceration penetrating muscle, bone, or supporting structure

B. Reduce or eliminate factors that contribute to the development or extension of pressure ulcers; refer to *High Risk for Impaired Skin Integrity related to immobility*

C. Prevent deterioration of the ulcer in stages I, II, and III

1. Wash reddened area gently with a mild soap, rinse area thoroughly to remove soap, and pat dry.
2. Gently massage healthy skin around the affected area to stimulate circulation; do not massage reddened area.
3. Protect the healthy skin surface with one or a combination of the following.
   a. Apply a thin coat of liquid copolymer skin sealant.
   b. Cover area with moisture-permeable film dressing.
   c. Cover area with a hydrocolloid wafer barrier and secure with strips of 1-inch microscope tape; leave in place for 2 to 3 days.
4. Increase dietary intake to promote wound healing.
   a. Initiate calorie count.
   b. Increase protein and carbohydrate intake to maintain a positive nitrogen balance: weigh the person daily and determine serum albumin level weekly to monitor status.
   c. Ascertain that daily intake of vitamins and minerals is maintained through diet or supplements (see Principles for recommended amounts).
   d. See *Altered Nutrition: Less Than Body Requirements* for additional interventions.

D. Devise plan for pressure ulcer management using principles of moist wound healing (Maklebust & Sieggreen, 1990)

1. Assess status of pressure ulcer. Measure size of wound bed for baseline data. Measure areas of tunneling or undermining. Assess color, odor and amount of drainage from wound. Also assess color of skin surrounding wound bed.
2. Debride necrotic tissue (collaborate with physician).
3. Flush ulcer base with sterile saline solution. Avoid use of harsh antiseptic solutions.
4. Protect granulating wound bed from trauma and bacteria. Insulate wound surface.
5. Cover pressure ulcer with a sterile dressing that maintains a moist environment over the ulcer base (*e.g.,* film dressing, hydrocolloid wafer dressing, moist gauze dressing). Do not occlude ulcers on immunocompromised patients.
6. Avoid the use of drying agents (heat lamps, Maalox, Milk of Magnesia).
7. Monitor for clinical signs of wound infection.
8. Measure pressure ulcer weekly to determine progress of wound healing.

E. Consult with nurse specialist or physician for treatment of necrotic, infected, or stage IV pressure ulcers

F. Initiate health teaching and referrals as indicated

1. Instruct person and family on care of ulcers.
2. Teach the importance of good skin hygiene and optimum nutrition.
3. Refer to community nursing agency if additional assistance at home is needed.

Oral Mucous Membrane, Altered

- ■ *Related to* **Inadequate Oral Hygiene or Inability to Perform Oral Hygiene**
- ■ *Related to* **(Specify) as Manifested by Stomatitis**

DEFINITION
Altered Oral Mucous Membrane: The state in which an individual experiences or is at risk of experiencing disruptions in the oral cavity.

DEFINING CHARACTERISTICS

Major (must be present)
Disrupted oral mucous membranes

Minor (may be present)

Coated tongue	Leukoplakia
Xerostomia (dry mouth)	Edema
Stomatitis	Hemorrhagic gingivitis
Oral tumors	Purulent drainage
Oral lesions	

RELATED FACTORS

Pathophysiologic
Diabetes mellitus
Oral cancer
Periodontal disease
Infection
Herpes simplex   Gingivitis

Treatment-related
NPO more than 24 hours
Radiation to head or neck
Prolonged use of steroids or other immunosuppressives
Antineoplastic drugs
Endotracheal tube
Nasogastric tube

Situational (personal, environmental)
Chemical trauma
Acidic foods   Alcohol
Drugs   Tobacco
Noxious agents

Mechanical trauma
    Broken or jagged teeth
    Ill-fitting dentures
    Braces
Malnutrition
Dehydration
Mouth breathing
Inadequate oral hygiene
Lack of knowledge
Fractured mandible

Diagnostic Considerations
See Impaired Tissue Integrity

Errors in Diagnostic Statements
See Impaired Tissue Integrity

Focus Assessment Criteria

Subjective Data

1. The person complains of
    Mouth pain, irritation, or burning
    Xerostomia (dry mouth)
    Bad taste or odor in mouth
    Chewing difficulties
    Change in tolerance to temperature of food (cold, hot)
    Change in tolerance to acidic or highly seasoned food
    Change in taste
    Poorly fitting dentures
2. History
    Medical/surgical
    Medication use (prescribed, over the counter)
    Use of tobacco
        Type (cigarettes, pipe, cigars, snuff)
        Frequency (packs per day, how many years)
    Use of alcohol
        Type
        Amount (daily, weekly)
3. Oral hygiene
    Frequency of dental checkups
    Personal hygiene
        "Describe your oral care procedure."
        Type of equipment (brush, floss)
        Frequency
    Possible barriers to performing oral care
        Unable to hold standard brush
        Unable to close hand
        Limited arm movement
        Semicomatose
        Lack of knowledge

4. Nutritional status (refer to *Altered Nutrition* for specific assessment criteria)

Daily intake of basic four food groups

Daily fluid intake

Difficulty in chewing or swallowing

Are certain foods avoided? Why?

Objective Data

1. Lips

Color

Presence of

Cracks	Blisters
Fissures	Ulcers/lesions

2. Tongue

Color

Presence of

Masses	Cracks, dryness
Lesions	Exudates
Hairy extensions	

3. Oral mucosa (gums, floor of mouth, inner cheeks, palate)

Color

Presence of

Bleeding	Plaques
Swelling	Lesions

4. Teeth

Presence of

Sharp edges	Looseness
Chips	Missing teeth
Cracks	

5. Dentures/prosthetics

Condition

Fit

Presence of

Sharp edges	Cracks
Loose parts	Chips

Principles and Rationale for Nursing Care

1. Oral health directly influences many activities of daily living (eating, fluid intake, breathing) and interpersonal relations (appearance, self-concept, communication).
2. The frequency of oral health maintenance will vary according to an individual's health status and self-care ability. All persons should have their teeth and mouths cleaned at least once after meals and at bedtime. High-risk persons (*e.g.,* persons with nasogastric tubes, cancer and poorly nourished persons) should have oral assessments daily. Persons in chronic care settings should have oral assessment *at least once* a week.
3. Factors that contribute to oral disease are alcohol and tobacco (excessive use), microorganisms, inadequate nutrition (quantity, quality), inadequate hygiene, and trauma (nasogastric tubes, ill-fitting dentures, sharp-edged teeth, sharp-edged prostheses, improper use of cleaning devices) (Harrell & Damon, 1989).
4. Many oral diseases begin quietly and are painless until significant involvement has taken place.
5. Plaque is microbial flora found in the mouth and is the primary factor contributing to

dental cavities and periodontal disease. Daily removal of plaque through brushing and flossing can help prevent dental decay and disease.

6. Decreased salivary flow and increased viscosity of saliva reduce the removal of debris (food, bacteria) from the mouth (Pettigrew, 1989).

7. Common causes of decreased salivation are dehydration, anemia, radiation treatment to head and neck, vitamin deficiencies, removal of salivary glands, allergies, and side-effects of drugs (*e.g.,* antihistamines, anticholinergics, phenothiazines, narcotics, chemotherapy).

8. Excessive use of hydrogen peroxide for mouth care may predispose to an oral yeast infection. Rinse afterward with normal saline (Pettigrew, 1989).

9. Lemon and glycerine swabs should be used only on clean, healthy mouths as a source of refreshment for an NPO client (Danielson, 1988).

10. Alcohol and tobacco are chronic irritants to oral mucosa and may lead to oral carcinoma.

Pediatric Considerations

1. Oral candidiasis (thrush) is common in the newborn. It can be acquired by person-to-person transmission, from a maternal vaginal infection during delivery, or from use of contaminated nipples or other articles (Whaley & Wong, 1989).

2. Teething may cause discomfort and make the gums appear red and swollen (Upton, 1989).

Gerontologic Considerations

1. Age-related changes in oral mucosa include loss of elasticity, atrophy of epithelial cells, and diminished blood supply to connective tissue (Miller, 1990).

2. Dry mouth and vitamin deficiencies in elderly persons increase vulnerability to oral ulcerations and infection (Miller, 1990).

3. Elderly persons commonly exhibit increased saliva viscosity and diminished saliva quantity (Lassila, 1987).

■ Altered Oral Mucous Membrane
Related to Inadequate Oral Hygiene or Inability to Perform Oral Hygiene

Assessment

Subjective Data

The person
Does not practice oral hygiene
Cannot perform oral hygiene

Objective Data

Pain
Burning
Coated tongue

Outcome Criteria

The person will
• Demonstrate integrity of the oral cavity
• Be free of harmful plaque to prevent secondary infection
• Be free of oral discomfort during food and fluid intake

Interventions

A. Assess for the presence of causative or contributing factors
   1. Lack of knowledge
   2. Lack of motivation
   3. Impairment of use of hands
   4. Fatigue
   5. Altered consciousness

B. Discuss the importance of daily oral hygiene and periodic dental examinations
   1. Explain the relationship of plaque to dental and gum disease.
   2. Evaluate the person's ability to perform oral hygiene.
   3. Allow person to perform as much of his oral care as possible.

C. Teach correct oral care
   1. Have person sit or stand upright over sink (if unable to get to sink, place an emesis pan under the chin).
   2. Remove and clean dentures and bridges daily.
      a. Fill wash bowl half full of water (place washcloth on bottom to keep denture from breaking if dropped).
      b. Brush dentures with a denture brush or stiff hard toothbrush inside and outside; rinse in cool water before replacing.
      c. Stains and odors can be removed from dentures by soaking them overnight in 8 oz of water and 1 teaspoon of laundry bleach (avoid bleach on any appliance with metal).
      d. Hard deposits can be removed by soaking dentures in white (not brown) vinegar overnight.
      e. If commercial liquid denture cleaners are used, brushing is still required.
   3. Floss teeth (every 24 hr).
      a. With a piece of dental floss approximately 25 inches long, floss each tooth by wrapping the floss around the second and third fingers of each hand.
      b. Beginning with the back teeth, insert the floss between each tooth gently to prevent injuring the gum.
      c. Wrap floss around tooth, making a C, and gently pull floss up and down over the back of each tooth.
      d. Repeat this in reverse to floss the front of the tooth.
      e. Remove the floss by either pulling straight up or by releasing one end and pulling the floss through (minor bleeding may occur).
      f. Allow the person to rinse.
      g. Floss holders can be used by the person or the nurse to make flossing easier (back teeth cannot be reached with a floss holder).

4. Brush teeth (after meals and before sleep).
   a. Use a soft toothbrush (avoid hard brushes) with a nonabrasive toothpaste or sodium bicarbonate (1 tsp in 8 oz of water; may be contraindicated in persons with sodium restrictions).
   b. Brush back and forth or in a small circle, starting at the back of the mouth and brushing one or two teeth at a time.
   c. Gently brush tongue and inner sides of cheeks.
   d. Rinse with water.
5. Inspect mouth for lesions, sores, or excessive bleeding.

D. Perform oral hygiene on person who is unconscious or at risk for aspiration as often as needed

1. Preparation
   a. Tell person what you are going to do.
   b. Turn person on his side, supporting back with pillow (protect bed with an absorbent pad).
   c. Place a tongue blade or bite block to keep mouth open.
   d. Wear gloves to protect hands.
2. Brushing procedure
   a. For persons with their own teeth, brush following the procedure outlined in Nos. 3 and 4 above.
   b. Use a solution instead of toothpaste: hydrogen peroxide and water (1:4), sodium bicarbonate (1 tsp:8 oz water), or normal saline solution (may be contraindicated in persons with sodium restrictions).
   c. For persons with dentures, remove dentures and clean according to procedure in C, No. 2.
   d. Leave dentures out for persons who are semicomatose and store in water (in denture cup).
   e. If gums are inflamed, use moist cotton-tipped applicators or soft foam Toothettes.
   f. Use a bulb syringe to rinse mouth; aspirate rinse with suction or use an aspirating toothbrush.
   g. Move tongue blade or bite block for access to other areas; do not put fingers on tops or edges of teeth.
   h. Brush tongue and inner cheek tissue gently.
   i. Pat mouth dry and apply lip lubricant.
   j. Gums and teeth should be lightly wiped four to six times a day to prevent drying (*e.g.*, swab with mineral oil or saline but use sparingly to prevent aspiration).

E. Initiate health teaching and referrals as indicated

1. Identify individuals who need toothbrush adaptations to perform own mouth care.
   a. Difficulty closing hand tightly (Danielson, 1988)
      • Tape a wide elastic band to toothbrush tightly enough to hold brush snugly in hand.
   b. Limited hand mobility
      • Enlarge toothbrush handle with a sponge hair roller, wrinkled aluminum foil, or a bicycle handbar grip attached with a small amount of plaster of paris.
   c. Limited arm movement
      • Extend handle of standard toothbrush by attaching handle of an old

toothbrush (after cutting off bristle end) to a new toothbrush with strong cord or plastic cement, or by attaching toothbrush to a plastic rod (the toothbrush can be curved by gently heating and then bending it).

2. Refer individuals with tooth and gum disorders to a dentist.
3. Teach parents to
   a. Provide their child with fluoride supplements if not present in concentrations over 0.7 parts per million (ppm) in drinking water.
   b. Avoid taking tetracycline drugs during pregnancy or giving to child during infancy.
   c. Refrain from putting an infant to bed with a bottle of juice or milk.
   d. Provide child with safe objects for chewing during teething.
   e. Replace toothbrushes frequently (every 3 mo).
   f. Schedule dental checkups every 6 months after the age of 2 years.
4. Teach child to
   a. Avoid highly sugared liquids, foods, and chewing gum.
   b. Drink water and extra fluid.
   c. Brush teeth using fluoride toothpaste.

■ Altered Oral Mucous Membrane
Related to (Specify) as Evidenced by Stomatitis

Stomatitis is inflammation of the mucous membrane of the mouth, ranging from redness to ulcerations to hemorrhage.

Assessment

Subjective Data
The person reports
   Oral burning or pain
   Change in tolerance to food temperatures (cold, hot)
   Change in tolerance to acidic or highly seasoned food

Objective Data
   Erythema of oral mucosa (mild)
   Small areas of ulcerations or white patches (moderate)
   White patches over 25% of oral mucosa (moderate to severe)
   Hemorrhagic ulcerations (severe)

Outcome Criteria

The person will
• Be free of oral mucosa irritation or exhibit signs of healing with decreased inflammation
• Demonstrate knowledge of optional oral hygiene

Interventions

A. Assess for the presence of causative or contributing factors
  1. Lack of oral hygiene
  2. Malnourishment
  3. History of high alcohol intake and tobacco use
  4. Chemotherapeutic drugs with mucous membrane toxicity
  5. Radiation to head or neck
  6. Immunosuppression
  7. Dehydration
  8. Steroid therapy

B. Teach individuals at risk to develop stomatitis preventive oral hygiene
  1. Refer to *Altered Oral Mucous Membrane related to inadequate oral hygiene* for specific instructions on brushing and flossing.
  2. Instruct person to
     a. Perform the regimen after meals and before sleep (if there is excessive exudate, perform regimen before breakfast also).
     b. Avoid mouthwashes with high alcohol content, lemon/glycerine swabs, or prolonged use of hydrogen peroxide.
     c. Rinse mouth with flavored saline solution.
     d. Apply lubricant to lips every 2 hours and PRN (*e.g.,* lanolin, A&D ointment, petroleum jelly).
     e. Inspect mouth daily for lesions and inflammation and report alterations.
  3. For person who is unable to tolerate brushing or swabbing, teach to irrigate mouth (every 2 hr and PRN).
     a. With normal saline, use an enema bag (labeled for oral use only) with a soft irrigation catheter tip.
     b. Place catheter tip in mouth and slowly increase flow while standing over a basin or having a basin held under chin.
     c. Remove dentures prior to irrigation and do not replace in person with severe stomatitis.
  4. Consult with physician for possible need of prophylactic antifungal or antibacterial agent.

C. Promote healing and reduce progression of stomatitis
  1. Inspect oral cavity three times daily with tongue blade and light; if stomatitis is severe, inspect mouth every 4 hours.
  2. Ensure that oral hygiene regimen is done every 2 hours while awake and every 6 hours (every 4 hours if severe) during the night.
  3. Use normal saline solution as a mouthwash.
  4. Floss teeth only once in 24 hours.
  5. Omit flossing if excessive bleeding occurs and use extreme caution with persons with platelet counts of less than 50,000.

D. Reduce oral pain and maintain adequate food and fluid intake
  1. Assess person's ability to chew and swallow.
  2. Administer mild analgesic q 3–4 hours as ordered by physician.
  3. Instruct individual to
     a. Avoid commercial mouth washes, citrus fruit juices, spicy foods, extremes in food temperature (hot, cold), crusty or rough foods, alcohol, mouth washes with alcohol.

   b. Eat bland, cool foods (sherbets).
   c. Drink cool liquids q 2 hours and PRN.
4. Consult with dietitian for specific interventions.
5. Refer to *Altered Nutrition: Less Than Body Requirements Related to Anorexia* for additional interventions.
6. Consult with physician for an oral pain relief solution.
   a. Xylocaine Viscous 2% oral swish and expectorant q 2 hours and before meals (if throat is sore, the solution can be swallowed; if swallowed, Xylocaine produces local anesthesia and may affect the gag reflex).
   b. Mix equal parts of Xylocaine Viscous, 0.5 aqueous Benadryl solution, and Maalox, swish and swallow 1 oz of mixture q 2–4 hours PRN.
   c. Mix equal parts of 0.5 aqueous Benadryl solution and Kaopectate; swish and swallow q 2–4 hours PRN.

E. Initiate health teaching and referrals as indicated
   1. Teach person and family the factors that contribute to the development of stomatitis and its progression.
   2. Teach diet modifications to reduce oral pain and to maintain optimal nutrition.
   3. Have individual describe or demonstrate home care regimen.

References/Bibliography

Allman, R. M. (1989). Pressure sores among the elderly. *New England Journal of Medicine, 320*(13), 850–853.

Allman, R., Laprade, C., Noel, L., Walker J., Moorer, C., Dear, M., & Smith C. (1986). Pressure sores among hospitalized patients. *Annals of Internal Medicine, 105*(3), 337–342.

Bergstrom, N., Demuth, P.J., & Braden, B.J. (1987). A clinical trial of the Braden Scale for predicting pressure sore risk. *Nursing Clinics of North America, 22*(2), 417–428.

Bergstrom, N., Braden, B.J., Laguzza, A., & Holman, V. (1987). The Braden Scale for predicting pressure sore risk. *Nursing Research, 36*(4), 205–210.

Cooper, D.M. (1990). Challenge of open wound assessment in the home setting. *Progression: Developments in Ostomy and Wound Care, 2*(3), 11–18.

Cooper, D. M. (1990). Optimizing wound healing: A practice within nursing's domain. *Nursing Clinics of North America, 25*(1), 165–180.

Dossey, L. (1983). The skin: What is it? In the integument. *Topics in Clinical Nursing, 5*(2), 1–4.

Doughty, D. (1990). Your patient: Which therapy? *Journal of Enterostomal Therapy, 17*(4), 154–159.

Fowler, E. (1982). Pressure sores: A deadly nuisance. *Journal of Gerontological Nursing, 8*(12), 680–685.

Gilchrist, B. A. (1982). Age-associated changes in skin. *Journal of the American Geriatric Society, 30,* 139–143.

Goldfarb, M. J., Ellis, C. N., & Voorhees, J. J. (1990). Dermatology. In Cassel, C. K., Riesenberg, D. E., Sorenson, L. B., & Walsh, J. R. *Geriatric medicine* (2nd ed.). New York: Springer-Verlag.

Gosnell, D. J. (1987).: Development of an instrument to assess client risk for pressure sores. In Waltz C.F., & Strickland, O. (Eds). *Measurement of clinical and educational nursing outcomes: A compendium of tools for research, education and practice.* New York: Springer.

Horsley, J. (1981). *Preventing decubitus ulcers.* CURN Project. New York: Grune & Stratton.

Hudson-Goodman, P., Girard, N., & Jones, M. B. (1990). Wound repair and the use of growth factors. *Heart and Lung, 19*(4), 379–384.

Hunsberger, M., & Wonnecott, E. (1989). Nursing strategies: The injured child. In Foster, R. l., Hunsberger, M. M. & Anderson, J. J. T. (Eds.). *Family-centered nursing care of children.* Philadelphia: W. B. Saunders, p. 2055.

Jeter, K., Faller, N., & Norton, C. (1990). *Nursing for continence.* Philadelphia: W. B. Saunders.

Krasner, D. (1990). Alterations in skin integrity related to continence management/incontinence: Some problems and solutions. *Ostomy/Wound Management, 28,* 62–63.

Krasner, D. (1990). *Chronic wound care: A clinical sourcebook for health care professionals.* Philadelphia: Health Management Publications.

Linder, R. M., & Morris, D. (1990). The surgical management of pressure ulcers: A systematic approach based on staging. *Decubitus, 3*(2), 32–38.

Low, A. W., (1990). Prevention of pressure sores in patients with cancer. *Oncology Nursing Forum, 17*(2), 179–184.

Macmillan, A. L. (1985). Aging and the skin. In Brocklehurst, J. C. (Ed.). *Textbook of geriatric medicine and gerontology.* Edinburgh: Churchill Livingstone.

Maklebust, J. (1987). Pressure ulcers: Etiology and prevention. *Nursing Clinics of North America, 22*(2), 359–377.

Maklebust, J. (1989). Pulling the plug on heatlamps. *RN, 52*(12), 79.

Maklebust, J., Brunckhorst, L., Cracchiolo-Caraway, A., Ducharme, M., Dundon, R., Panfilla, R., Parzuchowski, J., Sieggreen, M., & Walthall, S. (1988). Pressure ulcer incidence in high-risk patients managed on a special three layered air cushion. *Decubitus, 1*(4), 30–40.

Maklebust, J. A., Mondoux, L. C., & Sieggreen, M. Y. (1986). Pressure relief characteristics of various support surfaces used in prevention and treatment of pressure ulcers. *Journal of Enterostomal Therapy, 13*(3), 85–89.

Maklebust, J., & Sieggreen, M. (1990). *Pressure ulcers: Guidelines for prevention and nursing management.* West Dundee, Il: S-N Publications.

Maklebust, J., Sieggreen, M. Y., & Mondoux, L. (1988). Pressure relieving capabilities: A comparison of the SoF-Care cushion and the Clinitron bed. *Ostomy/Wound Management, 21,* 32–41.

Maklebust, J., Sieggreen, M. Y., Mondoux, L., LaPlante, J., Lenk, D., Singer, D., & Cameron, O. (1987). *Pressure ulcer guidelines: Nursing diagnoses and management* (2nd ed.). Detroit: Harper Grace Hospitals.

Matteson, M. A., & McConnell, E. S. (1988). *Gerontological nursing: Concepts and practice.* Philadelphia: W. B. Saunders.

National Pressure Advisory Panel. (1989). *Pressure ulcers: Incidence, economics, risk assessment. consensus development conference statement.* West Dundee, IL: S-N Publications.

Oot-Giromini, B., Gosnell, D., & Morris, J., (1990). Pressure ulcer prevention—Developing discharge criteria. *Continuing Care, 9*(6), 22–27.

Parish, L. C., Witkowski, J. A., Crissey, J. T. (1983). *The decubitus ulcer.* New York: Masson.

Petro, J. (1990). Ethical dilemmas of pressure ulcers. *Decubitus, 3*(2), 28–31.

Pinchcofsky-Devin, G. D., & Kaminski, M. V. (1986). Correlation of pressure sores and nutritional status. *Journal of the American Geriatric Society, 34*(3), 435–440.

Ravits, H. G. (1984, May). The skin in midlife. *Transition,* 13–17, 20–22.

Roe, D. A. (1990) Overview of effects of aging on nutrition. *Clinics in Geriatric Medicine, 6*(2), 319–333.

Schumann, D. (1982). The nature of wound healing. *AORN Journal, 35*(6), 1068–1077.

Sieggreen, M. Y. (1987). The healing of physical wounds. *Nursing Clinics of North America, 22*(2), 439–447.

Stotts, N. A. (1988). Predicting pressure ulcers in a surgical population. *Heart and Lung, 17*(6), 641–647.

Stotts, N. A., & Paul, S. M. (1988). Pressure ulcer development in surgical patients. *Decubitus, 1*(3), 24–30.

Upton, L. (1989). Growth and development of the infant. In Foster, R. L., Hunsberger, M. M., & Anderson, J. J. T. (Eds.). *Family-centered nursing care of children.* Philadelphia: W. B. Saunders, p. 224.

Watson, R. (1990). The benefits of excellence: A cost effective treatment program for pressure sores. *Professional Nurse, 5*(7), 356, 358, 360.

Whaley, L. F., & Wong, D. L. (1989). *Essentials of pediatric nursing* (3rd ed.). St. Louis: C. V. Mosby.

Willis, J. (1986). Extended wear contact lenses and corneal ulcers. In FDA Drug Bulletin, DHHS, FDA, Rockville, MD: *16*(1).

High Risk for Impaired Tissue Integrity

Bergstrom, N., Demuth, P. J., & Braden, B. (1987). A clinical trial of the Braden Scale for predicting pressure sore risk. *Nursing Clinics of North America, 22*(2), 417–428.

Bergstrom, N., Braden, B. J., Laguzza, A., & Holman, V. (1987). The Braden Scale for predicting pressure sore risk. *Nursing Research, 36*(4), 205–210.

Braden, B. J., & Bergstrom, N. (1987). A conceptual schema for the study of the etiology of pressure sores. *Rehabilitation Nursing, 12*(1), 8–12.

Ek, A. C., Unosson, M., & Bjurulf, P. (1989). The modified Norton Scale and the nutritional state. *Scandinavian Journal of Caring Sciences, 3*(4), 183–187.

Gosnell, D. J. (1973). An assessment tool to identify pressure sores. *Nursing Research, 22*(1), 55.

Gosnell, D. J. (1987) Development of an instrument to assess client risk for pressure sores. In Waltz, C. F., & Strickland, O. (Eds.). *Measurement of clinical and education nursing outcomes: A compendium of tools for research, education, and practice.* New York: Springer Publishing.

Gosnell, D. J. (1987). Assessment and evaluation of pressure sores. *Nursing Clinics of North America, 22*(2), 399–416.

Oral Mucous Membrane

Bennett, J. (1981). Oral health maintenance. In Carnevali, D., & Patrick, M. (Eds). *Nursing management for the elderly.* Philadelphia: J. B. Lippincott, pp. 111–135.

Buss, C. L., (1987). Nutritional support of cancer patients. *Primary Care, 13*(2), 317–335.

Daeffler, R. R: Oral hygiene measures for patients with cancer. *Cancer Nursing, 3*(10), 347–355, 1980; *3*(12), 427–432, 1980, *4*(2), 29–36, 1981.

Danielson, K. H. (1988). Oral care and older adults. *Journal of Gerontological Nursing, 14*(11), 6–10.

DeWys, W. (1985). Management of cancer cachexia. *Seminars in Oncology, 12*(3), 452–460.

Dudjak, L. A. (1987). Mouth care for mucositis due to radiation therapy. *Cancer Nursing, 10*(3), 131–140.

Eilers, J., Berger, A., & Petersen, M. (1988). Development, testing, application of the oral assessment guide. *Oncology Nursing Forum, 15*(3), 325.

Harrell, J. S., & Damon, J. F. (1989). Prediction of patient's need for mouth care. *Western Journal of Nursing Research, 11*(6), 748–756.

Knobf, M. T., Fischer, D. S., Welch-McCaffrey, M. (1984). *Cancer chemotherapy: Treatment and care.* Chicago: Year Book Medical Publishers.

Lassila, V. P. (1987). Stimulated saliva and microbial growth in older adults. *Special Care in Dentistry, 7*(4), 157–160.

Lawson, K. (1989). Oral-dental concerns of the pediatric oncology patient. *Issues in Comprehensive Pediatric Nursing, 12*(2/3), 199–206.

Meckstroth, R. L. (1989). Improving quality and efficacy in oral hygiene. *Journal of Gerontological Nursing, 15*(6), 38–44.

Miller, C. A. (1990). *Nursing care of older adults.* Glenview, IL: Scott, Foresman.

Napierski, G. E., & Danner, M. A. (1982). Oral hygiene for the dentulous total-care patient. *Special Care in Dentistry, 2*(6), 257–259.

Niehaus, C. S., Peterson, D. E., & Overholser, C. D. (1987). Oral complications in children during cancer therapy. *Cancer Nursing, 10,* 15.

Pettigrew, D. (1989). Investing in mouth care. *Geriatric Nursing, 10*(1), 22–24.

Ringsdorf, W., & Cheraskin, E. (1982). Vitamin C and human wound healing. *Oral Surgery, 53*(3), 231–236.

Ross, L. S. (1982). *Oral management of patients radiated to the head and neck.* Detroit: The Oral Cancer Detection Center, Michigan Cancer Foundation.

Roth P. T., & Creason, N. S. (1986). Nursing administered oral hygiene: Is there a scientific basis? *Journal of Advanced Nursing, 11,* 323.

Schweiger, J., Lang, J. W., Schweiger, J. W., et al. (1980). Oral assessment: How to do it. *American Journal of Nursing, 80,* 654–657.

Smith, R. (1989). Mouth stick design for the client with spinal cord injury. *American Journal of Occupational Therapy, 43*(4), 251–255.

Tissue Perfusion, Altered (Specify) (Renal, cerebral, cardiopulmonary, gastrointestinal, peripheral)

Tissue Perfusion, Altered Peripheral

Tissue Perfusion, Altered (Specify) (Renal, cerebral, cardiopulmonary, gastrointestinal, peripheral)

DEFINITIONS

Altered Tissue Perfusion: The state in which the individual experiences or is at high risk of experiencing a decrease in nutrition and respiration at the cellular level due to a decrease in capillary blood supply.

Diagnostic Considerations

See *Altered Peripheral Tissue Perfusion*

Errors in Diagnostic Statements

See *Altered Peripheral Tissue Perfusion*

Tissue Perfusion, Altered Peripheral

■ *Related to* **(Specify)**

DEFINITION

Altered Peripheral Tissue Perfusion: The state in which an individual experiences or is at high risk of experiencing a decrease in nutrition and respiration at the peripheral cellular level due to a decrease in capillary blood supply.

DEFINING CHARACTERISTICS

Major (must be present)

Presence of one of the following types (see Principles for definitions)
Claudication
Rest pain
Aching pain
Diminished or absent arterial pulses
Skin color changes
Pallor (arterial)
Cyanosis (venous)
Reactive hyperemia (arterial)
Skin temperature changes
Cooler (arterial)
Warmer (venous)
Decreased blood pressure changes (arterial)
Capillary refill greater than 3 seconds (arterial)

Minor (may be present)

Edema (venous)
Loss of sensory function (arterial)
Loss of motor function (arterial)
Tropic tissue changes (arterial)
Hard, thick nails
Loss of hair
Lack of lanugo (newborn)

RELATED FACTORS

Pathophysiologic

Vascular disorders
Arteriosclerosis
Hypertension
Aneurysm
Arterial thrombosis
Deep vein thrombosis
Collagen vascular disease
Rheumatoid arthritis
Leriche's syndrome
Raynaud's disease/syndrome
Varicosities
Buerger's disease
Sickle cell crisis
Cirrhosis
Alcoholism
Diabetes mellitus
Hypotension
Sympathetic stress response (vasospasm/vasoconstriction)
Blood dyscrasias (platelet disorders)
Renal failure
Cancer/tumor

Treatment-related

Immobilization
Presence of invasive lines
Pressure sites/constriction (Ace bandages, stockings)
Medications (diuretics, tranquilizers, anticoagulants)
Anesthesia
Blood vessel trauma or compression

Situational (personal, environmental)

Pregnancy
Heredity
Obesity
Diet (hyperlipidemia)
Anorexia/malnutrition
Dehydration
Dependent venous pooling
Hypothermia
Frequent exposure to vibrating tools/equipment
Tobacco use
Exercise
Trauma

Maturational

Neonate
    Immature peripheral circulation
    Rh incompatibility (erythroblastosis fetalis)
    Hypothermia
Elderly
    Sensory–perceptual changes
    Atherosclerotic plaques
    Capillary fragility

Diagnostic Considerations

Tissue perfusion depends on many physiologic factors within the body systems and in cellular structures and functions. A person's response to altered tissue perfusion can disrupt some or all functional health patterns and can cause physiologic complications. For example, a person with chronic renal failure will be at risk for fluid/electrolyte imbalances, acidosis, nutritional problems, edema, fatigue, pruritus, and self-concept disturbances. Does the diagnosis *Altered Renal Tissue Perfusion* describe these varied responses, or does it simply rename renal failure or renal calculi?

The use of any *Altered Tissue Perfusion* diagnosis other than *Peripheral* merely provides new labels for medical diagnoses, labels that do not describe the nursing focus or accountability. The following represent examples of *Altered Tissue Perfusion* diagnoses with associated goals from the literature:

- *Altered Tissue Perfusion related to hypovolemia secondary to GI bleeding*
  Goal: Tissue perfusion improves, as evidenced by stabilized vital signs
- *Altered Cerebral Tissue Perfusion related to increased intracranial pressure*
  Goal: ICP is ≤ 15 mm Hg and clinical signs of ICP are decreased
- *Altered Tissue Perfusion related to vasocclusive nature of sickling secondary to sickle cell crisis*
  Goal: Demonstrates improved tissue perfusion, as evidenced by adequate urine output, absence of pain, good orientation, strong peripheral pulses

All the above outcomes represent criteria that nurses will use to assess the client's status to determine the appropriate nursing and medical interventions indicated. Thus, these situations represent the following collaborative problems, respectively: *PC: GI bleeding, PC: Increased ICP* and *PC: Sickling crisis.*

The diagnosis *Altered Tissue Perfusion (Renal, cerebral, cardiopulmonary, gas-*

trointestinal) was approved by NANDA in 1980. Currently, it does conform to the NANDA definition approved in 1990 (refer to Chapter 2). When using these diagnoses, nurses cannot be accountable for prescribing the interventions for outcome achievement. Instead of using *Altered Tissue Perfusion,* the nurse should focus on the nursing diagnoses and collaborative problems applicable due to altered renal, cardiac, cerebral, pulmonary, or GI tissue perfusion.

Altered Peripheral Tissue Perfusion can be a clinically useful nursing diagnosis if used to describe chronic vascular insufficiency or potential thrombophlebitis. (In contrast, acute embolism and thrombophlebitis represent collaborative problems.) A nurse focusing on preventing thrombophlebitis in a postoperative client would write the diagnosis *High Risk for Altered Peripheral Tissue Perfusion related to postop immobility and dehydration.*

Errors in Diagnostic Statements

Altered GI Tissue Perfusion related to esophageal bleeding varices
Because, this diagnosis actually represents a situation that nurses monitor and manage with nursing and medical interventions, the diagnosis should be rewritten as the collaborative problem *Potential Complication: Hypovolemia related to esophageal bleeding varices.*
Altered Cerebral Tissue Perfusion related to cerebral edema secondary to intracranial infections
This diagnosis represents merely a new label for encephalitis, meningitis, or abscess. Instead, the nurse should specify collaborative problems to clearly describe and designate the nursing accountability: *Potential Complication: Increased intracranial pressure* and *Potential Complication: Septicemia.* In addition, certain nursing diagnoses may be indicated, *e.g., High Risk for Infection Transmission, Altered Comfort.*
Altered Peripheral Tissue Perfusion related to deep vein thrombosis
Deep vein thrombosis is a medical diagnosis that evokes responses for which nurses are accountable: monitoring for and managing, with physician- and nurse-prescribed interventions, physiologic complications (*e.g.,* embolism, stasis ulcers). This situation would be represented by collaborative problems such as *Potential Complication: Embolism* and *Potential Complications: Stasis ulcers.* In addition, the nurse would intervene independently to prevent complications of immobility and teach how to prevent recurrence, applying nursing diagnoses such as *High Risk for Disuse Syndrome* and *High Risk for Altered Health Maintenance related to insufficient knowledge of risk factors.*

Principles and Rationale for Nursing Care

Generic Considerations

1. Cellular nutrition and respiration depend on adequate blood flow through the microcirculation.
2. Adequate cellular oxygenation depends on the following processes:
   The ability of the lungs to exchange air adequately (O_2–CO_2)
   The ability of the pulmonary alveoli to diffuse oxygen and carbon dioxide across the cell membrane to the blood
   The ability of the red blood cells (hemoglobin) to carry oxygen
   The ability of the heart to pump with enough force to deliver the blood to the microcirculation
   The ability of intact blood vessels to deliver blood to the microcirculation

3. Hypoxemia (decreased oxygen content of the blood) results in cellular hypoxia, which causes cellular swelling and contributes to tissue injury.
4. Obstruction of blood flow can be a result of
   Clot formation (thrombus)
   Embolus (air, fat, thrombi, other)
   Blood vessel injury (*e.g.,* trauma)
   Pressure upon the vessels (*e.g.,* tourniquet, edema, tumor)
   Structural changes in the vessels (*e.g.,* arteriovascular disease)
   Vasospasm
5. *Arterial* blood flow is enhanced by a *dependent* position and inhibited by an *elevated* position (gravity pulls blood downward, away from the heart).
6. *Venous* blood flow is enhanced by an *elevated* position and inhibited by a *dependent* position (gravity pulls blood downward toward the heart).
7. Immobility and venous stasis predispose one to thrombus and embolus production.
8. Tissue perfusion depends on many physiologic factors within the systems of the body and in the structures and functions of the cells. When an alteration in peripheral tissue perfusion exists, the nurse must take into account the nature of the alteration in perfusion. The two major components of the peripheral vascular system are the arterial and the venous systems. Signs, symptoms, etiology, and nursing interventions are different for problems occurring in each of these two systems and are therefore addressed separately when appropriate.

Blood Pressure

1. Blood pressure (necessary for tissue perfusion) depends on two factors: the force of the flow of blood (cardiac output) and the diameter of the blood vessel.
2. Blood pressure is affected by the sympathetic and parasympathetic nervous systems. The *sympathetic nervous system increases blood pressure* by increasing heart rate and ventricular contraction (thereby increasing cardiac output and increasing the force of blood flow) and by controlling the diameter of the arterioles and resistance of blood vessels (*i.e.,* blood vessel constriction). The *parasympathetic nervous system decreases blood pressure* by relaxation of the vessel walls and by vagal stimulation, causing a decreased heart rate (thereby decreasing cardiac output and decreasing the force of blood flow).
3. Blood pressure depends on adequate circulating blood volume (*i.e.,* dehydration predisposes one to hypotension).
4. Constricted vessels cause a rise in blood pressure, while dilated vessels cause a drop in blood pressure.
5. *Systolic blood pressure* depends on cardiac stroke volume (pressure within the vessels while the heart is contracting).
6. *Diastolic blood pressure* depends on the condition of the vessels while the heart is at rest (vessel resistance).

Gerontologic Considerations

1. Age-related vascular changes include stiffened blood vessels, which cause increased peripheral resistance, impaired baroreceptor functioning, and diminished ability to increase organ blood flow (Adelman, 1988).
2. These age-related changes cause the veins to become thicker, more dilated, and less elastic. Valves of the large leg veins become less efficient in returning blood to the heart. Age-related reduction in muscle mass and inactivity further reduces peripheral circulation (Miller, 1990).
3. Physical deconditioning or lack of exercise accentuates the functional consequences

of age-related changes in cardiovascular functioning. Factors that can contribute to deconditioning include acute illness, mobility limitations, cardiac disease, depression, and lack of motivation (Miller, 1990).

Focus Assessment Criteria

(See Tables II–21 and II–22)

Subjective Data

Symptoms
  Pain (associated with, time of day)
  Temperature change
  Pallor, cyanosis, paresthesias
  Loss of motor function
Medical history
  See Related Factors
Risk Factors
  Smoking (none, quit, number of years)
  History of phlebitis
  Immobility
  Sedentary life-style
  Family history for heart disease, peripheral vascular disease, stroke, kidney
    disease or diabetes mellitus
  Stress
Medications
  Type
  Dosage
  Presence of side-effects

Table II–21 **Arterial Insufficiency vs. Venous Insufficiency:**
A Comparison of Subjective Data

Symptom	Arterial Insufficiency	Venous Insufficiency
Pain		
Location	Feet, muscles of legs, toes	Ankles, lower legs
Quality	Burning, shocking, prickling, throbbing, cramping	Aching, tightness
Quantity	Increase in severity with increased muscle activity	Varies with fluid intake, use of support hose, and decreased muscle activity
Chronology	Brought on predictably by exercise	Greater in evening than in morning
Setting	Use of affected muscle groups	Increases during course of day with prolonged standing or sitting
Aggravating factors	Exercise Extremity elevation	Immobility Extremity dependence
Alleviating factors	Cessation of exercise Extremity dependence	Extremity elevation Compression stockings or Ace wraps
Paresthesia	Numbness, tingling, burning, decreased sensation	No change unless arterial system or nerves are affected

Table II–22 **Arterial Insufficiency vs. Venous Insufficiency:
A Comparison of Objective Data**

Sign	Arterial Insufficiency	Venous Insufficiency
Temperature	Cool skin	Warm skin
Color	Pale on elevation, dependent rubor (reactive hyperemia)	Flushed, cyanotic Typical brown discoloration around ankles
Capillary filling	>3 sec	Nonapplicable
Pulses	Absent	Present unless there is concomitant arterial disease
Movement	Decreased motor ability with nerve and muscle ischemia	Motor ability unchanged unless edema is severe enough to restrict joint mobility
Ulceration	Occurs on foot at site of trauma or at tips of toes (most distal to be perfused) Ulcers are deep with well-defined margins Surrounding tissue is shiny and taut with thin skin	Occurs around ankle (area of greatest pressure from chronic venous stasis due to valvular incompetence) Ulcers shallow with irregular edges Surrounding tissue edematous with engorged veins

     Functional ability
       Occupation
       Role activities

Objective Data
   Skin
      Temperature (cool, warm)
      Color (pale, dependent rubor, flushed, cyanotic, brown discolorations)
      Ulcerations (size, location, description of surrounding tissue)
   Bilateral pulses (radial, posterior tibial, dorsalis pedis)
      Rate, rhythm
      Volume
          0 = Absent, nonpalpable
         +1 = Thready, weak, fades in and out
         +2 = Present but diminished
         +3 = Normal, easily palpable
         +4 = Aneurysmal
   Paresthesia (numbness, tingling, burning)
   Edema (location, pitting)
   Capillary refill (normal < 3 sec)
   Motor ability (normal, compromised)
   Diagnostic studies
   Noninvasive vascular studies
      Doppler ultrasound
      Exercise stress test
   Laboratory studies
      Serum lipid profile
      Platelet profile

■ Altered Peripheral Tissue Perfusion
Related to (Specify)

Statement Example: Altered Peripheral Tissue Perfusion related to insufficient circulation for ADL secondary to Diabetes Mellitus

Assessment

Rest pain (see preceding Defining Characteristics)
Diminished or absent arterial pulses

Outcome Criteria

The individual will
- Define own peripheral vascular problem in own words
- Identify factors that improve peripheral circulation
- Identify necessary life-style changes
- Identify medical regimen, diet, medications, activities that promote vasodilation
- Identify factors that inhibit peripheral circulation
- Report decrease in pain
- Describe when to contact physician/health care professional

---

Interventions

A. Assess causative and contributing factors
1. Underlying disease
2. Inhibited arterial blood flow
3. Inhibited venous blood flow
4. Fluid volume excess or deficit
5. Hypothermia or vasoconstriction
6. Activities related to symptom/sign onset

B. Promote factors that improve arterial blood flow
1. Keep extremity in a dependent position.
2. Keep extremity warm (do not use heating pad or hot water bottle, since the individual with a peripheral vascular disease may have a disturbance in sensation and will not be able to determine if the temperature is hot enough to damage tissue; the use of external heat may also increase the metabolic demands of the tissue beyond its capacity.
3. Reduce risk for trauma.
   a. Change positions at least every hour.
   b. Avoid leg crossing.
   c. Reduce external pressure points (inspect shoes daily for rough lining).
   d. Avoid sheepskin heel protectors (they increase heel pressure and pressure across dorsum of foot).
   e. Encourage range-of-motion exercises.

    f. Plan a daily walking program.
- Instruct individual in reasons for program.
- Teach individual to avoid fatigue.
- Instruct to avoid increase in exercise until assessed by physician for cardiac problems.
- Reassure individual that walking does not harm the blood vessels or the muscles; "walking into the pain," resting and resuming walking, assists in developing collateral circulation.

    g. Discuss cessation of smoking (see *Altered Health Maintenance Related to Tobacco Use*).

C. Promote factors that improve venous blood flow

1. Elevate extremity above the level of the heart (may be contraindicated if severe cardiac or respiratory disease is present).
2. Avoid standing or sitting with legs dependent for long periods of time.
3. Consider the use of Ace bandages or below-knee elastic stockings to prevent venous stasis.
4. Reduce or removal external venous compression, which impedes venous flow.
   a. Avoid pillows behind the knees or Gatch bed, which is elevated at the knees.
   b. Avoid leg crossing.
   c. Change positions, move extremities or wiggle fingers and toes every hour.
   d. Avoid garters and tight elastic stockings above the knees.
5. Measure baseline circumference of calves and thighs if individual is at risk for deep venous thrombosis, or if it is suspected.

D. Initiate health teaching as indicated

1. Teach to:
   a. Avoid long car or plane rides (get up and walk around at least every hour).
   b. Keep dry skin lubricated (cracked skin eliminates the physical barrier to infection).
   c. Wear warm clothing during cold weather.
   d. Wear cotton or wool socks.
   e. Use gloves or mittens if hands are exposed to cold (including home freezers).
   f. Avoid dehydration in warm weather.
   g. Give special attention to feet and toes.
   - Wash feet and dry well daily.
   - Do not soak feet.
   - Avoid harsh soaps or chemicals (including iodine) on feet.
   - Keep nails trimmed and filed smooth.
   h. Inspect feet and legs daily for injuries and pressure points.
   i. Wear clean socks.
   j. Wear shoes that offer support and fit comfortably.
   k. Inspect the inside of shoes daily for rough lining.
2. Teach risk factor modification.
   a. Diet
   - Avoid foods high in cholesterol.
   - Modify sodium intake to control hypertension.
   - Refer to dietitian.
   b. Relaxation techniques to reduce effects of stress
   c. Smoking cessation (see *Altered Health Maintenance Related to Tobacco Use*)
   d. Exercise program

3. Teach methods to relieve pain.
   a. Dependent position for ischemic pain
   b. Elevate extremities for relief of venous aching.
   c. Phantom pain after an amputation may be relieved by massaging or tapping stump or opposite limb.
   d. Use other nursing measures such as relaxation or distraction to assist in pain relief.
   e. If pain is not relieved by above methods, refer to a physician.
   f. Teach symptoms/signs of underlying disease and when to call the physician or health care professional.

References/Bibliography

Adelman, B. (1988). Peripheral vascular disease. In Rowe, J.W., & Besdive, R.W. (Eds.). *Geriatric medicine.* Boston: Little, Brown.

Appleton, D. L., & Laquaglia, J. D. (1985). Vascular disease and postoperative nursing management. *Critical Care Nurse 5,* 34.

Barnes, R. W. (1981). Managing peripheral vascular disease. *Journal of Cardiovascular Medicine, 6*(1), 33–40.

Bates, B. (1980). *A guide to physical examination.* Philadelphia: J. B. Lippincott.

Clochesy, J. M. (1984). Profound hypothermia. *Focus Critical Care, 11,* 19.

Craven, R. & Curry, T. (1981). When the diagnosis is Raynauds. *American Journal of Nursing, 81,* 1097.

Dennison, R. (1986). Cardiopulmonary assessment. *Nursing 86, 60,* 34.

Doyle, J. E. (1983). All leg ulcers are not alike: Managing and preventing arterial and venous ulcers. *Nursing, 13*(1), 58–62.

Doyle, J. E. (1981). If your legs hurt the reason may be arterial insufficiency. *Nursing, 4*(4), 74–79.

Fahey, V. (1988). *Vascular nursing.* Philadelphia: W. B. Saunders.

Goetter, W. (1986). Nursing diagnosis and interventions with the acute stroke patient. *Nursing Clinics of North America, 21,* 309.

Guyton AC: (1986). *Textbook of medical physiology* (6th ed.). Philadelphia: W. B. Saunders.

Herman, S. A. (1986). Nursing assessment and nursing diagnosis in patients with peripheral vascular disease. *Nursing Clinics of North America, 21,* 219.

Kim, M.J. McFarland, G.K. & McLane, A.M. (1987). *Pocket guide to nursing diagnoses* (2nd ed.). St. Louis: C. V. Mosby.

Luckenbaugh, P. R. (1983). An overview of nursing diagnosis and suggestions for use with chronic hemodialysis patients. *Nephrology Nurse, 5,* 58.

Luckmann, J. & Sorensen, K. C. (1987). *Medical-surgical nursing: A psychophysiologic approach* (3rd ed.). Philadelphia: W. B. Saunders.

Miller, C. A. (1990). *Nursing care of older adults.* Glenview, IL: Scott, Foresman.

Miller, K. A. (1978). Assessing peripheral perfusion. *American Journal of Nursing, 8*(10), 1673–1674.

Ng, L., & Warren, J. L. (1986). A critical care approach to the implementation of the standards of cardiovascular nursing practice. *Cardiovascular Nursing, 22,* 13.

Peterson, F. Y. (1983). Assessing peripheral vascular disease at the bedside. *American Journal of Nursing, 83,* 1549.

Scandrett, S., & Becker, S. (1986). Relaxation training. In Bulechek, G., & McCloskey, J. C. (Eds.). *Nursing interventions: Treatments for nursing diagnoses.* Philadelphia: W. B. Saunders.

Shpritz, D. W. (1983). Craniocerebral trauma. *Critical Care Nurse, 3,* 49.

Sieggreen, M. (1989). Nursing management of adults with arterial disorders, Nursing management of adults with venous and lymphatic disorders. In Beare, P., & Myers, J. *Principles and practice of adult health nursing.* St. Louis: C. V. Mosby.

Snow, C. J. & Carter, S. A. (1984). Is exercise therapy beneficial in intermittent claudication? *Vascular Diagnostics and Therapy, 5*(1), 20–25.

Thorn, G. W., Braunwald, J. E., Purrillo, J. E., Myerburg, R. J., & Castellanos, A. (1991). *Harrison's principles of internal medicine* (12th ed.). New York: McGraw-Hill

Turner, J. (1986). Nursing intervention in patients with peripheral vascular disease. *Nursing Clinics of North America, 21,* 233.

Ventura, M. R. Young, D., Feldman, M. J., et al. (1984). Effectiveness of health promoting interventions. *Nursing Research, 33*(3), 62–167.

Wagner, M. M. (1986). Pathophysiology related to peripheral vascular disease. *Nursing Clinics of North America, 21,* 195.

Warbinek, E., & Wyness, M. A. (1986). Designing nursing care for patients with peripheral arterial occlusive disease. Part 1: Update. *Cardiovascular Nursing, 22,* 1.

Warbinek, E., & Wyness, M.A. (1986). Peripheral arterial occlusive disease. Part 2: Nursing assessment and standard care plans. *Cardiovascular Nursing, 22,* 6.

West, C. M. (1986). Ischemia. In Carrieri, V. K., Lindsey, A.M., & West, C.M. (Eds.). *Pathophysiological phenomena in nursing: Human responses to illness.* Philadelphia: W. B. Saunders.

Unilateral Neglect

■ *Related to* **(Specify)**

DEFINITION

Unilateral Neglect: The state in which an individual is unable to attend to or "ignores" the hemiplegic side of the body and/or objects, persons, or sounds on the affected side of the environment.

DEFINING CHARACTERISTICS

Major (must be present)

Neglect of involved body parts and/or extrapersonal space (hemispatial neglect)
Denial of the existence of the affected limb or side of body (anosognosia)
Right parietal lobe lesion

Minor (may be present)

Left-sided hemiplegia, hemiparesis, and/or hemianesthesia
Left homonymous hemianopsia
Difficulty with spatial-perceptual tasks

RELATED FACTORS

Pathophysiologic

Neurologic disease/damage
Cerebrovascular accident (CVA)
Brain injury/trauma
Cerebral aneurysms

Diagnostic Considerations

Unilateral Neglect represents a disturbance in the reciprocal loop occurring most often in the right hemisphere of the brain. This diagnosis also could be viewed as a syndrome diagnosis, *Unilateral Neglect Syndrome.* As mentioned in Chapter 3, syndrome diagnoses encompass a cluster of nursing diagnoses related to the situation. The nursing interventions for *Unilateral Neglect Syndrome* would focus on *Self-Care Deficit, Anxiety,* and *High Risk for Injury.*

Errors in Diagnostic Statements

Unilateral Neglect related to lack of grooming and hygiene for right side of face, head, and right arm

Lack of grooming on one side of the body can be an indicator of *Unilateral Neglect* if neurologic disease or damage is present; it is not a related factor. When writing the diagnostic statement, the nurse should ask herself or himself "How does the nurse treat unilateral neglect?" Because the nursing focus is on teaching adaptive techniques, phasing the diagnosis *Unilateral Neglect related to lack of knowledge of adaptive techniques* would be appropriate. If *Unilateral Neglect* was viewed as a syndrome diagnosis, the appropriate diagnostic statement would be *Unilateral Neglect Syndrome*. No "related to" is needed with a syndrome diagnosis because the label includes the etiology. The interventions would have the same focus, reducing neglect by using adaptive techniques.

Focus Assessment Criteria

Subjective Data

The person does not verbalize or perceive a problem, but if asked will give an excuse such as:
"There is someone else in this bed."
"This arm does not belong to me."
"This arm is dead."
The person gives the affected limb a pet name.
The person will confabulate a reason for not walking or using the affected extremity.

Objective Data

1. Assess for presence of related factors
    Determine the extent of neurologic involvement
    Determine the person's dominance (handedness)
2. Assess for the presence of factors that complicate the neglect syndrome
    Sensory loss of involved body parts
    Allesthesia: Perception of stimuli delivered to the affected extremity (contra-lateral [opposite] to the lesion) as having been delivered to the unaffected side (ipsilateral [same side]) as the lesion (Booth, 1982)
    Hemiakinesia: Failure to move the affected extremity in the absence of, or out of proportion to, motor dysfunction (Booth, 1982)
    Apraxia: Inability to conceptualize, plan and execute skilled or nonhabitual motor patterns despite adequate muscle power, sensation, and coordination (Wyness, 1985)
    Visual field deficit (homonymous hemianopsia)
    Gaze preference away from the affected extremity
    Extinction to double simulataneous stimulation: The person will acknowledge only the stimulus delivered to the unaffected side (Booth, 1982)
    Impulsiveness
    Short attention span
    Lack of insight into extent of disability
    Diminished learning skills
    Overestimation of abilities
    Inability to recognize faces
    Concrete thinking (inability to abstract)
    Body schema changes
    Confusion
3. Assess the effect of the neglect on the person's ability to safely care for self in the environment
    Activities of daily living (ADLs)
        Bathing, grooming and hygiene
            Does the person:
                Wash the affected side of his body?

Shave both sides of his face?

Brush all his teeth?

Put dentures in straight?

Comb only part of his hair?

Apply makeup to both sides of face?

Put eyeglasses on straight?

Feeding

Does the person:

Pocket food on the affected side of his mouth?

Eat only half of his food (*e.g.*, eat only food on the unaffected side of plate/ tray?)

Dressing

Does the person:

Dress the affected limb(s)?

Mobility/positioning

When sitting in a wheelchair, does the person lean or tilt toward the un- affected side?

Does the affected arm dangle off the lapboard?

Are the head and eyes turned toward the unaffected side?

When propelling the wheelchair or when ambulating, does the person bump or run into objects on affected side?

Safety

Does the person

Attempt to walk or transfer out of the chair or bed when unable to ambulate?

Have sensation in the affected limb(s)?

Frequently injure the affected arm or hand (cuts, bumps, bruises)

Feel pain when injured?

Aware of when injury occurs?

Scan the entire visual field?

Turn head to the affected side to compensate?

Respond to stimuli presented from the affected side?

Does the affected arm dangle at the side and get caught in the wheelchair spokes, side rails, doorways, etc.?

Principles and Rationale for Nursing Care

Generic Considerations

1. Unilateral neglect is also called hemi-inattention, unilateral asomatognosia (uni- lateral spatial agnosia, Anton-Babinski syndrome), anosognosia and autopagnosia.
2. The most common cause of unilateral neglect is right hemispheric brain damage; specifically, lesions in the right parietal lobe cause this defect much more frequently than lesions in the left lobe (Heilman & Valenstein, 1972).
3. The neglect phenomena has been demonstrated with unilateral lesions in an area identified as the reciprocol loop (the cortico-limbic-reticular loop). Heilman and Van Den Abell (1980) postulated that any lesion that disrupts this system produces neglect, and that this neglect is a manifestation of a deficit in the orienting response, which is thought to be related to the reticular activiating system.
4. The right parietal lobe attends to stimuli presented to both the right and left sides; in a lesion of the left parietal lobe, the right parietal lobe could continue attending to the ipsilateral (same side) or (right-sided) stimuli. However, because the left parietal lobe

cannot attend to ipsilateral stimuli as well as the right parietal lobe can, lesions of the right parietal lobe more likely will induce a profound contralateral sensory inattention than lesions of the left parietal lobe (Heilman & Van Den Abell, 1980).

5. Severe and persistent neglect of the left hemisphere generally occurs after combined injury to frontal, parietal, and deep structures (Hier, Mondlock, & Caplan, 1983).

6. Unilateral neglect is characterized by an unawareness or denial of the affected half of the body, often extending to the extrapersonal space.

7. The extent of sensory loss does not correlate with the severity of neglect (Mitchell, Hodges, Muwaswes, & Walleck, 1988).

8. Homonymous hemianopsia (loss of vision on the contralateral side) usually occurs with unilateral neglect. But unilateral neglect and hemianopsia are two separate phenomena, and either can be present without the other. When they occur together, the person has more difficulty compensating for the loss.

9. Anosognosia (ignorance of paralysis) and dressing apraxia may occur in lesions of either hemisphere but have been observed more frequently in lesions of the nondominant hemisphere.

10. The person with a parietal lobe injury will demonstrate problems with body schema, spatial judgment, and sensory interpretation.

11. Additionally, the person with this type of brain injury may exhibit some or all of the following characteristics that complicate the neglect syndrome:
    a. Impulsiveness
    b. Short attention span
    c. Lack of insight into the extent of the disability
    d. Diminished learning skills
    e. Inability to recognize faces
    f. Decrease in concrete thinking
    g. Confusion

12. Prognosis for recovery from many of the behavioral abnormalities associated with right hemisphere stroke is more favorable after hemorrhage as opposed to after infarction (Hier, Mondlock, & Caplan, 1983).

13. Early recognition of the existence and extent of these syndromes allows more accurate planning of goals.

Pediatric Considerations

1. Children at greatest risk for developing unilateral neglect are those with acquired hemiplegia; *e.g.,* from stroke. Strokes may occur in children with congenital heart disease, sickle cell anemia, meningitis, or head trauma (Painter & Bergman, 1990).

Geriatric Considerations

1. Most persons who experience unilateral neglect are elderly, simply because the incidence of stroke is greatest in the elderly population.

■ Unilateral Neglect
Related to (Specify)

Outcome Criteria

The person will
- Demonstrate an ability to scan the visual field to compensate for loss of function/sensation in affected limb(s)
- Identify safety hazards in the environment
- Describe the deficit and the rationale for treatment

Interventions

A. Assist the person to recognize the perceptual deficit

1. Initially adapt the environment to the deficit:
   a. Position person, call light, bedside stand, television, telephone and personal items on the unaffected side.
   b. Position bed with unaffected side toward the door.
   c. Approach and speak to person from his uninvolved side.
   d. If you must approach person from affected side, announce your presence as soon as you enter the room to avoid startling the person.
   e. When working with the person's affected extremity, position the unaffected side near a wall to minimize distractions.
2. Gradually change the person's environment as you teach him to compensate and learn to recognize the forgotten field; move furniture and personal items out of the visual field.
3. Keep the room well-lighted and free of clutter.
4. Provide a full-length mirror to help with vertical orientation and to diminish the distortion of the vertical and horizontal plane, which manifests itself in the patient leaning toward the affected side.
5. Use verbal instructions rather than mere demonstrations. Keep instructions simple.
6. For a person in a wheelchair, obtain a lapboard (preferably Plexiglass); position the affected arm on the lapboard with the fingertips at midline. Encourage person to look for the arm on the board.
7. For an ambulatory person, obtain an arm sling to prevent the arm from dangling and causing shoulder subluxation.
8. When the person is in bed, elevate affected arm on a pillow to prevent dependent edema.
9. Constantly cue the person to the environment.

B. Assist the person with adaptations needed for self-care and other activities of daily living (ADLs)

1. Encourage to wear prescribed corrective lenses or hearing aids.
2. For bathing, dressing, and toileting
   a. Instruct to attend to affected extremity/side first when performing ADLs.

    b. Instruct client to always look for affected extremity when performing ADL, to know where it is at all times.

    c. Teach to perform dressing and grooming tasks in front of a mirror.

    d. Suggest color-coded markers sewn or placed inside shoes or clothes to help distinguish right from left.

    e. Encourage client to integrate affected extremity during bathing and to feel extremity by rubbing and massaging it.

    f. Utilize adaptive equipment as appropriate.

    g. Refer to *Self-Care Deficit* for additional interventions.

3. For feeding

    a. Set up meals with a minimum of dishes, food, and utensils.

    b. Instruct client to eat in small amounts and place food on unaffected side of mouth.

    c. Instruct client to use tongue to sweep out "pockets" of food from affected side after every bite.

    d. After meals/medications, check oral cavity for pocketed food/medication.

    e. Provide oral care tid and PRN.

    f. Initially place food in the person's visual field; gradually move food out of field and teach person to scan entire visual field.

    g. Utilize adaptive feeding equipment as appropriate

    h. Refer to *Self-Care Deficit: Feeding* for additional interventions

    l. Refer to *Altered Nutrition: Less Than Body Requirements related to swallowing difficulties* if person has difficulty in chewing and swallowing food.

C. Teach measures to prevent injury

1. Retrain person to scan his entire environment:

    a. Instruct to turn head past midline to view scene on the affected side.

    b. Perform activities that require turning the head.

    c. Remind client to scan when ambulating or propelling a wheelchair.

2. Use tactile sensation to reintroduce affected arm/extremity to the person.

    a. Have person stroke involved side with uninvolved hand and watch the arm or leg while stroking it.

    b. Rub different-textured materials to stimulate sensations (hot, cold, rough, soft).

3. Instruct the person to keep the affected arm and/or leg in view.

    a. Position arm on lapboard. (Plexiglass lapboards allow person to view affected leg and thereby, help to integrate the leg into the body schema.)

    b. Provide an arm sling for an ambulatory person.

    c. Instruct client to take extra care around sources of heat or cold, moving machinery or parts to protect affected side from injury.

D. Initiate health teaching and referrals

1. Assess to ensure that both person and family understand the purpose and rationale of all interventions.

2. Proceed with teaching as needed.

    a. Explain denial and its course (See Principles and Rationale for Nursing Care).

    b. Instruct family on how to facilitate the person's relearning techniques, *e.g.*, cueing, scanning visual field.

    c. Teach use of adaptive equipment, if appropriate.

    d. Teach principles of maintaining a safe environment.

References/Bibliography

Adams, R. D., & Victor, M. (1981). *Principles of neurology.* New York: McGraw-Hill.

Anderson, M. D., & Choy, E. (1970). Parietal lobe syndromes in hemiplegia. *The American Journal of Occupational Therapy, 24*(1), 13–18.

Booth, K. (1982). The neglect syndrome. *Journal of Neurosurgical Nursing, 14,* 38–43.

Burt, M. M. (1970). Perceptual deficits in hemiplegia. *American Journal of Nursing, 70,* 1026–1029.

Heilman, K. M., & Van Den Abell, T. (1980). Right hemisphere dominance for attention: The mechanism underlying hemispheric asymmetries of inattention (neglect). *Neurology, 30,* 327–330.

Heilman, K. M., & Valenstein, E. (1972). Frontal lobe neglect in man. *Neurology, 22,* 660–664.

Hier, D., Mondlock B., & Caplan, L. (1983). Behavioral abnormalities after right hemisphere stroke. *Neurology, 33,* 337–344.

Hier, D., Mondlock, B., & Caplan, L. (1983). Recovery of behavioral abnormalities after right hemisphere stroke. *Neurology, 33,* 345–350.

Hickey, J. V. (1986). *The clinical practice of neurologic and neurosurgical nursing* (2nd ed.). Philadelphia: J. B. Lippincott.

Hopkins, H. L., & Smith H. D. (1983). *Willard and Spackman's occupational therapy* (6th ed.). Philadelphia: J. B. Lippincott.

Licht, S. (1975). *Stroke and its rehabilitation.* Baltimore: Waverly Press.

Martin, N., Holt, N. B., & Hicks, D. (1981). *Comprehensive rehabilitation nursing.* New York: McGraw-Hill.

Mitchell, P. H., Hodges, L. C., Muwaswes, M., & Walleck, C. A. (1988). *AANN's neuroscience nursing.* Norwalk, CT: Appleton & Lange.

Mumma, C., (Ed.). (1987). *Rehabilitation nursing. Concepts and practice, a core curriculum* (2nd ed.) Evanston, IL: Rehabilitation Nursing Foundation.

Painter, M. J., & Bergman, I. (1990). Neurology. In Behrman, R. E., & Kliegman, R. (Eds.). *Nelson's essentials of pediatrics.* Philadelphia: W. B. Saunders.

Taylor J. W., & Ballenger, S. (1980). *Neurological dysfunctions and nursing interventions.* New York: McGraw-Hill.

Trombly, C. A. (1983). *Occupational therapy for physical dysfunction* (2nd ed.). London: Williams & Wilkins.

Wahburn, K. B. (1981). *Physical medicine and rehabilitation: Essentials of primary care.* Garden City, NY: Medical Examination Publishing.

Weinberg, J., Diller, L., Gordon, W., Gerstman, L., Lieberman, A., Lakin, P., Hodges G., & Erachi, O. (1979). Training sensory awareness and spatial organization in people with right brain damage, *Archives of Physical Rehabilitation, 60*(8), 491–496.

Wyness, M. A. (1985). Perceptual dysfunction: Nursing assessment and management. *Journal of Neuroscience Nursing, 17,* 105–110.

Urinary Elimination, Altered Patterns of

Maturational Enuresis*

Functional Incontinence

Reflex Incontinence

Stress Incontinence

Total Incontinence

Urge Incontinence

Urinary Retention

Urinary Elimination, Altered Patterns of

DEFINITION

Altered Patterns of Urinary Elimination: The state in which the individual experiences or is at risk of experiencing urinary elimination dysfunction.

DEFINING CHARACTERISTICS

Major (must be present)

Reports or experiences a urinary elimination problem

Urgency	Dribbling
Frequency	Bladder distention
Hesitancy	Incontinence
Nocturia	Large residual urine volumes
Enuresis	

*This diagnosis is not currently on the NANDA list but has been included for clarity and usefulness.

RELATED FACTORS

Pathophysiologic

Congenital urinary tract anomalies

    Strictures   Bladder neck contractures

    Hypospadias   Megalocystis (large capacity

    Epispadias   bladder without tone)

    Ureterocele

Disorders of the urinary tract

    Infection   Urethritis

    Trauma

Neurogenic disorders or injury

    Cord injury/tumor/infection   Diabetic neuropathy

    Brain injury/tumor/infection   Alcoholic neuropathy

    Cerebrovascular   Tabes dorsalis

    Demyelinating diseases   Parkinsonism

    Multiple sclerosis

Prostatic enlargement

Estrogen deficiency

    Atrophic vaginitis   Atrophic urethritis

Herpes zoster

Treatment-related

Surgical

    Postprostatectomy   Extensive pelvic dissection

Diagnostic instrumentation

General or spinal anesthesia

Drug therapy (iatrogenic)

    Antihistamines   Immunosuppressant therapy

    Epinephrine   Diuretics

    Anticholinergics   Tranquilizers

    Sedatives   Muscle relaxants

Postindwelling catheters

Situational (personal, environmental)

Loss of perineal tissue tone

    Obesity   Childbirth

    Aging

    Recent substantial weight loss

Irritation to perineal area

    Sexual activity   Poor personal hygiene

Pregnancy

Inability to communicate needs

Fecal impaction

Dehydration

Stress or fear

Decreased attention to bladder cues

    Depression   Confusion

    Intentional suppression (self-induced deconditioning)

Environmental barriers to bathroom

    Distant toilets   Bed too high

Poor lighting   Side rails
Unfamiliar surroundings
Impaired mobility

Maturational

Child: Small bladder capacity, lack of motivation
Elderly: Sensory losses, loss of muscle tone, inability to communicate needs, depression, mobility problems, dehydration

Diagnostic Considerations

Altered Patterns of Urinary Elimination probably is too broad a diagnosis for effective clinical use. For this reason, the nurse should use a more specific diagnosis, such as *Stress Incontinence*, whenever possible. When the etiologic or contributing factors for incontinence have not been identified, the nurse could temporarily write a diagnosis of *Altered Patterns of Urinary Elimination related to unknown etiology as evidenced by incontinence.*

The nurse performs a focus assessment to determine whether the incontinence is transient in response to an acute condition (*e.g.,* infection, medication side-effects) or established in response to various chronic neural or genitourinary conditions (Miller, 1990). In addition, the nurse should differentiate the type of incontinence: functional, reflex, stress, urge, or total. The diagnosis *Total Incontinence* should not be used unless all other types of incontinence have been ruled out.

Errors in Diagnostic Statements

Altered Patterns of Urinary Elimination related to surgical diversion

This diagnosis represents a new label for urostomy, and does not focus on the nursing accountability. A person with a urostomy should be assessed for its effect on functional patterns and on physiologic functioning. For this person, the collaborative problems *Potential Complication: Stomal obstruction,* and *Potential Complication: Internal urine leakage,* as well as nursing diagnoses such as *High Risk for Body Image Disturbance* and *High Risk for Altered Health Maintenance,* could be applicable.

Altered Patterns of Urinary Elimination related to renal failure

This diagnosis renames renal failure and is inappropriate as a nursing diagnosis. For this reason, the diagnosis *Fluid Volume Excess related to acute renal failure* also would be incorrect. Renal failure will cause or contribute to various actual or potential nursing diagnoses, such as *High Risk for Infection* and *High Risk for Altered Nutrition,* and collaborative problems, such as *Potential Complication: Fluid/electrolyte imbalances* and *Potential Complication: Metabolic acidosis.*

Total Incontinence related to effects of aging

The physiologic effects of aging on the urinary tract system can negatively influence functioning when other risk factors also are present, *e.g.,* mobility problems, dehydration, side-effects of medications, decreased awareness of bladder cues. This nursing diagnosis projects a biased view of anticipated incontinence in an elderly person, with associated use of indwelling catheters, diapers, and/or bed pads. When this equipment is used, the nurse is not treating incontinence but rather managing urine. The use of such equipment is a short-term solution. For these situations, *High Risk for Infection* and *High Risk for Impaired Skin Integrity* would apply. When an elderly person has an incontinent episode, the nurse should proceed cautiously before applying the nursing diagnosis label of "incontinence." If factors exist that increase the likelihood of recurrence and the client is motivated, the diagnosis *High Risk for Functional/Urge Incontinence related to* (specify—*e.g.,* dehydration, mobility difficulties, decreased bladder capacity) could apply. This diagnosis would focus nursing interventions on preventing incontinence rather than to expect it as inevitable. For an elderly person with the combination of functional and urge incontinence, the nurse would focus on assisting the person to increase bladder capacity and reduce barriers to bathrooms, using the diagnosis *Functional/Urge Incontinence related to age-related effects on bladder capacity, self-induced fluid limitations, and unstable gait.*

Focus Assessment Criteria

Many adults are uncomfortable discussing urinary elimination and/or may deny incontinence. To aid communication during assessment, the nurse should use understandable, nonembarrassing terms (*e.g.,* "Do you have difficulty going to the bathroom?").

Subjective Data

1. History of symptoms
   Complaints of
Lack of control	Frequency
Dribbling	Pain or discomfort
Hesitancy	Burning
Urgency	Change in voiding pattern

   Onset and duration
   Description
   Frequency
   Precipitated by what?
   Relieved by what?
   Aggravated by what?
   Restrictions on life-style
Social	Sexual
Occupational	Role responsibilities

2. Incontinence (adult)
   History of continence
      Is degree of continence acceptable?
      Age of attainment of continence?
      Previous history of enuresis?
      History of "weak" bladder?
      Family history of incontinence?
   Onset and duration (day, night, just certain times)
   Factors that increase incidence (Ruff & Reaves, 1989):
      Coughing
      Laughing
      Standing
      Turning in bed
      Delay in getting to bathroom
      When excited
      Leaving bathroom
   Perception of need to void
Present	Absent
Diminished	

   Ability to delay urination after urge
Present (how long)?	Absent

Sensations occurring before or during micturition
    Difficulty starting stream
    Difficulty stopping stream
    Painful straining (tenesmus)
    Need to force urine out
    Lack of sensation to void
Relief after voiding
    Complete
    Continued desire to void after bladder is emptied
Use of catheters, diapers, bed pads

3. Presence of risk factors
    Physiologic
        Dehydration (self-imposed, overuse of diuretics, caffeine, alcohol)
        Prostatic hypertrophy
        Bladder, vaginal infections
        Chronic illnesses (*e.g.,* diabetes, alcoholism, Parkinson's disease, Alzheimer's disease, multiple sclerosis, cerebrovascular accident, vitamin B_{12} deficiency)
        Metabolic disturbances (*e.g.,* hypokalemia, hypercalcemia)
        Fecal impaction/severe constipation
        Certain medications (diuretics, anticholinergics, antihistamines, sedatives, acetaminophen, amitriptyline, aspirin, barbiturates, chlorpropamide, clofibrate, fluphenazine, haloperidol, narcotics)
        Multiple or difficult deliveries
        Pelvic, bladder, or uterine surgery, disorders
    Functional ability
        Perception of bladder cues
        Walking, balance, manual dexterity
        Ability to reach toilet in time
    Environmental barriers
        Location of bathroom within 40 feet
        Stairs, narrow doorways
        Dim lighting
        Ability to locate bathroom in social settings

4. Enuresis (child)
    Onset and pattern (day, night)
    Toilet training history
    Family history of bed-wetting
    Response of others to child (parents, siblings, peers)

Objective Data

1. Urination stream
    Slow   Sprays
    Small   Starts and stops
    Drops   Slow or hard to start
    Dribble
2. Urine
    Color
        Yellow   Yellow brown
        Amber   Green brown
        Straw colored   Dark brown
        Red brown   Black

Odor

    Faint   Offensive

    Ammoniac   Acetonic

Appearance

    Clear   Cloudy

Reaction (normal, 4.6–7.5, or alkaline, >7.5)

Specific gravity

    Dilute (<1.003)

    Concentrated (>1.025)

    Normal (1.003–1.025)

Negative or positive for

    Glucose   Bacteria

    Protein   Red blood cells

    Ketone

3. Voiding and fluid intake patterns (record for 2–4 days to establish a baseline)

    What is daily fluid intake?

    When does incontinence occur?

4. Muscle tone

    Abdomen firm, or soft and pendulous?

    History of recent significant weight loss or gain?

5. Reflexes

    Presence or absence of cauda equina reflexes

        Anal   Bulbocavernosus

6. Bladder

    Distention (palpable)

    Can it be emptied by external stimuli? (Credé's method, gentle suprapubic tapping or warm water over the perineum, Valsalva, pulling of pubic hair, anal stretch)

    Capacity (at least 300–350 mL)

7. Residual urine

    None   Present in what amount?

8. Functional ability

    Get in/out of chair

    Walk alone to bathroom

    Maintain balance

    Manipulate clothing

9. Cognitive ability

    Asks to go to bathroom

    Initiates toileting with reminders

    Aware of incontinence

    Expects to be incontinent

10. Assess for presence of

    Constipation   Depression

    Fecal impaction   Mobility disorders

    Dehydration   Sensory disorders

11. Diagnostic studies

    Urinalysis; culture and sensitivity

    Blood (creatinine, urea nitrogen)

    Roentgenograms (intravenous pyelogram, kidney, ureters, bladder), cystometrogram

    Electromyography of the muscles of the external urinary sphincter and muscles of the pelvic floor

Principles and Rationale for Nursing Care

Generic Considerations

1. The three components of the lower urinary tract that assist to maintain continence are (Plymat & Turner, 1988)
   a. Detrusor muscle in the bladder wall, which allows bladder expansion to increase volume of urine
   b. Internal sphincter or proximal urethra which, when contracted, prevents urine leakage
   c. External sphincter, which by voluntary control provides added support during stressed situations (e.g., overdistended bladder)
2. Innervation of the bladder arises from the spinal cord at the sacral levels of 2,3, and 4. The bladder is under parasympathetic control. Voluntary control over urination is influenced by the cortex, midbrain, and medulla.
3. The female urethra is 3 cm to 5 cm long. The male urethra is approximately 20 cm long. Continence is maintained primarily by the urethra, but the cerebral cortex is the principal area for suppression of the desire to micturate.
4. Capacity of the normal bladder (without experiencing discomfort) is 250 mL to 400 mL. The desire to void occurs when there is 150 mL to 250 mL of urine in the bladder.
5. The sitting position for the female and the standing position for the male allow for optimal relaxation of the external urinary sphincter and perineal muscles.
6. Bladder tissue tone can be lost if the bladder is distended to 1000 mL (atonic bladder) or continuously drained (Foley catheter).
7. Mechanisms to stimulate the voiding reflex or Credé's method may be ineffective if the bladder capacity is less than 200 mL.
8. Alcohol, coffee, and tea have a natural diuretic effect and are bladder irritants.
9. Injury to the spinal cord above sacral 2,3,4 produces a spastic or reflex bladder tone. Injury to the spinal cord below sacral 2,3,4 produces a flaccid or atonic bladder.
10. Lesions affecting inhibitory centers in the brain or the pathways transmitting inhibitory impulses to the bladder result in an uninhibited bladder.

Infection

1. Stasis or pooling of urine contributes to bacterial growth. Bacteria can travel up the ureters to the kidney (ascending infection).
2. Recurrent bladder infections cause fibrotic changes in the bladder wall with resultant decrease in bladder capacity.
3. Urinary stasis, infections, alkaline urine, and decreased urine volume contribute to the formation of urinary tract calculi.
4. Dilute acid urine helps prevent infection and allows for solubility of inorganic materials.

Incontinence

1. Incontinence is transient in as many as 50% of individuals presenting with the problem, and of the remaining group, about two-thirds can be cured or markedly improved with treatment (Resnick & Yalla, 1985). There are many effective corrective measures for the management of urinary tract pathology in the elderly, and a positive approach should be taken to minimize the incidence of urinary incontinence.
2. The daily cost of caring for incontinence in nursing homes nationwide is $2.9 million. An estimated one-half of the 1.4 million home residents receiving Medicaid benefits are incontinent (Cella, 1988).
3. Incontinence can be transient or reversible. Causes of transient incontinence are

acute confusion, urinary tract infection, atrophic vaginitis, side-effects of medication, metabolic imbalance, impaction, and mobility problems (Wyman, 1988).

4. It is important to determine the natural history of the incontinence pattern. A new onset of incontinence is likely to be due to an external precipitating factor outside of the urinary tract (such as medications, acute illness, inaccessible toilets, impaired mobility preventing getting to the toilet on time, etc.) which can often be easily corrected. Incontinence can be either transient (reversible) or established (controllable). Controllable incontinence cannot be cured, but urine removal can be planned.

5. Continence training programs are either self-directed or caregiver-directed. Self-directed programs of bladder training, retraining, exercises are for motivated cognitively intact individuals. Caregiver-directed programs of scheduled toileting or habit training are appropriate for motivated caregivers of cognitively impaired persons (Miller, 1990).

6. The essential components of any continence training program (self-directed or caregiver-directed) include motivation, assessment of voiding and incontinent patterns, a regular fluid intake of 2000 to 3000 mL/day, timed voiding of 2- to 4-hour intervals in an appropriate place, and ongoing assessment (Miller, 1990).

7. Certain medications are associated with incontinence. Narcotics and sedatives diminish awareness of bladder cues. Adrenergic agents cause retention by increasing bladder outlet resistance. Anticholinergics (antidepressants, some antiparkinsonian medications, antispasmodics, antihistamines, antiarrhythmics, opiates) cause chronic retention with overflow. Diuretics rapidly increase urine volume and can cause incontinence if voiding cannot be delayed (Miller, 1990; Wyman, 1988).

8. Obstruction of the bladder neck that progresses to bladder distention and overflow (incontinence) can be caused by fecal impaction and enlarged prostate gland.

9. Persons with diabetes mellitus, which can contribute to increased residual urine, frequency, and urgency, may be less aware of bladder fullness.

10. Dehydration can cause incontinence by eliminating the sensation of a full bladder (the signal to urinate) and also by reducing the person's alertness to the sensation.

11. Social isolation of incontinent persons can be self-imposed because of fear and embarrassment or imposed by others because of odor and esthetics.

12. Depression can prevent the person from recognizing or responding to bladder cues and thus contributes to incontinence.

Intermittent Catheterization

1. Intermittent self-catheterization, periodic drainage of urine by the individual by the use of a catheter in the bladder, is indicated when a neurologic impairment impairs bladder emptying.

2. This method maintains the tonicity of the bladder muscle, prevents overdistention, and provides for complete emptying of the bladder.

3. Intermittent catheterization, when performed in a health care facility, should follow aseptic technique because the organisms present in such a facility are more virulent and resistent to drugs than organisms found outside. Persons at home can practice clean technique because of the lack of virulent organisms in the home environment.

4. The initial removal of more than 500 mL of urine from a chronically distended bladder can cause severe hemorrhage, which results when bladder veins, previously compressed by the distended bladder, rapidly dilate and rupture when bladder pressure is abruptly released. (After the initial release of 500 mL of urine, alternate the release of 100 mL of urine with 15-min catheter clamps).

5. An overdistended bladder reduces blood flow to the bladder wall, making it more susceptible to infection from bacterial growth.

6. The accumulation of more than 500 mL to 700 mL of urine in a bladder should not be permitted.
7. Intermittent catheterization provides for a decrease in morbidity associated with long-term use of indwelling catheters, increased independence, a more positive self-concept, and more normal sexual relations.

Urinary Retention

1. Urinary retention can be caused by three different entities: bladder outlet obstruction, detrusor inadequacy, and impaired afferent pathways.
2. Bladder outlet obstruction is commonly caused by impacted stool or an enlarged prostate. The impacted stool or enlarged prostate will compress the urethra so that urine is retained until the bladder distends, causing overflow incontinence.
3. Detrusor inadequacy is characterized by the pressure of uninhibited detrusor contractions sufficient to cause urinary incontinence. One cause of detrusor inadequacy is deconditioned voiding reflexes characterized by anxiety or discomfort associated with voiding. Another cause is central nervous system diseases.
4. Impaired afferent pathways occur when both the sensory and motor branches of the simple reflex arc are damaged. Therefore, there are no sensations to tell the individual the bladder is full or no motor impulses for emptying the bladder. Thus, the individual develops a neurogenic bladder (autonomous).
5. With this type of neurogenic bladder the individual is likely to dribble urine when the pressure in the bladder rises because of the bladder filling beyond its normal capacity or because of coughing, straining, or exercising.
6. Other common names for this type of bladder are lower motor neuron, hypotonic, flaccid, cord, tabetic, and atonic bladder.
7. External manual compression and/or abdominal straining are the most effective methods to empty a neurogenic bladder.

Reflex Incontinence

1. A lesion above the sacral cord segments (above T12) involving both motor and sensory tracts of the spinal cord will result in a reflex bladder. Other common names for this type of bladder dysfunction are spastic, supraspinal, hypertonic, automatic, and upper motor neuron bladder.
2. A lesion that does not completely transect the spinal cord can produce variable findings.
3. Control from higher cerebral centers is removed in the reflex neurogenic bladder. Therefore, micturition cannot be started or stopped in a voluntary manner.
4. The simple spinal reflex arc takes over the control of micturition.
5. A positive bulbocavernosus reflex suggests that the voiding reflex (spinal reflex arc) is intact.
6. Since the voiding reflex located in the sacral cord segments is spared, micturition can occur automatically after external cutaneous stimulation (manual triggering).
7. Individuals with reflex neurogenic bladders can learn methods for stimulating the reflex arc to stimulate bladder emptying.
8. Preferred cutaneous triggering methods are light, rapid suprapubic tapping, light pulling of pubic hairs, massage of the abdomen, and digital rectal stimulation.
9. Avoid the use of Credé's maneuver with a reflex bladder because the urethra may be damaged or vesicoureteral reflux may occur if the external sphincter is contracted.
10. If the opening of the urinary sphincter and the relaxation of the striated muscle surrounding the urinary sphincter are uncoordinated, there is a potential for large residual urine volumes after triggered voiding.

11. Autonomic dysreflexia (dysreflexia) is an abnormal hyperactive reflex activity that occurs only in spinal cord injured individuals with a lesion above T8. Most often, these individuals have an upper motor neuron bladder (reflex incontinence). This is a life-threatening situation in which the blood pressure rises to lethal levels. Autonomic hyperreflexia is most often set off by stimuli resulting from an overstretched bladder or bowel.

Stress Incontinence

1. Urinary continence is maintained by the junction of the bladder and the urethra, by support from the perineal floor, and by the muscle around the urethra.
2. Stress incontinence is the leakage of small amounts of urine when the urethral outlet is unable to control passage of urine in the presence of increased intra-abdominal pressure.
3. In stress incontinence, the pelvic floor muscles (pubococcygeus) and levator ani muscles have been weakened or stretched by childbirth, trauma, menopausal atrophy, or obesity.
4. Stress incontinence is usually made worse by the menopausal decrease in elasticity.
5. A trial of vaginal estrogen cream in the postmenopausal woman who exhibits a pale, atrophic vaginal vault may be helpful in reducing the incidence of incontinence.
6. Kegel exercises will strengthen and tone the muscles of the pelvic floor. They may provide enough augmentation or urethral pressure to prevent mild stress incontinence. They should be taught to all women as a preventive measure.
7. A stress test is used to help diagnose stress incontinence. It involves observation of the urethral meatus of a patient with a full bladder in the standing position while she coughs or strains. Short spurts of urine escaping simultaneously with cough or strain suggest a probable diagnosis of stress incontinence.
8. The patient with pure stress incontinence will have a normal cystometrogram.
9. The degrees of stress incontinence are designated as:
    a. Grade 1—Loss of urine with sudden increase in abdominal pressure, but never at night.
    b. Grade 2—Lesser degrees of physical stress such as walking, standing erect from a sitting position or sitting up in bed produce incontinence.
    c. Grade 3—In this stage, there is total incontinence, and urine is lost without any relation to physical activity or to position.

Urge Incontinence

1. Urge incontinence is an involuntary loss of urine associated with a strong desire to void. This is characterized by loss of large volumes of urine and may be triggered by emotional factors, body position changes, or the sight and sound of running water. This type of urge incontinence is commonly called bladder detrusor instability or vesical instability.
2. Detrusor instability is characterized by the presence of uninhibited detrusor contractions sufficient to cause urinary incontinence. Common causes include central nervous system disease, hyperexcitability of the afferent pathways, and deconditioned voiding reflexes.
3. Deconditioning of the voiding reflex can result in incontinence through self-induced or iatrogenic causes. Frequent toileting (more than every 2 hr) causes chronic low-volume voiding, which reduces bladder capacity and increases detrusor tone and bladder wall thickness, which potentiates incontinent episodes.
4. Iatrogenic causes include placing a person on the toilet after the incontinent episode or using uncomfortable equipment to make him continent.

5. A person with an uninhibited neurogenic bladder will have damage to the cerebral cortex affecting the ability to inhibit urination. Sensation of bladder fullness is also limited; this is manifested by urgency. There is little time between the sensation to void and the uninhibited contraction (CVA, Parkinson's disease, brain injury/tumor).
6. Factors that contribute to urgency include acute urinary tract infection, neurologic impairments, diuretics, diabetes mellitus, inadequate fluid intake, and habitual frequent voiding.
7. Older persons experience urgency owing to the bladder's limited capacity and their decreased ability to inhibit bladder contractions.
8. Warning time is the amount of time the individual can delay urination after the urge to void is felt.
9. Diminished warning time can cause incontinence if the individual is unable to reach a toilet in time.

Functional Incontinence

1. Functional incontinence is the inability or unwillingness of the person with a normal bladder and sphincter to reach the toilet in sufficient time.
2. Functional incontinence may be caused by conditions affecting the individual's physical and emotional ability to manage the act of urination.
3. Underlying psychologic problems can be a functional etiology of incontinence.
4. Environmental barriers such as unfamiliar surroundings, uncomfortable equipment, and/or lack of privacy may aggravate this situation.
5. Approximately 45% of all nursing home residents are incontinent. Of those with bladder incontinence, 82% are mobility limited.

Total Incontinence

1. The person may lose urine without warning; this may be a constant or periodic symptom.
2. The person may or may not be aware of incontinence.
3. Injury to the urethral smooth muscle sphincters may occur during prostatectomy or childbirth.
4. Congenital or acquired neurogenic diseases may lead to dysfunction of the bladder and incontinence.
5. This individual has tried methods to control the bladder and has been unsuccessful for a variety of reasons.
6. A cognitively impaired person with total incontinence requires caregiver-directed treatment. In institutional settings, indwelling and external catheters or disposal or washable diapers or pads are beneficial to the caregivers but detrimental to the incontinent person. Aids and equipment should be considered only after other means have been attempted. In the home setting, the caregiver's needs may take precedence over the cognitively impaired person's. Urinary incontinence is cited as the major reason for seeking institutional care for persons living at home (Miller, 1990).

Gerontologic Considerations

1. Urinary incontinence affects 5% to 15% of elderly people living in the community, and its prevalence increases to about 40% in hospitalized patients and 50% in the institutionalized patients (Resnick & Yalla, 1985). One of the major problems of incontinence in the elderly is that it may be overlooked and not adequately evaluated by professionals, and as a result, appropriate treatment is denied. Elderly people themselves may not admit to the problem because of attitudes about the inevitability of complications such as incontinence.

2. Age-related physiologic changes result in decreased bladder capacity, incomplete emptying, contractions during filling and increased residual urine (Miller, 1990).
3. Older adults can comfortably store 250 mL to 300 mL of urine, compared with a storage capacity of 350 mL to 400 mL in younger adults.
4. The sensation to void is delayed in older adults, which shortens the interval between the initial perception of the urge and the actual need to void, resulting in urgency (Miller, 1990). Any factor that interferes with the older adult's perception to void (*e.g.*, medications, depression, limited fluid intake, neurologic impairments) or delays his or her ability to reach the toilet can cause incontinence.
5. Other physiologic components of aging that contribute to incontinence are the diminished ability of kidneys to concentrate urine, decreasing muscle tone of the pelvic floor muscles, and the ability to postpone urination.
6. Frequent voiding out of habit or limiting fluids may contribute to urgency by impairing the neurologic mechanisms that signal the need to void, because the bladder is rarely fully expanded.
7. The diminished vision, impaired mobility, and decreased energy level that may accompany aging mean that increased time is needed to locate the toilet, which also requires the person to be able to delay urination.
8. In one study, incontinent elderly female subjects exhibited a history of vaginal deliveries, bacteriuria, and a greater number of functional impairments (Ouslander, Morishita, Blaustein, Orzech, Dunne, & Sayre, 1987).

Maturational Enuresis*

■ *Related to* **(Specify)**

DEFINITION
Maturational Enuresis: The state in which a child experiences involuntary voiding during sleep which is not pathophysiologic in origin.

DEFINING CHARACTERISTICS

Major (must be present)
Reports or demonstrates episodes of involuntary voiding during sleep

*This diagnosis is not currently on the NANDA list but has been included for clarity or usefulness.

RELATED FACTORS

Situational (personal, environmental)

Stressors (school, siblings)
Inattention to bladder cues
Unfamiliar surroundings

Maturational

Child

Small bladder capacity
Lack of motivation
Attention-seeking behavior

Diagnostic Considerations

Enuresis can be due to physiologic or maturational factors. Certain etiologies, such as strictures, urinary tract infection, nocturnal epilepsy, and diabetes, should be ruled out when enuresis is present. These situations do not represent nursing diagnoses.

When enuresis results from small bladder capacity, failure to perceive cues because of deep sleep, or inattention to bladder cues, or is associated with a maturational issue (*e.g.*, new sibling, school pressures), the nursing diagnosis *Maturational Enuresis* is appropriate. Psychologic problems usually are not the cause of enuresis, but may result from lack of understanding or insensitivity to the problem. Interventions that punish or shame the child must be avoided.

Errors in Diagnostic Statements

Maturational Enuresis related to stressors and conflicts

Rather than focus on etiology for maturational enuresis, the nurse should focus on teaching the child and parents management strategies. The nurse also should encourage parents to share their concerns and direct them away from punishing behaviors. Given this nursing focus, the diagnosis could be restated as *Maturational Enuresis related to unknown etiology, as evidenced by reported episodes of bed wetting*.

Focus Assessment

See *Altered Patterns of Urinary Elimination*

Principles and Rationale for Nursing Care

1. The newborn may void up to 20 times per day due to small bladder capacity (Whaley & Wong, 1989). As the child grows, bladder capacity increases and frequency of urination decreases (Chow, Durand, Feldman, & Mills, 1984).
2. Most children by age 4 to 5 have complete neuromuscular control of urination (Chow, Durand, Feldman, & Mills, 1984).
3. Foye and Sulkes (1990) define enuresis as urinary incontinence at any age when urinary control would be expected.
4. The etiology of enuresis is complex and not well understood. The following factors have been implicated:
   a. Developmental/maturational delay (*e.g.*, small functional bladder capacity, deep sleep, or mental retardation)
   b. Organic factors (*e.g.*, infection, sickle cell anemia, diabetes, and neuromuscular disorders)

c. Psychologic/emotional factors (*e.g.,* stressors such as birth of sibling, hospitalization, or divorce of parents) (VanCleve & Baldwin, 1989; Chow, Durand, Feldman, & Mills, 1984).

5. Children at risk for urinary retention include those who
   a. Have congenital anomalies of the urinary tract
   b. Are neurologically impaired (Whaley & Wong, 1989)
   c. Are postoperative (Hunsberger, 1989)

6. Enuresis is primarily a maturational problem and usually ceases between the ages of 6 and 8 years. It is more common in boys.

7. There is a high frequency of bed-wetting in children whose parents or other near relatives were bed-wetters.

■ Maturational Enuresis
Related to (Specify)

Assessment
See Defining Characteristics

Outcome Criteria

- The child will remain dry during the sleep cycle
- The child or family will be able to state the nature and causes of enuresis

---

Interventions

A. Assess for contributing factors
   1. Small bladder capacity
   2. Sound sleeper
   3. Response to stress (at school or at home, *e.g.,* new sibling)

B. Promote a positive parent–child relationship
   1. Explain the nature of enuresis to parents and child.
   2. Explain to parents that disapproval (shaming, punishing) is useless in stopping enuresis but can make child shy, ashamed, and afraid.
   3. Offer reassurance to child that other children wet the bed at night and he is not bad or sinful.

C. Reduce contributing factors if possible.
   1. Small bladder capacity: After child drinks fluids, encourage him to postpone voiding to help stretch the bladder.
   2. Sound sleeper
      a. Have child void prior to retiring.
      b. Restrict fluids at bedtime.

    c. If child is awakened later (about 11 P.M.) to void, attempt to awaken child fully for positive reinforcement.

  3. Too busy to sense a full bladder (if daytime wetting occurs)

    a. Teach child awareness of sensations that occur when it is time to void.

    b. Teach child ability to control urination (have him start and stop the stream; have him "hold" the urine during the day, even if for only a short time).

    c. Have child keep a record of how he is doing; emphasize dry days or nights (*e.g.,* stars on a calendar).

    d. If child wets, have him explain or write down, if he can, why he thinks it happened.

D. Initiate health teaching and referrals as indicated

  1. For children with enuresis

    a. Teach child and parents the facts about enuresis.

    b. Teach child and family techniques to control the adverse effects of enuresis (*e.g.,* use of plastic mattress covers, use of child's own sleeping bag (machine washable) when staying overnight away from home).

  2. Seek out opportunities to teach the public about enuresis and incontinence (*e.g.,* school and parent organizations, self-help groups).

Functional Incontinence

■ *Related to* **Age-Related Urgency Secondary to (Specify): High Risk for**

DEFINITION

Functional Incontinence: The state in which an individual experiences a difficulty or inability to reach the toilet in time due urgency, environmental barriers, decreased attention to cues and/or physical limitations.

DEFINING CHARACTERISTICS

Major (must be present)

Incontinence before or during an attempt to reach the toilet

RELATED FACTORS

Pathophysiologic

  Neurogenic disorders

    Brain injury/tumor/infection

    Cerebrovascular accident

Demyelinating diseases
Multiple sclerosis
Alcoholic neuropathy
Parkinsonism
Progressive dementia

Treatment-related

Drug therapy (iatrogenic)
Antihistamines
Epinephrine
Anticholinergics
Sedatives
Immunosuppressant therapy
Diuretics
Tranquilizers
Muscle relaxants

Situational (personal, environmental)

Impaired mobility
Stress or fear
Decreased attention to bladder cues
Depression
Confusion
Intentional suppression (self-induced deconditioning)
Environmental barriers to bathroom
Distant toilets
Poor lighting
Unfamiliar surroundings
Bed too high
Side rails

Maturational

Elderly: Loss of perineal muscle tone, inability to communicate needs, depression, diminished bladder capacity, mobility problems

Principles and Rationale for Nursing Care

See *Altered Patterns of Urinary Elimination*

■ # High Risk for Functional Incontinence
Related to Age-Related Urgency Secondary to (Specify)*

Assessment
See Defining Characteristics

Outcome Criteria

The person will
- Remove or minimize environmental barriers from home
- Utilize proper adaptive equipment to assist with voiding, transfers, and dressing
- Describe causative factors for incontinence

Interventions

A. Assess causative or contributing factors
   1. Determine if there is another cause contributing to incontinence (refer to Focus Assessment Criteria)
   2. Assess for
      a. Obstacles to toilet
         - Poor lighting, slippery floor, misplaced furniture and rugs, inadequate footwear, toilet too far, bed too high, side rails up
         - Toilet inadequate
           Too small for walkers, wheelchair, seat too low/high, no grab bars
         - Inadequate signal system for requesting help
         - Lack of privacy
      b. Sensory/cognitive deficits
         - Visual deficits (blindness, field cuts, poor depth perception)
         - Cognitive deficits due to aging, trauma, stroke, tumor, infection
      c. Motor/mobility deficits
         - Limited upper and/or lower extremity movement/strength (inability to remove clothing)
         - Barriers to ambulation (*e.g.,* vertigo, fatigue, altered gait, hypertension)

B. Reduce or eliminate contributing factors if possible
   1. Other causes of incontinence: Establish appropriate bladder reconditioning program (see *Total Incontinence*).
   2. Environmental barriers
      a. Assess path to bathroom for obstacles, lighting, and distance.

---

*Age-related urgency is caused by decreased bladder capacity, self-imposed fluid limitation, and/or frequent voiding, which decreases time between initial perception and actual need to void.

b. Assess adequacy of toilet height and need for grab bars.

c. Assess adequacy of room size.

d. Provide a commode between bathroom and bed, if necessary.

3. Sensory/cognitive deficits

a. For an individual with diminished vision

- Ensure adequate lighting.
- Encourage person to wear prescribed corrective lens.
- Provide clear, safe pathway to bathroom.
- Keep call bell easily accessible.
- If bedpan or urinal is used, make sure it is within easy reach in the same location at all times.
- Assess person for safety in bathroom.
- Assess person's ability to provide self-hygiene.

b. For an individual with cognitive deficits

- Offer toileting reminders every 2 hours, after meals, and before bedtime.
- Establish appropriate means to communicate need to void.
- Answer call bell immediately.
- Encourage wearing ordinary clothes.
- Provide a normal environment for elimination (use bathroom if possible).
- Allow for privacy while maintaining safety.
- Allow sufficient time for task.
- Reorient individual to where he is and what task he is doing.
- Be consistent in your approach to person.
- Give simple step-by-step instructions; use verbal and nonverbal cues.
- Give positive reinforcement for success.
- Assess person for safety in bathroom.
- Assess need for adaptive devices on clothing to make dressing and undressing easier.
- Assess person's ability to provide self-hygiene.

4. Motor/mobility deficits

a. For persons with limited hand function

- Assess person's ability to remove and replace clothing.
- Clothing that is loose is easier to manipulate.
- Provide dressing aids as necessary, *e.g.,* Velcro closures in seams for wheelchair patients, zipper pulls; all garments with fasteners may be adapted with Velcro closures.

C. Provide for factors that promote continence

1. Maintain optimal hydration.

a. Increase fluid intake to 2000 to 3000 mL/day, unless contraindicated.

b. Teach older adults not to depend on thirst sensations but to drink liquids even when not thirsty.

c. Space fluids every 2 hr.

d. Decrease fluid intake after 7 P.M. and provide only minimal fluids during the night.

e. Reduce intake of coffee, tea, dark colas, alcohol, and grapefruit juice because of their diuretic effect.

f. Avoid large amounts of tomato and orange juice because they tend to make the urine more alkaline.

g. Encourage cranberry juice to acidify urine.

2. Maintain adequate nutrition to ensure bowel elimination at least once every 3 days.
   a. Monitor elimination pattern; check for fecal impaction if indicated.
   b. Assess daily dietary intake for daily requirements of roughage, basic four food groups, and adequate fluids.
   c. See *Altered Nutrition* and *Constipation* for additional interventions.
3. Promote micturition.
   a. Ensure privacy and comfort.
   b. Use toilet facilities, if possible, instead of bedpans.
   c. Provide male with opportunity to stand, if possible.
   d. Assist person on bedpan to flex knees and support back.
   e. Teach postural evacuation (bend forward while sitting on toilet).
   f. Ensure safe access to facilities.
      • Provide person with access to urinal or bedpan.
      • Provide person with call light.
      • Reduce obstacles to toilet facilities (path that is well lighted and free of obstacles, bed at lowest level).
      • Modify path to bathroom with rails.
      • Modify bathroom with grab rails, elevated seats.
   g. Stimulate the cutaneous surface to trigger the voiding reflex.
      • Have person brush or stroke inner thigh or abdomen.
      • Pour warm water over perineum.
      • Give glass of water to drink while sitting on the toilet.
4. Promote personal integrity and provide motivation to increase bladder control.
   a. Encourage person to share his feelings about incontinence and determine its effect on his social patterns.
   b. Convey to him that incontinence can be cured or at least controlled to maintain dignity.
   c. Expect him to be continent, not incontinent (*e.g.,* encourage street clothes, discourage use of bedpans).
   d. Use protective pads or garments only after conscientious reconditioning efforts have been completely unsuccessful after 6 weeks.
   e. Work to achieve daytime continence before expecting nighttime continence.
   f. Encourage socialization.
      • Encourage and assist person to groom self.
      • If hospitalized, provide opportunities to eat meals outside bedroom (dayroom, lounge).
      • If fear or embarrassment is preventing socialization, instruct person to use sanitary pads or briefs temporarily until control is established.
      • Change clothes as soon as possible when wet to avoid indirectly sanctioning wetness.
      • Advise the oral use of chlorophyll tablets to deodorize urine and feces.
      • See *Social Isolation* and *Ineffective Individual Coping* for additional interventions, if indicated.
5. Promote skin integrity.
   a. Identify individuals at risk of developing pressure ulcers.
   b. Wash area, rinse, and dry well after incontinent episode.
   c. Use a protective ointment if needed (for area burns, use hydrocortisone cream; for fungal irritations, use antifungal ointment).
   d. See *High Risk for Impaired Skin Integrity* for additional information.

6. Promote personal hygiene
   a. Take showers rather than baths to prevent bacteria from entering urethra.
   b. Instruct women to cleanse the perineum and urethra from front to back after each bowel movement.

D. Teach prevention of urinary tract infections (UTI)
   1. Encourage regular complete emptying of the bladder.
   2. Ensure adequate fluid intake.
   3. Keep urine acidic; avoid citrus juices, dark colas, and coffee.
   4. Monitor urine pH.
   5. Teach individual to recognize abnormal changes in urine properties.
      a. Increase in mucus and sediment
      b. Blood in urine (hematuria)
      c. Change in color (from normal straw-colored) or odor
   6. Teach individual to monitor for signs and symptoms of UTI.
      a. Elevated temperature, chills, and shaking
      b. Changes in urine properties
      c. Suprapubic pain
      d. Painful urination
      e. Urgency
      f. Frequent small voids or frequent small incontinences
      g. Increased spasticity in spinal cord injured individuals
      h. Increase in urine pH
      i. Nausea/vomiting
      j. Lower back and/or flank pain

E. Explain age-related effects on bladder function and that urgency and nocturnia do not necessarily lead to incontinence. Initiate health teaching referral when indicated

F. Initiate referral to visiting nurse (occupational therapy department) for assessment of bathroom facilities at home

Reflex Incontinence

■ *Related to* **(Specify)**

DEFINITION

Reflex Incontinence: The state in which the individual experiences an involuntary loss of urine caused by damage to the spinal cord between the cortical and sacral (S1, S2, S3) bladder centers.

DEFINING CHARACTERISTICS

Major (must be present)
> Uninhibited bladder contractions
> Involuntary reflexes producing spontaneous voiding
> Partial or complete loss of sensation of bladder fullness or urge to void

RELATED FACTORS

Pathophysiologic
Cord injury/tumor/infection

Principles and Rationale for Nursing Care
See *Altered Patterns of Urinary Elimination*

■ Reflex Incontinence
Related to (Specify)

Assessment
See Defining Characteristics

Outcome Criteria

The person will
- Report a state of dryness that is personally satisfactory
- Have a residual urine volume of less than 50 mL
- Utilize triggering mechanisms to initiate reflex voiding

Interventions

A. Assess for causative and contributing factors
  1. Spinal cord lesion above T12
  2. Traumatic injury
  3. Infection
  4. Tumor
  5. Syringomyelia
  6. Multiple sclerosis
  7. Brown-Séquard syndrome
  8. Transverse myelitis
  9. Pernicious anemia

B. Explain to person rationale for treatment (see Principles and Rationale for Nursing Care)

C. Develop a bladder retraining or reconditioning program (see Interventions: Generic Considerations under *Total Incontinence*)

D. Teach techniques to stimulate reflex voiding
   1. Cutaneous triggering mechanisms
      a. Repeated deep, sharp suprapubic tapping (most effective)
      b. Instruct individual to:
         • Position self in a half-sitting position.
         • Tapping is aimed directly at bladder wall.
         • Rate is 7 to 8 times/5 seconds (50 single blows).
         • Use only one hand.
         • Shift site of stimulation over bladder to find most successful site.
         • Continue stimulation until a good stream starts.
         • Wait approximately 1 minute, repeat stimulation until bladder is empty.
         • One or two series of stimulations without response signifies that nothing more will be expelled.
      c. If the above is ineffective, instruct to perform each of the following for 2 to 3 minutes each, waiting 1 minute between facilitation attempts.
         • Stroking glans penis
         • Punching abdomen above inguinal ligaments (lightly)
         • Stroking inner thigh
      d. Encourage person to void or trigger at least every 3 hours.
      e. Indicate on intake and output sheet which mechanism was used to induce voiding.
      f. Persons with abdominal muscle control should use the Valsalva maneuver during triggered voiding.
      g. Teach person that if he increases his fluid intake he also needs to increase the frequency of triggering to prevent overdistention.
      h. Schedule intermittent catheterization program (see *Total Incontinence*).

E. Initiate health teaching as indicated
   1. Teach bladder reconditioning program (see *Total Incontinence*).
   2. Teach intermittent catheterization (see *Total Incontinence*).
   3. Teach prevention of urinary tract infections (see *Total Incontinence*).
   4. Teach about autonomic dysreflexia (see Principles and Rationale for Nursing Care).
   5. Instruct person in prevention of dysreflexia.
      a. Establish and maintain a scheduled fluid intake and bladder-emptying routine.
      b. Establish and maintain a regulated bowel-emptying program (see *Altered Bowel Elimination*).
      c. Establish and maintain a preventive skin care program (see *High Risk for Impaired Skin Integrity*).
   6. Instruct person in signs and symptoms of dysreflexia.
      a. Elevated blood pressure, decreasing pulse
      b. Flushing and sweating above the level of the lesion
      c. Cool and clammy below the level of the lesion
      d. Pounding headache
      e. Nasal stuffiness
      f. Anxiety, "feeling of impending doom"

        g. Goose pimples

        h. Blurred vision

   7. Instruct person in measures to reduce or eliminate symptoms.

        a. Elevate head

        b. Check blood pressure

        c. Rule out bladder distention; empty bladder by catheter (do not trigger); use lidocaine lubricant for catheter

        d. If condition persists after emptying bladder, check for bowel distention. If stool is present in the rectum, use a Nupercainal suppository to desensitize the area before removing stool.

   8. If condition persists or person has not been able to identify cause, notify physician immediately or seek help in an emergency room.

   9. Instruct person to carry an identification card that states signs, symptoms, and management in the event that the person would not be able to direct others.

Stress Incontinence

■ *Related to* **(Specify)**

DEFINITION

Stress Incontinence: The state in which an individual experiences an immediate involuntary loss of urine upon an increase in intra-abdominal pressure.

DEFINING CHARACTERISTICS

Major (must be present)

The individual reports

    Loss of urine (usually < 50 mL) occurring with increased abdominal pressure from standing, sneezing, or coughing

RELATED FACTORS

Pathophysiologic

    Congenital urinary tract anomalies

        Strictures

        Hypospadias

        Epispadias

        Ureterocele

        Bladder neck contractures

        Megalocystis (large-capacity bladder without tone)

Disorders of the urinary tract
>   Infection
>   Trauma
>   Urethritis
> Estrogen deficiency
>   Atrophic vaginitis
>   Atrophic urethritis

Situational (personal, environmental)

Loss of perineal tissue tone
>   Obesity
>   Aging
>   Recent substantial weight loss
>   Childbirth
> Irritation to perineal area
>   Sexual activity
>   Poor personal hygiene
> Pregnancy
> Stress or fear

Maturational

Elderly: loss of muscle tone

Principles and Rationale for Nursing Care

See *Altered Patterns of Urinary Elimination*

■ Stress Incontinence
Related to (Specify)

Assessment

See Defining Characteristics

Outcome Criteria

The person will
• Report a reduction or elimination of stress incontinence
• Be able to explain the cause of incontinence and rationale for treatment

---

Interventions

A. Assess for contributing factors
>   1. Loss of tissue or muscle tone due to:
>   a. Childbirth

    b. Obesity
    c. Aging
    d. Recent weight loss
    e. Cystocele
    f. Rectocele
    g. Prolapsed uterus
    h. Atrophic vaginitis or urethritis
 2. History of surgery of the bladder and urethra with adhesions to the vaginal wall
 3. Increased intra-abdominal pressure from:
    a. Pregnancy
    b. Overdistention between voidings
    c. Obesity

B. Assess pattern of voiding/incontinence and fluid intake

 1. Promote optimal hydration (see *Total Incontinence*).
 2. Assess voiding (see *Total Incontinence*).
 3. Instruct person to avoid fluids such as coffee, tea, dark colas, and alcohol, which act as diuretics and irritants.

C. Reduce or eliminate causative or contributing factors

 1. Loss of tissue and muscle tone
    a. Explain the effect of incompetent floor muscles on continence (see Principles and Rationale for Nursing Care).
    b. Teach to identify her pelvic floor muscles and strengthen them with exercise (Kegel exercises: 25 times, 4–6 sets a day); provide the following instructions:
       • "For posterior pelvic floor muscles, imagine you are trying to stop the passage of stool and tighten your anal muscles without tightening your legs or your abdominal muscles."
       • "For anterior pelvic floor muscles, imagine you are trying to stop the passage of urine, tighten the muscles (back and front) for 4 seconds and then release them; repeat ten times, four times a day." (Can be increased to four times an hour if indicated)
       • Stop and start the urine stream several times during voiding.
 2. Increased abdominal pressure with pregnancy
    a. Teach to avoid prolonged periods of standing.
    b. Teach the benefit of frequent voidings at least every 2 hours.
    c. Teach Kegel exercises.
 3. Increased abdominal pressure with obesity
    a. Instruct person to void every 2 hours.
    b. Avoid prolonged periods of standing.
    c. Explain the relationship of obesity and stress incontinence.
    d. Teach Kegel exercises.
    e. If person desires to lose weight, refer to *Altered Health Maintenance*.

D. Initiate health teaching for persons who continue to remain incontinent after attempts at bladder reconditioning or muscle retraining

 1. Promote personal integrity (see *Total Incontinence*)
 2. Promote skin integrity (see *Total Incontinence*)
 3. Schedule intermittent catheterization program, if appropriate (see *Total Incontinence*)
 4. Discuss use of incontinence briefs to contain incontinence.

Total Incontinence

■ *Related to* **(Specify)**

DEFINITION

Total Incontinence: The state in which an individual experiences continuous, unpredictable loss of urine.

DEFINING CHARACTERISTICS

Major (must be present)

> Constant flow of urine without distention
> Nocturia more than two times during sleep time
> Incontinence refractory to other treatments

Minor (may be present)

> Unaware of bladder cues to void
> Unaware of incontinence

RELATED FACTORS

Pathophysiologic

> Congenital urinary tract anomalies
>> Strictures
>> Hypospadias
>> Epispadias
>> Ureterocele
>> Megalocystis (large-capacity bladder without tone)
> Disorders of the urinary tract
>> Infection
>> Trauma
>> Urethritis
> Neurogenic disorders or injury
>> Cord injury/tumor/infection
>> Brain injury/tumor/infection
>> Cerebrovascular accident
>> Demyelinating diseases
>> Multiple sclerosis
>> Diabetic neuropathy
>> Alcoholic neuropathy
>> Tabes dorsalis

Treatment-related
Surgical
Postprostatectomy
Extensive pelvic dissection
General or spinal anesthesia
Postindwelling catheters

Situational (personal, environmental)
Inability to communicate needs
Dehydration
Stress or fear
Decreased attention to bladder cues
Depression
Confusion

Maturational
Elderly: Motor and sensory losses, loss of muscle tone, inability to communicate needs, depression

Principles and Rationale for Nursing Care
See *Altered Patterns of Urinary Elimination*

■ Total Incontinence
Related to (Specify)

Assessment
See Defining Characteristics

Outcome Criteria

The person will
- Be continent (specify during day, night, 24 hrs)
- Be able to identify the cause of incontinence and rationale for treatment

---

Interventions

A. Assess causative or contributing factors
1. Physiologic
a. Congenital abnormalities
b. Exstrophy of the bladder
c. Hypospadias/epispadias
2. Vesicovaginal fistula
3. Ectopic urethral orifice

4. Surgery
5. Neurogenic diseases
   a. Brain trauma/tumor/infection
   b. Cerebrovascular accident
   c. Coma
   d. Demyelinating disease
   e. Alzheimer's disease
6. Loss of tissue and muscle tone (grade III stress incontinence)
7. Psychologic
   a. Disorientation
   b. Depression

B. Reduce or eliminate causative and contributing factors when possible
   1. In persons who are unable to respond to bladder cues
      a. Establish method to communicate urge to void.
      b. Provide opportunity to void prior to person's usual time for incontinence.
      c. Offer opportunity to void in response to person's usual behavior prior to incontinence (restlessness, screaming).
      d. Wake person during the night and provide opportunity to void.
   2. If person is unable to void, institute intermittent catheterization.

C. Develop a bladder retraining or reconditioning program to include communication, assessment of voiding pattern, scheduled fluid intake, and scheduled voiding times
   1. Promote communication among all staff members and among individual, family, and staff.
      a. Provide all staff with sufficient knowledge concerning the program planned.
      b. Assess staff's response to program.
   2. Assess the person's potential for participation in a bladder retraining program.
      a. Cognition
      b. Desire to change behavior
      c. Ability to cooperate
      d. Willingness to participate
   3. Provide individual with rationale for plan and acquire his informed consent.
   4. Encourage individual to continue program by providing accurate information concerning reasons for success or failure.
   5. Assess voiding pattern (see Fig. II–5)
      a. Monitor and record intake and output.
      b. Time and amount of fluid intake
      c. Type of fluid
      d. Amount of incontinence; measure if possible or estimate amount as small, moderate, or large
      e. Amount of void, whether it was voluntary or involuntary
      f. Presence of sensation of need to void
      g. Amount of retention (retention is the amount of urine left in the bladder after an unsuccessful attempt at manual triggering or voiding)
      h. Amount of residual (residual is the amount of urine left in the bladder after either a voluntary or manual triggered voiding; also called a postvoid residual)
      i. Amount of triggered urine (triggered voiding is urine that is expelled after manual triggering [*e.g.,* tapping, Credé's method])

	Intake	Output						
Time	Type of Fluids	Incontinence	Void	Manual Trigger	Retention	Residual	Behavior/ Activity
12M							
01							
02							
03							
04							
05							
06							
07							
08							
09							
10							
11							
12N							
1							
2							
3							
4							
5							
6							
7							
8							
9							
10							
11							
Totals							

Fig. II-5 Chart used for the assessment of voiding patterns.

      j. Identify certain activities that precede voiding (*e.g.,* restlessness, yelling, exercise).
      k. Record in appropriate column.
  6. Schedule fluid intake and voiding times.
      a. Provide for fluid intake of 2000 mL each day unless contraindicated.
      b. Discourage fluids after 7 P.M.
      c. Initially, bladder emptying is done at least every 2 hours and at least twice during the night; goal is 2- to 4-hour intervals.
      d. If the person is incontinent before scheduled voids, shorten the time between voids.
      e. If the person has a postvoid residual greater than 100 ml to 150 mL, schedule intermittent catheterization.

D. Schedule intermittent catheterization program (ICP), if indicated
  1. Monitor intake and output.
  2. Fluid intake should be at least 2000 mL/day.
  3. Use sterile catheterization technique in the hospital, clean technique at home.

4. Desired catheter volumes are less than 500 mL.
5. Increase or decrease the interval between catheterization to obtain the desired catheter volumes.
6. Usual catheterization times are every 4 to 6 hours.
7. Urine volumes may increase at night; thus, it may be necessary to catheterize more frequently at night.
8. Encourage the individual to attempt to void before scheduled catheterization time.
9. Initially obtain postvoid residuals at least every 6 hours.
10. Terminate ICP when the bladder is consistently emptied voluntarily or by triggering with less than a 50-mL residual urine after each void.

E. Teach intermittent catheterization to person and family for long-term management of bladder (see Principles and Rationale for Nursing Care)
   1. Explain the reasons for the catheterization program.
   2. Explain the relationship of fluid intake and the frequency of catheterization.
   3. Explain the importance of emptying the bladder at the prescribed time regardless of circumstances because of the hazards of an overdistended bladder (*e.g.*, circulation contributes to infection, and stasis of urine contributes to bacterial growth).

F. Teach the individual about his bladder reconditioning program
   1. Explain rationale and treatments of bladder reconditioning program (see Principles and Rationale for Nursing Care).
   2. Explain the schedule of fluid intake, voiding attempts, manual triggering, and catheterization to control incontinence.
   3. Teach person and family the importance of positive reinforcement and adherence to program for best results.
   4. Refer to community nurses for assistance in bladder reconditioning if indicated.

G. If bladder retraining fails, consider use of an indwelling catheter
   1. For males, a catheter no larger than #16 Fr.
   2. For females, up to a #18 for routine use
   3. Teach care of indwelling catheter.
      a. Maintain 3000-mL fluid intake every day.
      b. Keep urine acidic.
      c. Change catheter at least every 2 weeks or when it does not drain properly.
      d. Tape catheter to prevent pulling.
         • Males—to suprapubic abdominal area
         • Females—to inner aspect of thighs
      e. Perform thorough cleaning of the meatus, distal catheter, and perineum at least twice a day.
      f. Maintain sterile drainage system at all times in the hospital; at home may use clean system.
      g. Know that the urine collection system should drain by gravity.
      h. Do not lift collection bag above the level of the bladder without pinching off the tubing to prevent backflow.
      i. Connect the catheter to a leg bag drainage system during the day.

H. Initiate health teaching
   1. If appropriate, teach intermittent catheterization.
   2. Instruct person in prevention of urinary tract infection.

3. Teach person how to change indwelling catheter.
4. For persons living in the community, initiate a referral to the visiting nurse for follow-up and/or regular indwelling catheter changes.

Urge Incontinence

■ *Related to* **(Specify)**

DEFINITION

Urge Incontinence: The state in which an individual experiences an involuntary loss of urine associated with a strong sudden desire to void.

DEFINING CHARACTERISTICS

Major (must be present)

Urgency followed by incontinence

RELATED FACTORS

See Altered Patterns of Urinary Elimination

Pathophysiologic

Disorder of the urinary tract
Infection
Trauma
Urethritis
Neurogenic disorders or injury
Brain injury/tumor/infection
Cerebrovascular accident
Demyelinating diseases
Diabetic neuropathy
Alcoholic neuropathy
Parkinsonism

Treatment-related

Diagnostic instrumentation
General or spinal anesthesia
Postindwelling catheters

Situational (personal, environmental)

Loss of perineal tissue
Obesity
Aging

Recent substantial weight loss
Childbirth
Irritation to perineal area
Sexual activity
Poor personal hygiene
Intentional suppression (self-induced deconditioning)

Maturational

Child: Small bladder capacity
Elderly: Decreased bladder capacity

Principles and Rationale for Nursing Care

See *Altered Patterns of Urinary Elimination*

■ Urge Incontinence
Related to (Specify)

Assessment
See Defining Characteristics

Outcome Criteria

The person will
- Report an absence or decreased episodes of incontinence (specify)
- Explain causes of incontinence

Interventions

A. Assess for causative or contributing factors
1. Bladder irritants
   a. Infection
   b. Inflammation
   c. Alcohol, caffeine, or dark cola ingestion
   d. Concentrated urine
2. Diminished bladder capacity
   a. Self-induced deconditioning (frequent small voids)
   b. Post-indwelling catheter
3. Overdistended bladder
   a. Increased urine production (diabetes mellitus, diuretics)
   b. Intake of alcohol and/or large quantities of fluids
4. Uninhibited bladder contractions due to neurologic disorder
   a. Cerebrovascular accident
   b. Brain tumor/trauma/infection
   c. Parkinson's disease

B. Assess pattern of voiding/incontinence and fluid intake
1. Maintain optimal hydration (see *Total Incontinence*).
2. Assess voiding pattern (see *Total Incontinence*).

C. Reduce or eliminate causative and contributing factors when possible
1. Bladder irritants
   a. Infection/inflammation
      • Refer to physician for diagnosis and treatment.
      • Initiate bladder reconditioning program (see *Total Incontinence*).
      • Explain the relationship between incontinence and intake of alcohol, caffeine and dark colas (irritants).
   b. Explain the risk of insufficient fluid intake and its relation to infection and concentrated urine.
2. Diminished bladder capacity
   a. Determine amount of time between urge to void and need to void (record how long person can hold off urination).
   b. For a person with difficulty prolonging waiting time, communicate to personnel the need to respond rapidly to his request for assistance for toileting (note on care plan).
   c. Teach person to increase waiting time by increasing bladder capacity.
      • Determine volume of each void.
      • Ask person to "hold off" urinating as long as possible.
      • Give positive reinforcement.
      • Discourage frequent voiding that is result of habit, not need.
      • Develop bladder reconditioning program (see *Total Incontinence*).
3. Overdistended bladder
   a. Explain that diuretics are given to help reduce the amount of water in the body; they work by acting on the kidneys to increase the flow of urine.
   b. Explain that in diabetes mellitus, insulin deficiency causes high levels of blood sugar. The high level of blood sugar pulls fluid from body tissues, causing osmotic diuresis and increased urination (polyuria).
   c. Explain that because of the increased urine flow, regular voiding is needed to prevent overdistention of the bladder. Explain that overdistention can result in loss of bladder sensation, which increases incontinent episodes (diabetic neuropathy).
   d. Assess voiding pattern (see *Total Incontinence*).
   e. Check postvoid residual; if greater than 100 mL, include intermittent catheterization in bladder reconditioning program.
   f. Initiate bladder reconditioning program (see *Total Incontinence*).
4. Uninhibited bladder contractions
   a. Assess voiding pattern (see *Total Incontinence*).
   b. Establish method to communicate urge to void (document on care plan).
   c. Communicate to personnel the need to respond rapidly to a request to void.
   d. Establish a planned voiding pattern.
      • Provide an opportunity to void upon awakening, after meals, physical exercise, bathing, and drinking coffee or tea, and before going to sleep.
      • Begin by offering bedpan, commode, or toilet every half-hour initially, and gradually lengthen the time to at least every 2 hours.
      • If person has incontinent episode, reduce the time between scheduled voidings.
      • Document behavior/activity that occurs with void or incontinence (see Assessment of voiding pattern in *Total Incontinence*).

- Encourage person to try to "hold" urine until see voiding time if possible.
- Refer to *Total Incontinence* for additional information on developing a bladder reconditioning program.

D. Initiate health teaching

Instruct person on prevention of urinary tract infections (see *Functional Incontinence*).

Urinary Retention

■ *Related to* (Specify)

DEFINITION

Urinary Retention: The state in which an individual experiences a chronic inability to void followed by involuntary voiding (overflow incontinence).

DEFINING CHARACTERISTICS

Major (must be present)

Bladder distention (not related to acute reversible etiology) or
Bladder distention with small frequent voids or dribbling (overflow incontinence)
100 mL or more residual urine

Minor (may be present)

The individual states that it feels like the bladder is not emptying after voiding

RELATED FACTORS

Pathophysiologic

Congenital urinary tract anomalies
   Strictures
   Ureterocele
   Bladder-neck contractures
   Megalocystis (large-capacity bladder without tone)
Neurogenic disorders or injury
   Cord injury/tumor/infection
   Brain injury/tumor/infection
   Cerebrovascular accident
   Demyelinating diseases
   Multiple sclerosis
   Diabetic neuropathy
   Alcoholic neuropathy
   Tabes dorsalis
Prostatic enlargement

Treatment-related

Surgical
    Postprostatectomy
    Extensive pelvic dissection
Diagnostic instrumentation
General or spinal anesthesia
Drug therapy (iatrogenic)
    Antihistamines
    Epinephrine
    Anticholinergics
    Theophylline
    Isoproterenol
Postindwelling catheters

Situational (personal, environmental)

Loss of perineal tissue tone
    Obesity
    Aging
    Recent substantial weight loss
    Childbirth
Irritation to perineal area
    Sexual activity
    Poor personal hygiene
Pregnancy
Inability to communicate needs
Fecal impaction
Dehydration
Stress or fear
Decreased attention to bladder cues
    Depression
    Confusion
    Intentional suppression (self-induced deconditioning)
Environmental barriers to bathroom
    Distant toilets
    Poor lighting
    Unfamiliar surroundings
    Bed too high
    Side rails

Maturational

Child: Small bladder capacity, lack of motivation
Elderly: Motor and sensory losses, loss of muscle tone, inability to communicate needs, depression

Principles and Rationale for Nursing Care

See *Altered Patterns of Urinary Elimination*

■ Urinary Retention
Related to (Specify)

Assessment
See Defining Characteristics

Outcome Criteria

The person will
- Empty the bladder using the Créde's and/or Valsalva maneuvers with a residual urine of less than 50 mL if indicated
- Void voluntarily
- Achieve a state of dryness that is personally satisfactory

Interventions

A. Assess for causative or contributing factors
   1. Factors that cause impaired afferent pathways
     a. Cerebrovascular accidents
     b. Demyelinating diseases
     c. Spinal cord injury/trauma/infection
     d. Peripheral nerve damage
       • Diabetic neuropathy
       • Alcoholic neuropathy
       • Pelvic fractures/extensive surgery
   2. Loss of bladder tone (detrusor weakness)
     a. Benign prostatic hypertrophy (postoperative)
     b. Spinal cord injury/tumor/infection
     c. Cerebrovascular accident
     d. Brain injury/tumor/infection
     e. Medications
       • Anticholinergics
       • Alpha-adrenergics
   3. Conditions contributing to bladder neck obstruction
     a. Strictures/contracture/spasms
     b. Edema (postsurgical, postpartum, vaginal or rectal packing)
     c. Prostatic hypertrophy

      d. Fecal impaction

      e. Tumor

      f. Congenital abnormalities

    4. Conditions that inhibit micturition

      a. Poor fluid intake

      b. Anxiety

B. Explain to the person the rationale for treatment (see Principles and Rationale for Nursing Care)

C. Develop a bladder retraining or reconditioning program (see *Total Incontinence*)

D. Instruct on methods to empty bladder

    1. Assist person to a sitting position.

      a. Teach abdominal strain and Valsalva maneuver; Instruct person to:

- Lean forward on thighs.
- Contract abdominal muscles if possible and strain or "bear down"; hold breath while straining (Valsalva maneuver).
- Hold strain or breath until urine flow stops; wait 1 minute and strain again as long as possible.
- Continue until no more urine is expelled.

      b. Teach Créde's maneuver; instruct person to:

- Place hands flat (or place fist) just below umbilical area.
- Place one hand on top of the other.
- Press firmly down and in toward the pelvic arch.
- Repeat six or seven times until no more urine can be expelled.
- Wait a few minutes and repeat to ensure complete emptying.

      c. Teach anal stretch maneuver; instruct person to:

- Sit on commode or toilet.
- Lean forward on thighs.
- Place one gloved hand behind buttocks.
- Insert one to two lubricated fingers into the anus to the anal sphincter.
- Spread fingers apart or pull to posterior direction.
- Gently stretch the anal sphincter and hold it distended.
- Bear down and void.
- Take a deep breath and hold it while straining (Valsalva maneuver).
- Relax and repeat the procedure until the bladder is empty.

    2. Instruct individual to try all three techniques or a combination of techniques to determine which is most effective in emptying the bladder.

    3. Indicate on the intake and output record which technique was used to induce voiding.

    4. Obtain postvoid residuals after attempts at emptying bladder; if residual urine volumes are greater than 100 mL, schedule intermittent catheterization program (see Interventions).

E. Initiate health teaching

    1. Teach bladder reconditioning program (see *Total Incontinence*).

    2. Teach intermittent catheterization (see *Total Incontinence*).

    3. Instruct person on prevention of urinary tract infections (see *Total Incontinence*).

References/Bibliography

Ashervath, J. (1990). Achieving continence in the confused elderly. *Advancing Clinical Care, 5*(4), 37–40.

Bavendam, T. G. (1990). Stress urinary incontinence in women. *Journal of Enterostomal Therapy, 17*(2), 57–66.

Burgio, L. Jones, L., & Engel, B. (1988). Studying incontinence in an urban nursing home. *Journal of Geriatric Nursing, 14*(4), 40–45.

Cella, M. (1988). The nursing costs of urinary incontinence in nursing home population. *Nursing Clinics of North America, 23*(1), 159–168.

Chow, M. P., Durand, B. A., Feldman, M. N., & Mills, M. A. (1984). *Handbook of pediatric primary care* (2nd ed.). New York: Wiley & Sons.

Foye, H., & Sulkes, S. (1990). Developmental and behavioral pediatrics. In Behrman, R. E., & Kliegman, R. (Eds.). *Nelson essentials of pediatrics.* Philadelphia: W. B. Saunders, p. 34.

Hunsberger, M. (1989). Principles and skills adapted to the care of children. In Foster, R. L., Hunsberger, M. M., & Anderson, J. J. T. (Eds.). *Family-centered nursing care of children.* Philadelphia: W. B. Saunders, p. 840.

Jacobs, M. & Geels, W. (1985). *Signs and symptoms in nursing: Interpretation and management.* Philadelphia: J. B. Lippincott.

Lockhart-Pretti, P. (1990). Urinary incontinence. *Journal of Enterostomal Therapy, 17*(3), 112–119.

Long, M. L. (1985). Incontinence. *Journal of Gerontological Nursing, 11*(1), 30–41.

McCormick, K. A., & Burgio, K. L. (1984). Incontinence: An update on nursing care measures. *Journal of Gerontological Nursing, 10*(10), 16–23.

Miller, C. A. (1990). *Nursing care of older adults.* Glenview, IL: Scott, Foresman.

Newman, D. K. (1989). The treatment of urinary incontinence in adults. *Nurse Practitioner, 14*(6) 21–32.

Niederpruem, M. S. (1984). Autonomic dysreflexia. *Rehabilitation Nursing, 9*(1), 29–31.

Ouslander, J.G., Morishita, L., Blaustein, J., Orzeck, S., Dunn, S., & Sayre, J. (1987). Clinical, functional and psychosocial characteristics of an incontinent nursing home population. *Journal of Gerontology, 42*(6), 631–637.

Pierson, C. A. (1984). Assessment and quantification of urine loss in incontinent women. *Nurse Practitioner, 9*(12), 18–30.

Plymat, K., & Turner, S. (1988, July/August). In-home management of urinary incontinence. *Home Healthcare Nurse, 6*(4), 30–34.

Ramphal, M. (1987). Urinary incontinence among nursing home patients: Issues in research. *Geriatric Nursing, 8*(5), 249–254.

Resnick, N., & Yalla, S. (1985). Management of urinary incontinence in the elderly. *New England Journal of Medicine, 5*(13), 800–805.

Ruff, C., & Reaves, E. (1989). Diagnosing urinary incontinence in adults. *Nurse Practitioner, 14*(6), 10–17.

Tunink, P. (1988). Alteration in urinary elimination. *Journal of Gerontological Nursing, 14*(4), 25–30.

Van Cleve, S. N., & Baldwin, S. E. (1989). Nursing strategies: Altered genitourinary function. In Foster, R.L., Hunsberger, M. M., & Anderson, J. J. T. (Eds.). *Family-centered nursing care of children.* Philadelphia: W. B. Saunders, p. 1486.

Voith, A. M. (1986). A conceptual framework for nursing diagnosis: Alteration in urinary elimination. *Rehabilitation Nursing, 11*(1), 18–21.

Wahlquist, G. I., McGuire, E., Greene, W., et al. (1983). Intermittent catheterization and urinary tract infection. *Rehabilitation Nursing, 8*(1), 18–41.

Whaley, L. F., & Wong, D. L. (1989). *Essentials of pediatric nursing* (3rd ed.). St. Louis: C. V. Mosby.

Williams, T. F. (1987). Aging or disease? *Clinical Pharmacology and Therapeutics, 42*(6), 663–665.

Wyman, J. F. (1988). Nursing assessment of the incontinent geriatric outpatient population. *Nursing Clinics of North America, 23*(1), 169–179.

Resources for the Consumer

Literature

The HIP Report, Help for Incontinent People
Katherine F. Jeter (Ed.)
PO Box 544
Union, SC 29379

Managing Incontinence: A Guide to Living With Loss of Bladder Control
Simon Foundation
Box 835
Wilmette, IL 60091
1-800-237-4599

Violence, High Risk for

■ *Related to* **(Specify)**

DEFINITION

High Risk for Violence: A state in which an individual has been, or is at high risk to be, assaultive toward persons or objects.

RISK FACTORS

Major (must be present)

Presence of Risk Factors
  See also Related Factors

RELATED FACTORS

Pathophysiologic

Temporal lobe epilepsy
Progressive central nervous system
  disorder
Deterioration (brain tumor)
Head injuries
Hormonal imbalance
Viral encephalopathy
Mental retardation
Minimal brain dysfunction
Toxic response to alcohol or drugs
Mania

Treatment-related

Toxic reaction to medication

Situational (personal, environmental)

History of overt aggressive acts
Physical immobility
Environmental controls
Perceived threat to self-esteem
Hallucination
Suspiciousness
Persecutory delusions
Verbal threats of physical assault
Low frustration tolerance
Poor impulse control
Feelings of helplessness
Excessively controlled, inflexible
Fear of the unknown
Response to catastrophic event
Rage reaction
Misperceived messages from others
Antisocial character
Dysfunctional communication patterns

Maturational

Adolescent: Role identity, peer pressure, separation from family
Elderly: Dementia

Diagnostic Considerations

The diagnosis *High Risk for Violence* describes a person who has been assaultive or because of certain factors (*e.g.*, toxic response to alcohol or drugs, hallucinations or delusions, brain dysfunction) is at high risk for assaulting others. In such a situation, the nursing focus is on decreasing violent episodes and protecting the person and others.

The nurse should not use this diagnosis to address underlying problems such as anxiety or poor self-esteem, but instead should refer to the diagnoses of *Anxiety* and/or *Ineffective Individual Coping* for a focus on the sources of the violence (spouse, child, elder). When domestic violence is present or suspected, the nurse should explore the diagnosis *Ineffective Family Coping: Disabling*. A person at risk for suicide would warrant the diagnosis *High Risk for Self-Harm*.

Errors in Diagnostic Statements

High Risk for Violence related to reports of abuse by wife

Reports of abuse by a spouse represents a family dysfunction, not a situation covered by *High Risk for Violence*. Spouse abuse is a complex situation necessitating individual and family therapy. The nursing diagnoses *Ineffective Family Coping: Disabling* and *Ineffective Individual Coping* for the abuser and the victim would be more clinically useful.

High Risk for Violence related to poor management of agitation by staff

This diagnostic statement is legally problematic and does not offer constructive strategies. In a situation in which staff inappropriately manage an agitated client, the nurse must treat this as a staff management problem, not a client problem. If the staff increased the client's agitation due to lack of knowledge, the nurse must outline specific do's and don'ts in the nursing care plan. In addition, an inservice program on identifying precursors to violence and agitation reduction strategies should be held for the staff. For the client, the nurse could rewrite the diagnosis as *High Risk for Violence related to mental dysfunction and persecutory delusions*.

Focus Assessment Criteria

(Refer also to Focus Assessment Criteria for *Ineffective Individual Coping, Ineffective Family Coping, Altered Thought Processes, Anxiety*.)

Subjective Data

1. Medical history

Epilepsy	Alcohol abuse
Head injury	Drug abuse
Brain disease	(amphetamines, PCP,
Hormonal imbalance	marijuana)
Present medication	

2. Psychiatric history

Previous hospitalizations	Outpatient therapy

3. History of emotional difficulties in individual and/or family

    Alcoholism   Parental brutality

    Cruelty to animals   Pyromania

4. Interaction patterns (note changes)

    Family   Coworkers

    Friends   Others

5. Coping patterns (past and present)

6. Sources of stress in current environment

7. Work/school history

    How does he function under   Employment

       stress?   Stable

    Level of education attained   Frequency of job changes

    Learning disabilities   Periods of unemployment

    Fights in school

8. Legal history

    Arrests and convictions for   Juvenile offenses for violent

       violent crimes   behavior

9. History of violence

    Assess recency, severity, and frequency

        "What is the most violent thing you have ever done?"

        "What is the closest you have ever come to striking someone?"

        "In what kinds of situations have you hit someone or destroyed property?"

        "When was the last time this happened?"

        "How often does this occur?"

        "Were you using drugs or alcohol when these episodes occurred?"

10. Present thoughts about violence

    Identify possible victim and weapon

        "How do you feel after an incident?"

        "Are you currently having thoughts about harming someone?"

        "Is there anyone in particular you think about harming?" (Identify the victim and the person's access to victim.)

        "Do you have a specific plan for how you might accomplish this?" (Identify plan, type of weapon, and availability of weapon.)

11. Thought content

    Helplessness   Fear of loss of control

    Suspiciousness or hostility   Persecutory delusions

    Perceived intention   Disorientation

       (*e.g.*, "He meant to hit me"

       in response to a slight bump)

Objective Data

1. Body language

    Posture (relaxed, rigid)   Hands (relaxed, rigid, clenched)

    Facial expression (calm,

       annoyed, tense)

2. Motor activity

    Within normal limits   Pacing

    Immobile   Agitation

    Increased

3. Affect

Within normal limits	Flat
Labile	Inappropriate
Controlled	

4. Diagnostic studies

Electrolyte levels	CT scans
Renal function	Blood glucose
EEG	Drug levels (blood, urine, gastric)
Blood gases	Blood alcohol levels

Principles and Rationale for Nursing Care

(Refer to *Ineffective Family Coping* for further information on spouse, elderly and child abuse.)

Generic Considerations

1. A central theme in violent individuals is helplessness. Assaultive behavior is a defense against passivity and helplessness.
2. Aggressive behavior is a defense against anxiety. This coping mechanism is reinforced, since it reduces anxiety by increasing the individual's sense of power and control. (Refer to Principles and Rationale for Nursing Care—*Anxiety* for further discussion of anger.) Interventions that encourage "acting out of anger" will reinforce assaultiveness, and thus are to be avoided.
3. Fear and anxiety can distort the individual's perception of external stimuli.
4. Violence usually occurs in response to dynamically significant stresses or situations and is not random.
5. When brain dysfunction is a prime or contributing factor in violent behavior, social and environmental variables still need to be evaluated. Organic impairment may interfere with an individual's ability to handle certain stresses. A person's normal behavior can be altered by exposure to or ingestion of toxic chemicals, such as lead and pesticides. Examples of violent behavior in brain dysfunction are biting, scratching, temper outbursts, and mood lability.
6. Alcohol and drug abuse/use impairs judgment and decreases internal controls over behavior.
7. Assaultive behavior tends to occur when conditions are crowded, are without structure, and involve staff-"demanded" activity (Harris & Varnley, 1986).
8. Suspicious, delusional patients may misinterpret the environment or the motives of staff or others.
9. Individuals who had a history of emotional deprivation in childhood are particularly vulnerable to attacks on their self-esteem.
10. Even though the individual may identify the person with whom he is angry, this may not be the real object of his aggression. Individuals often cannot allow themselves to express anger toward a person on whom they are dependent.
11. Staff frequently respond to violent individuals with actual fear or overreactions. This can lead to punitive sanctions such as heavier medication, seclusion, or attempts to cope by avoidance and withdrawal from the individual (Maier, Stava, Morrow, Van Rybroek, & Bauman, 1987).
12. Staff must identify their own reactions to violent individuals so that they can more effectively manage the situation. Trust your intuition that the person is potentially violent.
13. Staff activities may be counterproductive in managing aggressive behavior. Recogni-

tion and replacement of attitudes such as "I must be calm and relaxed at all times" with "No matter how anxious I feel, I will keep thinking and decide on the best approach" often will prevent escalation of aggression (Davies, 1989).

14. Although individuals may verbalize hostile threats and take a defensive stance, most are fearful of losing control and want assistance in maintaining their control (Lion, 1972).

15. A habitually violent person exhibits a wider-than-average body buffer zone (Davies, 1989).

16. Eye contact can increase arousal and be misinterpreted as hostility; the best approach is to maintain short periods of eye contact with no staring (Davies, 1989).

17. The least aggressive stance is at a 45° angle to the person versus face-to-face (Davies, 1989).

18. Crisis management techniques can help prevent escalation of aggression and help the person achieve self-control. The least restrictive safe and effective measure should be used (Sclafani, 1986).

19. Steps in crisis management include (Sclafani, 1986):
    a. Prevention through environmental considerations and attitudes
    b. Verbal intervention; first an individual, then a team, approach
    c. Pharmacologic intervention; rapid tranquilization can be accomplished using oral concentrations with some cooperative patients
    d. Mechanical restraint

20. Seclusion and restraint are options for a person exhibiting serious, persistent aggression. The person's safety must be protected at all times. Using the least restrictive measures allows the person the most opportunity to regain self-control (Ropor, Coutts, Sather, & Taylor, 1985).

21. Use of ambulatory waist restraints offers a less restrictive alternative to seclusion and restraint (Maier, Stava, Morrow, Van Rybroek, & Bauman, 1987).

■ High Risk for Violence
Related to (Specify)

Assessment
See Defining Characteristics

Outcome Criteria

The person will
- Demonstrate control of behavior with assistance from others
- Have a decreased number of violent responses
- Describe causation and possible preventive measures
- Explain rationale for interventions

Interventions

The nursing interventions for the diagnosis *High Risk for Violence* apply to any individual who is potentially violent regardless of related factors.

A. Promote interactions that will increase the individual's sense of trust

1. Acknowledge the individual's feelings. (*e.g.,* "You are having a rough time.")
   a. Be genuine and empathetic.
   b. Tell individual that you will help him control his behavior and not let him do anything destructive.
   c. Be direct and frank. ("I can see you are angry.")
   d. Be consistent and firm.
2. Set limits when individual presents a risk to others. Refer to *Anxiety* for further interventions on limit-setting.
3. Offer the individual choices and options. At times, it is necessary to give in on some demands to avoid a power struggle.
4. Encourage individual to express anger and hostility verbally instead of "acting out."
5. Encourage walking or exercise as activities that may diffuse aggression.
6. Maintain person's personal space.
   a. Do not touch the individual.
   b. Avoid feelings of physical entrapment of individual or staff.
7. Be aware of your own feelings and reactions.
   a. Do not take verbal abuse personally.
   b. Remain calm, if you are becoming upset, leave the situation in the hands of others, if possible.
   c. Following a threatening situation, ventilate your feelings with other staff.

B. Initiate immediate management of high-risk person

1. Allow the acutely agitated individual space that is five times greater than that for an individual who is in control. Do not touch the person unless you have a trusting relationship. Avoid physical entrapment of individual or staff.
2. Convey empathy by acknowledging the individual's feelings. Let him know you will not let him lose control.
3. Do not approach a violent individual alone. Often the presence of three to four staff members will be enough to reassure the individual that you will not let him lose control.
4. Give the individual control by offering him alternatives (*e.g.,* walking, talking).
5. Set limits. Use concise, easily understood statements.
6. When assault is imminent, quick, coordinated action is essential.
7. Approach individual in a calm, self-assured manner so as not to communicate your anxiety or fear.
8. Avoid using force in giving intramuscular injections when possible, since it serves to increase the person's sense of powerlessness. Use only when a clear danger to others or self exists.
9. If the person has a weapon, do not attempt to grab it. Instruct the person to put it down. Attempt to calm the person without risking bodily harm to yourself.

C. Establish an environment that reduces agitation

1. Decrease noise level.
2. Give short, concise explanations.
3. Control the number of persons present at one time.

    4. Provide single or semiprivate room.

    5. Allow individual to arrange personal possessions.

    6. Be aware that darkness can increase disorientation and enhance suspiciousness.

    7. Decrease situations in which the individual is frustrated.

D. Assist the individual in maintaining control over his behavior

    1. Establish the expectation that he can control his behavior, and continue to reinforce the expectation.

    2. Provide positive feedback when person is able to exercise restraint.

    3. Reassure individual that the staff will provide control if he cannot ("I am concerned about you, I will get [more staff, medications, etc.] to keep you from doing anything impulsive").

    4. Set firm, clear limits when individual presents a danger to self or others. ("Put the chair down.")

    5. Allow appropriate verbal expressions of anger. Give positive feedback.

    6. Set limits on verbal abuse. Do not take insults personally. Support others (clients, staff) who may be targets of abuse.

    7. Do not give attention to person who is being verbally abusive. Tell the person what you are doing and why.

    8. Assist with external controls, as necessary.

        a. Maintain observation every 15 to 30 minutes.

        b. Remove items that could be used as weapons (glass, sharp objects, etc.).

        c. Assess ability to tolerate off-unit procedures.

        d. If person is acutely agitated, be cautious with items such as hot coffee.

E. Plan for unpredictable violence

    1. Assess person's potential for violence and past history.

    2. Ensure availability of staff prior to potential violent behavior (never try to assist person alone when physical restraint is necessary).

    3. Determine who will be in charge of directing personnel to intervene in violent behavior if it occurs.

    4. Ensure protection for oneself (door nearby for withdrawal, pillow to protect face).

F. Utilize seclusion and/or restraint, if indicated

    1. Remove individual from situation if environment is contributing to aggressive behavior, using the least amount of control needed (*e.g.,* ask others to leave, and take individual to quiet room).

    2. Reinforce that you are going to help him control himself.

    3. Repeatedly tell the person what is going to happen before external control is begun.

    4. Protect individual from injuring self or others through use of restraints or seclusion.*

    5. When using seclusion, institutional policy will provide specific guidelines; the following are general.

        a. Observe individual at least every 15 minutes.

        b. Search the individual before secluding to remove harmful objects.

        c. Check seclusion room to see that safety is maintained.

---

* May require a physician's order.

    d. Offer fluids and food periodically (in nonbreakable containers).

    e. When approaching an individual to be secluded, have sufficient staff present.

    f. Explain concisely what is going to happen ("You will be placed in a room by yourself until you can better control your behavior") and give person a chance to cooperate.

    g. Assist person in toileting and personal hygiene (assess his ability to be out of seclusion; a urinal or commode may need to be used).

    h. If person is taken out of seclusion, someone must be present continually.

    i. Maintain verbal interaction during seclusion (provides information necessary to assess person's degree of control).

    j. When person is allowed out of seclusion, a staff member needs to be in constant attendance to determine whether person can handle additional stimulation.

  6. When using restraint, institutional policy will provide specifics. The following are general measures.

    a. A person in a 4-point or 2-point restraint must be in seclusion or with 1:1 nursing care for protection. Seclusion guidelines should be followed.

    b. Restraints must be loosened every hour (one limb at a time)

    c. Waist restraints must allow enough arm movement to enable eating/smoking and protecting self from falling.

    d. Restraints should be padded.

    e. Restraints never should be attached to side rails, but rather to the bed frame.

G. Assist individual in developing alternative coping strategies when crisis has passed and learning can occur

  1. Explore what precipitates the person's loss of control ("What was happening before you began to feel like hitting her?").

  2. Assist the person in recalling the physical symptoms associated with anger.

  3. Help person evaluate where in the chain of events change was possible.

    a. Use role play to practice communication techniques.

    b. Discuss how issues of control interfere with communication.

    c. Help the person recognize negative thinking patterns associated with low self-esteem.

  4. Practice negotiation skills with significant others and people in authority.

  5. Encourage an increase in recreational activities.

  6. Use group therapy to decrease sense of aloneness and increase communication skills.

    a. Instruct or refer for assertiveness training.

    b. Instruct or refer for negotiation skills development.

References/Bibliography

APA Task Force. (1974). *Clinical aspects of the violent individual.* Washington, D.C.: American Psychiatric Association.

Barash, D. (1984). Defusing the violent patient before he explodes. *RN, 47*(3), 35–37.

Davies, W. (1989). The prevention of assault of professional helpers. In Howells, K., & Hallin, C. (Eds.). *Clinical approaches to violence.* New York: John Wiley & Sons.

Grigson, J. (1984). Beyond patient management: The therapeutic use of seclusion and restraints. *Perspectives in Psychiatric Care, 22*(4), 137–142.

Harris, G. T., & Varnly, G. W. (1986). Assaults and assaulters in maximum security. *Research Reports, 3*(2), Mental Health Center, Penetanguishene, Ontario.

Knowles R. D. (1981). Dealing with feelings: Managing anger. *American Journal of Nursing, 81,* 2196–2197.

Lion, J. (1972). *Evaluation and management of the violent patient.* Springfield, IL: Charles C Thomas.

Maier, G., Stava, L., Morrow, B., Van Rybroek, G., & Bauman, K. (1987). A model for understanding and managing cycles of aggression among psychiatric inpatients. *Hospital and Community Psychiatry, 38*(5), 520–524.

Ropor, J., Coutts, A., Sather, J., & Taylor, R. (1985). Restraint and seclusion. *Journal of Psychosocial Nursing, 23*(6), 18–23.

Sclanfani, M. (1986). Violence and behavior control. *Journal of Psychosocial Nursing, 24*(1), 8–12.

Stewart, A. (1978). Handling the aggressive patient. *Perspectives in Psychiatric Care, 18*(3), 228–232.

Saunders, S., Anderson, A., & Hart, C. (Eds.). (1984). *Violent individuals and families: A handbook for practitioners.* Springfield, IL: Charles C Thomas.

Section III

Manual of Collaborative Problems

Introduction

This Manual of Collaborative Problems presents 37 specific collaborative problems grouped under eight generic collaborative problem categories. These problems have been selected because of their high incidence. Appendix XI provides a more comprehensive list. Information on each generic collaborative problem is presented under the following subheads:
- Physiologic Overview
- Definition
- Diagnostic Considerations: Discussion of the problem to clarify its clinical use
- Focus Assessment Criteria: Subjective and objective, guiding the nurse in data collection for client monitoring.
- Significant Laboratory Assessment Criteria: Laboratory findings useful in monitoring.

Discussions of the 37 specific collaborative problems cover the following information:
- Definition
- High-Risk Populations
- Nursing Goals: A statement specifying the nursing accountability for the collaborative problem
- Interventions: These specifically direct the nurse to:
  Monitor for onset or early changes in status
  Initiate physician-prescribed interventions as indicated
  Initiate nurse-prescribed interventions as indicated
  Evaluate the effectiveness of these interventions
- Rationale: A statement in parentheses explaining why a sign or symptom is present, or giving the scientific explanation for why an intervention will produce the desired response

Keep in mind that for many of the collaborative problems in Section III, associated nursing diagnoses can be predicted to be present. For example, a client with diabetes mellitus would receive care under the collaborative problem *PC: Hypo/Hyperglycemia* along with the nursing diagnosis *Potential Altered Health Maintenance related to insufficient knowledge of (specify);* a client with renal calculi would be under the collaborative problem *PC: Renal Calculi* and also the nursing diagnosis *Potential Altered Health Maintenance related to insufficient knowledge of prevention of recurrence, dietary restrictions, and fluid requirements.*

Potential Complication: Cardiac/Vascular

PC: Decreased Cardiac Output

PC: Dysrhythmias

PC: Pulmonary Edema

PC: Deep Vein Thrombosis

PC: Hypovolemic Shock

PC: Compartmental Syndrome

PC: Pulmonary Embolism

Cardiovascular System Overview

The cardiovascular system consists of the heart, arteries, arterioles, veins, venules, capillaries, and lymphatic vessels. The hollow, muscular heart pumps blood to tissues; blood supplies oxygen and other nutrients and carries away tissue waste products such as carbon dioxide back to the lungs. The liters per minute of blood pumped by the heart's ventricles during a given period—*cardiac output*—is affected by the amount of blood ejected with each heart beat—*stroke volume*. The cardiac index is the cardiac output divided by body surface area. Cardiac index reflects the heart's ability to meet body tissue demands. Any change in circulatory blood volume and/or in heart rate will affect cardiac index. The contractility or pumping action of the myocardium results from the stimulation of sympathetic and parasympathetic fibers supplying the heart. Additionally, the cardiac conduction system generates and sends electrical impulses throughout the myocardium. Problems that can alter these electrical impulses, leading to altered cardiac output, include cardiac muscle cell damage, tissue hypoxia, medications, and abnormal serum calcium or potassium levels. Disorders of the heart or circulatory system can cause serious, even fatal, hypoxic states.

Considered part of the circulatory system, the lymphatic system consists of capillaries, vessels, and nodes. This system contains and maintains the immune system, transports fluids and proteins from interstitial spaces back to the veins, and reabsorbs fats (chyme) from the small intestines.

Potential Complication: Cardiac/Vascular

DEFINITION

PC: Cardiac/Vascular: Describes a person experiencing or at high risk to experience various cardiac and/or vascular dysfunctions.

Diagnostic Considerations

The nurse can use this generic collaborative problem to describe a person at risk for several types of cardiovascular problems. For example, for a client in a critical care unit vulnerable to cardiovascular dysfunction, using *PC: Cardiovascular* would direct nurses to monitor cardiovascular status for various problems, based on focus assessment findings. Nursing interventions for this client would focus on detecting and diagnosing abnormal functioning.

For a client with a specific cardiovascular complication, the nurse would add the applicable collaborative problem to the client's problem list, along with specific nursing interventions for that problem. For example, a Standard of Care for a client postmyocardial infarction could contain the collaborative problem *PC: Cardiovascular*, directing nurses to monitor cardiovascular status. If this client later experienced a dysrhythmia, the nurse would add *PC: Dysrhythmia* to the problem list, along with specific nursing management information, *e.g., PC: Dysrhthymia related to myocardial infarction*. Even if the risk factors or etiology are not directly related to the primary medical diagnosis, the nurse still should add them, if known, *e.g., PC: Hypo/hyperglycemia related to diabetes mellitus* in a client who has sustained myocardial infarction.

Focus Assessment Criteria

Subjective Data

1. Chest discomfort (pain and/or pressure)
   a. Description (location, radiation, character, duration, severity, onset)
   b. Precipitating/aggravating factors (*e.g.*, activity, eating)
   c. Alleviating measures (*e.g.*, rest, medications)
   d. Associated symptoms (*e.g.*, nausea, vomiting, vertigo, diaphoresis)
2. Perception of heart rate (*e.g.*, too fast, skipping beats)
3. Complaints of
   a. Shortness of breath
   b. Lightheadedness
   c. Fatigue
   d. Nausea

Objective Data

1. Apical pulse
   a. Rate (normal, above 100 beats/min, below 60 beats/min)
   b. Rhythm (regular, irregular, pulse deficits)
   c. Apical-radial pulse deficit
   d. Heart sounds (normal, gallops, murmurs, friction rubs)
2. Jugular veins, at a 45° angle (nondistended or distended)
3. Blood pressure and pulse pressure, any postural changes
4. Bilateral pulses (radial, posterior tibial, dorsalis pedis, brachial, popliteal)
   a. Rate and rhythm
   b. Volume
      - 0 = Absent, nonpalpable
      - +1 = Thready weak, fades in and out
      - +2 = Present but diminished
      - +3 = Normal, easily palpable
      - +4 = Bounding
5. Skin
   a. Temperature (cool, warm)
   b. Color (pale, dependent rubor, flushed, cyanotic, mottled, brown discolorations)
   c. Ulcerations (size, location, description of surrounding tissue)
6. Edema (location, pitting or nonpitting)
7. Capillary refill time (normal, <3 sec)
8. Motor ability (normal or compromised)
9. Urine output
10. Level of orientation, anxiety

Significant Laboratory Assessment Criteria

1. Cardiac enzymes (elevated with cardiac tissue damage, *e.g.*, in myocardial infarction)
   a. Creatinine phosphokinase (CPK), isoenzymes
   b. Lactic dehydrogenase (LDH), isoenzymes
   c. LDH/LDH_2 ratio (LDH_2 is lower with MI)
2. Serum potassium (fluctuates with diuretic therapy, parenteral fluid replacement)
3. White blood cell count (elevated with inflammation)
4. Erythrocyte sedimentation rate (elevated with inflammation, tissue injury)
5. Arterial blood gas (ABG) values (lowered SaO_2 indicates hypoxemia; elevated pH, alkalosis; lowered pH, acidosis)
6. Coagulation studies (elevated with anticoagulant therapy or coagulopathies)
7. Hemoglobin and hematocrit (elevated with polycythemia, lowered with anemia)
8. ECG (ST segment changes, PR, QR, or QT interval changes, rate or rhythm changes)
9. Doppler ultrasonic flowmeter
10. Hemodynamic monitoring

PC: Decreased Cardiac Output

DEFINITION

PC: Decreased Cardiac Output: Describes a person experiencing or at high risk to experience inadequate blood supply for tissue needs due to insufficient blood pumping by the heart.

High-Risk Populations

- Acute myocardial infarction
- Aortic or mitral valve disease
- Cardiomyopathy
- Cardiac tamponade
- Hypothermia
- Septic shock
- Coarctation of the aorta
- Chronic obstructive pulmonary disease (COPD)
- Congenital heart disease
- Hypovolemia (e.g., due to severe bleeding or burns)
- Bradycardia
- Tachycardia
- Congestive heart failure
- Cardiogenic shock
- Hypertension

Nursing Goals

The nurse will manage and minimize episodes of decreased cardiac output.

Interventions

1. Monitor for signs and symptoms of decreased cardiac output/index:
   a. Increased and irregular pulse rate
   b. Increased respiratory rate
   c. Decreased blood pressure
   d. Abnormal heart/lung sounds
   e. Decreased urine output (<30 mL/hr)
   f. Changes in mentation
   g. Cool, moist, cyanotic, mottled skin
   h. Decreased capillary refill time
   i. Neck vein distention
   j. Weak peripheral pulses
   (Decreased cardiac output/index leads to an insufficient supply of oxygenated blood to meet the metabolic needs of tissues. Decreased circulating volume can result in hypoperfusion of the kidneys and decreased tissue perfusion with a compensatory response of decreased circulation to extremities and increased pulse and respiratory rates. Changes in mentation may result from cerebral hypoperfusion. Vasoconstric-

tion and venous congestion in dependent areas [*e.g.,* limbs] produce changes in skin and pulses.)

2. Initiate appropriate protocols or standing orders, depending on the underlying etiology of the problem affecting the function of the ventricles.
   (Nursing management will differ based on etiology, *e.g.,* measures to help increase preload for hypovolemia and to decrease preload for impaired ventricular contractility.)

3. Position the client with the legs elevated, unless ventricular function is impaired.
   (This position can help increase preload and enhance cardiac output.)

4. Avoid Trendelenburg's position.
   (This position increases pressure of abdominal organs on the diaphragm.)

5. During acute episodes, maintain absolute bed rest and minimize all controllable stressors. Administer IV morphine p.r.n. according to protocol. Use with caution if hypotensive.
   (These measures decrease metabolic demands.)

6. Assist the client with measures to conserve strength, such as resting before and after activities (*e.g.,* meals, baths).
   (Adequate rest reduces oxygen consumption and decreases the risk of hypoxia.)

7. In a client with impaired ventricular function, cautiously administer IV fluids. Consult with the physician if the ordered rate exceeds 125 mL/hr. Be sure to include any additional IV fluids (*e.g.,* antibiotics) when calculating the hourly allocation.
   (A client with poorly functioning ventricles may not tolerate increased blood volumes.)

8. If decreased cardiac output results from hypovolemia, septic shock, or dysrhythmia, refer to the specific collaborative problem in this section.

PC: Dysrhythmias

DEFINITION

PC: Dysrhythmias: Describes a person experiencing or at high risk to experience a disorder of the heart's conduction system that results in an abnormal heart rate, abnormal rhythm, or a combination of both.

High-Risk Populations

- Myocardial infarction
- Congestive heart failure
- Hypoendocrine or hyperendocrine status
- Increased intracranial pressure
- Electrolyte imbalance (calcium, potassium, magnesium)
- Atherosclerotic heart disease
- Digitalis therapy

- Medication side effects (*e.g.*, aminophylline, dopamine, stimulants, digoxin, β blockers, dobutamine, lidocaine, procainamide, quinidine, diuretics)
- COPD
- Cardiomyopathy
- Anemia
- Valvular heart disease
- Postoperative cardiac surgery

Nursing Goals

The nurse will manage and minimize dysrhythmic episodes.

Interventions

1. Monitor for signs and symptoms of dysrhythmias.
   a. Abnormal rate, rhythm
   b. Palpitations, chest pain
   c. Syncope
   d. ECG changes
   e. Hypotension
   (Ischemic tissue is electrically unstable, causing dysrhythmias, certain congenital cardiac conditions and electrolyte imbalances. Medications can also cause disturbances in cardiac conduction.)
2. Initiate appropriate protocols depending on the type of dysrhythmia; this may include
   a. Paroxysmal atrial tachycardia: vagal stimulation (direct or indirect), IV calcium channel blockers, digoxin (IV), synchronized cardioversion, overdrive pacing
   b. Atrial fibrillation: electrical cardioversion
   c. Premature ventricular contractions, ventricular tachycardia: IV lidocaine, IV procainamide, IV bretylium
   d. Ventricular tachycardia: oxygen, lidocaine, procainamide, bretylium, synchronized cardioversion
   e. Bradycardia or heart blocks: atropine, pacing, isuprel
   f. Ventricular fibrillation: CPR defibrillation, epinephrine, lidocaine, bretylium
   g. Electromechanical dissociation: CPR, epinephrine, rule out cause
   h. Asystole: CPR, epinephrine, atropine
3. Administer supplemental oxygen, if indicated.
   (Supplemental oxygen therapy increases circulating oxygen levels.)
4. Monitor serum electrolyte levels (*e.g.*, sodium, potassium, calcium, magnesium).
   (High or low electrolyte levels may exacerbate a dysrhythmia.)
5. Evaluate the client's response to treatment.

PC: Pulmonary Edema

DEFINITION
PC: Pulmonary Edema: Describes a person experiencing or at high risk to experience insufficient gas exchange due to accumulation of fluid related to left-sided heart failure.

High-Risk Populations
- Hypertension
- Dysrhythmias
- Myocardial infarction
- Congestive heart failure
- Cardiomyopathy
- Coronary artery disease
- Cardiac valve disease
- Diabetes mellitus
- Inhalation of toxins
- Drug overdose
- Smoking
- Aortic stenosis
- Mitral valve regurgitation

Nursing Goals
The nurse will manage and minimize episodes of pulmonary edema.

Interventions
1. Monitor for signs and symptoms of pulmonary edema.
   a. Dyspnea
   b. Tachycardia
   c. Adventitious breath sounds, moist rales
   d. Persistent cough
   e. Productive cough with frothy, pink-tinged sputum
   f. Cyanosis
   g. Abnormal ABGs
   h. Decreased O_2 saturation via pulse oximetry
   i. Decreased cardiac output
   (Impaired pumping of left ventricle accompanied by a decreased cardiac output and increased pulmonary venous pressure and pulmonary artery pressure produces pulmonary edema.)
2. If indicated, administer oxygen as prescribed.
   (A high rate could depress ventilatory drive.)
3. Initiate appropriate treatments according to protocol, which may include
   a. Diuretics, to decrease preload
   b. Vasodilators, to decrease afterload

    c. Positive inotropics (*e.g.,* digitalis), to increase ventricular contractions
    d. Morphine, to decrease anxiety, decreased preload and afterload, and lower metabolic demands
4. Evaluate hydration status based on urine specific gravity and serum osmolality values.
(These tests can help early detection of fluid deficit or excess.)
5. Take steps to maintain adequate hydration while avoiding overhydration.
(Adequate hydration helps liquefy pulmonary secretions; overhydration can increase preload.)
6. Change the client's position every 2 hours. Determine which position provides optimum oxygenation by analyzing ABG values in samples obtained with the client in various positions.
(Limiting time the client spends in positions that compromise oxygenation will improve PaO_2.)
7. Place the client in high Fowler's position with legs dependent if severely dyspneic.
(This positioning will help decrease venous return, increase venous pooling, and decrease preload.)
8. Minimize controllable stressors (*e.g.,* noise, long series of tests and procedures) and explain all procedures and treatments.
(These measures may reduce anxiety, which can help decrease metabolic demands.)
9. Continue monitoring cardiovascular status—vital signs, ABG values, cardiac output, fluid balance, weight.
(This monitoring helps evaluate the client's response to treatment.)

PC: Deep Vein Thrombosis

DEFINITION
PC: Deep Vein Thrombosis: Describes a person experiencing venous clot formation due to blood stasis, vessel wall injury, or altered coagulation.

High-Risk Populations
- Immobility
- Extremity paralysis
- Fractures
- Chemical irritation of vein
- Blood dyscrasias
- Orthopedic, urologic, or gynecologic surgery
- History of venous insufficiency
- Obesity
- Oral contraceptive use
- Malignancy
- Heart failure

Nursing Goals

The nurse will manage and minimize complications of deep vein thrombosis.

Interventions

1. Monitor the status of venous thrombosis, noting
   a. Diminished or absent peripheral pulses
      (Insufficient circulation causes pain and diminished peripheral pulses.)
   b. Unusual warmth and redness or coolness and cyanosis
      (Unusual warmth and redness points to inflammation; coolness and cyanosis indicate vascular obstruction.)
   c. Increasing leg pain
      (Leg pain results from tissue hypoxia.)
   d. Sudden severe chest pain, increased dyspnea, tachypnea
      (Obstructed pulmonary circulation causes sudden chest pain and dyspnea.)
   e. Positive Homans' sign.
      (In a positive Homans' sign, dorsiflexion of the foot causes pain, due to insufficient circulation.)
2. Consult physician for use of antiembolic stockings or sequential pressure devices.
   (These will reduce venous stasis and promote venous return.)
3. Evaluate hydration status based on urine specific gravity and serum osmolality. Take steps to ensure adequate hydration.
   (Increased blood viscosity and coagulability and decreased cardiac output contribute to thrombus formation.)
4. Encourage the client to perform isotonic leg exercises.
   (Isotonic leg exercises promote venous return.)
5. Elevate the affected extremity above the level of the heart.
   (This positioning can help reduce interstitial swelling by promoting venous return.)
6. Discourage the person from smoking.
   (Nicotine can cause vasospasms.)
7. Administer anticoagulant therapy as the physician prescribes, and monitor blood coagulation results daily.
   (Anticoagulant therapy prevents extension of a thrombosis by delaying the clotting time of blood.)
8. For a client receiving anticoagulant therapy, monitor for early signs of abnormal bleeding (*e.g.,* hematuria, bleeding gums, ecchymoses, petechiae, epistaxis).
   (Prolonged clotting time can increase the risk of bleeding.)
9. Administer analgesics for leg pain as ordered.

PC: Hypovolemic Shock

DEFINITION

PC: Hypovolemic Shock: Describes a person experiencing or at high risk to experience inadequate cellular oxygenation and inability to excrete waste products of metabolism secondary to decreased fluid volume (*e.g.,* from bleeding, plasma loss, prolonged vomiting or diarrhea).

High-Risk Populations

- Intraoperative status
- Postoperative status
- Anaphylactic shock
- Trauma
- Bleeding
- Diabetic ketoacidosis
- Prolonged vomiting or diarrhea
- Infants, children, elderly
- Acute pancreatitis
- Major burns
- Disseminated intravascular coagulation
- Rupture of esophageal varices
- Dissecting aneurysms

Nursing Goals

The nurse will manage and minimize hypovolemic episodes.

Interventions

1. Monitor fluid status; evaluate
   a. Intake (parenteral and oral)
   b. Output and other losses (urine, drainage, and vomiting)
      (Early detection of fluid deficit enables interventions to prevent shock.)
2. Monitor the surgical site for bleeding, dehiscence, and evisceration.
   (Careful monitoring allows early detection of complications.)
3. Teach the client to splint the surgical wound with a pillow when coughing, sneezing, or vomiting.
   (Splinting reduces stress on the suture line by equalizing pressure across the wound.)
4. Monitor for signs and symptoms of shock.
   a. Increased pulse rate with normal or slightly decreased blood pressure
   b. Urine output <30 mL/hr
   c. Restlessness, agitation, decreased mentation
   d. Increased respiratory rate
   e. Diminished peripheral pulses
   f. Cool, pale, moist, or cyanotic skin

g. Thirst

h. Decreased Hb/Hct

(The compensatory response to decreased circulatory volume aims to increase oxygen delivery through increased heart and respiratory rates and decreased peripheral circulation [manifested by diminished peripheral pulses and cool skin]. Decreased oxygen to the brain results in altered mentation. Decreased circulation to the kidneys leads to decreased urine output.)

5. If shock occurs, place the client in the supine position with legs elevated unless contraindicated (*e.g.,* if he has a head injury).

(This position increases blood return [preload] to the heart.)

6. Insert an IV line; use a large-bore catheter if blood replacement is anticipated. Initiate appropriate protocols for shock (*e.g.,* vasopressin therapy). Refer also to *PC: Acidosis* or *PC: Alkalosis,* if indicated, for more information.

(Protocols aim to increase peripheral resistance and elevate blood pressure.)

7. Collaborate with the physician to replace fluid losses at a rate sufficient to maintain urine output >0.5 mL/kg/hr.

(This measure promotes optimal tissue perfusion.)

8. Restrict the client's movement and activity.

(This helps decrease tissue demands for oxygen.)

9. Provide reassurance, simple explanations, and emotional support to help reduce anxiety.

(High anxiety increases metabolic demands for oxygen.)

PC: Compartmental Syndrome

DEFINITION

PC: Compartmental Syndrome: Describes a person experiencing or at high risk to experience inadequate tissue perfusion in a muscle, usually in the forearm or leg.

High-Risk Populations

- Muscle trauma
- Fracture
- Cast or constrictive dressing
- IABP therapy

Nursing Goals

The nurse will manage and minimize compartmental syndrome.

Interventions

1. Instruct the client to report any changes in sensation or appearance, even if slight. Determine whether these changes are new and different.

(Neurovascular compromise often begins as minor sensations or as loss of sensation; early detection enables prompt intervention to prevent serious complications.)

2. Elevate the affected extremity and apply ice for the first 24 to 48 hours after injury. (This will help reduce edema.)

3. If signs of compartmental syndrome develop, discontinue elevation. (Elevation will impede arterial flow.)

4. Assess peripheral circulation at least every hour for the first 24 hours. (Refer to Focus Assessment Criteria, page 882, for specific criteria.)

5. Monitor for signs and symptoms of compartmental syndrome.
   a. Unrelieved or increasing pain
   b. Swelling
   c. Color change (cyanosis or pallor)
   d. Cool skin (distal)
   e. Tingling or numbness
   f. Diminished or absent pulse
   g. Compromised movement of fingers or toes
   (These signs and symptoms point to venous or arterial obstruction and nerve compression.)

6. Warn the client not to mask pain with analgesics until the exact cause has been identified.
   (Identifying the location and nature of pain assists in differential diagnosis.)

7. Perform gentle range-of-motion exercises on the affected limb. Instruct the client to move the fingers or toes of the limb every 30 minutes.
   (Movement enhances circulation and muscle tone and reduces venous stasis.)

8. Notify the physician of any early signs and symptoms of neurovascular compromise.
   (The physician will evaluate the cause and determine the necessary treatment, *e.g.*, cast-splitting, removal of medical anti-shock trousers [MAST], removal of IABP, surgery [*e.g.*, fasciotomy].)

PC: Pulmonary Embolism

DEFINITION

PC: Pulmonary Embolism: Describes a person experiencing or at high risk to experience obstruction of one or more pulmonary arteries from a blood clot, air or fat embolus.

High-Risk Populations

- Prolonged immobilization
- Prolonged sitting/traveling
- Varicose veins
- Vascular injury
- Tumor

- Increased platelet count (*e.g.,* from polycythemia, splenectomy)
- Thrombophlebitis
- Vascular disease
- Presence of foreign bodies (*e.g.,* IV or central venous catheters)
- Heart disease (especially congestive heart failure)
- Surgery or trauma (especially of hip, pelvis, spine, lower extremities)
- Postoperative state
- Pregnancy
- Postpartum state
- Diabetes
- COPD
- History of previous pulmonary embolism or thrombophebitis
- Obesity
- Oral contraceptive use, estrogen therapy
- Acute spinal cord injury
- Thrombus formation in heart from cardioversion, bacterial endocarditis, atrial fibrillation, or myocardial infarction

For air embolism
- Central line insertion or removal
- Central line tubing changes

Nursing Goals

The nurse will manage and minimize complications of pulmonary embolism.

Interventions

1. Consult with the physician for low-dose heparin therapy for a high-risk client until ambulatory.
   (Heparin therapy will decrease blood viscosity and platelet adhesiveness, reducing the risk of embolism.)
2. Refer to the nursing diagnosis *High Risk for Altered Peripheral Tissue Perfusion* in Section II for information on preventing deep vein thrombosis.
3. Monitor for signs and symptoms of pulmonary embolism
   a. Acute, sharp chest pain
   b. Dyspnea, restlessness
   c. Cyanosis
   d. Tachycardia
   e. Neck vein distention
   f. Hypotension
   g. Acute right ventricular dilation without parenchymal disease (on chest x-ray)
   h. Confusion
   i. Cardiac dysrhythmias
   (Occlusion of pulmonary arteries impedes blood flow to the distal lung, producing a hypoxic state.)
4. If these manifestations occur, promptly initiate protocols for shock.
   a. Establish an IV line (for medication and fluid administration).
   b. Administer fluid replacement therapy according to protocol.
   c. Insert an indwelling urinary (Foley) catheter (to monitor circulatory volume through urine output).
   d. Initiate ECG monitoring and invasive hemodynamic monitoring (to detect dysrhythmias and guide therapy).

    e. Administer vasopressins to increase peripheral resistance and raise blood pressure.

    f. Administer sodium bicarbonate as indicated (to correct metabolic acidosis).

    g. Administer digitalis glycosides and IV diuretics and antiarrhythmic agents, as indicated.

    h. Administer small IV doses of morphine (to reduce anxiety and decrease metabolic demands).

    i. Refer to *PC: Hypovolemic Shock* for additional interventions.

    j. Prepare for angiography and/or perfusion lung scans (to confirm diagnosis and detect the extent of atelectasis).

    (Because death from massive pulmonary embolism commonly occurs in the first 2 hours after onset, prompt intervention is crucial.)

5. Initiate oxygen therapy via nasal cannula.
    (This measure will rapidly increase circulating oxygen levels.)

6. Monitor serum electrolyte levels, ABG values, blood urea nitrogen (BUN), and complete blood count results.
    (These laboratory tests help determine perfusion and volume status.)

7. Initiate thrombolytic therapy (*e.g.*, urokinase, steptokinase) per physician's orders.
    (Thrombolytics can cause lysis of emboli and increase pulmonary capillary perfusion.)

8. When prescribed after thrombolytic infusion, initiate heparin therapy (continuous IV infusion or intermittent). Monitor clotting times during heparin therapy.
    (Heparin can slow or halt the underlying thrombotic process, helping prevent clot extension or recurrence.)

For *PC: Air Embolism*

1. Before central line catheter insertion and tubing changes, place the client in Trendelenburg's position and instruct him to perform Valsalva's maneuver during the procedure.
    (These measures increase intrathoracic pressure and help prevent air from entering the catheter.)

2. Secure the proximal catheter connection with a Luer-Lok IV set, and tape all connections securely.
    (These measures will help prevent accidental tubing disconnection, the most common cause of air embolism.)

3. Tape a loop of IV tubing to the client's chest (Thielen, 1990).
    (This measure eliminates traction on the catheter, which can enlarge the insertion site and increase the risk of air entry.)

4. Use only clamps designed for central lines. If tubing is difficult to disconnect during changes, *do not* use hemostats—instead, try using a rubber tourniquet with ends wrapped around the tubing to improve your grip.
    (These measures can help prevent damage to the tubing and resultant air leaks.)

5. Explain the potential problems associated with tubing disconnection, and instruct the client to crimp the tubing near the entry site if separation occurs.
    (Immediate action can prevent air embolism.)

6. Before IV catheter removal, place the client in Trendelenburg's position and instruct him to perform Valsalva's maneuver or at least hold his breath during the procedure. After removal, immediately apply direct pressure to the catheterization site, then apply a sterile nonpermeable dressing. Leave the dressing in place for 24 to 48 hours.
    (These measures will help prevent air entry.)

7. Monitor for signs and symptoms of air embolism during dressing and IV tubing changes and after any accidental separation of IV connections.

    a. Sucking sound on insertion

b. Dyspnea

c. Tachypnea

d. Wheezing

e. Substernal chest pain

f. Anxiety

(Air embolism can occur with IV tubing changes, with accidental tubing separation, and during catheter insertion and disconnection. [For example, a client can aspirate as much as 200 mL of air from a deep breath during subclavian line disconnection.] Entry of air into the circulatory system can block blood flow and cause cardiac arrest.)

8. If air embolism is suspected

a. Place the client in steep Trendelenburg's position on the left side.

(This position allows air to be displaced away from the pulmonary valve and prevents more air from entering [Thielen, 1990].)

b. Administer oxygen via face mask according to protocol.

(This promotes diffusion of nitrogen, which will compress an air embolism in about 80% of cases.)

c. Initiate protocols for shock if indicated.

References/Bibliography

Bousquet, G. L. (1990). Congestive heart failure: A review of nonpharmacologic therapies. *Journal of Cardiovascular Nursing, 4*(3), 35–46.

Chulay, M. (1988). Arterial blood gas changes with a hyperinflation and hyperoxygenation suctioning interventions in surgical patients. *Heart & Lung, 17*(6), 654–661.

Curie, D. (1990). Pulmonary embolism: Diagnosis and management. *Critical Care Nursing Quarterly, 13*(2), 41–49.

Dillon, J. (1987). Rapid initiation of thrombolytic therapy for acute MI. *Critical Care Nursing, 9*(2), 55–61.

Hudak, C., Gallo, B., & Benz, J. (1990). *Critical care nursing* (5th ed.). Philadelphia: J. B. Lippincott.

Kleven, M. (1988). Comparison of thrombolytic agents: Mechanism of action, efficacy, and safety. *Heart & Lung, 17*(6), Suppl., 750–755.

Mahoney, E., & Flynn, J. (1986). *Handbook of medical-surgical nursing*. New York: John Wiley & Sons.

Miccolo, M. A. (1988). Management of patient with sudden cardiac death caused by ventricular dysrhythmias. *Journal of Cardiovascular Nursing, 3*(1), 1–13.

Rice, V. (1987). Acid-base derangements in the patient with cardiac arrest. *Focus on Critical Care, 14*(6), 53–61.

Thelan, L., Davie, J., & Urden, L. (1990). *Textbook of critical care nursing*. St. Louis: C. V. Mosby.

Thielen, J. B. (1990). Air emboli: A potentially lethal complication of central venous lines. *Focus on Critical Care, 17*(5), 374–383.

Potential Complication: Respiratory

PC: Hypoxemia

PC: Atelectasis/Pneumonia

PC: Tracheobronchial Constriction

PC: Pneumothorax

Respiratory System Overview

Respiratory functioning primarily depends on two systems: the conducting system and the respiratory center in the brain stem. Consisting of the upper airway (nose, nasal mucosa, pharynx, larynx, epiglottis) and lower airway (trachea, bronchi, bronchioles, alveoliar ducts), the conducting system conducts and filters air, traps foreign bodies to be expectorated or swallowed, and warms and humidifies inspired air. The lungs consist of three lobes on the right side and two lobes on the left side. Oxygen (O_2) is exchanged with carbon dioxide (CO_2) across the alveolar capillary membrane by simple diffusion, and wastes are removed by alveolar macrophages. Surfactant, a phospholipid secreted by the alveoli, prevents lung collapse by reducing surface tension of the lungs. Blood supply to the lung consists of pulmonary circulation and bronchial circulation.

Located in the medulla oblongata in the brain stem, the respiratory center increases or decreases respiratory rate in response to CO_2 and hydrogen ion (H^+) concentrations in the cerebrospinal fluid.

The diaphragm is the major muscle of respiration. Additional respiratory muscles are the external intercostals, the scaleni, and the sternocleidomastoid. Normally expiration is passive. Diaphragmatic movement during inspiration and expiration changes the space in the thoracic cavity, allowing the lungs to expand and deflate.

The right and left pulmonary arteries transport deoxygenated blood from the right side of the heart to the lungs. The pulmonary veins transport oxygenated blood to the left side of the heart to be pumped through the body. The bronchial circulation supplies the lungs with oxygenated blood for nutrition of the pulmonary nerves and ganglia, arteries, and veins, pleura, and connective tissue.

The mechanics of respiration can be adversely affected by various factors, including foreign body obstruction, excessive or thickened secretions, edema, and poor positioning. Respiratory muscle movements may be impeded due to fatigue, mechanical ventilation, or depression of the respiratory center. Perfusion at the alveolar level can be impaired by compromised cardiac functioning, inadequate blood supply, inadequate oxyhemoglobin levels, or abnormalities in the alveoli (*e.g.*, excessive mucus, tumor).

Potential Complication: Respiratory

DEFINITION

PC: Respiratory: Describes a person experiencing or at high risk to experience various respiratory problems.

Diagnostic Considerations

The nurse uses the generic collaborative problem *PC: Respiratory* to describe a person at risk for several types of respiratory problems and to identify the nursing focus—monitoring respiratory status for detection and diagnosis of abnormal functioning. Nursing management of a specific respiratory complication is then described under the appropriate collaborative problem for that complication. For example, a nurse using *PC: Respiratory* for a client who later develops hypoxemia would then add *PC: Hypoxemia* to the client's problem list. If the risk factors or etiology were not directly related to the primary medical diagnosis, the nurse would add this information to the diagnostic statement, *e.g., PC: Hypoxemia related to COPD* in a client with COPD (chronic obstructive pulmonary disease) who experiences respiratory problems after gastric surgery.

For a person vulnerable to respiratory problems due to immobility or excessive tenacious secretions, the nurse should apply the nursing diagnosis *High Risk for Altered Respiratory Function related to immobility* rather than *PC: Respiratory.*

Focus Assessment Criteria

Subjective Data

1. History of
   a. Allergies
   b. Bronchitis
   c. Asthma
   d. Emphysema
   e. Tuberculosis
   f. Respiratory infection
   g. Heart disease
   h. Sarcoidosis
   i. Exposure to environmental inhalants (chemical dusts, fumes, asbestos)
2. Medication use (prescribed and over-the-counter, immunizations)
3. Tobacco use (type, amount, length of time)
4. Complaints of
   a. Shortness of breath (related to activity, during sleep)
   b. Weight loss
   c. Fatigue

　　d. Fever and chills
　　e. Anorexia
　　f. Cough (dry or productive, sputum, frequency)

Objective Data
1. Thoracic expansion (symmetrical or asymmetrical)
2. Diaphragmatic excursion (normal: descends 3–6 cm; abnormal: descends <3 or >6 cm, equal bilaterally vesicular/bronchial)
3. Breath sounds in all lung fields (Figure III-1) (normal [vascular], rales, rhonchi, wheezes, pleural friction rub)
4. Ability to cough (effective or ineffective)
5. Effect of coughing on rhonchi

Significant Laboratory Assessment Criteria
1. Blood pH (elevated in alkalosis, lowered in acidosis)
2. Arterial blood gas (ABG) values
　　a. pH (elevated in alkalemia, lowered in acidemia)
　　b. PCO_2 (elevated in pulmonary disease, lowered in hyperventilation)
　　c. PO_2 (lowered in pulmonary disease)
　　d. CO_2 content (elevated in COPD, lowered in hyperventilation)

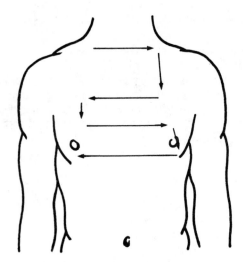

Fig. III-1 Sequence for chest auscultation.

PC: Hypoxemia

DEFINITION
PC: Hypoxemia: Describes a person experiencing or at high risk to experience insufficient plasma oxygen saturation (PO_2 less than normal for age) due to alveolar hypoventilation, pulmonary shunting, or ventilation–perfusion inequality.

High-Risk Populations
- COPD
- Pneumonia
- Atelectasis
- Pulmonary edema
- Adult respiratory distress syndrome (ARDS)
- Central nervous system depression
- Medulla or spinal cord disorders
- Guillain-Barré syndrome
- Myasthenia gravis
- Muscular dystrophy
- Obesity
- Compromised chest wall movement (*e.g.,* trauma)
- Drug overdose
- Head injury
- Near-drowning

Nursing Goals
The nurse will manage and minimize complications of hypoxemia.

Interventions
1. Monitor for signs of acid–base imbalance
   a. ABG analysis: pH <7.35, $PaCO_2$ >48 mm Hg
   (ABG analysis helps evaluate gas exchange in the lungs. In mild to moderate COPD, the client may have a normal $PaCO_2$ level as chemoreceptors in the medulla respond to increased $PaCO_2$ by increasing ventilation. In severe COPD, however, the client cannot sustain this increased ventilation, and the $PaCO_2$ value gradually increases.)
   b. Increased and irregular pulse, and increased respiratory rate initially, followed by decreased rate
   (Respiratory acidosis develops due to excessive CO_2 retention. A client with respiratory acidosis from chronic disease at first experiences increased heart rate and respirations in an attempt to compensate for decreased oxygenation. After a while, the client breathes more slowly and with prolonged expiration. Eventually, his respiratory center may stop responding to the higher CO_2 levels, and breathing may stop abruptly.)

   c. Changes in mentation (somnolence, confusion, irritability)
    (Changes in mentation result from cerebral tissue hypoxia.)
   d. Decreased urine output (<30 mL/hr); cool, pale, or cyanotic skin.
    (The compensatory response to decreased circulatory oxygen aims to increase blood oxygen by increasing heart and respiratory rates and to decrease circulation to the kidneys and to the extremities [marked by decreased pulses and skin changes].)

2. Administer low-flow (2 L/min) oxygen as needed via a mask or nasal cannula, if indicated.
(Oxygen therapy increases circulating oxygen levels. High flow rates increases CO_2 retention in persons with COPD. Using a cannula rather than a mask may help reduce the client's fears of suffocation.)

3. Evaluate the effects of positioning on oxygenation, using ABG values as a guide. Change the client's position every 2 hours, avoiding those positions that compromise oxygenation.
(This measure will promote optimal ventilation.)

4. Ensure adequate hydration. Teach the client to avoid dehydrating beverages (*e.g.,* caffeinated drinks, grapefruit juice).
(Optimal hydration will help liquefy secretions.)

5. Teach the client effective coughing technique.
(Effective coughing moves mucus from the lower airways to the trachea for expectoration.)

6. If the client cannot expectorate secretions, use coughing and/or chest physiotherapy to move secretions up from the trachea for suctioning.
(Suctioning is effective only at the tracheal level.)

7. Administer supplemental oxygen before and after suctioning.
(This measure helps prevent a decrease in PO_2 due to suctioning.)

8. Obtain a sputum sample for culture and sensitivity and Gram stain testing.
(Sputum culture and sensitivity determine whether an infection is contributing to symptoms.)

9. Eliminate smoke and strong odors from the client's room.
(Irritation of the respiratory tract can exacerbate symptoms.)

10. Monitor the ECG for dysrhythmias secondary to altered oxygenation.
(Hypoxemia may precipitate cardiac dysrhythmias.)

11. Monitor for signs of right-sided congestive heart failure
   a. Elevated diastolic pressure
   b. Distended neck veins
   c. Peripheral edema
   d. Elevated central venous pressure (CVP)
(The combination of arterial hypoxemia and respiratory acidosis acts locally as a strong vasoconstrictor of pulmonary vessels. This leads to pulmonary arterial hypertension, increased right ventricular systolic pressure, and, eventually, right ventricular hypertrophy and failure.)

12. Refer to the nursing diagnosis category *Activity Intolerance* in Section II for specific adaptive techniques to teach a client with chronic pulmonary insufficiency.

PC: Atelectasis, Pneumonia

DEFINITION

PC: Atelectasis, Pneumonia: Describes a person experiencing impaired respiratory functioning due to alveolar collapse, which can result in pneumonia.*

High-Risk Populations

- Postoperative status (abdominal or thoracic surgery)
- Immobilization
- Decreased level of consciousness
- Nasogastric feedings
- Chronic lung disease
- Debilitation
- Decreased surfactant production
- Compression of lung tissue (*e.g.,* from cancer, abdominal distention, obesity, pneumothorax)
- Airway obstruction

Nursing Goals

The nurse will manage and minimize complications of atelectasis or pneumonia.

Interventions

1. Monitor respiratory status and assess for signs and symptoms of inflammation.
   a. Increases respiratory rate
   b. Fever and chills (sudden or insidious)
   c. Productive cough
   d. Diminished or absent breath sounds
   e. Pleuritic chest pain
   f. Tachycardia
   g. Marked dyspnea
   h. Cyanosis
   (Tracheobronchial inflammation, impaired alveolar capillary membrane function, edema, fever, and increased sputum production disrupt respiratory function and compromise the blood's oxygen-carrying capacity.)
2. Monitor for signs and symptoms of infection.
   a. Fever of 101°F (39.4°C) or higher
   b. Chills
   c. Tachycardia
   d. Manifestations of shock: restlessness or lethargy, confusion, decreased systolic blood pressure

*The nurse should use the nursing diagnosis category *Potential Altered Respiratory Function* for persons at high risk for atelectasis and pneumonia, to focus on prevention. The collaborative problem *PC: Atelectasis, Pneumonia* is applicable only if the condition occurs.

(Bacteria can act as a pyrogen by raising the hypothalamic thermostat through the production of endogenous pyrogens, which may mediate through prostaglandins. Chills can occur when the temperature set-point of the hypothalamus changes rapidly. High fever increases metabolic needs and oxygen consumption. The impaired respiratory system cannot compensate; tissue hypoxia results.)

3. If fever occurs, provide cooling measures (*e.g.,* reduced clothing and bed linen, tepid baths, increased fluids, hypothermia blanket).
   (Reducing body temperature is necessary to lower metabolic rate and reduce oxygen consumption.)

4. Monitor for signs and symptoms of septic shock.
   a. Subnormal body temperature
   b. Hypotension
   c. Decreased level of consciousness
   d. Weak, rapid pulse
   e. Rapid, shallow respirations
   f. Cold, clammy skin
   g. Oliguria
   (Septic shock may develop in a client with pneumonia if treatment is delayed or if the causative organism is drug resistant.)

5. Evaluate the effectiveness of cough suppressants and expectorants.
   (A dry, hacking cough interferes with sleep and affects energy. Cough suppressants should be used judiciously, however, because complete depression of the cough reflex can lead to atelectasis by hindering movement of tracheobronchial secretions.)

6. Maintain oxygen therapy, as prescribed, and monitor its effectiveness.
   (Oxygen therapy may help prevent dyspnea and also reduce the risk of pulmonary edema.)

7. Provide respiratory physiotherapy (*e.g.,* chest percussion, postural drainage) to move thick, tenacious secretions along the tracheobronchial tree.
   (Exudate in the alveoli and bronchospasms linked to increased bronchopulmonary secretions can decrease ventilatory effort and impair gas exchange.)

8. Teach the client how to do diaphragmatic breathing.
   (This technique increases tidal volume by maximizing diaphragmatic descent.)

9. Refer to *PC: Hypoxemia* for additional interventions.

PC: Tracheobronchial Constriction

DEFINITION

PC: Tracheobrochial Constriction: Describes a person experiencing or at high risk to experience airflow limitations through the tracheobronchial tree due to asthma, bronchitis, emphysema, and/or allergic reaction.

High-Risk Populations
- COPD
- Allergies
- Asthma
- Chronic bronchitis

Nursing Goals
The nurse will manage and minimize episodes of tracheobronchial constriction.

Interventions
1. Monitor respiratory status continuously during acute exacerbation; evaluate
   a. Use of accessory muscles
   b. Respiratory rate, pulse rate, blood pressure
   c. Breath sounds (*e.g.,* wheexing)
   d. ABG values
   e. Peripheral perfusion (skin color, pulses)
   f. Level of consciousness.
   (A client's respiratory status can change rapidly, with specific changes depending on response to treatments, level of fatigue, and severity of the episode.)
2. Administer oxygen via nasal cannula at a rate of 2 to 3 L/min.
   (Oxygen therapy reduces hypoxemic effects; using a cannula rather than a mask may help minimize feelings of suffocation.)
3. Ensure adequate hydration either orally or intravenously.
   (Good hydration status helps prevent tenacious, impacted mucus.)
4. During acute episodes, stay with the client and have him breathe using pursed-lip or diaphragmatic breathing.
   (A panicky, dyspneic client will need a nurse's constant presence to help him gain control over his breathing.)
5. Maintain the client in an upright position.
   (The upright position promotes optimal lung expansion.)
6. Initiate physician-prescribed interventions, which may include bronchodilators, β-adrenergic agents, theophylline preparations, or corticosteroids.
7. Avoid administering narcotics and sedatives.
   (Sedation depresses respiratory drive.)
8. Monitor for medication side effects (*e.g.,* dysrhythmias, hypotension, hypertension, vomiting, theophylline blood levels).
   (Early detection of side effects enables prompt intervention to minimize their seriousness.)
9. Monitor for early signs of status asthmaticus (Summers, 1985).
   a. Previous severe asthma attack
   b. Little or no response to bronchodilator therapy after 1 hour
   c. Altered level of consciousness
   (Status asthmaticus is not relieved by usual treatment for an acute asthmatic episode and requires IV corticosteroids.)
10. Consult with the physician for possible intubation if the work of breathing becomes increasingly difficult for the client.
   (Exhaustion brought on by excessive respiratory effort can lead to pulmonary arrest.)
11. When indicated, initiate health teaching, using the nursing diagnosis *Potential Altered Health Maintenance related to insufficient knowledge of (specify)*.

PC: Pneumothorax

DEFINITION

PC: Pneumothorax: Describes a person experiencing or at high risk to experience accumulation of air in the pleural space due to lung injury.

High-Risk Populations

- Severe blunt or penetrating chest injury
- Postoperative status (cardiac or thoracic surgery)
- Mechanically ventilated with PEEP

Nursing Goals

The nurse will manage and minimize complications of pneumothorax.

Interventions

1. Monitor for signs and symptoms of pneumothorax.
   a. Acute pleuritic chest pain
   b. Dyspnea, tachypnea, tachycardia
   c. Hyperresonant percussion sounds with loss of breath sounds over the affected side
   d. Shifting of trachea
   (Early detection and prompt intervention are necessary to prevent serious complications.)
2. Administer oxygen, if indicated. If chronic CO_2 retention occurs, limit the liter flow rate to no more than 2 L/min.
   (Higher flow rates can depress ventilatory drive.)
2. Prepare for stat chest x-ray.
4. Evaluate the need for analgesics to manage thoracic pain.
   (Pain will interfere with lung expansion on inspiration, compromising oxygenation.)
5. Position the client with the head of the bed elevated, unless contraindicated.
   (This position helps maximize lung expansion.)
6. Reposition the client every 2 hours, keeping the unaffected lung in the dependent position.
   (This position limits pain and improves oxygenation by better equalizing ventilation and perfusion [Thelan, Davie, & Urdan, 1990].)
7. Explain and supervise deep breathing with sustained maximum inspiration.
   (Deep breathing expands the lungs and evacuates air from the pleural space into the chest drainage system [if present].)
8. Instruct the person to avoid coughing except when necessary to clear secretions.
   (Coughing increases pain.)
9. Minimize environmental stimuli, provide emotional support, and offer simple explanations for all procedures.
   (These measures may help reduce anxiety, which will increase respiratory rate.)

10. If use of a chest drainage system is indicated, follow institutional protocols for setup, assessment, and maintenance.

References/Bibliography

Brown, L. H. (1990). Pulmonary oxygen toxicity. *Focus on Critical Care, 17*(1), 68–75.

Capps, J. S. (1988). Work of breathing: Clinical monitoring and considerations in the critical care setting. *Critical Care Nursing Quarterly, 11*(3), 1–11.

Demers, R. R. (1987). Down with the good lung casualty [Editorial]. *Respiratory Care, 32*(10), 849.

Fontaine, D. K. (1989). Positioning as a nursing therapy in trauma care. *Critical Care Nursing Clinics of North America, 9*(2), 105–121.

Hudak, C., Gallo, B., & Benz, J. (1990). *Critical care nursing* (5th ed.). Philadelphia: J. B. Lippincott.

Mahoney, E., & Flynn, J. (1986). *Handbook of medical-surgical nursing.* New York: John Wiley & Sons.

Mims, B. C. (1989). Fat embolism syndrome, a variant of ARDS. *Orthopedic Nursing, 8*(3), 22–27.

Pfister, S. M. (1989). Arterial blood gas evaluation: Metabolic acidemia. *Critical Care Nurse, 9*(1), 70–72.

Preusser, B., Stone, K., Gonyon, S., & Winningham, M. L. (1988). Effects of two methods of preoxygenation on mean arterial pressure, cardiac output, peak airway pressure, and postsuctioning hypoxemia. *Heart & Lung, 17*(3), 290–299.

Reischman, R. R. (1988). Impaired gas exchange related to intrapulmonary shunting. *Critical Care Nurse, 8*(8), 45–49.

Summers, W. R. (1985). Status asthmaticus. *Chest* (Suppl.), *1*(2), 87s–89s.

Thelan, L., Davie, J., & Urden, L. (1990). *Textbook of critical care nursing.* St. Louis: C. V. Mosby.

Potential Complication: Metabolic/Immune/ Hematopoietic

PC: Hypo/Hyperglycemia

PC: Negative Nitrogen Balance

PC: Electrolyte Imbalances

PC: Septicemia

PC: Acidosis (Metabolic, Respiratory)

PC: Alkalosis (Metabolic, Respiratory)

PC: Allergic Reaction

PC: Thrombocytopenia

PC: Immunodeficiency

Metabolic/Immune/Hematopoietic System Overview

Metabolic functioning influences all physical and chemical changes occurring within the body. *Catabolism* refers to the breakdown of ingested substances into simpler substances (*e.g.,* food); *anabolism* refers to the conversion of ingested substances to protoplasm for cellular activities and tissue growth and repair.

For proper metabolic functioning, adequate amounts of carbohydrates, protein, fats, vitamins, electrolytes, minerals, and trace elements are needed. These nutrients are digested and absorbed into circulating blood and lymph.

Carbohydrates provide the preferred source of energy for cellular activity and are broken down into glucose, fructose, and galactose. Serum glucose levels are controlled primarily by the pancreatic hormones, insulin and glucagon. Insulin facilitates glucose transport into cells. Glucagon, which stimulates the conversion of liver glycogen to glucose, is available for release when the blood glucose level falls below normal.

Proteins provide the structural basis of all lean body mass and are required for visceral functions, initiation of chemical reactions, transportation of apoproteins, preservation of immune function, maintenance of osmotic pressure, and blood neutrality (Thelan, 1990). Proteins are broken down by gastric and pancreatic digestion into amino acids. About half the amino acids digested come from ingested foods (essential); the other half is derived from enzymes secreted into the intestine and from desquamated mucosal cells (nonessential). Nonessential amino acids cannot be manufactured if the supply of essential amino acids is inadequate. Nitrogen remains after protein is metabolized and must be excreted by the kidneys.

Lipids or fats (fatty acids, triglycerides, phospholipids, cholesterol, cholesterol esters) are responsible for insulation, structure and temperature control, and the manufacture of prostaglandins, and serve as carriers of fat-soluble vitamins. Lipids also are a stored source of energy when glucose supply is low (*e.g.*, an overnight fast).

Dietary fats are hydrolyzed in the small intestine to form short-chain and long-chain fatty acids. Bile from the gallbladder emulsifies the fat so that pancreatic lipase can break down the fat more effectively. Short-chain fatty acids are absorbed and transported to the liver; long-chain fatty acids are transported by the lymphatic system to the liver and other tissues. When fatty acids are utilized for energy, ketones are produced. Large amounts of circulating ketones can cause metabolic acidosis.

Endocrine glands—the pituitary, adrenals, thyroid, parathyroids, and parts of the pancreas—secrete various hormones into the bloodstream. These hormones control metabolic functions such as rate of chemical reaction in cells, transport of substances across cell membranes, and growth and secretion. Chemical and neurologic stimuli regulate the release of hormones. Chemical control is accomplished by negative feedback *e.g.*, rise or fall of one blood level of a hormone causes a corresponding rise or fall of the blood level of another hormone.

Neurologic stimuli are controlled by the autonomic and central nervous systems (CNS). For example, the autonomic system regulates blood pressure via glandular secretions and release of renin. In response to stimuli, the CNS activates the hypothalamus, which in turn activates the pituitary. Depending on the problem, the pituitary can then activate various other glands. Altered endocrine functions include hypofunction, hyperfunction, secondary failure, functional disorders, end-stage organ failure, abnormal hormone production, inborn errors of metabolism, ectopic hormone secretion, and organ-induced endocrine dysfunction.

The hematopoietic system encompasses the functions of blood and blood-forming processes. A type of connective tissue, blood contains plasma and cellular components. Plasma is composed of ions, proteins (*e.g.*, albumin, globulins), nonprotein nitrogen, glucose, and electrolytes. Albumin maintains an osmotic force that keeps fluid within the vascular space. Globulins are varied and have distinct purposes (*e.g.*, gamma globulins are antibodies). Cellular components of blood include erythrocytes, leukocytes, platelets, and fat droplets (chylomicrons). In the interior of spongy bones and the central cavity of long bones, red bone marrow produces blood cells.

The primary functions of the hematopoietic system include blood cell production (bone marrow); oxygen transport to tissues (erythrocytes; clot formation (platelets); defense against bacterial, viral (*e.g.*, lymphocyte B cell), fungal, and parasitic infections, cancer, and foreign tissue invasion (lymphocyte T cell); and providing anticoagulation (basophils).

Potential Complication: Metabolic/Immune/Hematopoietic

DEFINITION

PC: Metabolic/Immune/Hematopoietic: Describes a person experiencing or at high risk to experience various endocrine, immune, or metabolic dysfunctions.

Diagnostic Considerations

The nurse can use this generic collaborative problem to describe a person at risk for several types of metabolic and immune system problems. For example, for a client with pituitary dysfunction, who is at risk for various metabolic problems, using *PC: Metabolic/Immune* will direct nurses to monitor endocrine system function for specific problems, based on focus assessment findings. Under this collaborative problem, nursing interventions would focus on monitoring metabolic status to detect and diagnose abnormal functioning. If the client developed a specific complication, the nurse would add the appropriate specific collaborative problem, along with nursing management information, to the client's problem list. For a client with diabetes mellitus, the nurse would add the diagnostic statement *PC: Hypo/Hyperglycemia*. For a client receiving chemotherapy, the nurse would use *PC: Immunodeficiency,* a collaborative problem that encompasses leukopenia, thrombocytopenia, and erythrocytopenia. If thrombocytopenia were an isolated problem, it would warrant a separate diagnostic statement *i.e., PC: Thrombocytopenia.*

For a client with a condition or undergoing a treatment that produces immunosuppression (*e.g.,* AIDS, graft versus host disease, immunosuppressant therapy), the collaborative problem *PC: Immunosuppression* would be appropriate. When conditions have or possibly could have affected coagulation (*e.g.,* chronic renal failure, alcohol abuse, anticoagulant therapy), a collaborative problem such as *PC: Hemolysis* or *PC: Erythrocytopenia* would be indicated. If the risk factors or etiology were not directly related to the primary medical diagnosis, they could be added, *e.g., PC: Immunosuppression related to chronic corticosteroid therapy* in a client who has sustained a myocardial infarction.

Focus Assessment Criteria

Subjective Data

1. Complaints of change in appearance of face, hair (distribution, growth, texture), skin (pigmentation, dryness) eyesight, weight (gain or loss)
2. Complaints of headaches, change in libido and/or menses, excessive sweating, easy bruising, poor wound healing, sensitivity to cold or heat, nausea, anorexia, excessive urination, excessive thirst, excessive appetite, diarrhea, constipation, easy fatigability, frequent infections

Objective Data

1. Temperature
2. Pulse, respiration
3. Blood pressure
4. Urine: ketones, specific gravity
5. Weight for height
6. Ability to eat
7. Diet: calories and protein adequate to meet metabolic demands

Significant Laboratory Assessment Criteria

1. Serum amylase (elevated in acute pancreatitis, lowered in chronic pancreatitis)
2. Serum albumin (lowered in malnutrition)
3. Lymphocyte count (lowered in malnutrition)
4. Serum calcium (elevated in hyperparathyroidism, certain cancers, and acute pancreatitis, lowered in hypoparathyroidism)
5. Blood pH (elevated in alkalosis, lowered in acidosis)
6. Serum glucose (elevated in diabetes mellitus and pancreatic insufficiency, lowered in pancreatic islet cell tumors)
7. Urine acetone (present in diabetes mellitus)
8. Urine glucose (present in diabetes mellitus)
9. Urine ketone bodies (present in uncontrolled diabetes)
10. Platelets (elevated in polycythemia and chronic granulocytic leukemia, lowered in anemia and acute leukemia)
11. Immunoglobins (elevated in autoimmune disease)
12. Coagulation tests (elevated in thrombocytopenia, purpura, and hemophilia)
13. Prothrombin time (elevated in anticoagulant therapy, cirrhosis, and hepatitis)
14. RBC count (lowered in anemia, leukemia, and renal failure)

PC: Hypo/Hyperglycemia

DEFINITION

PC: Hypo/Hyperglycemia: Describes a person experiencing or at high risk to experience a blood glucose level that is too low or too high for metabolic function.*

High-Risk Populations

- Diabetes mellitus
- Parenteral nutrition
- Sepsis

---

*If the person is not at risk for both, the diagnosis should specify the problem (e.g., PC: Hyperglycemia related to corticosteroid therapy).

- Enteral feedings
- Corticosteroid therapy
- Neonate of diabetic mother
- Small for gestational age neonate
- Neonate of narcotic-addicted mother
- Thermal injuries (severe)
- Pancreatitis (hyperglycemia), cancer of pancreas
- Addison's disease (hypoglycemia)
- Adrenal gland hyperfunction
- Liver disease (hypoglycemia)

Nursing Goals

The nurse will manage and minimize episodes of hypoglycemia or hyperglycemia.

Interventions

For Hypoglycemia

1. Monitor serum glucose level at the bedside before administering hypoglycemic agents and/or before meals and hour of sleep.
   (Serum glucose is a more accurate parameter than urine glucose, which is affected by renal threshold and renal function.)
2. Monitor for signs and symptoms of hypoglycemia.
   a. Blood glucose <70 mg/dL
   b. Pale, moist, cool skin
   c. Tachycardia, diaphoresis
   d. Jitteriness, irritability
   e. Headache, slurred speech
   f. Incoordination
   g. Drowsiness, confusion
   h. Visual changes
   i. Hunger, nausea, abdominal pain
   (Hypoglycemia [insufficient glucose levels] can result from excessive insulin, insufficient food intake, or excessive physical activity. A rapid drop in blood glucose level stimulates the sympathetic system to produce adrenaline, which causes diaphoresis, cool skin, tachycardia, and jitteriness. A slowly falling blood glucose level depresses the CNS, causing problems such as headaches, slurred speech, incoordination, drowsiness, and visual changes. Insufficient glucose levels also can cause hunger and GI distress.)
3. If the client can swallow, give him 1/2 cup of orange juice, cola, or ginger ale every 15 minutes until his blood glucose level reaches >69 mg/dL.
   (Simple carbohydrates are metabolized quickly.)
4. If the client cannot swallow, administer glucagon hydrochloride subcutaneously or 50 mL of 50% glucose in water IV, according to protocol.
   (Glucagon causes glycogenolysis in the liver in the presence of adequate glycogen stores. In a client in critical condition who has been in a coma for some time, glycogen stores likely have already been used up, and IV glucose will be the only effective treatment.)
5. Recheck blood glucose level 1 hour after an initial blood glucose reading of >69 mg/dL.
   (Regular monitoring detects early signs of high or low levels.)
6. If indicated, consult with a dietitian to provide a complex carbohydrate snack at bedtime.
   (This measure can help prevent hypoglycemia during the night.)

For Hyperglycemia
1. Monitor for signs and symptoms of ketoacidosis.
   a. Blood glucose >300 mg/dL
   b. Positive plasma ketone, acetone breath
   c. Headache
   d. Kussmaul's respirations
   e. Anorexia, nausea, vomiting
   f. Tachycardia
   g. Decreased BP
   h. Polyuria, polydipsia
   i. Decreased serum sodium, potassium, and phosphate levels
   (When insulin is not available, blood glucose levels rise and the body metabolizes fat and protein for energy-producing ketone bodies. Excessive ketone bodies cause headaches, nausea, vomiting, and abdominal pain. Respiratory rate and depth increase in an attempt to increase CO_2 excretion and reduce acidosis. Glucose inhibits water reabsorption in the renal glomerulus, leading to osmotic diuresis with severe loss of water, sodium, potassium, and phosphates.)
2. If ketoacidosis occurs, initiate appropriate protocols to reverse dehydration, restore the insulin-glucagon ratio, treat circulatory collapse, ketoacidosis and electrolyte imbalance (Thelan, 1990):
   a. IV of physiologic saline or half-strength sodium chloride
   (Infusion rate will be adjusted according to urinary output to achieve rapid hydration.)
   b. IV infusion of 5% dextrose when serum glucose is 250 to 300 mg/dL
   (This will replenish glucose stores and prevent cerebral edema.)
   c. Insulin in IV fluids (approximately 6–10 units/hr)
   (Insulin is needed to facilitate entry of glucose in cells.)
   d. IV potassium and phosphate supplements
   (Deficits may occur as potassium and phosphate returns to the cells due to insulin.)
   e. IV bicarbonate
   (For severe acidosis (pH >7), bicarbonate >5 mEq/L.)
3. Continue to monitor hydration status every ½ hour, assess skin moisture and turgor, urine output and specific gravity, and fluid intake.
   (Accurate assessments are needed during the acute stage (first 10–12 hr) to prevent overhydration or underhydration.)
4. Continue to monitor blood glucose levels every ½ hour until stable.
   (Careful monitoring enables early detection of medication-induced hypoglycemia or continued hyperglycemia.)
5. Monitor serum potassium, sodium, and phosphate levels.
   (Acidosis will cause hyperkalemia and hyponatremia. Insulin therapy promotes potassium and phosphate return to the cells, causing serum hypokalemia and hypophosphatmia).
6. Monitor neurologic status every hour.
   (Fluctuating glucose levels, acidosis, and fluid shifts can affect neurologic functioning.)
7. Carefully protect the client's skin from microorganism invasion, injury, and shearing force; reposition every 1 to 2 hours.
   (Dehydration and tissue hypoxia increase the skin's vulnerability to injury.)
8. Do not allow a recovering client to drink large quantities of water. Give a conscious client ice chips to quench thirst.
   (Excessive fluid intake can cause abdominal distention and vomiting.)

9. Monitor for signs and symptoms of hyperosmolar hyperglycemic nonketotic (HHNK) coma
   a. Blood glucose 600 to 2000 mg/dL
   b. Serum sodium normal or elevated
   c. Serum potassium normal or elevated
   d. Serum osmolality >350 mOsm/kg
   e. Hypotension
   f. Dehydration
   g. Altered sensorium
   (A state of excessive hyperglycemia precipitated by insufficient insulin, increased endogenous glucose, or increased exogenous glucose, HHNK coma can occur in response to acute stress (*e.g.,* from myocardial infarction, burns, severe infection, dialysis, or hyperalimentation). Persons with type II insulin-resistant diabetes who experience marked dehydration are especially at risk. Glucose inhibits water reabsorption in the renal glomerulus, leading to osmotic diuresis with loss of water, sodium, potassium, and phosphates. Cerebral impairment results from intracellular dehydration in the brain.)
10. Monitor cardiac function and circulatory status; evaluate
    a. Rate, rhythm
    b. Skin color
    c. Capillary refill time
    d. Peripheral pulses
    e. Serum potassium
    (Severe dehydration can cause reduced cardiac output and compensatory vasoconstriction. Cardiac dysrhythmias can result from potassium imbalances.)
11. Follow protocols for ketoacidosis, as indicated.
12. Investigate for causes of ketoacidosis or hypoglycemia and teach prevention and early management, using the nursing diagnosis *High Risk for Altered Health Maintenance related to insufficient knowledge of (specify)* (see Section II).

PC: Negative Nitrogen Balance

DEFINITION

PC: Negative Nitrogen Balance: Describes a person experiencing or at risk to experience tissue breakdown occurring faster than the body's ability to repair it.

High-Risk Populations

- Severe malnutrition
- Prolonged NPO state
- Elderly with chronic disease
- Uncontrolled diabetes

- Digestive disorders
- Prolonged use of glucose or saline IV therapy
- Inadequate enteral replacement
- Excessive catabolism (*e.g.,* due to cancer, infection, burns)
- Anorexia nervosa, bulimia
- Critical illness
- Chemotherapy
- Sepsis

Nursing Goals
The nurse will manage and minimize negative nitrogen balance.

Interventions
1. Establish the client's optimum weight for height.
   (This establishes baseline goals.)
2. Weight the client daily at the same time, wearing same amount of clothes, same scale, and same bedding.
   (Monitoring weight will help detect excessive catabolism.)
3. Monitor for signs of negative nitrogen balance.
   a. Weight loss
   b. 24-hour urine nitrogen balance below zero
   (Cachexia results from the increased metabolic demands, insufficient replacement, and anorexia. Impaired carbohydrate metabolism causes increased metabolism of fats and protein, which—especially in the presence of metabolic acidosis—can lead to negative nitrogen balance and weight loss.)
4. Monitor for signs and symptoms of hypoalbuminemia, which can have a rapid or insidious onset
   a. Emotional depression, fatigue
   (These effects result from decreased energy supplies.)
   b. Muscle wasting
   (This results from insufficient protein available for tissue repair.)
   c. Poorly healing wounds
   (See b. above.)
   d. Edema
   (Edema results from a plasma to interstitial fluid shift due to insufficient vascular osmotic pressure.)
5. Monitor laboratory values.
   a. Serum albumin and transferrin
   (These values evaluate viscera/protein.)
   b. Blood urea nitrogen (BUN)
   (This value measures kidney clearance ability.)
   c. Creatinine/height index
   (This indicates the degree of protein depletion.)
   d. Electrolytes, osmolality
   (These values help assess kidney function.)
   e. Total lymphocyte count
   (Lymphocyte production requires protein.)
6. Continually reevaluate the client's energy/protein requirements. Consult with a registered dietitian for evaluation (*e.g.,* indirect calorimetry test, anthropometric measures).
   (The person's calorie/protein requirements will change depending on metabolic demands *e.g.,* from stress, fever, or infection.)

7. Administer total parenteral solutions, intralipid fat emulsions, and/or enteral formulas as prescribed by the physician and in accordance with appropriate procedures and protocols.
   (This client's increased caloric requirements for tissue repair cannot be met with routine IV therapy.)
8. For specific nursing interventions to increase oral nutrient intake, refer to the nursing diagnosis *Altered Nutrition: Less than Body Requirements* (see Section II).

PC: Electrolyte Imbalances*

■ *PC:* **Hypokalemia**

■ *PC:* **Hyperkalemia**

■ *PC:* **Hyponatremia**

■ *PC:* **Hypernatremia**

■ *PC:* **Hypocalcemia**

■ *PC:* **Hypercalcemia**

■ *PC:* **Hypophosphatemia**

■ *PC:* **Hyperphosphatemia**

■ *PC:* **Hypomagnesemia**

■ *PC:* **Hypermagnesemia**

■ *PC:* **Hypochloremia**

■ *PC:* **Hyperchloremia**

DEFINITION

PC: Electrolyte Imbalances: Describes a person experiencing or at risk to experience a deficit or excess of one or more electrolytes.

---

* For a person experiencing or at high risk to experience a deficit or excess in a single electrolyte, the diagnostic statement should specify the problem (*e.g., PC: Hypocalcemia related to diuretic therapy*).

High-Risk Populations

For Hypokalemia
- Crash dieting
- Metabolic or respiratory alkalosis
- Excessive intake of licorice
- Diuretic therapy
- Loss of GI fluids (through excessive NG suctioning, nausea, vomiting, or diarrhea)
- Steroid use
- Estrogen use
- Hyperaldosteronism
- Severe burns
- Decreased potassium intake
- Liver disease with ascites
- Renal tubular acidosis
- Malabsorption
- Severe catabolism
- Salt depletion
- Hemolysis
- Hypoaldosteronism
- Rhaldomyolysis

For Hyperkalemia
- Renal failure
- Excessive potassium intake (oral or IV)
- Cell damage (*e.g.,* from burns, trauma, surgery)
- Crushing injuries
- Potassium-sparing diuretic use
- Metabolic acidosis
- Transfusion of old blood
- Internal hemorrhage

For Hyponatremia
- Water intoxication (oral or IV)
- Renal failure
- Gastric suctioning
- Vomiting, diarrhea
- Burns
- Potent diuretic use
- Excessive diaphoresis
- Excessive wound drainage
- CHF
- Hyperglycemia
- Malabsorption syndrome
- Syndrome of inappropriate ADH (resulting from CNS disorders, major trauma, malignancies, or endocrine disorders)

For Hypernatremia
- Elderly, infants
- Inadequate fluid intake
- Heat stroke
- Diarrhea
- Severe insensible fluid loss (*e.g.,* through hyperventilation or sweating)
- Diabetes insipidus
- Excessive sodium intake (oral, IV, medications)

- Hypertonic tube feeding
- Coma

For Hypocalcemia
- Renal failure ($\uparrow$ phosphorus)
- Protein malnutrition (*e.g.,* due to malabsorption)
- Inadequate calcium intake
- Diarrhea
- Burns
- Malignancy
- Hypoparathyroidism
- Vitamin D deficiency
- Excessive antacid use

For Hypercalcemia
- Excessive vitamin D intake
- Hyperparathyroidism
- Decreased hypophosphatemia
- Bone tumors
- Cancers (Hodgkin's disease, myeloma, leukemia)
- Prolonged use of thiazide diuretics
- Paget's disease
- Parathyroid hormone–secreting tumors (*e.g.,* lung, kidney)
- Hemodialysis
- Multiple fractures
- Prolonged immobilization

For Hypophosphatemia
- Diabetic ketoacidosis
- Prolonged use of IV dextrose solutions
- Malabsorption disorders
- Renal wasting of phosphorus
- Low phosphate diet (oral, TPN)
- Rickets
- Excessive use of phosphate binders

For Hyperphosphatemia
- Excessive vitamin D intake
- Renal failure
- Healing fractures
- Bone tumors
- Hypoparathyroidism
- Hypocalcemia
- Phosphate laxatives
- Excessive IV or PO phosphate
- Chemotherapy
- Catabolism
- Lactic acidosis

For Hypomagnesemia
- Malnutrition
- Prolonged diuretic use
- Chronic alcoholism
- Excessive lactation
- Severe diarrhea, NG suctioning
- Cirrhosis
- Severe dehydration

- Ulcerative colitis
- Toxemia
- Prolonged IV therapy without magnesium

For Hypermagnesemia
- Renal failure
- Severe dehydration with oliguria
- Excessive intake of magnesium-containing antacids, laxatives
- Thiazide use

For Hypochloremia
- Loss of GI fluids (*e.g.,* through vomiting, diarrhea, suctioning)
- Metabolic alkalosis
- Diabetic acidosis
- Prolonged use of IV dextrose
- Excessive diaphoresis
- Excessive diuretic use
- Ulcerative colitis
- Fever
- Acute infections
- Severe burns

For Hyperchloremia
- Metabolic acidosis
- Severe diarrhea
- Excessive parenteral isotonic saline solution infusion
- Urinary diversion
- Renal failure
- Cushing's syndrome
- Hyperventilation
- Eclampsia
- Anemia
- Cardiac decompensation

Nursing Goals

The nurse will manage and minimize episodes of electrolyte imbalance.

Interventions

Identify the electrolyte imbalance(s) for which the client is vulnerable, and intervene as follows. (Refer to High-Risk Populations under the specific imbalance.)

PC: Hypo/hyperkalemia

1. Monitor for signs and symptoms of hyperkalemia.
   a. Weakness to flaccid paralysis
   b. Muscle irritability
   c. Paresthesias
   d. Nausea, abdominal cramping, or diarrhea
   e. Oliguria
   f. ECG changes: tall, peaked T wave, bradycardia, wide QRS complex, prolonged PR interval and flat or absent P wave
   (Hyperkalemia can result from the kidney's decreased ability to excrete potassium or from excessive potassium intake. Acidosis increases the release of potassium from cells. Fluctuations in potassium level affect neuromuscular transmission, producing cardiac dysrhythmias, and reducing action of GI smooth muscle.)

2. For a client with hyperkalemia
   a. Restrict potassium-rich foods, fluids, and IV solutions with potassium.
      (High potassium levels necessitate a reduction in potassium intake.)
   b. Provide range-of-motion (ROM) exercises to extremities.
      (ROM improves muscle tone and reduces cramps.)
   c. Per physician orders or protocols give medications to reduce serum potassium levels, *e.g.,*
      • IV calcium
        (To temporarily block effects on the heart muscle)
      • Sodium bicarbonate, glucose, insulin
        (To force potassium back into cells)
      • Cation-exchange resins (*e.g.,* kayexalate, hemodialysis)
        (To force excretion of potassium)
3. Monitor for signs and symptoms of hypokalemia.
   a. Weakness or flaccid paralysis
   b. Decreased or absent deep tendon reflexes
   c. Hypoventilation, change in consciousness
   d. Polyuria
   e. Hypotension
   f. Paralytic ileus
   g. ECG changes: U wave, flat or inverted T wave, dysrhythmias, and prolonged QT interval
   (Hypokalemia results from losses associated with vomiting, diarrhea, or diuretic therapy, or from insufficient potassium intake. Hypokalemia impairs neuromuscular transmission and reduces the efficiency of respiratory muscles. Kidneys are less sensitive to antidiuretic hormone [ADH] and thus excrete large quantities of dilute urine. Gastrointestinal smooth muscle action also is reduced. Abnormally low potassium levels also impair electrical conduction of the heart.)
4. For a client with hypokalemia
   a. Encourage increased intake of potassium-rich foods.
      (An increase in dietary potassium intake helps ensure potassium replacement.)
   b. If parenteral potassium replacement (always diluted) is instituted, do not exceed 20 mEq/hr in adults. Monitor serum potassium levels during replacement.
      (Excessive levels can cause cardiac dysrhythmias.)
   c. Observe the IV site for infiltration.
      (Potassium is very caustic to tissues.)

PC: Hypo/hypernatremia

1. Monitor for signs and symptoms of hyponatremia.
   a. CNS effects ranging from lethargy to coma, headache
   b. Weakness
   c. Abdominal pain
   d. Muscle twitching or convulsions
   (Hyponatremia results from sodium loss through vomiting, diarrhea, or diuretic therapy; excessive fluid intake; or insufficient dietary sodium intake. Cellular edema, caused by osmosis, produces cerebral edema, weakness, and muscle cramps.)
2. For a client with hyponatremia, initiate IV sodium chloride solutions and discontinue diuretic therapy, as ordered.
   (These interventions will prevent further sodium losses.)
3. Monitor for signs and symptoms of hypernatremia with fluid overload.
   a. Thirst, decreased urine output

b. CNS effects ranging from agitation to convulsions

c. Elevated serum osmolality

d. Weight gain

(Hypernatremia results from excessive sodium intake or increased aldosterone output. Water is pulled from the cells, causing cellular dehydration and producing CNS symptoms. Thirst is a compensatory response to dilute sodium.)

4. For a client with hypernatremia

a. Initiate fluid replacement in response to serum osmolality levels, as ordered. (Rapid reduction in serum osmolality can cause cerebral edema and seizures.)

b. Monitor for seizures. (Sodium excess causes cerebral edema.)

5. Monitor I & O, weight (This will evaluate fluid balance.)

PC: Hypo/hypercalcemia

1. Monitor for signs and symptoms of hypocalcemia.

a. Altered mental status

b. Numbness or tingling in fingers and toes

c. Muscle cramps

d. Seizures

e. ECG changes: prolonged QT interval, prolonged ST segment, and dysrhythmias (Hypocalcemia can result from the kidney's inability to metabolize vitamin D [needed for calcium absorption]. Retention of phosphorus causes a reciprocal drop in serum calcium level. A low serum calcium level produces increased neural excitability, resulting in muscle spasms [cardiac, facial, extremities] and CNS irritability [seizures]. It also causes cardiac muscle hyperactivity, as evidenced by ECG changes.)

2. For a client with hypocalcemia

a. Per physician orders for acute hypocalcemia, administer calcium via IV bolus infusion.

b. Consult with the dietitian for a high-calcium, low-phosphorus diet. (Lower serum calcium level necessitates dietary replacement.)

c. Assess for hyperphosphatemia or hypomagnesemia. (Hyperphosphatemia inhibits calcium absorption; in hypomagnesemia, the kidneys will excrete calcium to retain magnesium.)

d. Monitor for ECG changes: prolonged QT interval, irritable dysrhythmias, and AV conduction defects. (Calcium imbalances can cause cardiac muscle hyperactivity.)

3. Monitor for signs and symptoms of hypercalcemia.

a. Altered mental status

b. Anorexia, nausea, vomiting, constipation

c. Numbness or tingling in fingers and toes

d. Muscle cramps

(Insufficient calcium level reduces neuromuscular excitability resulting in decreased muscle tone, numbness, anorexia, and mental lethargy.)

4. For a client with hypercalcemia

a. Initiate normal saline IV therapy and loop diuretics, as ordered; avoid thiazide diuretics. [IV fluids will dilute serum calcium. Loop diuretics enhance calcium excretion; thiazide diuretics inhibit calcium excretion.]

b. Per physician's order, administer phosphorus preparations and mithramycin

(contraindicated in clients with renal failure.) (These will increase bone deposition of calcium.)
c. Monitor for renal calculi (see PC: Renal Calculi).

PC: Hypo/hyperphosphatemia

1. Monitor for hypophosphatemia.
   a. Muscle weakness, pain
   b. Bleeding
   c. Depressed white cell function
   d. Confusion
   e. Anorexia
   (Phosphorus deficiency impairs cellular energy resources and oxygen delivery to tissues and also causes decreased platelet aggregation.)
2. For a client with hypophosphatemia, per physician order replace phosphorus stores slowly via oral supplements, discontinue phosphate binders.
   (This helps prevent precipitation with calcium.)
3. Monitor for signs and symptoms of hyperphosphatemia.
   a. Tetany
   b. Numbness or tingling in fingers and toes
   c. Soft tissue calcification
   (Hyperphosphatemia can result from the kidneys' decreased ability to excrete phosphorus. Elevated phosphorus does not cause symptoms in itself but contributes to tetany and other neuromuscular symptoms in the short term and to soft tissue calcification in the long term.)
4. For a client with hyperphosphatemia
   a. Administer phosphorus-binding antacids, calcium supplements, or vitamin D and restrict phosphorus-rich foods.
   (Supplements are needed to overcome vitamin D deficiency and to compensate for a calcium-poor diet. High phosphate decreases calcium, which increases parathyroid hormone [PTH]. PTH is ineffective in removing phosphates due to renal failure but causes calcium reabsorption from bone and decreases tubular reabsorption of phosphate.)

PC: Hypo/hypermagnesemia

1. Monitor for hypomagnesemia
   a. Dysphagia, nausea, anorexia
   b. Muscle weakness
   c. Facial tics
   d. Athetoid movements (slow, involuntary twisting movements)
   e. Cardiac dysrhythmias, flat or inverted T waves, prolonged Q-T intervals
   f. Confusion
   (Magnesium deficit causes neuromuscular changes and hyperexcitability.)
2. For a client with hypomagnesemia, initiate magnesium sulfate replacement (dietary for mild deficiency, parenteral for severe deficiency), as ordered.
3. Initiate seizure precautions.
   (This will protect from injury.)
4. Monitor for hypermagnesemia.
   a. Decreased blood pressure, bradycardia, decreased respirations
   b. Flushing
   c. Lethargy, muscle weakness
   d. Peaked T waves

(Magnesium excess causes depression of central and peripheral neuromuscular function, producing vasodilation.)
5. If respiratory depression occurs, consult with the physician for possible hemodialysis. (Magnesium-free dialysate will cause excretion.)

PC: Hypo/hyperchloremia

1. Monitor for hypochloremia.
   a. Hyperirritability
   b. Slow respirations
   c. Decreased blood pressure
   (Hypochloremia occurs with metabolic alkalosis which results in loss of calcium and potassium which produces the symptoms.)
2. For a client with hypochloremia, see *PC: Alkalosis* for interventions.
3. Monitor for hyperchloremia.
   a. Weakness
   b. Lethargy
   c. Deep, rapid breathing
   (Metabolic acidosis causes loss of chloride ions.)
4. For a client with hyperchloremia, see *PC: Acidosis* for interventions.

PC: Septicemia

DEFINITION

PC: Septicemia: Describes a person experiencing or at high risk to experience a systemic response to the presence of pathogenic bacteria, viruses, fungi, or their toxins in the blood.

High-Risk Populations

- Burns
- Infection (GI, urinary, biliary tract)
- Immunosuppression
- Invasive lines (urinary, arterial, or central venous catheter)
- AIDS
- Disseminated cancer
- Pressure ulcers
- Extensive slow-healing wounds
- Surgical wound infection (gram-negative)
- Diabetes mellitus
- Malnutrition
- Postpartum status
- Cirrhosis
- Chronic illness

Nursing Goals

The nurse will manage and monitor the complications of septicemia.

Interventions

1. Monitor for signs and symptoms of septicemia:
   a. Temperature >101°F (38.3°C) or <98.6°F (37°C)
   b. Tachycardia and tachypnea
   c. Pale, cool skin
   d. Decreased urine output
   e. WBCs and bacteria in urine
   f. Positive blood culture
   g. Change in level of consciousness
   h. Abnormal arterial blood gases
   (Response to sepsis results in massive vasodilatation with hypovolemia, resulting in tissue hypoxia and decreased renal function and cardiac output. This in turn triggers a compensatory response of increased heart rate and respirations to correct hypoxia and acidosis.)
2. Per physician orders, initiate IV antimicrobial therapy.
   (This treatment combats gram-negative or gram-positive organisms.)
3. If indicated refer to *PC: Hypovolemic Shock* for more information.

PC: Acidosis (Metabolic, Respiratory)*

DEFINITION

PC: Acidosis: Describes a person experiencing or at high risk for experiencing an acid–base imbalance due to increased production of acids or excessive loss of base.

High-Risk Populations

For Respiratory Acidosis
- Hypoventilation
- Acute pulmonary edema
- Airway obstruction
- Pneumothorax
- Sedative overdose
- Severe pneumonia
- COPD
- Asthma

* When indicated, the nurse should specify the diagnosis as either *PC: Metabolic Acidosis* or *PC: Respiratory Acidosis*.

For Metabolic Acidosis
- Diabetes mellitus
- Lactic acidosis
- Late-phase salicylate poisoning
- Uremia
- Methanol or ethylene glycol ingestion
- Diarrhea
- Intestinal fistulas
- Intake of large quantities of isotonic saline or ammonium chloride

Nursing Goals

The nurse will manage and minimize complications of acidosis.

Interventions

For Metabolic Acidosis
1. Monitor for signs and symptoms of metabolic acidosis.
   a. Rapid, shallow respirations
   b. Headache
   c. Nausea and vomiting
   d. Negative base excess
   e. Behavior changes, drowsiness
   f. Increased serum potassium
   g. Increased serum chloride
   h. $PCO_2 < 35$ to 40 mm Hg
   i. Decreased HCO_3
   (Metabolic acidosis results from the kidney's inability to excrete hydrogen ions, phosphates, sulfates, and ketone bodies. Bicarbonate loss results when the kidney reduces its reabsorption. Metabolic acidosis is aggravated by hyperkalemia, hyperphosphatemia, and decreased bicarbonate levels. Excessive ketone bodies cause headaches, nausea, vomiting, and abdominal pain. Respiratory rate and depth increase to increase CO_2 excretion and reduce acidosis. Acidosis affects the CNS and can increase neuromuscular irritability because of the cellular exchange of hydrogen and potassium.)
2. For a client with metabolic acidosis
   a. Initiate IV fluid replacement as ordered, depending on the underlying etiology. (Dehydration may result from gastric and urinary fluid losses.)
   b. If the etiology is diabetes mellitus, refer to *PC: Hypo/Hyperglycemia* for interventions.
   c. Assess for signs and symptoms of hypocalcemia, hypokalemia, and alkalosis as acidosis is corrected.
   (Rapid correction of acidosis may cause rapid excretion of calcium and potassium and rebound alkalosis.)
   d. Correct, per physician orders, any electrolyte imbalances. Refer to *PC: Electrolyte Imbalances* for specific interventions for each type of electrolyte imbalance.
   e. Monitor ABG values, urine pH.
   (These values help evaluate the effectiveness of therapy.)

For Respiratory Acidosis
1. Monitor for signs and symptoms of respiratory acidosis.
   a. Tachycardia
   b. Dysrhythmias
   c. Diaphoresis

 d. Nausea and/or vomiting
 e. Restlessness
 f. Dyspnea
 g. Increased respiratory effort
 h. Decreased respiratory rate
 i. Increased PCO_2
 j. Normal or decreased PO_2
 k. Increased serum calcium
 l. Decreased sodium chloride
(Respiratory acidosis can occur when an impaired respiratory system is unable to remove CO_2, or when compensatory mechanisms that stimulate increased cardiac and respiratory efforts to remove excess CO_2 are overtaxed. An elevated $PaCO_2$ is the chief criterion. Elevated $PaCO_2$ increases cerebral blood flow, which decreases perfusion to heart, kidneys, and GI tract.)
 4. For a client with respiratory acidosis
  a. Improve ventilation by
   • Positioning with head of bed up
    (To promote diaphragmatic descent)
   • Coaching in deep-breathing with prolonged expiration
    (To increase exhalation of CO_2)
   • Aiding expectoration of mucus followed by suctioning, if needed
    (To improve ventilation perfusion)
  b. Consult with the physician for possible use of mechanical ventilation if improvement does not occur after the above interventions.
  c. Administer oxygen after the client is breathing better.
   (Use of oxygen is of no value if the client is not breathing effectively [Thelan, 1990].)
  d. Promote optimal hydration.
   (This helps liquefy secretions and prevent mucus plugs.)
  e. Limit use of sedatives and tranquilizers.
   (Both can cause respiratory depression.)
  f. Initiate Interventions 2a–2e to correct acidosis.

PC: Alkalosis (Metabolic, Respiratory)*

DEFINITION

PC: Alkalosis: Describes a person experiencing or at high risk for experiencing an acid–base imbalance due to excessive bicarbonate or loss of hydrogen ions.

---

 *When indicated, the nurse should specify the diagnosis as either *PC: Metabolic Alkalosis* or *PC: Respiratory Alkalosis.*

High-Risk Populations
For Respiratory Alkalosis
- Hyperventilation
- Severe infection
- Asthma
- Overlyvigorous mechanical ventilation
- Restricted diaphragmatic movement (*e.g.,* due to obesity, pregnancy)
- Inadequate oxygen in inspired air
- Congestive heart failure
- Alcohol intoxication
- Cirrhosis
- Thyrotoxicosis
- Paraldehyde, epinephrine, early salicylate overdose
- Overrapid correction of metabolic acidosis

For Metabolic Alkalosis
- Prolonged vomiting, gastric suctioning, diarrhea
- Use of potent diuretics (*e.g.,* thiazides), with resultant hydrogen and potassium loss
- Corticosteroid therapy
- IV replacement with potassium-free IV solutions
- Primary and secondary hyperaldosteronism
- Adrenocortical hormone disease
- Prolonged hypercalcemia or hypokalemia
- Excessive correction of metabolic acidosis

Nursing Goals
The nurse will manage and minimize complications of alkalosis.

Interventions
For Metabolic Alkalosis
1. Monitor for early signs and symptoms of metabolic alkalosis:
   a. Tingling of fingers, dizziness
   b. Hypertonic muscles (tremors)
   c. Hypoventilation (to conserve carbonic acid)
   d. Increased HCO_3
   e. Slightly increased PCO_2
   f. Decreased serum chloride
   g. Decreased serum potassium
   h. Decreased serum calcium
   (A decrease in ionized calcium produces most symptoms.)
2. For a client with metabolic alkalosis
   a. Initiate physician order for parenteral fluids.
      (To correct sodium, water, chloride deficits.)
   b. Monitor carefully the administration of ammonium chloride if ordered.
      (Ammonium chloride increases the amount of circulating hydrogen ions, which result in a decrease in pH. Treatment can cause too-rapid decrease in pH and hemolysis of RBCs.
   c. Evaluate renal and hepatic function prior to administration of ammonium chloride.
      (Impaired renal or hepatic function cannot accommodate increased hemolysis.)
   d. Administer sedatives and tranquilizers cautiously, if ordered.
      (Both depress respiratory function.)

    d. Monitor ABG values, urine pH, serum electrolyte levels, and BUN.
       (These values help evaluate response to treatment and detect rebound metabolic acidosis resulting from too-rapid correction.)

For Respiratory Alkalosis

1. Monitor for respiratory alkalosis.
   - Lightheadedness
   - Numbness
   - Tingling
   - Muscle weakness
   - Normal or decreased HCO_3
   - Decreased PCO_2
   - Decreased serum potassium
   - Increased serum chloride
   - Decreased serum calcium

(Decrease in plasma carbonic acid content causes vasoconstriction, decreased cerebral blood flow, and decreased ionized calcium.)

4. For a client with respiratory alkalosis
   a. Determine the cause of hyperventilation.
      (Different etiologies will warrant different interventions, *e.g.,* anxiety versus incorrect mechanical ventilation.)
   b. Calm the anxious person by maintaining eye contact and remaining with him or her.
      (Anxiety will increase respiratory rate and CO_2 retention.)
   c. Instruct the person to breathe slowly with you.
      (This will increase CO_2 retention.)
   d. Alternatively, have the anxious person breathe into a paper bag and rebreathe from the bag.
      (This will increase $PaCO_2$ as the person rebreathes his own exhaled CO_2.)
   e. If anxiety is causative, refer to the nursing diagnoses *Anxiety* and *Ineffective Breathing Patterns* in Section II for additional interventions.
   f. Consult with the physician for use of sedation as necessary.
      (Sedation can help reduce respiratory rate and anxiety.)
   g. Monitor ABG values and electrolyte levels (*e.g.,* potassium, calcium).
      (Monitoring these values helps evaluate the client's response to treatment.)
   h. As necessary, refer to *PC: Electrolyte Imbalances* for specific management of electrolyte imbalance.

PC: Allergic Reaction

DEFINITION

PC: Allergic Reaction: Describes a person experiencing or at high risk to experience hypersensitivity and release of mediators to specific substances (antigens).

High-Risk Populations

- History of allergies
- Asthma
- Immunotherapy
- Individuals exposed to high-risk antigens:
  Insect stings (*e.g.,* bee, wasp, hornet, ant)
  Animal bites/stings (*e.g.,* stingray, snake, jellyfish)
  Radiologic iodinated contrast media (*e.g.,* used in arteriography, intravenous pyelography)
  Transfusion of blood and blood products
- High-risk individuals exposed to
  High-risk medications (*e.g.,* aspirin, antibiotics, tetanus, opiates, local anesthetics, animal insulin, chymopapain)
  High-risk foods (*e.g.,* peanuts, chocolate, eggs, seafood, shellfish, strawberries, milk)
  Chemicals (*e.g.,* floor waxes, paint, soaps, perfume)

Nursing Goals

The nurse will manage and minimize complications of allergic reactions.

Interventions

1. Carefully assess of history of allergic responses (*e.g.,* rashes, difficulty breathing). (Identifying a high-risk client allows precautions to prevent anaphylaxis.)
2. If the client has a history of allergic response, consult with the physician regarding skin tests, if indicated.
   (Skin testing can confirm hypersensitivity.)
3. Monitor for signs and symptoms of localized allergic reaction.
   a. Wheals, flares (due to histamine release)
   b. Itching
   c. Nontraumatic edema (perioral, periorbital)
   (These early manifestations can indicate the beginning of a continuum of localized reaction to systemic reaction to anaphylactic shock.)
4. At the first sign of hypersensitivity, consult with the physician for pharmacologic intervention, such as antihistamines.
   (Antihistamines are commonly used to treat mild localized reactions by inhibiting histamine release.)

5. Monitor for signs and symptoms of systemic allergic reaction and anaphylaxis.
    a. Skin flushing and slight hypotension (resulting from histamine-induced vaso-dilation)
    b. Wheezing, hoarseness, dyspnea, and chest tightness (due to smooth muscle contraction from prostaglandin release)
    c. Irregular, increased pulse and decreased blood pressure (due to leukotriene release, which constricts airways and coronary vessels)
    d. Decreased level of consciousness, respiratory distress, and shock (resulting from severe hypotension, respiratory insufficiency, and tissue hypoxia)
    (Within minutes, such reactions can progress to severe hypotension, decreased level of consciousness, and respiratory distress and can prove rapidly fatal.)
6. Promptly initiate emergency protocol for anaphylaxis and/or stat page physician.
    a. Start an IV line.
    (For rapid medication administration)
    b. Administer epinephrine IV or endotracheally.
    (To produce peripheral vasoconstriction, which raises blood pressure and acts as a β-agonist to promote bronchial smooth muscle relaxation, and to enhance ino-tropic and chronotropic cardiac activity)
    c. Administer oxygen, establish a patent airway if indicated. Oropharyngeal intu-bation may be required.
    (Larynegeal edema will interfere with breathing.)
7. Administer other medications, as ordered, which may include
    a. Corticosteroids
    (To inhibit enzyme and WBC response to reduce bronchoconstriction)
    b. Aminophylline
    (To produce bronchodilation)
    c. Vasopressins
    (To counter profound hypotension)
    d. Diphenhydramine
    (To prevent further antigen–antibody reaction)
8. Frequently evaluate response to therapy; assess
    a. Vital signs
    b. Level of consciousness
    c. Lung sounds
    d. Cardiac function
    e. Intake and output
    f. ABG values
    (Careful monitoring is necessary to detect complications of shock and identify the need for additional interventions.)
9. After recovery, discuss with the client and family preventive measures for an-aphylaxis and the need to carry an anaphylaxis kit, which contains injectable epinephrine and oral histamines for use in self-treating allergic reaction.

PC: Thrombocytopenia

DEFINITION

PC: Thrombocytopenia: Describes a person experiencing or at high risk to experience insufficient platelet content in blood.

High-Risk Population

Decreased Platelet Production due to
- Chemotherapy
- Radiation therapy
- Bone marrow invasion by tumor
- Leukemia
- Heparin therapy
- Toxins
- Severe infection
- Alcoholism
- Aplastic anemia

Increased Platelet Destruction due to
- Antibodies
- Aspirin
- Alcohol
- Quinine, quinidine
- Digoxin
- Sulfonamides
- Entrapment in large spleen
- Infections (bacteremia, postviral infections)
- RDS
- Posttransfusion status

Increased Platelet Utilization due to
- Disseminated intravascular coagulation
- Thrombotic thrombocytopenic purpura
- Liver disease
- Administration of several units of non–platelet-containing fluids

Nursing Goals

The nurse will manage and minimize complications of decreased platelets.

Interventions

1. Monitor CBC, hemoglobin, coagulation tests, and platelet counts.
   (These values help evaluate response to treatment and risk for bleeding. Platelet count $<20,000$ mm^3 indicates a high risk for intracranial bleeding.)
2. Assess for other factors that may lower platelet count in addition to the primary cause, such as
   a. Abnormal hepatic function

   b. Abnormal renal function
   c. Infection, fever
   d. Anticoagulant use
   e. Alcohol use
   f. Aspirin use
   g. Administration of several units of non–platelet-containing fluids (*e.g.*, packed RBCs)
   (Assessment may identify factors that could be controllable [McNally, Stair, & Smernilly, 1985].)
3. Monitor for signs and symptoms of spontaneous or excessive bleeding.
   a. Spontaneous petechiae, ecchymoses, hematomas
   b. Bleeding from nose or gums
   c. Prolonged bleeding from invasive procedures such as venipunctures or bone marrow aspiration
   d. Hematemesis or coffee-ground emesis
   e. Hemoptysis
   f. Hematuria
   g. Vaginal bleeding
   h. Rectal bleeding
   i. Gross blood in stools
   j. Black, tarry stools
   k. Change in vital signs
   l. Change in neurologic status (blurred vision, headache, disorientation)
   m. Urine, feces, and emesis positive for occult blood
   n. High pad count for menstruating females
   (Constant monitoring is needed to ensure early detection of bleeding episodes [McNally, Stair, & Smernilly, 1985].)
4. Assess for systemic signs of bleeding and hypovolemia.
   a. ↑ Pulse, ↑ respirations, ↓ blood pressure
   b. Changes in neurologic status (*e.g.*, subtle mental status changes, blurred vision, headache, disorientation)
   (Changes in circulatory oxygen levels will produce changes in cardiac, vascular, and neurologic functioning.)
5. If hemorrhage is suspected, refer to *PC: Hypovolemic Shock* for specific interventions. Anticipate platelet transfusion.
6. Apply direct pressure for 5 to 10 minutes, then a pressure dressing, to all venipuncture sites. Monitor carefully for 24 hours.
   (These measures promote clotting and reduce blood loss.)
7. Treat nausea aggressively to prevent vomiting.
   (Severe vomiting can cause GI bleeding.)
8. Minimize rectal probing.
   (This will avoid injury to rectal tissue and bleeding.)
9. Using the nursing diagnosis *High Risk for Injury related to bleeding tendency* (see Section II), implement nursing interventions and teaching to reduce the risk of trauma (*e.g.*, use of soft toothbrushes).

PC: Immunodeficiency

DEFINITION
PC: Immunodeficiency: Describes a person experiencing or at high risk to experience immune system dysfunction.

High-Risk Population
- Immunosuppressive therapy (chemotherapy, antibiotics)
- Malignancy
- Septicemia
- AIDS
- Nutritional deficits
- Burns
- Trauma
- Extensive pressure ulcers
- Radiation therapy (long bones, skull, sternum)
- Elderly with chronic illness
- Drug/alcohol addiction

Nursing Goals
The nurse will manage and minimize complications of immunodeficiency.

Interventions
1. Monitor CBC, WBC differential (neutrophils, lymphocytes), and absolute neutrophil count (WBC × neutrophil).
   (These values help evaluate response to treatment.)
2. Monitor for signs and symptoms of primary or secondary infection.
   a. Slightly increased temperature
   b. Chills
   c. Adventitious breath sounds
   d. Cloudy or foul-smelling urine
   e. Complaints of urinary frequency, urgency, or dysuria
   f. Presence of WBCs and bacteria in urine
   g. Redness, change in skin temperature, swelling or unusual drainage in any area of disrupted skin integrity, including previous and current puncture sites
   h. Irritation or ulceration of oral mucous membrane
   i. Complaints of perineal or rectal pain and any unusual vaginal or rectal discharge
   j. Increased hemorrhoidal pain, redness, or bleeding
   k. Painful, pruritic skin lesions (herpes zoster), particularly in cervical or thoracic area
   l. Change in WBC count, especially an increase in immature neutrophils
   (In a client with severe neutropenia, the usual inflammatory responses may be decreased or absent.)
3. Obtain culture specimens (*e.g.*, urine, vaginal, rectal, mouth, sputum, stool, blood, skin lesions), as ordered.
   (Testing will determine the type of causative organism and guide treatment.)

4. Monitor for signs and symptoms of septicemia.
   (Gram-positive and gram-negative organisms can invade open wounds, causing septicemia. A debilitated client is at increased risk. Sepsis produces massive vasodilation, resulting in hypovolemia and subsequent tissue hypoxia. Hypoxia leads to decreased renal function and cardiac output, triggering a compensatory response of increased respirations and heart rate in an attempt to correct hypoxia and acidosis. Bacteria in urine or blood indicates infection.)
5. Monitor for therapeutic and nontherapeutic effects of antibiotics.
6. Monitor for signs and symptoms of opportunistic protozoal infections.
   a. *Pneumocystis carinii* pneumonia: dry, nonproductive cough, fever, gradual to severe dyspnea
   b. *Toxoplasma gondii* encephalitis: headache, lethargy, seizures
   c. *Cryptosporidium* enteritis: watery diarrhea, nausea, abdominal cramps, malaise.
   (Immunodeficient clients are at risk for secondary diseases of opportunistic infections; protozoal infections are the most common and serious.)
7. Monitor for signs and symptoms of opportunistic viral infections.
   a. Herpes simplex oral or perirectal abscesses: severe pain, bleeding, rectal discharge
   b. Cytomegalovirus (CMV) retinitis, colitis, pneumonitis, encephalitis, or other organ disease
   c. Progressive multifocal leukoencephalopathy: headache, decreased mentation
   d. Varicella zoster, disseminated (shingles)
8. Monitor for signs and symptoms of opportunistic fungal infections.
   a. *Candida albicans* stomatitis and esophagitis: exudate, complaints of unusual taste in mouth
   b. *Cryptococcus neoformans* meningitis: fever, headaches, blurred vision, stiff neck, confusion
9. Monitor for signs and symptoms of opportunistic bacterial infections, which commonly affect the pulmonary system.
   a. *Mycobacterium avium* (intracellular disseminated)
   b. *Mycobacterium tuberculosis* (extrapulmonary and pulmonary)
10. Emphasize the need to report symptoms promptly.
    (Early treatment of adverse manifestations often can prevent serious complications [*e.g.*, septicemia] and also increases the likelihood of a favorable response to treatment.)
11. Explain the need to balance activity and rest and to consume a nutritious diet.
    (Rest and nutritious diet provide the client with energy to heal and to enhance the body's defense system.)
12. Avoid or minimize invasive procedures (*e.g.*, urinary catheterization, arterial or venous punctures, injections, rectal tubes, suppositories).
    (This precaution helps prevent introduction of microorganisms.)
13. Refer to the nursing diagnosis *High Risk for Infection* in Section II for interventions to prevent introduction of microorganisms and to increase resistance.

References/Bibliography

Champagne, M., & Ashley, M. (1989). Nutritional support in the critically ill elderly patient. *Critical Care Nursing Quarterly, 12*(1), 15–25.

Cohen, F. (1989). Immunologic impairment, infection and AIDS in the aging patient. *Critical Care Nursing Quarterly, 12*(1), 38–45.

Hudak, C., Gallo, B., & Benz, J. (1990). *Critical care nursing* (5th ed.). Philadelphia: J. B. Lippincott.

Isley, W., & Hamburger, S. (Eds.). (1990). Endocrine/metabolic disorders. *Critical Care Nursing Quarterly, 13*(3), 1–88.

Mahoney, E., & Flynn, J. (1986). *Handbook of medical-surgical nursing.* New York: John Wiley & Sons.

McNally, J., Stair, J. C., & Smernilly, E. (1985). *Guidelines for cancer nursing practice.* Orlando: Grune & Stratton.

Pfister, S. M. (1989). Arterial blood gas evaluation: Metabolic acidemia. *Critical Care Nurse, 9*(1), 70–72.

Sabo, C. E. (1989). Diabetic ketoacidosis: Pathophysiology, nursing diagnoses, and nursing interventions. *Focus on Critical Care, 16*(1), 21–28.

Schneiderman, E. (1990). Thrombocytopenia in the critically ill patient. *Critical Care Nursing Quarterly, 13*(2), 1–6.

Thelan, L., Davie, J., & Urden, L. (1990). *Textbook of critical care nursing.* St. Louis: C.V. Mosby.

Tribett, D. (Ed.). (1989). The immunocompromised patient. *Critical Care Nursing Clinics of North America, 1*(4), 723–724.

Potential Complication: Renal/Urinary

PC: Acute Urinary Retention
PC: Renal Insufficiency
PC: Renal Calculi

Renal and Urinary System Overview

The kidneys and urinary system have related functions but also very distinct purposes. The kidneys regulate fluid and electrolyte balance, acid–base balance, and excretion of metabolic waste products. They also regulate arterial blood pressure, erythropoiesis, and vitamin D metabolism. Highly vascular, the kidneys receive the entire circulatory volume 20 times each hour to regulate body fluid composition. Factors affecting renal clearance include age, fluid volume, renal blood flow, glomerular membrane permeability, blood pressure, and cardiac output.

The urinary system (ureters, bladder, urethra) serves as a reservoir and conduit for urine from the kidney to elimination through urination. Factors that can affect this function are infections, prostate enlargement, neurogenic bladder, and tumors.

Potential Complication: Renal/Urinary

DEFINITION

PC: Renal/Urinary: Describes a person experiencing or at high risk to experience various renal or urinary tract dysfunctions.

Diagnostic Considerations

The nurse can use this generic collaborative problem to describe a person at risk for several types of renal or urinary problems. For such a client (*e.g.*, a client in a critical care unit, who is vulnerable to a variety of renal/urinary problems), using *PC: Renal/Urinary* will direct nurses to monitor renal and urinary status, based on the focus assessment, in order to detect and diagnose abnormal functioning. Nursing management of a specific renal or urinary complication would be addressed under the collaborative problem applying to the specific complication. For example, a standard of care for a client recovering from coronary bypass surgery could contain the collaborative problem *PC: Renal/Urinary,* directing the nurse to monitor renal and urinary status. If this client developed urinary retention, the nurse would add *PC: Urinary retention* to the problem list, along with specific nursing interventions to manage this problem. If the risk factors or etiology were not directly related to the primary medical diagnosis, the nurse still would specify them in the diagnostic statement, *e.g., PC: Renal insufficiency related to chronic renal failure* in a client who has sustained a myocardial infarction.

Keep in mind that the nurse must differentiate those problems in bladder function that can be treated independently by nurses as nursing diagnoses (*e.g.,* incontinence, chronic urinary retention) from those that nurses manage using both nurse-prescribed and physician-prescribed interventions (*e.g.,* acute urinary retention).

Focus Assessment Criteria

Subjective Data

1. History of symptoms
   a. Onset and duration
   b. Description
   c. Frequency
   d. Precipitating factors
   e. Alleviating factors
2. Weight (gain, loss, fluctuations)
3. Complaints of
   a. Pain, aching (costovertebral angle, urethral, bladder, scrotum/vulva, constant, with voiding)
   b. Dry, scaly skin
   c. Fatigue
   d. Inability to concentrate
   e. Fever
   f. Edema
4. History of
   a. Renal disease (family history)
   b. Hypertension
   c. Diabetes mellitus
   d. Lupus erythematosus
   e. Renal calculi
5. Medication use (prescribed and over-the-counter)

Objective Data

1. Urine characteristics
   a. Color
   b. Odor
   c. Appearance
   d. Specific gravity
   e. Presence of glucose, protein, ketones, red blood cells

Significant Laboratory Assessment Criteria

1. Blood
   a. Albumin (lowered in renal disease)
   b. Amylase (elevated with renal insufficiency)
   c. pH, base excess, bicarbonate (lowered in metabolic acidosis, elevated in metabolic alkalosis)
   d. Calcium (lowered in uremic acidosis)
   e. Chloride (elevated with renal tubular acidosis)
   f. Creatinine (elevated with kidney disease)
   g. Magnesium (lowered in chronic nephritis)
   h. Phosphorus (elevated with chronic glomerular disease, lowered with renal tubular acidosis)
   i. Potassium (elevated in renal failure, lowered with chronic diuretic therapy, renal tubular acidosis)
   j. Proteins (total, albumin, globulin) (lowered in nephritic syndrome)
   k. Sodium (elevated with nephritis, lowered with chronic renal insufficiency)
   l. Blood urea nitrogen (BUN) (elevated in acute or chronic renal failure)
   m. Uric acid (elevated with chronic renal failure)
   n. White blood cell (WBC) count (elevated, lowered with acute and chronic infections)
2. Urine
   a. Blood (present with hemorrhagic cystitis, renal calculi, renal, bladder tumors)
   b. Creatinine (elevated in acute/chronic glomerulonephritis, nephritis, lowered in advanced degeneration of kidneys)
   c. pH (elevated with metabolic acidosis, lowered with metabolic alkalosis)
   d. Specific gravity (elevated with dehydration, lowered with overhydration, renal tubular disease)
   e. WBC count (elevated with urinary tract infections)

PC: Acute Urinary Retention

DEFINITION

PC: Acute Urinary Retention: Describes a person experiencing or at high risk to experience an acute abnormal accumulation of urine in the bladder and the inability to void due to a temporary situation (*e.g.*, postoperative status) or to a condition reversible with surgery (*e.g.*, prostatectomy) or medications.

High-Risk Populations

- Postoperative status (*e.g.*, surgery of the perineal area, lower abdomen)
- Postpartum status
- Anxiety

- Prostate enlargement
- Medication side effects (*e.g.,* atropine, antidepressants, antihistamines)
- Postarteriography status

Nursing Goals

The nurse will manage and minimize acute urinary retention episodes.

Interventions

1. Monitor a postoperative client for urinary retention.
   (Anesthesia produces muscle relaxation, affecting the bladder. As muscle tone returns, spasms of the bladder sphincter prevent urine outflow, causing bladder distention.)
2. Observe for
   a. Bladder distention
   b. Urine overflow (30–60 mL of urine every 15–30 min)
   (When urine retention increases intravesical pressure, the sphincter releases urine.)
3. Instruct the client to report bladder discomfort or inability to void.
   (Bladder discomfort and failure to void may be early signs of urinary retention.)
4. Monitor for urinary retention in postpartum women.
   (Labor and delivery can temporarily slacken the tone of the bladder wall, causing urinary retention.)
5. Encourage the client to void within 6 to 8 hours after delivery.
   (The desire to void may be diminished because of an increased bladder capacity related to reduced intra-abdominal pressure after delivery.)
6. In a postpartum client, differentiate between bladder distention and uterine enlargement; keep in mind that
   a. A distended bladder protrudes above the symphysis pubis.
   b. When the nurse massages the uterus to return it to its midline position, the bladder will protrude further.
   c. Percussion and palpation can distinguish between a rebounding bladder (due to fluid) and a firm uterus.
   (A distended bladder can push the uterus upward and to the side and can cause uterine relaxation.)
7. If the client does not void within 8 to 10 hours after surgery or complains of bladder discomfort, take the following steps.
   a. Warm the bedpan.
   b. Encourage the client to get out of bed to use the bathroom, if possible.
   c. Instruct a male client to stand when urinating, if possible.
   d. Run water in the sink as the client attempts to void.
   e. Pour warm water over the client's perineum.
   (These measures may help promote relaxation of the urinary sphincter and facilitate voiding.)
8. After the first voiding postdelivery or postsurgery, continue to monitor and encourage the client to void again in an hour or so.
   (This first voiding usually does not empty the bladder completely.)
9. If the client still cannot void after 10 hours, follow protocols for straight catheterization, as ordered by the physician.
   (Straight catheterization is preferable to indwelling catheterization because it carries less risk of urinary tract infection from ascending pathogens.)
10. For a client with chronic urinary retention, refer to the nursing diagnosis *Urinary Retention* in Section II.

PC: Renal Insufficiency

DEFINITION
PC: Renal Insufficiency: Describes a person experiencing or at high risk to experience a decrease in glomerular filtration rate that results in oliguria or anuria.

High-Risk Populations
- Renal tubular necrosis due to ischemic causes
    - Excessive diuretic use
    - Pulmonary embolism
    - Burns
    - Intrarenal thrombosis
    - Renal infections
    - Peritonitis
    - Sepsis
    - Congestive heart failure
    - Myocardial infarction
- Renal tubular necrosis due to toxicity (Thelan, 1990)
    - Nonsteroidal anti-inflammatory drugs (NSAIDs)
    - Gout
    - Hypercalcemia
    - Certain street drugs (*e.g.*, PCP)
    - Gram-negative infection
    - Radiocontrast media
    - Aminoglycoside antibiotics
    - Antineoplastic agents
    - Methanol
    - Rhabdomyolysis
    - Carbon tetrachloride
    - Phenacetin-type analgesics
    - Heavy metals
    - Insecticides
    - Aminoglycosides
- Diabetes mellitus
- Primary hypertensive disease
- Hemolysis (*e.g.*, from transfusion reaction)

Nursing Goals
The nurse will manage and minimize complications of renal insufficiency.

Interventions
1. Monitor for early signs and symptoms of renal insufficiency:
    a. Sustained elevated urine specific gravity, elevated urine sodium levels
    b. Sustained insufficient urine output (<30 mL/hr), elevated blood pressure

   c. Elevated BUN, serum creatinine, potassium, phosphorus, and ammonia; decreased creatinine clearance

   d. Dependent edema (periorbital, pedal, pretibial, sacral)

   (Early detection of clinical manifestations enables prompt treatment to prevent serious renal dysfunction. These manifestations result from various mechanisms. Sustained elevated urine specific gravity and elevated urine sodium are linked to the decreased ability of the renal tubules to reabsorb electrolytes. Decreased glomerular filtration rate eventually causes insufficient urine output and stimulates renin production, resulting in elevated blood pressure in an attempt to increase blood flow to the kidney. Decreased excretion of urea and creatinine in the urine elevates BUN and creatinine levels. Dependent edema results from increased plasma hydrostatic pressure, salt and water retention, and/or decreased colloid osmotic pressure due to plasma protein losses.)

2. Weigh the client daily at a minimum; more often, if indicated. Ensure accurate findings by weighing at the same time each day, on the same scale, and with the client wearing the same amount of clothing.
   (Daily weights and intake and output records help evaluate fluid balance and guide fluid intake recommendations.)

3. Maintain strict intake and output records: determine the net fluid balance and compare with daily weight loss or gain for correlation. (A 1-kg [2.2-lb] weight gain correlates with excess intake of 1 liter.)

4. Explain prescribed fluid management goals.
   (The client's and family's understanding may enhance cooperation.)

5. Adjust the client's daily fluid intake so it approximates fluid loss plus 300 to 500 mL/day.
   (Careful replacement therapy is necessary to prevent fluid overload.)

6. Distribute fluid intake fairly evenly throughout the entire day and night. It may be necessary to match fluid intake with loss every 8 hours or even every hour if the client is critically imbalanced.
   (Maintaining a constant fluid balance, without major fluctuations, is essential. Allowing toxins to accumulate due to poor hydration can cause complications such as nausea and sensorium changes.)

7. Encourage the client to express feelings and frustrations; give positive feedback.
   (Fluid and diet restrictions can be extremely frustrating. Emotional support can help reduce anxiety and may improve compliance with the treatment regimen.)

8. Consult with a dietitian regarding the fluid and diet plan.
   (Important considerations in fluid management, requiring a specialist's attention, include the fluid content of nonliquid food, appropriate amount and type of liquids, liquid preferences, and sodium content.)

9. Administer oral medications with meals whenever possible. If medications must be administered between meals, give with the smallest amount of fluid necessary.
   (This measure avoids using parts of the fluid allowance unnecessarily.)

10. Avoid continuous IV fluid infusion whenever possible. Dilute all necessary IV drugs in the smallest amount of fluid that is safe for IV administration. Use small IV bags and an IV controller or pump, if possible, to prevent accidental infusion of a large volume of fluid.
   (Extremely accurate fluid infusion is necessary to prevent fluid overload.)

11. Monitor for signs and symptoms of metabolic acidosis.

   a. Rapid, shallow respirations

   b. Headaches

   c. Nausea and vomiting

    d. Negative base excess

    e. Behavioral changes, drowsiness

(Acidosis results from the kidney's inability to excrete hydrogen ions, phosphates, sulfates, and ketone bodies. Bicarbonate loss results from decreased renal reabsorption. Metabolic acidosis is aggravated by hyperkalemia, hyperphosphatemia, and decreased bicarbonate levels. Excessive ketone bodies cause headaches, nausea, vomiting, and abdominal pain. Respiratory rate and depth increase in an attempt to increase CO_2 excretion and thus reduce acidosis. Acidosis affects the CNS and can increase neuromuscular irritability due to the cellular exchange of hydrogen and potassium.)

12. For a client with metabolic acidosis, ensure adequate caloric intake while limiting fat and protein intake. Consult with a dietitian for an appropriate diet.

    (Restricting fats and protein helps prevent accumulation of acidic end products.)

13. Assess for signs and symptoms of hypocalcemia, hypokalemia, and alkalosis as acidosis is corrected.

    (Rapid correction of acidosis may cause rapid excretion of calcium and potassium and result in rebound alkalosis.)

14. Consult with the physician to initiate bicarbonate/acetate dialysis if the above measures do not correct metabolic acidosis:

    a. Bicarbonate dialysis for severe acidosis: Dialysate – $NaHCO_3$ = 100 mEq/L

    b. Bicarbonate dialysis for moderate acidosis: Dialysate – $NaHCO_3$ = 60 mEq/L

    (The acetate anion, converted by the liver to bicarbonate, is used in dialysate to combat metabolic acidosis. Bicarbonate dialysis is indicated for clients with liver impairment, lactic acidosis, or severe acid–base imbalance.)

15. Monitor for signs and symptoms of hypernatremia with fluid overload:

    a. Extreme thirst

    b. CNS effects ranging from agitation to convulsion

    (Hypernatremia results from excessive sodium intake or from increased aldosterone output. Water is pulled from the cells, causing cellular dehydration and producing CNS symptoms. Thirst is a compensatory response aimed at diluting sodium.)

16. Maintain prescribed sodium restrictions.

    (Hypernatremia must be corrected slowly to minimize CNS deterioration.)

17. Monitor for electrolyte imbalances.

    a. Potassium

    b. Calcium

    c. Phosphorus

    d. Sodium

    e. Magnesium

    (Refer to *PC: Electrolyte Imbalance* for specific signs and symptoms and interventions.)

    (Renal dysfunction can result in hyperkalemia, hypernatremia, hypocalcemia, hypermagnesemia, or hyperphosphatemia. Diuretic therapy can cause hypokalemia or hyponatremia.)

18. Monitor for GI bleeding. (Refer to *PC: GI Bleeding* for more information and specific interventions.)

    (Bleeding may be aggravated by the poor platelet aggregation and capillary fragility associated with high serum levels of nitrogenous wastes. Heparinization required during dialysis in the presence of gastric ulcer disease also may precipitate GI bleeding.)

19. Monitor for manifestations of anemia:

    a. Dyspnea

    b. Fatigue

    c. Tachycardia, palpitations
    d. Pallor of nail beds and mucous membranes
    e. Low hemoglobin and hematocrit levels
    f. Easy bruising
    (Chronic renal failure results in decreased RBC production and survival time due to elevated uremic toxins.)
20. Avoid unnecessary collection of blood specimens.
    (Some blood loss occurs with every blood collection.)
21. Instruct the client to use a soft toothbrush and avoid vigorous nose blowing, constipation, and contact sports.
    (Trauma should be avoided to reduce the risk of bleeding and infection.)
22. Demonstrate the pressure method to control bleeding should it occur.
    (Applying direct, constant pressure on a bleeding site can help prevent excessive blood loss.)
23. Monitor for manifestations of hypoalbuminemia.
    a. Serum albumin level <3.5 g/dL; proteinuria (<100–150 mg protein/24 hr)
    b. Edema formation: pedal, facial, sacral
    c. Hypovolemia
    d. Increased hematocrit and hemoglobin levels.
    (Refer to *PC: Negative Nitrogen Balance* for more information and interventions.) (When albumin leaks into the urine due to changes in the glomerular electrostatic barrier or due to peritoneal dialysis, the liver responds by increasing production of plasma proteins. However, when the loss is great, the liver cannot compensate, and hypoalbuminemia results.)
24. Monitor for hypervolemia. Evaluate daily
    a. Weight
    b. Fluid intake and output records
    c. Circumference of the edematous part(s)
    d. Laboratory data: hematocrit, serum sodium, and plasma protein in specific serum albumin
    (As glomerular filtration rate decreases and the functioning nephron mass continues to diminish, the kidneys lose the ability to concentrate urine and to excrete sodium and water, resulting in hypervolemia.)
25. Monitor for signs and symptoms of congestive heart failure and decreased cardiac output.
    a. Gradual increase in heart rate
    b. Increasing dyspnea
    c. Diminished breath sounds, rales
    d. Decreased systolic blood pressure
    e. Presence of or increase in S_3 and/or S_4 heart sounds
    f. Gallop rhythm
    g. Peripheral edema
    h. Distended neck veins
    (Congestive heart failure can occur due to increased cardiac output, hypervolemia, dysrhythmias, and hypertension, resulting in reduced ability of the left ventricle to eject blood and consequent decreased cardiac output and increased pulmonary vascular congestion.)
26. Encourage adherence to strict fluid restrictions: 800 to 1000 mL/24 hours or 24-hour urine output plus 500 mL.
    (Fluid restrictions are based on urine output. In an anuric client, restriction generally is 800 mL/day, which accounts for insensible losses from metabolism, the GI tract, perspiration, and respiration.)

27. Collaborate with the physician or dietitian in planning an appropriate diet. Encourage adherence to a low-sodium diet (2–4 g/day).
(Sodium restrictions should be adjusted based on urine sodium excretion.)
28. If hemodialysis or peritoneal dialysis is initiated, follow institutional protocols.

PC: Renal Calculi

DEFINITION

PC: Renal Calculi: Describes a person with or at high risk to develop calculi in the urinary tract.

High-Risk Populations
- History of renal calculi
- Urinary infection
- Urinary stasis
- Immobility
- Hypercalcemia (dietary)
- Conditions that cause hypercalcemia
    Hyperparathyroidism
    Renal tubular acidosis
    Myeloproliferative disease (leukemia, polycythemia vera, multiple myeloma)
- Excessive excretion of uric acid
- Inflammatory bowel disease

Nursing Goals

The nurse will manage and minimize complications of renal calculi.

Interventions

1. Monitor for signs and symptoms of calculi.
    a. Increased or decreased urine output
    b. Sediment in urine
    c. Flank or loin pain
    d. Hematuria
    e. Abdominal pain, distention, nausea, diarrhea
    (Stones in the urinary tract can produce obstruction, infection, and edema, manifested by loin or flank pain, hematuria, and dysuria. Calculi in the renal pelvis may increase urine production. GI symptoms can result from calculi stimulating renointestinal reflexes.)
2. Strain urine to obtain a stone sample; send samples to the laboratory for analysis.
    (Acquiring a stone sample confirms stone formation and enables analysis of stone constituents.)

3. If the client complains of pain, consult with the physician for aggressive therapy (*e.g.*, narcotics, antispasmodics).
   (Calculi can produce severe pain from spasms and proximity of the nerve plexus.)
4. Track the pain by documenting location, any radiation, duration, and intensity (client rating on a scale of 0 to 10).
   (This measure helps evaluate movement of calculi.)
5. Instruct the client to increase fluid intake, if not contraindicated.
   (Increased fluid intake promotes increased urination, which can help facilitate stone passage and flush bacteria and blood from the urinary tract.)
6. Monitor for signs and symptoms of pyelonephritis.
   a. Fever, chills
   b. Costovertebral angle (CVA) pain (a dull, constant backache below the 12th rib)
   c. Leukocytosis
   d. Bacteria and pus in urine
   e. Dysuria, frequency
   (Urinary tract infections can be caused by urinary stasis or irritation of tissue by calculi. Signs and symptoms reflect various mechanisms. Bacteria can act as a pyrogen by raising the hypothalamic thermostat through the production of endogenous pyrogen, which may mediate through prostaglandins. Chills can occur when the temperature set-point of the hypothalamus changes rapidly. CVA pain results from distention of the renal capsule. Leukocytosis reflects an increase in leukocytes to fight infection through phagocytosis. Bacteria and pus in urine indicate a urinary tract infection. Bacteria can irritate bladder tissue, causing spasms and frequency.)
7. Monitor for early signs and symptoms of renal insufficiency. (Refer to *PC: Renal Insufficiency.*)

References/Bibliography

Chambers, J. K. (1987). Fluid and electrolyte problems in renal and urologic disorders. *Nursing Clinics of North America, 22*(4), 815–822.

Coe, F. L., & Parks, J. H. (1987). Recurrent renal calculi: Causes and prevention. *Hospital Practice, 21*(3A), 49–57.

Hudak, C., Gallo, B., & Benz, J. (1990). *Critical care nursing* (5th ed.). Philadelphia: J. B. Lippincott.

Johnson, D. L. (1989). Nephrotic syndrome: A nursing care plan based on current pathophysiologic concepts. *Heart & Lung, 18*(1), 85–93.

Mahoney, E., & Flynn, J. (1986). *Handbook of medical-surgical nursing*. New York: John Wiley & Sons.

Norris, M. K. G. (1989). Acute tubular necrosis: Preventing complications. *Dimensions in Critical Care Nursing, 8*(1), 16–26.

Sillix, D. H., & McDonald, F. D. (1987). Acute renal failure. *Critical Care Clinics, 5*(4), 909–914.

Thelan, L., Davie, J., & Urden, L. (1990). *Textbook of critical care nursing*. St. Louis: C. V. Mosby.

Potential Complication: Neurologic/Sensory

PC: Increased Intracranial Pressure

PC: Seizures

PC: Increased Intraocular Pressure

Neurologic/Sensory System Overview

The neurologic system, in conjunction with the endocrine system, controls all body functions. Composed of the brain and spinal cord, the *central nervous system* (CNS) is divided into three major functional units: the spinal cord, the lower brain level, and the higher brain level or cortical function.

The brain contains four major structures. The *cerebrum* is divided into two hemispheres with four lobes in each (frontal, parietal, temporal, and occipital). Its functions include maintaining consciousness and controlling memory, mental processes, sensations, emotions, and voluntary movements. Included in these functions are speech, auditory recognition of written and spoken language, and vision. Located under the occipital lobe, the *cerebellum* controls balance and coordination. The *diencephalon* consists of the right and left thalamus, which function as conducting pathways for sensory impulses to the cerebral cortex, and the hypothalamus, which controls the autonomic nervous system, body temperature, and water balance and influences appetite and wakefulness.

Brainstem structures include the midbrain, pons, and medulla. The midbrain serves as a nerve pathway of the cerebral hemispheres and the lower brain. All but two of the cranial nerves originate from the brainstem. Cranial nerves III and IV originate from the midbrain; V, VI, VII, and VIII originate from the pons; and IX, X, XI, and XII originate from the medulla. The medulla contains the vasomotor center controlling heart rate and blood pressure. Respiratory centers are located throughout the brainstem (Hickey, 1986).

Consisting of 31 segments, the *spinal cord* provides conduction pathways to and from the brain and serves as the center for reflex actions.

In the *peripheral nervous system,* cranial and spinal nerves and ganglia control movements (descending pathways) and sensations (ascending pathways). The *autonomic nervous system* controls involuntary functions via the sympathetic and parasympathetic nervous systems. Sympathetic system responses include increased cardiovascular response, vasodilation, pupillary dilatation, decreased peristalsis, temperature regulation, blood glucose increases, rectal and bladder sphincter contraction, and increased secretion of sweat glands and thick saliva. The parasympathetic nervous system acts to constrict blood vessels, constrict pupils, slow heart rate, increase peristalsis, increase secretion of thin saliva, and relax rectal and bladder sphincters.

The sensory system comprises vision, hearing, olfaction, taste, and proprioception.

The eye consists of external structures, extraocular muscles, internal structures, refractory structures, and an anterior chamber. The external structures (orbit, eyelid, glands of eyelid, conjunctiva, lacrimal gland, and duct) protect and lubricate the eye. The sclera, an internal structure, provides rigid structure. The cornea allows passage of images to the retina, another internal structure. The uveal tract (choroid, ciliary body, and iris) prevents internal reflection of light, changes the shape of the lens for focusing, and controls the amount of light reaching the retina. The retina consists of the macula, retinal periphery, and optic disc. The macula provides color vision and differentiates fine details; the retinal periphery detects moving objects; and the optic disc carries impulses to the brain via the optic nerve. The refractory structures are the cornea, aqueous humor, lens, and vitreous humor. The cornea allows passages of images to the retina, and the lens performs the function of accommodation. The aqueous humor refracts light, supplies nutrients to the refractory structures, and maintains internal pressure. The vitreous humor also refracts light and maintains the spherical shape of the eyeball. The anterior chamber produces an aqueous fluid and regulates its flow, thus maintaining intraocular pressure.

The ear consists of three components: the external, middle, and inner ear. The external ear receives sound waves and directs them to the middle ear. The middle ear amplifies the waves and transmits sound to the inner ear; it also equalizes pressure. The inner ear is the receptor end organ of hearing and equilibrium; it also contains the acoustic nerve, which connects the inner ear with the brain.

The senses of olfaction and taste are discussed under the nursing diagnosis of *Altered Nutrition*. Proprioception is discussed under *Potential for Injury*.

Potential Complication: Neurologic/ Sensory

DEFINITION

PC: Neurologic/Sensory: Describes a person experiencing or at high risk to experience various neurologic or sensory dysfunctions.

Diagnostic Considerations

The nurse can use this generic collaborative problem to describe a person at risk for several types of neurologic or sensory problems (*e.g.*, a client recovering from cranial surgery or one who has sustained multiple trauma). For such a person, using *PC: Neurologic/Sensory* will direct nurses to monitor neurologic and sensory function based on focus assessment findings. Should a complication occur, the nurse would add the applicable specific collaborative problem (*e.g.*, *PC: Increased Intracranial Pressure*) to the client's problem list to describe nursing management of the complication.

If the risk factors or etiology were not directly related to the primary medical diagnosis or treatment, the nurse could add this information to the diagnostic statement. For example, for a client with a seizure disorder admitted for abdominal surgery, the nurse would add *PC: Seizures related to epilepsy* to the problem list.

In addition to the collaborative problem, the nurse should assess for other actual or potential responses that can compromise functioning. Some of these responses may represent nursing diagnoses (*e.g., High Risk for Injury related to poor awareness of environmental hazards secondary to decreased sensorium*).

Focus Assessment Criteria

Subjective Data
1. Complaints of
   a. Headaches (precipitating factors, location, duration, frequency, relieving factors)
   b. Vision problems (loss, double, blurred)
   c. Eye pain
   d. Numbness, tingling, paralysis
   e. Swallowing problems (liquids or solids)
   f. Speech problems (initiating, expressing)
   g. Memory problems (remote, recent)
   h. Ability to comprehend
   i. Changes in taste, smell, hearing
   j. Inability to sense hot, cold with hands, feet
   k. Unstable gait
2. History of seizures (type, precipitating factors, duration, progression of symptoms)

Objective Data
1. Mental status
   a. Alert
   b. Receptive aphasia
   c. Poor memory
   d. Oriented to person, place, and time
   e. Confused
   f. Combative
   g. Unresponsive
2. Speech
   a. Normal
   b. Slurred
   c. Garbled
   d. Expressive aphasia
   e. Language barrier
3. Pupils
   a. Equal or unequal size
   b. Reactive to light (left, right, yes, no/specify)
4. Eyes
   a. Clear
   b. Draining
   c. Reddened
   d. Other

5. Glasgow coma scale
   a. Eyes open: spontaneously, to speech, to pain, not at all
   b. Best verbal response: oriented, confused, inappropriate words, incomprehensible sounds, no response
   c. Best motor response: obeys verbal commands, localizes pain, abnormal flexion withdrawal to pain, abnormal extension to pain, no response
6. Balance and gait
   a. Steady
   b. Unsteady
   c. Description
7. Hand grasp
   a. Bilateral equality
   b. Strength
   c. Weakness/paralysis
8. Leg muscles
   a. Bilateral equality
   b. Strength
   c. Weakness/paralysis
9. Sensory acuity
   a. Visual
   b. Auditory
   c. Tactile
   d. Olfactory/gustatory
10. Cranial nerve function
   a. I (olfactory): ability to smell with each nostril
   b. II (optic): visual acuity
   c. III (oculomotor): pupillary constriction, accommodation, extraocular movements, and elevation of eyelids
   d. IV (trochlear): extraocular movements
   e. V (trigeminal): facial sensation
   f. VI (abducens): extraocular movements
   g. VII (facial): voluntary facial movements, symmetry, taste on anterior two-thirds of tongue
   h. VIII (acoustic): hearing acuity
   i. IX (glossopharyngeal): pharynx, speech quality
   j. X (vagus): pharynx, speech quality
   k. XI (spinal accessory): shoulder movement, sternocleidomastoid
   l. XII (hypoglossal): voluntary tongue movements, symmetry

Significant Laboratory Assessment Criteria

1. Cerebrospinal fluid
   a. Protein (increased in meningitis)
   b. WBC count (increased in meningitis)
   c. Albumin (elevated with brain tumors)
   d. Glucose (decreased with bacterial meningitis)
2. Blood
   • WBC count (elevated with bacterial infection, decreased in viral infection)

PC: Increased Intracranial Pressure

DEFINITION

PC: Increased Intracranial Pressure: Describes a person experiencing or at high risk to experience increased pressure (>15 mm Hg) exerted by cerebrospinal fluid within the brain's ventricles or the subarachnoid space.

High-Risk Populations

- Intracerebral mass (lesions, hematomas, tumors, abscesses)
- Blood clots
- Blockage of venous outflow
- Head injuries
- Reye's syndrome
- Meningitis
- Premature birth

Nursing Goals

The nurse will manage and minimize episodes of increased intracranial pressure (ICP).

Interventions

1. Monitor for signs and symptoms of increased ICP.
   a. Assess the following:
      - Best eye opening response: spontaneously, to auditory stimuli, to painful stimuli, or no response
      - Best motor response: obeys verbal commands, localizes pain, flexion–withdrawal, flexion–decorticate, extension–decerebrate, or no response
      - Best verbal response: oriented to person, place, and time; confused conversation; inappropriate speech; incomprehensible sounds; or no response

      (Cerebral tissue is compromised by deficiencies of cerebral blood supply caused by hemorrhage, hematoma, cerebral edema, thrombus, or emboli. These responses evaluate the client's ability to integrate commands with conscious and involuntary movement. Cortical function can be assessed by evaluating eye opening and motor response. No response may indicate damage to the midbrain.)
   b. Assess for changes in vital signs.
      - Pulse changes: slowing rate to 60 beats/min or lower or increasing rate to 100 beats/min or higher
      - (Bradycardia is a late sign of brainstem ischemia. Tachycardia may indicate hypothalamic ischemia and sympathetic discharge.)
      - Respiratory irregularities: slowing rate with lengthening apneic periods (Respiratory patterns vary depending on the site of impairment. Cheyne-Stokes breathing [a gradual increase followed by a gradual decrease, then period of apnea] points to damage in both cerebral hemispheres, midbrain, and upper pons. Central neurogenic hyperventilation occurs with midbrain

and upper pontine lesions. Ataxic breathing [irregular with random sequence of deep and shallow breaths] indicates pontine dysfunction. Hypoventilation and apnea occur with medullary lesions.)
- Rising blood pressure and/or widening pulse pressure
- Cushing's triad: bradycardia, increased systolic blood pressure, and increased pulse pressure
(These are a late sign of brainstem ischemia leading to cerebral herniation.)

c. Assess pupillary responses.
(Pupillary changes indicate pressure on oculomotor or optic nerves.)
- Inspect the pupils with a flashlight to evaluate size, configuration, and reaction to light. Compare both eyes for similarities and differences.
(Pupil reactions are regulated by the oculomotor nerve [cranial nerve III] in the brain stem.)
- Evaluate gaze to determine whether it is conjugate (paired, working together) or if eye movements are abnormal.
(Conjugate eye movements are regulated from parts of the cortex and brain stem.)
- Evaluate the ability of the eyes to adduct and abduct.
(Cranial nerve VI, or the abducent nerve, regulates abduction and adduction of the eyes. Cranial nerve IV, or the trochlear nerve, also regulates eye movement.)

d. Note any other signs and symptoms.
- Vomiting
(Vomiting results from pressure on the medulla, which stimulates the brain's vomiting center.)
- Headache (constant, increasing in intensity, or aggravated by movement or straining)
(Compression of neural tissue increases ICP and causes pain.)
- Subtle changes (*e.g.,* lethargy, restlessness, forced breathing, purposeless movements, changes in mentation)
(These signs may be the earliest indicators of cranial pressure changes.)

2. Elevate the head of the bed 30° to 45° unless contraindicated.
(Slight head elevation can aid venous drainage to reduce cerebrovascular congestion, thereby decreasing ICP.)

3. Avoid the following situations or maneuvers, which can increase ICP.
a. Carotid massage
(This slows the heart rate and reduces systemic circulation, which is followed by a sudden increase in circulation.)
b. Neck flexion or extreme rotation
(This inhibits jugular venous drainage, which increases cerebrovascular congestion and ICP.)
c. Digital anal stimulation, breath-holding, straining
(These can initiate Valsalva's maneuver, which impairs venous return by constricting the jugular veins, thus increasing ICP.)
d. Extreme flexion of the hips and knees
(Flexion increases intrathoracic pressure, which inhibits jugular venous drainage, increasing cerebrovascular congestion and, thus, ICP.)
e. Rapid position changes

4. Teach the client to exhale during position changes.
(This helps prevent Valsalva's maneuver.)

5. Consult with the physician for stool softeners, if needed.
(Stool softeners prevent constipation and straining during defecation, which can trigger Valsalva's maneuver.)

6. Maintain a quiet, calm, softly lit environment. Schedule several lengthy periods of uninterrupted rest daily. Cluster necessary procedures and activities to minimize interruptions.
(These measures promote rest and decrease stimulation, both of which can help decrease ICP.)

7. Avoid sequential performance of activities that increase ICP (*e.g.*, coughing, suctioning, repositioning, bathing).
(Research has validated that such sequential activities can cause a cumulative increase in ICP [Mitchell, 1986].)

8. Monitor temperature. As indicated, initiate external hypothermia or hyperthermia measures according to the physician's orders and institutional protocol.
(Impaired hypothalamic function can interfere with temperature regulation, necessitating intervention. Hypothermia may reduce ICP, whereas hyperthermia may increase it [Marshall, 1990].)

9. Limit suctioning time to 10 seconds at a time; hyperoxygenate and hyperventilate the client both before and after suctioning.
(These measures help prevent hypercapnia, which can increase cerebral vasodilation and raise ICP and prevent hypoxia, which may increase cerebral ischemia.)

10. Consult with the physician about administering prophylactic lidocaine before suctioning.
(This measure may help prevent acute intracranial hypertension [Thelan, 1990].)

11. Maintain optimal ventilation through proper positioning and regular suctioning.
(These measures help prevent hypoxemia and hypercapnia.)

12. Monitor arterial blood gas (ABG) values.
(ABG values help evaluate gas exchange in the lungs and determine the circulating oxygen level and arterial CO_2. It is recommended that arterial O_2 be in the range of 90–100 torr, and that arterial CO_2 be in the range of 25–30 torr, to prevent cerebral ischemia and cerebrovascular congestion, which increase ICP.)

13. If indicated, initiate protocols or collaborate with the physician for drug therapy, which may include the following (Thelan, 1990):
   a. Sedation, barbiturates
   (These drugs reduce cerebral metabolic rate, contributing to decreased ICP.)
   b. Anticonvulsants
   (These agents help prevent seizures, which increase cerebral metabolic rate.)
   c. Osmotic diuretics
   (These agents draw water from brain tissue to the plasma to reduce cerebral edema.)
   d. Nonosmotic diuretics
   (These agents draw sodium and water from edematous areas to reduce cerebral edema.)
   e. Steroids
   (These drugs can reduce capillary permeability, limiting cerebral edema.)

14. Carefully monitor hydration status; evaluate fluid intake and output, serum osmolality, and urine specific gravity and osmolality.
(Dehydration from diuretic therapy can cause hypotension and decreased cardiac output.)

15. If IV fluid therapy is prescribed, carefully administer IV fluids via an infusion pump.

(Careful IV fluid administration is necessary to prevent overhydration, which will increase ICP.)
16. If using an intracranial pressure monitoring device, refer to the procedures manual for guidelines.

PC: Seizures

DEFINITION
PC: Seizures: Describes a person experiencing or at high risk to experience paroxysmal episodes of involuntary muscular contraction (tonus) and relaxation (clonus).

High-Risk Populations
- Family history of seizure disorder
- Cerebral cortex lesions
- Head injury
- Infectious disorder (*e.g.,* meningitis)
- Cerebral circulatory disturbance (*e.g.,* stroke)
- Brain tumor
- Alcohol overdose or withdrawal
- Drug overdose or withdrawal
- Electrolyte imbalances
- Disorders of carbohydrate metabolism (*e.g.,* diabetes mellitus)
- High fever

Nursing Goals
The nurse will manage and minimize seizure episodes.

Interventions
1. Determine whether the client senses an aura before onset of seizure activity. If so, reinforce safety measures to take when an aura is felt (*e.g.,* lie down, pull car over to roadside and shut off ignition).
2. If seizure activity occurs, observe and document the following (Hickey, 1986):
   a. Where seizure began
   b. Type of movements, parts of body involved
   c. Changes in pupil size or position
   d. Urinary or bowel incontinence
   e. Duration
   f. Unconsciousness (duration)
   g. Behavior postseizure
   h. Weakness, paralysis postseizure

   i. Sleep postseizure (postictal period)
      (Progression of seizure activity may assist in identifying the anatomic focus of the seizure.)
3. Provide privacy during and after seizure activity.
   (To protect the client from embarrassment)
4. During seizure activity, take measures to ensure adequate ventilation (*e.g.,* loosen clothing). *Do not* try to force an airway or tongue blade through clenched teeth, however.
   (Strong clonic/tonic movements can cause airway occlusion. Forced airway insertion can cause injury.)
5. During seizure activity, gently guide movements to prevent injury. Do not attempt to restrict movements.
   (Physical restraint could result in musculoskeletal injury.)
6. If the client is sitting when seizure activity occurs, ease him to the floor and place something soft under his head.
   (These measures will help prevent injury.)
7. After seizure activity subsides, position the client on his side.
   (This position helps prevent aspiration of secretion.)
8. Allow the person to sleep after seizure activity; reorient upon awakening.
   (The person may experience amnesia; reorientation can help him regain a sense of control and can help reduce anxiety.)
9. If status epilepticus occurs, initiate emergency protocols (*e.g.,* airway maintenance, oxygen therapy, IV line).
   (Status epilepticus is a medical emergency because of the associated severe systemic and cerebral hypoxia.)
10. Keep the bed in a low position with the side rails up, and pad the side rails with blankets.
    (These precautions help prevent injury from fall or trauma.)
11. If the client's condition is chronic, evaluate the need for teaching self-management techniques. Use the nursing diagnosis *High Risk for Altered Health Maintenance related to insufficient knowledge of condition, medication regimen, safety measures, and community resources* (see Section II).

PC: Increased Intraocular Pressure

DEFINITION

PC: Increased Intraocular Pressure: Describes a person experiencing or at high risk to experience increased aqueous humor production or resistance to outflow, which can cause compression of nerve fibers and blood vessels in the optic disk.

High-Risk Population
- Glaucoma
- Corneal transplant
- Radiation therapy
- Eye trauma
- Ophthalmic surgery

Nursing Goals
The nurse will manage and minimize increased intraocular pressure.

Interventions
1. Reinforce prescribed postoperative activity restrictions, which may include avoiding the following:
   a. Bending at the waist
   b. Making sudden head movements
   c. Valsalva maneuver, *e.g.*, straining during bowel movements
   (These activities can increase intraocular pressure.)
2. Reinforce the need to wear eye protection (patch and shield).
   (These protect the eye from trauma.)
3. Monitor for bleeding, dehiscence, and evisceration.
   (Ocular tissue is vulnerable to these problems because of its high vascularity and fragile vessels.)
4. Monitor for severe, unrelieved eye pain. Differentiate between discomfort and pain.
   (Severe pain may indicate increased intraocular pressure.)
5. Administer an antiemetic if nausea develops.
   (Vomiting increases intraocular pressure and must be avoided.)
6. Monitor visual acuity and note any changes (*e.g.*, halos around lights).
   (Factors that can alter vision include blood in the vitreous or from the incision, infection, dislocation of the lens implant, redetachment of the retina, and increased intraocular pressure.)
7. Position the client on his back with the head elevated; turn on the unaffected side.
   (This positioning can help reduce pressure in the affected eye.)
8. Maintain a quiet environment; limit external stimuli and activities.
   (These measures can help reduce stress and may promote decreased intraocular pressure.)

References/Bibliography

Drummond, B. (1990). Preventing increased intracranial pressure. *Focus on Critical Care, 17*(21), 116–122.

Henneman, E. A. (1989). Clinical assessment and neurodiagnostics. *Critical Care Nursing Clinics of North America, 1*(1), 131–142.

Hickey, J. V. (1986). *The clinical practice of neurological and neurosurgical nursing.* Philadelphia: J. B. Lippincott.

Hudak, C., Gallo, B., & Benz, J. (1990). *Critical care nursing* (5th ed.). Philadelphia: J. B. Lippincott.

Lee, S. (1989). Intracranial pressure changes during positioning of patients with severe head injury. *Heart & Lung, 18*(4), 411–414.

Little, M. T. (1989). Complications of multiple trauma. *Critical Care Nursing Clinics of North America, 1*(1), 75–84.

Mahoney, E., & Flynn, J. (1986). *Handbook of medical-surgical nursing.* New York: John Wiley & Sons.

Mitchell, P. H. (1986). Intracranial hypertension: Influence of nursing care activities. *Nursing Clinics of North America, 21*(4), 563–567.

Thelan, L., Davie, J., & Urden, L. (1990). *Textbook of critical care nursing.* St. Louis: C. V. Mosby.

Walleck, C. A. (1989). Controversies in the management of the head-injured patient. *Critical Care Nursing Clinics of North America, 1*(1), 67–74.

Potential Complication: Gastrointestinal/ Hepatic/Biliary

PC: Paralytic Ileus

PC: GI Bleeding

PC: Hepatic Dysfunction

PC: Hyperbilirubinemia

Gastrointestinal, Hepatic, and Biliary Systems Overview

A tube extending from the mouth to anus, the gastrointestinal (GI) system also includes the esophagus, stomach, and small and large intestines. Its functions include ingesting and breaking down food particles into small molecules for digestion, absorbing the small molecules into the blood stream, and eliminating undigested and unabsorbed foodstuffs and other body wastes. Specific hormones (*e.g.*, gastrin, secretin) and enzymes (*e.g.*, pepsin, hydrochloric acid), as well as large volumes of fluid, are needed for digestion, absorption, and elimination. Blood supply to the GI tract, via the thoracic and abdominal arteries, comprises about 20% of the total cardiac output—more after eating.

The body's largest gland, the liver, performs various regulatory, digestive, and other biochemical functions. Important functions include carbohydrate metabolism, fat metabolism, protein metabolism, phagocytosis (Kupffer cells), bile formation, vitamin storage (A, D, B complex), iron storage, and formulation of coagulation factors (fibrinogen, prothrombin, acceleration globulin, and factor VII). About 75% of the blood that perfuses the liver comes from the portal vein; this blood is rich with nutrients from the GI tract. The remaining hepatic blood supply comes via the hepatic artery and is oxygen rich. The hepatic vein provides the only exit pathway. Hepatic dysfunction can involve local enlargement and portal hypertension, as well as systemic effects such as altered blood coagulation and nutritional and metabolic problems.

A small, pear-shaped organ attached to the liver's inferior surface, the gallbladder stores bile for release into the intestines, where it acts in fat emulsification. The hepatic duct from the liver and the cystic duct from the gallbladder join to form the common bile duct to the duodenum.

Potential Complication: Gastrointestinal/ Hepatic/Biliary

DEFINITION

PC: Gastrointestinal/Hepatic/Biliary: Describes a person experiencing or at high risk to experience compromised function in the GI, hepatic, or biliary systems. (Note: These three systems are grouped together for classification purposes. In a clinical situation, the nurse would use either *PC: Gastrointestinal, PC: Hepatic,* or *PC: Biliary* to specify the applicable system.)

Diagnostic Considerations

The nurse can use these generic collaborative problems to describe a person at risk for various problems affecting the GI, hepatic, or biliary systems. Doing so focuses nursing interventions on monitoring GI, hepatic, or biliary status to detect and diagnose abnormal functioning. Should the person develop a complication, the nurse would add the applicable specific collaborative problem (*e.g., PC: GI Bleeding, PC: Hepatic Dysfunction*) to the problem list, specifying appropriate nursing management.

In most cases, along with these collaborative problems, the nurse will treat other associated responses, using nursing diagnoses (*e.g., Altered Comfort related to accumulation of bilirubin pigment and bile salts*).

Focus Assessment Criteria

Subjective Data
1. Alcohol use (past and present)
2. IV drug use (past and present)
3. Exposure to toxins (environmental, travel, occupational)
4. History of
   a. Hepatitis
   b. Cirrhosis
   c. Peptic ulcer
   d. Renal failure
5. Complaints of
   a. Anorexia, indigestion
   b. Pruritus, jaundice
   c. Nausea, vomiting
   d. Constipation
   e. Diarrhea
   f. Bleeding, easy bruising
   g. Tarry or clay-colored stools

    h. Abdominal distention
    i. Tea-colored urine

Objective Data

1. Height and weight, general nutritional status
2. Bowel sounds
3. Stool color, presence of occult blood
4. Presence of jaundice (yellowed skin, sclera)

Significant Laboratory Assessment Criteria

1. Serum albumin (lowered in chronic liver disease)
2. Serum amylase (elevated in biliary tract disease)
3. Bilirubin (elevated in hepatic disease, newborn hyperbilirubinemia)
4. Potassium (lowered in liver disease with ascites, vomiting, diarrhea)
5. Blood urea nitrogen (BUN) (increased in hepatic failure)
6. Prothrombin time (elevated in cirrhosis, hepatitis)
7. Hemoglobin, hematocrit (decreased with bleeding)
8. Sodium (decreased with dehydration)
9. Platelets (decreased with liver disease or bleeding)

PC: Paralytic Ileus

DEFINITION

PC: Paralytic Ileus: Describes a person experiencing or at high risk to experience neurogenic or functional bowel obstruction.

High-Risk Populations

- Postoperative status (bowel, retroperitoneal, or spinal cord surgery)
- Hypokalemia
- Postshock status
- Hypovolemia
- Post-trauma (*e.g.,* spinal cord)

Nursing Goals

The nurse will manage and minimize complications of paralytic ileus.

Interventions

1. In a postoperative client, monitor bowel function, looking for
    a. Bowel sounds in all quadrants returning within 24–48 hours of surgery
    b. Flatus and defecation resuming by the second or third postoperative day

(Surgery and anesthesia decrease innervation of the bowels, reducing peristalsis and possibly leading to transient paralytic ileus.)

2. Do not allow the client any fluids until bowel sounds are present. When indicated, begin with small amounts. Monitor the client's response to resumption of fluid and food intake, and note the nature and amount of any emesis or stools.
   (The client will not tolerate fluids until bowel sounds resume.)

3. Monitor for signs of paralytic ileus—primarily pain, typically localized, sharp, and intermittent.
   (Intraoperative manipulation of abdominal organs and the depressive effects of narcotics and anesthetics on peristalsis can cause paralytic ileus, typically developing between the third and fifth postoperative day.)

4. If paralytic ileus is related to hypovolemia, refer to *PC: Hypovolemia* for more information and specific interventions.

PC: GI Bleeding

DEFINITION

PC: GI Bleeding: Describes a person experiencing or at high risk to experience GI bleeding.

High-Risk Populations

- Disorders of GI, hepatic, and biliary systems
- Transfusion of 5 units (or more) of blood
- Recent stress (*e.g.,* trauma, surgery, sepsis), prolonged mechanical ventilation
- Esophageal varices
- Peptic ulcer
- Colon cancer
- Diverticular disease
- Ulcerative colitis
- Platelet deficiency
- Coagulopathy

Nursing Goals

The nurse will manage and minimize complications of GI bleeding.

Interventions

1. Monitor for signs and symptoms of GI bleeding:
   a. Nausea
   b. Hematemesis
   c. Blood in stool

    d. Decreased hematocrit or hemoglobin

    e. Hypotension, tachycardia

    f. Diarrhea or constipation

    g. Anorexia

    (Clinical manifestations will depend on the amount and duration of GI bleeding. Early detection enables prompt intervention to minimize complications.)

2. Examine stools and vomitus for both gross and occult blood.
   (See Intervention 1 above.)
3. Monitor vital signs often, particularly blood pressure and pulse.
   (Careful monitoring can detect early changes in blood volume.)
4. If nasogastric (NG) intubation is prescribed, use a large-bore (18-gauge) tube and follow protocols for insertion and client care.
   (An NG tube can remove irritating gastric secretions, blood, and clots and can reduce abdominal distention.)
5. Follow the protocol for gastric lavage, if ordered.
   (Lavage provides local vasoconstriction and may help control GI bleeding.)
6. Monitor hemoglobin, hematocrit, red blood cell count, platelets, PT, PTT, and BUN values.
   (These values reflect the effectiveness of therapy.)
7. If hypovolemia occurs, refer to *PC: Hypovolemia* for more information and specific interventions.
8. Prepare for transfusion per physician order.
   (To re-establish volume status.)

PC: Hepatic Dysfunction

DEFINITION

PC: Hepatic Dysfunction: Describes a person experiencing or at high risk to experience progressive liver dysfunction.

High-Risk Populations

- Cirrhosis
- Renal failure
- Hepatitis
- Nutritional deficiencies
- Drug or chemical toxicity (*e.g.*, ethanol, carbon tetrachloride, chloroform, phosphorus, arsenicals)
- Hyperbilirubinemia
- Cystic fibrosis

- Thalassemia
- Rh incompatibility
- Ingestion of raw fish

Nursing Goals

The nurse will manage and minimize the complications of hepatic dysfunction.

Interventions

1. Monitor for signs and symptoms of hepatic dysfunction.
   a. Anorexia, indigestion
      (GI effects result from circulating toxins.)
   b. Jaundice
      (Yellowed skin and sclera result from excessive bilirubin production.)
   c. Petechiae, ecchymoses
      (These skin changes reflect impaired synthesis of clotting factors.)
   d. Clay-colored stools
      (This can result from decreased bile in stools.)
   e. Elevated liver function tests (*e.g.,* serum bilirubin, serum transaminase)
      (Elevated values indicate extensive liver damage.)
   f. Prolonged prothrombin time
      (This reflects reduced production of clotting factors.)
2. With hepatic dysfunction, monitor for hemorrhage.
   (Hepatic dysfunction results in impaired synthesis of clotting factors, which increases the risk of bleeding. Obstructed hepatic blood flow results in dilated vessels prone to hemorrhage [*e.g.,* esophageal varices].)
3. Teach the client to report any unusual bleeding (*e.g.,* in the mouth after brushing teeth).
   (Mucous membranes are prone to injury due to their high surface vascularity.)
4. Monitor for signs and symptoms of hypokalemia.
   (Overproduction of aldosterone causes sodium and water retention and increased potassium excretion)
5. Monitor for portal systemic encephalopathy by assessing
   a. General appearance and behavior
   b. Orientation
   c. Speech patterns
   d. Laboratory values: blood pH and ammonia level
   (Liver dysfunction results in high serum ammonia level, possibly leading to hepatic coma.)
6. Assess for side effects of medications. Avoid administering narcotics, sedatives, and tranquilizers and exposing the client to ammonia products.
   (Liver dysfunction results in decreased metabolism of certain medications [*e.g.,* opiates, sedatives, tranquilizers], increasing the risk of toxicity from high drug blood levels. Ammonia products should be avoided because of the client's already high serum ammonia level.)
7. Monitor for signs and symptoms of renal failure. (Refer to *PC: Renal Failure* for more information.)
   (Obstructed hepatic blood flow results in decreased blood to the kidneys, impairing glomerular filtration and leading to fluid retention and decreased urinary output.)
8. Monitor for hypertension.
   (Fluid retention and overload can cause hypertension.)

9. Teach the client and family to report signs and symptoms of complications, such as
   a. Increased abdominal girth
      (Increased abdominal girth may indicate worsening portal hypertension.)
   b. Rapid weight loss or gain
      (Rapid weight loss points to negative nitrogen balance; weight gain, to fluid retention.)
   c. Bleeding
      (Unusual bleeding indicates decreased prothrombin time and clotting factors.)
   d. Tremors
      (Tremors can result from impaired neurotransmission due to failure of the liver to detoxify enzymes that act as false neurotransmitters.)
   e. Confusion
      (Altered mentation can result from cerebral hypoxia caused by high serum ammonia levels due to the liver's impaired ability to convert ammonia to urea.)

PC: Hyperbilirubinemia

DEFINITION

PC: Hyperbilirubinemia: Describes a neonate with or at high risk of developing excessive serum bilirubin levels (>0.15 mg/dL).

High-Risk Neonates

- ABO incompatibility
- Rh-negative mother
- Polycythemia
- Small for gestational age
- Preterm status
- Large for gestational age

Nursing Goals

The nurse will manage and minimize complications of hyperbilirubinemia.

Interventions

1. Prevent cold stress.
   (Metabolism of brown adipose tissue releases nonesterified free fatty acids, which compete with bilirubin for albumin-binding sites.)
2. Ensure adequate hydration.
   (Optimal fluid balance facilitates bilirubin excretion.)

3. Monitor for signs of hyperbilirubinemia.
   a. Jaundice
      (Yellowed skin and sclera reflect excessive bilirubin production.)
   b. Manifestations of CNS depression (*e.g.,* lethargy, absent Moro reflex, poor sucking reflex) or excitation (*e.g.,* tremors, twitching, high-pitched cry).
      (CNS effects result from deposition of unconjugated bilirubin in brain cells.)
4. Initiate phototherapy according to protocol, if indicated.
   (Phototherapy breaks down bilirubin into water-soluble products that can be excreted.)
5. If phototherapy is performed, ensure optimal hydration. Weigh the infant daily to assess fluid status.
   (Phototherapy increases fluid loss through diaphoresis.)
6. Protect the infant's eyes during phototherapy treatment. Use plexiglass shields; ensure that lids are closed before applying shields. Provide periods out of light with eye shields removed.
   (These precautions help ensure safe treatment.)
7. Monitor for eye discharge, excessive pressure on lids, and corneal irritation.
   (These complications may result from use of eye shields.)
8. Turn the infant frequently during phototherapy.
   (Any areas not exposed to the light will remain jaundiced.)
9. Monitor temperature, checking it at least every 4 hours.
   (A nude infant is vulnerable to hypothermia; use of radiant warmers increases the risk of hyperthermia.)

References/Bibliography

Berk, J. E. (Ed.). (1985). *Gastroenterology.* Philadelphia: W. B. Saunders.

Guenter, P., & Slown, B. (1983). Hepatic disease: Nutritional implications. *Nursing Clinics of North America, 18*(1), 71–82.

Hudak, C., Gallo, B., & Benz, J. (1990). *Critical care nursing* (5th ed.). Philadelphia: J. B. Lippincott.

Groenwald, S., Frogge, M., Goodman, M., & Yarbro, C. (1990). *Cancer nursing: Principles and practice* (2nd ed.). Boston: Jones & Bartlett.

Littleton, M. T. (1989). Complications of multiple trauma. *Critical Care Nursing Clinics of North America, 1*(1), 75–84.

Mahoney, E., & Flynn, J. (1986). *Handbook of medical-surgical nursing.* New York: John Wiley & Sons.

Peck, S. N. (1988). Reducing portal hypertension and variceal bleeding. *Dimensions in Critical Care Nursing, 7*(5), 269–279.

Peppercorn, M. A. (1987). Acute gastrointestional hemorrhage. *Consultant, 27*(6), 61–70.

Thelan, L., Davie, J., & Urden, L. (1990). *Textbook of critical care nursing.* St. Louis: C. V. Mosby.

Potential Complication: Muscular/Skeletal

PC: Pathologic Fractures

PC: Joint Dislocation

Musculoskeletal System Overview

Providing the support structure for the body and housing all body systems, the skeletal system contains 206 bones, as well as ligaments (which provide stability to joints) and tendons (which connect bone to muscle). Besides their structural function, bones also provide a site for red blood cell production and mineral—especially calcium—storage. Joints, the unions between two or more bones, are classified as fibrous (*e.g.,* distal tibiofibular junction), cartilaginous (*e.g.,* symphysis pubis), or synovial (*e.g.,* wrist bones). Cartilage, a connective tissue, provides support and facilitates movement in joints, while also absorbing shock.

Skeletal muscles serve important functions in movement, posture, and heat production. Each skeletal muscle is composed of many elongated multinucleated muscle fibers, through which run slender protein threads known as myofibrils. Motor impulses transmitted from the brain via peripheral motor nerves trigger neurochemical mechanisms—acetylcholine release, calcium release, adenosine triphosphate (ATP) release—that in turn control muscle contraction and relaxation.

Musculoskeletal injuries are common and range from mild to severe. Although not usually life-threatening, disorders of this system—especially when chronic—can adversely affect a person's ability to perform all activities of daily living.

Potential Complication: Muscular/Skeletal

DEFINITION

PC: Muscular/Skeletal: Describes a person experiencing or at high risk to experience various musculoskeletal problems.

Diagnostic Considerations

The nurse can use this generic collaborative problem to describe persons at risk for several types of musculoskeletal problems (*e.g.*, all clients who have sustained multiple trauma). This collaborative problem focuses nursing management on assessing musculoskeletal status to detect and diagnose any abnormalities.

For a client exhibiting a specific musculoskeletal problem, the nurse would add the applicable collaborative problem (*e.g., PC: Pathologic Fractures*) to the problem list. If the risk factors or etiology were not directly related to the primary medical diagnoses, this information would be added to the diagnostic statement (*e.g., PC: Pathologic Fractures related to osteoporosis*).

Because musculoskeletal problems typically affect daily functioning, the nurse must assess the client's functional patterns for evidence of impairment. Findings may have significant implications; for instance, a casted leg that prevents a woman from assuming her favorite sleeping position and impairs her ability to perform housework. After identifying any such problems, the nurse should use nursing diagnoses to address specific responses of actual or potential altered functioning.

Focus Assessment Criteria

Subjective Data

1. Complaints of
   a. Pain, tenderness (site, precipitating factors, relieving factors)
   b. Change in shape and/or size of extremity
   c. Paresthesias, paralysis
   d. Swelling, stiffness (site, precipitating factors, alleviating factors)
   e. Fatigue (pattern, alleviating factors)
   f. Difficulty moving (pattern)
2. History of
   a. Osteoporosis
   b. Joint disease
   c. Fractures
   d. Orthopedic surgery
   e. Tick bite (possibility of Lyme disease)
3. Medication use (prescribed and over-the-counter)

Objective Data

1. Balance and gait
2. Restrictive devices (*e.g.*, cast, brace)
3. Range of motion (flexion, extension, adduction, abduction, external rotation, internal rotation) in
   a. Neck
   b. Shoulders
   c. Elbows, wrists, hands, and fingers
   d. Hips
   e. Knees, ankles, feet, and toes
4. In all extremities
   a. Pulses
   b. Color and temperature
   c. Thermal sensation

    d. Sensitivity (light touch, two-point discrimination)
    e. Strength
    f. Presence of edema, atrophy

Significant Laboratory Assessment Criteria
1. Serum calcium (decreased in osteoporosis)
2. Serum phosphorus (decreased in osteoporosis)

PC: Pathologic Fractures

Definition
PC: Pathologic Fractures: Describes a person experiencing or at high risk to experience a fracture unrelated to trauma due to defects in bone structure.

High-Risk Populations
- Osteoporosis
- Cushing's syndrome
- Malnutrition
- Long-term corticosteroid therapy
- Osteogenesis imperfecta
- Bone tumors (primary or metastatic)
- Paget's disease
- Prolonged immobility

Nursing Goals
The nurse will manage and minimize complications of pathologic fractures.

Interventions
1. Monitor for signs and symptoms of pathologic fractures
    a. Pain in the back, neck, or extremities
    b. Visible bone deformity
    c. Crepitation on movement
    d. Loss of movement or use
    e. Localized soft tissue edema
    f. Skin discoloration
    (Detection of pathologic fractures enables prompt intervention to prevent or minimize further complications.)

2. In a client with osteoporosis, monitor for signs and symptoms of vertebral, hip, and wrist fractures, such as
   a. Pain in the lower back, neck, or wrist
   b. Localized tenderness
   c. Pain radiating to abdomen and flank
   d. Spasm of paravertebral muscles
   (Bones with high amounts of trabecular tissue [*e.g.,* hip, vertebrae, wrist] are more readily affected by progressive osteoporosis.)
3. Promote weight-bearing activities as soon as possible.
   (Weight-bearing prevents bone demineralization.)
4. Teach measures to help prevent injury and promote weight-bearing, such as
   a. Using smooth movements to avoid pulling or pushing on limbs
   b. Supporting the extremities when turning in bed
   c. Lifting the buttocks up slightly when sitting to provide weight-bearing to the legs and arms
5. Monitor x-ray results and serum calcium levels.
   (These diagnostic findings help evaluate the client's risk for fractures.)
6. If a fracture is suspected, maintain proper alignment and immobilize the site using pillows or a splint; notify the physician promptly.
   (Timely, appropriate intervention can prevent or minimize soft tissue damage.)
7. Teach the client and family measures to prevent or delay bone demineralization, using the nursing diagnosis *Health-Seeking Behaviors: Prevention of osteoporosis.*

PC: Joint Dislocation

DEFINITION
PC: Joint Dislocation: Describes a person experiencing or at high risk to experience displacement of a bone from its position in a joint.

High-Risk Populations
- Total hip replacement
- Total knee replacement
- Fractured hip, knee, shoulder

Nursing Goals
The nurse will manage and minimize complications of joint dislocation.

Interventions

1. After hip fracture, monitor for signs and symptoms of hip joint displacement, such as
   a. External rotation of affected leg
   b. Shortening of affected leg
   c. Increased pain
   (Damaged tissue and muscles may not provide adequate support of the hip joint, resulting in displacement.)
2. After replacement surgery, monitor for signs of joint dislocation, such as
   a. Shortening of leg
   b. Inability to move
   c. Misalignment
   d. Abnormal rotation
   e. Bulge at the surgical site
   (Until the surrounding muscles and joint capsule heal, joint dislocation may occur if positioning exceeds the limits of the prosthesis, as in flexing or hyperextending the knee or abducting the hip more than 45°.)
3. Maintain bed rest as ordered. Keep the affected joint in a neutral position with rolls, pillows, or specified devices.
   (Bed rest typically is ordered for 1–3 days after surgery to allow stabilization of the prosthesis.)
4. Turn the client to the unaffected side only; limit the use of Fowler's position.
   (Pressure on the affected side can disrupt the prostheses in the acetabular component. Prolonged assumption of Fowler's position can lead to prosthesis dislocation.)

References/Bibliography

Gleit, C. J., & Graham, B. A. (1985). The role of calcium and estrogen in osteoporosis. *Orthopedic Nursing, 4*(3), 13–18.

Hallal, J. C. (1985). Osteoporotic fractures exact a toll. *Journal of Gerontological Nursing, 11*(8), 13–18.

Groenwald, S., Frogge, M., Goodman, M., & Yarbro, C. (1990). *Cancer nursing: Principles and practice* (2nd ed.). Boston: Jones & Bartlett.

Hudak, C., Gallo, B., & Benz, J. (1990). *Critical care nursing* (5th ed.). Philadelphia: J. B. Lippincott.

Mahoney, E., & Flynn, J. (1986). *Handbook of medical-surgical nursing*. New York: John Wiley & Sons.

McCullough, F. L. (1989). Skeletal trauma in children. *Orthopedic Nursing, 8*(2), 41–46.

Thelan, L., Davie, J., & Urden, L. (1990). *Textbook of critical care nursing*. St. Louis: C. V. Mosby.

Potential Complication: Reproductive

PC: Prenatal Bleeding

PC: Preterm Labor

PC: Pregnancy-Associated Hypertension

PC: Fetal Distress

PC: Postpartum Hemorrhage

Reproductive System Overview

The female reproductive system is composed of external genitalia (mons pubis, labia majora, labia minora, clitoris, vestibule) and internal genitalia (ovaries, fallopian tubes, uterus, vagina). Neuroendocrine interactions control the reproductive cycle. In this cycle, the ovarian follicle grows into the graafian follicle in response to secretion of follicle-stimulating hormone (FSH) and luteinizing hormone (LH) by the anterior pituitary. The preovulatory phase involves the maturation of graafian follicle and rising estrogen production. Anterior pituitary secretion of LH then stimulates ovulation. The graafian follicles release the ovum, then form the corpus luteum, which secretes increased amounts of estrogen and progesterone to stimulate endometrial growth. If the ovum is not fertilized, the corpeus luteum regresses and decreases secretion of estrogen and progesterone, and menstruation—uterine discharge of blood, epithelial cells, fluid, and mucus—occurs.

The male reproductive system also consists of external genitalia (scrotum, testes, penis, epididymis) and internal genitalia (vas deferens, spermatic cord, inguinal canal, ejaculatory ducts, urethra). Accessory glands—seminal vesicles, prostate gland, and Cowper's glands—secrete substances that contribute to semen volume.

Androgens, especially testosterone, control differentiation of fetal external genitalia, development of secondary male sex characteristics, maturation of sperm, and growth and development of male sex organs. The anterior pituitary secretes FSH, which stimulates production of spermatogenesis, and interstitial cell–stimulating hormone, which stimulates production of spermatogenesis and activates cells of Leydig to produce testosterone.

Factors that can cause problems with male or female reproductive system function include hormone imbalances, trauma, tumors, vascular and structural defects, and bacterial and viral infections.

Potential Complication: Reproductive

DEFINITION

PC: Reproductive: Describes a person experiencing or at high risk to experience a problem in reproductive system functioning.

Diagnostic Considerations

This generic collaborative problem provides a category under which to classify more specific collaborative problems affecting the reproductive system. Unlike the other generic collaborative problems (*e.g., PC: Respiratory, PC: Cardiac*), it is of little clinical use by itself. So instead of adding this generic collaborative problem to a client's problem list, the nurse should use the appropriate specific collaborative problem, such as *PC: Fetal Distress* or *PC: Postpartum Hemorrhage.*

Focus Assessment Criteria

Subjective Data

1. Menses (usual, change, midcycle, bleeding)
2. Pregnancy history
2. Contraceptive history
4. If pregnant, date of last menstrual period, presence of cramping, bleeding, or spotting
5. Complaints of
   a. Discomfort or pain with intercourse and/or urination
   b. Penile or vaginal discharge
   c. Breast discharge, lumps, other changes
   d. Stress incontinence
   e. Rectal pain or itching
   f. Difficulty starting or stopping urinary stream
   g. Genital rashes, lesions, or growths
   h. Testicular swelling, pain
   i. Warm or hot flushes

Objective Data

1. Vital signs (fetal heart rate, rhythm)
2. Presence of edema (peripheral, facial)
3. Presence of discharge
4. Breast examination findings
5. Female genital examination findings
6. Male genital examination findings
7. Postpartum monitoring
   a. Vital signs
   b. Urine output

   c. Uterine fundus (height, size, tone)
   d. Perineum
   e. Lochia
   f. Breast assessment

Significant Laboratory Assessment Criteria
1. Gram stain for diplococci (positive in gonorrhea)
2. Venereal Disease Research Laboratory (VDRL) test (positive in syphilis)
3. Cervical, urethral smears (positive in infections)
4. Pap smear (positive in dysplasia, carcinoma]
5. Fetal pH (lowered hypoxia)

PC: Prenatal Bleeding

DEFINITION
PC: Prenatal Bleeding: Describes a woman experiencing or at high risk to experience bleeding during pregnancy.

High-Risk Populations
   • Spontaneous therapeutic abortion
   • Ectopic pregnancy
   • Hydatidiform mole
For Placenta Previa
   • Multiparity
   • Previous placenta previa
   • Uterine abnormalities
   • Increased maternal age
   • Multiple pregnancy
   • Previous cesarean section
For Abruptio Placentae
   • Shortened umbilical cord
   • Trauma
   • Precipitous labor
   • Uterine abnormalities
   • Hypertension
   • Folic acid deficiency
   • Compression of vena cava
   • History of abruption
   • High multiparity
   • Oxytocin induction
   • Second born of multiple births, e.g., twins, triplets

Nursing Goals

The nurse will manage and minimize complications of prenatal bleeding.

Interventions

1. Teach the client to report unusual bleeding immediately.
2. If bleeding occurs, monitor
   a. Amount
   b. Presence of pain or tenderness
   c. Vital signs
   d. Urine output
3. Monitor fetal heart tones. (Refer to *PC: Fetal Distress* for specific guidelines.)
4. Maintain the client in a supine position.
   (This position reduces compression on the vena cava, which increases perfusion to the fetus.)
5. Administer oxygen via face mask at a rate of 8 L/min, as indicated.
   (Supplemental oxygen therapy increases maternal circulating oxygen to the fetus.)
6. If signs of shock occur, refer to *PC: Hypovolemic shock* for more information on nursing management.

PC: Preterm Labor

DEFINITION

PC: Preterm Labor: Describes a woman experiencing or at high risk to experience expulsion of a viable fetus between the 20th and 38th weeks of gestation.

High-Risk Population

- Low socioeconomic status
- Maternal medical conditions (*e.g.*, infection)
- Premature membrane rupture
- Multiple gestation
- Previous premature birth
- Uterine anomalies
- Cervical incompetency
- Closely spaced pregnancies
- Low weight, small stature mother
- Heavy work outside home

Nursing Goals

The nurse will manage and minimize complications of premature labor.

Interventions

1. Teach the client to watch for and report
   a. Menstrual-like cramps
   b. Low backache
   c. Pelvic pressure
   d. Change in character of vaginal secretions
   (Early detection of impending premature labor enables interventions to ensure successful delivery and decrease the risk of complications.)
2. Once labor begins, stay with the client and provide emotional support. (Reassurance and support can help the client prepare for and cope with premature birth.)
3. Maintain constant bed rest and ensure optimal hydration (oral and/or IV). (These measures help expand blood volume and inhibit oxytocin release.)
4. Monitor fetal heart rate and rhythm.
5. Anticipate the use of tocolytic agents (*e.g.*, progestins, antioxytocins, β-sympathomimetics, prostaglandin inhibitors). After administration, monitor for side effects in the mother and newborn.
6. Anticipate delivery of a preterm neonate and intervene as appropriate.

PC: Pregnancy-Associated Hypertension

DEFINITION

PC: Pregnancy-Associated Hypertension: Describes a woman experiencing or at high risk to experience vasoconstriction, hypertension, proteinuria, and edema during pregnancy.

High-Risk Populations

- Under age 20 years
- Over age 35 years
- Preexisting renal disease
- Diabetes mellitus
- Multiple gestation
- Hydatidiform mole
- Chronic hypertensive disease

Nursing Goals

The nurse will manage and minimize complications of hypertension.

Interventions

1. Monitor blood pressure and compare readings to those taken earlier in the pregnancy.
   (Midway through pregnancy, blood pressure commonly is lower than the woman's usual reading; thus, any elevation—even if readings still are within normal limits—may be significant.)
2. Monitor daily weights.
   (Sudden weight gain of 2 lb or more can indicate tissue or occult edema.)
3. Monitor for edema, particularly in the ankles, fingers, and face.
   (Edema results from sodium retention related to decreased glomerular filtration.)
4. Monitor laboratory results for proteinuria.
   (Peripheral arterial vasoconstriction leads to decreased glomerular filtration.)
5. Instruct the client to report headaches, visual disturbances, vomiting, or decreased urine volume.
   (Headaches, visual disturbances, and vomiting may point to cerebral edema; oliguria may indicate renal insufficiency.)
6. Teach a client exhibiting mild hypertension with minimal or no edema or proteinuria to
   a. Restrict activities and rest in bed most of the day
   b. Increase dietary protein intake to compensate for losses in urine
   c. Measure and record intake, output, and weight daily
7. For a client with progressive or severe hypertension and/or proteinuria, hospitalization may be indicated with
   a. Complete bed rest
   b. Daily weight, intake, and output monitoring
   c. Daily urinalysis for protein and casts
   d. Sedation
   e. Magnesium sulfate therapy
8. For a client receiving magnesium sulfate, monitor for signs and symptoms of hypermagnesemia.
   a. Complaints of flushing, extreme thirst, diaphoresis
   b. Diminished deep tendon reflexes (knee, radial biceps)
   c. CNS depression
9. If hypermagnesemia occurs, monitor vital signs and intake and output.
   (Hypermagnesemia can cause CNS depression, respiratory depression, and circulatory collapse.)
10. Ensure ready availability of calcium gluconate (10% solution).
    (Calcium gluconate administration can reverse respiratory depression and heart block.)
11. Ensure that the client gets as much undisturbed rest as possible.
    (Adequate rest promotes relaxation and may help reduce hypertension and decrease the risk of seizure activity.)
12. If seizures occur, refer to *PC: Seizures* for nursing interventions.

PC: Fetal Distress

DEFINITION

PC: Fetal Distress: Describes a fetus experiencing or at high risk to experience hypoxia.

High-Risk Populations

Fetal Factors
- Prematurity
- Intrauterine growth retardation
- Atresia of umbilical cord
- Cord compression
- Placental insufficiency
- Infection
- Multiple gestation
- Congenital anomalies
- Dysmaturity
- Acute hemolytic crisis
- Prolonged labor
- Prolonged rupture of membranes

Maternal Factors
- Chronic hypertension
- Pregnancy-associated hypertension
- Diabetes mellitus
- Third trimester bleeding
- Maternal hypoxia (*e.g.,* respiratory insufficiency)
- Seizures, hypotension
- Prolonged uterine activity
- Abruptio placentae
- Cardiovascular disease
- Drug addiction
- Malnutrition

Nursing Goals

The nurse will manage and minimize episodes of fetal distress.

Interventions

1. Determine baseline fetal heart tones and evaluate if normal as:
   a. Rate of 120 to 160 beats/min
   b. Presence of beat-to-beat variation (normal fetal rate has a fine irregularity of >5–10 beats/min)
   c. Early decelerations (transient slowing of fetal heart rate with compression of the contraction causing parasympathetic stimulation)

2. Monitor for abnormal fetal heart rate or rhythm, including
   a. Decreased variability (<6 beats/min)
   b. Tachycardia (>160 beats/min)
   c. Bradycardia (<110 beats/min)
   d. Late decelerations (a drop in fetal heart rate of 15–45 beats/min after the contraction)
   e. Variable decelerations, caused by compression of the umbilical cord
   f. Sinusoidal pattern (repetitive undulation of baseline)
   (The fetal heart is very sensitive to the effects of disturbed gas exchange.)
3. If tachycardia occurs, assess
   a. Maternal temperature
      (Fetal tachycardia occurs when maternal core temperature rises. It may increase before the mother's temperature can be measured orally or rectally.)
   b. Maternal intake, output, and urine specific gravity
      (Maternal dehydration can cause fetal tachycardia.)
   c. Maternal anxiety level
      (Severe anxiety can increase fetal heart rate.)
   d. Maternal medication use
      (Certain medications used by the mother can cause increased fetal heart rate, *e.g.*, atropine, ritodrine hydrochloride, scopolamine.)
4. Increase maternal hydration.
   (Maternal dehydration can cause fetal tachycardia.)
5. Notify the physician of the situation and your assessment findings.
6. Position the mother on her left side.
   (This position decreases occlusion of the inferior vena cava by the uterus, promoting venous return to the heart.)
7. If decreased variability occurs evaluate possible causes, which can include
   a. Sleeping fetus
   b. Effects of narcotics or sedatives
   c. Fetal hypoxia
   d. Maternal position
8. If bradycardia, decreased variability, or late decelerations continue, notify the physician and take the following steps.
   a. Keep the mother in a left side-lying position.
      (See Intervention 6 above.)
   b. Administer oxygen via face mask at a flow rate of 8 L/min according to protocol.
      (This will increase oxygen delivery to the fetus.)
   c. Acquire a fetal scalp blood sample according to protocol.
      (To evaluate fetal pH and metabolic status)
   d. Discontinue oxytocin infusion, if indicated, according to protocol.
9. Initiate electronic fetal monitoring according to protocol, if indicated.
10. Remain with the mother and partner, provide information, and give them opportunities to share concerns and fears.
    (This ensures constant monitoring and also may help reduce the mother's anxiety.)
11. If the mother's condition worsens or if fetal pH is 7.2 or below, anticipate a cesarean section and assist as indicated.
12. If mild variable decelerations occur, change the mother's position from supine to lateral or from one side to the other. If fetal heart rate does not improve, see Intervention 13.
    (Position shifts may relieve cord compression.)

13. If severe variable decelerations occur, take the following steps.
    a. Notify the physician.
    b. Discontinue oxytocin infusion per protocol.
    c. Perform a vaginal examination to assess for cord prolapse.
    d. Shift the mother's position to left side-lying and evaluate fetal heart rate; if not improved, turn the mother on her right side.
    e. If these position changes do not improve fetal heart rate, or if cord is prolapsed, help the mother assume a knee-chest position, which will reduce pressure on the cord and increase perfusion to the fetus.
    f. Administer oxygen via face mask at a rate of 8 L/min, according to protocol, to increase oxygen delivery to the fetus.
14. Anticipate an emergency vaginal delivery or cesarean section if the mother's condition worsens, if cord prolapase occurs, and/or if fetal pH is 7.2 or lower.

PC: Postpartum Hemorrhage

DEFINITION

PC: Postpartum Hemorrhage: Describes a woman who is experiencing or is at high risk to experience acute blood loss greater than 500 mL within the first 24 hours postpartum.

High-Risk Populations

- Problematic third stage of labor
- Overdistended uterus (*e.g.,* due to hydramnios, large fetus, multiple gestation)
- Prolonged labor
- Precipitous labor
- Oxytocin induction
- Multiparity
- Maternal exhaustion
- Instrument delivery
- History of uterine atony
- History of blood dyscrasias
- Excessive analgesic use
- Pregnancy-associated hypertension
- Retained placental fragments

Nursing Goals

The nurse will manage and minimize postpartum bleeding.

Interventions

1. Assess the uterine fundus every 5 minutes for the first hour postpartum and p.r.n. thereafter for the first 24 hours; evaluate
   a. Height (normally should be at the level of the umbilicus after delivery)
   b. Size (when contracted, should be about the size of an apple)
   c. Consistency (should feel firm)
   (A boggy or relaxed uterus will not control bleeding by compression of the uterine muscle fibers.)
2. If the uterus is relaxed or relaxing, massage it with firm but gentle circular strokes until it contracts.
   (Massage will stimulate the uterine muscle to contract.)
3. Avoid routine massage or overmassaging the uterus.
   (Unnecessary massage can cause pain and muscle fatigue, with subsequent uterine relaxation.)
4. Monitor blood pressure and pulse every 15 minutes for 1 hour, then every 30 minutes for the next hour, and then once every hour until the mother's condition stabilizes.
   (Careful vital sign monitoring provides accurate evaluation of hemodynamic status.)
5. Monitor perineal blood loss. Keep a record of the number of pads used and the amount of saturation.
   (Continuous seepage of blood with a firm uterus can indicate cervical or vaginal lacerations. Bleeding after the first 24 hours can indicate retained placental fragments or subinvolution.)
6. Monitor bladder size and urine output with the same frequency as for vital signs (see Intervention 4 above).
   (A distended bladder can displace the uterus and increase uterine atony.)
7. If bleeding becomes excessive, if the uterus fails to contract, or if vital sign changes occur, notify the physician.
8. If the woman exhibits signs of shock, refer to *PC: Hypovolemic Shock* for nursing interventions.

References/Bibliography

Bennett, N., & Bott, J. (1989). New strategies for preterm labor. *Nurse Practitioner, 14*(4), 27–38.

Babson, S., Gorham, S., & Benson, R. (1980). *Management of high-risk pregnancy and intensive care of the neonate*. St. Louis: C.V. Mosby.

Groenwald, S., Frogge, M., Goodman, M., & Yarbro, C. (1990). *Cancer nursing: Principles and practice* (2nd ed.). Boston: Jones & Bartlett.

Haubrich, K. L. (1990). Amnioinfusion: A technique for the relief of variable deceleration. *Journal of Obstetric, Gynecologic, and Neonatal Nursing, 19*(4), 299–303.

Hudak, C., Gallo, B., & Benz, J. (1990). *Critical care nursing* (5th ed.). Philadelphia: J. B. Lippincott.

May, K., & Mahlmeister, L. (1990). *Comprehensive maternity nursing*. Philadelphia: J. B. Lippincott.

Sala, D. J., & Moise, K. (1990). The treatment of preterm labor using a portable subcutaneous terbutaline pump. *Journal of Obstetric, Gynecologic, and Neonatal Nursing, 19*(2), 108–115.

Thelan, L., Davie, J., & Urden, L. (1990). *Textbook of critical care nursing*. St. Louis: C. V. Mosby.

Whitley, N. (1985). *Manual of clinical obstetrics*. Philadelphia: J.B. Lippincott.

Appendixes

Appendix I: Adult Assessment Guide

This guide directs the nurse to collect data to assess functional health patterns* of the individual and to determine the presence of actual, high risk, or possible nursing diagnoses. Should the person have medical problems, the nurse will also have to assess for data in order to collaborate with the physician in monitoring the problem.

As with any printed assessment tool, the nurse must determine whether to collect or defer certain data. The symbol Δ identifies data that should be collected on hospitalized persons. The collection of data in sections not marked with Δ probably should be deferred with most acutely ill persons or when the information is irrelevant to the particular individual.

As the nurse interviews the person, significant data may surface. The nurse should then ask other questions (focus assessment) to determine the presence of a pattern. Each diagnosis in Section II has a focus assessment to help the nurse gather more pertinent data in a particular functional area.

For example, the client reports during the initial interview that she has a problem with incontinence. The nurse should ask specific questions utilizing the focus assessment for *Altered Patterns of Urinary Elimination* to determine which incontinence diagnosis is present. After the nurse has identified the factors, the plan of care can be initiated.

Adult Data Base Assessment Format

1. Health Perception–Health Management Pattern
   a. Health management
      "How would you usually describe your health?"

Excellent	Fair
Good	Poor

      "How would you describe your health at this time?"
      Review the daily health practices of the individual

Dental care	Exercise regime
Food intake	Leisure activities
Fluid intake	Responsibility in the family

      Use of

Tobacco	Drugs (over-the-counter,
Salt, sugar, fat products	prescribed)
Alcohol	

      Knowledge of safety practices

Fire prevention	Automobile (maintenance, seat
Water safety	belts)
Children	Bicycle
	Poison control

---

*The functional health patterns have been adapted from Gordon, M. (1982). *Nursing diagnosis: Application and process.* New York: McGraw-Hill.

Knowledge of disease and preventive behavior
  Specific disease (*e.g.,* heart disease, cancer, respiratory disease, childhood
    diseases, infections, dental disease)
  Susceptibility (*e.g.,* presence of risk factors, family history)
  "What do you do to keep healthy and to prevent disorders in yourself? In your
    children?"

Adequate nutrition	Professional examinations
Weight control	(gynecologic,
Exercise program	dental)
Self-examinations (breast,	Immunizations
testicular)	

b. Developmental history*
  Family history

Maternal grandparents		Paternal grandparents
Mother	Patient	Father
Spouse	Children	Siblings

  Assess for achievement of developmental tasks
  Young adult
    (Intimacy vs. isolation)
    Accepting himself and stabilizing self-concept
    Establishing independence from parental home and financial aid
    Becoming established in a vocation or profession that provides personal
      satisfaction, economic independence, and a feeling of making a worth-
      while contribution to society
    Learning to appraise and express love responsibility through more than
      sexual contexts
    Establishing an intimate bond with another, either through marriage or
      with a close friend
    Establishing and managing a residence/home
    Finding a congenial social group
    Deciding whether or not to have a family
    Formulating a meaningful philosophy of life
    Becoming involved as a citizen in the community
  Middle age
    (Generactivity vs. stagnation)
    Developing a sense of unity and abiding intimacy with mate
    Helping growing and grown children become happy and responsible
      adults—relinquishing central position in their life
    Taking pride in accomplishments of self and spouse
    Finding pleasure in generativity and recognition in work
    Balancing work with other roles
    Preparing for retirement
    Role reversal with parents/parental loss
    Achieving mature social and civic responsibility
    Developing or maintaining active organizational membership
    Accepting and adjusting to changes of middle age (physical)
    Socialization with new and old friends
    Use of leisure time

*Source: Nursing History Guide. Nursing Dept, Southeastern Missouri University, Cape
Girardeau, MO

Older adult
(Integrity vs. despair)
Deciding how and where to live out remaining years
Continuing supportive, close, and warm relationship with significant others, including a satisfying sexual relationship
Satisfactory living arrangements—safe, comfortable household routine
Supplemental retirement income, if possible
Maintaining maximum level of self-health care
Maintaining interest in people outside of family
Maintaining social, civic, and political responsibility
Pursuing interests
Finding meaning in life after retirement
Facing inevitable illness and death of self and significant others
Formulating a philosophy of life
Finding meaning to life through philosophy/religion
Adjusting to death of spouse or loved one

c. Health perception

Δ Reason for and expectations of hospitalization (and previous hospital experiences)

Δ "Describe your illness"

Cause	Onset

Δ "What treatments or practices have been recommended?"

Diet	Surgery
Weight loss	Cessation of smoking
Medications	Exercises

Δ "Have you been able to follow the prescribed instructions?" If not, "What has prevented you?"

Δ "Have you experienced or do you anticipate a problem with caring for yourself (your children, your home)?"

Mobility problems	Financial concerns
Sensory deficits (vision, hearing)	Structural barriers (stairs, narrow doorway)

Δ Are there any problems that could contribute to falls or accidents?
Unfamiliar setting
Decreased sensorium (vertigo, confusion)
Sensory deficits (visual, auditory, tactile)
Motor deficits (gait, tremors, coordination)
Urinary/bowel urgency

Δ 2. Nutritional–Metabolic Pattern
"What is the usual daily food intake (meals, snacks)?"
"What is the usual fluid intake (type, amounts)?"
"How is your appetite?"

Indigestion	Vomiting
Nausea	Sore mouth

"What are your food restrictions or preferences?"
"Any supplements (vitamins, feedings)?"
"Has your weight changed in the last 6 months?" If yes, "Why?"
"Any problems with ability to eat?"

Swallow liquids	Chew
Swallow solids	Feed self

Skin
"What is the skin condition?"

Color, temperature, turgor

Edema (type, location)

Lesions (type, description, location)

Pruritus (location)

Are there any factors present that could contribute to pressure ulcer development?

Immobility
Dehydration
Malnourishment
Decreased circulation
Sensory deficits

Δ 3. Elimination Pattern

a. Bladder
"Are there any problems or complaints with the usual pattern of urinating?"

Oliguria

Retention

Polyuria

Burning

Dysuria

Incontinence

Dribbling

"Are assistive devices used?"

Intermittent catheterization

Incontinence briefs

Catheter (Foley, external)

Cystostomy

b. Bowel
"What is the usual time, frequency, color, consistency, pattern?"
"Assistive devices (type, frequency)?"

Ileostomy

Cathartics

Colostomy

Laxatives

Enemas

Suppositories

4. Activity–Exercise Pattern
"Describe usual daily/weekly activities of daily living"

Occupation

Exercise pattern (type, frequency)

Leisure activities

Δ "Are there any limitations in ability?"

Ambulating (gait, weight-bearing, balance)

Dressing/grooming (oral hygiene)

Bathing self (shower, tub)

Toileting (commode, toilet, bedpan)

"Are there complaints of dyspnea or fatigue?"

Δ Are there factors present that could interfere with self-care after discharge?

Motor deficits
Cognitive/sensory deficits
Emotional deficits
Environmental barriers
Lack of knowledge
Lack of resources

Δ 5. Sleep–Rest Pattern
"What is the usual sleep pattern?"

Bedtime

Sleep aids (medication, food)

Hours slept

Sleep routine

"Any problems?"

Difficulty falling asleep

Not feeling rested after sleep

Difficulty remaining asleep

Δ 6. Cognitive–Perceptual Pattern

"Any deficits in sensory perception (hearing, sight, touch)?"

Glasses   Hearing aid

"Any complaints?"

Vertigo

Insensitivity to superficial pain   Insensitivity to cold or heat

"Able to read and write?"

7. Self-Perception Pattern

Δ "What are you most concerned about?"

"What are your present health goals?"

Δ "How would you describe yourself?"

"Has being ill made you feel differently about yourself?"

"To what do you attribute the following?"

Becoming ill

Getting better

Maintaining health

8. Role–Relationship Pattern

Δ Communication

Any hearing deficits? (hearing aids, lip-reading)

What language is spoken?

Is speech clear? Relevant?

Assess ability to express self and understand others (verbally, in writing, with gestures)

Relationships

"Do you live alone?" "If not, with whom?"

"To whom do you turn for help in time of need?"

Assess family life (members, educational level, occupations)

Cultural background   Decision-making

Activities (lone or group)   Communication patterns

Roles, discipline   Finances

"Any complaints?"

Parenting difficulties   Marital difficulties

Difficulties with relatives,   Abuse (physical, verbal,

(in-laws, parents)   substance)

9. Sexuality–Sexual Functioning Pattern

"Has there been or do you anticipate a change in your sexual relations because of your condition?"

Fertility   Pregnancy

Libido   Contraceptives

Erections   History

Menstruation

Assess knowledge of sexual functioning

10. Coping–Stress Management Pattern

Δ "How do you make decisions (alone, with assistance, who)?"

Δ "Has there been a loss in your life in the past year (or changes—moves, job, health)?"

"What do you like about yourself?"

"What would you like to change in your life?"

"What is preventing you?"

"What do you do when you are tense or under stress (*e.g.*, problem-solve, eat, sleep, take medications, seek help)?"

Δ "What can the nurses do to provide you with more comfort and security during your hospitalization?"

11. Value–Belief System

"With what (whom) do you find a source of strength or meaning?"

"Is religion or God important to you?"

"What are your religious practices (type, frequency)?"

"Have your values or moral beliefs been challenged recently? Describe."

Δ "Is there a religious person or practice (diet, book, ritual) that you would desire during hospitalization (institutionalization)?"

12. Physical Assessment (objective)

a. General

Age

Height

Weight (actual/approximate)

General appearance

Temperature, pulse, blood pressure, respirations

b. Cognitive–emotional

Language spoken

Ability to read English

Ability to communicate

Ability to comprehend

Level of anxiety

Interactive skills

c. Respiratory–circulatory

Quality, cough, breath sounds

Right/left pedal pulse

d. Metabolic–integrumentary

Skin

Color, temperature, turgor, edema, lesions, bruises

Tubes

Mouth

Gums, teeth

Abdomen

Bowel sounds, distended

e. Neurosensory

Mental status

Speech

Pupils (size, reactivity to light)

Eyes (appearance, drainage)

f. Muscular–skeletal

Functional ability (mobility and safety)

Dominant hand

Use of right and left hands, arms, legs

Strength, grasp

Range of motion

Gait (stability)

Use of aids (wheelchair, braces, cane, walker)

Weight-bearing (full, partial, none)

Appendix II: Adult Psychiatric Assessment Guide*

Shadowed Areas—To be completed by Admitting Nurse
White Areas—To be completed within 48 hrs of Admission by Primary Nurse

1. DEMOGRAPHIC INFORMATION

| ADM/TRANS DATE | / / | TIME | am | pm | AGE | SEX ☐ Male | ☐ Female |

| HAIR COLOR: | ☐ White | ☐ Blond | ☐ Brown | ☐ Red | ☐ Auburn |
| | ☐ Black | ☐ Gray | ☐ Other | | |

EYE COLOR: ☐ Blue ☐ Brown ☐ Green ☐ Hazel ☐ Other

ETHNIC ORIGIN: ☐ Caucasian ☐ Am. Indian ☐ Hispanic ☐ Afr Amer ☐ Asian ☐ Other

ADMITTED FROM: ☐ Home ☐ Hospital ☐ Nursing Home ☐ Group Home ☐ Other

ADMITTED WITH: ☐ Family ☐ Friend ☐ Other

HOME CARE AGENCY PTA:

INFO OBTAINED FROM: ☐ Spouse ☐ Family ☐ Friend ☐ Patient ☐ Other

MARITAL STATUS: ☐ Single ☐ Married ☐ Divorced ☐ Separated ☐ Widow ☐ Widower

EMERGENCY CONTACT:
    Name   Address   Relationship   Telephone @ Home @ Work
1.

2.

3.

PARENT/GUARDIAN:
    Name   Address   Relationship   Telephone @ Home @ Work

REASON FOR ADMISSION:

PREVIOUS OR CURRENT HEALTH PROBLEMS ☐ No ☐ Yes. Describe: _____

*Developed by the Psychiatric Nursing Practice Council, Department of Pediatric, Perinatal, Psychiatric Nursing, University of Michigan Medical Center, Ann Arbor, Michigan. Used with permission.

PREVIOUS PSYCHIATRIC TX/HOSPITALIZATION: ☐ No ☐ Yes. Describe: _____

_____

_____

_____

2. ORIENTATION TO UNIT

☐ Patient Room ☐ Bathroom ☐ Showers ☐ Telephones ☐ Dining Room

☐ Community Rooms ☐ Staff Areas ☐ Other _____

EXPLANATION OF PATIENT'S RIGHTS BOOKLET

☐ Yes, by _____ ☐ No. Explain why not. _____

BELONGINGS SEARCHED

☐ No ☐ Yes. By Whom? _____ Items Removed: _____

Articles were: ☐ Sent Home ☐ Stored

Money deposited in Cashier's Office ☐ No ☐ Yes Amount $ _____

EXPLANATION OF PROHIBITED ARTICLES

☐ Safety Razors ☐ Razor Blades ☐ Scissors ☐ Weapons

☐ Glass Articles ☐ Other Sharps ☐ Cigarettes ☐ Pipe

☐ Chewing Tobacco ☐ Matches ☐ Lighter ☐ Medications

☐ Drugs ☐ Alcohol ☐ Cameras ☐ Recording Devices

☐ Televisions

ORIENTATION TO UNIT COMPLETED BY R.N. Signature _____

3. HEALTH-PERCEPTION/HEALTH MANAGEMENT

HEIGHT	WEIGHT	TEMP	RESP	ALLERGIES

ALLERGIES

Drugs	Food	Other

B/P — RIGHT — LEFT

☐ Lying _____
☐ Sitting _____
☐ Standing _____

☐ PCN ☐ Chocolate ☐ Tape
☐ SULFA ☐ Shellfish ☐ Cosmetics
☐ ASA ☐ Milk Products ☐ Wool

☐ Others _____

PULSE — RIGHT — LEFT

☐ Lying _____
☐ Sitting _____
☐ Standing _____

ALLERGIC REACTIONS

☐ Rash ☐ N/V ☐ Diarrhea

☐ Anaphylaxis ☐ Upper Respiratory

☐ Other _____

ALLERGY TREATMENT

_____

MEDICATIONS (Last 3 months)

NAME OF MEDICATION	DOSE	SCHEDULE	LAST DOSE	REASON	HOW LONG?

SUBSTANCES

Caffeine: ☐ No ☐ Coffee ☐ Tea ☐ Cola ☐ Chocolate

How much _____ How long? _____

Tobacco: ☐ No ☐ Cigarettes ☐ Cigars ☐ Pipe ☐ Chewing Tobacco

How much _____ How long? _____

DRUGS: ☐ No ☐ Marijuana ☐ Cocaine ☐ Heroin ☐ LSD

☐ Designer ☐ Amphetamines ☐ Barbiturates ☐ Other _____

How much/How long? _____

Last ingestion _____ How much? _____

Do you think you have a problem related to your drug intake? ☐ No ☐ Yes

ALCOHOL ☐ No ☐ Beer ☐ Liquor ☐ Wine

How much? _____

How long? _____ Frequency _____ Last drink _____ How much? _____

SYMPTOMS ☐ No ☐ Miss work ☐ Miss school ☐ Pass out

☐ Drink alone ☐ Drink with others ☐ Loss of memory

Family history of ETOH abuse? ☐ No ☐ Yes. Describe: _____

_____

Do you think you have a drinking problem? ☐ No ☐ Yes. Describe: _____

_____

KNOWN EXPOSURE TO COMMUNICABLE DISEASES: ☐ No ☐ Yes. Describe: _____

_____

CURRENT ILLNESS/INFECTIONS: ☐ No ☐ Yes. Describe: _____

_____

CHRONIC ILLNESS/INFECTION ☐ No ☐ Yes. Describe: _____

_____

PAST ACCIDENT/INJURIES: ☐ No ☐ Yes. Describe: _____

_____

_____

GENERAL APPEARANCE:

☐ Clean ☐ Neat ☐ Unkempt ☐ Dirty ☐ Disheveled ☐ Odorous

☐ Well-nourished ☐ Obese ☐ Thin ☐ Emaciated

SELF-CARE (Dress/bathing)

☐ Independent ☐ Dependent ☐ Assistance. Describe _____

4. COPING/STRESS MANAGEMENT

What are the main concerns in your life right now? _____

How are you managing these concerns? _____

How do you manage your anger? _____

SIGNIFICANT/RECENT CHANGES	NO	YES	DESCRIBE
School			
Work			
Family Unit			
Health			
Finances			
Home			
Own illness			
Death of a significant other			
Marital status/relationship			
Retirement			

What makes you tense or nervous? _____

What do you do when you are feeling tense or nervous? _____

Does it help relieve your tension? ☐ No ☐ Yes   Are you impulsive? ☐ No ☐ Yes

Do you feel depressed? ☐ No ☐ Yes

Are you able to talk about your feelings? ☐ No ☐ Yes

SUICIDE POTENTIAL	NO	YES	DESCRIBE
1. Do you feel you have control over the events in your life?			
2. Feel like giving up?			
3. Feel guilty?			
4. Current thoughts of harming self?			

	NO	YES	DESCRIBE
5. Past attempts at harming self?			
6. Past thoughts of suicide?			
7. Past suicide attempts?			
8. Current thoughts of suicide?			
Plan for suicide?			
Ability to contract			
9. Recent suicide attempt?			
10. Attempt in the hospital?			
11. Family history of suicide?			
POTENTIAL FOR AGGRESSION	**NO**	**YES**	**DESCRIBE**
1. Have you ever hurt someone?			
2. Have you ever broken things/destroyed property?			
3. Are you having thoughts of hurting someone?			
4. Do you plan to hurt someone?			

5. NUTRITION-METABOLIC

TEETH ☐ Normal ☐ Dentures ☐ Upper
☐ Lower ☐ Partial ☐ Braces

ORAL
SYMPTOMS ☐ None ☐ Bleeding Gums ☐ Sores/Patches
☐ Swelling ☐ Decay ☐ Halitosis ☐ Other

SKIN INTEGRITY ☐ Intact ☐ Turgor Normal ☐ Diaphoretic ☐ Turgor Poor

☐ Cool ☐ Hot ☐ Moist ☐ Dry

Skin Breakdown. Describe: _____

Reddened areas. Describe: _____

Ecchymosis. Describe: _____

Lesions. Describe: _____

Warts. Describe: _____

MEAL PATTERN

Number meals/day 1 2 3 4 5 Meal times _____

With family ☐ Yes ☐ No Meals include 4 basic food groups: ☐ Yes ☐ No

Food restrictions/diet _____

SELF-CARE
(feeding) ☐ Independent ☐ Dependent ☐ Assistance. Describe: _____

PROBLEMS WITH EATING
OR WEIGHT ☐ No ☐ Yes. Describe _____

SYMPTOMS ☐ No ☐ Recent loss of ☐ Difficulty ☐ Nausea ☐ Vomiting
                 appetite   swallowing

Describe problems: _____

FEEDING AIDS ☐ No ☐ Yes ☐ Tubes ☐ Special Utensils. Describe: _____

6. ELIMINATION

BOWEL HABITS: Last BM _____ # Stools/Day 0 1 2 3 4 ☐ Other _____

SYMPTOMS ☐ No ☐ Diarrhea ☐ Constipation ☐ Gas

☐ Cramping ☐ Bleeding ☐ Hemorrhoids ☐ Involuntary stooling

☐ Use of laxatives ☐ Other. Describe: _____

TREATMENT _____

BOWEL SOUNDS ☐ Active ☐ Inactive ☐ Hyperactive ☐ Sluggish

URINARY DIFFICULTIES ☐ No ☐ Yes

SYMPTOMS ☐ Frequency ☐ Burning ☐ Pain ☐ Bleeding

☐ Incontinence ☐ Hesitancy ☐ Dribbling ☐ Urgency

☐ Stress

☐ Enuresis - Nocturnal - Daytime. Describe: _____

TREATMENT _____

ASSISTIVE DEVICES ☐ No ☐ Colostomy ☐ Urinary Device

☐ Catherizations ☐ Other. Describe _____

Self Care: ☐ Independent ☐ Dependent ☐ With Assistance. Describe: _____

7. SEXUALITY/REPRODUCTION

ONSET OF MENARCHE/MENOPAUSE _____ LMP _____

SEXUALLY ACTIVE? ☐ No ☐ Yes | CURRENTLY PREGNANT? ☐ No ☐ Yes

SYMPTOMS ☐ No ☐ Dysmenorrhea ☐ Heavy menstrual flow ☐ Irregular cycle

CONTRACEPTIVES

☐ No ☐ Yes TYPE: ☐ Birth Control Pills ☐ Vaginal Spermicides

☐ Condoms ☐ Cervical cap ☐ Diaphragm ☐ Rhythm Method

☐ Other. Describe: _____

NUMBER: PREGNANCIES ____ LIVE BIRTHS ____ MISCARRIAGES ____ ABORTIONS ____

SELF BREAST EXAM ☐ No ☐ Yes ☐ Deferred

SELF TESTICULAR EXAM ☐ No ☐ Yes ☐ Deferred

SYMPTOMS ☐ No ☐ Painful intercourse ☐ Open sores/lesions

☐ Drainage ☐ Odor ☐ Other _____

Recent change in sexual behavior? ☐ No ☐ Yes. Describe: _____

Have any sexual/reproductive concerns? ☐ No ☐ Yes. Describe: _____

KNOWN EXPOSURE TO STD? ☐ No ☐ Yes. See Below

☐ AIDS ☐ Syphilis ☐ Herpes ☐ Gonorrhea ☐ Chlamydia ☐ Hepatitis B

☐ Other. Describe: _____

8. ACTIVITY/REST

ENERGY LEVEL ☐ Usual ☐ High ☐ Low

☐ Tires easily ☐ Lethargic ☐ Daily Variation

Describe _____

AMBULATION: ☐ Independent ☐ Dependent ☐ Assistance

CLIMB STAIRS: ☐ Independent ☐ Dependent ☐ Assistance

ASSISTIVE AIDS: ☐ No ☐ Cane ☐ Walker

☐ Crutches ☐ W/C ☐ Prosthesis

Describe problems: _____

ROM: ☐ Full ☐ Partial. Describe: _____

BALANCE/GAIT: ☐ Steady ☐ Unsteady. Describe: _____

ROUTINE EXERCISE PATTERN: Describe: _____

SYMPTOMS	NO	YES	WITH EXERTION	WITHOUT EXERTION	DESCRIBE
Chest pain					
Shortness of breath					
Coughing					
Palpitations					
Pedal edema					
Chest tightness					
Dizziness					
Joint pain					
High blood pressure					
Other					

ACTIVITY RESTRICTIONS ☐ No ☐ Yes. Describe: _____

HOBBIES/INTERESTS/EXTRA CURRICULAR ACTIVITIES Describe: _____

_____

9. SLEEP/REST

Hrs. Sleep/Night _____ Hrs. Sleep/Daytime _____ Bedtime _____ Wake-up time _____

Feel rested? ☐ No ☐ Yes

BEDTIME RITUALS ☐ Reading ☐ Snacks ☐ T.V. ☐ Prayer ☐ Bath

☐ Exercise ☐ Nightlight ☐ Other. Describe: _____

SLEEPING AIDS
(Medications/Others) ☐ No ☐ Yes. Describe: _____

SYMPTOMS ☐ Awake easily ☐ Nightmares ☐ Night Sweats

☐ Insomnia - Early - Middle - Late   ☐ Recent Change   ☐ Fear Associated with sleep.

Describe: _____   ☐ Other. Describe: _____

10. COGNITIVE/PERCEPTUAL

EDUCATION   Last grade completed _____   College _____

Can patient read? ☐ No ☐ Yes   Can patient write? ☐ No ☐ Yes

PRIMARY LANGUAGE SPOKEN: ☐ English ☐ Other

VISION			HEARING		
R L		VISION CORRECTED WITH:	R L		PATIENT CAN:
☐☐ Normal	☐ Glasses		☐☐ Normal		☐ Use Sign Language
☐☐ Impaired	☐ Contacts		☐☐ Impaired		☐ Lip read
☐☐ Cataracts	☐ Prosthesis		☐☐ Deaf		☐ Other: _____
☐☐ Glaucoma	☐ Other. Describe: _____		☐☐ Hearing Aid	_____	
☐☐ Blind	_____		☐☐ Other. Describe: _____		
☐☐ Blurred			_____		
☐☐ Other. Describe: _____					

DISCOMFORT/PAIN ☐ No ☐ Yes. Location _____ Treatment _____

DISTRACTABILITY/ATTENTION SPAN

☐ Able to attend   ☐ Unable to attend   ☐ Easily distracted

☐ Other. Describe: _____

MOOD   *How would you describe your usual mood?*

☐ Pleasant	☐ Happy	☐ Shameful
☐ Irritable	☐ Euphoric	☐ Labile
☐ Recent change	☐ Anxious	☐ Helpless/Hopeless
☐ Calm	☐ Fearful	☐ Sad
☐ Guilty	☐ Other	

Describe: _____

AFFECT

☐ Appropriate	☐ Flat	☐ Restricted
☐ Blunted	☐ Expansive	

SPEECH RATE

☐ Normal	☐ Fast	☐ Slow
☐ Stutter	☐ Hesitant	☐ Pressured

SPEECH PRODUCTION

☐ Normal	☐ Loud	☐ Soft
☐ Clear	☐ Mumbling	☐ Slurred
☐ Monotone	☐ Mute	

COGNITION

Recent memory change? ☐ No ☐ Yes. Describe: _____

Persistent, bothersome or fearful thoughts that you cannot stop? ☐ No ☐ Yes.

Describe: _____

_____

Rituals or practices that you feel compelled to do or cannot stop from doing? ☐ No ☐ Yes.

Describe: _____

_____

_____

THOUGHT CONTENT

DELUSIONS	NO	YES	DESCRIBE
Persecutory			
Grandiose			
Religious			
Self-accusatory			
HALLUCINATIONS			
Auditory			
Visual			
Tactile			
Olfactory			

ABSTRACTIONS (proverbs, similarity/differences)   ☐ Within normal range

☐ Altered. Describe: _____

_____

_____

_____

JUDGMENT (describe patient's answer)

1. "Stamped, addressed, sealed envelope" _____

_____

2. "Smoke in theater" _____

_____

INSIGHT

What is your understanding about why you are in the hospital? _____

_____

_____

_____

_____

MINI MENTAL STATUS EXAM

ORIENTATION		Score	Points
1. What is the	Year?	_____	1
	Season?	_____	1
	Date?	_____	1
	Day?	_____	1
	Month?	_____	1
2. Where are we?	State?	_____	1
	County?	_____	1
	Town or		
	City?	_____	1
	Hospital?	_____	1
	Floor?	_____	1

REGISTRATION

3. Name three objects, taking one second to say each. Then ask the patient all three after you have said them. Give one point for each correct answer. Repeat the answers until the patient learns all three. _____ 3

ATTENTION AND CALCULATION

4. Serial sevens, give one point for each correct answer. Stop after 5 answers. Alternate: Spell WORLD backwards. _____ 5

RECALL

5. Ask for names of three objects learned in question 3. _____ 3

LANGUAGE	Score	Points
6. Point to a pencil and a watch. Have the patient name them as you point.	_____	2
7. Have the patient repeat "No ifs, ands or buts."	_____	1
8. Have the patient follow a three stage command: "Take the paper in your right hand. Fold the paper in half. Put the paper on the floor."	_____	3
9. Have the patient read and obey the following: "CLOSE YOUR EYES."	_____	1
10. Have the patient write a sentence of his/her choice.	_____	1
11. Have patient copy design.	_____	1
12. Total	_____/30	

THOUGHT FLOW

☐ spontaneous   ☐ sequential   ☐ appropriate   ☐ indecisive

☐ slowed response   ☐ loose associations   ☐ flight of ideas   ☐ thought blocking

☐ thought insertion   ☐ thought withdrawal   ☐ circumstantial   ☐ tangential

☐ poverty of thought   ☐ illusion   ☐ Other. Describe: _____

11. SELF PERCEPTION

What do you like about yourself? _____

What don't you like about yourself? _____

Do you want to change?   ☐ No   ☐ Yes. Do you think you can change?   ☐ No   ☐ Yes

What do you think you will be doing in three years? Describe: _____

12. ROLE RELATIONSHIP

INTERACTIONS WITH SIGNIFICANT OTHERS:

Code:

A. Relaxed
B. Supportive
C. Tense
D. Argumentative
E. Abusive
F. Withdrawn
G. Other

SIGNIFICANT PEOPLE

NAME	AGE	RELATIONSHIP	INTERACTIONS (Use Code)

Who or what is your greatest support system? _____

_____

Family concerns regarding your hospitalization: _____

_____

13. VALUE/BELIEF

Is there a spiritual belief system that is important to you?

☐ No ☐ Yes. Describe: _____

Are there any practices within your spiritual system that are important for you during your hospitalization?

☐ No ☐ Yes. Describe: _____

Is your spiritual belief organized around a particular religion?

☐ No ☐ Yes. Describe: _____

What is most important to you in your life? Describe: _____

14. SIGNATURES

ADMITTING NURSE   R.N. SIGNATURE _____, R.N. _____
DATE/TIME

PRIMARY NURSE   R.N. SIGNATURE _____, R.N. _____
DATE/TIME

ADDITIONAL OBSERVATIONS: _____

_____

_____

_____

_____

_____

R.N. SIGNATURE

Appendix III: Pediatric Assessment*

This assessment tool contains questions useful for screening and for more specific focused questions. The focused questions should not be asked of all parents but are useful if indicated. The symbol Δ represents those questions that should be asked of most parents and children.

I. Identifying Information

Child's initials _____
Birthdate _____   Age _____
Sex _____
Weight _____   Percentile _____
Length of height _____   Percentile _____
Head circumference (if appropriate) _____   Percentile _____
Allergies _____

II. Data Base Assessment*

A. Health Perception–Health Management Pattern
   1. For all children
      a. How is your child's health in general?
      b. How is your child's health today?
      c. What do you do to keep your child well?
         • Nutrition
         • Opportunities for exercise and play
         • Professional health care
         • Immunization status
         • Any regular medications? What are they? What is their purpose?
   2. For the hospitalized or ill child
      a. Why was your child admitted to the hospital?
         • What caused the illness/injury?
         • When did the illness begin?
      b. What treatment is your child receiving?
      What is your understanding of the purpose of the treatment?
      How do you think the treatment is working?
      c. Has your child ever been hospitalized before? For what reason? How did that go for you and the child?
      d. What expectations do you have about this hospitalization?
      e. Do you anticipate any problems in caring for your child when he goes home?
      What are the anticipated problems?

*Developed by Susan Ross, RN, MS, and Linda H. Snow, RN, MS, Assistant Professors, Department of Nursing, American International College, Springfield, MA, March 1985. Used with permission. Adapted from Appendix I, Adult Assessment Guide.

3. For both well and ill children: complete for all children under 24 months of age and when appropriate because of related problems (*e.g.,* developmental disabilities, complications of prematurity, etc.).
   a. Did the mother have prenatal care? How long?
   b. Did the mother take any medications during pregnancy?
   c. Were there any complications during pregnancy?
   d. What were the infant's birth weight and length?
   e. What was the length of gestation?
   f. Were there any complications with the infant during the first month of life?

B. Nutritional–Metabolic Pattern

Δ 1. How is the child's appetite?
Δ 2. Describe a typical day for your child in terms of what he eats and drinks at meals and snacks.
   a. Breast-fed
      • How often?
      • How long at each feeding?
      • Any difficulties?
      • Plans for continuing or weaning
   b. Formula-fed
      • Name of formula
      • Number of feedings in 24 hours
      • Amount of formula at each feeding
      • Any difficulties perceived
      • Plans for continuing or weaning
   c. Solid foods
      • When begun
      • Food groups that child eats
      • Approximate amounts at each meal
      • Describe a typical after-school snack
   Δ d. General
      • Are there any food restrictions or special diet due to allergies, intolerances, other health problems, or religious practice?
      • What vitamins and/or supplements does the child take?
      • How much milk does the child drink in 24 hours?
      • Does the child use a bottle or cup?
Δ 3. What are the child's special food likes and dislikes?
4. How often does the child go to "fast-food" restaurants? What does he usually order?
5. How much candy, other sweets, processed snack foods, and soda does your child eat/drink?
6. What, if any, concerns do you have about your child's appetite, feeding behavior, or diet?

C. Elimination Pattern

1. Bowel
   Δ a. How many stools does your child have daily?
   Δ b. What is the color, amount, and consistency?
   Δ c. Is he toilet trained?
   Δ d. Does he ever need laxatives, enemas, or suppositories? How often? How do you decide that one of the above is necessary?
   Δ e. What is the usual colostomy/ileostomy care (if applicable)?

2. Bladder
  Δ a. Does your child have any problems with urination?
- Bed-wetting (enuresis)
- Burning or other dysuria
- Dribbling
- Oliguria
- Polyuria
- Urinary retention

    b. Are any assistive devices used?
- Intermittent catheterization
- Indwelling catheter
- Stoma for urinary drainage—describe routine of care

  Δ c. Is the child toilet trained?
- Daytime
- Nighttime
- Accidents?

Δ 3. Skin—Does your child ever have any trouble with his skin (*e.g.*, itching, swelling, rashes, sores, acne, color, or temperature changes)? Describe.

D. Activity–Exercise Pattern

1. Gross motor abilities
  a. When did your child roll over? Sit unsupported? Walk alone? Climb stairs? Ride tricycle? (etc.) (Obtain information appropriate to child's age and developmental abilities.)
  b. What sports/exercise does your child enjoy and participate in?
  Δ c. What, if any, concern do you have about your child's abilities in these areas?
2. Fine motor abilities
  a. Does your baby reach for things? Grasp? Transfer objects from one hand to another? Use his fingers to pick up objects? Feed himself a cracker? Use a spoon?
  b. What hobbies does your child have?
  c. What, if any, concerns do you have about your child's abilities to use his hands?
3. Self-care abilities or activities
  Δ a. How independent is your child in feeding himself? Describe the help he needs, if any.
  Δ b. How much help does your child need with toileting? If assistive devices are used, is child independent or does he need help? Describe. Does child use diapers, a potty chair, or toilet?
  Δ c. How much help does your child need with dressing (buttons, ties, zippers, etc.)?
  Δ d. How much help does your child need with hygiene practices (bathing, brushing teeth, etc.)? Does he prefer a shower or tub?

E. Sleep–Rest Patterns

Δ 1. How many hours does the child sleep each 24 hours?
  a. At night
  b. Naps
Δ 2. What is the child's usual sleep routine?
  a. Bedtime
  b. Naptime

      c. Rituals (stories, drink, etc.)
      d. Security object(s)
    Δ 3. Are there any problems related to sleep?
      a. Nightmares, night terrors
      b. Difficulty falling asleep
      c. Refusal at bedtime
      d. Waking up during night

F. Cognitive–Perceptual Pattern

    Δ 1. Does the child have any sensory perception deficits (hearing, smell, sight, touch) Describe.
      2. What grade in school is child?
      a. How does he do in school?
      b. What, if any, problems are perceived by parent, teacher, or child relative to school achievement?

G. Self-Perception Pattern

    Δ 1. How has your child's illness made you feel? What are you most concerned about?
    Δ 2. For school-age and adolescent child: How does your illness (injury) make you feel? What are you most concerned about?
      3. For well older school-age child and adolescent: How do you feel about yourself?

H. Role–Relationship Pattern

    1. Communication
      a. Language development
        • When did child coo? Babble? Say words? Phrases? Sentences? Use pronouns?
        (Use questions appropriate to child's age and developmental abilities.)
        Δ• Does the child use language appropriate for his age?
        Δ• What, if any, concerns do you have about your child's language development or characteristics of speech?
      b. What language is spoken at home?
    2. Relationships
      a. Describe family life
        Δ• Composition of household (family members, ages)
        Δ• Cultural background
        Δ• Roles
        Δ• Occupations and educational background of adults
        Δ• Decision-making patterns
        Δ• Communication patterns
        Δ• Discipline
        Δ• Problems (*e.g.,* finances, family violence, problems with parenting, marital problems)
      b. Peer relationships
        Δ• Does your child play with other children? Describe the quality of the child's play (*e.g.,* solitary, parallel, interactive, cooperative, aggressive).
        Δ• Does the child have a "best friend" of the same sex? Belong to a "gang"?
        Δ• Does your child prefer playmates who are older, younger, same age?
        Δ• Does your child have imaginary playmates?
        Δ• What concerns, if any, do you have about your child's relationships with others?

I. Sexuality–Sexual Functioning Pattern

  Δ 1. What interest does your child show in sexuality/sexual function? How do you feel about this? How do you handle your child's curiosity and behavior?
  2. For adolescent, assess:
    a. Knowledge of sexual functioning
    b. Sexual activity
    c. Use of contraceptives
    d. History of pregnancy
    e. Feelings about opposite sex

J. Coping–Stress Management Pattern

  1. How do you make decisions? (alone? with whom?)
  Δ 2. Have there been any losses or changes in your life in the past year? In your child's? (e.g., move, death of significant other or pet, loss of parental job)
  Δ 3. To whom do your turn for support and help when you are feeling stressed?
  4. How do you manage child care, housework, and other responsibilities? For the teenager: How do you manage school work, sports and other activities, and work responsibilities?
  5. What can the nurses do to help you during this hospitalization?

K. Value–Belief System

  Δ 1. What religious affiliation or preference do you hold?
  Δ 2. Is there a religious person or practice (diet, book, ritual) that you desire during your child's hospitalization?

L. Physical Assessment (objective)

  1. General appearance
  2. Temperature (note whether oral, rectal, or axillary)
  3. Skin
    a. Color
    b. Temperature
    c. Turgor
    d. Lesions
    e. Edema
    f. Excoriations
  4. Head
    a. Size, shape
    b. Fontanelles and cranial sutures
  5. Neck
  6. Eyes (appearance, drainage)
    a. Pupils (size, equal, reactive to light)
    b. Vision
      • Responds to visual stimulus
      • Wears glasses
  7. Mouth and pharynx
    a. Mucous membranes (color, moisture, lesions)
    b. Teeth (number, primary and/or secondary, condition, orthodontic devices)
    c. Pharynx (redness, exudate, tonsils)
  8. Ears (appearance, drainage)
    a. TMs

b. Responds to auditory stimulus
c. Uses hearing aids

9. Pulses (radial, apical, peripheral)
   a. Rate
   b. Rhythm
   c. Quality
10. Blood pressure (note if by palpation, Doppler)
11. Respirations
    a. Rate
    b. Quality (include signs of respiratory distress)
    c. Breath sounds
12. Abdomen
    a. Bowel sounds
    b. Scars
    c. Prostheses
13. Genitalia
14. Functional ability (mobility and safety)
    a. Presence/absence of primary reflexes
    b. Gross and fine motor ability
    c. Dominant hand
    d. Mobility and use of four extremities
    e. Strength, grasp
    f. Use of aids (*e.g.,* wheelchair, braces, crutches)
    g. Weight-bearing
15. Mental status
    a. Orientation (time, person, place, events)
    b. Level of consciousness
    c. Pain (presence/absence, location, description)
    d. Affect
    e. Eye contact
    f. Use of language (ability and amount)
    g. Personal-social abilities (*e.g.,* self-care, nonverbal communication)
    h. Growth and development
       • Cognitive development
           Objective data
           Stage of development according to Piaget
       • Psychosocial development
           Objective data
         State of development according to Erikson

Appendix IV: Older Adult Assessment Guide*

Marian Villa Nursing Assessment Tool

Date: _____

Admitted from: ☐ Home alone   ☐ Home with relative   ☐ Long-term care facility
                 ☐ Home with _____ ☐ Other _____
Mode of Arrival: ☐ Wheelchair   ☐ Ambulance
Reason for Coming to Marian Villa:
_____
_____

Past Medical History:
_____
_____

Medication (over the counter):	Dosage	Last Dose	Frequency

Health Maintenance Perception Pattern (from Resident's Viewpoint): "_____"

USE OF TOBACCO: ☐ None   ☐ Quit (Date) _____ ☐ Pipe   ☐ Cigar
                  ☐ <1 pk/day   ☐ 1 - 2 pks/day   ☐ > 2 pks/day   Pks/Year history _____
USE OF ALCOHOL: ☐ None   Type _____ Amount _____ /day _____ /week ____/month
OTHER DRUGS: ☐ Yes   ☐ No   Type _____ Use _____
ALLERGIES (drugs, food, tape, dyes):   ☐ Yes   Type _____ Reaction _____

Activity/Exercise Pattern (from Resident's Viewpoint): "_____"

SELF-CARE ABILITY	Independent	Assistive Device	Assistance from Others	Assistance from Others & Equipment	Dependent/ Unable
Eating/Drinking					
Bathing					
Dressing/Grooming					
Toileting					
Bed Mobility					
Transferring					
Ambulating					
Stair Climbing					

Assistive Devices: ☐ None   ☐ Crutches   ☐ Walker   ☐ Cane   ☐ Bedside Commode
                  ☐ Splint/Brace   ☐ Wheelchair   ☐ Other _____

Nutrition/Metabolic Pattern (from Resident's Viewpoint): "_____"
Special diet/supplements: _____
Previous Dietary Instructions: ☐ Yes   ☐ No
Appetite: ☐ Normal   ☐ Increased   ☐ Decreased   ☐ Decreased taste sensation   ☐ Nausea
☐ Vomiting   ☐ Stomatitis

CODE: (1) Non-applicable, (2) Unable to acquire, (3) Not a priority at this time, (4) Other - specify in notes.

*Used with permission of St. Joseph's Health Centre, London, Ontario, Canada. This form, which has since been integrated into the General Admission Data Base, was developed by Nancy A. Bols, R. N., M. S. N., when a clinical specialist at St. Joseph's Health Centre. She is currently a clinical specialist at Parkwood Hospital, London, Ontario, Canada.

Weight Fluctuations last 6 months:	☐ None	☐ Gained	☐ Lost	Lbs. _____
Swallowing Difficulty (Dysphagia):	☐ None	☐ Solids	☐ Liquids	
Dentures:	☐ Upper ( ) Partial ( ) Full		☐ Lower ( ) Partial ( ) Full	
History of Skin/Healing Problems:	☐ None	☐ Abnormal Healing	☐ Rash( )	☐ Dryness
	☐ Excess Perspiration			

Elimination Pattern (from Resident's Viewpoint): "_____"

Bowel Habits:	_____ # BMs/day _____	Date of last BM		
	☐ Within Normal Limits	☐ Constipation ☐ Diarrhea	☐ Incontinence	
	☐ Ostomy: Type:_____	Appliance _____	Self Care ☐ Yes	☐ No
Bladder Habits:	☐ WNL ☐ Frequency	☐ Dysuria ☐ Nocturia	☐ Urgency	☐ Hematuria
	☐ Retention			
Incontinency:	☐ Yes ☐ No	_____ Total ☐ Daytime	☐ Nighttime	☐ Occasional
	☐ Difficulty delaying voiding	☐ Difficulty reaching toilet		
Assistive Devices:	☐ Intermittent catheterization	☐ Indwelling catheter	☐ External catheter	
	☐ Incontinent briefs	☐ Penile implant _____	Type	

Sleep/Rest Pattern (from Resident's Viewpoint): "_____"

Habits:	_____hrs/night ☐ AM nap	☐ PM nap	Feel rested after sleep	☐ No	☐ Yes
Problems:	☐ None ☐ Early waking	☐ Insomnia	☐ Nightmares		

Cognitive-Perceptual Pattern (from Resident's Viewpoint): "_____"

Hearing:	☐ WNL ☐ Impaired ( ) Right ( ) Left	☐ Deaf ( ) Right ( ) Left	
	☐ Hearing Aid ☐ Tinnitus		
Vision:	☐ WNL ☐ Eye Glasses ☐ Contact Lens		
	☐ Impaired ( ) Right ( ) Left	☐ Blind ( ) Right ( ) Left	☐ Cataract ( ) Right ( ) Left
	☐ Glaucoma ☐ Prostheses ( ) Right ( ) Left		
Vertigo:	☐ Yes ☐ No		
Discomfort/Pain:	☐ None ☐ Acute	☐ Chronic ☐ Description	_____
Pain Management:	_____		

Coping Stress Tolerance/Self-Perception/Self-Concept Pattern
What do you think about moving to Marian Villa?
_____
_____

Major loss/change in past year:	☐ Yes	☐ No

_____

Affection/Reproduction Pattern

Are you an affectionate person?	☐ Yes	☐ No
Is your skin sensitive to touch?	☐ Yes	☐ No
Last Pap smear date:	_____	

Role/Relationship Pattern
What does your family think about your move to Marian Villa?
_____
_____

What do your friends think about your move?
_____
_____

CODE: (1) Non-applicable, (2) Unable to acquire, (3) Not a priority at this time, (4) Other - specify in notes.

List Family Members:

_____   _____
_____   _____
_____   _____

List Friends:

_____   _____
_____   _____
_____   _____

Past Occupations:

_____   _____
_____   _____

Value/Belief Pattern

Religion: ☐ Roman Catholic   ☐ Protestant   ☐ Jewish   ☐ Other (specify) _____

Religious Rituals: ☐ Yes   ☐ No   Contact: _____

Physical Assessment (Objective)

CLINICAL DATA   Age _____ Height _____ Weight _____ (Actual/Approximate)

    Temperature: _____

    Pulse: ☐ Strong   ☐ Weak   ☐ Regular   ☐ Irregular

    Blood Pressure: Right Arm _____ Left Arm_____ Sitting_____ Lying_____

RESPIRATORY/CIRCULATORY

Rate:

    Quality: ☐ WNL   ☐ Shallow   ☐ Rapid   ☐ Labored   ☐ Other _____

    Cough: ☐ Yes   ☐ No   Describe_____

METABOLIC-INTEGUMENTARY

Skin Color: ☐ WNL   ☐ Pale   ☐ Cyanotic   ☐ Ashen   ☐ Jaundice   ☐ Other

    Temperature: ☐ WNL   ☐ Warm   ☐ Cool

    Turgor: ☐ WNL   ☐ Poor

    Edema: ☐ Yes   ☐ No   Description/Location _____

    Lesions: ☐ Yes   ☐ No   Description/Location _____

    Bruises: ☐ Yes   ☐ No   Description/Location _____

    Reddened: ☐ Yes   ☐ No   Description/Location _____

    Pruritus: ☐ Yes   ☐ No   Description/Location _____

    Tubes: Specify   _____

Mouth Gums: ☐ WNL   ☐ White plaque ☐ Lesions   ☐ Other _____

    Teeth: ☐ WNL   ☐ Other _____

NEURO/SENSORY

    Mental Status: ☐ Alert   ☐ Receptive Aphasia   ☐ Poor Historian ☐ Oriented   ☐ Confused

                      ☐ Combative   ☐ Unresponsive

    Speech: ☐ Normal   ☐ Slurred   ☐ Garbled   ☐ Expressive Aphasia

                      Spoken Language: _____ Interpreter: _____

    Pupils: ☐ Equal   ☐ Unequal

    Eyes: ☐ Clear   ☐ Draining   ☐ Reddened   ☐ Other _____

MUSCULAR-SKELETAL

    Range of motion: ☐ Full   ☐ Other _____

    Balance and Gait:☐ Steady   ☐ Unsteady

    Hand grasps: ☐ Equal   ☐ Strong   ☐ Weakness/Paralysis ( ) Right ( ) Left

    Leg Muscles: ☐ Equal   ☐ Strong   ☐ Weakness/Paralysis ( ) Right ( ) Left

Signature/Title_____ Date:_____

Appendix V: Maternal Assessment Guide

This data base is divided into four sections. Section I directs the initial data collection on admission to the labor and delivery unit. Section II focuses on the collection of specific data during the immediate postdelivery period. Section III, organized under the functional health patterns, focuses on the collection of data on the family unit after the immediate postdelivery period. In Section III, the nurse can choose to defer the collection of certain data that are determined to be inappropriate. Section IV represents a Parental-Infant Interaction Assessment that is initiated during labor and delivery and is continued on the postpartum unit.

I. Intrapartal Assessment

1. Support person present
2. Childbirth preparation classes (type, location)
3. Prenatal history
   Estimated date of confinement (EDC)
   Past/present medical problems

Hospitalizations	Diabetes mellitus
Infections	Hypertension

4. Health history
   Contact with communicable disease (gonorrhea, herpes, rubella, measles, hepatitis, mumps, AIDS)
   Medications taken during pregnancy
   Gravida, para (abortions, cesarean-sections, miscarriages, premature)
   Previous labor history (length, medications, problems)
   Tobacco, alcohol, drug use
5. Labor history
   When labor became apparent
   Character and amount of show
   Membranes (intact, ruptured, color)
   Contractions (frequency, character)
6. Last food intake (time, type)
7. Last bowel movement
8. Present status

Rested	In control
Alert	Fearful
Tired	Out of control
Excited	Anxious
Exhausted	

9. Physical assessment
   Vital signs
   Cervix (effacement, dilatation)
   Contractions (frequency, character)
   Urine (glucose, acetone)
   Fetal heart sounds

II. Immediate Postdelivery Assessment
1. Physical assessment

Vital signs	Breasts
Uterine involution (position in cm)	Bowel sounds
Lochia (amount, color)	Bladder (voiding, distention,
Perineal area (episiotomy,	incontinence)
lacerations)	

2. Present status (mother, significant other)

Emotional status (describe)	Discomforts (describe)

III. Postpartum Assessment
Assess each pattern for usual functioning and evaluate its impact on parenting, child care, and lactation as indicated. Proceed with health teaching under each pattern when indicated.

1. Health Perception–Health Maintenance Pattern
   "How would you usually describe your health?"
   "Do you have any chronic illness?"
   "How would you describe your health at this time?
   Review the daily health practices of the individual (adults, children)

Dental care	Exercise regimen
Food intake	Leisure activities
Fluid intake	Responsibilities in the family

   Use of

Tobacco	Drugs (over-the-counter,
Salt, sugar, fat products	prescribed)
Alcohol	

   Knowledge of safety practices

Fire prevention	Automobile (maintenance, seat
Water safety	belts, infant seats)
Children/infants	Bicycle
Poison control	

   Knowledge of infant care
   Nutrition (bottle, breast-feeding)
   Clothing needs
   Hygiene needs
   Sleep needs
   Developmental needs

2. Nutritional–Metabolic Pattern
   "What is the usual daily food intake (meals, snacks)"
   "What is the usual fluid intake (type, amounts)?"
   "How is your appetite?"

Indigestion	Vomiting
Nausea	Sore mouth

   "What are your food restrictions or preferences?"
   "Any supplements (vitamins, feedings)?"
   "Has your weight changed prior to pregnancy?" If yes, "Why?"

3. Elimination Pattern
   Bladder
   "Are there any problems or complaints with the usual pattern of urinating?"

Oliguria	Retention

Polyuria

Burning

Dysuria

Stress incontinence

Dribbling

Bowel

"What is the usual time, frequency, color, consistency, pattern?"

"Assistive devices (type, frequency)?"

Enemas

Cathartics

Laxatives

Suppositories

4. Activity–Exercise Pattern

"Describe usual daily/weekly activities of daily living."

Occupation

Exercise pattern (type,

Leisure activities

frequency)

"Do you work outside the home?"

"Are there factors present that could interfere with activities at home (self-care, home care)?"

Lack of knowledge

Lack of resources

5. Sleep–Rest Pattern

"What is the usual sleep pattern?"

Bedtime

Sleep aids (medication, food)

Hours slept

Sleep routine

"Any problems?"

Difficulty falling asleep

Not feeling rested after sleep

Difficulty remaining asleep

6. Cognitive–Perceptual Pattern

"Any deficits in sensory perception (hearing, sight, touch)?"

Glasses

Hearing aid

"Any complaints?"

Vertigo

Insensitivity to cold or heat

Insensitivity to superficial pain

"Able to read and write?"

7. Self-Perception Pattern

"What are you most concerned about?"

"What are your present health goals?"

"How would you describe yourself?"

"How do you think your life will change with this baby?"

8. Role–relationship pattern

Relationships

"To whom do you turn for help in time of need?"

Assess family life (members, educational level, occupations)

Cultural background

Decision-making

Activities (lone or group)

Communication patterns

Roles

Finances

"Any complaints?"

Parenting difficulties

Marital difficulties

Difficulties with relative

Abuse (physical, verbal,

(in-laws, parents)

substance

9. Sexuality–Reproductive Pattern

Age at menarche

Contraceptive use (type, years of use)

Leukorrhea, vaginal itching, postcoital bleeding, pain, or cystitis

Sexual activities
"Have you been satisfied with the quality and quantity of your sexual activities (your partner)?"
"Any pain or discomfort with intercourse?"
"Has there been or do you expect a change in your sexual relations (related to pregnancy, child care, breast feeding)?"

10. Coping–Stress Pattern
Δ "How do you make decisions (alone, with assistance, with whom)?"
Δ "Has there been a loss in your life in the past year (or changes—moves, job, health)?"
"What do you like about yourself?"
"What would you like to change in your life?"
"What is preventing you?"
"What do you do when you are tense or under stress (*e.g.*, problem-solve, eat, sleep, take medication, seek help)?"

11. Values–Belief Pattern
"With what (whom) do you find a source of strength or meaning?"

12. Physical Assessment
General appearance
Weight and height
Eyes (appearance, drainage)
  Pupils (size, equal, reactive to light)
  Vision (glasses)
Mouth
  Mucous membrane (color, moisture, lesions)
  Teeth (condition, loose, broken, dentures)
Hearing (hearing aids)
Pulses (radial, apical, peripheral)
  Rate, rhythm, volume
Respirations
  Rate, quality, breath sounds (upper and lower lobes)
Blood pressure
Temperature
Skin (color, temperature, turgor)
  Lesions, edema, pruritus
Uterine involution (position in cm)
Lochia (amount, color)
Perineal area (episiotomy, lacerations)
Breasts
Bowel sounds
Bladder (voiding, distention, incontinence)

IV. Parental–Infant Interaction Assessment

Place check marks in front of data that are present. Add additional data as indicated.

A. Delivery room assessment

1. Attempts to see infant as soon as delivered
2. Response

Happy	Angry
Disappointed	Ambivalent
Apathetic	Sad

3. Holds and talks to infant
4. Uses baby's name
5. Response to partner

Happy	Angry
Ignores him	Indifferent

B. Postpartum assessment

1. Verbal responses of mother
   Verbalizes positive feelings
   Seeks proximity by holding infant closely; touches and hugs
   Smiles and gazes at infant; seeks eye-to-eye contact
   Seeks family resemblance (*i.e.,* "has my eyes," "sleeps like his father")
   Refers to infant by name and sex
   Expresses interest in learning infant care
   Performs nurturing behavior (*i.e.,* feeding, changing)
2. Requests that baby be taken to nursery
3. Complains about baby
4. Does not refer to baby by name
5. Nonverbal responses of mother*

Looks, reaches out to baby	Tenses face, arms
Hugs, kisses baby	Turns head from baby
Smiles at baby	Unresponsive to partner/nurse
Positive eye contact with partner	Doesn't touch baby
Holds hand of partner	Doesn't look at baby
Breast-feeds baby	Pushes baby away
Sleepy, not drug-induced	Cries unhappily

Comments:

_____

_____

* Source: Neeson, J. D., & May, K. A. (1986). *Comprehensive maternity nursing*. Philadelphia: J. B. Lippincott, p. 646.

Appendix VI: Noninvasive Pain Relief Techniques

Noninvasive pain relief techniques are external measures that influence the person's internal response to pain.

General Principles
1. Convey to the person that you believe that the pain is present.
2. Explain the relationship of stress and muscle tension to pain.
3. Explain the various methods of relief and allow the person to choose one or two.
4. Attempt to teach the method when pain is absent or mild.
5. Perform the technique with the person to coach him and encourage him to focus on details of the distraction.
6. Encourage the person to practice the technique when the pain is mild.
7. Teach the person to use the technique before feeling pain (if the pain can be anticipated) and to increase the complexity of the distraction as the pain increases in intensity (*e.g.,* increase the volume of music via earphones as discomforts increase during a bone-marrow aspiration).
8. Inform others (staff, family) about the technique and its purpose.
9. Explain that noninvasive pain relief can be utilized with medications and usually increases their effects.

Specific Techniques
- Distraction
- Cutaneous stimulation
- Relaxation

Distraction
Distraction is the deliberate focusing of attention on stimuli other than the pain sensation. The ability to be distracted from pain does not denote that the pain is nonexistent or mild. Even persons with severe pain can choose to be distracted from their pain.

Distraction can be taught to children. (Caution parent not to confuse this therapeutic distraction technique that the child chooses to practice with the surprise distraction of a child prior to painful events. This latter technique serves only to produce feelings of mistrust and fear in children.)

Distraction cannot usually be practiced for very long periods. After the distraction ends, the person may have an increased awareness of the pain and fatigue.
1. Examples of distraction methods
   a. Visual distractions
      - Counting objects (flowers on wallpaper, spots on wall, animals in picture, someone's blinks)
      - Describe objects (pictures, slides)
   b. Auditory distractions (songs, tapes)

    c. Tactile kinesthetic distractions (holding, stroking, rocking, rhythmic breathing)

    d. Guided imagery (see Appendix X)

2. Breathing techniques

    a. Slow rhythmic

- Have person take slow deep breaths through nose and exhale through mouth
- Try to slow rate to nine breaths a minute if possible
- Instruct person to take extra breaths if needed

    b. Heartbeat breathing (McCaffery, 1979). Teach person to

- Take a slow deep breath
- Count pulse on wrist
- Inhale as you count two beats
- Exhale as you count the next three beats

    c. He-who breathing (McCaffery, 1979). Instruct person to

- Take a slow deep breath
- Inhale and say *he* on inhaling
- Exhale and say *who* on exhaling
- Rate can be increased (should not exceed 40 min) if pain increases

Cutaneous Stimulation

Cutaneous stimulation is stimulation of the skin's surface. Examples of methods follow.

1. Massage

    Rub with warm lubricant over painful part or over the opposite adjacent part if the actual painful part cannot be massaged (*e.g.,* if a fractured left leg is casted, the person can massage the fracture site on the right leg)

2. Application of cold

    a. The therapeutic effects of cold are (Lehmann, 1974)

- Reduces small-diameter nerve conduction, which lessens the perception of pain
- Decreases the inflammatory response of tissues
- Decreases blood flow
- Decreases edema

    b. The use of cold is indicated with

- Trauma (first 24–48 hr)
- Fractures
- Insect bites
- Hemorrhage
- Muscle spasms
- Rheumatoid arthritis (if relief is acquired)
- Pruritus
- Headaches

    c. The use of cold is contraindicated

- With Raynaud's disease
- With cold allergy
- 48 hours after trauma

    d. Guidelines for use of cold

- Protect skin from cold burn (*e.g.,* layers of cloth between skin and cold source)
- Caution its use with persons with limited communication ability or decreased sensorium (infants, sedated persons)
- Caution its use on areas with impaired sensation (*e.g.,* diabetic's foot)

    e. Examples of cold application methods

- Towel or washcloth soaked in ice water and wrung out

- Ice bags (Zip-loc plastic bag filled with ice water or frozen)
- Reusable gel pak (stored in refrigerator or freezer)
- Massage of painful site with ice

3. Application of heat
  a. The therapeutic uses of heat are
    - Slows small-diameter nerve conduction, which lessens the perception of pain
    - Increases the inflammatory response of stress
    - Increases blood flow
    - Increases edema
  b. The use of heat is indicated with
    - Trauma (past 48 hr)
    - Cystitis
    - Hemorrhoids
    - Backache
    - Arthritis (if relief is attained)
    - Bursitis
  c. The use of heat is contraindicated with
    - Trauma (first 24–48 hr)
    - Edema/hemorrhage
    - Vascular insufficiency
    - Malignant sites
    - Pruritus
  d. Examples of heat application methods
    - Towel or washcloth soaked in warm water and wrung out (cover cloth with plastic around area to trap heat longer)
    - Heating pads (moist or dry)
    - Warm bath or shower
    - Sunbathing
    - Moist heat pack (commercially available)

4. External analgesic preparations (McCaffery, 1979)
  a. External analgesic preparations—ointments, lotions, liniments—produce a sensation (usually warmth) that may persist for several hours
  b. Guidelines for use
    - Do not use on broken skin
    - Do not apply to mucous membranes (anus, vagina)
    - Always skin-test each product before using
    - Follow directions and use sparingly or painful burning may occur
  b. Examples of external analgesic preparations
    - Products with methyl salicylate (oil of wintergreen)
    - Products with menthol

Relaxation

Relaxation is a state of relief from skeletal muscle tension that the person achieves through the practice of deliberate techniques

1. The therapeutic effects of relaxation are that it
  - Decreases anxiety
  - Provides the person with some control over pain
  - Decreases skeletal muscle tension
  - Serves as a distraction from pain

2. Examples of relaxation techniques
  - Biofeedback

- Yoga
- Meditation
- Progressive relaxation exercises (see Appendix X)

References/Bibliography

Benson, H. (1976). *The relaxation response*. New York: Avon Books.

Breeden, S. A., & Kondo, C. (1975). Using biofeedback to reduce tension. *American Journal of Nursing, 75,* 2010–2012.

Brown, B. (1977). *Stress and the art of biofeedback*. New York: Bantam Books.

Donovan, M. (1980). Relaxation with guided imagery: A useful technique. *Cancer Nursing, 3*(1), 27–32.

Flynn, P. A. R. (1980). *Holistic health*. Maryland: Robert J Brady.

Lehmann, J. F., Warren, C. G., & Scham, S. M. (1974). Therapeutic heat and cold. *Clinical Orthopaedics and Related Research, 99,* 207–245.

McCaffery, M. (1977). Pain relief for the child: Problem areas and selected non-pharmacological methods. *Pediatric Nursing, 3*(4), 11–16.

McCaffery, M. (1977). Technique to help a patient relax. *American Journal of Nursing, 77,* 794–795.

McCaffery, M. (1979). *Nursing management of the patient with pain* (2nd ed). Philadelphia: J. B. Lippincott.

McCoy, P. (1977). Further proof that touch speaks louder than words. *RN, 40*(11), 43–46.

Mennell, J. M. (1975). The therapeutic use of cold. *American Osteopathic Journal, 74,* 1146–1158.

Michelsen, D. (1978). Giving a back rub. *American Journal of Nursing, 78,* 1197–1199.

Petrello, J. M. (1973). Temperature maintenance of hot moist compresses. *American Journal of Nursing, 73,* 1050–1051.

Simonton, C., Mathews-Simonton, S, & Creighton, J. (1978). *Getting well again: A step-by-step self-help guide to overcoming cancer for patients and their families*. Los Angeles: J. P. Tarcher.

Wilson, R. L. (1976). An introduction to yoga. *American Journal of Nursing, 76,* 261–263.

Appendix VII: Guidelines for Problem-Solving and Crisis Intervention

The two basic coping behaviors in response to problems are emotion-focused behaviors and problem-focused behaviors.*

Emotion-Focused Behaviors

1. *Minimization* occurs when the seriousness of a problem is minimized. This may be useful as a way to provide needed time for appraisal, but it may become dysfunctional when it precludes appraisal.
2. *Projection, displacement,* and *suppression of anger* occur when anger is attributed to or expressed toward a less threatening person or thing, which may reduce the threat enough to allow an individual to deal with it. Distortion of reality and disturbance of relationships may result, which further compound the problem. Suppression of anger may result in stress-related physical symptoms.
3. *Anticipatory preparation* is the mental rehearsal of possible consequences of behavior or outcomes of stressful situations, which provides the opportunity to develop perspective as well as to prepare for the worst. It becomes dysfunctional when the anticipation creates unmanageable stress, as, for example, in anticipatory mourning.
4. *Attribution* is the finding of personal meaning in the problem situation, which may be religious faith or individual belief. Examples are fate, the will of the divine, luck. Attribution may offer consolation but becomes maladaptive when all sense of self-responsibility is lost.

Problem-Focused Behaviors

1. *Goal-setting* is the conscious process of setting time limitations on behaviors, which is useful when goals are attainable and manageable. It may become stress-inducing if unrealistic or short-sighted.
2. *Information-seeking* is the learning about all aspects of a problem, which provides perspective and, in some cases, reinforces self-control.
3. *Mastery* is the learning of new procedures or skills, which facilitates self-esteem and self-control, *e.g.,* self-care of colostomies, insulin injection, or catheter care.
4. *Help-seeking* is the reaching out to others for support. Sharing feelings with others provides an emotional release, reassurance, and comfort, as, for example, with Weight Watchers and other self-help and support groups.

Problem-Solving Techniques

1. Identify the problem
    What is wrong?
    What are the causes?
    Refer to pertinent literature, individuals, and organizations for more knowledge about the problem, if indicated.

---

*Lazarus, R. S., & Folkman, S. (1980). Analysis of coping in a middle-age community sample. *Journal of Health and Social Behavior, 21*(9), 219–239.

2. Find the cause
 Who or what is responsible for the problem?
 How have you contributed to the problem?
 Put yourself in the place of each person and consider the problem from his perspective.
3. Discover the options
 What are your goals?
 What do you want to accomplish?
 What are the goals of the others involved in the problem?
 List all possible options for dealing with the problem (including not doing anything).
4. List advantages and disadvantages for each option
 What will happen if you do nothing?
 What is the worst thing that could happen with each option?
5. Choose an option and a plan
 What preparation do you need before implementing the plan?
 How do others fit into the plan?
 How will you know if the plan is working or not?

Guidelines for Crisis Intervention

1. Assist the victim to confront reality (*e.g.*, encourage viewing of dead body).
2. Encourage persons involved to display emotions of crying and anger (within limits).
3. Do not encourage the person to focus on all the implications of the crisis at once—*e.g.*, divorce, death—for they may be too overwhelming.
4. Avoid giving false reassurances such as "It will be all right" or "Don't worry."
5. Clarify fantasies with facts; encourage verbalization to assist with catharsis and to identify misinformation.
6. Avoid encouraging person or family to blame others but allow ventilation of anger (*e.g.*, rape).
7. Encourage person or family to seek help and validate its acceptability (*e.g.,* "A friend of mine found the American Cancer Society very helpful").
8. Assist person or family to identify resources (agencies, people) to help with everyday tasks of living until resolution is attained.

Appendix VIII: Guidelines for Submission of Nursing Diagnoses*

I. Newly Proposed Diagnosis

The North American Nursing Diagnosis Association (NANDA) solicits newly proposed nursing diagnoses for review by the Association. Such proposed diagnoses undergo a systematic review process for inclusion in NANDA's approved list of diagnoses. Approval indicates that NANDA endorses the diagnosis for clinical testing and continuing development by the discipline.

To assist with submission of proposed diagnoses, the NANDA Diagnosis Review Committee has prepared a set of guidelines. These guidelines are designed to promote the consistency, clarity, and quality of submissions. Diagnoses that are submitted but do not meet the guidelines will be returned to the submitter for appropriate revision. Questions regarding the submission process may be forwarded to the NANDA office.

Nursing Diagnosis Defined (Approved at 9th Conference)

A nursing diagnosis is a clinical judgment about individual, family, or community responses to actual or potential health problems/life processes. Nursing diagnoses provide the basis for selection of nursing interventions to achieve outcomes for which the nurse is accountable.

Actual Nursing Diagnosis

1. *Label:* The label provides a name for the diagnosis, a concise phrase or term which represents a pattern of related cues. Diagnostic labels may include but *are not limited* to the following qualifiers:

   Altered—A change from baseline

   Impaired—Made worse, weakened; damaged, reduced; deteriorated

   Depleted—Emptied wholly or partially; exhausted of

   Deficient—Inadequate in amount, quality, or degree; defective; not sufficient; incomplete

   Excessive—Characterized by an amount or quantity that is greater than is necessary, desirable, or useful

   Dysfunctional—Abnormal; incomplete functioning

   Disturbed—Agitated; interrupted, interfered with

   Ineffective—Not producing the desired effect

   Decreased—Lessened, lesser in size, amount or degree

   Increased—Greater in size, amount or degree

   Acute—Severe but of short duration

   Chronic—Lasting a long time; recurring; habitual; constant

   Intermittent—Stopping and starting again at intervals; periodic; cyclic

2. *Definition:* The definition of the diagnosis provides a clear, precise description. The definition delineates its meaning and helps differentiate this diagnosis from similar diagnoses.

*Source: North American Nursing Diagnosis Association, 3525 Caroline Street, St. Louis, MO 63104, (314) 577–8954.

3. *Defining characteristics:* Defining characteristics are clinical cues that cluster as manifestations of a nursing diagnosis. Diagnostic cues are clinical evidence that describe a cluster of behaviors or signs and symptoms that represent a diagnostic label. Diagnostic cues are concrete and measurable through observation or client/group reports. Diagnostic cues are separated into major and minor.

Major diagnostic cues are critical indicators of the diagnosis. Minor diagnostic cues are supporting indicators that are not always present but they complete the clinical picture and increase the diagnostician's confidence in making the diagnosis (Gordon, 1982). Differentiation of major from minor characteristics should be logically defended. If appropriate, the submitter may designate major as occurring 80% to 100% of the time and minor as occurring 50% to 79% of the time.

4. *Related Factors:* Related factors are conditions or circumstances that can cause or contribute to the development of a diagnosis. Related factors that are associated with the proposed diagnosis must be listed and supported by an accompanying literature review.

5. *Literature/Clinical Validation:* A narrative review of the relevant literature is required to support the rationale for the diagnosis, the defining characteristics and the related factors. If the diagnosis is similar to an approved NANDA diagnosis, the reason for its usefulness must be addressed. Literature citations for defining characteristics are required and should be cited for each cue. If defining characteristics are not supported by the literature, an explanation for their inclusion is required. In addition, the designation of major versus minor defining characteristics must be supported by clinical data. These data can be derived from case studies, nurse consensus, retrospective chart reviews and/or other appropriate validation methods. A sample 3-part (label, related factors and signs and symptoms) nursing diagnostic statement with the associated outcome criteria and nurse-prescribed interventions must accompany the submission.

Sample:

Activity Intolerance related to deconditioned status as evidenced by inability to wash body or body parts without tachycardia, dyspnea and fatigue.

Outcome Criteria

Bathes independently without tachycardia or dyspnea

Interventions

Position to minimize energy requirements; assist to recondition; teach energy conservation techniques—pacing techniques; provide assistance as indicated

II. High Risk Nursing Diagnosis

(NANDA-approved diagnoses currently designated as Potential will be labeled "High Risk for" in 1992)

A high risk nursing diagnosis is a clinical judgment that an individual, family, or community is more vulnerable to develop the problem than others in the same or similar situation. High risk nursing diagnoses are supported by risk factors that guide nursing interventions to reduce or prevent the occurrence of the problem.

1. *Label:* The label provides a name for the diagnosis, a concise phrase or term which represents a pattern of related cues. Diagnostic labels may include but *are not limited* to the following qualifiers:

Altered—A change from baseline

Impaired—Made worse, weakened; damaged, reduced; deteriorated

Depleted—Emptied wholly or partially; exhausted of

Deficient—Inadequate in amount, quality, or degree; defective; not sufficient; incomplete

Excessive—Characterized by an amount or quantity that is greater than is necessary, desirable, or useful

Dysfunctional—Abnormal; incomplete functioning

Disturbed—Agitated; interrupted, interfered with

Ineffective—Not producing the desired effect

Decreased—Lessened, lesser in size, amount or degree

Increased—Greater in size, amount or degree

Acute—Severe but of short duration

Chronic—Lasting a long time; recurring; habitual; constant

Intermittent—Stopping and starting again at intervals; periodic; cyclic

2. *Definition:* The definition of the label provides a clear, precise description. The definition delineates its meaning and helps differentiate this diagnosis from all others.
3. *Risk Factors:* Risk factors identify behaviors, conditions or circumstances that render an individual, family, or community more vulnerable to a particular problem than others in the same or similar situation. There are no signs and symptoms for high risk diagnoses.
4. *Literature/Clinical Validation:* A narrative review of literature is required to support the rationale for the diagnosis and the risk factors. Literature citations for each risk factor are required. If the diagnosis is similar to an approved NANDA diagnosis, the reason for its usefulness must be addressed. The submission must include a sample 2-part (including label and risk factors) high risk nursing diagnostic statement with related outcome criteria and nursing-prescribed interventions.

Sample:

High Risk for Injury: Fall related to fatigue and altered gait
Outcome Criteria
    Describes or demonstrates necessary safety measures
Interventions
    Teach measures to prevent falls; instruct to request assistance when needed

III. Wellness Nursing Diagnosis

A wellness nursing diagnosis is a clinical judgment about an individual, family or community in transition from a specific level of wellness to a higher level of wellness.

1. *Label:* The term "Potential for Enhanced" will be the designated qualifier. Enhanced is defined as made greater, to increase in quality, or more desired. Wellness diagnoses will be one-part statements.
2. *Definition:* The definition of the label provides a clear, precise description. The definition delineates its meaning and helps differentiate this diagnosis from all others.
3. *Literature/Clinical Validation:* A narrative review of literature is required to support the rationale for the diagnosis. A sample one-part wellness nursing diagnostic statement with related outcome criteria and nursing-prescribed interventions must accompany the submission.

Sample:

Potential for Enhanced Parenting
Outcome Criteria
    Will practice listening without advice-giving with children
Interventions
    Describe active listening; differentiate between listening and advice-giving

IV. Revision of NANDA-Approved Nursing Diagnoses

Changes can be proposed for the label, the definition, and/or the defining characteristics. In order for any NANDA-approved nursing diagnosis to be refined or revised, the proposal must contain:

1. A narrative describing the rationale for the proposed change.
2. Research findings to support the proposed changes. These findings can be the results of research by the submitter or from research reported in the literature.

V. Deletion of NANDA-Approved Nursing Diagnoses

Proposals can be submitted to delete a NANDA-approved nursing diagnosis. The proposal must contain a narrative describing the rationale for the proposed deletion. The rationale must be supported by:

1. Logical justification and
2. Research findings and/or relevant literature review

VI. Diagnosis Review Committee Review Cycle

1. Submission Deadline: March 1 (year prior to conference, *e.g.*, 1991, 1993, 1995).
2. Initial review by DRC Chairperson for inclusion of required components.
3. Incomplete submissions returned with a re-submission deadline date of July 1.
4. Submissions with all the required components will be reviewed by the Diagnosis Review Committee. One of the following decisions will be made for each submission:
   a. *Not Accepted*—The proposed diagnosis has not been accepted for review by the Expert Advisory Panel. Reasons for "not accepted" are:
      • Represents a medical diagnosis
      • Represents a treatment or procedure
      • Did not represent a human response
      • Defining characteristics for actual nursing diagnosis are not cues or signs/ symptoms
      • Defining characteristics for high risk nursing diagnosis are not risk factors
   b. *Hold for Revisions*—This proposed diagnosis will be returned to the submitter for revisions. Examples of needed revisions are:
      • Research population was not representative for conclusions drawn
      • Inadequate literature support for proposed diagnosis
   c. *Accepted for Expert Advisory Panel Review*
5. After the Expert Advisory Panel and the DRC review, each proposed diagnosis or proposal (revisions or deletions) will receive one of the following designations:
   a. *Returned to Be Developed (TBD)*—This decision delineates submitted work as promising but requires substantive development. This work will require re-submission in its entirety to the DRC. This category acknowledges promising work in need of substantive revisions.
   b. *Conditional Accept*—This category indicates a provisional acceptance of the submitted work pending receipt of revisions agreed on by the committee and the submitter.
   c. *Accepted*—This category indicates the submitted work is accepted.
6. Accepted diagnoses or proposals for revisions/deletions will be forwarded to the Board of Directors for approval.
7. Board-approved proposed diagnoses or proposals for revisions/deletions will be presented at the NANDA Conference and will be subject to membership mail vote.

Reference

Gordon, M. (1982). *Nursing diagnosis: Process and application.* New York: McGraw-Hill.

Appendix IX: Guidelines for Play Therapy

Play is a natural means of expression for children and is essential to their mental, emotional, and social well-being. The need for play during stress (*e.g.,* developmental, illness, treatments) is essential to provide the child with an outlet for emotional release and a sense of mastery over the situation. Play provides parents and professionals with opportunities to assess the mood, words, and actions of a child and identify the child's present perception of the situation.

A. General
  1. Professionals and parents use play to assist the child to
     a. Recognize her feelings
     b. Cope with a new concept
     c. Identify his fears
     d. Understand threatening or unknown events
     e. Clarify distortions received from others (parents, peers)
     f. Gain a sense of mastery
  2. Play can be used to diagnose the child's perception of the situation, his perception of caregivers, and his mental responses to events
  3. Guidelines for therapeutic play
     a. Promote spontaneity by reflecting only what the child expresses
     b. Avoid forcing the child to participate
     c. Allow sufficient time without interruption
     d. Identify when it is appropriate to encourage child to share concerns
     e. Play for the child who cannot play for himself
     f. Allow child to work freely on her project without direction or adult comment
     g. Allow child to engage in violent nondestructive acts

B. Types of play
  1. Drawing and painting
     a. Supplies: Crayons, paint, brushes, paper
        • Artwork usually requires little direction
        • Older children can be asked to draw what they like or do not like about the hospital
        • An old sheet can cover the bed clothes of a child confined to bed
        • Ask child to explain picture when it is done
        • Clarify misconceptions
  2. Dramatic play
     b. Supplies: Puppets, dolls, stuffed animals, replicas of hospital equipment, actual hospital equipment, miniature hospital furniture
        • Assign roles to the child and to the doll or puppet ("Mary, you are the nurse and the puppet is you")
        • Ask child to administer a treatment to the puppet or doll
        • Supervise the child when playing with equipment

3. Needle play (dramatic play)
   c. Supplies: Doll, stuffed animals, clean syringes and needles, alcohol wipes, water vial, Band-Aids, miniature IV sets (tubing, tourniquets, tongue blade for arm board)
      - Introduce immediately after or in between the child's experiences
      - Expect reluctance to touch syringe
      - Demonstrate injection and ask the child to help you push the fluid in
      - Allow child to give injections on the doll anywhere and however he wants to
      - Make appropriate sounds of crying and protest to show the child that crying is permitted
      - Show child how to give the doll love after the injection
      - Encourage child to talk about why injections are needed
      - Use group play to encourage participation
      - Overly aggressive children should be shown acceptance

Bibliography

Axline, V. (1969). *Play therapy.* New York: Ballantine Books.

Brooks, M. (1970). Why play in the hospital? *Nursing Clinics of North America, 5,* 431–441.

Levinson, P., & Ousterhout, D. (1980). Art and play therapy with pediatric burn patients. *Journal of Burn Care and Rehabilitation, 1*(5), 42–46.

Oehler, J. (1981). The frog family books: Color the pictures sad or glad. *Maternal-Child Nursing Journal, 6,* 281–283.

Petrillo, M., & Sanger, S. (1980). *Emotional care of hospitalized children* (2nd ed.). Philadelphia: J. B. Lippincott.

Smallwood, S. (1988). Preparing children for surgery. *AORN Journal, 47*(1), 177–182.

Taylor, M., & Williams, H. (1980). Use of therapeutic play in the ambulatory pediatric hematology clinic. *Cancer Nursing, 3,* 433–437.

Resources for Parents and Children

Literature

Books that help children deal with a hospital experience (Publication number 017-031-00020-1)

When your child goes to the hospital (Publication number 793-30092)

A reader's guide for parents of children with mental, physical, or emotional disabilities. (Publication number [HSA]77-5290). An annotated reference on basic reading, books on teaching and playing at home, books that deal with particular issues, and books written by parents and children.

The above three titles are available from the U.S. Government Printing Office, Washington, DC 20402

Preparing children and families for health care encounters. A compilation of articles for parents and professionals on various aspects of preparation. Available from the Association for the Care of Children's Health, 3615 Wisconsin Avenue NW, Washington, DC 20016

Appendix X: Stress Management Techniques

The following techniques can be taught to provide an individual with an opportunity to control his response to stressors and, in turn, increase his ability to manage stress constructively. Suggested readings are listed at the end to provide more specific information.

Progressive Relaxation Technique

Progressive relaxation is a self-taught or instructed exercise that involves learning to constrict and relax muscle groups in a systematic way, beginning with the face and finishing with the feet. This exercise may be combined with breathing exercises that focus on inner body processes. It usually takes 15 to 30 minutes and may be accompanied by a taped instruction that directs the person concerning the sequence of muscles to be relaxed.

1. Wear loose clothing; remove glasses and shoes.
2. Sit or recline in a comfortable position with neck and knees supported; avoid lying completely flat.
3. Begin with slow, rhythmic breathing.
   a. Close your eyes or stare at a spot and take in a slow deep breath.
   b. Exhale the breath slowly.
4. Continue rhythmic breathing at a low steady pace and feel the tension leaving your body with each breath.
5. Begin progressive relaxation of muscle groups.
   a. Breathe in and tense (tighten) your muscles and then relax the muscles as you breathe out.
   b. Suggested order for tension-relaxation cycle (with tension technique in parentheses)
      - Face, jaw, mouth (squint eyes, wrinkle brow)
      - Neck (pull chin to neck)
      - Right hand (make a fist)
      - Right arm (bend elbow in tightly)
      - Left hand (make a fist)
      - Left arm (bend elbow in tightly)
      - Back, shoulders, chest (shrug shoulders up tightly)
      - Abdomen (pull stomach in and bear down on chair)
      - Right upper leg (push leg down)
      - Right lower leg and foot (point toes toward body)
      - Left upper leg (push leg down)
      - Left lower leg and foot (point toes toward body)
6. Practice technique slowly.
7. End relaxation session when you are ready by counting to three, inhaling deeply, and saying, "I am relaxed."

Self-coaching

Self-coaching is a procedure to decrease anxiety by understanding one's own signs of anxiety (such as increased heart rate or sweaty palms) and then coaching oneself to relax.

For example, "I am upset about this situation but I can control how anxious I get. I will take things one step at a time, and I won't focus on my fear. I'll think about what I must do to finish this task. The situation will not be forever. I can manage until it is over. I'll focus on taking deep breaths."

Thought Stopping

Thought stopping is a self-directed behavioral procedure learned to gain control of self-defeating thoughts. Through repeated systematic practice, a person does the following:
1. Says "Stop" when a self-defeating thought crosses the mind (*e.g.,* "I'm not smart enough" or "I'm not a good nurse")
2. Allows a brief period—15 to 30 seconds—of conscious relaxation (because of an increased focus on negative thoughts, it may seem at first that self-defeating thoughts increase; however, eventually the self-defeating thoughts will decrease)

Assertive Behavior

Assertive behavior is the open, honest, empathetic sharing of your opinions, desires, and feelings. Assertiveness is not a magical acquisition but a learned behavioral skill. Assertive persons do not allow others to take advantage of them and thus are not victims. Assertive behavior is not domineering but remains controlled and nonaggressive. An assertive person

Does not hurt others
Does not wait for things to get better
Does not invite victimization
Listens attentively to the desires and feelings of others
Takes the initiative to make relationships better
Remains in control or uses silences as an alternative
Examines all the risks involved before asserting
Examines personal responsibilities in each situation before asserting

Refer to suggested readings for specific techniques or participate in an assertiveness training course led by a competent instructor. Assertive behavior is best learned slowly in several sessions rather than in one lengthy session or workshop.

Guided Imagery

This technique is the purposeful use of one's imagination in a specific way to achieve relaxation and control. The person concentrates on the image and pictures himself involved in the scene. The following is an example of the technique.
1. Discuss with person an image he has experienced that is pleasurable and relaxing to him, such as
   a. Lying on a warm beach
   b. Feeling a cool wave of water
   c. Floating on a raft
   d. Watching the sun set
2. Choose a scene that will involve at least two senses.
3. Begin with rhythmic breathing and progressive relaxation.
4. Have a person travel mentally to the scene.
5. Have the person slowly experience the scene; how does it look? sound? smell? feel? taste?

6. Practice the imagery.
   a. Suggest tape-recording the imagined experience to assist with the technique.
   b. Practice the technique alone to reduce feelings of embarrassment.
7. End the imagery technique by counting to three and saying, "I am relaxed" (if the person does not utilize a specific ending, he may become drowsy and fall asleep, which defeats the purpose of the technique).

Bibliography

Alberti, R. E., & Emmons, L. (1974). *Your perfect right: A guide to assertive behavior* (2nd ed.). San Luis Obispo, CA: Impact.

Benson, H. (1976). *The relaxation response*. New York: Avon Books.

Bloom, L, Coburn, K., & Pearlman, J. (1976). *The new assertive woman*. New York: Dell.

Chenevert, M. (1978). *Special techniques in assertiveness training for women in the health professions*. St. Louis: C. V. Mosby.

Gridano, D., & Everly G. (1979). *Controlling stress and tension*. Englewood Cliffs, NJ: Prentice-Hall.

Herman, S. (1978). *Becoming assertive: A guide for nurses*. New York: Van Nostrand.

Hill, L., & Smith, N. (1985). *Self-care nursing*. Englewood Cliffs. NJ: Prentice-Hall (especially Part II, Self-care primarily associated with the mind)

McCaffery, M. (1979). *Nursing management of the patient with pain* (2nd ed.). Philadelphia: J. B. Lippincott (especially Chapter 9, Relaxation; Chapter 10, Imagery).

Appendix XI: Collaborative Problems*

Potential Complication: Cardiac/Vascular
PC: Decreased Cardiac Output Index
PC: Dysrhythmias
PC: Pulmonary Edema
PC: Cardiogenic Shock
PC: Thromboemboli/Deep Vein Thrombosis
PC: Hypovolemic Shock
PC: Peripheral Vascular Insufficiency
PC: Hypertension
PC: Congenital Heart Disease
PC: Disseminated Intravascular Coagulation
PC: Angina
PC: Pulmonary Embolism
PC: Spinal Shock
PC: Ischemic Ulcers

Potential Complication: Respiratory
PC: Hypoxemia
PC: Atelectasis/Pneumonia
PC: Tracheobronchial Constriction
PC: Pleural Effusion
PC: Tracheal Necrosis
PC: Ventilator Dependency
PC: Pneumothorax
PC: Laryngeal Edema

Potential Complication: Renal/Urinary
PC: Acute Urinary Retention
PC: Renal Insufficiency
PC: Bladder Perforation
PC: Renal Calculi

Potential Complication: Gastrointestinal/Hepatic/Biliary
PC: Paralytic Ileus/Small Bowel Obstruction
PC: Hepatic Failure
PC: Hyperbilirubenia
PC: Evisceration
PC: Hepatosplenomegaly
PC: Curling's Ulcer
PC: Ascites
PC: GI Bleeding

*Frequently used collaborative problems are represented on this list. Other situations not listed here could qualify as collaborative problems.

Potential Complication: Metabolic/Immune/Hematopoietic

PC: Hypoglycemia/Hyperglycemia
PC: Negative Nitrogen Balance
PC: Electrolyte Imbalances
PC: Thyroid Dysfunction
PC: Hypothermia (severe)
PC: Hyperthermia (severe)
PC: Septicemia
PC: Acidosis (metabolic, respiratory)
PC: Alkalosis (metabolic, respiratory)
PC: Hypo/Hyperthyroidism
PC: Allergic Reaction
PC: Donor Tissue Rejection
PC: Adrenal Insufficiency
PC: Anemia
PC: Thrombocytopenia
PC: Immunodeficiency
PC: Polycythemia
PC: Sickling Crisis

Potential Complication: Neurologic/Sensory

PC: Increased Intracranial Pressure
PC: Stroke
PC: Seizures
PC: Spinal Cord Compression
PC: Autonomic Dysreflexia
PC: Meningitis
PC: Cranial Nerve Impairment (specify)
PC: Paralysis
PC: Peripheral Nerve Impairment
PC: Increased Intraocular Pressure
PC: Corneal Ulceration
PC: Neuropathies

Potential Complication: Muscular/Skeletal

PC: Osteoporosis
PC: Joint Dislocation
PC: Compartmental Syndrome
PC: Pathologic Fractures

Potential Complication: Reproductive

PC: Fetal Distress
PC: Postpartum Hemorrhage
PC: Pregnancy-Associated Hypertension
PC: Hypermenorrhea
PC: Polymenorrhea
PC: Syphilis
PC: Prenatal Bleeding
PC: Preterm Labor

Appendix XII: Self-Reporting Oncology Nursing Assessment*

This questionnaire is designed for the client or significant other to complete prior to an interview with the professional nurse. During the interview the nurse will review the answers with the client and significant other. Additional data obtained during the interview are recorded in the column on the right.

SELF-REPORTING PATIENT HEALTH QUESTIONNAIRE
(Please complete this questionnaire by checking off the appropriate word that fits your situation or writing in the information where space is provided. When you are not certain about a question put a "?" beside it. The nurse will discuss this with you privately during your interview.)

	INTERVIEW INFORMATION
PART I: ADMISSION DATA Date: __/__/__ Age: __ yrs. Male __ Female __ Name you prefer _____ 　　　　d m y If we are unable to reach you, whom could we contact on your behalf? 1. _____ Phone (___) - ____ 2. _____ Phone (___) - ____ What languages do you speak? _____ Who is your family doctor? _____ Which pharmacy/drugstore do you use? _____ Phone (___) - ____	
PART II: PATIENT HISTORY 1. What is the health problem that has brought you here today? _____ _____ 2. What tests, surgeries or medical consultations have you had in the past 6 weeks? _____ _____ 3. What treatment(s) are you receiving at this time? _____ _____	

(left vertical label: HEALTH MAINTENANCE)

(continued)

*Developed by Rosemary Allaster, R.N., B.A.; Eunice Anderson, R.N., M.Sc.N.; Mary Liz Bland, R.N., B.Sc.N.; Maureen Brock, R.N., B.Sc.N.; Gwen Flegel, R.N.; Bonnie Hall, R.N., M.Sc.N.; Maria Jefferies, R.N., M.S.N.; Sue Kudirka, R.N.; Marcia Langhorn, R.N.; Linda D. Riehl, R.N.; Heather Ryan, R.N., M.Sc.N.; and Marilyn Semple, R.N., of the Nursing Department, London Regional Cancer Centre, London, Ontario, Canada. Used with permission.

HEALTH PERCEPTION

4. List your past health history (major illness/operations/injuries/accidents with dates):

_____

_____

5. a. Do you smoke? Yes___ No___ b. Did you ever smoke? Yes___ No___

   If Yes, indicate type, amount, for how long, and when you quit: _____

_____

6. Have you had any experience with cancer (yourself, relative, or a friend)?

   Yes___ No___

   If yes, specify person, relationship and type of cancer: _____

_____

_____

7. Do you take any medications? Yes___ No___ If yes, please list the prescription medications and over-the-counter medications you now take. Please include the dose—how many mg or mL you take, why you need to take the drug.

_____

_____

_____

8. Do you have a drug plan? Yes___ No___

9. Do you have any ALLERGIES? Yes___ No___ If yes, please list the cause of your allergy and the allergic reaction that you have.

_____

_____

10. Please check the services you are now using: None___   Home Care___

    Visiting nurse ___ VON___ Public Health Nurse ___ Cancer Society ___

    Other (specify) _____

NUTRITION–METABOLIC

11. Please check the word to describe your diet: Regular___ Soft___ Liquid___

    Diabetic___ Other: _____

12. Do you take a diet supplement? Yes___ No___

    If yes, please specify: _____

13. Do you drink alcohol (beer, wine, liquor)? Yes___ No___

14. Place a check beside the word, if you are having problems with:

    Loss of appetite___ Nausea___ Vomiting___ Indigestion___

    Swallowing___ Chewing___ Meal preparation___ Mouth sores___

INTERVIEW INFORMATION

(continued)

		INTERVIEW INFORMATION
	Swelling (hands, ankles)___ Skin problems___ Dental problems___ Weight Loss___ Weight gain ___ 15. Do you have dentures? Yes___ No___ Upper___ Lower___ Partial___	
ELIMINATION	16. Place a check beside the word(s) if you are having problems with your urinary bladder: No problem___ Frequency___ Burning___ No control___ Not starting___ Other_____ 17. Are these problems new? Yes___ No___ If yes, explain _____ _____ 18. Place a check beside the word(s) if you are having problems with bowel function: No problem___ Constipation___ Diarrhea___ Hemorrhoids___ Other_____ 19. Are these problems new? Yes___ No___ If yes, explain _____ _____	
ACTIVITY–EXERCISE	20. Place a check beside the word(s) if you are having any problems with: Bruising___ Bleeding___ Swelling___ Leg pain ___ Shortness of breath___ 21. Do you have a cough? Yes___ No___ Does your cough produce sputum? Yes___ No___ 22. Do you use oxygen? Yes___ No___ 23. Place a check beside the word(s) if you have noticed a change in your energy level when: Eating___ Bathing___ Dressing___ Walking___ Doing housework___ Preparing meals___ Shopping___ Doing your job___ Exercising___ Doing hobbies 24. Are these changes recent? Yes___ No___	
SLEEP–REST	25. Do you have any problems sleeping? Yes___ No___ If yes, explain _____ 26. Do you feel rested after sleep? Yes___ No___ If no, explain _____ 27. Do you take anything to help you sleep? Yes___ No___ If yes, explain _____	

COGNITIVE– PERCEPTUAL	28. Do you wear: Glasses? Yes___ No___
	             Contacts? Yes___ No___
	             Hearing Aid? Yes___ No___
	
	29. Place a check deside the word(s) if you are having problems with:
	Eyes___ Ears___ Nose___ Tongue___ Sight___ Hearing___ Smell___
		(continued)

Taste___ Numbness___ Tingling___ Dizziness___ Seizures___

Headaches___

COGNITIVE–PERCEPTUAL

30. Are any of these problems new? Yes___ No___ If yes, explain:

_____

31. Do you have pain? Yes___ No___ If yes, where and when do you have

pain? _____

_____

_____

Check the words that describe your pain: Piercing___ Shooting___

Burning___ Cramping___ Stinging___ Dull ache___ Constant___

Comes and goes___ Other_____

32. Is your pain controlled? Yes___ No___

CONCEPT

33. Please check the words that describe how you are feeling.

Anxious___ Hopeful___ Content___ Angry___ Scared___

Depressed___ Other _____

ROLE–RELATIONSHIP

34. Marital status _____ Number of children _____

35. Do you live: Alone___ With spouse___ With family ___ Other_____

36. What is your occupation? _____

Full time___ Part time___ Retired___ Student___

37. Are you working? Yes___ No___

If yes, where _____ Phone (___) ___-____

38. If you are not working, do you plan to return to work? Yes___ No___

39. Are you receiving sick benefits? Yes___ No___

SEXUALITY–REPRODUCTIVE

40. Do you use birth control? Yes___ No___

41. Are you planning to have a family in the future? Yes___ No___

FEMALE:
42. Are you still having menstrual periods? Yes___ No___

43. If yes, how long is your cycle? ___ days

If no, what age did you stop? ___ yrs

44. When was your last PAP test? _____

45. Do you practice breast self-examination? Yes___ No___

MALE:

46. Do you practice testicular self-examination? Yes___ No___

INTERVIEW
INFORMATION

(continued)

		INTERVIEW INFORMATION
COPING STRESS-TOLERANCE	47. Have you experienced any recent stressful events in addition to your illness? Yes___ No___ If yes, explain _____ _____ 48. What helps you to manage when you feel stressed? _____ _____ 49. Who is most helpful in talking things over? _____ _____	
BELIEF VALUES	50. Do you have any religious or cultural beliefs that we should be aware of during your treatment? Yes___ No___ If you wish, please explain _____	
	51. Is there anything you wish to discuss while you are here? Yes___ No___ If you wish, please explain _____	

PATIENT'S SIGNATURE: _____

DATE: _____

NURSE'S SIGNATURE/INITIALS: _____

DATE: _____

IF COMPLETED BY SOMEONE OTHER THAN PATIENT:

_____

(Name and relationship to patient)

Index

Page numbers in italics *indicate illustrations; page numbers followed by t indicate tables. Capitalized entries indicate nursing diagnoses.*

GREATEST MOMENTS
IN
LSU
FOOTBALL HISTORY

EDITED BY FRANCIS J. FITZGERALD

From the sports pages of the

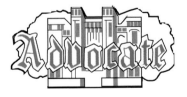

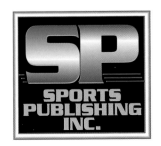

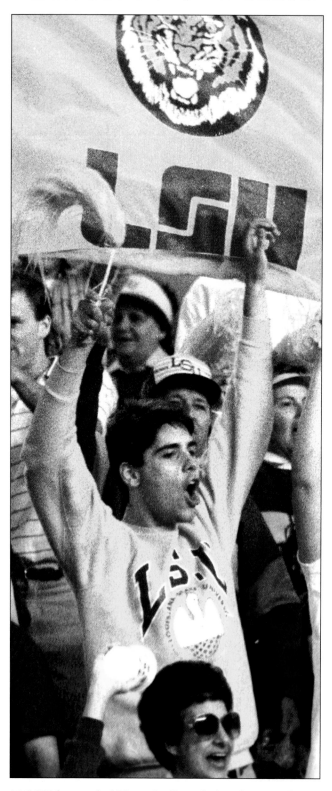

■ LSU fans rocked Tiger Stadium during the Bengals' 1988 victory over Auburn. A campus seismograph proved it to be the loudest stadium in the country.

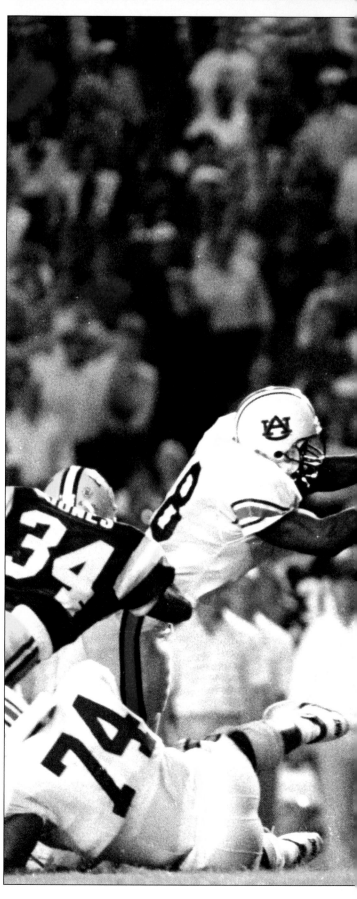

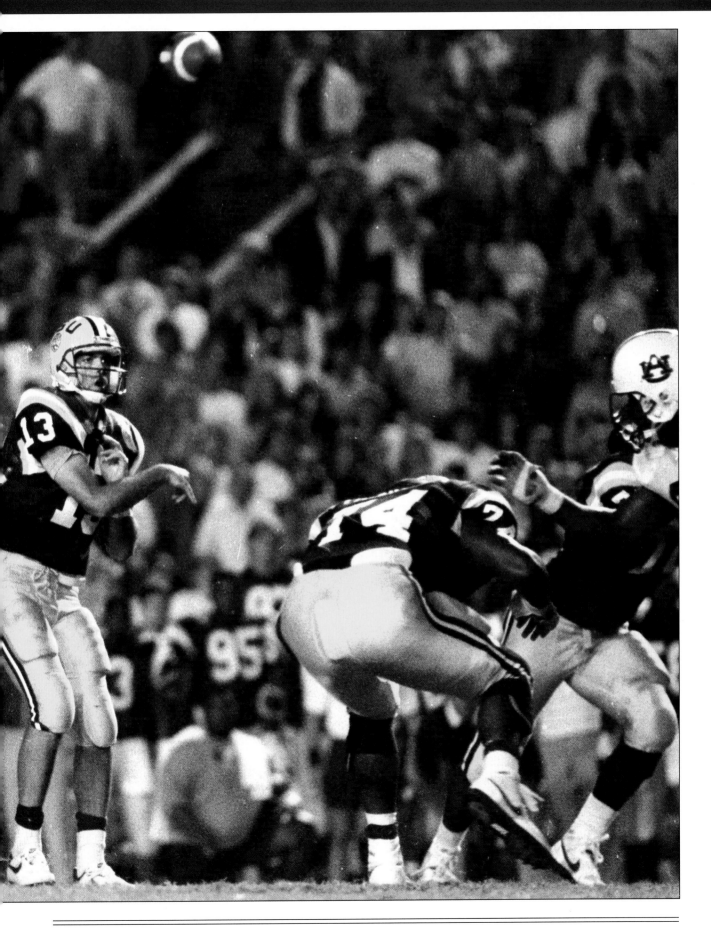

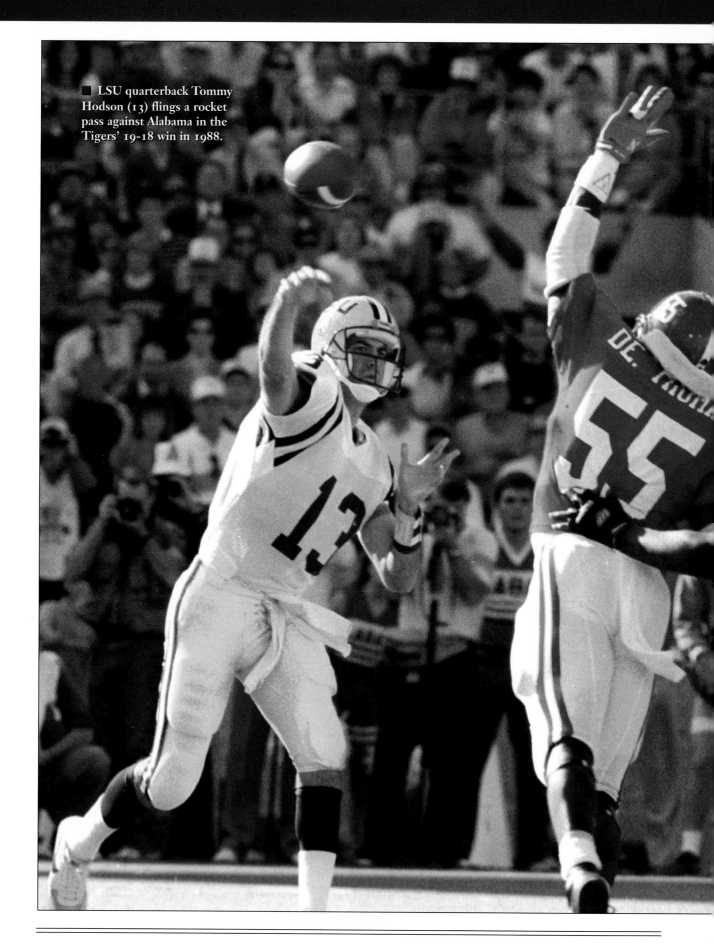

LSU quarterback Tommy Hodson (13) flings a rocket pass against Alabama in the Tigers' 19-18 win in 1988.

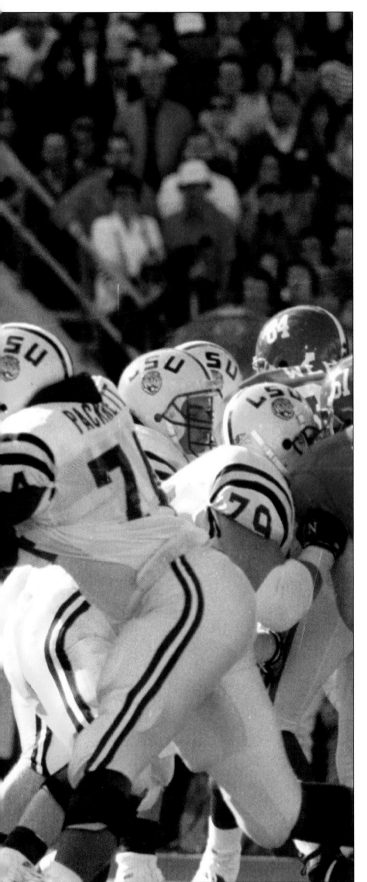

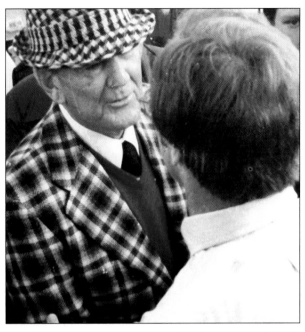

■ Jerry Stovall is congratulated by Alabama coach Paul (Bear) Bryant after LSU's 20-10 win in 1982.

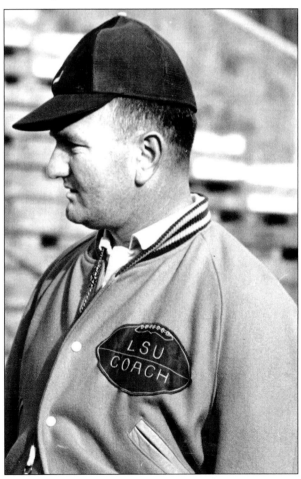

■ Charlie McClendon is LSU's winningest coach with a record of 137-59-7 during 18 seasons.

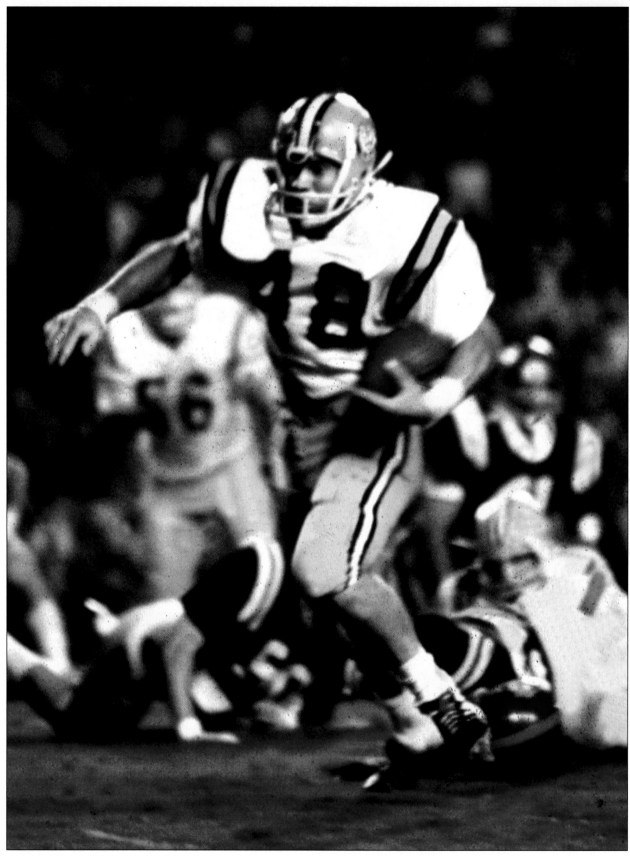

■ **THE NIGHT THE CLOCK STOPPED:** LSU's 17-16 win over Ole Miss in 1972.

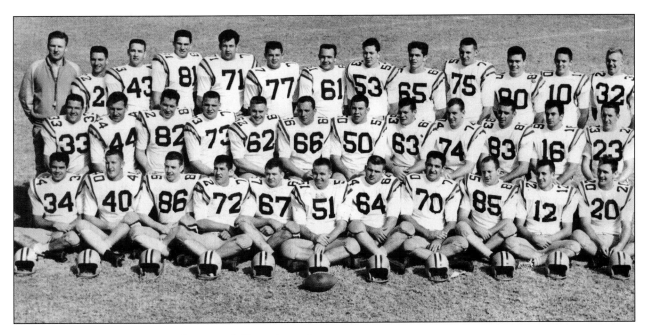

■ The 1958 Tigers were named National Champions after an 11-0 season.

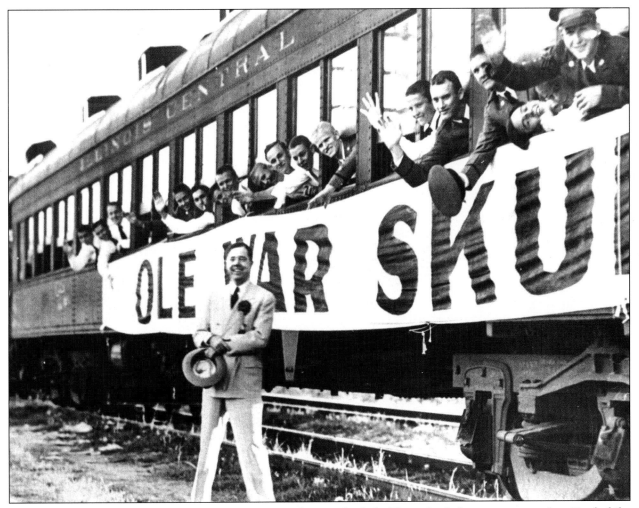

■ Governor Huey Long took five trains and 5,000 students to back the Tigers in their 1934 game against Vanderbilt.

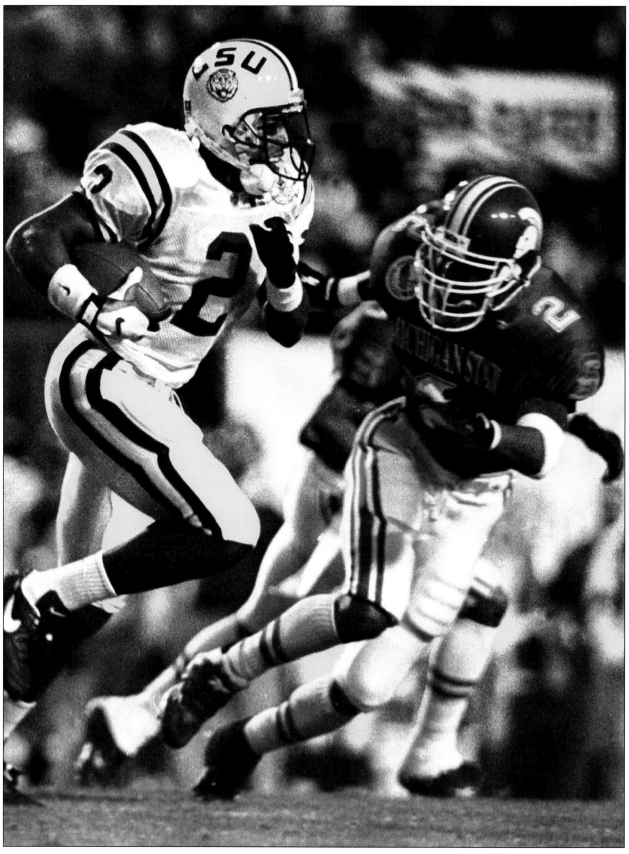

■ The Tigers defeated Michigan State, 45-26, in the 1995 Independence Bowl to cap Gerry DiNardo's first season.

Table of Contents

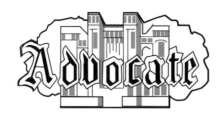

PUBLISHER: DAVID C. MANSHIP
EXECUTIVE EDITOR: LINDA C. LIGHTFOOT
MANAGING EDITOR: JIM WHITTUM
EXECUTIVE SPORTS EDITOR: BUTCH MUIR
SPORTS EDITOR: SAM KING
DIRECTOR OF PHOTOGRAPHY: MICHAEL HULTS
LIBRARY DIRECTOR: JILL ARNOLD
GRAPHICS EDITOR: PAUL SANDAU
MARKETING DIRECTOR: LINDA WUNSTEL

ACKNOWLEDGEMENTS: This book would not have been completed on time without the hard work and resource-ful efforts of Jill Arnold, The Advocate's library director, and her top notch staff — Laurie Christensen, Judy Jumonville, Christopher Miller, Sheila Varnado, Margaret Forrest and Dianne Muchow — who assisted me in finding the difficult pho-tos in their archives and the microfilm newspaper stories that were not easy to locate at other libraries, and Butch Muir's excellent sports staff — Sam King, Scott Rabalais, Robin Fambrough, Scott Gremillion, Joe Macaluso, Sheldon Mickles, Joseph Schiefelbein, Glenn Guilbeau, Tony Brown, Gary English, Matt Randolph, Ben Reed, Bonner Ridgeway, T.J. Simoneaux and David Constantine. Also, the Southwestern Bell Cotton Bowl, the FedEx Orange Bowl, the Nokia Sugar Bowl, the Chick-Fil-A Peach Bowl, the CompUSA Florida Citrus Bowl, The Birmingham News, The South Bend Tribune and T.J. Ribs who assisted in providing key photos for this book, and Herb Vincent and his media relations staff at LSU.

ISBN: 1-58261-018-5 (trade edition)

Produced by Epic Sports, Birmingham, Ala.
Cover and Book Design by Richard Epps, Detroit.
Photo imaging by Philip Webb, Detroit.

Typefaces: Janson, Giza

Published in association with The Advocate by:

Sports Publishing Inc.
804 North Neil Street
Suite 100
Champaign, IL 61820
(217) 359-5940
http://www.sportspublishinginc.com

The LSU Fighting Tigers' ever-growing football program enters its 105th year with high expectations and hopes of making history repeat on this the 40th anniversary of its 1958 national championship team.

Since the days when Charles F. Coates, a professor of chemistry, brought football to the campus until this present era of Gerry DiNardo, there have been many thrills, victories and happy and glorious moments.

There have been some good days and some bad days, but the bad is outnumbered by far by the good — especially the great hours and nights spent in Tiger Stadium, which enters its 75th season of showcasing its beloved Tigers.

In its illustrious history, LSU has posted a 603-341-47 won-loss record (.632) and is 276-224-30 (.549) in the Southeastern Conference. The Tigers have won one national championship (1958), made 31 bowl appearances, won seven SEC titles and, prior to the founding of the SEC in 1933, claimed one Southern Intercollegiate Conference title and three Southern Intercollegiate Athletic Association championships. It has produced 118 All-SEC first team players, 32 of whom claimed the honor two or more times with placekicker David Browndyke, cornerback Tommy Casanova and tailback Dalton Hilliard being honored three times. Quarterback Tommy Hodson stands alone as the only four-time, All-SEC first-team member in the history of the school.

There have been 38 Tigers to claim All-American's honors, including six two-time All-Americas — tailback Charles Alexander (1977-78), halfback Billy Cannon (1958-59), linebacker Warren Capone (1972-73), split end Wendell Davis (1986-87), center Marvin (Moose) Stewart (1935-36) and end Gaynell Tinsley (1935-36). Safety Tommy Casanova is LSU's only three-time All-America (1969-70-71).

There have been scores of great games and hundreds of spectacular performances by players that have made LSU's program one of the tops in the nation and the place in which they play — Tiger Stadium, aka "Death Valley" — possibly the very best in the land. Recently ESPN concluded, "There is no better place to be on planet Earth on a Saturday night than LSU's Tiger Stadium" — something Tiger fans have known for scores of years.

The fans throng to this stadium to cheer on their Tigers, their home attendance ranking in the Top 10 thirty-four times since 1957, including 32 straight years (1957-88). Tiger Stadium's largest crowd ever (82,390) was on Sept. 24, 1983, when LSU defeated Washington, 40-14.

The program has grown from its inconspicuous start with little or no money, to a multi-million dollar business that helps finance a total of 20 sports that are showcased and supported by many state of the art facilities and programs.

For all these thousands of athletes, for all their great performances, for so many great games, The Advocate and its sister newspaper, The State-Times, were on hand to deliver its readers and LSU fans their accounts, reports and features about the team they so loyally cheered and supported. The State-Times, established in 1907 after being founded as The Democratic Advocate in 1843, was purchased by Capital City Press in 1909. A morning newspaper, The Morning Advocate, was established by Capital City Press in 1925. Since that time The State-Times, The Morning Advocate and now The Advocate have provided coverage of a team and a program that takes a backseat to none in the nation.

In *Greatest Moments in LSU Football History*, readers will be able to relive some of the most glorious moments in Tiger football history from the game reports of former sports editors W.I. Spencer, Bud Montet, Dan Hardesty and numerous football beat writers — as well as rekindle memories with an unforgettable selection of photographs.

It covers great moments such as, "The Night the Tigers Moved the Earth," on Oct. 8, 1988, when Tommy Hodson's pass to Eddie Fuller defeated Auburn, Billy Cannon's fabled 89-yard, Halloween night run in 1959 against Ole Miss, LSU's 56-0 victory over the University of Havana in college football's first international game on Dec. 25, 1907, as well as more than 40 other great game stories.

On this the 40th anniversary of LSU's lone national championship team, you can relive that great 1958 season, in a story, "1958: The Year LSU Owned the College Football World," by present Advocate sports editor Sam King, who also takes a look at the mystique of Tiger Stadium in another story. Staffer Scott Rabalais recounts the days of "The Kingfish," Gov. Huey Long, and his involvement in LSU football in another story.

The Advocate believes LSU football is every bit as important as its 100,000-plus readers do and strives to cover it the very best way possible. At least three writers and two photographers now staff every road game with the numbers increasing for home contests, depending upon the opponent and the importance of the game. Executive sports editor Butch Muir directs and leads a highly-efficient and talented staff in designing pages and presenting stories and photographs in the very best package possible to the readers of The Advocate and the fans of LSU.

In short, it is one outstanding team being covered by another outstanding team for the benefit of a great team — LSU's fans and the readers of The Advocate.

Sam King
The Advocate, *Sports Editor*

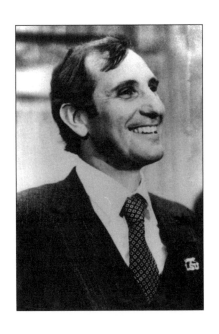

DEDICATION

This book is dedicated to Bo Rein, who never had the opportunity to coach in Tiger Stadium.

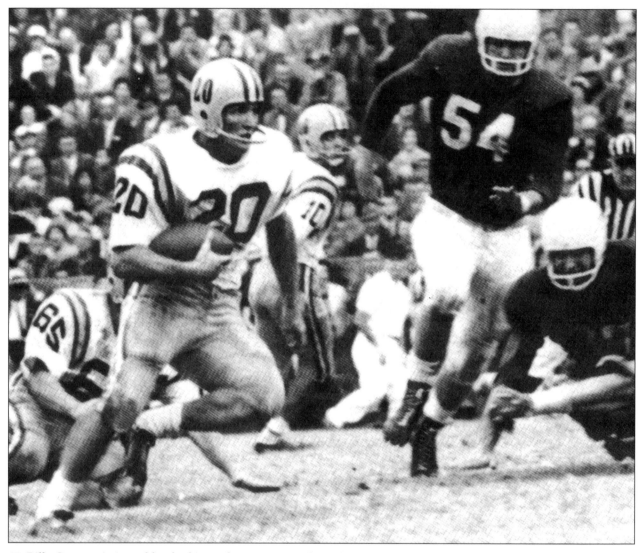

■ Billy Cannon (20) rambles for big yardage against arch-rival Tulane.

1958: When LSU Owned the College Football World

BY SAM KING
The Advocate

Except for the passing of summer and the arrival of football, there was little to cheer about in Louisiana in the early days of September 1958. Forty years ago, it seemed like Louisiana led the nation in everything bad and brought up the rear in all that was good. Air conditioning was a household pipe dream; television was still a nightly attraction in show rooms of furniture stores across the state.

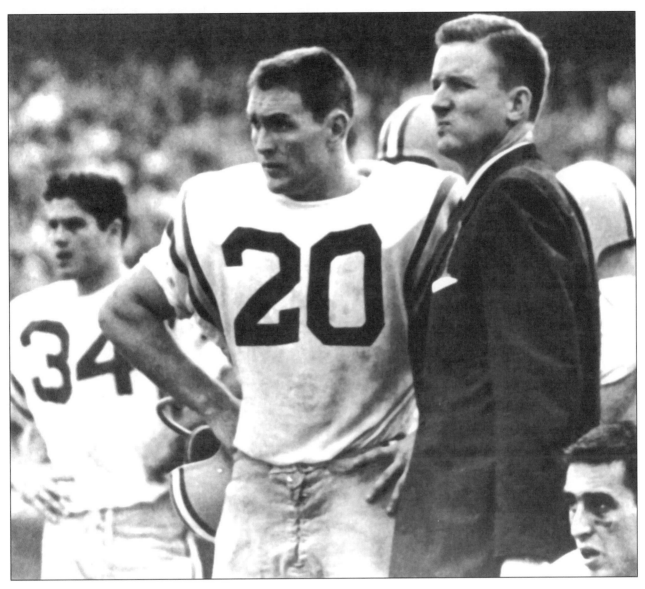

■ **LSU coach Paul Dietzel and his star halfback, Billy Cannon.**

Football might have been bad, but politics was worse. The governor (Earl Long) was teetering between stripping and "flipping" — trying to stay with stripper Blaze Starr and stay out of a mental institution — being admitted to the latter on June 15, 1959.

The economy was down, but promised to get better. You couldn't say the same for LSU's football team.

The Tigers had lost four of their final five games in 1957, marking their fourth straight losing season and third under 34-year-old coach Paul Dietzel, who likely questioned his job security at the time. LSU was ranked no better than No. 37 (UPI) and No. 33 (AP) in the major polls and was young and inexperienced. It had 31 underclassmen and only two seniors who would play. It sorely lacked depth.

Not only did Dietzel have to replace All-America fullback Jimmy Taylor, but the entire right side of the offensive line. He had some outstanding players for his first team, but after that, only some who could play offense and others who could play only defense.

"Frankly, it takes a different type of player for offense and defense," said Dietzel. "On offense, you need kids that are smart, that aren't too fast, but are quick. On defense, you need players that are semi-wild, very aggressive and very fast."

He wanted to be two teams deep, but that seemed unlikely. Dietzel and his staff huddled. They made a decision that would stand the football world on its kicking tee. They would have three teams. The starters, the best players, would play both ways and be on the White Team. The remainder would compose the Go Team, which played only offense, and the others were the wild defensive specialists who composed the famed and ever-so popular Chinese Bandits.

Dietzel and Tigers everywhere loved those Chinese Bandits,

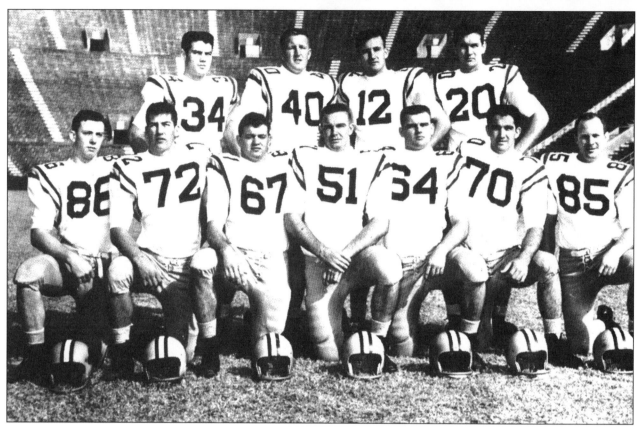

■ **The White Team: LSU's 1958 starting offensive and defensive team.**

who entered the game to the tune of a specially written song.

"The White team was good, but allowed the opponent 3.2 yards per carry," said Dietzel. "But, the Bandits gave up only .9 yards per carry.

"They really weren't that good, but they didn't know it. They were so wound up and were s-o-o-o wild. I never understood why there was so much gang tackling, but their speed was all the same and they all got to the ball at the same time."

And a tip of the coolie hat to you.

Coach Charles McClendon, who was in charge of the defense (there were no coordinators in those days), said, "the Bandits just got stronger and stronger and stronger.

"They didn't know they weren't a good football team — nobody ever told them. They were 100 percent go-getters."

Dietzel said he had been thinking about a move to provide more depth since Ole Miss thrashed the Tigers, 46-17, in 1956.

"That's what got us going. We could not play both ways with just one team. They just wore us out," said Dietzel. "Our first team could play them to a standstill, but got tired. We just didn't have enough depth.

"Now, everybody was very alert because they knew they had to play," said Dietzel. "The morale was fantastic because of that."

Possibly the greatest asset was the unbelievable amount of Louisiana talent that migrated to LSU. Then, if you were worth your salt, you didn't even consider going out of state to play. If you left, your family and just about everyone who liked

you were ostracized. Schools and communities, no matter how small or how large, took great pride in the fact that one of their own was playing at LSU.

Unquestionably, this team was Louisiana's — and would become its proudest possession.

"There was a tremendous feeling about what that team brought to the state," recalled Chinese Bandits defensive back Merle Schexnaildre during the 30-year celebration of the championship.

"The team was everybody's and everyone who was there knows and understands what I'm talking about.

"It was a source of pride for our state. There's not a day that goes by when someone or something doesn't remind me of that year."

Dietzel struck a mother lode of talent, the type that comes along only once every three or four generations. He put it to use very wisely.

The 33 spots on the 1958 Tiger squad were filled with 24 players from Louisiana, including three starters — Istrouma and University High halfbacks Billy Cannon and Johnny Robinson and Baton Rouge High quarterback Warren Rabb — in the backfield who grew up in the shadows of Tiger Stadium.

"That was one of the most unique things I've ever seen," said Dietzel recently. "Having three starting backs from one town is almost unbelievable — and they were all outstanding.

"Robinson," he surmised, "was the most underrated football player we had. He was such a good athlete. He was overshadowed by the fact Cannon was an All-American and won the

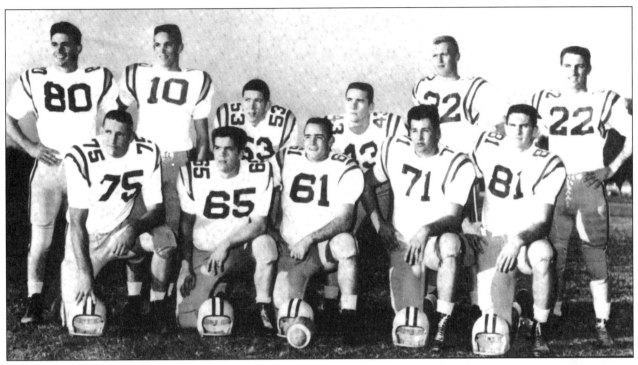

■ **The Chinese Bandits were a specialized defensive team who held opposing offenses to .9 yards per carry in 1958.**

Heisman Trophy — but Billy deserved that."

The three-team concept wasn't all the innovative Dietzel improvised.

The success Ole Miss had experienced with the winged-T offense had Dietzel thinking about yet another change. He had already swapped the Tigers offense from the Split-T to the double winged-T.

After hearing Iowa coach Forest Evashevski speak at a spring coaching clinic here, Dietzel was convinced to go to the winged-T. Evashevski loaned Dietzel his Iowa game film and helped install the offense.

Ironically, when the season unfolded it was LSU that beat out Iowa for the No. 1 honor.

And what a year it was — the year of all years, a season to always remember.

Cannon would become everybody's All-American. Dietzel would become National Coach of the Year. The Chinese Bandits would become a legend in their own time and Tiger Stadium became Death Valley, deafening and frightening to all opponents — none of whom left victorious the next two years.

The LSU bandwagon picked up a crowd in a hurry, playing to sellout crowds later in the season. It was Mardi Gras and New Year's Eve all rolled into one.

"When it started, it was more or less a routine season," recalled Hart Bourque, a Chinese Bandit back. "As the season went on, the enthusiasm and attention grew. People got more and more involved. They not only came (to the games), but they got more into the playing of the games. It was great."

Although it was three or four games into the season before the hysteria and hoopla really began, LSU's home attendance jumped from an average of 49,659 per game the previous year to 59,315.

It was hard-working people in a hard-working community pulling hard for their Tigers — and they were THEIR Tigers in every sense of the word.

"Baton Rouge was always a blue collar community," recalls Cannon. "There were some rich and affluent people, but basically it was blue collar. The fans were just fantastic.

"In our era they dressed up to go to the ball games. Football season was a social season. It coincided with Halloween, Thanksgiving and Christmas. It was a very good time of the year."

Cannon stopped and laughed a little.

"I thought it was pretty good then, but they're making movies about that era now and telling me it was better than I thought," said Cannon.

The incredible happenings early in the season may have left players and coaches wondering what was going to unfold. Lightning struck and injured some players and trainer Marty Broussard a week before the first game. The stands would collapse in the second quarter of a game against Alabama in Mobile, Ala., and Rabb's father would die late in the morning just hours before LSU's first home game.

It began on the Saturday before LSU opened at Rice, when a bolt of lightning struck in Bernie Moore Stadium and knocked the fillings out of the teeth of three freshmen. Across the street at Alex Box Stadium, the "big" bolt hit.

"I could see it coming from the side of my eyes. It came through the goal posts and I just felt myself being raised up. It hit me and knocked me about 30 yards," recalled Broussard, who was knocked unconscious, had two discs ruptured, sus-

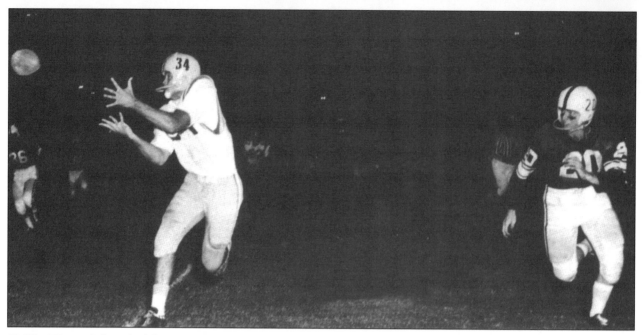

■ **The Tigers defeated Alabama and their new coach, Paul (Bear) Bryant, 13-3, in 1958.**

tained a broken fibula in his left leg and suffered scalp blisters when his cap burned up.

LSU was impressive in a 26-6 win in the opener against Rice, its offense having its way with the Owls and the defense extremely aggressive. It marked Dietzel's first win over the Owls in four tries.

Coach Paul (Bear) Bryant, who was just starting to rebuild Alabama's football fortunes and met LSU the next week, watched the game.

"I was impressed by the quarterback play of LSU and the fine running of little Don Purvis. Of course, Cannon is always a threat and tough to contain," said Bryant.

LSU vaulted to No. 13 in the AP poll and No. 16 in the UPI poll with the triumph.

The play of the Chinese Bandits led LSU to its 13-3 victory over Alabama a week later. Dietzel put the Bandits in after Alabama recovered a fumble near the goal. Thrice they denied the Tide any ground and forced a field goal into the north stadium seats — which collapsed seconds later sending hundreds of fans into a heap.

Bandit lineman Emile Fournet called the contest, "The game in which the Chinese Bandits were born."

"Bear Bryant had a heck of a team and Alabama recovered a fumble deep in our territory. Instead of leaving the Go Team in on defense, Dietzel sent in the Bandits," said Fournet, of Bogalusa.

"Alabama had the ball with first-and-goal at the three and we stopped them. That convinced the coaches and everyone else that we could play."

LSU moved to No. 13 in the AP poll, but slipped to No. 17 in the UPI.

A damper was put on the home opener for Rabb, whose dad, Amos, died late that morning. However, Rabb played — and played superbly, completing 5 of 6 passes for 88 yards and

ran for a 9-yard touchdown as LSU posted the 20-6 victory.

"Warren played the finest football of his career. I know he wanted to. He had made up his mind to do it for his dad," said Dietzel.

LSU was still unable to crack the Top 10 of either poll, standing at No. 11 in the AP and No. 15 in the UPI poll.

A strong Miami team awaited LSU in the Sunshine State. An obviously much stronger Tiger team went in and knocked the wind out of the Hurricanes, 41-0.

Andy Gustafson said following the shelling. "Paul Dietzel told me a year ago that he was building for 1959. It looks like they've arrived a year early."

Indeed they had.

"That's the game that really started it (LSU's drive to a national championship)," recalls Dietzel. "It convinced us we had a pretty good football team. Everything worked well."

It was the first time LSU had won its first four games since 1937 and the loss was the worst for Miami since 1944. It was the first time Miami had been shutout since 1927.

"We went down there and the game was supposed to be a tossup," Bourque said. "The way we beat a team that was supposed to be our equal was the high point up until that time."

Cannon had noted, "After we beat Miami, the Eastern press realized we were a good football team."

Respect at last! LSU vaulted to No. 9 in both polls. LSU fans couldn't wait for the next game. LSU was for real. A record 65,000 fans would turn Tiger Stadium into the Death Valley we now know when LSU went against Kentucky, which lost by only 8-0 to No. 1-ranked and defending national champion Auburn the previous week. LSU's offense was awesome; its defense overwhelming.

"We just wilted down," said Kentucky coach Blanton Collier, whose team experienced the problems felt by the

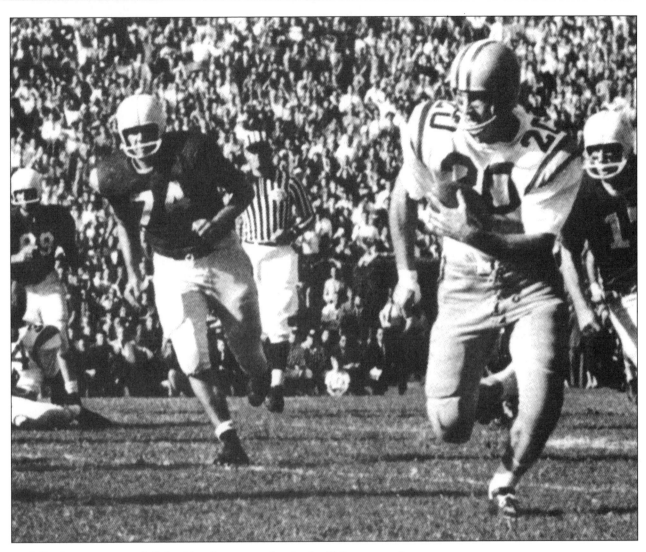

■ **Billy Cannon sweeps left, looking for an opening in the Tulane secondary.**

Tigers only a year earlier.

"I don't know if anyone could beat LSU unless it had an off night," said Kentucky Gov. Happy Chandler after the Tigers' 32-7 romp.

LSU moved to No. 5 in the UPI poll and zoomed to No. 3 in the AP poll — the highest a Tiger team had climbed since 1937.

Depth-laden Florida gave LSU all it could handle a week later in Gainesville, however. Billy Cannon's 1-yard smash helped keep it even with Tommy Davis' 26-yard field goal, providing the winning margin in the 10-7 victory with only 2:59 remaining.

It's hard-fought victory helped LSU to its first No. 1 ranking in the AP poll, although it remained No. 5 in the UPI poll.

That set the scene for one of the wildest weeks in LSU history.

Arch-rival Ole Miss, undefeated, untied and ranked No. 6 in both polls, would come calling. It truly was one of those weeks in which "you had to be there" to believe the excitement and electricity.

Go Team center Max Fugler once recalled "that entire week

before the Ole Miss game was terrific.

"We were thinking of the Southeastern Conference championship, not the national championship. The way the entire student body, the community and the state got behind us was something I'll never forget," he said. "The students kept a fire burning on top of two mounds in front of the Field House the entire week. The game itself is indelible probably due to the crowd noise and the intensity. It was the only time I ever really heard the crowd noise while I was playing."

Ticket scalping flourished. Advertisements seeking tickets filled the papers and airwaves.

"Go to Hell, Ole Miss," banners were displayed throughout the city. Graffiti reading the same message was on walls, plate glasses and auto windows. The message was also blared on all radio stations. Coolie hats were all over the town. Football fever was rampant. It was all part of what was to be known as "Ole Miss Week" for years.

The LSU campus was bombed by "Go to Hell, LSU" pamphlets dropped from an airplane (a maneuver credited by the innovative Dietzel to fire up students, fans and his team). It worked.

Several thousand students rushed over to cheer the Tigers in practice. The next day, Ole Miss students cheered their team at practice in Oxford.

Ole Miss threatened first in the game, but one of LSU's many great south end zone goal-line stands denied the Rebels, who had first-and-goal to go on the LSU 2, and three chances to put it in from one foot away, but couldn't.

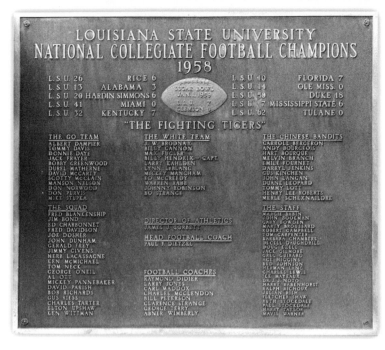

Only Tulane stood between LSU and a national championship, since the polls would be announced prior to the bowl games.

The game was no runaway early. LSU led by only 6-0 — but then scored 56 points in the final 30 minutes for a 62-0 romp in Sugar Bowl Stadium before the largest football crowd ever (85,000) in the South.

White Team guard Larry Kahlden said his highlight of the year "had to be the Ole Miss game. We stopped them four times on the goal line."

Fugler echoed the same thought as for his highlight in the championship season.

"The goal line stand easily," he quipped. "They started at the (LSU) 2 and ended up on the (LSU) 4."

LSU recovered a fumble and drove a short 21 yards for the first touchdown. Rabb looked for a receiver, but decided to run on fourth down at the five. He was met on the 2 by one Rebel, but was then hit by another player from behind who drove him into the end zone.

Durel Matherne, the Go Team quarterback, rolled in for the final score to ice away the 14-0 victory.

The win strengthened LSU's grip on No. 1 in the AP poll, but the coaches shunned LSU in the UPI poll, putting Army No. 1.

However, even the coaches couldn't deny LSU a No. 1 ranking the next week after the Tigers flattened Duke and quarterback Bob Brodhead, 50-18. It was a brilliant day for all the Tiger backs who helped LSU score 50 points for the first time since 1908.

The SEC title was now within reach, but the Tigers were only one slip away from failing. The water-logged field of Hinds Stadium against Mississippi State would have been an appropriate place to slip the following week.

It was one of the games which Dietzel still remembers vividly.

"We were in ankle-deep mud. It was one of the worst playing fields I've ever seen. We were literally up to our ankles in water," said Dietzel.

Recovering a Bulldogs' fumble, LSU trudged from the 34 to the 5 where the Tigers faced fourth down. Rabb hit Hendrix as he sloshed to the sideline for the touchdown. Davis' extra point provided the narrow 7-6 triumph over State.

It was the most points scored by LSU since 1936 when the Tigers slammed USL by 93-0.

The Go team and Chinese Bandits performed too well, particularly in the last quarter and Dietzel had to send the White team, the starters in for the final portion of the game.

"Tulane fans thought we had run the score up, but we were trapped by the substitution rule," said Dietzel. "Half way through the fourth quarter we had to play the White Team — so, here goes Cannon and Robinson and the others in.

"I didn't say run it up, but everything they did, they scored," said Dietzel.

Cannon, on the other hand, had a good laugh talking about that game. "Someone speared Scooter (Purvis) and I was the only 'live' back on the bench. He (Dietzel) had to send me in.

"He said, 'I want you to go out there and tell Durel (quarterback Matherne) to run the clock out, take the ball and fall on it,'" said Cannon. "I went in, called a toss left — to me — and went on in to make it 62-0.

"It was so funny," continued Cannon, "(Wave coach Andy) Pilney was on one sideline cussing Dietzel for everything in the book for running up the score. Dietzel was standing on the other (sideline) screaming, 'It wasn't me. I didn't call it.'"

On Dec. 1, LSU was proclaimed national champion. The appropriate celebrations for such an honor ensued with parties and celebrations and the production and sale of national championship license plates, bumper stickers, Coolie hats and trinkets of all kinds to commemorate the occasion. It was a crowning achievement for Dietzel and assistants Charles McClendon, George Terry, Carl Maddox, Larry Jones, Abner Wimberly and Bill Peterson.

The hard-earned 7-0 victory over Clemson in the Sugar Bowl would only be icing for the biggest cake in college football.

It was truly a year to remember.

Billy Cannon Wins Heisman Trophy

New York — *Dec. 9, 1959*

LSU's Billy Cannon, the two-time All-American, joined gridiron's immortal greats today when he was awarded the 25th Heisman Memorial Trophy, which is symbolic of the nation's outstanding football player of the year.

Vice President Richard Nixon made the presentation at The Downtown Athletic Club, which sponsors the award.

Cannon won the award on the vote of nearly 1,000 sportswriters throughout the nation. He received 1,929 votes while the runnerup, Richie Lucas of Penn State, was awarded with 613 votes.

The Tiger star topped all five sections in the voting and won by one of the largest margins in the history of the Heisman Trophy.

In making the award, Vice President Nixon said, "LSU had more than a Cannon; they had an atomic Cannon, the ultimate in weapons. He was the chief weapon in Tiger coach Paul Dietzel's arsenal of football weapons that included the White team and the Chinese Bandits."

The Vice President also said he watched Syracuse play UCLA and after checking records found out that they had the best offense and the best defense and were No. 1.

"In fact, they had everything but a Billy Cannon."

In presenting the trophy, Vice President said he was glad Cannon was a weight lifter so he could carry the trophy. The replica of the Heisman Trophy weighs 36 pounds and was silver plated this year in honor of its 25th year.

In accepting the award Cannon stated: It is a great honor but one I couldn't have gained without a lot of help and so I would like to thank my high school coach, Big Fuzzy Brown, who started me in football and taught me how to win and what it meant to win.

"I would also like to thank my mother and father, and my wife who put up with me during the football seasons.

"And most of all. I would like to thank my teammates who made it possible for me to get this honor and it was through their great efforts that I was able to win it."

Prior to the presentation of the award, Gen. Troy Middleton, the president of LSU, spoke briefly and said that LSU was proud of Cannon who was a fine athlete and a great young man who appreciated all that had been done for him.

Coach Paul Dietzel spoke briefly and said, "The coaching staff at LSU is proud of Cannon who had the tremendous desire to excel at everything he played. He also showed great humility and was a great pleasure to coach."

Attending the presentation award was Mr. and Mrs. Harvey Cannon, parents of the Tiger star, and his wife, Mrs. Dorothy Cannon.

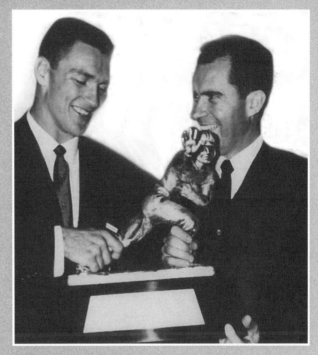

■ **Vice President Richard Nixon and Billy Cannon.**

The presentation ceremonies were attended by a host of sports figures from all over the nation. The ceremonies were broadcast over a national network.

Cannon joins a host of former stars who gained the top recognition, including Jay Berwanger of Chicago, Doak Walker of SMU, Johnny Lujack of Notre Dame, Army stars Glenn Davis and Doc Blanchard and others.

For Cannon, the award climaxed a fabulous career that started at Istrouma High where he won All-American prep fame before entering LSU.

At LSU, Cannon became an all-time backfield great, rolling up a record rushing yardage for the Bengals in three years and twice gaining All-American honors.

Among the nationally known sportswriters were Tom Meany of New York, and Mel Allen, famed radio and TV broadcaster.

Cannon returns to Baton Rouge where he'll resume training with his Tiger teammates for their Sugar Bowl clash with Ole Miss.

Following his performance in the Sugar Bowl, Cannon will go to Honolulu to play in the Hula Bowl there on Jan. 10.

Cannon was recently drafted by the Los Angeles Rams of the National Football League and has announced his intentions to join that pro club. He was also drafted by Houston of the American Football League.

Hendrix & Davis Give LSU Edge Over Miss. St., 7-6

By Ted Castillo

The Advocate

Jackson, Miss. — *Nov. 15, 1958*

The LSU Golden Bengals had to take advantage of a fumble to come from behind and eke out a 7-6 victory over the rough and tough Mississippi State Maroons here tonight to protect their unblemished record, the only perfect record among the nation's collegiate greats.

State proved a tough and capable foe, scoring early in the second quarter after being thrust back three times by the valiant Tigers in the first period.

The Maroons went into the half with a 6-0 lead but LSU came back early in the third period to take advantage of Bubber Trammell's fumble on the State 34 to move for their touchdown in seven plays and Tommy Davis booted the extra point for what proved the winning margin.

Warren Rabb, the hard working Tigers quarterback, pitched the telling blow for the touchdown when he hit Red Hendrix in the end zone on fourth down for the touchdown.

Like State, LSU passed up earlier opportunities to score as they played most of the second quarter deep in the Maroons' territory.

The game, which kept the fans on their feet was climaxed in the fourth quarter with both elevens passing up scoring opportunities.

State had the first chance when J.E. Logan recovered a Billy Cannon fumble on the Tiger 16. The Maroons marched to the Bengal 10 and on fourth down Bobby Tribble missed a field goal, his second missed field goal of the night.

Billy Stacy, State's great quarterback, twice gave LSU scoring opportunities late in the fourth quarter. Once he fumbled on his 39 and LSU Hendrix recovered for the Bengals. A few minutes later, Stacy fumbled going through the middle and this time Rabb recovered for LSU at the Maroon 27.

This time a 15-yard penalty stymied the Tigers and the LSU first eleven held State deep in their own territory to windup the tingling gridiron fray.

It was the nation's No. 1 eleven's poorest performance of the season as they could never get a sustained drive going at any time in the game and they fumbled the wet and soggy ball at crucial times.

The Maroons were ready for the vaunted Bengals and their big mobile forward wall gave LSU trouble all night as they spilled the Tiger halfbacks before they could get going off their tricky winged-T attack.

LSU edged the Maroons in rushing yardage with 140 to 134 but the Maroons picked up 57 yards to 16 for LSU in the air to take the edge in total offense with 191 yards to 156 for LSU.

Tonight's game was played on a soggy and slick field that gave the passers trouble all night. A steady downpour a half hour before the game drenched the already soggy field.

Some 26,000 fans, a capacity turnout, witnessed the fumbling, bumbling, but hard fought play.

Tiger coach Paul Dietzel was forced to play his first team out for more minutes than in any other game this season and Coach Wade Walker of the Maroons kept his top unit in the game for the most part.

Billy Cannon, who was bothered all night keeping the ball under control, ran 13 times for 57 yards while big Tommy Davis picked up 35 yards on nine plays. Red Brodnax ran six times for 35 yards.

Bubber Trammell, the left halfback of the Maroons, was the top carrier for State with 44 yards in 10 carries.

The expected aerial duel between the Bengals' Rabb and the Maroons' Stacey failed to materialize as both teams stuck to the ground. Rabb connected on three of six passes for 16 yards but it was his telling scoring pass in the third period that put LSU back in the game.

Stacey completed three of 10 passes for 57 yards but was heavily rushed by the valiant Tigers' forward wall all night.

Both elevens put themselves in the hole time after time again with fumbles, both losing the ball three times during the fray.

The expected kicking duel between State's Gil Peterson and LSU's Tommy Davis also failed to materialize as both were kicking deep in the foes territory and both had several kicks to roll over the goal. Cannon also kicked for LSU.

Probably the standout play for the Bengals was the hustle of Hendrix, who snagged the scoring pass from the hands of State defender and who recovered a crucial fumble.

Score by Periods

LSU	0	0	7	0 —	7
Mississippi State	0	6	0	0 —	6

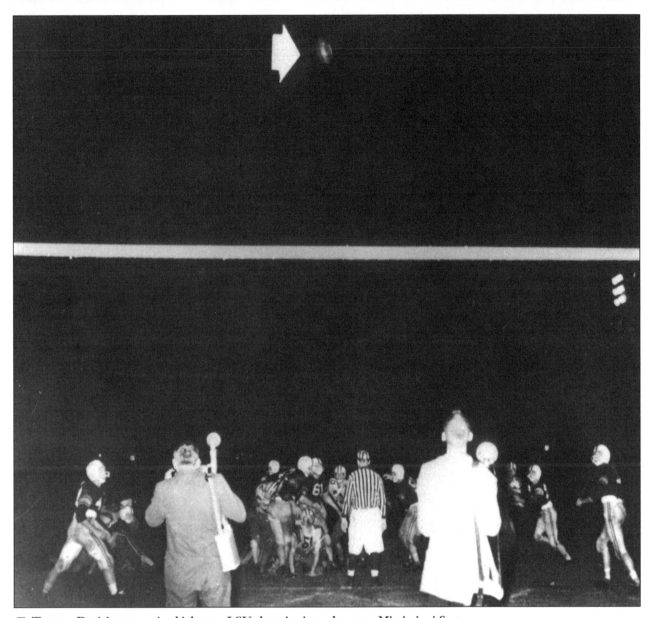

■ **Tommy Davis' extra-point kick gave LSU the winning edge over Mississippi State.**

The game opened with State getting a chance when Davis punted short to his 46 and Stacy returned the Tiger 32, State drove to the Bengal 3 where a 15-yard penalty stymied them but only after Stacy had hit Jack Batte with a 20-yard pass to put the Maroons back on the Tigers doorstep at the LSU 3. A fourth-down pass by Gil Peterson failed to click.

A few minutes later, State took a short Tiger punt and rolled again from the LSU 38, this time to the Tiger 7 before they failed.

As the first quarter ended, State got still another try when Cannon fumbled on his 21 and State's Willie Daniels recovered. However, LSU held as the period ended and on the first play of the second quarter Tribble failed to kick his first try for a field goal.

State scored a few plays later when Donnie Dave fumbled on the Tiger 22 and the Maroons recovered. This time State moved

in for their score, getting a first down at the 13. After Peterson picked up two yards, Stacy rolled out to his left and picked up good blocking to speed over the Tiger goal line after an 11-yard jaunt.

However, the Tigers finally cashed in on a break when Brodnax recovered Trammell's fumble on the State 34.

On a fine fake, Brodnax roared down the middle for 14 yards for a first down at the State 20. LSU moved the ball on short dashes to the 5. On fourth down, Rabb hit Hendrix in the end zone for the tying score. Davis kicked the extra point to give LSU its 7-6 win, but not before both elevens threatened in the final period.

It was LSU's 10th win in a row and their ninth straight this season.

The Tigers have only Tulane left as an obstacle to their first undefeated and untied record since 1908, some 50 years ago.

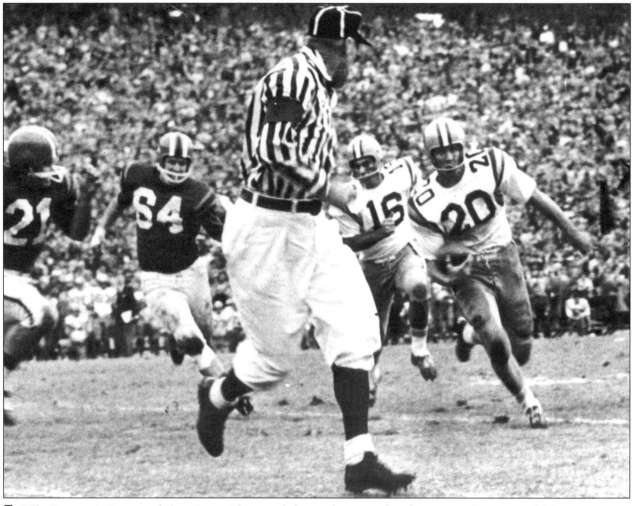

■ Billy Cannon (20) sweeps left against a Clemson defense who spent the afternoon trying to corral him.

Cannon's TD Pass to Mangham Seals LSU Win

By Bud Montet
The Advocate

New Orleans, La. — *Jan. 1, 1959*

The LSU Tigers, the nation's No. 1 football power, were hard pressed to protect their unblemished record today as an inspired and hard-hitting Clemson eleven held the vaunted Baton Rouge collegians to a 7-0 decision.

Clemson, who was a two to three-touchdown underdog prior to the game, gave the 25th Silver Anniversary Sugar Bowl turnout its best game in the past few years as they held the vaunted Bengals well in check most of the game and managed to stage the game's longest drive right after LSU scored.

For LSU the victory gave them their 12th straight victory, the longest winning streak in modern LSU history. It was also LSU's first Sugar Bowl win in five attempts. In previous Sugar Bowls, LSU lost to TCU, Santa Clara, twice, and Oklahoma.

Clemson kept the pressure on the Bengals throughout the game and LSU had to use a break late in the third period to get its lone score.

The scoring play came when on fourth down Clemson's center passed the ball back poorly on an attempted punt play and LSU's Duane Leopard recovered the ball at the Clemson 11.

LSU moved to the nine in two plays and then Durel Matherne handed off to Billy Cannon, who raced to his right and pitched to Mickey Mangham in the end zone for the score. Cannon added the extra point to put the Tigers up, 7-0, and that completed the scoring for the afternoon.

LSU missed the services of its All-SEC quarterback, Warren Rabb, who sustained a broken right hand near the end of the first half. With Rabb out, Tiger coach Paul Dietzel used Matherne the entire second half on his offensive units.

The fleet LSU attack was bothered by the slippery turf in the Sugar Bowl Stadium and Bengal backs slipped down a number of times. However, it was their inability to hang onto the ball in the first half that stymied LSU on a number of scoring opportunities.

Clemson's big forward wall gave the Bengals plenty of trouble all afternoon and their short plunges by a half dozen backs enabled the South Carolina Tigers to outgain the No. 1 eleven on the ground.

However, Clemson made but two sustained drives, moving to the LSU 26 where a fumble by George Usry halted the drive as LSU's Bo Strange recovered.

In the fourth period, Clemson made a determined bid to tie the game when they drove from their 16-yard line to the Tiger 24 where they gave up the ball on downs and LSU kept possession until the final whistle.

On the play before the final one of the game, a mild melee started among the players but was quickly broken up by the officials.

In the battle of the figures, Clemson gained an edge on LSU, picking up 195 yards on the ground to 134 for LSU. The Baton Rouge Bengals hit on four passes for 68 yards while Clemson hit on two for 23 yards.

Clemson didn't throw a pass until the fourth period as they were content to run for short gains behind their huge line.

LSU and Clemson both lost a pair of fumbles.

The Bengals lost three scoring opportunities in the second period with fumbles marring a pair of chances. Late in the first period, LSU drove from their 25 to the Clemson 25 for the first sustained drive of the game.

However, on the first play of the second half, Matherne fumbled and end Ray Masneri recovered for Clemson to end the threat.

A few minutes later the Bengals got another scoring chance when Clemson's Charlie Horne had a punt partially blocked and lost two yards on the boot with LSU getting possession on the Clemson 29-yard line.

LSU drove down to the Clemson 12 where Rabb missed on four straight passes.

The third time didn't prove lucky for LSU for a few minutes later they drove from their 44 to the Clemson 1-yard line where Red Brodnax fumbled going over the goal line. However, the officials ruled he had fumbled while still in the playing field and Clemson recovered in the end zone for a touchback and the South Carolina eleven got the ball back out on their 20.

Billy Cannon, LSU's great All-American back, was held well in check by the big Clemson line and the fleet Tiger gained

Score by Periods

LSU	0	0	7	0 —	7
Clemson	0	0	0	0 —	0

only 51 yards on 13 tries but it was his clutch touchdown pass to Mangham that gave LSU its victory.

Cannon won The Digby-Miller Memorial Trophy as the game's Most Valuable Player for his efforts.

LSU's Bo Strange, a sophomore tackle — playing against tackles that outweighed him 20 and 30 pounds — turned in a fine defensive game for LSU.

Also outstanding for the Bengals were center Max Fugler, end Mangham and Durel Matherne, who replaced the injured Rabb in the second half.

Clemson's hard driving backs — Rudy Hayes, Usry, Bob Morgan and Charlie Horne — all played well in sparking the Clemson attack. Up front, Jim Padgett and Lou Cordileone, a pair of huge tackles, stood out for the Mountain Tigers.

The first period was spent in a punting duel with LSU's Cannon getting the edge. Later in the period, LSU started their first drive from their 25. With the Go Team in the game, LSU marched steadily with Davis getting the drive going with an 11-yard plunge. Later, Matherne pitched to Scotty McClain for 26 yards and a first down at the Clemson 30.

LSU got to the Clemson 25 as the quarter ended and then on the first play of the second period Matherne fumbled and Masneri recovered for Clemson.

A few minutes later, LSU drove from the Clemson 29 to the 12. Taking the ball after a poor Clemson partially blocked kick at the 29, Brodnax rambled for nine yards and then Rabb hit Cannon with an eight-yard pass for a first down at the Clemson 12. Here Rabb missed on four passes in a row.

Midway in the period, LSU staged its longest sustained drive. Taking over on their 44, Rabb pitched 23 yards to Mangham to get the drive going.

The pass play gave LSU a first down at the Clemson 33. Rabb then kept for 15 yards and combined with Brodnax for 11 yards and a first down at the Clemson 8. Cannon got to the Clemson 1 on two tries and then Brodnax fumbled on the goal line.

In the third period, Clemson made it's first big march to the LSU 26 before fumbling. Then LSU came back to get their score but Clemson wasn't finished as they drove in the fourth period from their 16 to the Tiger 24 before giving up the ball.

LSU failed to exhibit the sharp winged-T attack that featured their play all season. No doubt the loss of Rabb proved a stunning blow.

For the first time this season Coach Dietzel mixed up his playing units.

Strange enough, LSU ended the season with but one able quarterback, Matherne, as Daryl Jenkins, the Bandit quarterback, didn't suit out, and Rabb was lost after the first half.

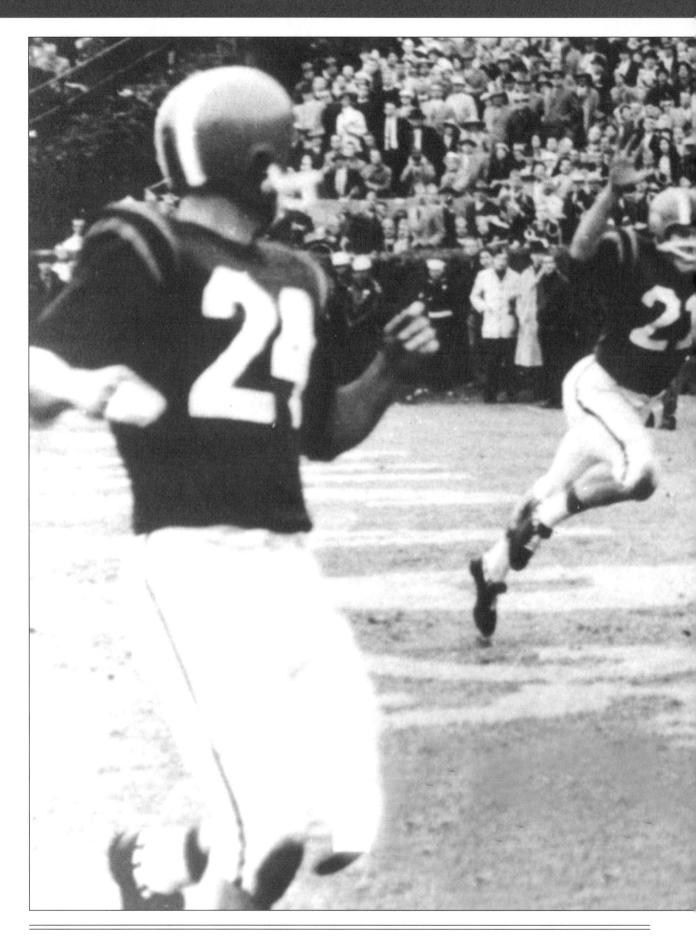

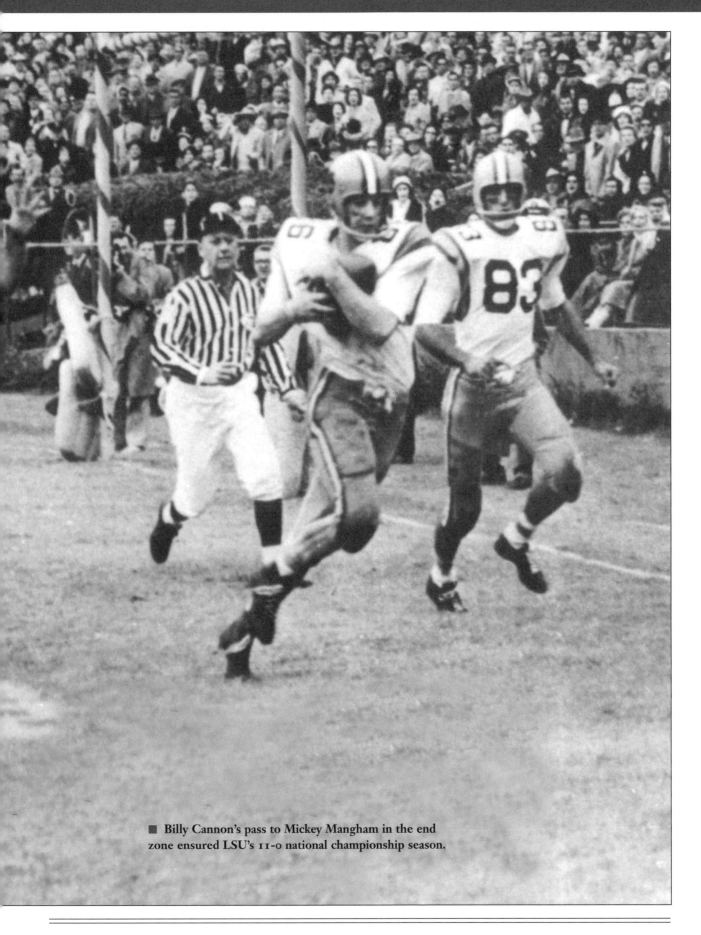

■ Billy Cannon's pass to Mickey Mangham in the end
zone ensured LSU's 11-0 national championship season.

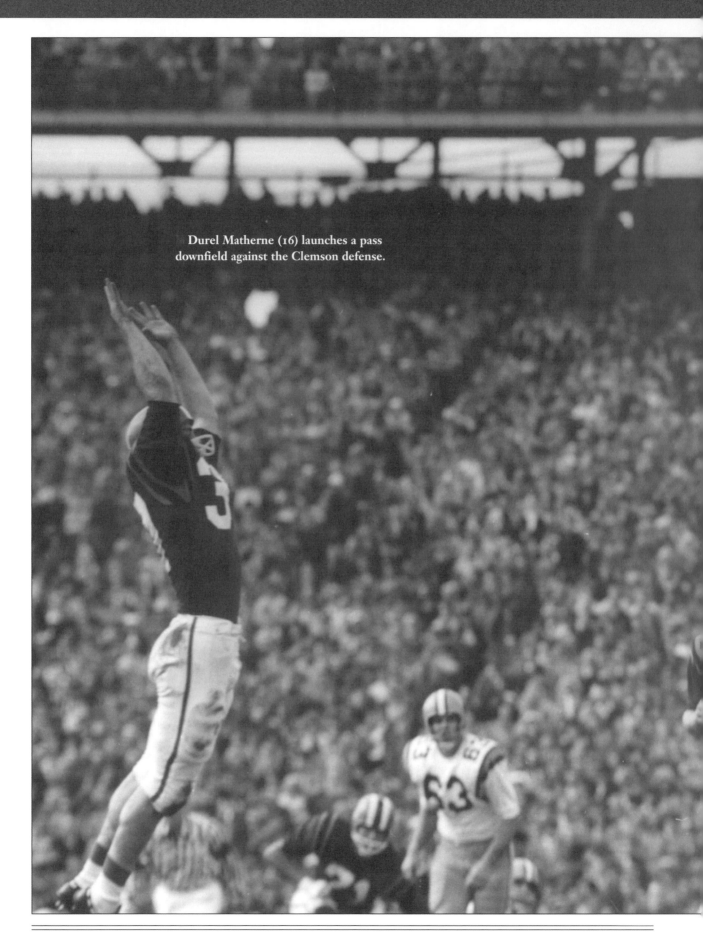

Durel Matherne (16) launches a pass downfield against the Clemson defense.

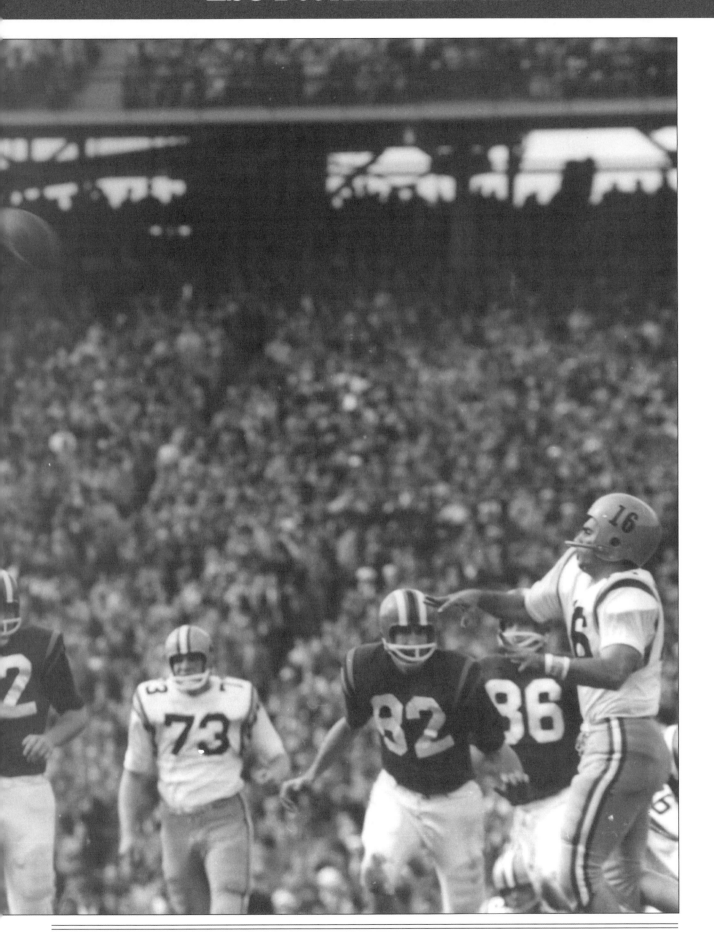

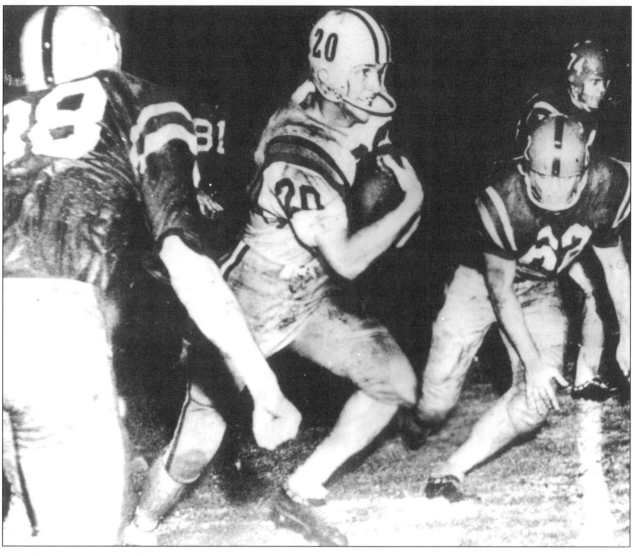

■ Billy Cannon's 89-yard punt return on Halloween night 1959 will forever be part of LSU folklore.

Cannon Gallops Past Rebs For 7-3 LSU Win

BY BUD MONTET
The Advocate

Baton Rouge, La. — *Oct. 31, 1959*

The defending national champion LSU Tigers proved to be a brilliant "clutch" eleven tonight when they roared with Billy Cannon to come from behind and hand Ole Miss a 7-3 setback — their first loss of the season. It was LSU's 19th straight victory without a loss.

Battling from behind all the way, LSU overcame the three-point deficit with 10 minutes left in the game when All-American Cannon grabbed a Jake Gibbs punt on his 11-yard line and, starting slowly, picked his way to the sidelines and twisted past a quartet of Ole Miss defenders to break loose at midfield and gallop on over for the lone touchdown of the game. It was a twisting, coolly-calculated run by the big Tiger back who finally broke loose to the roaring of 67,000 fans who jammed Tiger Stadium for Homecoming.

But Cannon's run just set the stage for the most thrilling 10 minutes of the game as the Rebels took the kickoff and marched from their 21 to inside the Tiger 2-yard line where the Tigers held them on fourth down with 18 seconds left in the game.

Coach Paul Dietzel had to call on his tired but game White eleven to go in and halt the threatening Rebels.

The Tiger's goal line stand of holding the Rebels from their seven with four downs to go duplicated their great stand of last year when they hurled back the Rebels to protect their lead.

Santa Claus looked as if he was coming early to the Ole Miss Rebels when LSU gave the Mississippians a "gift" of five scoring chances in the first half. Three fumbles paved the way for the Rebels to threaten, a questionable pass interference gave the visitors a chance, and a poor kick by Bandit end Gus Kinchen also gave the Rebs a shot at the Tiger goal.

Each time LSU threw back the challenge, but early in the first quarter the Rebs moved from their 40 to the Tiger 3 and Bobby Khayat booted a 23-yard field goal squarely through the uprights. It was Khayat's fourth field goal in 10 tries this season.

Later, Kinchen's 27-yard punt out of bounds gave the Rebels a shot and this time they were held at the 30.

The second quarter found the Rebs moving to the Tiger 22 where LSU center Johnny Langan knocked down a Rebel fourth down pass.

Ole Miss drove from their 39 to the LSU 22 a few minutes later and this time LSU halted a flurry of passes to take the ball away.

Big Earl Gros fumbled near the end of the first half on the LSU 29 to give the Rebels another shot and this time LSU rose up and halted the Mississippians on their eight.

LSU spent the entire third period in Rebel territory, moving to the Ole Miss 31 once before Wendell Harris missed a 37-yard attempt at a field goal. Later LSU moved to the 19 with big Gros missing a first down try by inches.

LSU came back to drive to the Rebel 35 where Cannon tried a fake punt and run on fourth down and was hauled down for a yard loss.

Then the Bengals exploded midway in the fourth period with Cannon making his sensational gallop, answering the Ole Miss critics who were rating their big fullback Charlie Flowers over the brilliant Cannon.

Cannon answered the critics with the greatest run in his Tiger career. It also allowed LSU to capture its 19th straight

Score by Periods

Ole Miss	3	0	0	0 —	3
LSU	0	0	0	7 —	7

victory, their seventh of this season, and probably kept the Bengals at the top the national rankings.

But while Cannon's long 89-yard gallop was the offensive fireworks it remained for the valiant goal line stand of the White Team to really climax the fierce battle, which was rated as the nation's number-one game of the week.

LSU's frequent fumbles in the first half — they lost the ball three times in four fumbles — kept the Bengals from getting under way.

Ole Miss picked up 160 yards on the ground to LSU's 142. In the air, LSU gained 29 yards and Ole Miss 19.

Cannon was the "big gun" for the Tigers in more ways than one. While it remained for his long touchdown gallop to prove the deciding factor, the hard-working youth packed the ball 12 times for 48 yards, which edged him over his rival Flowers, who carried for 35 yards in 10 tries.

Cannon proved a timely and clutch punter, booting four times for a 42-yard average.

Defensively, the Bengals played probably their greatest game of the year. Time after time they rose up to hurl back the Rebels within the shadow of their goal and their great "clutch" goal-line stand that saved the game was one of their finest efforts.

LSU started off brilliantly, moving from their 27 after the opening kickoff to the Rebel 40 where Donnie Daye fumbled and Ole Miss' Billy Brewer recovered for the Rebs at the 44-yard line. It was the first of three recoveries for Brewer, a fine defensive back.

Ole Miss senior quarterback, Bobby Franklin, set up the first Ole Miss threat when he booted 43 yards out on the Tiger 5-yard line.

Cannon ran the ball out to the 21 but fumbled and again Brewer pounced on it.

This time the Rebels moved in short dashes to the LSU 3-yard line where LSU held and Ole Miss coach Johnny Vaught sent in his kicking specialist, Khayat, who booted the field goal and gave the Rebels a 3-0 lead.

Ole Miss kept coming at the Tigers for the rest of the half, once moving to the 30 after a poor kick by Kinchen.

The tables turned in the third period with LSU's Cannon giving the Bengals a chance when he intercepted a Jake Gibbs' pass on the LSU 48 and returned it to the Rebel 36. LSU moved to the 31 where a passing flurry failed.

Again LSU moved this time with the Go Team performing steady and moving from their 3 to the Ole Miss 19, where Gros missed a first-down try by inches.

Still later in the period, the Bengals moved from their 49 to

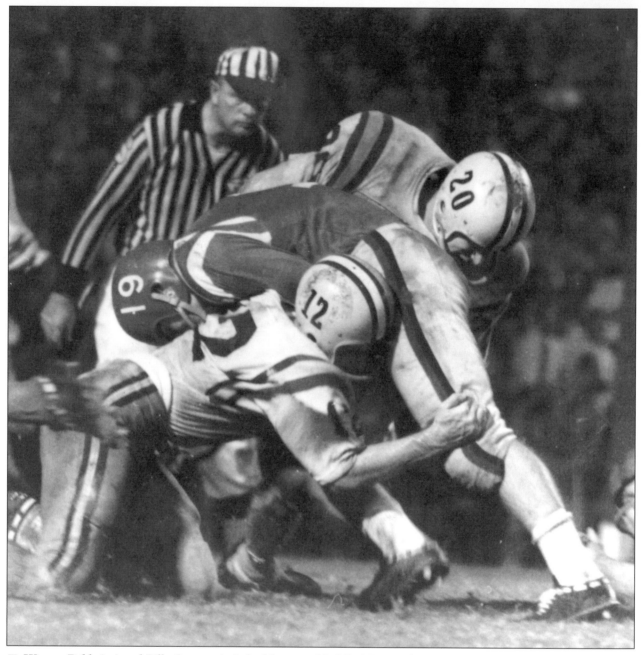

■ **Warren Rabb (12) and Billy Cannon (20) double-team Ole Miss' Doug Elmore at the 1-yard line.**

the Rebel 35 where Cannon's fourth down fake punt play failed.

Despite the drama of the first three quarters it remained for the final 10 minutes to unroll as great a gridiron drama as ever witnessed in Tiger Stadium.

With defeat staring them in the face, the Tigers kept going and then Cannon changed the outlook with his sensational gallop, one of the greatest ever seen on a Tiger gridiron.

Then came the brilliant try by Ole Miss to keep going and get back in the game.

Ole Miss took their kickoff on their 32 and in steady marches, with Cowboy Woodruff furnishing most of the impetus,

moved to the LSU 7 for a first down. The Bengal White Team rose up and held Ole Miss' George Blair for a two-yard gain. Fleet Doug Elmore on a keeper play sped to the Tiger 2 and then Jimmy Anderson gained a half yard on third down.

Ole Miss' Elmore rolled out to the left but a trio of Bengals closed in on him at the LSU 1 and smashed him to the turf to halt the threat and save the game.

Hysteria gripped the 67,000 fans who jammed Tiger Stadium as only 18 seconds remained in the game and once again LSU had pulled one out of the fire.

Never in LSU history have the Bengal gridders treated their homecoming fans to such a drama packed contest.

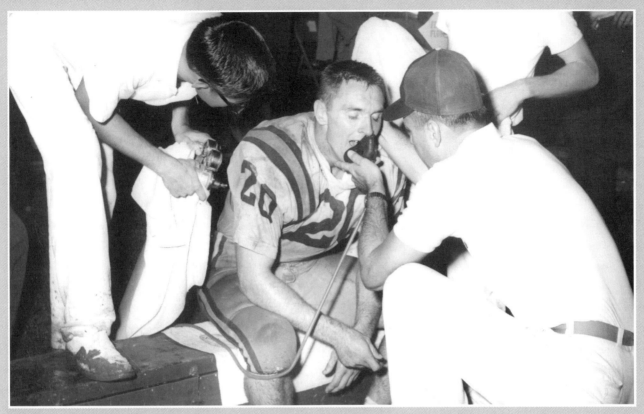

■ Following his epic punt return, Billy Cannon was administered oxygen on the sideline.

'But Big Billy Kept Going,' Tigers Recall

BY TED CASTILLO
The Advocate

Baton Rouge, La. — *Oct. 31, 1959*

"I thought Billy (Cannon) was down, then I looked up and that big animal was still going," declared LSU tackle Bo Strange after the Tiger All-American had pulled LSU off the floor with an 89-yard scoring sprint to give the Bengals their only touchdown in a 7-3 cliffhanger with Ole Miss tonight at Tiger Stadium.

"He ran over five men," Strange shouted above the dressing room din. "They thought he was down but big Billy kept going. When you need it, he's there. He won't get a hundred touchdowns against Podunk but he'll get one on somebody like Ole Miss."

Strange, like some other members of the White Team such as Ed McCreedy, Warren Rabb and Johnny Robinson said they felt they would hold the Rebels in the final minutes.

"I knew they'd have to pass to score," Robinson said, "but in a situation like that you don't know if you want them to come your way or go the other."

But Cannon and Mickey Mangham weren't as confident as their teammates.

"I was mighty afraid," Cannon said. And Mangham echoed his sentiments.

"They had me worried," the Tiger first-team terminal stated. "Ole Miss had the best line we've faced. TCU's backs were just as good but Ole Miss' line was better. I thought (Warren) Rabb played a whale of a game. He made the stop on their quarterback on fourth down when they got so close."

Describing part of his touchdown run while holding an ice pack to a bruised forehead, Cannon praised the blocking of this teammates.

"They really blocked for me, Johnny Robinson and Lynn LeBlanc and Scotty McClain and two or three others ... That's all I saw, all I could think about was hold that ball and don't fumble again," said the big Bengal back, who hugged the sidelines for more than half of his long gallop after breaking into the clear around the LSU 35. "I was mighty close to those chalklines," Cannon added.

Rebs Tie LSU on Late Field Goal, 6-6

By Bud Montet

The Advocate

Oxford, Miss.— *Oct. 29, 1960*

A last minute Ole Miss passing attack clutched victory right out of the hands of the gritty and determined LSU Tigers and Allen Green, the Rebels kicker, booted a 41-yard field goal with 13 seconds left in the game to give the vaunted Mississippians a 6-6 deadlock with the surprising Tigers.

Until the final minute and a half the Bengals covered the All-American prospect Jake Gibbs like a blanket but it was Gibbs' clutch passing that set up the field goal.

For LSU it was again a game of frustration as they watched the Rebels get two field goals to tie the score. It was the fourth game in a row where field goals either tied the score or won it for the opposition.

The Bengals stuck to the ground — they threw only two aerials — and pounded out 216 yards to 107 for the Rebs in rushing for their best ground offensive showing of the season.

Ole Miss struck through the air to pile up a net 107 yards — 52 yards of that came in the final two minutes of the game.

LSU threw just two passes, hitting on one for five yards.

The sparkling feature of the game was the running of the sophomore Go Team for LSU and the spirited defensive play of all Tiger gridders who held Ole Miss without a touchdown for the first time this season.

Gibbs, ranked as a crack runner as well as passer, was so well covered by the Bengals that he finished with a minus 13 yards.

While the Bengals turned in their season's top effort, again it was glaring errors that cost them the game. They drove to the Ole Miss 3 in the opening minutes of the first quarter when Wendell Harris missed an easy try at a field goal.

Then the Tigers' Earl Gros fumbled on the first scrimmage play of the second half to set up Green's first field goal. The Rebs moved to the Tiger 22 and Green booted his 38-yard kick to give the Rebels a 3-0 lead.

Green had previously missed one from the Tiger 13, the ball barely going wide of the posts.

Late in the game a questionable unsportsmanship 15-yard

Score by Periods

LSU	0	0	6	0 —	6
Ole Miss	0	0	3	3 —	6

penalty by LSU gave the Rebels a chance to drive deep but they failed. The Rebs got moving when LSU attempted to kill the clock and Jerry Stovall punted with one minute and 21 seconds left in the game.

Gibbs then came through to move the ball to the Tiger 25 and Green kicked the field goal that tied the game.

Often accused of being fangless, the Tigers rose up to answer their critics with their snarling offensive play. Stovall, the gifted sophomore halfback, led the squad with a net 96 yards on seven carries.

Charles Cranfield, the sophomore fullback, picked up 30 yards in six carries and once tumbled over the line to land on his feet and keep going for extra yardage. His fake into the middle on the Bengal touchdown was one of the finest of the afternoon as he teamed with Lynn Amedee to completely fool the Ole Miss defense.

Wendell Harris picked up 22 yards on nine carries and Donnie Daye garnered 24 in seven tries.

Ole Miss' top runner was Art Doty, a fast moving youth, who garnered 46 yards in 12 tries.

Gibbs continued his fine passing with seven completions in 18 attempts for 89 yards and almost half came on the clutch drive that enabled the Rebels to tie the score.

For the third straight year LSU has proven to be a spoiler of the Rebels. In 1958, they halted an undefeated Rebel eleven and again in 1959 they handed the Rebels their first defeat.

This year they couldn't quite match those efforts but they put a tie blot on the Rebel record after losing four straight games.

The Bengals, who haven't tasted victory since their season's opener against Texas A&M, weren't overly impressed with the Rebels' No. 2 ranking on the nation's grid lists. Against LSU, they turned in their finest offensive effort of the season but once more they were denied after getting within striking distance.

LSU had two opportunities in the opening quarter when they drove 77 yards to the Rebel 3 the first time they got their hands on the ball only to fail on the field goal try.

It was a fine 32-yard gallop by Stovall that set up this drive. On the first LSU scrimmage play he broke over left guard and cut back to his right and scooted to the Rebel 38 before he was hauled down.

Then in short bursts Stovall and Harris carried the ball to the Ole Miss 3 where the Rebels halted them and Harris missed the field goal attempt on fourth down.

A few minutes later Gene Sykes recovered Bill Roy Adams' fumble on the Rebel 32 and here the Rebels' Jim Dunaway broke through and blocked Harris' second attempt at a field goal.

Ole Miss got but one chance in the first half as they drove from the Tiger 48 to the five where LSU held them and Green missed his first try.

However, the big boy more than made up for it later with his two clutch field goals that kept the Rebels in the undefeated class.

The opening plays of the second half set the keynote as far as the Rebels were concerned. When Gros fumbled, his only appearance carrying the ball, Bookie Bolin, a Reb guard, recovered at the Tiger 24.

Ole Miss failed on two running plays and then Gibbs missed a pass into the end zone before Green stepped back and delivered a 39-yard field goal.

Stung by three straight losses as the results of field goals, the Bengals stormed back late in the period and drove to their 48 to score, their lone touchdown.

Tommy Neck set up the drive when he returned Gibbs' punt 22 yards to the Tiger 48. After missing a pass, Amedee handed off to Ray Wilkins, who gained a yard, and then Amedee stepped down the right sidelines for 15 yards and a first down at the Rebel 32.

Cranford danced through the middle for 10 yards and another first down, then picked up five more yards. Amedee followed up with a 5-yard pass to Wilkins — the Bengals' lone pass completion of the game — and on the final play of the third period Cranford drove to the Ole Miss 7.

Wilkins shook off tacklers for a six-yard gallop to the Rebel 2 and Cranford dove to the one. Then Amedee faked to Cranford, who made a great jump high onto the pile in the middle and the ball was handed off to Wilkins who scored over left tackle. Harris missed the extra point, which proved a crucial miss.

Ole Miss made one threat before they managed to get their

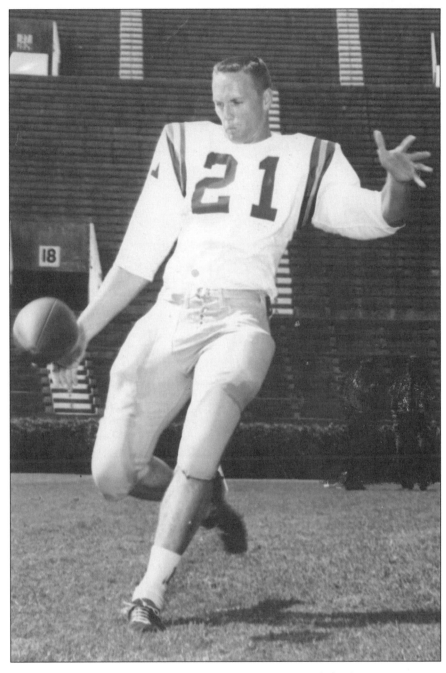

■ **The close contest between LSU and Ole Miss mirrored the fierce punting duel between Jerry Stovall and the Rebels' Jake Gibbs.**

tying field goal, but LSU halted them on their 37 when three of Gibbs' passes went astray.

The Bengals apparently had the game sewed up when Gibbs ran back Stovall's punt to his 31 with a minute and 21 seconds left.

Gibbs then tossed to Crespino for 15 yards to get the drive going He lost six when hit hard by Billy Booth. However, Gibbs came back and connected on a pass to Crespino at the Rebel 49. He then tossed to Ralph Smith for 14 yards and a first down at the Tiger 35.

Gibbs' next pass to Crespino set the stage for Green's game-tying boot.

Feisty Bengals Swat Yellow Jackets, 10-0

By Bud Montet
The Advocate

Baton Rouge, La.— *Oct. 7, 1961*

A supposedly toothless Tiger ripped the hide off No. 3-ranked Georgia Tech's Yellow Jackets to take a stirring 10-0 victory tonight at Tiger Stadium before 66,000 roaring fans.

LSU dominated the game in the first half as they piled up a 10-point lead and then smashed all Tech efforts to come back.

After holding the Jackets to one first down in the first half, the Bengals went to sleep on a fake kick early in the third period and allowed Tech to complete a 44-yard pass from Bill Lothridge to Billy Williamson to mount a threat.

However, the Bengals rose up on their 1-foot line to toss Tech fullback Mike McNames for a two-yard loss on fourth down and Tech never threatened that close again.

All the scoring came in the second period when LSU exchanged fumbles with the Jackets. The Bengals drove to the Tech 19 early in the second period but Bo Campbell then fumbled and Williamson recovered for Tech at the 15.

The Jackets moved a bit but on fourth down Billy Lothridge went back to kick and dropped the ball and a host of Tigers swarmed him under on the Tech 16.

LSU went to work and big Earl Gros slammed over right guard for 12 yards and a first down at the Tech 4. Gros hit the middle for three yards and on the next play Jimmy Field faked to Gros and then sped off right tackle for the Tigers' touchdown.

Wendell Harris, the senior right half, added the extra point as the Tigers took a 7-0 lead with 6:02 left in the period.

LSU's next threat was set up a few minutes later when sophomore fullback, Buddy Hamic, intercepted a Stan Gann

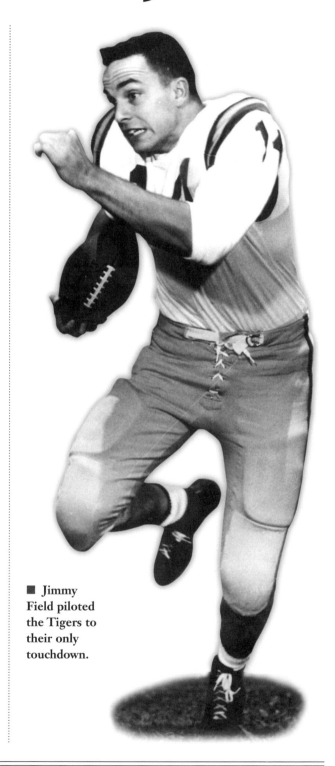

■ Jimmy Field piloted the Tigers to their only touchdown.

Score by Periods

Georgia Tech	0	0	0	0 —	0
LSU	0	10	0	0 —	10

pass at midfield and raced it back for 21 yards to the Tech 29.

Lynn Amedee and the Go Eleven went to work and the ex-Istrouma High youth hit Ray Wilkins with a nine-yard pass and then kept for three yards and a first down at the Tech 17.

Amedee then pitched two straight ones into "left field," missing his receivers by tens of feet. Amedee gained eight yards and then Gros hit off the middle for four yards and a first down at the Jacket five.

LSU couldn't move and with time running out, Wendell Harris rushed into the game and booted a 22-yard field goal to give LSU a 10-0 lead.

Only nine seconds were left in the half when Harris booted the ball through the uprights.

The second half was mainly a punting duel between Jerry Stovall of the Bengals and Billy Lothridge of the Yellow Jackets.

LSU's defense completely halted the vaunted Tech's offense which had completely smothered Southern Cal and the Rice Owls, a team that humbled the Bengals in their opener.

It was the third time in the history of the rivalry that LSU has been able to trim the Yellow Jackets. It was LSU's second victory over Tech at Tiger Stadium, the first coming in 1957.

The Bengals completely dominated the game with the exception of Tech's drive at the start of the second half.

LSU piled up 11 first downs to nine for Tech and picked up a net rushing of 145 yards against 86 for Tech. LSU picked up 66 yards on the air and Tech got 70.

LSU pitched 11 aerials and completed five while Tech, supposedly a "hot" passing combine, pitched only 16 passes and completed six.

While the Bengals turned in their best offensive efforts of the season, it was their superb defensive work against the tricky Tech offense that eventually spelled victory.

The Bengals ends and linebackers turned in their best efforts of the season as they handled Tech's sprint-out and rolled-out passes in good shape.

Big Roy Winston turned in his best effort of the season as he consistently broke through to haul down Gann, the tricky Tech quarterback.

Also, Jack Gates, Billy Booth, Monk Guillot and Bob Flurry turned in fine defensive efforts as did the entire Chinese Bandit unit which had been below par during the two opening games.

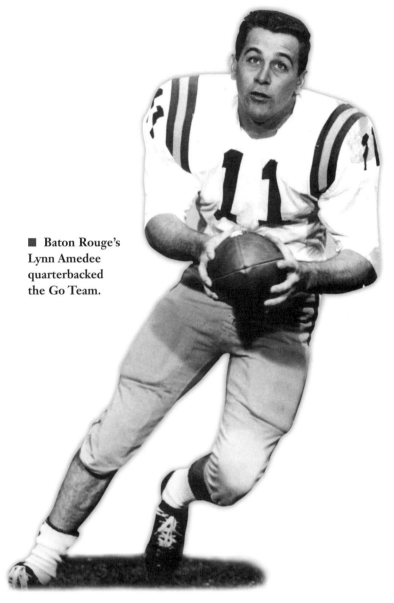

■ Baton Rouge's Lynn Amedee quarterbacked the Go Team.

Others who looked good were Dan Hargett, Rodney Guillot and a host of other Tigers.

Big Earl Gros proved to be a hard-running fullback in the game as he led the Tiger rushers with 37 yards in eight tries while Harris picked up 30 yards in four tries and Wilkins got 24 in 5 tries.

Wilkins also proved the top Tiger pass receiver, grabbing three passes for 26 yards.

Mike McNames, the big fullback, was the top Tech ground-gainer who picked up 37 yards in nine tries. Williamson gained 32 yards in seven tries.

The touted Gann was held to three completions in eight tries his worst passing performance of the season. His completions gained but five yards.

His understudy, Lothridge, completed three of eight passes for 65 yards — most coming on his fake punt deal that was good for 44 yards to Williamson.

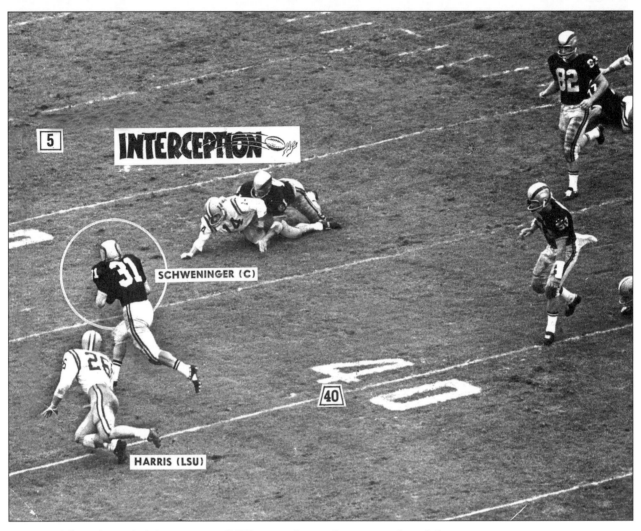

■ Loren Schweninger (31) intercepts an LSU pass and races for a 54-yard touchdown.

Tiger Defense Buries Colorado in Orange Bowl

BY BUD MONTET
The Advocate

Miami, Fla. — *Jan. 1, 1962*

With sheathed claws and hidden fangs the LSU Tigers still had a surprisingly easy time in downing the Colorado Buffaloes, 25-7, today before a crowd of only 62,391 fans who braved slight showers throughout the game.

Tossing away scoring chances time after time, the Bengals nevertheless managed to get three touchdowns, a field goal and a safety.

LSU had to come from behind after building up an early lead of 5-0 on Wendall Harris' field goal and a safety on a blocked kick by Gary Kinchen.

Colorado's lone touchdown came early in the second quarter when Loren Schweninger, the Buffalo fullback, grabbed a wobbly-tossed Jimmy Field pass on his 41 and sped unmolested down the sideline for 59 yards and the touchdown to take a 7-5 lead.

However, LSU came right back to march 82 yards for their first touchdown, with Charles Cranford going over from the Colorado 1 for the touchdown. On the extra-point play, LSU failed but they held a 11-7 first-half lead and were never threatened after that.

LSU scored twice in the third quarter as they built up their lead. Early in the period, LSU scored on a short 43-yard jaunt with Field going over from the Colorado 9 on a keeper play.

Late in the period, LSU backed the Buffaloes up to their goal line and Gene Sykes broke through to block Chuck McBride's attempted punt in the end zone and then fell on the ball for the third Tiger touchdown.

The Bengals didn't display their usual fine offensive effort and threw away several scoring chances.

Defensively, the Tigers lived up to their billing as they held the All-American end, Jerry Hillenbrand, well in check as a pass receiver and completely stopped the vaunted running of Colorado's Ted Woods and Bill Harris.

Colorado took to the air in an effort to best the Bengals and tossed 39 passes, a new Orange Bowl record.

But only once did the passing attack seriously threaten the Bengals.

It was LSU's second Orange Bowl victory and their third post-season triumph in the school's history.

Coach Paul Dietzel, who's rumored to leave Tigerland for West Point shortly, was carried off the field on the shoulders of his victorious youths.

Colorado failed to live up to its notice as an explosive football eleven and its All-Americans, guards Joe Romig and end Hillenbrand, didn't bother the Bengals.

LSU displayed an erratic passing game, hitting at will at times and then tossing interceptions.

It was no contest in the game statistics as LSU netted 206 yards on the ground to 30 for the Buffaloes and picked up 109 yards in the air to 105 for Colorado.

Colorado was able to complete only 12 of their 39 passes and most of those came late in the game when LSU sought to contain the long passes and gave the Buffs the short ones.

Ironically, not a single Colorado back netted yardage in double figures with their fullback Schweninger getting a net nine yards in five carries.

LSU's rushing was sparked by big Earl Gros who picked up 55 yards in ten carries. Field got 36 yards in eight attempts and

Score by Periods

Colorado		0	7	0	0 — 7
LSU		5	6	14	0 — 25

Harris got 26 yards in six tries.

Lynn Amedee connected on six of 12 passes for LSU while Field was successful on two of 6 tosses.

Weidner was the top aerial artist of the Buffs as he tossed 36 passes and connected on 11 for 98 yards.

LSU sputtered in the first quarter as they took the opening kickoff from their own 33 to the Colorado 14 where they bogged down and Harris booted a 30-yard field goal.

Colorado couldn't move the first time they got their hands on the ball and Kinchen's rush and block of McBride's punt resulted in a safety as the ball rolled out of the end zone.

LSU missed another scoring opportunity late in the first quarter when they drove to the Buffs' 28 and faltered.

Colorado came to life although they scored their lone touchdown before they got their first down.

In the first three minutes of the second quarter Field was trapped trying to pass, then uncorked a wobbly "wounded pigeon" that was gathered in by the fleet Schweninger, who scampered down the sidelines for 59 yards and a touchdown without anyone laying a hand on him.

LSU came right back to drive 78 yards with a 37-yard pass from Amedee to Ray Williams. It was the clutch play of the drive.

Wendell Harris set up the touchdown with a 14-yard scamper to the Buffs' 1-yard line. Cranford dove over on the next play for the Tigers' first score.

LSU got a quick touchdown in the first minutes of the third quarter when they almost blocked McBride's punt and the resulting punt rolled dead on the Colorado 42.

Moving on the ground, LSU got to the Colorado 21 where Field raced 12 yards around right end. He then added nine more on a sweep around left end for the Tigers' second touchdown.

LSU got another scoring chance late in the quarter when Woods fumbled and Sammy Odom recovered for LSU at the Colorado 49. The Bengals then marched to the Buffaloes' 19 where they gave up the ball, but a few seconds later Sykes made his great play and recovery on McBride's punt in the end zone and that wrapped up the scoring for both teams.

Colorado made their only sustained scoring threat early in the fourth quarter when they drove from their 42 where Woods recovered Gros' fumble. Colorado drove to the Tiger 11 where the threat failed.

It was LSU's second Orange Bowl victory and their third post-season triumph in the school's history.

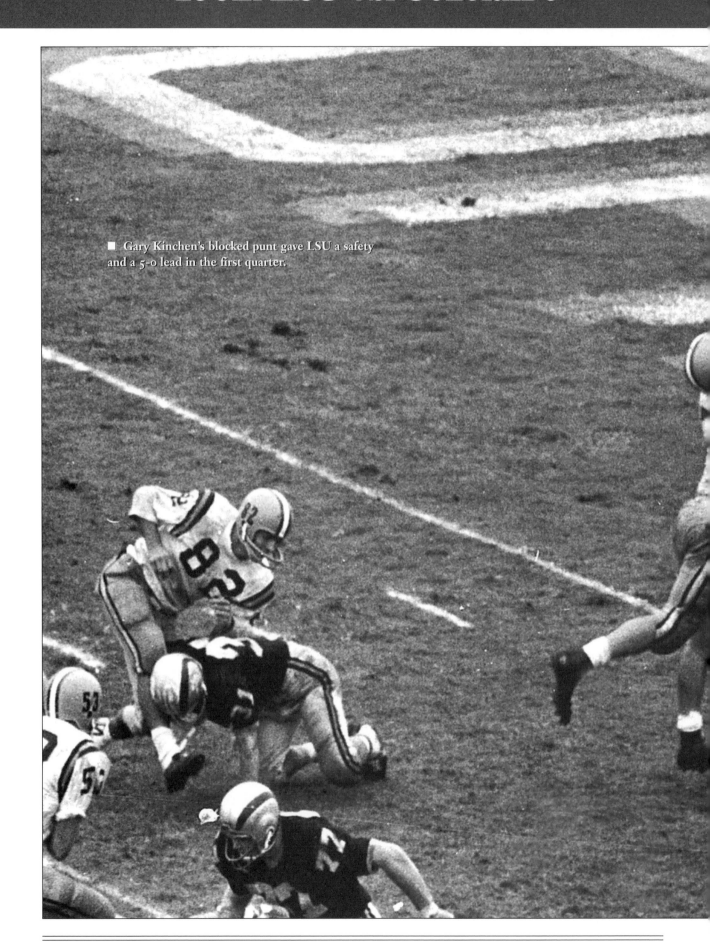

■ Gary Kinchen's blocked punt gave LSU a safety and a 5-0 lead in the first quarter.

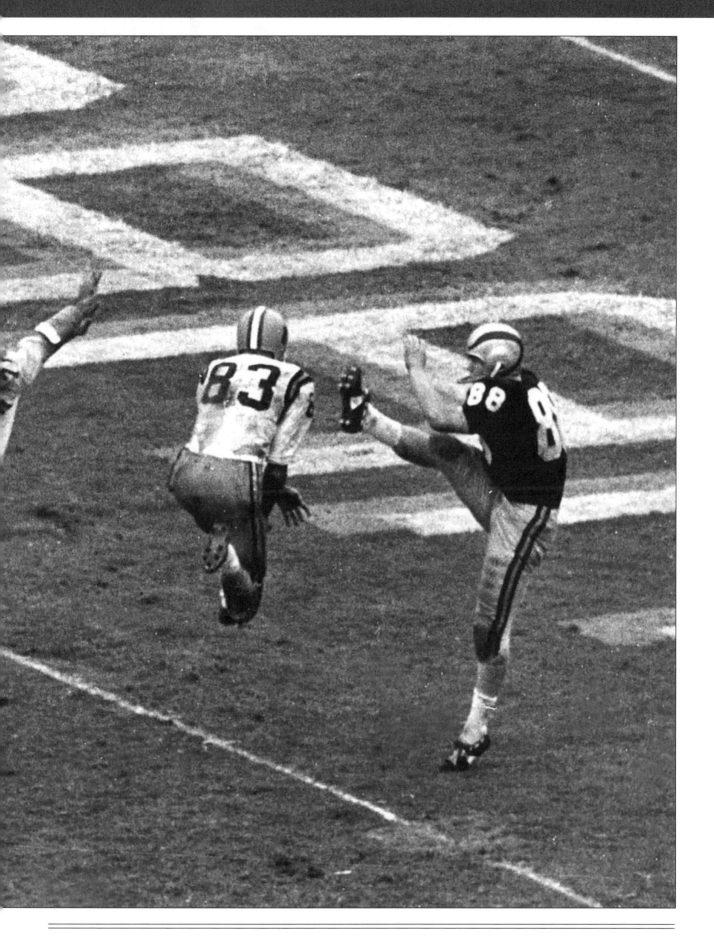

Tigers Tame Longhorns, 13-0 in Cotton Bowl

BY BUD MONTET
The Advocate

Dallas, Tex.— *Jan. 1, 1963*

An alert LSU fighting Tiger eleven capitalized on fumble recoveries and pass interceptions to trounce the Texas Longhorns, 13-0, in a bruising battle that developed more offensive fireworks than anticipated.

It was the Bengals' second bowl victory in a row and was a fitting climax to Tigers coach Charlie McClendon finishing up his first year as head mentor of the LSU eleven.

Although Texas threatened twice in the game, LSU stayed in command from the time Lynn Amedee booted a 23-yard field goal. Amedee came back to get another field goal in the fourth period, this time a 37-yarder.

LSU's lone touchdown came on Jimmy Field's 23-yard gallop around left end after being rushed trying to find a receiver.

Amedee, the outstanding back of the game, proved to be the workhorse of the Tigers as his accurate toe accounted for the two field goals which now give him the all-time LSU record with seven in one year.

The Cotton Bowl record was a 22-yard field goal.

The lithe Baton Rougean also fired up the Tigers air with nine completions in 13 tries for 93-yards without an interception.

LSU's Jerry Stovall was a marked man as the tough Texas defenses keyed on him constantly. However, Stovall halted the final threat when he intercepted a Tommy Wade aerial deep in Tiger territory.

After that, Stovall managed to pick up 36 yards in 12 carries and played with all three units at one time or another.

Amedee, the Go Unit quarterback, walked off with the outstanding back of the game honors and joined Texas' Johnny Treadwell, the outstanding lineman, as the game's heroes.

Amedee, who for three years led the Bengals in total offense, finished his career in fine fashion. In the first half, Amedee hit on seven of nine passes for 74 yards.

In the scribes' voting, Amedee received 37 votes to four for Stovall and two for Jimmy Field, the White Team quarterback.

Treadwell received 20 votes while Bengals who received lineman votes were Jack Gates, another Tiger senior who

Score by Periods

LSU	0	3	7	3 —	13
Texas	0	0	0	0 —	0

played a fine game, Fred Miller, Ruffin Rodrique, Bill Truax, Jim Turner and Dennis Gaubatz.

The usual LSU defensive units played their usual hard-hitting ball and the host of White-shirted Bengals kept the Longhorns at bay most of the game.

Gates and Miller, along with Gaubatz, Rodrique, Buddy Hamic, Stovall, Gene Sykes, Dwight Robinson, and a host of others were responsible for the blanking of the Texas eleven.

Ironically, Stovall was in poor punting form but got some fine "LSU" bounces and came up with a brilliant 44-yard average.

His kicking rival, Ernie Koy of the famed Texas Koy family, averaged 47 yards and was largely instrumental in keeping the score down.

Koy kicked the Bengals back into the hole time after time.

LSU's other senior quarterback, Jimmy Field, had one of his finest days, scoring the lone touchdown and pitching four for eight passes for 39 yards. The Bengals' prime target was junior end Bill Truax, who grabbed three passes for 49 yards and late in the game caught a touchdown pass from Amedee but the play was nullified when LSU was caught with an ineligible receiver downfield.

LSU's win completed the SEC sweep of the New Year classics as Alabama downed Oklahoma and Ole Miss defeated Arkansas.

The first quarter wasn't five minutes old when LSU started a long drive from their 2 to the Longhorn 42 where they bogged down and had to kick.

Stovall and Koy then engaged in a fine kicking duel although LSU managed late in the period to get down to the Longhorns' 30-yard line.

Texas started the fireworks in the second quarter as they showed their best offensive drive of the day, going from their 15 to the Tiger 25 from where Tony Crosby tried a long field goal and missed badly.

LSU came right back to show their best offensive series of the game as they drove 80 yards and fought the fading seconds of the clock to get their first field goal with eight seconds left in the first period.

On the drive, Amedee's passing was the big factor and his

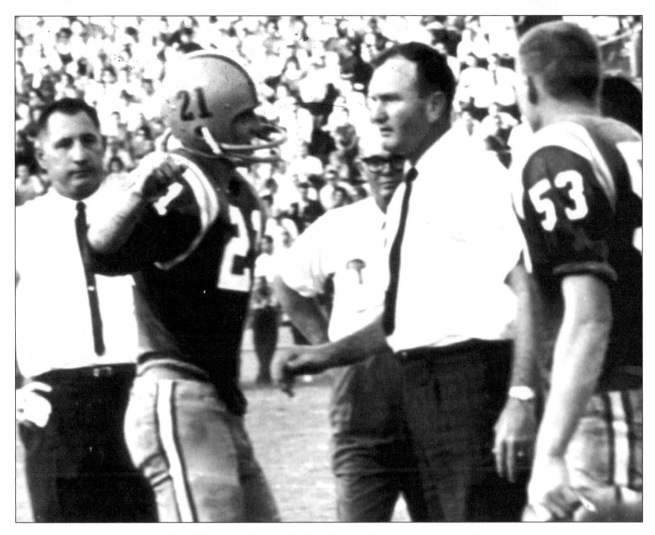

■ **LSU halfback Jerry Stovall huddles with his coach, Charlie McClendon, on the sidelines.**

22-yard toss to Truax set up the field goal.

After the Bengals moved to the Longhorns' 5, Amedee calmly booted the ball through the uprights with the clock ticking away.

LSU got a break on the second-half kickoff and made the most of it. Texas' Jerry Cook returned the punt back but was hit hard at his 34 and Amedee fell on the ball at that point.

An 11-yard Field-to-Gene Sykes pass set up the drive and two plays later Field faded to his right, seeking a receiver, but whirled and reversed his field, and raced to his left to go 22 yards for the lone touchdown of the game. On the sprint, Field made Texas' Joe Dixon miss him at the Longhorns' 5 as he neatly changed pace and side-stepped.

Amedee added the point-after, and LSU had a 10-0 lead.

Texas roared back and drove from their 32 to the Tiger 38 when a Johnny Genung passing attack failed.

The Bengals got a break near the end of the third period when a lineman tipped a Tommy Wade pass and Rodrique grabbed the ball for LSU at the midfield stripe.

LSU marched right down to the Longhorns' 7 with Jack

Gates making a sensational diving catch of a Field-thrown aerial. However, LSU lost on successive plays as the period ended.

Texas started a march early in the fourth period as they moved to the LSU 32, where Hamic intercepted a Wade pass at the LSU 30.

The Bengals then took over and with Amedee pitching the ball moved to Texas' 22, where the Tiger star flipped a scoring pass to Truax only to have it nullified.

However after the penalty, Amedee ended the game's scoring with his second field goal for the afternoon.

Late in the fourth quarter, Koy kicked 72 yards dead on the LSU 2 to put the Bengals in a hole. After a short Stovall kick, the Longhorns drove to the Tiger 30 where Stovall intercepted a wild pass and LSU retained possession of the ball to the end of the game.

Following the game, tackle Red Estes and halfback Stovall signed pro contracts with the St. Louis Cardinals. LSU's convincing victory was a sweet one to Tigers coach McClendon and after the game the veteran mentor, serving his first year as LSU's head coach, had nothing but praise for his squad.

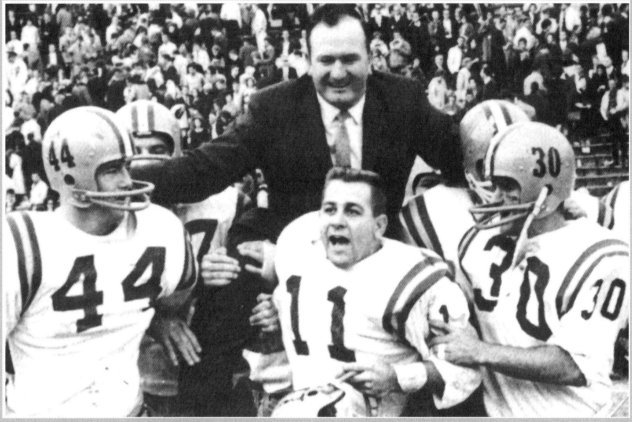

■ Charlie McClendon enjoys a victory ride following the Tigers' 13-0 win over Texas.

Two Minutes Told the Tale

By The Associated Press
The Advocate

Dallas— *Jan. 1, 1963*

"Two minutes in which Louisiana State scored 10 points proved the turning point of the Cotton Bowl football game," LSU coach Charlie McClendon observed today.

Louisiana State beat Texas, 13-0, and the victory was decisive since the Longhorns never got closer to LSU's goal line than the 25.

But it was that 2-minute period — part in the second quarter and part in the third — that vaulted LSU to its triumph.

LSU got another field goal late in the game, but Texas by then had been beaten down and disheartened by its mistakes and the unexpected strong LSU offense.

"I never felt safe with a 10-point lead going into the fourth quarter, because Texas has come back many times this year," said McClendon.

But it wasn't in the books this afternoon.

Texas coach Darrell Royal said, "I just didn't expect them to pass and catch like that. Their passing was tremendous and their receiving was great. They played fine football."

LSU tried 21 passes and completed 13 — an unusual output for the defense-minded Tigers.

But it was fumbling and pass interceptions that took the toll of the Longhorns' morale, Texas players admitted.

Bobby Gamblin, the Texas guard, said, "Anytime you fumble it's a mental letdown. But generally I don't think we played as well as we could."

McClendon declined to cite any one of his players as outstanding. "They were all outstanding and there were 18 seniors I was real proud of," he declared.

He said LSU passed more because of Texas' tight inside defense, which he praised. But he added that he thought Texas would pass more.

Pat Culpepper, the Texas linebacker, said the Tigers were the top team the Longhorns faced in quite a while.

Lynn Amedee, the LSU quarterback who was voted outstanding back of the game, said he was more sure of his second field goal than his first. He kicked a 23-yarder in the second period and a 37-yarder in the fourth quarter.

"I thought somebody might have tipped that first one," he said. This bettered the Cotton Bowl record by a yard.

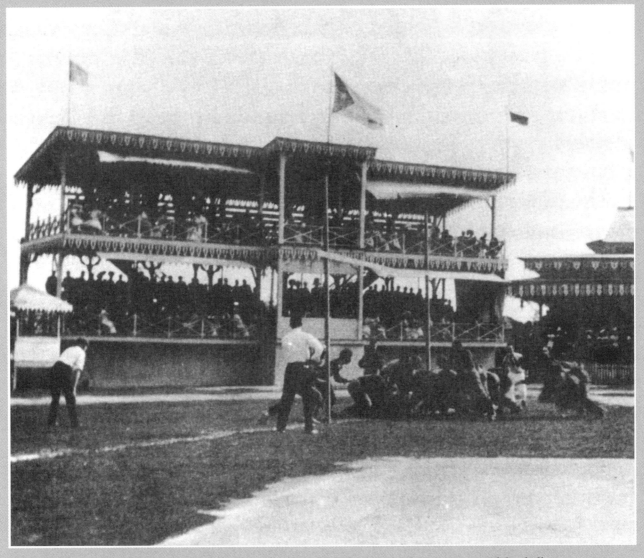

■ LSU coach Edgar Wingard brought his Tigers to Havana to play in the first international football game.

LSU Routs Havana in Holiday Game

BY THE ASSOCIATED PRESS
The Advocate

Havana, Cuba— *Dec. 25, 1907*

The cadets of Louisiana State University, who are still on campus, not having gone home to spend the Christmas holidays with their families, are celebrating after receiving a cablegram from here, which announced that LSU had defeated the University of Havana, 56-0.

The LSU players expected and were confident that they would defeat the Havana team, but they did not expect to be able to pile up such a large score against the Cubans. The University of Havana is the largest institution of learning in Cuba. It has a number of former American players on its team and for this reason it should have been able to put up a good defense against LSU.

This game is the first international college football game ever played by an American team on foreign soil, the result was awaited with much interest. LSU draws thirty or forty students every year from Cuba.

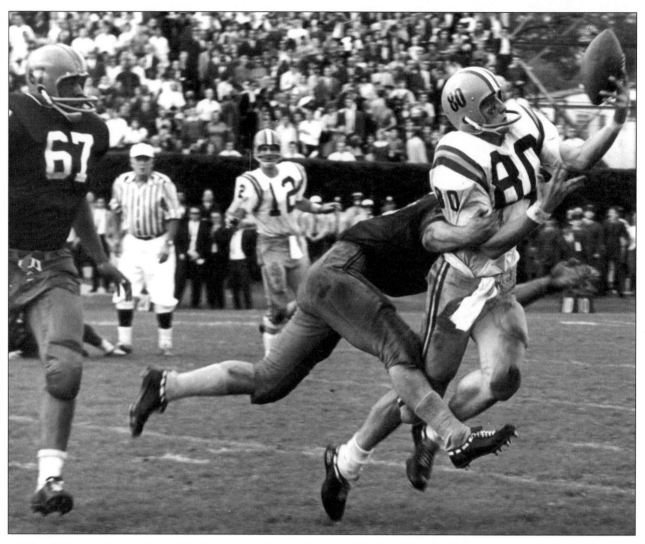

■ Doug Moreau (80) pulls in a Pat Screen pass during the second half against the Orangemen.

Moreau Boots Tigers To 13-10 Win Over Syracuse

BY BUD MONTET
The Advocate

New Orleans, La. — *Jan. 1, 1965*

The gifted left toe of Doug Moreau spelled a hard-earned 13-10 victory for the LSU Tigers over the stubborn Syracuse Orangemen here today before 65,000 fans ... .

Moreau's 14th field goal of the season, an accurate 28-yarder with less than four minutes left in the game, broke a 10-all deadlock and gave LSU its second Sugar Bowl victory in seven appearances.

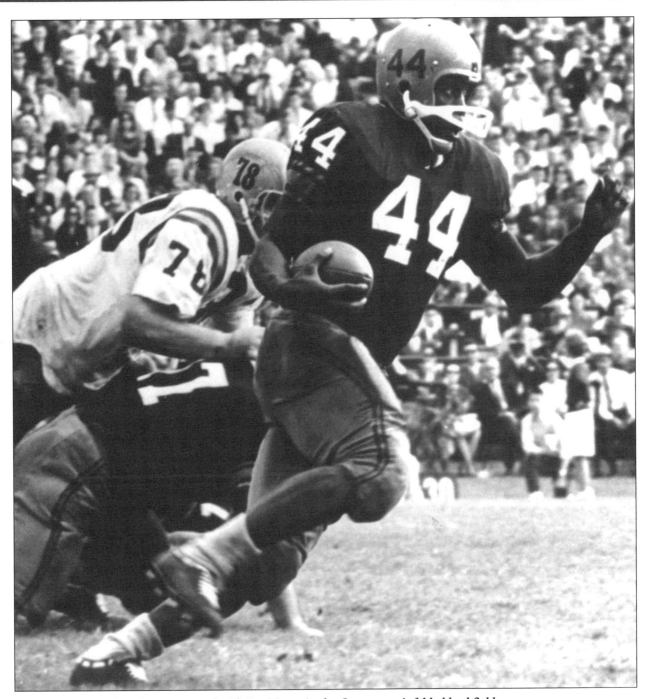

■ Syracuse's Floyd Little (44) teamed with Jim Nance in the Orangemen's fabled backfield.

The Tiger flanker set up his game winning effort by hauling down a long heave from quarterback Billy Ezell that was good for the Tigers' touchdown midway in the third quarter that tied the game when Ezell came right back to hit Joe Labruzzo with a "two-pointer" pass.

Moreau's fine efforts gained him the annual Fred Digby Most Valuable Player Award.

The Tigers played the first half with their usual disinterest in Sugar Bowl proceedings, and trailed, 10-2, going in at halftime.

Reversing their attitude in the second half the Bengals came

Score by Periods

	1	2	3	4	
LSU	2	0	8	3	— 13
Syracuse	10	0	0	0	— 10

to life and the first time they got their hands on the ball they marched 75 yards in seven plays and sustained the long drive despite a 15-yard penalty that threatened to mar their effort.

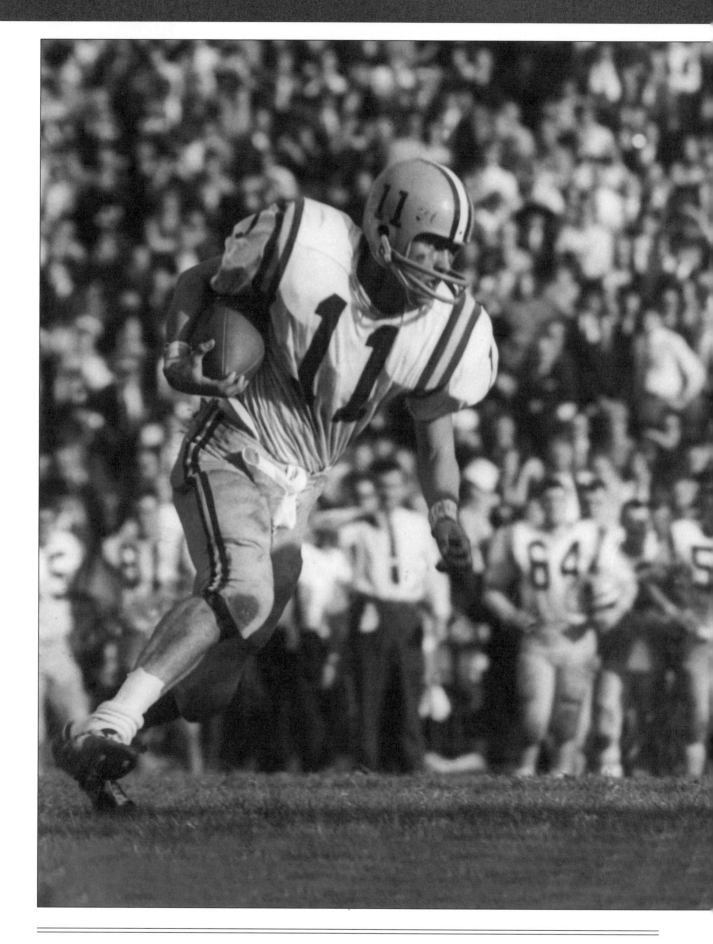

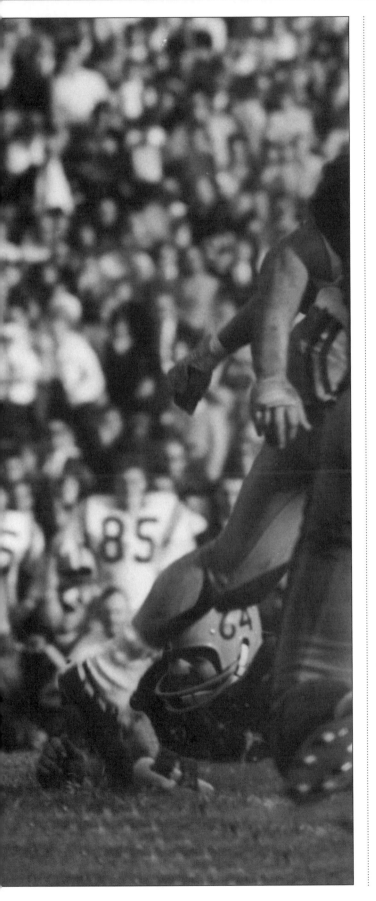

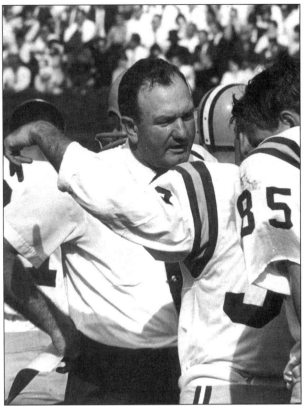

■ On the sidelines, LSU coach Charlie McClendon listens to strategy from one of his players.

Syracuse's strong defensive tactics kept the Tiger running game completely bottled up in the first half and their good rushes forced the Tiger quarterbacks to hurry their throws with resulting poor efforts.

In the second half, the Bengals moved the big Orangemen to get their ground game going.

After LSU tied the game, Syracuse came back and sustained their longest drive to threaten to go ahead. The Orangemen drove from their 22 to the Tiger 13 where White Graves intercepted a Walley Mahle pass at the Bengals' 6.

In getting their winning three points, LSU drove from their 28 to the Syracuse 11 where a penalty marred the drive and Moreau then booted his 22-yarder for the victory.

Syracuse opened the game with a drive from midfield to the Tiger 7 where a 15-yard penalty pushed them back and Roger Smith booted a 23-yard field goal to put the Orangemen out in front, 3-0.

The Orangemen took advantage of a break near the end of the first period when their Dennis Reilly broke through and blocked a Buster Brown punt on the Tiger 45 and Syracuse's end, Brad Clarke, scooped up the ball on the Tiger 35 and raced over for the score. After the touchdown Smith added the point-after kick.

Between the two Syracuse scores, LSU managed to get a safety with big George Rice breaking through and hauling fleet Floyd Little down in the end zone.

■ LSU quarterback Billy Ezell (11) sprints for a first down.

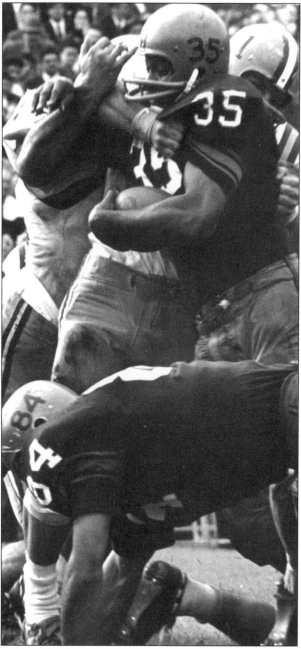

■ **NO PLACE TO GO: Jim Nance (35) runs into a roadblock of LSU Tigers.**

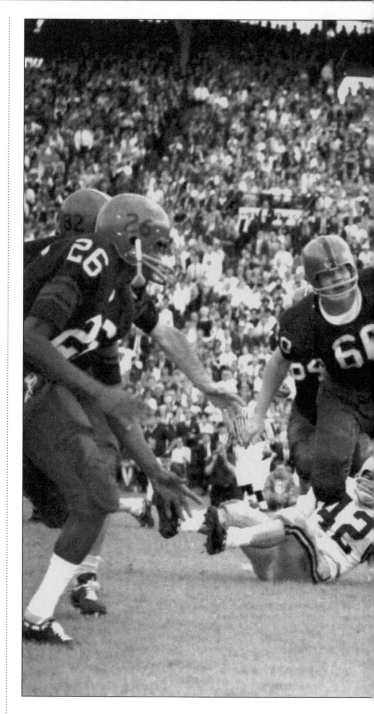

Brown's boot dead at the Syracuse 3 set up the play for the Tigers.

The Bengals held a slim lead in rushing with a net 161 yards to 151 for the Orangemen but picked up 199 yards in the air to only 52 for the Orangemen.

LSU hit on six of 15 aerials but two proved to be key plays, Ezell's long pass to Moreau for the Tiger touchdown and Pat Screen's 36-yard toss to Joe Labruzzo late in the final period set up the game-winning field goal.

Ezell's "two-pointer" pitch to Labruzzo also proved a key aerial in the game.

LSU passed up an early scoring opportunity when

Syracuse's Mahle fumbled on his 43-yard line and Richard Granier recovered for the Bengals midway through the period.

In the second quarter, a pair of short kicks by Syracuse's Rich King gave the Bengals good field position that they failed to exploit.

LSU's long touchdown drive featured short dashes by Labruzzo and fullback Don Schwab and a crucial first down 9-yard pass from Ezell to Labruzzo.

After marching to the Syracuse 40, LSU was guilty of a holding penalty and pushed back to their 43. On the next play, Ezell faked a pitch down the middle and then picked up Moreau at the Syracuse 30 and the fleet Tiger flanker gathered

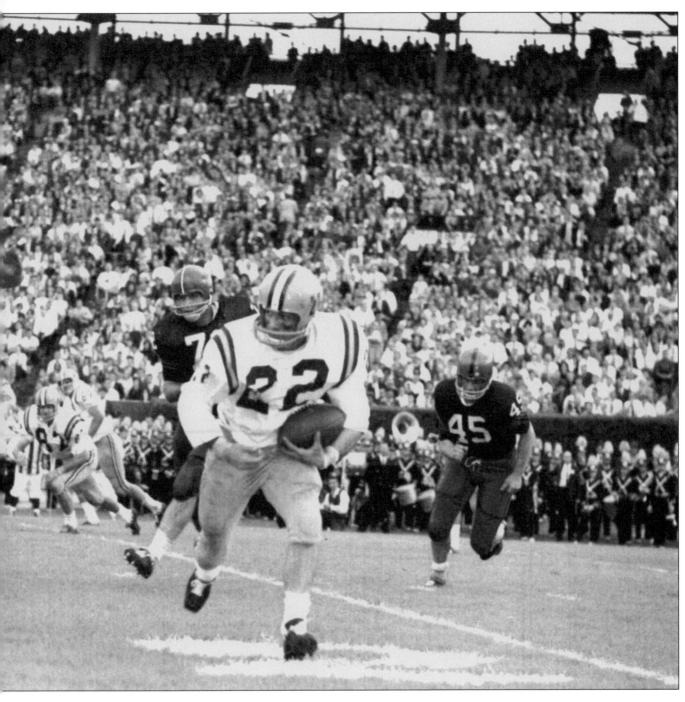

■ Joe Labruzzo (22) sweeps outside against Syracuse. Labruzzo's running set up the game-winning field goal.

in the pass without breaking stride and moved quickly to the Syracuse goal line. Moreau had beaten his defender by yards.

LSU's Schwab once again proved the workhorse of the backfield carrying the ball 17 times for a net 81 yards to outgain the fabled pair of Jim Nance and Floyd Little.

Gawain DiBetta ran 13 times and netted 18 yards while Labruzzo carried the ball 10 times and netted 25.

Ezell completed two of five passes for 67 yards and Screen pitched 10 passes and hit on four for 47.

Big Nance proved an erratic runner but managed to net 70 yards on 15 carries.

Syracuse's regular quarterback, Mahle, started the game at right half and proved a troublesome runner, picking up a net 23 yards on seven carries.

The victory was a sweet one for the Bengals who have had their troubles in the Sugar Bowl in the past. It was the first meeting between LSU and Syracuse.

The Tigers' win was the second bowl victory for LSU coach Charlie McClendon in three tries as a head grid mentor.

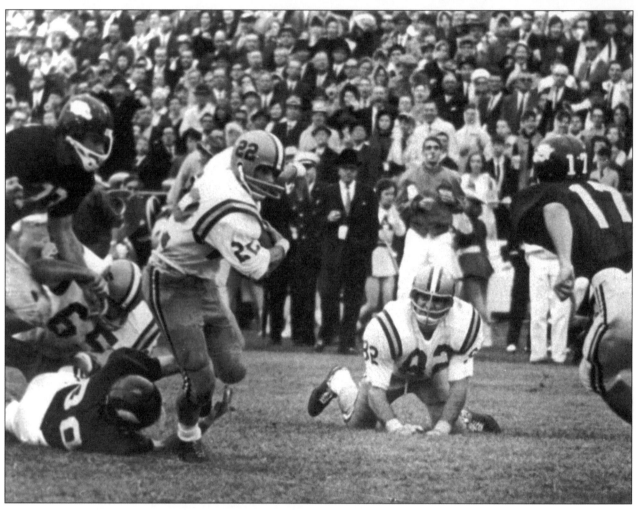

■ Joe Labruzzo (22) scored both of the Tigers' touchdowns in the second quarter.

LSU Halts Hogs in Cotton Bowl, 14-7

BY BUD MONTET
The Advocate

Dallas, Tex.— *Jan. 1, 1966*

The Fighting Tigers of LSU who made a practice crusade of "Never 23" made good on the slippery turf of the Cotton Bowl when they bested the Arkansas Porkers, 14-7, and broke their win streak at 22.

Score by Periods

LSU	0	14	0	0	— 14
Arkansas	7	0	0	0	— 7

The clutch running of Joe Labruzzo, who scored both Bengal touchdowns in the second quarter, some fine offensive blocking by big Tiger tackle Dave McCormick and a sticky defense that never gave up although constantly threatened by the fleet Hogs were the big factors in the Bengals' upset victory.

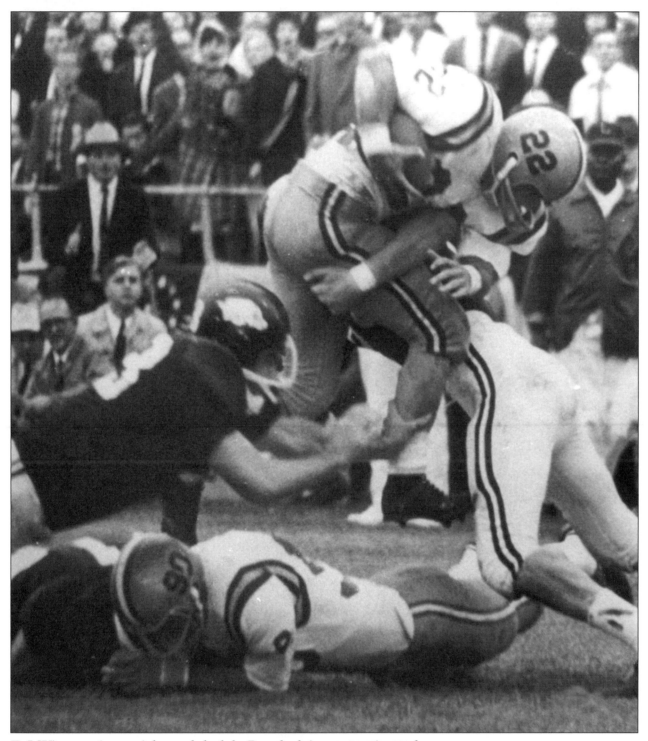

■ **LSU's 14-7 win over Arkansas halted the Razorbacks' 22-game win streak.**

All during the pre-game practice sessions LSU coach Charlie McClendon dressed out his redshirt squads in red jerseys, numbered 23, a constant reminder that the mighty Porkers were trying for their 23rd straight victory in the Cotton Bowl.

Arkansas, ranked No. 2 in both major polls, constantly threatened during the game but were able to get but one touchdown, a 19-yard aerial, from Jon Brittenum to Bobby Crockett.

The score came in the first period to give the Porkers a 7-0 lead.

The Bengals struck back the hard way early in the second period when they drove 80 yards, sticking on the ground and overcoming a costly 15-yard roughing penalty.

Nelson Stokely, the Tiger sophomore quarterback who has been sidelined with injuries, got the drive under way and moved the Bengals from their 20 to the Porkers' 43 where he reinjured his knee and had to leave the game.

On the drive, Stokely hit Schwab with an 18-yard pass for a first down and turned in two runs of four and seven yards.

On this drive, LSU got a first down at the Porkers' 9 and in three carries Labruzzo punched the ball over for the first score and Doug Moreau added the point-after kick to tie the score.

The Bengals moved into the lead a few minutes later when Ronnie South and Nix fumbled on an attempted handoff and Bill Bass recovered for LSU at the Hogs' 34.

LSU moved on in to score in seven plays. Labruzzo got the Bengals a first down at the Porkers' 16, carried to the five on a fine 11-yard gallop and then bulled over left tackle behind blocks by McCormick in three plays. Moreau's extra-point boot was good and LSU led, 14-7, at intermission.

Although they remained behind, the Porkers continued to threaten. Early in the third period they moved to the Bengals' 15 where Ernest Magoire pulled probably the weirdest defensive stunt of the season to halt the drive.

Lindsey, on a counter, got behind Magoire, who desperately swung his leg out and Lindsey tripped over it for a seven-yard loss. This drive finally ended with South missing on an attempted 46-yard field goal try.

LSU failed to make a single first down in the third period but they came back at the start of the final period to stage a 54-yard drive to the Porkers' 2-yard line, where Moreau missed an easy 19-yard try for a field goal, which at the time looked like a costly mistake.

Arkansas took to the air and drove from their 20 to the Tiger 36 with Brittenum tossing strikes to Crockett for eight, 16, and 18 yards before Jerry Joseph broke up the threat at the Tiger 20 when he made a fine interception of a Brittenum pass.

With less than three minutes left in the game, Brittenum again mounted a drive that carried to the Tiger 24 before the final whistle caught the Porkers. The unhappy Hogs were a disappointed group marching off the field.

Arkansas' 22-game win streak was the longest of the current season.

The victory kept the Bengals' Cotton Bowl record intact — the Tigers having never lost a Cotton Bowl fray. In their first one — 1947, they tied the Arkansas Porkers, and in 1963 they bested Texas, 13-0.

Today's win was a sweet one for Coach McClendon, who was highly criticized midway during the regular season when he lost his No. 1 quarterback, Stokely, and quickly dropped resounding games to Ole Miss and Alabama.

However, McClendon pulled Pat Screen back into action and the plucky New Orleans youth played his first game of the year against the Porkers.

Screen called a fine game, keeping possession of the ball and risking passes only when he had to gain a first down.

Labruzzo's great clutch running was a potent factor as was the all-around defensive play.

LSU did just what Coach McClendon predicted they would — not stop the potent Arkansas offense but blunt it enough to

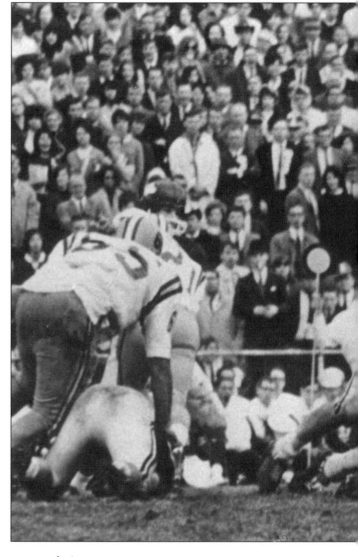

go on and win.

Labruzzo's running gained for him the outstanding back award. Others who received votes were Screen 10, and Arkansas' Harry Jones four.

Dave McCormick, the LSU tackle, gained the outstanding lineman award over Hog end Bobby Crockett in a close vote, 22-18.

Labruzzo carried the ball 21 times and netted 69 yards. Jim Dousay had a fine afternoon with 14 carries and a net 38.

Jones, one of the quickest backs in America, proved the toughest Hog for the Bengals to handle. The fleet back ran 10 times and netted 79 yards for a 7.9 average. The Porkers hard running Bobby Burnett, picked up 44 yards on 12 carries.

For LSU big George Rice, Mike Robichaux, John Garlington, Mike Duhon and David Strange played outstanding ball.

LSU's linebacking duo of Mike Vincent and Bill Bass turned in their finest effort of the season.

The Bengals rushed for a net of 166 yards and passed for 100

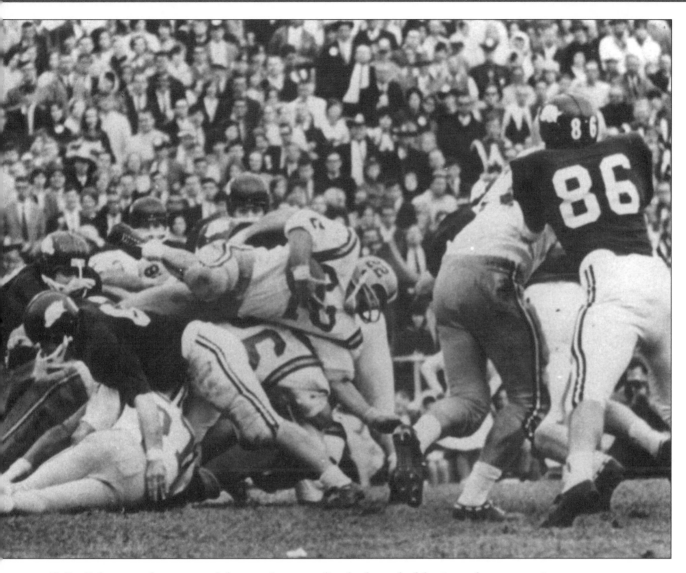

■ Joe Labruzzo, who was voted the game's outstanding back, rushed for 69 yards on 21 carries.

yards for a total offensive effort of 266 yards. Arkansas rushed for 129 yards but passed for 177 in the air for a total of 306.

The Porkers' Crockett caught 10 passes to set a new Cotton Bowl record for receptions.

LSU was the victim of several costly penalties that threatened to stymie them.

In the first period, when the Bengals were trying to get back in the game after the Porker score, Screen scrambled all over the field and finally tossed a 47-yard pass to Moreau at the Porkers' 20 but the Bengals had an ineligible receiver downfield.

Coming back with their tying touchdown, the Tigers had to overcome a 15-yard penalty that set them back.

Screen hit on seven of 10 pass attempts while rival Brittenum hit on 15 of 24.

Masters was the top LSU receiver with four receptions for 45 yards. Arkansas' Crockett caught 10 for 129 yards and a touchdown.

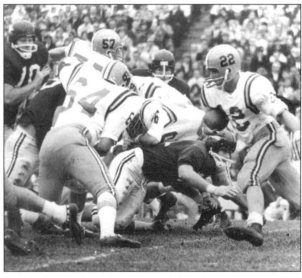

■ LSU outrushed the Hogs, 166 yards to 129.

MAC: 'Made 'Em Play Our Way'

BY THE ASSOCIATED PRESS

The Advocate

Dallas, Tex.— *Jan. 1, 1966*

"We slowed them down and made them play our type of game," explained Tigers coach Charlie McClendon, after Louisiana State snapped Arkansas' 22-game winning streak with a 14-7 Cotton Bowl triumph.

"I told you writers before the game that we couldn't match their speed, and we couldn't. But we played control ball and came up with the big play.

"Our kids followed instructions right to the end."

McClendon called the upset on this gloomy New Year's Day his greatest thrill since his playing days with Kentucky and the Wildcats' Sugar Bowl victory over Oklahoma.

That triumph severed a 32-game Oklahoma winning streak.

McClendon said he didn't think his Tigers made a single wrong decision and "We didn't have a fumble or single pass interception."

"There were times when it looked like we should pass," he continued. "But we weren't going to put the ball into the air and give them the chance for that interception. They'll kill you."

McClendon had promised that his thrice-beaten Bengals would have a couple of surprises for the second-ranked Razorbacks.

However, this generally was restricted to fluctuating offensive formations and defensive plays."

"I just told Pat Screen (LSU quarterback) before the game, 'Let's go after them with everything we've got.' He said, 'Coach, I think I'm ready.' "

McClendon said he could not pinpoint a single play as the turning point in the game, although the fourth-period interception by Jerry Joseph was a chillier.

The junior halfback said LSU shifted from a man-to-man pass defense to a half man-to-man and half zone to contain Arkansas Bobby Crockett.

"He'd been going wide on me," Joseph said. "I decided the next time he came down wide, I was going to cut in front of him. He did, and I cut in front and got it."

The interception came at the LSU 20 and punctured a spirited Arkansas scoring threat.

Doug Moreau, who missed what could have been a critical 19-yard field goal attempt in the final period, said he had no excuses.

"I just missed it," he said. "Nervousness didn't have anything to do with it."

McClendon had noted that a successful kick by Moreau would have iced the game for LSU.

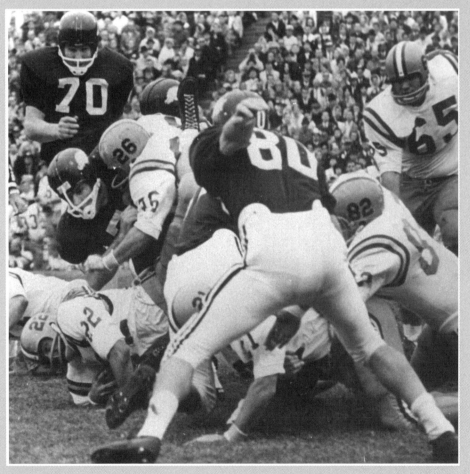

■ The Tigers' solid defense was the key in LSU's upset win.

1966 Cotton Bowl Remembered

BY SAM KING
The Advocate

Baton Rouge, La. — *Nov. 18, 1995*

Today's Southeastern Conference "no-contest" between LSU and Arkansas couldn't have been more fitting for the 30-year reunion of the 1965 LSU football team.

Heavy underdogs, outmanned and lightly regarded, coach Charles McClendon's team defied all odds and upset Arkansas, 14-7, in the fabled Jan. 1, 1966, Cotton Bowl.

The victory cost the undefeated Razorbacks, who had won 22 straight games, a possible national championship.

More importantly, however, McClendon says the upset created an unbelievable bond among members of the Tigers, who have reunions virtually every year.

Forty-seven players and coaches from that '65 team gathered this weekend and relived their memories, prior to, during and after the present Tigers' 28-0 rout of No. 14 Arkansas.

In fact, they made their entrance into Tiger Stadium, walked beneath the goal post and formed lines for the Tigers to run through onto the field. It was quite a salute for a deserving group.

"This group is the tightest football team I've ever known," McClendon said. "This is what winning a tough game like that does.

"It is amazing how it affected all of these players," McClendon said. "I don't know what the word for it is, but it really brought them together. They were together all year, but the way they came together for that game was unbelievable."

McClendon repeated one of his favorite stories about the game. Because LSU's record was 7-3 and the Razorbacks were hogging the national spotlight, McClendon said Arkansas and Texas fans and the media felt LSU shouldn't even be playing in the Cotton Bowl.

"We had a situation where some Arkansas fans, the night before the game, poked fun at the Tigers as we walked up some stairs," McClendon said. "I can still see these ladies all dressed in red looking at them and one of them exclaimed, 'Well, they

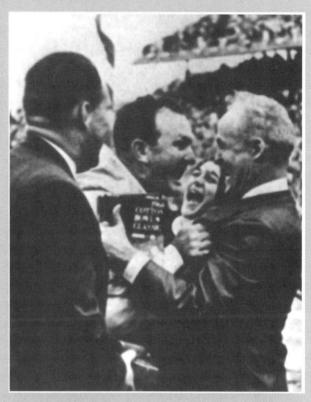

■ **Charlie McClendon and LSU athletic director Jim Corbett celebrate the Tigers' win.**

did show up.'

"You don't embarrass an injured Tiger," McClendon said. "You don't play games with them."

Then came game day.

"They came out and they were dedicated to doing their jobs," he said. "They really had fire in their eyes. They were ready to take on King Kong. It's amazing how it brought everybody together.

"I knew, somewhere down the line, something good was really going to come out of what happened to that team," McClendon said. "It's amazing how they feel this way. They'll feel the same way 20 years from now.

"They'll still be getting together. I wish I could say I'd be around, but I can't.

"I told them one thing, though," he said. "I may not be here at your next reunion, but you can count on one thing, I'm going to be looking over your shoulders to hear what you have to say about me."

Tigers Foil Dietzel's Return

By Bud Montet
The Advocate

Baton Rouge, La. — *Sept. 17, 1966*

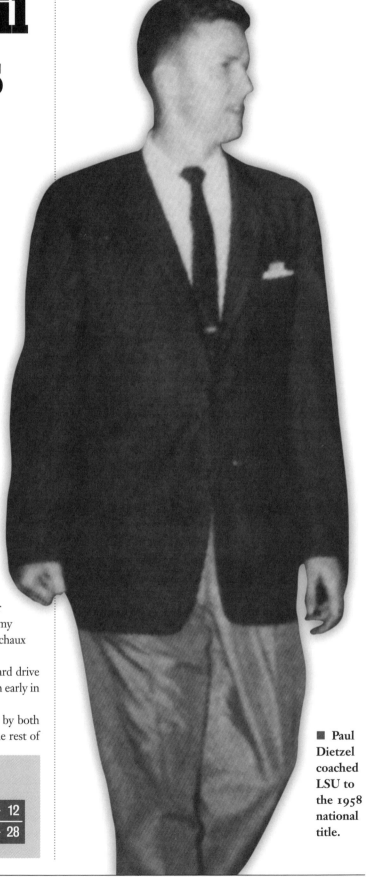

■ Paul Dietzel coached LSU to the 1958 national title.

Coach Charlie McClendon stepped out of the shadows tonight at Tiger Stadium as his gridders presented him with a 28-12 victory over his old boss Paul Dietzel and his South Carolina Gamecocks, before 67,512 rabid Bengal fans.

LSU's partisan rooters also gave Dietzel a personal setback when the Dietzel-inspired "longest boo in history ... " failed to materialize when the former Tiger coach brought his eleven on the field.

The Bengals scored the second time they got their hands on the ball with brilliant little Nelson Stokley going eleven yards around right end and Steve Daniels' placement gave the Bengals a 7-0 lead which they never lost.

South Carolina came right back to go 76 yards for their long sustained drive of the night with their Jimmy Killen going over from the Gamecock 1. Mike Robichaux blocked the try for the extra point.

LSU soon moved ahead as they sustained an 80-yard drive that was climaxed by Gawain DiBetta's two-yard punch early in the second period.

This trio of long drives ended the sustained effort by both teams who then turned to weird football to pile up the rest of

Score by Periods

South Carolina	6	0	6	0	— 12
LSU	7	7	7	7	— 28

the points on the scoreboard.

Midway in the third period LSU got their third score when Carolina's Jeff Jowers attempted to punt and fumbled the pass from center, ran to the sidelines where he tried a running punt, only to have big Jack Dyer of LSU block the effort and knock the ball over the goal line where George Bevan, LSU's sophomore linebacker, fell on it for the touchdown.

Trailing, 21-6, South Carolina got back into the game when their Bobby Bryant took a 46-yard Mitch Worley punt on his 23 and raced for a 77-yard touchdown jaunt as the clock expired for the third period, the first of the touchdowns to be scored as time ran out.

In an odd fourth period South Carolina was held deep in its own territory and on three occasions tried to run out of trouble on fourth down.

The first time their desperate gamble failed, LSU took over on the Gamecock 27 but after making a first down at the 15 Stokley tossed an interception.

Late in the game with 1:06 left in the fray, Carolina gambled and lost with big Mike Robichaux tossing Mike Fair for a six-yard loss and the Bengals taking over on the Gamecock 18.

This time little Freddie Haynes dove over the goal line as the game expired. Ronnie Manton's boot for the extra point gave LSU its 28-12 victory. The Bengals dominated the erratic contest that was heralded as one of the top games of the opening day of the 1966 season.

LSU gained 283 yards on the ground but completed only one pass in seven attempts.

The usually cautious Dietzel let his quarterback, Fair, toss 17 passes and the junior star hit on six for 71 yards.

South Carolina gained a net of 101 on the ground.

Dietzel, who built the game up as a vendetta on the part of the Tiger coaches and gridders, surprised all of his old Baton Rouge followers when he gambled constantly on fourth down in the opening minutes.

The blond mentor, who was making his debut with Carolina, also pulled out his "shotgun" offense early in the fray with his star, Fair, moving back and taking direct passes from the center.

It was a sweet victory for Coach McClendon who has coached LSU to four straight bowl appearances, but has been under the shadow of his former boss at LSU.

Dietzel, who built the game up as a vendetta on the part of the Tiger coaches and gridders, surprised all of his old Baton Rouge followers when he gambled constantly on fourth down in the opening minutes. The blond mentor, who was making his debut with Carolina, also pulled out his "shotgun" offense early in the fray with his star, Fair, moving back and taking direct passes from the center.

The Bengal mentors uncovered some fine bright young prospects in Tommy (Trigger) Allen and Maurice LeBlanc. Allen carried 12 times and piled up 40 yards while LeBlanc, still slowed down from a pulled muscle, stepped through for 63 net yards in 12 tires.

However, it remained for the plucky little Stokley to lead the squad's rushing attack with a net 78 yards in 15 carries.

Fullback Gawain DiBetta piled up 53 yards on 12 carries.

Defensively, the Bengals of LSU showed flashes of their vaulted form that has made them feared in southern grid circles, but they broke down badly on kickoff and punt return coverage.

South Carolina's Bryant returned three punts for 89 yards with his long one, the 77-yard touchdown jaunt, coming after he picked up a fine block at midfield from teammate Wally Orrel.

Only one Tiger had a shot at Bryant and DiBetta was too far out of the play to make a stop although he desperately dove at the flying Gamecock safety at the goal line.

Bryant returned two kickoffs for 67 yards and South Carolina's Benny Galloway returned a pair of kickoffs for 48 yards.

LSU's first sustained drive, the second time they got their hands on the ball, was sparked by the fine running of Allen, DiBetta and then Stokley, who took over at the 25 and lugged the ball over the goal line in two tries. Stokley and DiBetta started the second sustained scoring drive and LeBlanc, making his debut as a Bengal, came in to contribute runs of eight, six and eight yards again.

Only in their first quarter drive did the Gamecocks show consistency, although they hung on throughout the game and took advantage of Tigers mistakes to halt threatening drives.

Defensively, after their first lapse in the first period, the Bengals showed a stiffened attitude and flankmen John Garlington and Robichaux constantly harried Fair and his teammates and Mike Pharis made key tackles as well as blocking one of the two blocked Carolina punts.

Big John Demarie, the defensive tackle, made several key tackles to halt Carolina in Tiger territory. Tommy Fussell, always a ball hawk for the Tigers, recovered a fumble to halt a Carolina threat.

The game ends the current series between the Carolina Gamecocks and the Tigers.

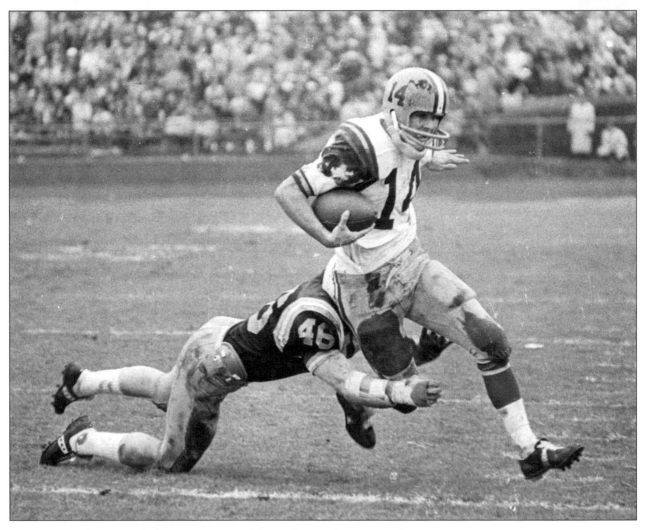

■ **Nelson Stokely (14) eludes a Wyoming tackler in the Cowboys' secondary.**

Tigers Rally to Lasso Wyoming, 20-13

By Bud Montet
The Advocate

New Orleans, La. — *Jan. 1, 1968*

The "Comeback" LSU Tigers did it again today as they spotted the Wyoming Cowboys a 13-point first half lead before storming back to grab a 20-13 victory in their eighth Sugar Bowl Classic appearance.

The Cowboys' stubborn defense completely halted the Tigers in the first half as the Bengals were able to make just one first down, only 33 yards on the ground, and five yards in the air.

The victory was the third time a Charlie McClendon-led Bengal eleven has humbled an unbeaten eleven in a bowl appearance.

Wyoming, ranked sixth by one major wire service, were riding a 14-game win streak.

Tiger elevens halted a long Texas Longhorns streak in the Cotton Bowl and three years ago handed the Arkansas Porkers a Cotton Bowl defeat to halt a Frank Broyles' streak of 22 games.

The game was McClendon's fifth appearance in a bowl in his six-year tenure as head grid mentor.

LSU got two scoring opportunities in the first period but the Cowboys held them at bay with jarring tackles and alert defensive play.

Jim Kiick, Wyoming's co-captain, opened the second quarter when he broke away from a host of Tigers to score from one yard out and Jerry Depoyster's boot put the Cowboys out in front, 7-0.

Depoyster then got field goals of 24 and 49 yards — the 49-yarder a new Sugar Bowl record. Depoyster set another record when he kicked four times for an average 49.0 yards per boot.

After LSU went in front, 20-13, with but 4 minutes and 32 seconds left, the Cowboys fought back and threatened as the result of a freak 54-yard pass play.

With less than a minute to play, Paul Toscano, the Cowboy quarterback, tossed a long pass to the Tiger 35 where a pair of Bengals batted the ball forward and the Cowboys' George Anderson grabbed the ball and headed for the Tiger goal. But, he was hauled down on the Bengal 17-yard line by Barton Frye. On the final play of the game, Toscano hit his favorite receiver, Gene Huey, who was pulled down on the Tiger five by Kent, who was injured on the play.

LSU's Glenn Smith, a sophomore tailback, who put new life in the Tiger attack in the second half with some fine running, was chosen as the game's Most Valuable Player.

Smith carried 16 times and netted 74 yards for a 4.7 average.

LSU's senior linebacker, Benny Griffin, intercepted two Toscano aerials and was a standout for the Bengals on defense.

It was Griffin's second interception and his 17-yard run back to the Wyoming 31 set-up the winning score for the Tigers.

Another Tiger standout was Tommy Morel, the fleet Tiger end, who grabbed two touchdown passes — his second the winning score, a 16-yard grab between a pair of Wyoming defenders.

The Bengals managed to finish the game with a net 151 yards running and net 91 in the air, while the Cowboys picked up 167 yards on the ground and 239 in the air.

Stokley hit on only six passes in 20 attempts while Toscano hit on 14 of 23.

LSU's Glenn Smith, a sophomore tailback, who put new life in the Tiger attack in the second half with some fine running, was chosen as the game's Most Valuable Player.

Score by Periods

LSU	0	0	7	13	— 20
Wyoming	0	13	0	0	— 13

However, the little Bengal pitched a pair of scoring aerials and climaxed his first full-time season with a creditable performance.

Coach Charlie McClendon reached deep into his reserve crew today and had a half dozen reserves in the lineup when the Tigers marched 80 yards for their first score with Smith going over from the 1-yard line.

On this drive, it was Smith's clutch running and Stokley's pitching that kept the drive alive.

A few minutes later, LSU drove 52 yards for the deadlocking score with Stokley pitching to Morel for eight yards and the score.

Roy Hurd, who booted the first Tiger extra point, missed the second and left the game tied at 13-all with 11:39 left in the game.

LSU had a chance in the final seven minutes when Tommy Youngblood intercepted Kiick's halfback pass at the Tiger 35, but the Bengals couldn't move.

Then came the Griffin interception, the second of the day for the Tiger linebacker, and LSU moved in for the victory after Griffin's runback to the Cowboy 31 set up the drive.

Smith hit off right end for 16 yards and a first down at the Wyoming 15 and then made two yards before Stokley found Morel in the end zone and hit him with a fine pitch. Hurd's boot gave the Bengals a 20-13 lead with 4:32 left but the Cowboys never quit and came back to end the game with the ball on the Tiger 5.

Before the Cowboys made their desperate last-second drive to tie the game or win, LSU's Youngblood hit Toscano hard on a driving tackle, forcing a fumble, and Tiger defensive end Johnny Garlington recovered for LSU at the Cowboy 43.

The Bengals attempted to run out the clock but Wyoming used their remaining timeouts to stop the ticking clock and LSU was forced to punt with 45 seconds left to play.

Then came the fluke pass that almost cost LSU a victory when Tiger defenders batted the ball into Anderson's hands and the play was a 54-yard aerial after Frye bumped the big end on the Tiger 17.

Depoyster lived up to his great kicking reputation, despite having his first field goal blocked by Tiger Fred Michaelson.

Depoyster's 49-yard field goal broke the old Sugar Bowl mark of 48 yards set by Alabama's Tim Davis' old mark of 48-plus set in 1964.

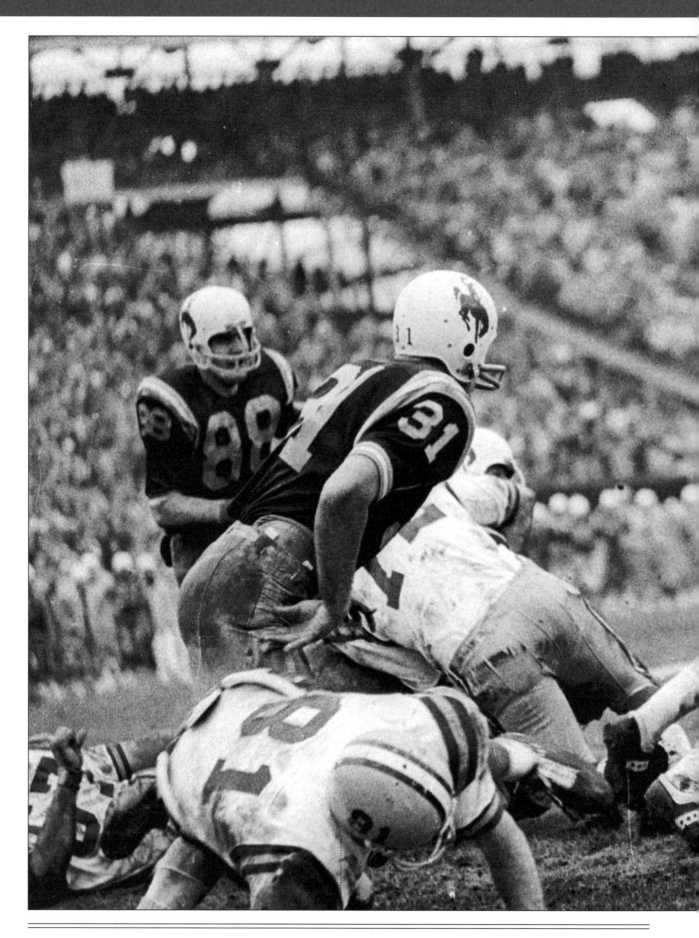

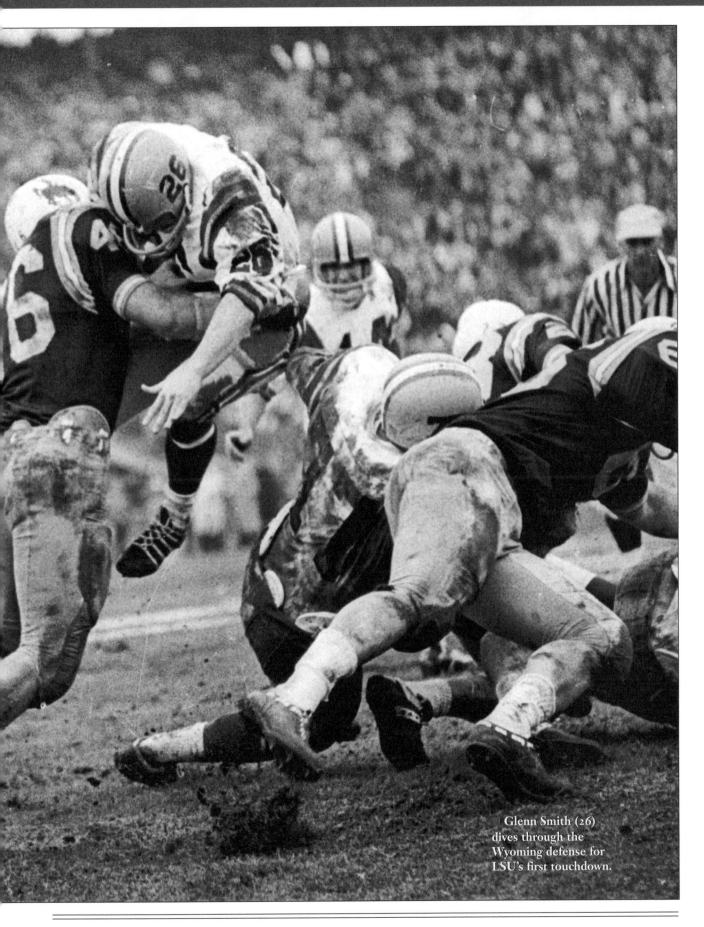

Glenn Smith (26) dives through the Wyoming defense for LSU's first touchdown.

Tigers Come From Behind to Defeat Oregon, 13-14

The Advocate

Baton Rouge, La. — *Dec. 14, 1934*

Snapping back with flashy scoring thrusts after being out-classed for nearly half the game and with defeat staring starkly at them, LSU's gridmen overcame a two-touchdown lead today to defeat Oregon, 14-13.

The accurate extra-point kicking toe of Ernie Seago, the brilliant Abe Mickal's understudy kicker, and Oregon derision, that put misjudged faith in a pass instead of a kick for the extra point, directly accounted for LSU's triumph.

Oregon's emerald-jerseyed warriors, playing smart, fast football, and led by the dashing backs, Frank Michek and Maurice Van Vilet, hammered and passed two touchdowns in the first and second periods to lead LSU, 13-0.

Early in the second period, Van Vilet, as if to make up for the missed extra point, broke through left guard from the Tiger 26-yard line and dodged LSU tacklers to the Tiger goal line.

Score by Periods

LSU	0	7	0	7 —	14
Oregon	6	7	0	0 —	13

This time V. Walker, a substitute end, kicked the extra point.

Then LSU coach Biff Jones, after sending in his reserves, who fought viciously, kept the Oregonians at bay for a while, thus allowing his first stringers to get a new strategy and shot them back in. From then on it was a different game.

Mickal began zipping passes to Jeff Barrett, the LSU end and crack receiver, and drove to the Oregon 4-yard line. From there, Mickal slipped a flat one to Barrett over the goal line. Seago kicked the extra point.

With the end of the game nearing, and with Mickal out, Jesse Fatheree, the race-horse of the Tiger squad, tore around left end for 39 yards and a touchdown. Seago's point-after kick sealed the win.

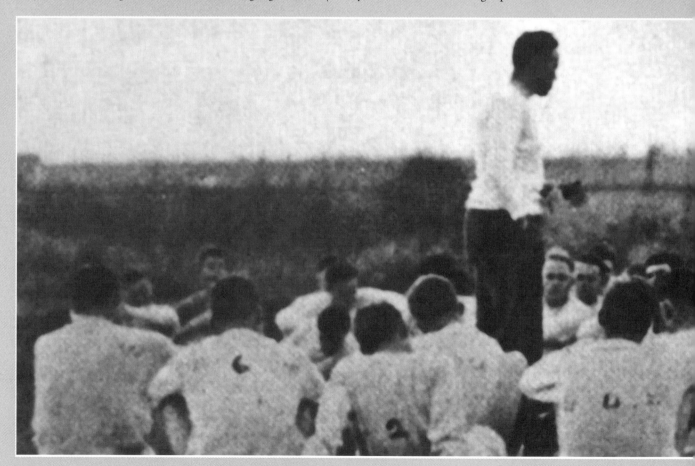

Jones & Huey at Odds, LSU Coach Rumored to Resign

The Advocate

Baton Rouge, La. — *Dec. 14, 1934*

Lawrence (Biff) Jones, the LSU football coach said tonight he had "nothing to say" about reports that he had resigned after today's game with the University of Oregon.

Reports were rampant in Baton Rouge tonight that Jones, an army captain and former football coach at West Point, had resigned after an argument with Senator Huey P. Long.

"Have you resigned because of any difficulty with Senator Long?" he was asked.

"I have nothing to say," was his only reply.

Senator Long this year has been an exuberant booster of the LSU grid team and at one time financed a trip for almost the entire LSU student body to the game with Vanderbilt at Nashville, Tenn.

Last month, he masterminded the holding of a mock election on the university campus in which Abe Mickal, the star LSU halfback, was named a "state senator."

Long had made all the plans for Mickal to take a "seat" in the senate during the last special session but Coach Jones conferred with Long and the elaborate "induction" ceremony was called off.

When efforts were made by telephone to reach Senator Long at his hotel for comment, attendants at his suite announced he had retired for the night and could not be disturbed until morning.

Jones appeared angry as he received questions regarding his reported resignation.

"It's too late to talk," he asserted. "I have nothing to say. I've had a hard season and I'm tired."

Athletic Director T.F. Heard of LSU said he knew nothing of the reported resignation. "I've very sorry, but I don't know anything about it," he declared.

Jones refused to talk to newsmen who sought to interview him at his home, other than to repeat he had "nothing to say."

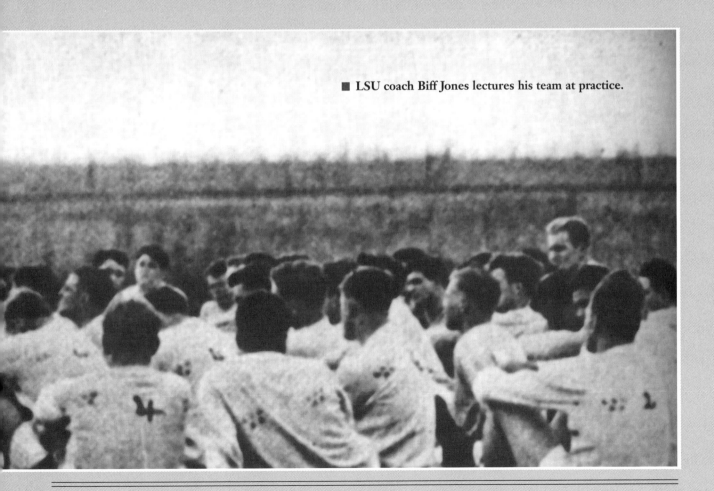

■ LSU coach Biff Jones lectures his team at practice.

The Kingfish, Biff & the Golden Thirties

BY SCOTT RABALAIS
The Advocate

A benevolent dictator. A demagogue. A consummate politician. And the most ardent and powerful LSU football fan of all time.

Huey Pierce Long was all those things. And from the late 1920's until his assassination in 1935, Louisiana was his state, LSU was his university, and the Tigers were his football team.

When it came to LSU, nothing was too audacious for Long. He recruited players then invited them to live in the governor's mansion. He even once tried to make one of his favorite Tigers a state senator. He transformed the school's band from a small military outfit to a marching musical army. He railroaded the railroads into providing low-cost transportation for LSU students to away games, and bluffed a circus into altering its schedule so it wouldn't draw fans away from a crucial home game.

Huey Long could do it all because he had all the power. His power came from the common people, the ones in later years to whom he preached "Share our wealth," and the people loved football. It is, and was even in Long's day, one of the few spectacles that can draw tens of thousands of people to one place at one time, and the game's popularity, energy and excitement captivated Long.

Though a one-time Tulane law student, Long became a devoted LSU fan. He immersed himself in football and in the Tigers, ecstatic in their victories and laid low by their defeats.

Huey became, as former LSU All-American and later coach Gus Tinsley once recalled, quite well versed in the intricacies of the game. Once in a chance meeting with Tinsley on the state capitol steps following the 1934 season, Long began drawing plays on the slabs of stone with a pencil. His ideas were, Tinsley remembered, very good for someone without a coach or player's knowledge of the game.

In 1928, Long was a newly elected governor and Russ Cohen was LSU's new head football coach, having succeeded Mike Donahue. Cohen's Tigers got off to a superb 4-0 start and were preparing for their then annual battle with Arkansas in Shreveport when Long arrived at the practice fields.

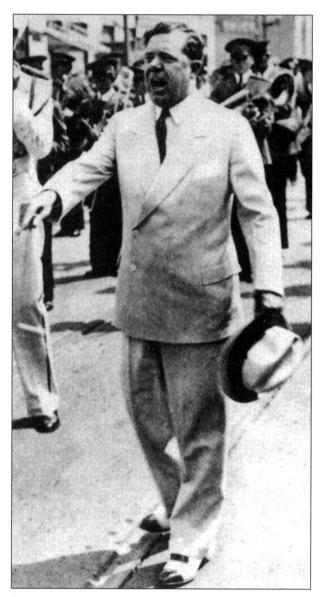

■ **Huey Long enjoys his favorite pastime, leading the LSU band.**

Long came to explain to Cohen the importance of the game in terms of how it affected the Kingfish. He hated everyone in Shreveport, Long told Cohen, and everyone in Shreveport hated him. Therefore, to Long's way of thinking, the Tigers simply had to win.

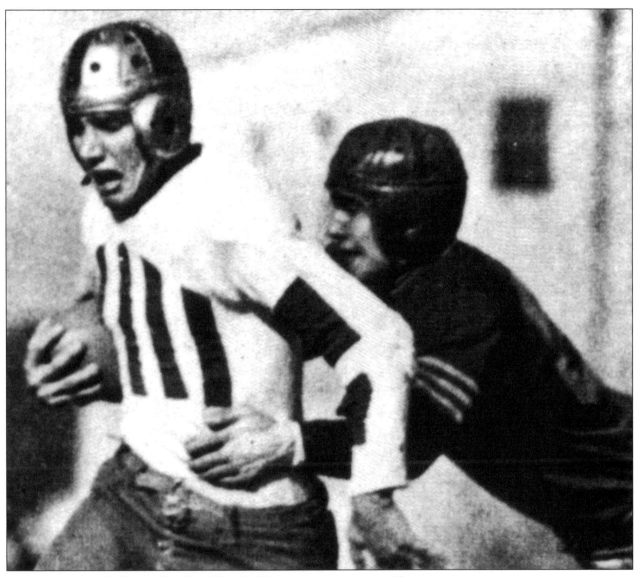

■ **LSU legendary halfback Abe Mickal led the Tigers to a 23-3-3 record from 1933-1935.**

They didn't, falling 7-0, but Long wasn't in a mood to call for Cohen's head. He was at this stage of his political life not entirely caught up in calling the shots at LSU, but would grow into that role soon enough.

Long did quickly become a recruiter for the Tigers. Shortly after Huey came to power, Cohen told him that he was interested in a hot prep prospect named Joe Almokary. According to Dan Hardesty's book, *The Louisiana Tigers*, this was the gist of Huey's recruiting pitch:

Long: "Are you going to come to LSU?"

Almokary: "I don't know. I think maybe I'll go to Centenary (which had a strong football program at the time)."

Long: "What in the world would you want to go to Centenary for? They can't teach you anything but the Bible, and I know more about the Bible than they do. If you come to LSU you can get any kind of education you want. What do you want to be when you finish college?"

Almokary: "I would like to be a lawyer."

Long: "You want to be a lawyer. I don't think you would be a good lawyer. You look to me like you would make a good engineer. They can't teach you engineering at Centenary. You're good at mathematics, aren't you?"

Almokary: "Yes, sir."

Long: "You're good at algebra?"

Almokary: "Yes, sir."

Long: "Geometry?"

Almokary: "Yes, sir."

Long: "Good in calculus?"

Almokary: "Yes, sir."

Long: "You see, I told you that you would make a good engineer. You certainly should come to LSU."

Almokary admitted afterward he didn't have much idea what Long was talking about, but was scared to say so. He lettered at LSU for three years.

Late in 1930, Long's growing grip on LSU football and the state was becoming quite evident. That fall he was elected to the U.S. Senate, although he served out his term as governor and did not officially take his senate seat until 1932.

Meanwhile, the Tigers had slipped to an indifferent 6-3 record with a 33-0 thrashing by Alabama, and the LSU Board of Supervisors voted to move Cohen from the job of football coach to the athletic director's office. However, the new coach had to be approved by the school's newly appointed president, James Monroe Smith, and Governor Long.

LSU's 1930 finale was a narrow 12-7 loss to a strong Tulane team. But instead of sealing Cohen's demise, the game gave him new life. The Monday following the Tulane game, Cohen signed a new three-year contract in the Governor's Mansion. Cohen was the only man in Louisiana, Long informed him, that had his name on a contract without first providing Huey with his undated resignation.

Long delighted in providing LSU with players, and with providing certain favored players with all the comforts the mansion had to offer.

One such player was Art Foley, a brilliant halfback from Oklahoma. Foley's stay in Baton Rouge was brief — he played just one game before a lung ailment forced him to leave Louisiana's humid climate — but while he was with the team he was Huey's house guest.

So were Tigers Ed Khoury, LSU's team captain in 1931, Billy Butler and Sid Bowman. They feasted on steak, cornbread, turnip greens and pineapple upside down cake twice a day and washed it down with soured milk (for some reason, Huey believed milk was best if it had been allowed to sit out until it turned sour).

But all of Huey's efforts as a cheerleader, power broker and training table expert turned out to be in vain. Cohen's Tigers struggled through a 5-4 campaign, culminating with a 34-7 pounding by Rose Bowl-bound Tulane. Cohen was out, and Huey was on the search for a new coach.

Finding quality candidates for the job wasn't easy because of one thing: Huey's intrusive presence. They had reason to worry, given Lewis Gottlieb's description of the coaching search in *The Louisiana Tigers*, a search that resulted in the hiring of Lawrence (Biff) Jones:

"I was on the athletic council at the time, but I had absolutely no part in his selection," Gottlieb said. "Nobody really did but Huey. We didn't know anything about it until we were told that Jones was going to be the new coach. He had a good record and nobody complained about the choice, but I'm not sure that it would have done any good if anybody had complained."

Jones had been head coach at Army from 1927-29 and was at the time assistant athletic director at West Point. It took some convincing and a personal request to General Douglas MacArthur, then the Army chief of staff, but Jones finally became LSU's head coach. So that he didn't have to resign from the Army to take the job, the new coach was detailed to LSU as a military science instructor.

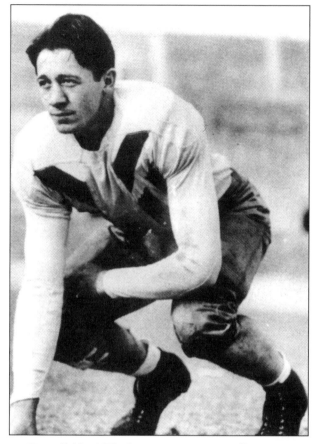

■ **Gaynell (Gus) Tinsley was a two-time All-American in 1935 and 1936.**

One of Jones' first acts as head coach was to convince Long to stay out of the pep talk business. For once, Huey listened to someone else's wishes and kept any desires to make emotional pleas to the team to a minimum — for the time being.

Satisfied that he had a good coach capable of building him a winner, Huey began to turn his attention toward improving the LSU marching band — and becoming its bandleader. For the Tigers first road game of 1932, an Oct. 1 trip to Houston, Long led a 150-cadet formation through the downtown streets. Sometimes he was drum major, other times cheerleader, always in control.

"Huey loved the band, LSU and the football team," said Lew Williams, LSU's real drum major from 1929 to 1934. "He did everything he could to help us."

LSU's record in 1932 was a modest 6-3-1, though it did include a 14-0 victory over its most despised rival, Tulane. Among Tiger fans, including Long, optimism reigned as LSU became one of 13 schools to form the Southeastern Conference in 1933.

That year the Tigers enjoyed their most successful season since the perfect 10-0 campaign of 1908. LSU posted the odd-looking record of 7-0-3 and 3-0-2 in the SEC, finishing percentage points behind 5-0-1 Alabama for the league's first title. Expectations rose even high for 1934.

The schedule would prove to be too tough for LSU to post

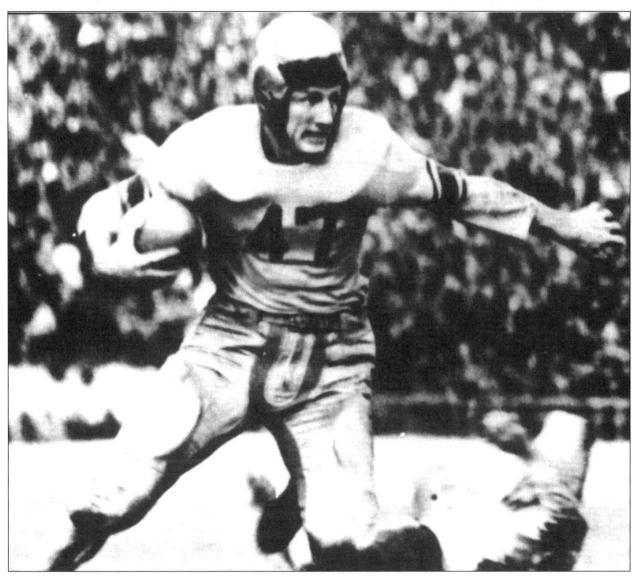

■ **George (Pinky) Rohm was a stellar halfback for the Tigers from 1935-37.**

a brilliant record, though the Tigers went 7-2-2. However, Huey was in unprecedented form, his antics the equivalent of an undefeated season in their own right.

From the outset, Long had Jones squirming with boasts to sportswriters that LSU had the best team in the country, and could back up his claim by taking on national contenders Alabama and Minnesota on the same day. The statement may have been laughable, but the Kingfish wasn't joking when, according to T. Harry Williams definitive biography, *Huey Long*, the senator looked into the eyes of an assistant coach and said: "LSU can't have a losing team because that'll mean I'm associated with a loser."

After a season-opening 9-9 tie at Rice, the Tigers prepared for their Oct. 6 home opener against Southern Methodist. Despite LSU's successes ticket sales were sluggish. This was a particularly sticky problem, since athletic director T.P. Heard had to offer SMU a large $10,000 guarantee to make the trip from Dallas.

Long asked Heard what he thought the problem was.

Heard replied that the famous Barnum & Bailey Circus was making an appearance in Baton Rouge that night and was apparently making a big dent in the advance ticket sales. Huey sprang to action like a circus tiger. Before Barnum & Bailey could move its production from Texas to Baton Rouge, Long and an assisting law student looked through Louisiana's sanitary code to find something useful. They did: an obscure cattle dipping law which Huey seized upon to use to his advantage.

Long asked for a meeting with Barnum & Bailey's advance man. To the visitor's astonishment, Huey informed him of the dipping law and Long's intention to enforce it. For vivid effect, Long asked the man if his circus had ever dipped one of its tigers, much less an elephant. All Barnum & Bailey had to do was cancel the Saturday night show.

The circus decided it unwise to call Huey's bluff on so important a matter as LSU football. The performance was canceled, ticket sales surged and Heard made more than enough profit to cover the guarantee to SMU, which battled LSU to a 14-14 tie.

Huey's circus act was just a warmup to bigger stunts in the weeks ahead. As LSU's Oct. 27 game at Vanderbilt approached, the Kingfish decided that he should bring LSU to Nashville, or at least as much of it as could be arranged.

"No student should miss this trip because of a lack of funds," Huey announced, and then set about the task of transporting most of LSU's student body to Tennessee.

The first hurdle was to talk the Illinois Central into providing those students with an affordable fare. Naturally, the railroad balked at slashing the price of what was then a $19 round trip ticket. So Huey responded by suggesting to railroad officials that it would be sad indeed for them if the Louisiana legislature — Huey's legislature — should raise the tax assessment on the railroad's bridges across the state from their current level of $100,000 to their rightful value of $4 million.

Like so many others who squared off against Huey, the Illinois Central backed down. The fare was slashed to $6.

This was still a considerable sum for many students. So Long emptied his wallet in a visit to the campus and later doled out thousands from his suite at the old Heidelberg Hotel. All they had to do was provide their name — or any name as the case might be — and add it to the list headed "I. O. Huey." Many of them borrowed the train fare and $1 for meals.

"I'm expecting most of this money back within a year," Huey said. Months later, he remarked that indeed most of the loans had been repaid, although retired Advocate sports editor Bud Montet didn't remember it that way. "I don't recall anyone who did," said Montet, who was a junior at LSU when he made the trip. "It wasn't like Huey was standing on the street corner."

By Friday afternoon some 5,000 people were ready to make the trip, including a 125-piece band and 1,500 ROTC students. Five trains of 14-cars each pulled out of Baton Rouge, each with a color designation: Red for cadets; white for players, the band and coaches (Huey and his party had their own car on this train); blue for non-military students and co-eds; green and orange for more regular students and fans.

While money was tight enough that many of them needed to borrow money from Huey, there was still enough discretionary income on board to keep craps games going in virtually every car.

"You had nickel, quarter, four bits and dollar games," Montet said. "It was the middle of the depression in '34, so the craps limits were pretty low. It was all quite a show, one not lost upon the media of the day, as told in Harnett Kane's book *Louisiana Hayride*:

"Huey's football shows could not be kept out of the newspapers, no matter how much the newspapers hated Huey. They were spectacles in the Billy Rose-Roxy tradition: 2,000 cadets, 200 musicians, 50 'purple jackets' — co-eds in white pleats, blazers and 50 smiles — octets of dancing boy and girl cheerleaders and 50 sponsors in a row. And the star of the troupe, Huey, swinging, roaring, hightailing it at the head of the march. He led his boys and girls down the main streets of the invaded towns,

razzled-dazzled over the field between halves and, remained, as usual, perilously close to the players during the game."

He had hardly slept when the train arrived in Nashville at 9 a.m. Saturday. Nonetheless the Kingfish, accompanied by bodyguards who had hastily been deputized as Tennessee game wardens so they could carry weapons, jumped from the train ready to lead his cadets on a two-mile march through downtown Nashville. The townsfolk responded with wild cheers and the headline across the front page of The Nashville Banner summed up the moment quite appropriately: "Nashville Surrenders to Huey Long."

A few hours later, Vanderbilt surrendered to LSU, 29-0. About the only disappointment the day may have held for some was that Huey did not announce his candidacy for president as had been rumored.

While Huey was not yet ready to run for the White House, he returned home ready to make LSU's star quarterback a state senator. During one of many special legislative sessions he called during his reign, Long arranged to honor quarterback Abe Mickal as a "de facto" state senator.

The fact Mickal was underage to hold office, wasn't even a Louisiana resident (he was from McComb, Miss.) and that the whole business infuriated Biff Jones because of what he feared it would do to team morale didn't faze Huey. When T.P. Heard relayed Jones' feelings to Long, the Kingfish offered to make all the Tigers state senators. At last, when it was pointed out that the $10 a day paid to senators might jeopardize a player's amateur status, Long finally relented, and "Senator" Mickal was removed from office. By season's end, it was Biff Jones who was removing himself from office.

A bitter 13-12 loss to Tulane left the Kingfish declaring that Jones might not be the worst coach around, "but he sure ain't the best." Apparently, Huey had forgotten the 18-game unbeaten streak LSU had enjoyed under Jones going into the Tulane game.

A 19-13 loss at Tennessee a week later didn't improve the senator's mood, especially when Jones played a battered Mickal against Huey's wishes. It set the scene for cold relations on a cold December day when Oregon visited LSU in the season finale.

LSU played listlessly in the first half and trailed, 13-0, at halftime. As Jones was about to address his players, Long appeared at the dressing room door asking to talk to the team. According to Peter Finney's *The Fighting Tigers*, this was the exchange between coach and senator:

Long: "Can I talk to the team?"

Jones: "No."

Long: "Who's going to stop me?"

Jones: "Well, you're not going to talk."

Long: "Well, I'm sick of losing and tying games. You'd better win this one."

Jones: "Well, Senator, get this: win, lose or draw, I quit."

Long: "That's a bargain."

For the first time as LSU's coach, Jones then asked his Tigers to win one for him. They did, 14-13, but it did little to soothe the situation, especially once word of Jones' resignation reached

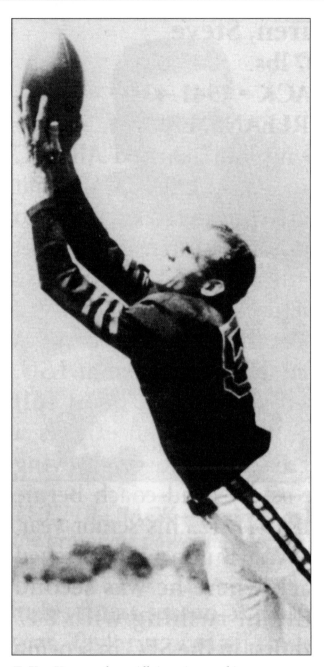

■ **Ken Kavanaugh, an All-American end in 1939.**

the press. Both men thought badly of their encounter but neither one wanted to back down publicly. In the end, Jones and Long reached an amicable parting, but the fact remained that once again LSU was in the market for a football coach.

After his row with Jones, Huey boasted of bringing in a big-name coach, so big that he would make everyone forget Biff Jones. Indeed it was a big name, Alabama's Frank Thomas, whom the Kingfish set his sights on, and in late 1934 the two hammered out a secret deal that would have paid Thomas $15,000 a year. Thomas' only stipulation was that their agreement stay out of the press he prepared the Crimson Tide for a trip to the Rose Bowl.

But as the days passed, Huey became converted by recommendations that he hire Bernie Moore, a long-time assistant of Jones and Cohen who also coached LSU to the 1933 NCAA track and field championship. Long had dispatched Heard to Southern California to keep tabs on Thomas, but when Heard arrived in Los Angeles he picked up a paper which told him: "Kingfish Appoints Moore Head Coach."

Some felt Moore was a political choice, and Moore suffered the loss of some of his friends by way of the association.

Huey kept quiet publicly after Moore's hiring. At the time he was also deeply involved in the LSU band, having "kidnapped" Castro Carazo from his job as orchestra leader at New Orleans' Roosevelt Hotel to become leader of the school's marching band. It was Carazo who helped the Kingfish write the song that would become his anthem, *Every Man a King*, as well as one of LSU's fight songs, *Touchdown for LSU*.

Not long after he appointed Moore, Huey consulted retired Vanderbilt coach Dan McGugin for a can't miss play. McGugin gave Long a play he called "Number 88," which Long passed on to his new coach. LSU may have been working on "Number 88" the last time Huey ever saw his beloved Tigers.

It was Sept. 3, and Long had stopped to watch practice after a cross-country speaking tour that was a prelude to a likely third-party presidential campaign in 1936. The senator had returned to Baton Rouge to preside over yet another special session whose sole purpose was to rubber stamp whatever legislation the Kingfish wanted passed.

Five days later, during a late-night session at the state capitol, Dr. Carl Austin Weiss stepped from the shadows and pointed a .32 automatic pistol at Long. Whether Weiss actually fired the bullet that struck Long or whether it came from one of Long's bodyguards when they saw the young doctor draw his weapon will always remain the subject of conjecture.

Whatever happened, the facts were Weiss was shot to death on the spot and Long was mortally wounded. He would die early on the morning of Sept. 10 at the age of 42. Two days later, with drums muffled, Carazo's LSU band played "Every Man a King" in dirge-like fashion as Long was laid to rest in the gardens fronting the capitol.

"Number 88" went to the grave with Huey, as Moore never felt obliged to call it with the Kingfish no longer patrolling the sidelines. But even if Moore hadn't used the play, Long would have loved what he would have seen from the Tigers in 1935. LSU won the first of two straight Southeastern Conference titles and made the first of three consecutive trips to the Sugar Bowl.

So ended the Huey Long era of LSU football. The Tigers would go on to greater glories in years to come and in the 1960's and 70's became the darlings of another governor's eye, a governor named John McKeithen.

But never again would one governor be able to politically afford to lavish the money and attention on LSU and its football program that Huey Long directed toward them. If Long wanted to make every man a king, the LSU Tigers were the jewels in the crown.

LSU Breaks Aggie Win-Streak

By Bud Montet
The Advocate

Baton Rouge, La. — *Sept. 21, 1968*

The LSU Tigers had to come from behind a 12-point deficit to continue their jinx over the Texas A&M Aggies at Tiger Stadium tonight as they staged a fourth-quarter comeback and grabbed a 13-12 thriller that wasn't decided until the final two seconds before 68,000 hysterical fans.

The victory once again proved the Tigers are fast becoming the best "streak" stoppers in collegiate football.

The Aggies entered the game with a seven-game win streak only to see the Bengals stop it. Less than nine months ago the Tigers beat the Wyoming Cowboys in the Sugar Bowl and ended their 1967 undefeated streak.

Coach Charlie McClendon and his Tigers also halted the Arkansas Razorbacks' 22-game win streak in the 1966 Cotton Bowl and in his first effort as head coach of the Bengals, McClendon halted a long Texas Longhorns' streak.

Texas A&M grabbed the first nine points in a minute and 36 seconds when a booming Steve O'Neal boot of 46 yards bounced out of bounds on the Tiger one-foot line.

The Aggies got their first two points when Mickey Christian, a defensive end turned snapper, tossed the ball over Eddie Ray's head in the end zone on an attempted kick.

The safety gave the Aggies a two-point lead with 4:09 left in the first period.

In less than two minutes, the Aggies picked up their lone touchdown when they drove 46 yards in four plays. A Tiger roughing penalty against an Aggie punt returner set up the drive. The Aggies' Edd Hargett pitched 19 yards to Barney

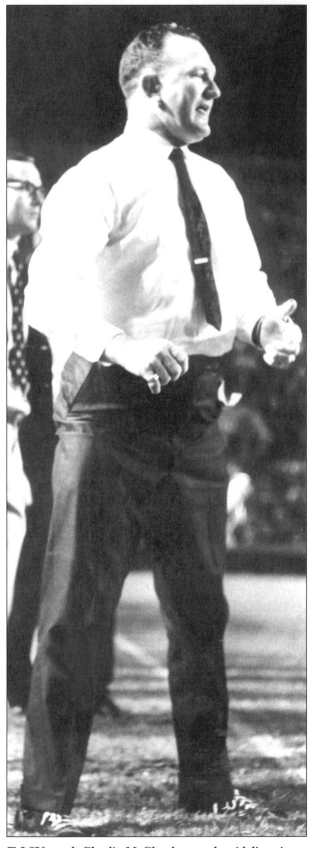

■ **LSU coach Charlie McClendon on the sidelines in Tiger Stadium.**

Harris at the Tiger 32, and came back to hit Bob Long with a 25-yard pass for another first down at the LSU 3.

After Larry Stegent was held for no gain, Hargett pitched to Long in the Tiger end zone for the touchdown and Riggs' extra-point boot gave the Aggies a 9-0 lead.

A poor 17-yard punt by Eddie Ray of the Tigers in the fading minutes of the second quarter gave the Aggies a chance to add a field goal.

The Aggies took over on the LSU 35 and moved to the nine where a penalty caught them and they had to be satisfied with a 31-yard field goal by Riggs.

LSU stormed back to go 80 yards in nine plays with Haynes leading the charge to the Aggie 34 where Jimmy Gilbert, playing his first game at quarterback for LSU, moved the Bengals on in.

Gilbert pitched to Bob Hamlett for 16 yards and a first down at the Aggie 18 and after Kenny Newfield drove for eight yards, Gilbert came back to sweep seven yards around right end for a first own at the A&M 3.

Frank Matte, the Tiger "utility" man, then drove over right guard for a touchdown but Mark Lumpkin missed the point after and LSU had to be satisfied with a 12-6 score at the intermission.

The fourth quarter was one of the wildest ever seen in Tiger Stadium. The Aggies started it off when Riggs missed an attempted 43-yard field goal.

Maurice LeBlanc set up the Tigers' winning march when he returned a 51-yard O'Neal punt 16 yards to the LSU 46.

Haynes then took over and drove the Bengals downfield to score in 10 plays. The winning touchdown came on a pitchout from Haynes to West around left end with the fleet West getting a great block from Tommy (Trigger) Allen to spring him over the goal line.

This time Lumpkin booted the extra-point kick and LSU held a slim 13-12 lead with 7:47 left in the game. The Aggies roared back with Hargett pitching to Stegent and the Aggies gaining the ball at their 48 when Gerry Kent, the Tiger defensive back, was ruled interfering with the receiver.

A 15-yard penalty pushed the Aggies back to their 34 and Hargett was tossed for a nine-yard loss back to the Aggie 25. Hargett then hit Jimmy Adams with a 47-yard aerial for a first down at the LSU 28.

Hargett came right back to hit Long with a 23-yarder and a first down at the LSU 5. After LSU stopped Stegent for no gain, Hargett pitched out to Long who fumbled over the goal line. The play was ruled a touchback and LSU gained possession at their 20.

Haynes put the clincher on the game by keeping a drive

Score by Periods

LSU	0	6	0	7	— 13
Texas A&M	9	3	0	0	— 12

going to the Aggie 37, making the drive eat up the clock time by staying on the ground.

Three times Haynes picked up crucial first down yardage to keep the drive going. However, with less than a minute left, Haynes fumbled at the Aggie 36 and Bill Hobbs recovered for the Aggies with seconds left.

Hargett hit Long with a pass to the Tiger 46 for a first down and, with ten seconds left, Hargett killed the clock with an out of bounds pass.

Hargett then pitched a long pass out of bounds. With two seconds left, Long attempted a 61-yard field goal that fell short and was fielded by LSU as the game ended.

The defeat was a heart-rending one for Coach Gene Stallings and his Aggies. The Aggies haven't downed the Bengals in Tiger Stadium since 1956 and Stalling has yet to post a victory over the Tigers since taking over the head job at Aggieland.

The Tigers' Haynes sparked the Bengals' touchdown drives, getting the first underway before turning the job over to Gilbert and engineering the second and winning scoring push. Haynes also teamed with Allen to slowly drive downfield in the waning minutes to wipe time off the clock and put the Aggies in the hole although a fumble gave them a last second desperate chance to pull the game from a loss to a victory.

Haynes pitched 11 times and hit on five passes for 64 yards and teamed with Allen as the workhorses of the Tiger offense.

Allen accounted for 56 yards on 20 carries.

The Aggies' touted Hargett passed 28 times and hit on 13 passes for 220 yards and one touchdown. His longest pass play was a 47-yarder in the fading seconds.

However, the Aggies' best weapon was the great kicking of O'Neal who punted nine times for a sensational 47.4 average which bettered LSU's Eddie Ray, who turned in a 39.6 average effort.

Not only did O'Neal keep the Tigers in the hole much of the first half, it was his booming boot out of bounds on the Tiger one-foot line that shook the Bengals and allowed the Aggies to get nine points in less than two minutes.

The Bengals edged the Aggies in total offense with 283 yards to 225 for the visitors. LSU gained 203 yards on the ground and 80 in the air while the Aggies netted but 46 yards on the ground and 220 in the air.

The defeat was a heart-rending one for Coach Gene Stallings and his Aggies. The Aggies haven't downed the Bengals in Tiger Stadium since 1956 and Stalling has yet to post a victory over the Tigers since taking over the head job at Aggieland.

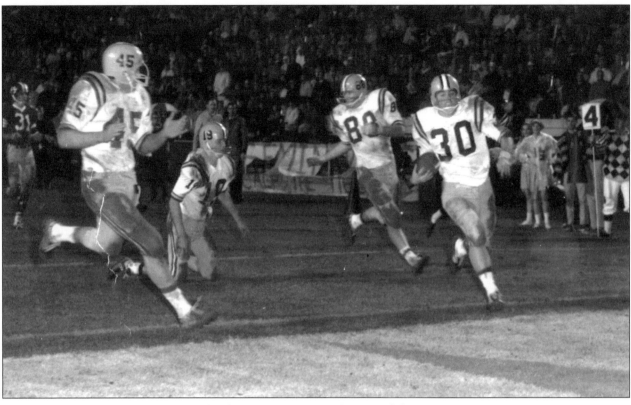

■ LSU's Craig Burns (30) returns a Florida State interception for a touchdown.

LSU Scalps Seminoles, 31-27

By Bud Montet
The Advocate

Atlanta, Ga. — *Dec. 30, 1968*

The LSU Tigers spent the night trying to find the handle on the football and Florida State's Bill Cappleman spent three quarters trying to find his ace receiver, Ron Sellers, and when the searches were over LSU won, 31-27, in the inaugural Peach Bowl victory.

The game was played in a steady shower that started an hour before the game. Some 35,545 fans braved the 40 degree weather to watch an exciting see-saw battle.

Score by Periods

LSU	0	10	14	7 —	31
Florida State	7	6	0	14 —	27

Tonight's victory was Coach Charlie McClendon's fifth bowl win in six tries. It was also doubly sweet as McClendon led the Tigers' win over former LSU assistant, Bill Peterson of Florida State.

LSU lost the football on fumbles three times in the opening quarter, opening the game with a fumble by Mark Lumpkin on the initial kickoff.

Florida State scored on their first scrimmage play with the Seminoles' Tom Bailey going 36 yards for the touchdown.

The Bengals then spent the rest of the first period march-

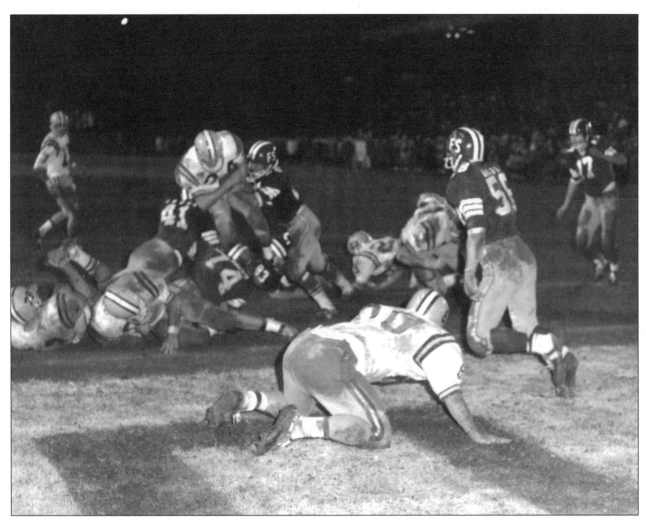

■ **Maurice Leblanc (34) scored LSU's winning touchdown on a 3-yard dive.**

ing on the Seminoles unable to reach the Florida State goal line due to fumbles and interceptions.

The Tigers managed to get over their fumbles after the first period though they had a relapse in the final period when Glenn Smith fumbled on a kickoff to give Cappleman and FSU a chance to go ahead, 27-24.

But the fumbling Bengals failed to give up and marched 61 yards in the fading minutes to score the winning touchdown with Maurice Leblanc going over from the FSU 3 to give LSU its 31-27 victory.

Florida State's Cappleman had trouble finding his ace receiver, the nation's top receiver, Sellers, who caught but one pass for 18 yards in the first half.

However, Cappleman found Sellers in the second half and hit him seven times in the final half. Sellers grabbed eight aerials for 76 yards and two went for touchdowns.

LSU's Mike Hillman, who outpitched

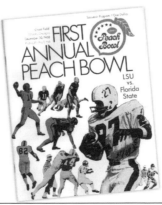

Cappleman, hit 16 receivers in 29 tries for 229 yards and two scores.

The hard working lefty also set up the winning touchdown when he staged a beautiful fake and raced around right end for 11 yards to the Seminoles' 3. Hillman had but one pass intercepted.

His great work gained him the Clint Castleberry Trophy as the outstanding offensive player.

Buddy Millican, a late starter for the Bengals, turned in a superb defensive end performance and this gained him the Smiley Johnson Award as the outstanding defensive player.

Millican constantly harassed Cappleman and tossed him for big losses a number of times.

Cappleman hit on 21 of 41 aerials for 221 yards and three scores.

The Tigers dominated the game, rolling up 22 first downs to 19 for the Seminoles. LSU netted 151 yards on the ground to 92 for the Seminoles.

In passing the Bengals netted 233 yards to 221 for Florida State.

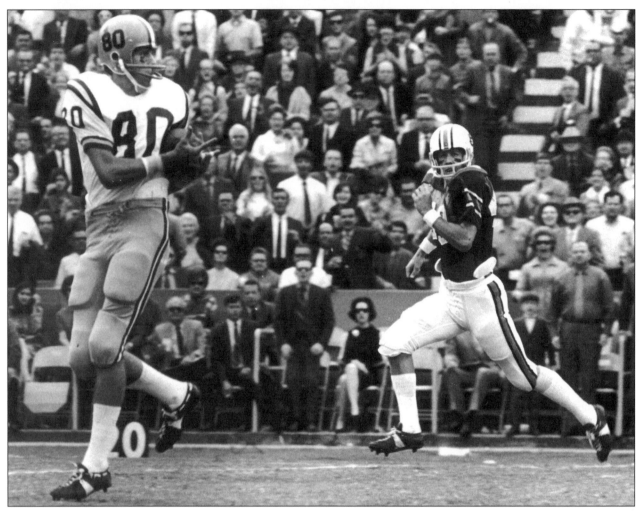

■ Andy Hamilton (80) scored his 62-yard touchdown on the first play of the game.

Bevan Blocks Auburn Kick in Tigers' 21-20 Win

By Bud Montet
The Advocate

Baton Rouge,La. — *Oct. 25, 1969*

The LSU Tigers managed to stay undefeated by the "foot" as Mark Lumpkin's three points after touchdown and Eddie Ray's booming punts in the second half gave the Bengals a 21-20 victory over the bruising and hard-hitting Auburn Tigers.

LSU scored on the first scrimmage play of the game when quarterback Mike Hillman pitched to tailback Jimmy Gilbert who hurled a pass to Andy Hamilton in the open and the fleet wide receiver raced over for the 62-yard touchdown.

For the next 62 minutes Auburn throttled the LSU offense and the Bengals didn't make another first down for the next 26 minutes.

Auburn came right back to tie the score when Pat Sullivan pitched a 12-yard scoring pass to Micky Zofko and John Riley tied the game with his point-after kick.

For the first time this season LSU slipped behind when Auburn's Buddy McClinton recovered an Eddie Ray fumble and moved 39 yards in five plays with a Sullivan to Connie Frederick aerial play for 33 yards — the key play in the drive. Wallace Clark went over from the LSU 2 and Riley added the extra point.

It was the only time this year the Bengals found their side of the scoreboard with a smaller figure than the opposition. Auburn protected their 14-7 lead until 23 seconds of the first half when LSU scored with Hillman pitching to Jim West.

West made a fine catch and Hillman, hotly badgered by a host of visiting Tigers, made a great effort to get the ball off.

Again Lumpkin came through with the point-after kick to tie the game at 14-all.

It was Gilbert's 29- and 15-yard gallops, back to back, that got the Tigers in scoring position.

LSU moved 75 yards in 11 plays the first time they got the football at the start of the second half. Stumpy Allen Shorey sliced through left guard for the touchdown and this time Lumpkin booted his third straight extra point — the one that later proved the difference.

Auburn got back in the game at the start of the fourth period when Sullivan hit Zofko with a 14-yard scoring pass.

Riley's extra-point kick to tie the game was blocked by George Bevan. Bill Thomason earlier had blocked a Riley field-goal attempt.

LSU had another chance to score midway in the fourth period when they moved from their 38 to the Auburn 12 but a penalty stopped the scoring drive and Lumpkin missed on an attempted 28-yard field goal.

In the fading seconds, Auburn tried a fourth down pass but Craig Burns batted the ball out of bounds and LSU killed the clock in two plays.

The victory gave the Bengals a 6-0 record and was their second Southeastern Conference victory.

It was Auburn's second loss and their second in conference play.

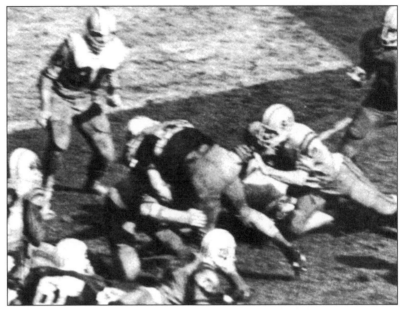

■ **Auburn's Wallace Clark dives over for a touchdown.**

The vaunted Auburn sophomore, Pat Sullivan, harried the LSU secondary defenses with his precision-thrown aerials. The slim sophomore hit on 13 of 34 passes for 221 yards. Sullivan had a pair intercepted.

LSU netted 149 yards on the ground and picked up 157 in the air for a total offense effort of 306 yards against the Auburn eleven that was leading the nation in total defense.

The game figures were about equal as Auburn rushed for 76 yards and passed for 221 for a total offense effort of 297 yards.

Big Ray who fumbled twice in the game made up for it with his great punting. Ray booted nine times for a 44-yard average and in the second half he booted one out on the five and kicked one dead on the two.

With the game hanging in the balance and a minute and 20 seconds left, Ray booted to the Auburn goal line — a 54 yard kick, and LSU held the return to 10 yards. Auburn then tried its final flurry of passes in an attempt to get back in front.

The game reminded one of famed past battles as the two Tiger elevens hit with authority all afternoon. Late in the game Mike Demarie of the Bengals had to leave the field of play.

Early in the game, Auburn kept the Bengals backed up against their goal line by some great kicking by Frederick.

LSU had possession at their 15, 12 and eight in the first half.

Hillman hit on five of 15 passes for 91 yards and one a scoring pass. Tight end Bill Strober was the chief target, grabbing four passes. Gilbert, with 61 yards in 10 carries, was the top Bengal ball carrier. Ray picked up 35 tough yards in 14 carries and Shorey got 22 in 12 carries.

Tommy Casanova had 88 kick return yards in three attempts during the afternoon.

The meeting was the first between the two Tiger elevens since 1942 when Auburn won.

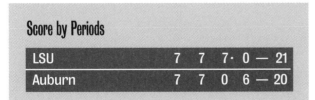

Score by Periods

LSU	7	7	7 · 0 — 21	
Auburn	7	7	0	6 — 20

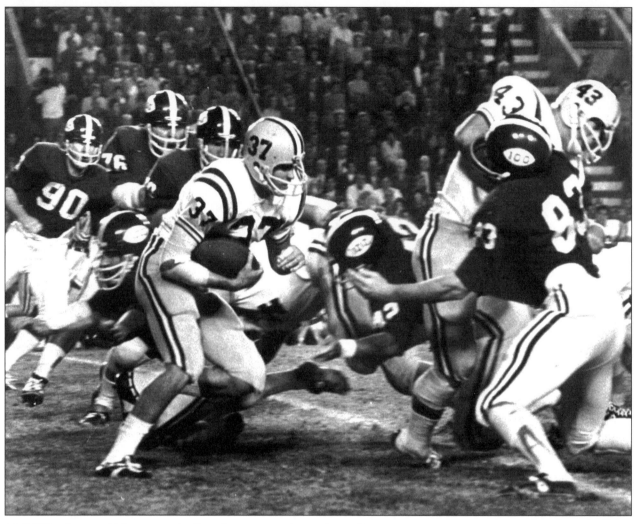

■ LSU's win over Alabama was its first since a 13-3 victory in 1958.

Tigers Break Loose Against Tide For 20-15 Win

By Bud Montet

The Advocate

Baton Rouge, La. — *Nov. 8, 1969*

LSU's erratic Bengals pulled out a 20-15 victory over the Alabama Crimson Tide, their first victory since 1958 and the first that Coach Charlie McClendon has won over his old coach, Paul (Bear) Bryant.

The victory was a hard fought one as LSU was constantly plagued by penalties and several times had ball carriers slopping down to stymie promising drives.

After the first half ended in a 3-3 deadlock, LSU came out at the start of the second half and drove 76 yards to score and take a 10-3 lead. They were never behind, although the Tide constantly threatened on the long bombs tossed by Alabama's Scott Hunter, who set two Tide school records with his great performance against the Bengals.

Alabama's two touchdowns came in the fourth period on long passes by Hunter. After LSU took their 10-3 lead. Hunter fired a 36-yard pass to Hunter Husband, a tight end, for a touchdown to get within four points of the Bengals.

LSU moved well out in front again with a 51-yard drive with Allen Shorey going over from the one — his second one-yard scoring jaunt of the game.

Trailing, 20-9, Alabama came right back with Hunter pitching five completions on the drive. The touchdown pass was a 34-yard shot to David Bailey, a sophomore split end, who beat Tiger James Earley to the end zone.

Mark Lumpkin put the Tigers in front in the second period with a 30-yard field goal but Alabama's Oran Buck tied the game at 3-all with his 26-yarder with 36 seconds left in the first half.

The Bengals blasted the Alabama ground defenses as stocky little Shorey raced for 118 yards in 26 carries and two touchdowns. Big Tiger fullback Eddie Ray gained 102 yards on 16 carries. It was the first time this season that an LSU back has netted more than 100 yards from scrimmage.

Hunter had his greatest night passing since he challenged Ole Miss's Archie Manning several weeks ago. The Alabama junior hit on 18 of 35 passes for 284 yards and two touchdowns.

However, he failed to get help from his rushers as LSU held the Alabama Tide to a net 47 yards on the ground.

LSU moved by rushing with 239 yards on the ground and 138 in the air. In total offense LSU totaled 377 yards and Alabama 331.

Aside from the many penalties, most coming in the first half, and other mistakes, the Bengals dominated the game with only Hunter's scoring bombs giving the Bengals trouble.

Tiger quarterback Mike Hillman used the aerials sparingly and pitched but 18 passes and hit on nine for 113 yards.

Split end Lonnie Myles was the chief Tiger receiver with five catches for 69 yards. Ken Kavanaugh Jr., the son of LSU's famed All-American Ken Kavanaugh, caught two aerials.

But the Bengals victory was achieved by blasting the Tiger lines with Shorey and Ray doing most of the carrying.

LSU threatened early in the game when midway in the first period they drove from their 13 to the Tide 39 where Hillman was tossed for a 13-yard loss and Butch Duhe missed on an attempted 47-yard field goal.

Alabama threatened at the start of the second quarter when they drove to the Tiger 21 where LSU held.

Midway in the second quarter, LSU drove from their four-yard line to the Tide 6 where a five-yard penalty set the Tigers back and LSU had to settle for Lumpkin's 30-yard field goal that put them in front.

Alabama got back into the game when Hunter pitched to George Ranager for 47 yards to the Tiger 24 and Alabama then had to settle for a field goal by Buck, a 26-yarder.

Ray and Shorey teamed at the start of the second half to put LSU in front to stay. It was Shorey's one-yard dive that gave LSU its first touchdown.

LSU got a break after the kickoff when Alabama's Phil Chaffin fumbled on his 35 and Bozeman recovered for LSU. The Bengals failed to score a touchdown when on the Tide 5 quarterback Buddy Lee slipped down on a third down play and LSU had to be satisfied with a 25-yard field goal by Lumpkin.

LSU came right back to threaten again and moved to the Tide 35 where Hillman laid a perfect pass on Andy Hamilton's hands on the Alabama 5-yard line but the fleet Bengal dropped the ball.

Alabama started the fourth period with a great Hunter to Bubba Seay pass for 57 yards. However, the Tide couldn't capitalize on the threat as Ranager, a flanker, fumbled on a reverse and the Bengals' Tommy Casanova recovered for LSU at the Tiger 5.

Alabama then struck with the bomb with Hunter pitching to Husband for 37 yards and a touchdown.

Alabama gambled with an onside kick and LSU took over at their 49 and moved on in to get their second touchdown of the game with Shorey again going over from the one.

Alabama came right back as LSU went into their "prevent" defense but were unable to keep the Tide from crossing their goal line, with the score coming on Hunter's 34-yard pass to Bailey.

Hunter had to settle for new records as the Bengals took the game victory.

The hard-throwing Tide junior set a new mark of 1,592 yards for the season, breaking his old mark of 1,471 yards set last year.

Hunter also set a new Alabama season total offense mark with 1,594 yards which breaks the old mark set by Steve Sloan, now a member of the Alabama coaching staff.

Kicker Mark Lumpkin set a new LSU mark of 52 points by extra-point conversions which broke the old mark of Doug Moreau of 51, set in 1963-64.

For Coach McClendon the game itself must have been as frustrating as his past efforts against his old tutor, Bryant. Time after time it appeared as if the Bengals were going to break the game wide open, only to slip up with a glaring mistake.

The victory gave LSU a 7-1 record to date and it was the third loss for the Crimson Tide.

Alabama hasn't lost three games in a single season since 1958 when they lost four encounters.

Score by Periods

LSU	0	3	10	7 —	20
Alabama	0	3	0	12 —	15

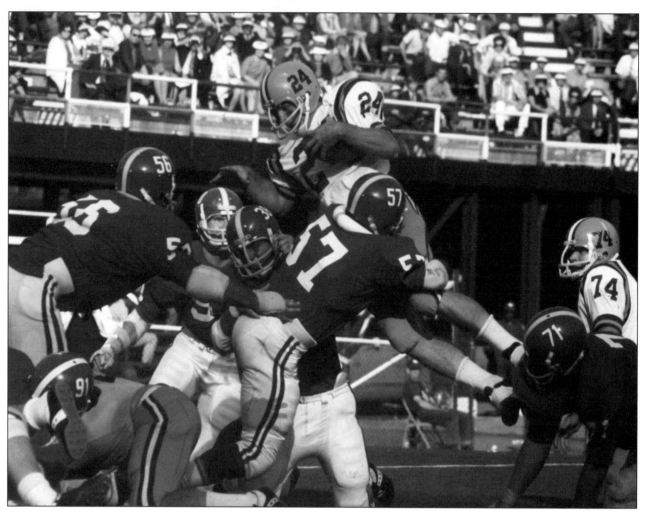

■ **LSU tailback Art Cantrelle (24) dives for a touchdown in the second quarter.**

Tigers Make It Two in a Row Against Tide, 14-9

By Bud Montet
The Advocate

Birmingham, Ala. — *Nov. 7, 1970*

The LSU Tigers put back-to-back victories together over standout Alabama elevens as they humbled the Alabama Crimson Tide, 14-9, here before 70,371 fans to follow their upset win over Auburn two weeks ago.

The win wasn't an easy one as the Bengals had to stave off a last-minute threat by the Tide which was attempting to strike back late in the game.

The victory was the second in successive years for the Bengals over the Tide, a feat they haven't been able to accomplish since the mid-fifties.

It was also the first Tiger win over Alabama in Birmingham since 1909.

After the Tide jumped into a first quarter 3-0 lead on Richard Cieminy's 23-yard field goal, LSU came back to get a touchdown with Art Cantrelle diving over from the two.

LSU scored their second touchdown in the third period on a long 37-yard sustained drive, one of the longest of the season for the Tigers. Buddy Lee pitched a two-yard pass to little Jimmy LeDoux for the score.

Alabama got its lone touchdown of the game in the fourth period when Scott Hunter pitched 10 yards to David Bailey.

LSU's defenses once again held a grid eleven from scoring a touchdown on the rush — their tenth straight performance in that department.

The last time a rusher scored against the Bengals was in last year's Ole Miss game when Archie Manning, now injured and out for the season, tallied on a sprint-out.

The Tigers missed scoring opportunities but their defensive unit made the 14 points stand up for victory.

Once again Coach Charlie McClendon of the Bengals bested his old grid boss, Paul (Bear) Bryant.

At the opening of the game the Tigers, playing their first game on artificial turf, stumbled numerous times before they became accustomed to the footing.

The Bengals' defense was sparked by a brilliant performance by Craig Burns, who intercepted two passes and ran them back ... to put the Bengals within striking distances and the burly safety raced back two punts for a total of 51 yards.

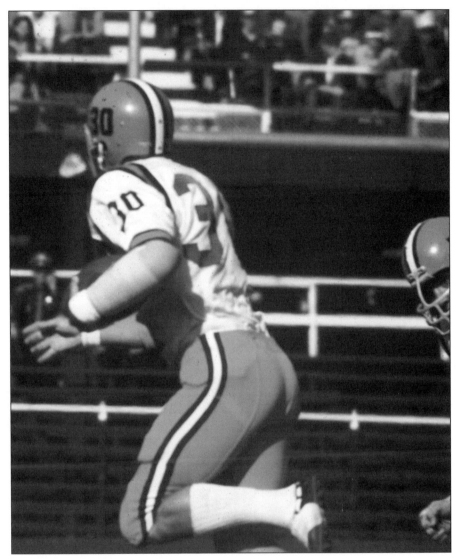

■ **Allen Shorey's touchdown attempt from the Tide 2 failed in the fourth quarter.**

Early in the second quarter, Burns took a Frank Mann punt and raced it back 33 yards to the Tide 23 and LSU moved on in to score in five plays, with Cantrelle getting the touchdown.

A few minutes later, Burns intercepted a Scott Hunter pass and raced it back 17 yards to the Tide 35, but Bert Jones slipped down after two plays and lost 14 yards to stymie the drive.

Early in the third period, Burns grabbed a Hunter pass and raced it back 25 yards to the Tide 12 but Alabama held again.

Burns set up another Tiger threat midway in the fourth period when he ran back a Mann punt 28 yards to the Tide 42 and LSU moved to inside the 2-yard line where they failed on a sweep by Allen Shorey.

The play set up a weird set of situations when Dantin fumbled and the ball was recovered by Ed Hines, who then fumbled when hit hard by several Tigers.

The ball then bounded into the end zone where a Tiger dove on it but the ball squirted from his grasp and was recovered by the Tide's Lanny Norris.

Score by Periods

LSU	0	7	7	0 —	14
Alabama	3	0	0	6 —	9

The officials, after making several signals, finally determined that LSU had given the impetus to the ball over the goal and it was called a touchback and Alabama gained possession at their 20 and moved on in to score their lone touchdown.

Oddly enough with the exception of two technical calls of pass interference, which is labeled a penalty at the spot of infraction, there wasn't any other penalties called in the hard hitting game.

LSU lost the services of Andy Hamilton for most of the game as he was hit on the head and was groggy the rest of the way.

Tommy Casanova missed part of the third and fourth periods when he suffered a knock on the head.

John Sage also was knocked out early in the game but returned to the action.

Up front, the Tiger foursome and trio of linebackers turned in an excellent game in containing the vaunted Johnny Musso. Musso, who had averaged 99 yards a game until today, was held to 44 yards in 18 carries, the best job done against him this season.

While the Bengals allowed Hunter the short passes they managed to keep the receivers within hand, Hunter hit on 19 of 37 passes for 207 yards and one score. LSU intercepted four of his tosses.

Ned Hayden pitched seven passes and hit on four for 42 yards.

Alabama netted but 79 yards on the ground but it picked up 249 in the air for a total offense of 238 yards while LSU netted 107 on the ground and 138 in the air for 245 yards total offense.

The key to the game according to Coach McClendon was the kicking game. Sophomore Wayne Dickinson booted an average of 40.3 yards while the touted Mann booted for 43.8 yards.

But LSU had a total of 155 yards in returns while Alabama was held to only five yards.

Once again, hard working Art Cantrelle was the chief LSU ball carrier with 82 yards in 23 carries and one score. Cantrelle picked up 24 on one jaunt for his longest run. Once the tailback slipped into the open and was seemingly going for long yardage when he stumbled and was nailed down.

Lee hit on seven of eight passes for 49 yards while Jones hit on three of six for 89 yards.

LSU couldn't get out of their own territory in the first period and failed to make a first down and netted but seven yards on the ground and none in the air.

However, the Bengals started to move at the start of the second quarter and drove from their 15 where Bill Norsworthy intercepted a Hunter pass. The Bengals moved to the Tide 8 with Jones tossing a 57-yard pass to fleet Al Coffee. Coffee caught the ball on the Tide 15 but stumbled as he tried to get going which enabled the Tide's Norris to haul him down at the eight.

LSU tried a field goal but Jones fumbled a poor pass from center and Mark Lumpkin tried to run the ball but was nailed at the 10.

Burns' 33-yard punt return gave the Bengals a chance to go ahead and they held a 7-3 halftime lead.

Early in the third quarter, the Bengals drove 87 yards in 12 plays to get their insurance score. On the drive, Cantrelle put the Bengals within reach with a 24-yard gallop to the Tiger 14

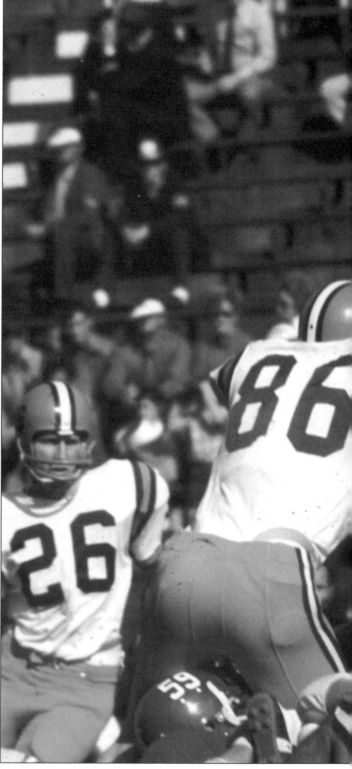

and LSU picked up the touchdown on Lee's pass to LeDoux.

On the Alabama touchdown drive Tiger James Earley was judged interfering with receiver George Ranager at the Tiger 22 and LSU drew a 36-yard penalty on the play.

With little over a minute to play Hunter tried to pitch the Tide back in the game but Louis Cascio picked off a pass at mid-

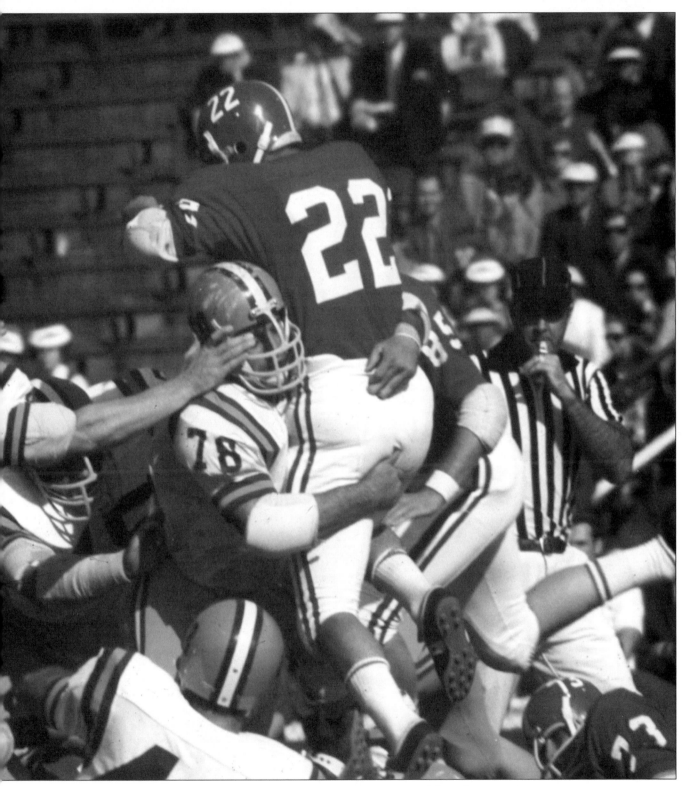

■ **Alabama All-American halfback Johnny Musso (22) is denied a touchdown by LSU's Ron Estay (78).**

field and Lee took two losses to run out the clock.

Up front the Tiger rush was sparked by Ronnie Estay, the junior tackle, who was credited with eight clean tackles. His teammate, John Sage, picked up six tackles and two assists despite missing part of the game.

Burns added to his laurels making six tackles in the secondary. Big Mike Anderson was credited with a half dozen and Cascio got four.

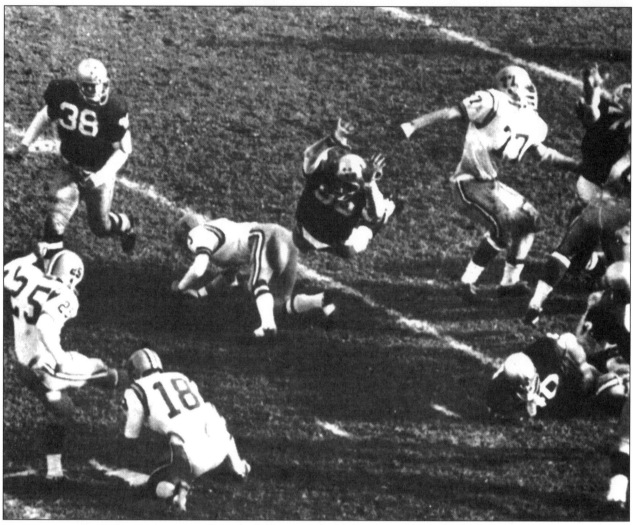

■ Mark Lumpkin's fourth-quarter field goal attempt was blocked by the Irish's Bob Neibart.

Irish Field Goal Defeats Tigers, 3-0

By Bud Montet

The Advocate

South Bend, Ind. — *Nov. 21, 1970*

The "bowling" Notre Dame Fighting Irish had to take advantage of a pass interference and a possible interception in the end zone that was dropped to take a 3-0 victory over the LSU Fighting Tigers in the final two minutes and 54 seconds, keeping their win streak going at nine in a row.

Scott Hempel booted the 24-yard field goal that gave the Irish their slim win over a gallant band of Bayou Bengals who blunted the nation-leading offense all afternoon.

Notre Dame got its chance on a short Wayne Dickinson punt midway the fourth period and the Irish's Mike Crotty returned the ball six yards to the Tiger 36.

On the first play, Ed Gulyas moved to the Tiger 17 where the officials judged James Earley interfered and Notre Dame had its chance.

On the third down, Joe Theismann tried a pass into the end zone and Tommy Casanova got a hand on it but failed to hold the ball, giving the Irish their chance at the field goal.

Earlier, LSU got a chance when the Tigers' Bill Norsworthy grabbed a pass that bounded out of the hands of Bill Barz and Norsworthy was there to grab it at the Irish 34. LSU moved to the 17-yard line of the Irish and after LSU halted them Mark Lumpkin came in to try a 34-yard field goal and Bob Neibart broke through to block the attempt.

A few minutes later the Irish got their chance.

Notre Dame, which led the nation in total offense for a game average of 540.1 yards was held to 227 yards — 78 on the ground (25 of those coming with a 26-yard jaunt by Theismann, the Irish's brilliant quarterback after the Irish went ahead) and 149 in the air.

While the Bengals' offense was spotty, the Tigers rushed for 83 yards, mostly gained by Art Cantrelle, and picked up 82 in the air for a total offense of 165 yards, their lowest of the season.

The game was a hard-fought battle from start to finish and LSU did a fine job of rushing Theismann and dumped him for considerable losses several times.

Theismann was able to connect on 14 of 30 aerials for 149 yards and had one intercepted.

The Bengals contained Theismann on his keeper with the one exception in the fourth period and also halted the running of the Irish running backs.

Notre Dame, which had announced prior to the game, that they wouldn't make the bowl decision until some time Sunday, were almost knocked out of the ranks as the "most desirable" bowl foes for 1970.

In the first half the Tigers held the Irish to 55 yards on the ground and 55 in the air while they picked up 29 yards on the ground and 122 in the air.

However, the bruising first half battle was just a prelude to the fierce encounter in the second half.

Both elevens had several breaks for chances to move into the end zone but were never able to capitalize until the Irish got their chance once too often.

Early in the game LSU got a break when Early grabbed a fumble by Dennis Allan. However, Notre Dame threw

Score by Periods

LSU	0	0	0	0 —	0
Notre Dame	0	0	0	3 —	3

Cantrelle and Buddy Lee for successive nine-yard losses to blunt the chance.

Several minutes later the Irish got a chance when Ralph Stepaniak intercepted a Lee pass and returned 16 yards to midfield.

A 34-yard pass from Theismann to his tight end for 34 yards to the Tiger 13. LSU was backed to their three-yard line when Lloyd Frye hit Darryll Dewan hard, causing a fumble and Richard Picou recovered for LSU at the four.

The Irish moved into Tiger territory several times in the second quarter but the tough Tiger defense held them at bay.

Midway in the period, Lumpkin tried a 49-yard field goal, but was far short of the cross bar. In the third period, Notre Dame got into LSU territory only twice — once to the 44 and once to the 45.

In the fourth period, the Bengals missed their chance on the Norsworthy pass interception and the resulting miss of the short field goal by Lumpkin.

Notre Dame's tremendous rush on the Tiger passers cut down on the effectiveness of Lee and Bert Jones, as both got only three completions.

Once again Cantrelle proved the workhorse of the Tiger backfield, going for a net 94 yards in 23 tries. His longest gain was for 15 yards. Chris Dantin got 42 yards in nine attempts.

Notre Dame's top runner Gulyas was held to a net 25 yards in nine carries.

The Irish's favorite receiver, Tom Gatewood, was held to four receptions for 21 yards. His longest catch was for nine yards. Most of the time, Gatewood was covered by Casanova, who turned in a fine effort in stymieing the fine Irish receiver.

The Tiger front four and linebackers all played superb defensive football, Buddy Millican, John Sage, Ronnie Estay, Art Davis, Mike Anderson, Louis Cascio and Picou.

Davis tossed Theismann for a loss of 18 yards and Bobby Joe King came through for losses of nine and three yards. Estay got to the quarterback for a sack of seven yards.

The Irish, who were held to a 10-7 score last week by Georgia Tech and then had to scramble for their 3-0 win over LSU, are favored to take a Cotton Bowl bid. At the end of the game, LSU was still in doubt whether it would get a major bowl bid or any bowl bid at all.

The close loss was the second of the season for LSU against seven victories. The Bengals meet Tulane and Ole Miss in their next two outings.

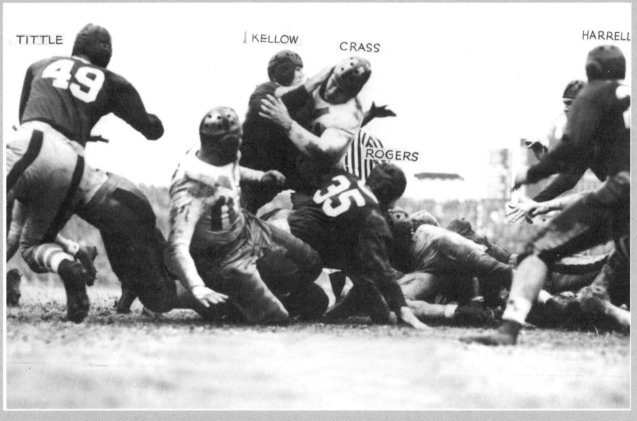

TITTLE · 49 · KELLOW · CRASS · HARRELL · ROGERS · 35

■ TCU's defense stopped LSU's Bill Crass at the goal line in the second quarter.

Manton Kicks No. 1 Frogs to 3-2 Win

By W.I. Spencer
The Advocate

New Orleans, La. — *Jan. 1, 1936*

The low scoring jinx that has hung over two previous football games between Louisiana State and Texas Christian extended through their Sugar Bowl classic here this afternoon with the worst "football weather" of the year, spoiling the New Year's fete for some 35,000 spectators. Taldon Manton's accurate toe booted a field goal late in the second quarter that gave the Horned Frogs a 3-2 victory.

LSU, by fiercely rushing Sammy Baugh, the great TCU quarterback, in the second quarter as he attempted a daring pass behind his own goal line, forced the Frog field general back of his own end line for a safety, as he futilely tried to get rid of the ball.

TCU scored shortly after the safety as the second quarter's minutes were ebbing away.

Willie Walls, the best Horned Frog on the field today, covered Bill Crass' fumble on the LSU 45-yard line. Jimmy Lawrence, a hard-running back and pass receiver for the Texans, crossed up the Tiger defense by hurling a fine pass to this same "thorn in the Tiger side," Walls. The TCU end was cleanly tackled on the LSU 13-yard line by Junior Bowman.

The Tigers threw the Frogs back four yards after three plays. Manton, the big fullback who played a whale of a game backing up the line and was always good for gaining yardage through the line, then dropped back to the LSU 28, where he booted a perfect field goal from a slight angle and into the teeth of a good northern wind.

LSU threatened in the fourth quarter, when Crass led a smashing drive from the TCU 31-yard line, following a Baugh fumble that had been recovered by Bernie Dumas.

The Bengals moved to a first down on the TCU 8-yard line, and after a six-yard swing around right end by Junior Bowman, the touchdown the Tigers wanted so much seemed in sight.

But TCU stiffened, halted Crass on three successive plays and the ball went over.

The Horned Frogs threatened in the closing minutes, when Baugh broke away for 42 yards around left tackle, with Gaynell Tinsley finally bringing the Frog down with a hard, diving tackle on the Tiger 4-yard line, and drew a penalty to the LSU 1-yard line for unnecessary roughness.

But here Marvin Stewart, Ernest Seago, Justin Rukas, Tinsley and the rest of the Tigers showed their greatness, and in four plays smeared the Frogs back on the LSU 10 to take the ball on downs.

Playing what probably was the greatest game of this career, Baugh was an All-American back in every sense of the word. His passing was good — what he did of it. But his punting was masterly, his blocking and ball-carrying brilliant and better than anything else he did, his defensive work was superb. On more than one occasion, Baugh stopped what looked like a sure LSU touchdown. And intercepting a couple of Tiger passes deep in TCU territory, he saved nobody knows what else for his team.

Jimmy Lawrence, Drew Ellis, Wison Groseclose, Bob Harrell, Darrell Lester, Walter Roach, Willie Walls and L.D. Meyer also contributed to the great Frog defense — one of the gamest and most durable seen here in a long time.

One of TCU's "threshold" stands against LSU cost the services of the great Lester, twice an All-American center. He was hurt stopping a plunge over center by Bill Crass in the second period — stopping Crass' charge on the one-foot line.

You might say the "breaks" went against first one side and then the other to cause the points.

But there really was nothing lucky about the 32-yard return of a punt by Bowman from midfield to TCU's 18-yard line. Nor had there been anything lucky about the fine punt Bill Crass had put out of bounds on TCU's 6-yard line on a previous play to force this danger zone punt.

No luck either, attached to the fine pass from Bill Crass to Jeff Barrett to put the ball on the TCU 2-yard line. Though you might have called it bad luck for LSU that the Frogs had Sam Baugh playing safety instead of somebody else. Because when Baugh tackled a

Score by Periods

LSU	0 2 0 0	— 2
TCU	0 3 0 0	— 3

man, that man stayed tackled.

The Tigers fought themselves to a standstill trying to find a way through the TCU line. But they couldn't. And they finally lost the ball on downs at the TCU 6-yard line

Sam Baugh, backed up to the crowd in the end zone, faked a punt and then shot a pass which slipped out of his fingers and fell incomplete in the end zone. Gaynell Tinsley had crowded Baugh and had made him dodge and that probably accounted for the poor pass.

Anyhow, it put the ball out on the 20-yard line and the Tigers had a two-point margin. But not for long.

A bad break against them came a few minutes later. Bowman had run the kickoff back 15 yards to the LSU 45-yard line but on the first play Crass fumbled and Willie Walls carved a niche for himself in TCU's hall of fame by recovering the ball.

A few seconds later, Walls turned the niche into an alcove when he gathered in a fine pass from Jimmy Lawrence for a gain of 23 yards to put the ball on LSU's 17-yard line.

There the Old Gold and Purple held as it never had before. It pushed the Frogs back on three plays.

With one shell left in their gun, the Frogs decided to gamble on Manton and when that young man dropped back to the LSU 26-yard line and booted a "liner" through the goal posts even the LSU rooters cheered him.

It was a "money" kick — one that Manton probably never will forget.

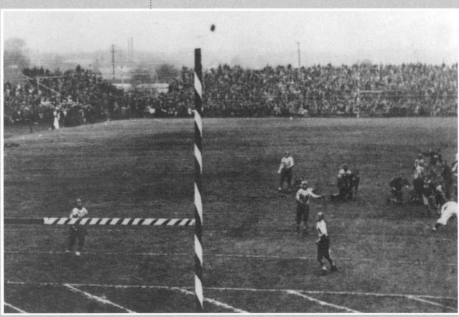

■ **Taldon Manton's field goal ensured the Horned Frogs' victory.**

LSU Romps Over Rebs, Wins SEC Title

By Ted Castillo

The Advocate

Baton Rouge, La. — *Dec. 5, 1970*

L SU's student body pelted the field with oranges and the Tiger football team belted Ole Miss, 61-17, tonight at Tiger Stadium before 67,590 keyed-up mostly Tiger fans. The surprisingly one-sided victory not only sends the Bengals on to a New Year's night Orange Bowl date with Big 8 champion Nebraska but also made LSU the Southeastern Conference champion for the first time since 1961.

Coming against an arch rival and one LSU had not beaten since 1964, the sweeter-than-sugar victory gave Tiger coach Charlie McClendon's team a 5-0 SEC slate and a 9-2 season record.

The loss left Ole Miss with a 4-2 record in the SEC and 7-3 overall for its Gator Bowl date with Auburn on Jan. 2.

A crippled Archie Manning, who wore a protective covering on his left arm, was unable to rally the Rebels as he had done for two previous years against LSU.

Manning left the game midway in the third period. A report later indicated that his right arm was injured. The protective gear of the Reb whiz was okayed by umpire Cliff Norvell, prior to the 8:30 kickoff of the regionally telecast game.

Manning threw a 9-yard pass to Jim Poole for the game's first score, set up by one of LSU's three first-period fumbles, all of which the Rebels recovered. But after that the hampered Manning was practically stymied.

LSU scored so many touchdowns it was hard to keep count. The Tigers erased an early Ole Miss 7-0 lead on a 20-yard pass from soph quarterback Bert Jones to Jimmy LeDoux.

After Poole's 21-yard field goal tipped the balance back in the Rebels favor, 10-7, the Tigers went to work and scored again on Buddy Lee's 46-yard bomb to Andy Hamilton.

Tommy Casanova's first dazzling punt return, for 61 yards, accounted for the next Tiger TD and Ronnie Estay's dumping of Manning in the end zone left the Bengals with a 23-10 halftime lead.

Mark Lumpkin's 21st LSU field goal, a new career record, followed and then Craig Burns scampered 61 yards with a punt.

Score by Periods

Ole Miss	7	3	7	0	— 17
LSU	7	16	10	28	— 61

Shug Chumbler directed Ole Miss to its second touchdown and the third quarter closed with LSU showing a 33-17 margin.

But the dam really broke in the final quarter. Tailback Art Cantrelle stepped 55 yards for one score; Casanova returned another punt all the way for 74 yards and a touchdown; Jones' pass to Ken Kavanaugh Jr. for 13 yards added another; and LeDoux streaked nine yards around the left side for the final marker.

LSU's total was the highest ever collected by either team in the series while the setback was the most one-sided in the heated rivalry since a 52-7 Tiger victory in 1917.

Individually and collectively, LSU set a number of records. The three punt returns for touchdowns tied an all-time NCAA record.

In the individual departments, Cantrelle, who jetted 117 yards on 25 carries, broke Steve Van Buren's 1943 rushing record of 847 yards with a total of 892 on the season. Hamilton caught three passes for 98 yards and smashed Ken Kavanaugh's most yards gained on receptions mark of 1,075, set in 1937-39. With another year left, Hamilton has 1,141 career reception yards.

Lumpkin broke the field goal mark of 20 set by Doug Moreau in 1963-65 and Lee, with 177 yards on passes, moved into third place on LSU's all-time passing list behind Y.A. Tittle and Mike Hillman. Lee has 1,641 yards passing in his career.

The courageous Manning was limited to 82 yards and 12 completions in 27 attempts by one of the best Tiger pass rushes in years, and some excellent secondary defense as well. Manning was intercepted twice and dumped four times for losses of 28 yards.

Manning finished with a minus 25 yards rushing. Chumbler connected on 6 of 17 passes for 50 yards and was intercepted three times.

The Rebs managed only 2 yards rushing against the nation's top rushing defense while the Tigers had 214 yards rushing plus 291 yards passing. Lee missed only three of 10 passes and Jones connected on 7 of 14 passes for 114 yards. Jones threw the only Tiger interception and it set up an Ole Miss field goal.

LSU crammed 28 points into the final quarter and scored every way a team can in the game, including eight touchdowns, a like number of conversions, Lumpkin's 24-yard field goal, and a safety.

Tigers Stun Ole Miss, Orange Bowl Brass

BY BERNELL BALLARD
The Advocate

Baton Rouge, La. — *Dec. 5, 1970*

There never was an LSU victory like this one.

Orange Bowl officials looked stunned as LSU chalked up a record 61-17 win over Ole Miss before a capacity crowd at Tiger Stadium and a regional television audience.

"It was one of the most tremendous football games I have ever seen," stated W. Keith Phillips Jr., the president of the Orange Bowl. "It was unbelievable and certainly a great individual victory for Coach McClendon. And it assures the Orange Bowl the best bowl game ever, not only of those bowls this New Year's but ever. With Nebraska, the fine offensive team, and LSU's great defense and all-around team, we should have it made."

And oranges, hundreds of them, sailed onto the field all night as fantastically fired-up LSU fans tossed them from the stands until finally warned to stop by the public address announcer or LSU would suffer a penalty.

Still, after LSU's touchdowns mounted and mounted, more oranges came until one Ole Miss player, in utter frustration, finally jumped up from his stance, picked up an orange, and tossed it back toward the LSU stands.

After Jimmy LeDoux streaked nine yards for LSU's final touchdown with only 42 seconds remaining, the Tigers got another chance when Bill Norsworthy intercepted Shug Chumbler's pass and returned it 30 yards to the Ole Miss 16-yard line with 14 seconds still remaining.

But 10,000 LSU fans stormed onto the field in wild jubilation, preventing any possible attempt for the Tigers to add any more points to the staggering victory total.

Police had to assist the LSU players from the field as fans mobbed the Tiger gridders en masse.

It was the biggest LSU win over Ole Miss since 1917 when the Tigers beat the Rebels, 52-7.

And it's pretty certain it was like hell for Ole Miss, who was greeted with "Go to hell, Ole Miss, go to hell," from start to finish by screaming Bengal fans.

"This is the greatest thing I ever envisioned could happen," said an overwhelmed LSU coach Charles McClendon, "I've been to bowl games before, but that was the most important victory of my life."

All will agree, McClendon can rest assured, it was a big one.

"Our kids played a football game which compliments our entire coaching staff. Togetherness is the name of the game. You can't imagine how I feel. Our kids are probably able to live with this better than I ever will," McClendon said.

Not only did the victory establish an all-time scoring mark against Ole Miss, but it also added to the ever-growing list of records on the LSU record books.

Tommy Casanova's two punt returns for touchdowns, a 61-yarder and a 74-yarder, made him the first SEC player ever to accomplish the feat. And Casanova became only the third college player in NCAA history to run back two punts for touchdowns in a game.

The other, a 61-yard punt return for touchdown by Craig Burns, coupled with Casanova's two, gave LSU a new SEC punt return yardage record of 205 yards for a single game, wiping out the old conference mark of 203 by Vanderbilt in 1948.

Those three punt returns for scores also tied another NCAA mark of most touchdowns by a team by punt returns in one game.

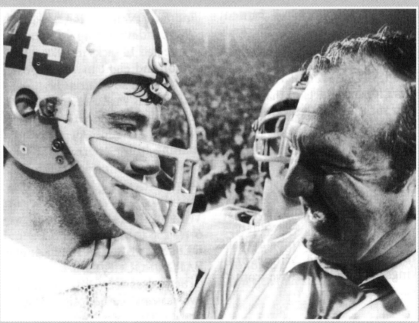

■ **All-American linebacker Mike Anderson and Charlie McClendon enjoy recounting a big play in the Tigers' 61-17 win over Ole Miss.**

Bengals Blast Irish, 28-8, in Tigerland

BY BUD MONTET
The Advocate

Baton Rouge — *Nov. 20, 1971*

T he Sun Bowl-bound LSU Fighting Tigers gained sweet revenge when they took a 28-8 victory over the Fighting Irish of Notre Dame before 68,000 rabid-Cajun fans at Tiger Stadium tonight.

After building a 14-0 first-half lead, the Tigers went to work on the Irish records. They picked up touchdowns in the third and fourth periods, breaking the Irish streak of holding its 1971 foes scoreless in second-half play and the string of 20 games in which the Irish have held their foes scoreless in the final quarter of play.

The Bengals added the final crushing blow to the mighty Irish when, following the lone Notre Dame score, they took over at midfield and moved in for the final score of the game, a Paul Lyons to Andy Hamilton 12-yard pass play.

With a second left on the clock some LSU fans swarmed through the field fence to surround the players. The final second was never played.

The victory gave the Bengals a 7-3 record for the season and was the second setback for the Irish. LSU has only Tulane left on its 1971 regular season schedule

LSU will later clash with Iowa State in the Sun Bowl on Dec. 18. The Irish voted earlier in the week to skip any bowl appearance this season.

Surprise starter Bert Jones of the Bengals pitched to his cousin, Andy Hamilton, for the first two LSU scores, with one aerial going 36 yards, the first touchdown, and the second traveling 32 yards. Jones scored the third period touchdown with a five-yard keeper. Lyons' 12-yard pitch to Hamilton accounted for the final Tiger score.

The lone Notre Dame touchdown came in the fourth quarter with Cliff Brown pitching to Tom Gatewood for seven yards.

Although they held a 14-0 advantage at halftime, the Bengals spent most of the half defending their goal line with tactics that reminded of the Chinese Bandits of the 1958 National Championship eleven.

LSU, despite giving away a tremendous weight advantage, managed to rush for 143 yards and pitch for 156 for a total offense of 299 yards. The Irish rushed for 172 yards against the stubborn Tiger defense and passed for 151 for a total offense of 323 yards.

Jones hit on seven of nine aerials for 143 yards and his chief target, Hamilton, caught seven for 153 yards and three touchdowns.

Art Cantrelle figured in the only other Tiger pass completion, a three yarder.

The Irish's Brown put the ball in the air 29 times and hit on 13 for 151 yards. Gatewood was his chief target with seven catches for 75 yards.

The Bengals' fierce defense honors had to be shared by all. Ronnie Estay picked up 13 individual tackles and four assists.

Richard Picou and John Weed picked up seven individual tackles.

Warren Capone picked off two Brown passes, one halting a Notre Dame drive and the other setting up the second LSU score in the second period.

In the third period, the Irish were on the Tiger 32 when Capone wrestled a Brown pass from the Irish receiver, halting the threat.

LSU scored the first time they got their hands on the football in the first period, moving 77 yards with Jones pitching to Hamilton for 36 yards and the score.

LSU was moving again when they ran into trouble of their own making with Jones fumbling and giving up the ball at the Tiger 37.

Notre Dame marched to the Tiger 1-foot line where the Bengals stopped Andy Huff short of the goal and the first down.

Early in the second period, the Irish moved to the Tiger 1-yard line where Norman Hodgins pulled down Brown on a keeper play and forced the Irish to turn over the ball.

A few minutes later the Irish drove to the Tiger 3 where a fourth down Brown pass failed.

LSU took command in the second half but early in the fourth period Casanova's interception in the end zone stifled one Irish threat but midway in the period the Irish put together the long scoring strike.

While the Bengals were spoiling some Notre Dame streaks, their own gridders were setting new Tiger standards.

Paul Lyons, who served as the backup quarterback, set a new season mark of 16 touchdowns scored, which broke the old mark of 15 which Lyons shared with Y.A. Tittle.

Score by Periods

	1	2	3	4	Total
Notre Dame	0	0	0	8	8
LSU	7	7	7	7	28

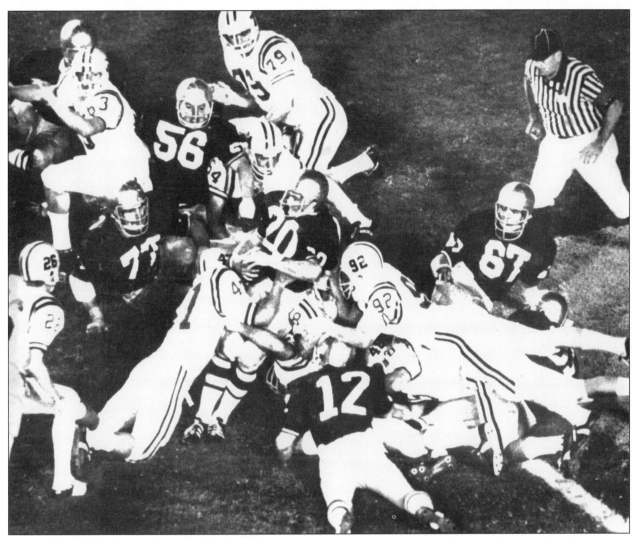

■ **The LSU defense stopped Notre Dame's Andy Huff (20) at the goal line in the first quarter.**

Lyons has scored six touchdowns and passed for 10.

Andy Hamilton's three touchdown grabs tied the LSU record of touchdown receptions in a game. The old mark is held by Ken Kavanaugh Sr., set against Holy Cross in 1939. Kavanaugh's son is a Tiger tight end.

Hamilton also tied another old record held by Kavanaugh — seven touchdown passes in a single season. Kavanaugh set his mark in 1939.

Hamilton's 16 career touchdowns record ties the old mark held by Kavanaugh.

The fleet Tiger wide receiver has the Tulane game left in which to break Kavanaugh's old records.

Tonight's game wound up the brief two-game series. Notre Dame won, 3-0, last year at South Bend.

For most of the game it appeared that LSU would hold the Irish scoreless, a feat none have accomplished since Miami blanked the Irish in 1965.

LSU put together two drives for two scores and took advantage of breaks to get their other two scores. Capone's interception and 32-yard runback gave the Tigers the impetus for their second touchdown.

Norman Hodgins' recovery of a Brown fumble at the Irish 33 gave LSU its chance for the third touchdown.

LSU's Cantrelle was the workhorse on the ground with 18 carries for a net 53 yards.

Dantin carried nine times for 36 yards and Allen Shorey six times for 25.

Huff was the top ball carrier for the Irish with 13 carries for 42 yards. Ed Gulyas carried 15 for 39 yards.

The Bengals who have been plagued all season with costly mistakes on offense seemed destined to have to live through it all over again.

After fighting off a trio of Irish threats in the first half LSU took the second half kickoff and marched from their 41 to the Irish 31 when Cantrelle fumbled and the Irish took over.

From that point, the Bengals took command of the game, until the Notre Dame scoring drive early in the fourth period.

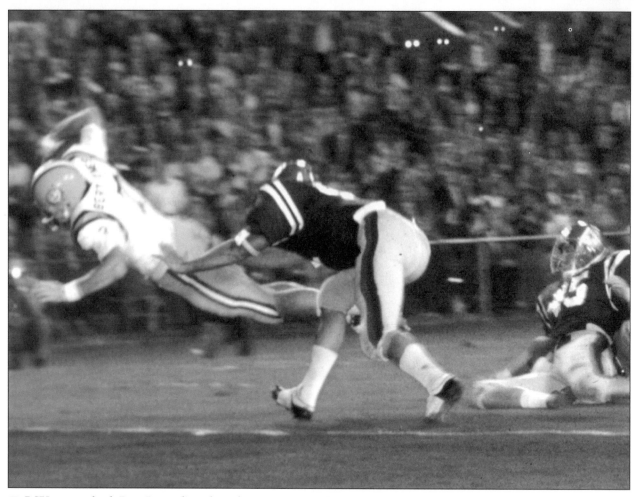

■ LSU quarterback Bert Jones dives for a first-quarter touchdown.

LSU Wins Wild Thriller Over Rebs, 17-16

BY JOE PLANAS
The Advocate

Baton Rouge, La. — *Nov. 4, 1972*

A teenage blonde cried in the end zone, an elderly gentleman asked for some nitroglycerin pills, and Heisman Trophy candidate Bert Jones compressed football history into a mere second tonight.

About 70,502 fans — some of them not able to believe the spectacle — watched as soph Brad Davis hugged deliriously a Bert Jones pass tossed to him after the final gun in LSU's unbelievable 17-16 triumph over Ole Miss.

Jones, who had set a few records in total offense and number of touchdowns responsible for, had started to march LSU the necessary 80 yards with 3:02 left in the game after a determined LSU defense forced the Rebs to punt after three offensive plays. With last-down-and-everything facing him, Jones threw to Davis in the flat and the former Hammond High sparkler sparkled by making the grab that was reminiscent of Doug Moreau's two-point catch in the end zone in LSU's 11-10 win over the Rebels in 1964. There was one second left on

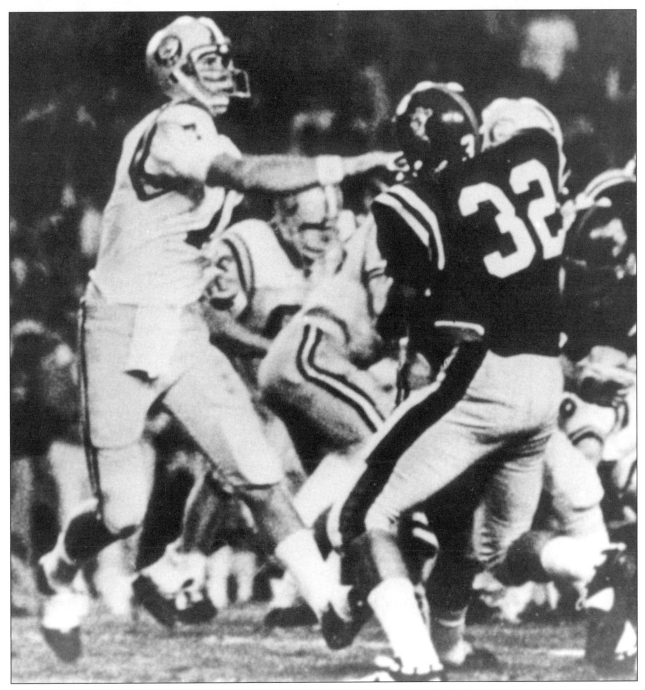

■ **Bert Jones unleashed his touchdown pass with no time left on the scoreboard clock.**

the clock when Jones got the snap and the horn sounded before Jones pumped his arm. If there was ever a finer finish in a football game, it had to have happened in Utopia, or somewhere like that.

A pass interference call against the Rebs after LSU had taken its last timeout with 10 seconds left had elevated Tiger hearts and advanced the ball from the Reb 20 to their 10. But, with four seconds left, those same hearts went down deeper into chest cavities when little Jimmy LeDoux watched Reb Mickey Fratesi bat away a Jones aerial. Then came the one-sec-

Score by Periods

	1	2	3	4		
Ole Miss	3	3	7	3	—	16
LSU	7	3	0	7	—	17

ond confrontation, Jones' response to it, and the still hard-to-believe final outcome. The pass was really a two-point play but LSU got 300 percent out of it.

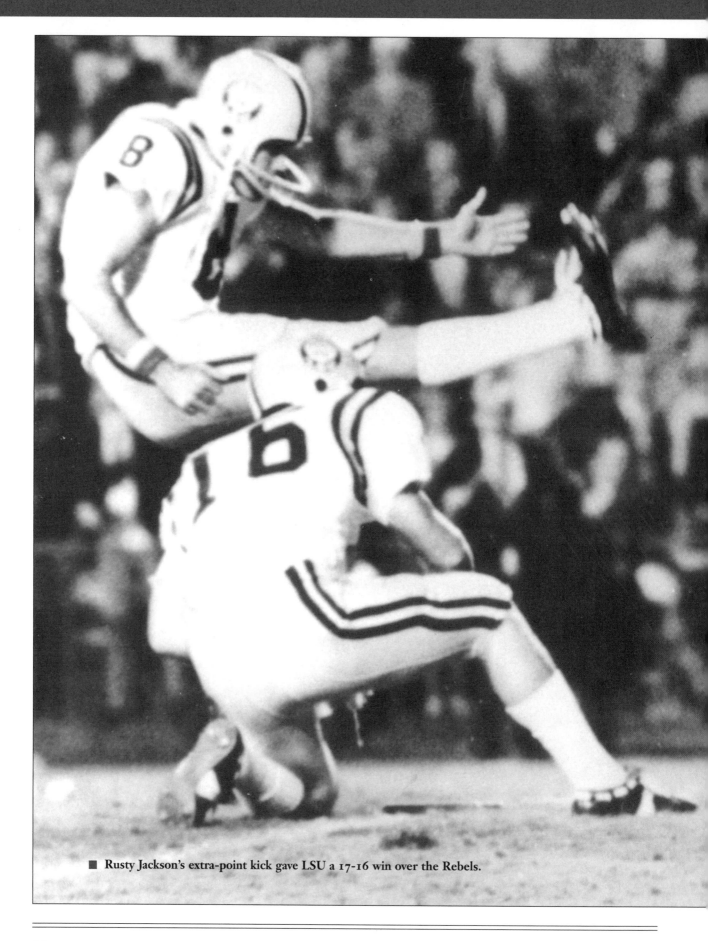

■ Rusty Jackson's extra-point kick gave LSU a 17-16 win over the Rebels.

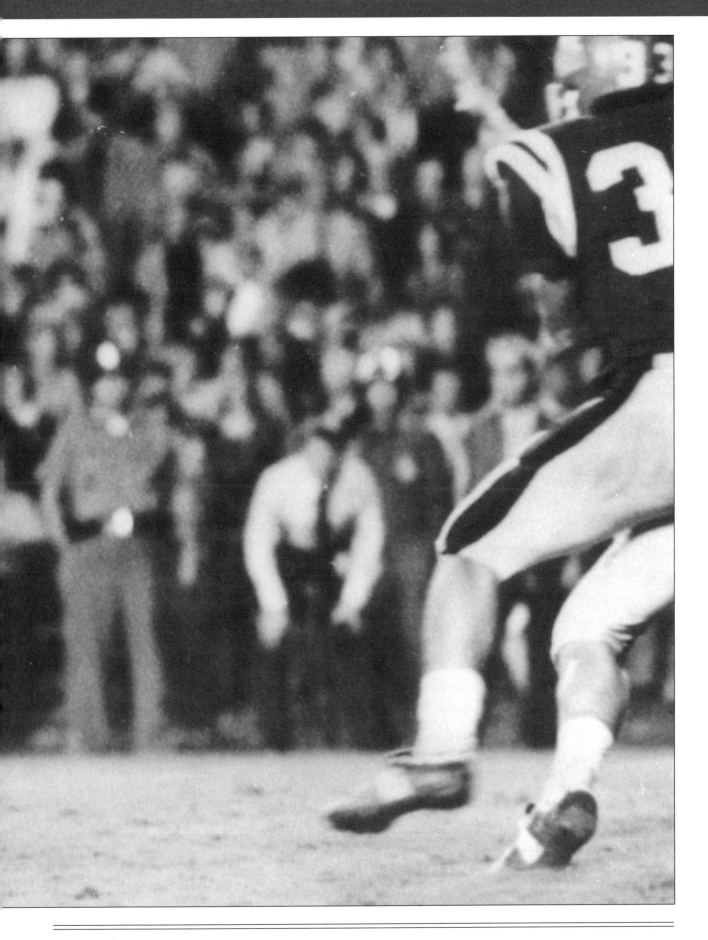

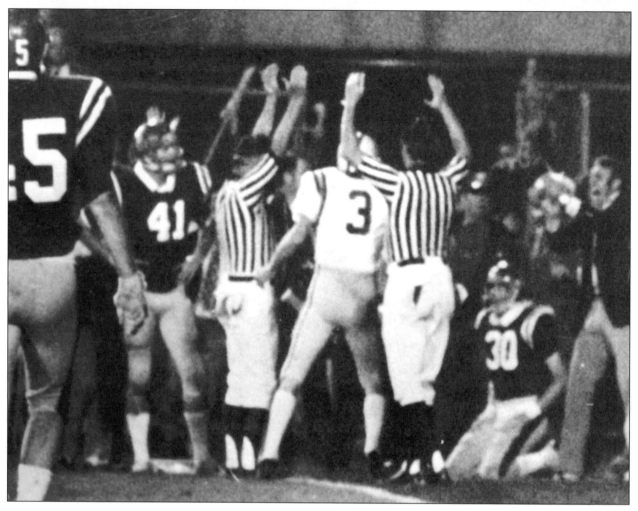

■ **In the end zone, the official signaled the results of Brad Davis' catch.**

For 59 minutes and 59 seconds, Ole Miss had been the superior football club. But, it only takes a second — they say. Jones had started LSU on the 13-play, 80-yard caper with 3:02 left in the game. He didn't waste a minute, or, for that matter, even a second. Rusty Jackson's kick was a formality the fans expected.

"I just fell over the flag," offered a wet Davis who still had shaving lather on his face and was trying to be polite by not letting water from his shower spill on a sports writer's coat. "The pass was meant for me and I just grabbed for it. I think I've caught only two others this season." The 10-yard reception was the only catch Davis made all night. The other two he had caught prior to the Ole Miss game were good for minus-one yard.

Davis, who brilliantly led Oscar Lofton's Hammond Tors to many football victories, also looked good running the ball. He finished the evening with 56 yards in 15 carries — his longest run being for 15 yards. Chris Dantin, whose longest gainer was for 16 stripes, was LSU's leading rusher with 60 yards in a dozen trips.

"We only had one second left and only one play left," Jones said. "I knew I had to get rid of the ball quickly to let somebody get a chance at catching it. I thought Brad lost it somewhere up there in the lights but I guess he found it. Yes, I do think we're ready for Alabama."

Jones was on target 14 of the 21 times (167 yards.) He threw for 67 percent and had one intercepted. The completion total gave him a career mark of 181 completions, breaking Mike Hillman's total of 171. Though utilized for losses of 20 yards in all, Jones upped his total offense figures to 2,726 yards, cracking Tittle's total of 2,694. He also eased past Tittle's touchdowns-responsible-for mark of 30 by shoving his own to 31. Not bad for a country boy from Ruston.

"In all my years here I don't think I remember an LSU team winning with no time on the clock," a joyous Charley McClendon said. "Can you imagine what we did? Our defense stopped 'em from getting their first down with under five minutes left to go, and then we go and take it right to 'em and win. I'd rather fight any football team in America than that clock. That clock, fellows, just doesn't give you any consideration."

McClendon was happily interrupted by former LSU gridders R.B. Nunnery and O.J. Ferguson, who patted him on the back and said how great the win was. "You're part of it, you know, R.B. and O.K. You fellows are all part of it."

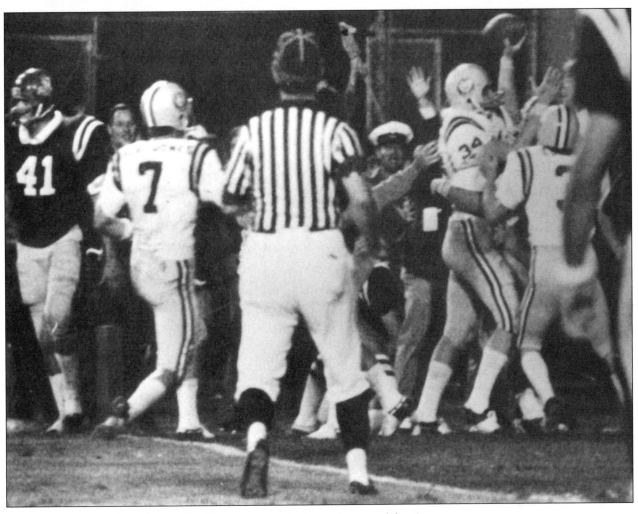

■ **Wasting no time, Bert Jones joins his teammates in the end zone celebration.**

McClendon turned his praise on Jones and Davis and rugged, play-for-forever Warren Capone. "When you work under adversities, that's what Heisman trophy winners are drawn from," Mac noted. "And you'd have to say Bert was working under adversity in those last seconds. It was a great game for Jones and should raise his stock in the Heisman voting."

Did Mac call the play:

"That was coach 'Charlie Pevy's play,'" McClendon noted. "He deserves credit for calling that one. Yes, Davis was the primary receiver on that one, but we send three receivers out just in case. Brad was a splitback and just went out in the flat. He's a dutch player you know, sorta has a star on his forehead."

Then McClendon started thinking defense. "You know Warren Capone had a fantastic game for us." Jolly Cholly remarked. "Someone told me he had 13 individual tackles and seven assists, but fellows, I knew he had played a whale of a football game before I heard those statistics."

How much of a thrill was it in beating Ole Miss?

"You'd have to call this one victory one of the all-time thrills in Tiger football history," Mac opined. "Ole Miss played excellent, smart football. I guess you could say the only mistakes

they made were missing that field goal and getting that costly pass-interference call. You know as a coach you preach to kids that as long as there's a second left you've got hope. We had hope and it came through for us."

Mac had more praise for Ole Miss. "They played excellent football and seem to bring out the best in the Tigers," Mac said. "They controlled the football — lot more than we wanted them to and that Norris Weese from Chalmette is one fine football player. But then, he always plays well against us."

In the shower room, other LSU players chanted "Go to Hell, Ole Miss." Earlier, Dantin and Paul Lyons had embraced and following that, someone kissed Davis on the flank. "You deserve to be kissed after a catch like that," the donator said.

Coach Dave McCarty said he didn't believe the win. He was that excited.

An aging sports writer admitted his ticker couldn't stand "many more like this baby."

"It was beautiful," said an old lady who lingered with the crowd outside the LSU dressing room. "Simply beautiful," she added.

Now all Mac has to do is beat Ole Miss every year through 1976 to play .500 ball against the Rebs.

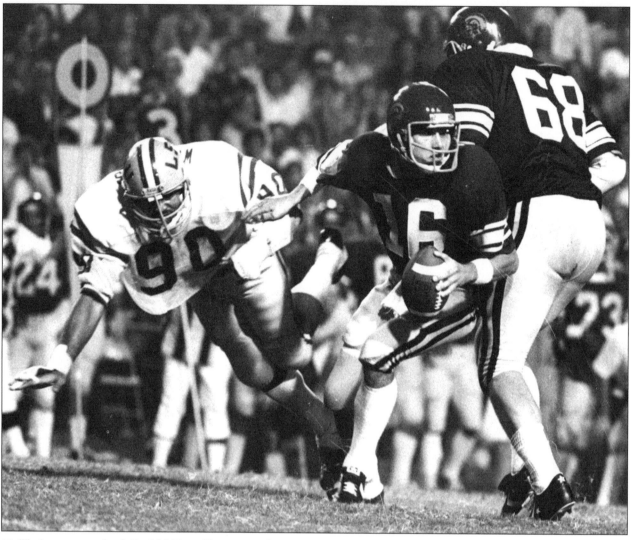

■ Trojans quarterback Paul McDonald connected on 14 passes for 145 yards against LSU.

No. 1 Trojans Stage Late Comeback to Defeat LSU

By Bud Montet

The Advocate

Baton Rouge, La. — *Sept. 29, 1979*

Hailed as THE football team of the final quarter century, the Southern California Trojans had to stage a desperate 79-yard march in the fading minutes to overtake the LSU Tigers and win, 17-12 before the second largest turnout at Tiger Stadium today before 78,322 fans.

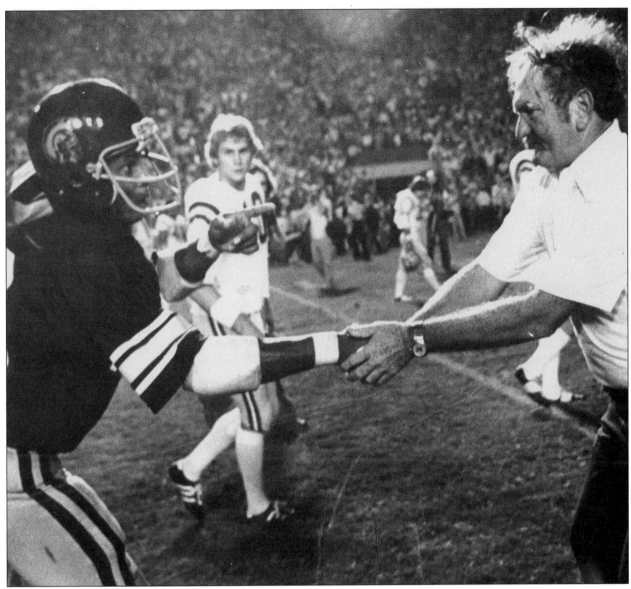

■ **Tigers coach Charlie McClendon congratulates USC tailback Charles White after the game.**

LSU grabbed a 9-3 halftime lead and added three points in the third period to grab a 12-3 lead but the mighty Trojans scored twice in the fourth period to grab the victory and keep their string going at four games and protect their No. 1 ranking in the nation.

Heavily favored prior to the contest, the visitors, meeting LSU for the first time, were hard put in the early stages.

LSU's stubborn defenses, led by middle guard George Atiyeh, harassed the Trojans throughout, although Heisman Trophy candidate Charlie White netted 185 yards in 31 carries.

LSU held White from the goal line until late in the fourth period when the All-American plunged over from the four-yard line and put the Trojans within striking distance.

Southern Cal put points on the board first when Eric Hipp booted a 32-yard field goal in the first quarter with 4:58 left.

In the second quarter, LSU drove 60 yards in eight plays to

Score by Periods

	1	2	3	4		Total
Southern Cal	3	0	0	14	—	17
LSU	0	9	3	0	—	12

move in front with Steve Ensminger pitching to LeRoid Jones for 14 yards and a touchdown.

With only 2:16 left in the half, Tiger walk-on kicker Don Barthel booted a 32-yard field goal to give LSU a 9-3 lead at the intermission.

Near the end of the third period the Bengals missed a chance to widen the margin with a touchdown when they moved to the Trojan 2-yard line and four downs to make the score.

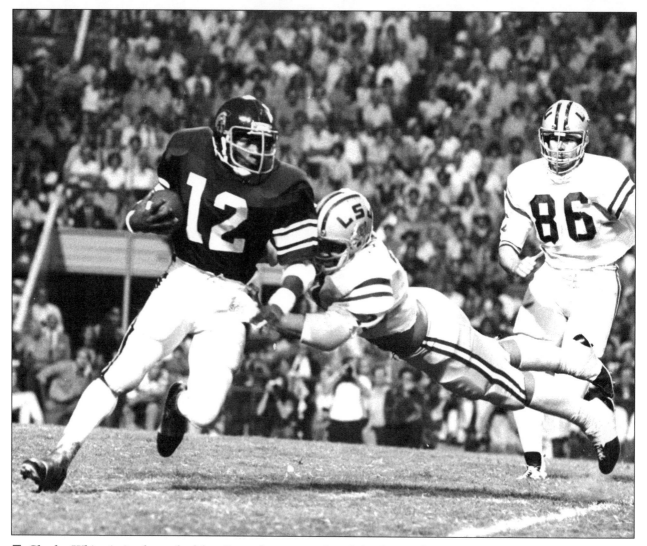

■ **Charles White (12), who rushed for 185 yards on 31 carries, shakes loose of a LSU defender before turning upfield.**

An attempted end around with Tracy Porter carrying the ball backfired and lost nine yards. Carlos Carson dropped a pass in the end zone and LSU had to settle for a 28-yard field goal by Barthel that gave them a 12-3 lead.

The fourth period belonged to the Trojans as they drove 56 yards in a half dozen plays to score their first touchdown with White going over from the four.

LSU missed a chance to put the game away midway the fourth period when freshman Alvin Thomas recovered a Marcus Allen fumble at the Trojan 17. On their first play, LSU tried a double reverse pass play and drew a 15-yard penalty that stymied the threat.

The Trojans got the ball at their 21 and with 4:16 left in the game moved to the Tiger 8-yard line. From there, Paul McDonald pitched to Kevin Williams for the winning score.

LSU kept coming after the kickoff with only 32 seconds left in the game. A 15-yard penalty gave LSU possession at their 42 and an Ensminger pass to Robert DeLee to the Trojan 30 set up two desperation passes by Ensminger into the Trojan end zone and both failed.

The vaunted Trojan offense didn't eclipse the Bengals by any great margin. Coach John Robinson's team piled up 396 yards while LSU totaled 272 yards.

Southern Cal netted 251 yards on the ground with White getting 185 yards of that total. In the air, the Trojans picked up 145 yards as McDonald connected on 14 aerials.

The Tigers picked up a net 169 yards on the ground and 103 in the air.

LSU suffered a crippling blow in the first half when their starting tailback, Hokie Gajan, was injured and missed the entire second half. Gajan carried the ball 10 times in the first half before he was injured.

LeRoid Jones came in for Gajan at the tailback slot and picked up 67 yards in nine attempts to lead the Tiger rushers. Fullback Jude Hernandez was also injured in the first half but came back to play in the second half and netted 40 yards in five carries.

Atiyeh with superb play in the middle forced the Trojans to move White. Atiyeh got seven solo tackles and four assists.

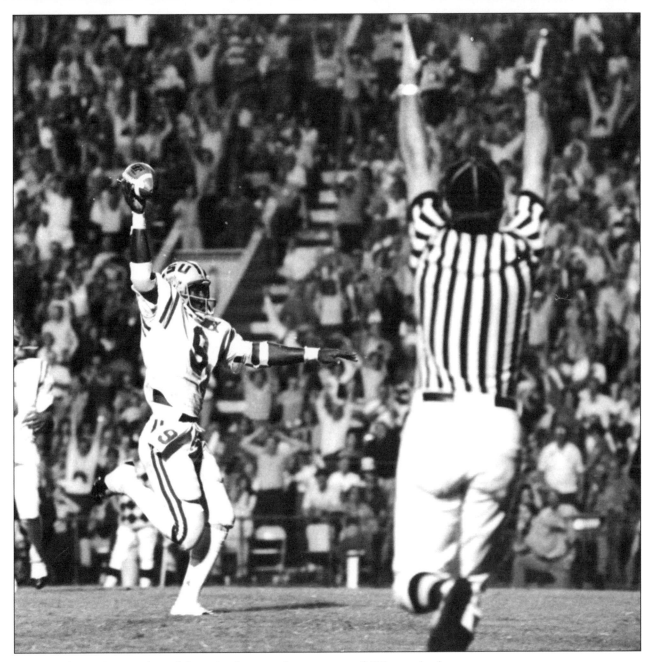

■ **LeRoid Jones' 14-yard touchdown in the second quarter gave LSU a 7-0 lead.**

Linebacker Jerry Hill brought back memories of former linebacking greats at LSU when he netted nine solos and five assists for his outstanding performance of the season.

Marcus Quinn, who was injured during the week played a standout defensive game, getting six solo tackles and seven assists.

USC's speedy defense slowed down the Tiger passing game which probably was the key to the contest. David Woodley and Ensminger had trouble getting away from the Trojans' pass rush. Woodley was tossed for 20 yards in losses while trying to throw.

Swift Chris Williams kept the Trojans at bay in the first period when he made a grab of a McDonald pass on the 2-yard line, bobbled it and then gained possession in the end zone.

A Tiger mistake gave the Trojans their chance to get on the board. First, when Jeff Fisher intercepted Woodley's pass at the Tiger 33 and USC went on to get their field goal.

It was Ensminger who came off the bench to get the Tigers rolling, leading them on their 6-yard scoring drive. On the drive, Ensminger connected on three passes.

Williams' pass interception in the first period was his 13th career interception and set a new Tiger record. The interception was the first thrown by McDonald this season.

After two victories over non conference foes and their loss to the Trojans, LSU swings into SEC play next Saturday when they entertain the Florida Gators at Tiger Stadium.

LSU Sends Mac Out A Winner, 34-10

BY JOHN ADAMS
The Advocate

Orlando, Fla. — *Dec. 22, 1979*

The end was much like the beginning for LSU coach Charles McClendon here tonight as his LSU Tigers — his last LSU Tigers — rolled up 24 points in the first half and charged to a 34-10 victory over the Wake Forest Deacons in the 31st Tangerine Bowl.

McClendon, the winningest coach in LSU history, was riding high-on the shoulders of his players after posting his 137th career victory. His first victory came 17 years ago against Texas A&M in the 1962 season opener.

His assistant coaches, most of whom were also coaching their final game at LSU, were given free rides, too, after the Tigers had erased the "Miracle" from Wake Forest's "Miracle" Deacons.

Wake Forest, which went from 1-10 to 8-3 in one year, matched up more to those 1-10 days against a Tiger team that played perhaps it best game of the year.

Of all the Tigers, senior quarterback David Woodley was the one who played the best. He ran for two touchdowns and passed for another — all in the first half — as LSU boosted its record to 7-5.

Woodley, who completed 11 of 19 passes for 199 yards, was named the game's Most Valuable Player. Jerry Murphree who caught five passes for 60 yards and one touchdown, was the offensive player of the game while Tiger tackle Benjy Thibodeaux was selected as the game's best defensive player.

"We broke a bunch of jinxes tonight," said Tiger center John Ed Bradley, one of 17 LSU seniors playing his final game. "People said we couldn't win on the road and we couldn't beat a good team. We did that tonight. I'm proud to end my career

Score by Periods

LSU	14	10	0	10 —	34
Wake Forest	0	3	7	0 —	10

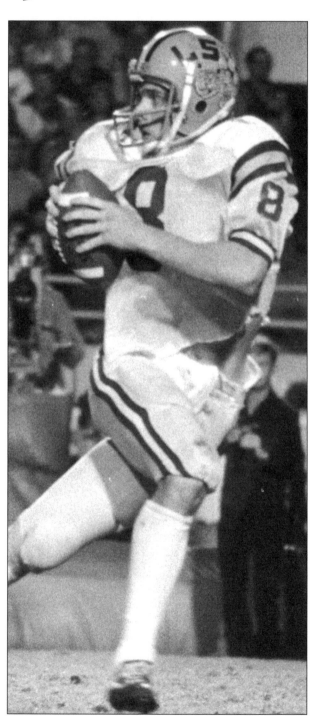

■ David Woodley completed 11 of 19 passes for 199 yards and was named the game's MVP.

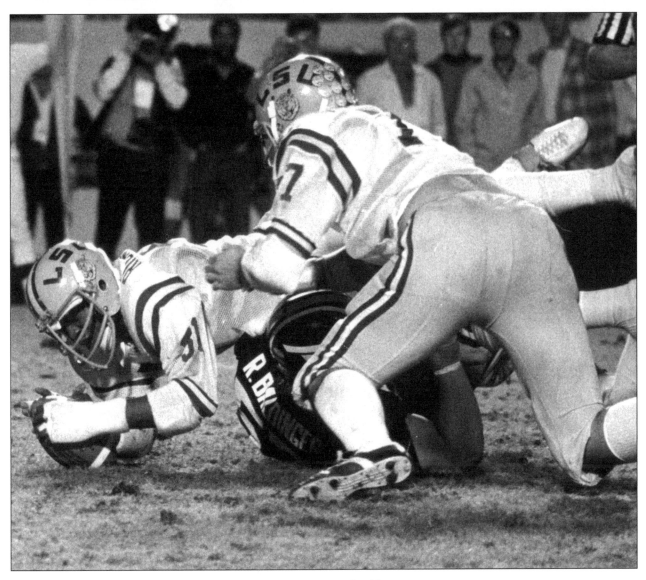

■ **A pair of LSU defenders scramble to recover a Wake Forest fumble.**

like that. We're going out winners. It's time to go out and tie one on."

Wake Forest, now 8-4, was just tied up. Quarterback Jay Venuto, the Atlantic Coast Conference player of the year, was intercepted three times, and was repeatedly harried by the Tigers' strong pass rush, led by Thibodeaux and defensive end Lyman White.

"LSU played well throughout the game," said Wake Forest coach John Mackovic. "Their offense did a good job controlling the game and their pass rush was tremendous.

"We dropped some passes in the first half and that hurt us. They just outmanned us in spots. They came to win, there's no question about that."

After Woodley directed LSU to three first-half touchdowns and a field goal by Don Barthel, the Deacons finally scored on the last play of the half on a 43-yard field goal by Phil Denfeld.

That seemed to spark the Deacons in the second half. Wake

Forest, which overcame an 18-point first-half deficit in a regular-season victory over Auburn, moved for a touchdown on its first possession of the second half.

Venuto, who completed 10 of 20 passes for 165 yards, drove the Deacons 80 yards, with the final 34 yards coming on a pass to split end Wayne Baumgardner.

However, the Deacons lost their momentum when they failed to take advantage of a Hokie Gajan fumble — one of three Tiger turnovers — on the Deacon 38.

They had another opportunity moments later when Venuto teamed up with Baumgardner for a 16-yard completion to the LSU 38. Fullback Bob Ventresca followed with a 15-yard run to the Tiger 17.

Then, Venuto — pressured by defensive end John Adams — attempted to throw the ball away before he was sacked near the sideline. His throw away landed in Thibodeaux's lap, and the Tigers had the football on their own 29.

"When the Venuto pass was intercepted we had a great opportunity to score and they sort of stopped us on that play," said Mackovic. "At the half, we determined that we had to come out and play with more intensity and I thought we did a good job early in the second half. We lost a great deal of momentum on that one play."

Woodley then passed 48 yards to Tracy Porter on the second play of the fourth quarter. After the Tiger quarterback was sacked twice and LSU lost another five yards for delay of game, Barthel kicked a 41-yard field goal.

On LSU's next possession, Steve Ensminger completed three straight passes in leading the Tigers on a 43-yard touchdown march. Ensminger got the final score of the evening on a 4-yard run with 8:32 to play.

"I really don't feel anything right now," said McClendon, who is being replaced by Bo Rein after 18 years as LSU's head coach. "We came out at the beginning of the game certainly ready to play. I believe that had to be the best first half we've had all season."

The Deacons wouldn't argue that point.

After the first half, the 12,000 Wake Forest fans that followed their team to Orlando, must have been asking one another, "We waited for this?"

The Deacons, who hadn't been to a bowl game in 31 years, spent the first 30 minutes of the game assisting LSU in adding lots of footage to its 1979 highlight film.

Not until Phil Denfeld booted his 43-yard field goal with no time showing on the scoreboard clock did Wake Forest have any reason to think a bowl game was supposed to be fun. If the Deacons had been bowling for dollars, they would have owed money at the end of the first half.

With Woodley having the best half of his three-year career at LSU, the Tigers amassed 17 first downs and 306 yards in total offense in rolling to a 24-3 lead. Another drive was blunted by a Jesse Myles fumble at the Deacon goal line and a second was cut short when the Tigers were stopped on a fourth-and-one situation at the Deacon 31.

In the first quarter, there was no stopping Woodley or the Tigers. On LSU's first possession, Woodley completed four of five passes — one was dropped — for 44 yards, and then ran 13 yards for a touchdown in the 80-yard, 12-play march.

Jerry Murphree had two catches, the first on third-and-2 at the LSU 28, to add more fuel to the drive. His second reception — for 13 yards — gave LSU a first down at the Deacon 21.

Fullback Jude Hernandez then broke through the middle for 8 yards to the Deacon 13, setting up Woodley's scoring run. Guard John Watson contributed a key block on Woodley's TD.

Moments later, the Tigers were in scoring position again. After McDonald had gained 19 yards on a third-down draw play, Tiger safety Marcus Quinn intercepted Venuto's pass on the Deacon 35.

Woodley struck quickly hitting Orlando McDaniel for a 15-

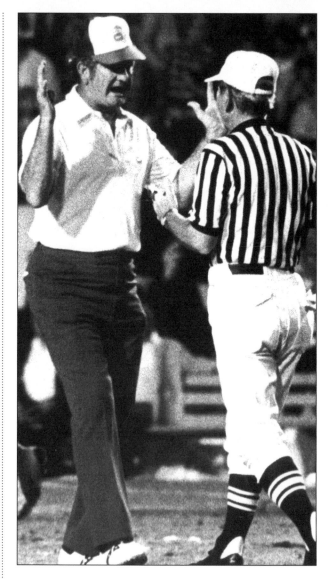

■ **Charlie McClendon argues with an official about the scoreboard clock.**

yard gain to the 20. Then facing a third-and-8 at the Deacon 12, Woodley — who was unaffected by noseguard James Parker pulling on his leg — lobbed a 6-yard completion to Carlos Carson.

On fourth-and-2, Woodley — aided by a Hernandez block — scampered 9 yards around the right side for a first down. On the next play, he rolled left, then cut between two would-be tacklers at the goal line for the second Tiger score.

With Steve Ensminger taking over at quarterback on the next possession, LSU again appeared on its way to a touchdown.

The Tigers' offensive line continued to control the line of scrimmage, as Ensminger, freshman Jesse Myles and Danny Soileau took turns riddling the Deacon defense.

After a pass interference call against Deacon defensive back Derek Crocker, who was covering Murphree in the end zone,

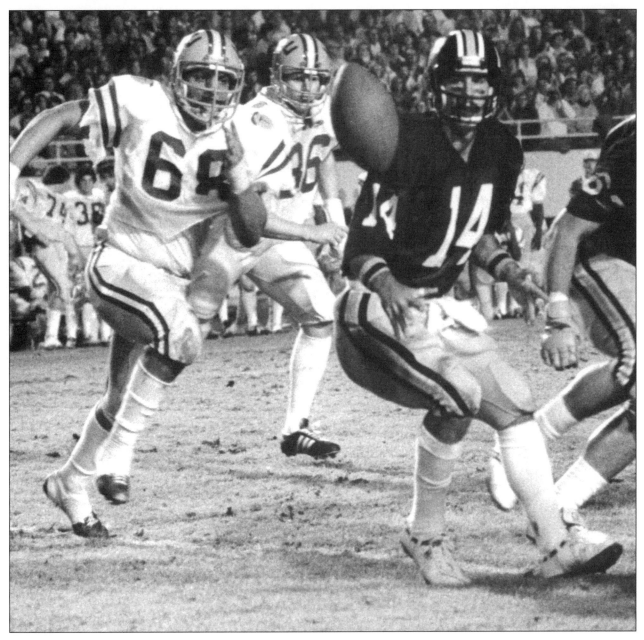

■ **Jay Venuto, who completed 10 of 20 passes for 165 yards, was constantly under attack by the LSU defense.**

the Tigers had a first down at the Deacon 1. However, on second down, Myles fumbled as he was hit at the goal line and Wake Forest's Eddie Green recovered.

Another Tiger drive was halted at the Wake Forest 31 before Woodley returned to engineer a 90-yard scoring drive. A 30-yard completion to Carson, open on the sideline when defender Lewis Owens fell down, accounted for most of the yardage. Two plays later, Woodley passed 19 yards to Murphree, who made a diving catch in the end zone for LSU's third TD of the evening.

The Tigers missed another scoring opportunity when Albert Richardson recovered an Albert Kirby fumble on the Wake Forest 20. After a 9-yard Woodley-to-Lionel Wallis

completion, LSU was pushed back 5 yards on an illegal procedure penalty. Two passes fell incomplete before the Tigers turned to Don Barthel, who responded with a 31-yard field goal.

Wake Forest came to life in the final minute of the first half after Landon King intercepted a Woodley pass on the Wake Forest 34.

Sophomore David Webber then replaced Venuto at quarterback and completed a 15-yard pass to tight end Mike Mullen. A 16-yard completion to Baumgardner seconds later gave the Deacons a first down on LSU's 27.

On the final play of the half, Denfeld put the Deacons on the scoreboard with his 43-yard field goal.

In A Difficult Hour, the Torch Is Passed

BY MARVIN WEST
Special to The Advocate

I t is a strange, strange story, a chilling mystery, a haunting twist of fate ... one man's heart was broken, another man died. Another, after dreaming 15 years and being denied, saw his dream come true.

This is the stunning story of how Jerry Lane Stovall became head football coach at Louisiana State University.

Stovall, a Tiger halfback two decades ago, wanted to be the coach where he had played. He prepared properly, touched all the bases, knew the time was near.

On a day when the date could just as easily have been set, Jerry Stovall got the coldest message of his life. Paul Dietzel, back in Baton Rouge as athletic director of LSU, was playing with a different deck of cards. The game had changed. Jerry didn't fit the criteria imposed on Dietzel by the school's Board of Supervisors.

Stovall is smart. He learns quickly. In a matter of minutes, some twenty years ago, he realized he'd never be the boss of the Bengals. Oh, how that hurt!

About the same time, Charles Y. McClendon was twisting in the wind. After all those good years in Tigertown, between the time Dietzel left and returned Cholly Mac was told to go, that he was finished, that his time had expired.

Well, he could stay as head coach through 1979.

Stovall, forced to choose between an apprenticeship in athletic administration, a far more lucrative business offer or dying on the vine as a McClendon assistant on the field, made a wise decision. He went on down the road with Dietzel.

After all, it was Dietzel who first put him on the path, played him as running back, receiver and safety, gave his such a chance, Jerry fell only a few votes short of the Heisman Trophy.

Dietzel training helped Stovall play as pro. When his fun and games ended in the NFL, it was Dietzel who took Stovall into coaching, as an aide at South Carolina, and told him some day he'd be a head coach.

That was good but Columbia, SC., wasn't home and when Jerry got a chance, he rushed back to Baton Rouge, to assist McClendon, to give back some of the things he had learned as a Tiger, to further prepare for the time when the top job would be his.

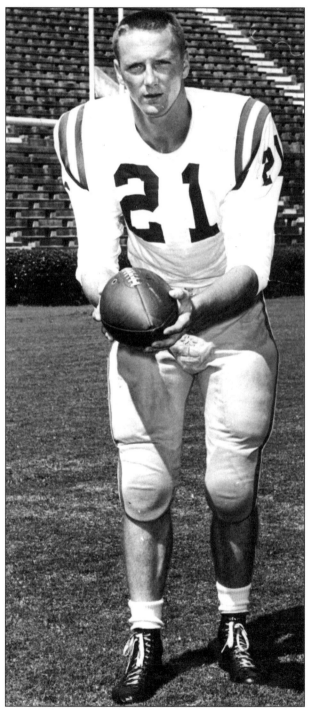

■ Jerry Stovall, a 1962 All-American halfback for the Tigers, became LSU's coach after Bo Rein's death.

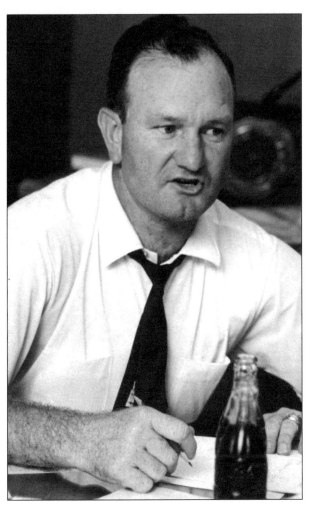

■ Charlie McClendon served as an assistant to Paul Dietzel and later coached the Tigers for 18 seasons.

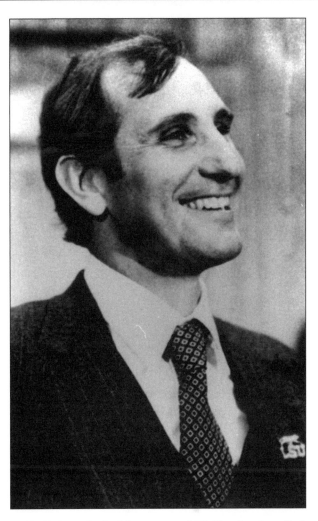

■ Bo Rein took the job to succeed McClendon, but died in a plane crash while on a recruiting trip 42 days later.

Then, the whole dream was gone ... but Dietzel was still there.

Dietzel lashed unfairly by some for allegedly undercutting Cholly Mac, only did what the LSU administration had dictated when he returned. McClendon was to be phased out, as gracefully as possible, and an established head coach be found to replace him.

That requirement knocked out the bridge for Stovall. He had never been a head coach. It didn't matter that he was Dietzel's down-deep choice, that they had a father-son relationship, that Paul was sure Jerry would be an inspiring leader.

Dietzel spent more than a year in a serious search. LSU faithful split into factions. Some wanted new life for McClendon. Some wanted Ara Parseghian, Lou Holtz or Bobby Bowden. Some thought Dietzel should attempt a comeback, try to again catch lightning in a jar, as he did with the national championship Tigers of 1958 the time of Billy Cannon.

Dietzel is too smart for that. He hired Bo Rein, 34, a former Ohio State wingback, and four years the head coach at North Carolina State, with a record of 27-17-1, two bowl teams and

one Atlantic Coast Conference championship.

Yes, Bo Rein was the man. He had no Tiger ties. He could unify the family. He was enthusiastic, energetic, a tireless recruiter. Rein brought seven helpers from his Raleigh staff, came to town while the McClendon team was still milling around the office, and hit the road to round up prep talent.

"This man has the look of an eagle," Dietzel said of Rein. "I liked him when I saw him, and, of course, when I hired him. Now that I have seen him at work, I like him even better."

Rein logged thousands of miles for LSU in 42 days. That's how long he was head coach of the Tigers.

On a Thursday night, Jan. 9, 1980, with pilot Lewis Benscotter, in a sophisticated corporate plane, on loan to LSU football, the coach was flying to home base from a recruiting trip in Shreveport, La.

A storm line near Alexandria may have forced the pilot to change his course, but that should not have been a problem. The almost new Cessna Conquest, owned by Nichols Construction Company, was a twin turbo prop, pressurized to be safe at 33,000 feet, and equipped with a radar transponder that automatically

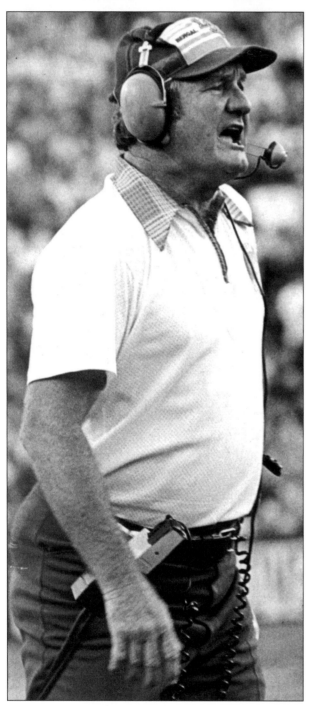

■ **Charlie McClendon took his teams to 13 bowl games in 18 seasons.**

returned it to a charter course after any pilot adjustment.

But for some strange reason, still unexplained, the Rein plane didn't follow its "mind." The pilot had requested clearance of Fort Worth air control to 25,000 feet but controllers, watching the blip on their screen, saw it ease on up to 29,000 and turn northeast toward Memphis instead of southeast to Baton Rouge.

An FAA report says the Forth Worth tracking crew tried to establish radio contact but failed.

The Air Force Rescue Center near St. Louis dispatched two F-4 fighter planes from Seymour-Johnson Air Force Base, near Raleigh to seek information — standard procedure when an event so puzzling is in progress. The jet pilots spotted the Cessna, but saw no cabin lights, no sign of life aboard. Again, radio contact efforts failed.

Many find it ironic, if not spooky, that the Rein plane flew near Raleigh, where he had worked three years for Holtz and four on his own, where the family home hadn't been sold, where the Rein daughters, nine and 13, were still staying with relatives.

Why Raleigh?

Another Air Force jet, an F-106, went up from Langley AFB near Norfolk, Va., to see what it could see. This pilot reported "close fly-bys," said he blinked landing lights and fired an afterburner in a bid to attract the Cessna's attention. Nothing happened.

Something finally did. The Rein ride went on, as high as 41,000 feet and more than 1,000 miles in the wrong direction, until it crashed, apparently out of fuel, about 120 miles off the Virginia coast, into the Atlantic Ocean. The Coast Guard reported the plane hit, with great impact in an area past the continental shelf, where water is up to 6,000 feet deep.

The tragedy rocked LSU to the foundations. What would happen to the young family? How about the assistant coaches who had followed Rein to Tigertown and now had no leader? What about the LSU football program, so long struggling with instability? The recruiting race was about to peak.

Dietzel, up through a night of anxiety, into a morning of shock, started home from the office at 5:45 a.m. Something had to be done in a hurry.

"I remember my prayer ... 'Lord, what do we do now? Please guide my decision. It is in Your hands now.' "

After two hours rest, Dietzel rushed to the office of Chancellor Paul W. Murrill. They agreed the loss was terrible, that Rein's staff was devastated, that chaos was near. There was not time for another search. The school had an obligation to McClendon's assistants until June and to Rein's for a year. It could not, with any logic, hire another established coach with another staff and pay three!

Yes, Dietzel said, he could have a recommendation for a Saturday Board of Supervisor's meeting.

Stovall was the only solution, the only man who would stick his finger into the dike with a chance to stop the leak.

"Jerry Stovall was absolutely and completely qualified in every way," says Dietzel, looking back. "He is young, tough, aggressive, articulate, a great recruiter, the best I ever had.

"He is highly intelligent, professionally trained, with superior integrity. He knew LSU through and through and, of all the people I could think of, he knew Bo's staff best."

Stovall, working as LSU fund-raiser out of Dietzel's office, knew the assistants far better than did the athletic director. Stovall had seen them come into the state, meet people they had never seen, go to towns with names they couldn't pro-

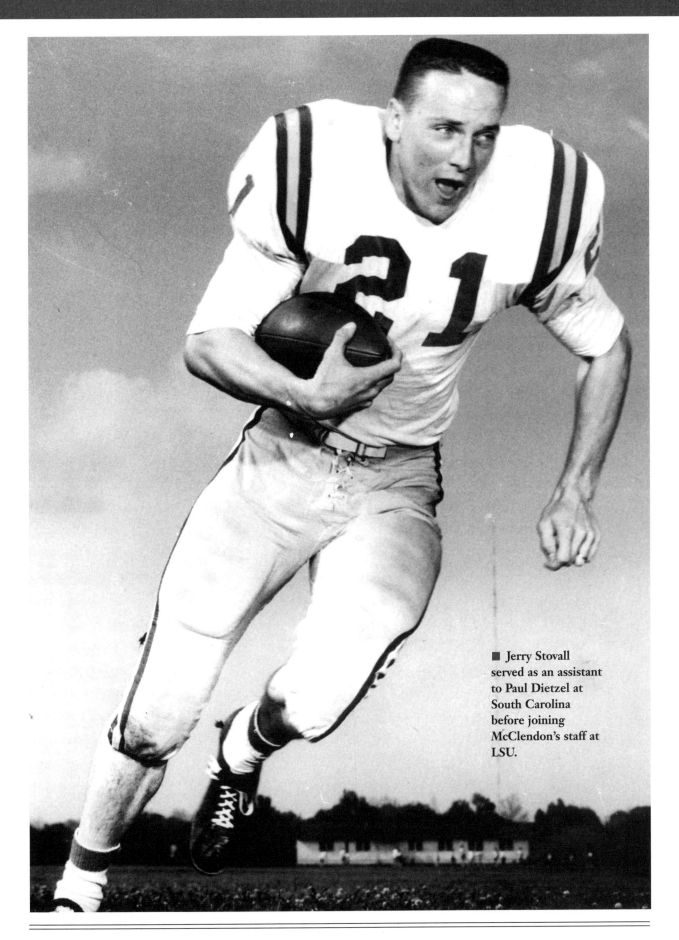

■ Jerry Stovall served as an assistant to Paul Dietzel at South Carolina before joining McClendon's staff at LSU.

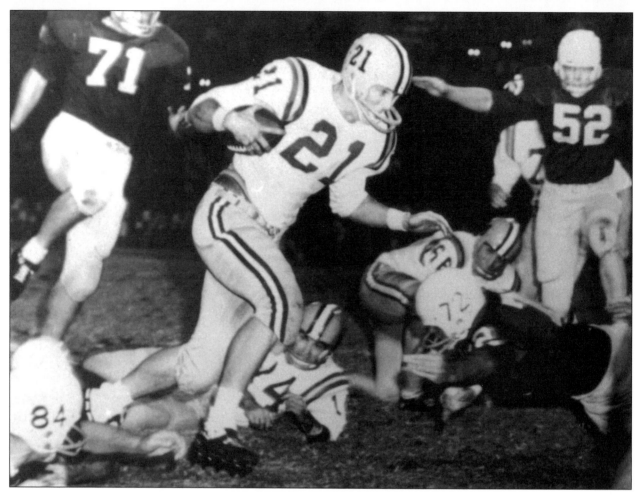

■ **Jerry Stovall was a runner-up for the Heisman Trophy in 1962.**

nounce and do a job for LSU. He had escorted them, individually, to booster club meetings in their new recruiting territories.

Stovall would take the head coaching responsibility and keep all the assistants that wanted to stay.

Why the haste? Did it have to be Saturday, one day and a few hours after the ill-fated flight?

"We were already getting calls with suggestions on who we ought to hire this time," recalls Dietzel. "The division was beginning again. For the sake of LSU, it had to be stopped. Jerry Stovall was the obvious solution."

And so, Dietzel advanced the name he would have liked in the first place, had the supervisors not demanded a coach with a name already in lights.

Jerry Stovall, the only choice in a time of great crisis, got the job he couldn't get when there was a year to evaluate. It's like asking a man to leave the mansion when dinner is about to be served and then calling his name in desperation when the roof is on fire.

Stovall responded with sadness ... and perfectly normal delight.

"I would gladly surrender this job, and any other, and my

right arm if Bo Rein could still be here," said Stovall, a sincere man, a Christian.

"Yes, this is a dream come true," he would say later. "I am so happy to have the opportunity but I regret deeply the circumstances that gave me the job. It involved tragedy in others' lives. I am keenly aware of the hurt Sue Rein and her family are going through. I wouldn't wish than on anyone.

"But there's no way on God's Earth I am going to hang my head and say I backed into this job. I am the head coach at LSU and I am proud to have been chosen. I would like to think I was the person who could plug the dike. I don't know how many others could. I do know Paul Dietzel could have done it."

Stovall started dreaming this dream in 1964.

"That's when Judy and I started dreaming it. I say 'we' because we are a team. And it is Judy and Jerry, if anybody asks. We are not Mr. And Mrs. Stovall, we are Mrs. and Mr. I couldn't do anything that requires the time and energy of coaching by myself. It takes both of us to do the job."

"Both of us" resigned from dental school in St. Louis in 1964 and made the commitment to coaching. "Both of us" wanted to come back to Baton Rouge when Coach Mac had an opening.

"Both of us" were broken-hearted when they discovered

there was no end to the rainbow, that Judy and Jerry couldn't be head coach when Coach McClendon was through.

"We talked about it, decided the Good Lord does not close one door to you without opening another. A good friend in Birmingham, Ala., offered us a job in Denver at a lot more money.

"I was very, very disappointed by what happened at LSU but I didn't really want to leave. We had to face that 'Never be head coach' and live with it. We cried. We wanted it so badly, you don't get over such a trauma in a week."

When Judy and Jerry decided they'd stay, they put the hurt behind them and went back to work, just as hard for LSU. Such is the character of the new head coach.

Can Stovall compete?

"I believe in Jerry Stovall," said Jerry. "I've stolen enough good ideas from Coach Dietzel and others to be good.

"You want to go to the blackboard with chalk in hand and do X's and O's? Let's go.

"You want to hit the road and recruit? I'll do it against anybody.

"You want to talk about motivation? Hey, I'll go head-to-head."

Stovall says the experience of not getting the LSU job in the beginning may have better prepared him when it came.

"I had to accept the facts. I found out that part of my prayer — Your will be done, Lord — was very real. I had been living life pretty much my way, the way I wanted it to go. When it headed off in the other direction, I wondered, for a minute, if the old ship would sink. But, there was that old verse about all things working for good for those who love the Lord."

What was a Stovall way back then, that we might get a clue to what is a Stovall today?

"LSU signed 52 the year I came in. I was No. 51. I came with minimal talent, marginal skills. My best 100 (-yard dash time) was 10.2, in living color. One sportswriter, generous to a fault, called me a 'slender youngster from West Monroe.' I was a skinny runt.

"The only real asset I had was the fact that I would try. Then and now, you may whip me but you better bring a big stick and a sack lunch to the fight ... because it's going to last a while!

"I'm not very fast or quick or strong or big ... but I will try."

Can a coach be so religious?

"I've been mixing faith and football a long time, now. I can keep doing it. I will not compromise my principles to get through this jungle. I can win without cheating.

"There are still too many good people working very hard at raising children in the right way, so they'll be quality people, positive people, with genuine values when they grow up.

"We just need 30."

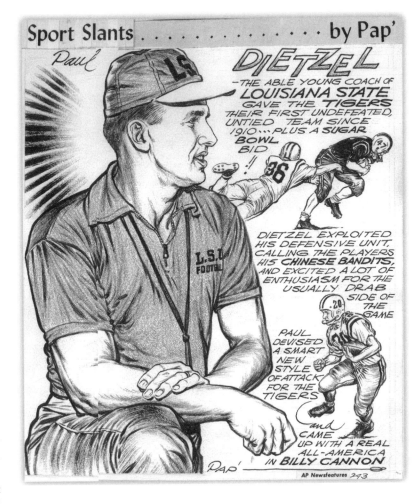

Stovall, after being selected as the new coach, attended a memorial service in Raleigh for Bo Rein on Sunday, Jan. 12. He met with Rein's coaches, told them he wanted them, told them they were better qualified, by six weeks, to help LSU through the crisis than anyone else in America.

"I told them I am a Christian, that they needed to understand that. They needed to know what I stand for, why I want to do what is right. I told them if they didn't agree with that basic concept, they should not consider returning to LSU.

"I saw some questions on some faces. They wondered what the words meant. Will he let me coach hard? Is he tough enough to win? What will he do if others cheat on the player I am recruiting? Does he have enough guts to get on the phone and do something about it?

"This is a place where you can not only win, you can dominate! I'm not interested in winning 10 of 11. I want to win 'em all. I don't want to go out there and whip you a little. I want to stop your will to compete against me.

"It's not a question of whether we'll win or lose. It's how badly we are going to whip you, on the scoreboard and physically. We're gonna stick those yellow headgears in some ears."

This article was originally published in Fall 1980.

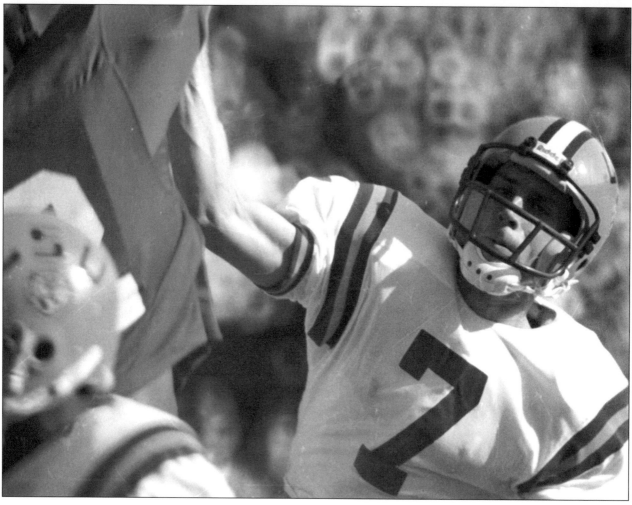

■ Alan Risher completed 13 of 16 first-half passes against the Crimson Tide.

Risher & Tigers Upset Alabama, 20-10

By Jimmy Hyams
The Advocate

Birmingham, Ala. — *Nov. 6, 1982*

After 12 years of bondage, the LSU Tigers finally freed themselves. The cage was opened. The chains were unbuckled. No longer are they "owned" by Bama and the Bear.

Their Moses was a feeble-looking, yet heady player named Alan Risher, who orchestrated miracle after miracle with his right arm and wiggly feet to end more than a decade of frustration.

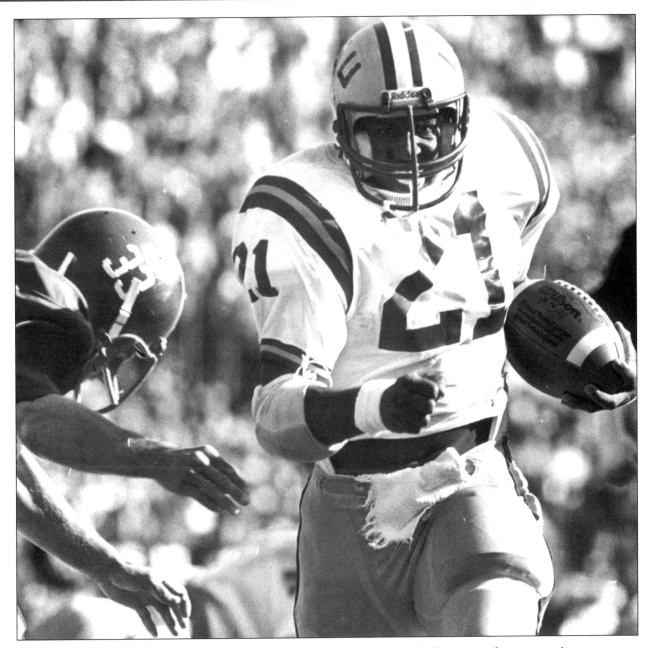

■ Dalton Hilliard (21) only rushed for 30 first-half yards, but turned in a dazzling 33-yard pass reception.

LSU's senior quarterback parted the Crimson Tide with 20 completions and scrambled for numerous crucial first downs to lead the No. 10 Tigers to one of their most brilliant victories in LSU football history, a 20-10 upset over No.7-ranked Alabama before 77,230 fans in Legion Field this afternoon

So dominant was LSU's performance, it had Alabama coach Bear Bryant, the winningest coach in college history, talking retirement.

"I think this is the biggest win for anyone associated with LSU in the last 12 years," said Risher, who threw for 182 yards and one touchdown. "This ends 12 years of suffering as a fan and player."

The usually reserved Risher even did a little "victory dance" on the field after he'd picked up a first down with four minutes

Score by Periods

LSU	0	17	0	3	— 20
Alabama	0	0	10	0	— 10

to go. "I was just real happy," He said.

So was LSU coach Jerry Stovall, who had downplayed LSU's earlier victory over then No. 4-ranked Florida.

"Without a doubt, this is the biggest victory I've ever had as a coach," said Stovall, who gave the game ball to his wife, Judy. "It's been a long, long time. You can't understand what it's like to get hit in the mouth 11 years in a row."

It was LSU delivering the knockout punch today, though, using a wide open offense and a stingy defense as its 1-2 punch. The Tigers erupted for 17 second-quarter points on Dalton Hilliard's 16-yard run, Risher's 3-yard pass to Malcolm Scott and Juan Carlos Betanzos' 23-yard field goal. And the defense held on in the second half after the Tide had cut the margin to 17-10.

LSU is now 7-0-1 on the season and second in the Southeastern Conference with a 4-0-1 mark. The Tigers had hoped to move into the SEC lead, but first place Georgia (5-0) bombed Florida, 44-0. However, the Tigers are still in the thick of the race for the Sugar Bowl, which automatically goes to the conference champion.

Georgia plays its final conference game at Auburn next Saturday while LSU visits Mississippi State in Starkville, Miss. Also its league finale.

Alabama which has won or tied for the SEC title nine of the last 11 years in now 7-2 and 3-2.

"I think that's the best beating we've had since the 1960's," said Bryant, whose team was outgained 321 yards to 119. "LSU had the superior team and I know that they had the best coach. They were better prepared."

It appeared that way from the beginning.

Using a more simplistic scheme than in the last two years to stop the wishbone, LSU's Bandit defense held the Crimson Tide without a first down and only 32 total yards in the first half. The Bandits contained Alabama quarterback Walter Lewis so well, he was benched in favor of Ken Coley in the last five minutes of the first half.

Lewis, who is second on Alabama's all-time single-season total yardage list was held to 21 yards rushing and 74 yards passing. The Tide managed only 45 yards rushing against the nation's No. 1-rated defense.

"I think our game plan was just super," said LSU senior linebacker Albert Richardson, explaining that LSU had at least two men assigned to the fullback, quarterback and pitch man on each play.

So frustrated was the Tide offense, Bryant had them running plays before the start of the third quarter. The Tide did show more spunk in the second half, but it wasn't enough.

"Lewis has beaten everybody they've played this year," said LSU linebackers coach Buddy Nix, who served as a graduate assistant at Alabama in 1961-62. "We had different ways to take him (the quarterback) out of plays if we needed them — and we did. Alabama discovers what you're doing on the first series and they hone in on it. We just rotated which man had who on their option."

But even Nix, who calls LSU's defensive signals, was surprised at LSU's first half success, which included holding Alabama to 10 yards on 15 carries. The Tide was averaging more than 300 yards rushing per game.

"If somebody had told me we'd hold them without a first down in the first half, I'd have said they were crazy," admitted Nix, who lost to Alabama five straight years while he was a defensive assistant at Auburn (1976-80).

"I've been coaching a long time (21 years) and that's the

sweetest (win) I've ever been around," he said.

Not only was LSU's defensive game plan a marvel, the offense showed a series of different sets and new plays which kept Alabama off balance for all but the first quarter. LSU dominated time of possession, holding the ball for 39 minutes and 30 seconds against a team noted for its ball control. The Tigers also converted 14 of 26 third downs while Alabama was 0-for-11.

"The game plan worked probably exactly like we wanted it to," said LSU quarterbacks coach Mack Brown, who also calls the plays. "We felt like we had to break all of our tendencies and throw about 50 percent of the time on first down — Alabama has done such a great job coaching against tendencies."

Brown also had high praise for Risher, who hit 13 of 16 first half passes and had 218 total yards in the game.

"Alan has come 10,000 miles since the first of the year," said Brown, who has added flare to the Tiger offense in his first season at LSU. "He's as good a quarterback mentally as any in the country."

Risher, however, lost his smarts for a few moments during a brutal defensive struggle in the first quarter. He sat out two plays and one series before re-entering in the second quarter.

"I just got my bell rung." Said Risher, who holds 15 LSU records. "I got hit in the head by one of their linebackers. I just wanted to come out and get my head together."

During the series Risher missed, LSU missed an excellent scoring opportunity. Cornerback Eugene Daniel recovered a Lewis fumble at the Alabama 24 with 6:03 left in the first period. But reserve quarterback Timmy Byrd was sacked on consecutive plays for minus-20 yards and the Tigers ended up punting from the 43.

Alabama, the SEC's No. 1 scoring team, couldn't take advantage of two first-half breaks. The second low punt-snap from center Curt Gore of Fairhope, Ala., gave the Crimson Tide possession on the Tiger 40. And Eddie Lowe recovered a Garry James fumble at the Tide 46 five minutes later. On both occasions, Alabama was stifled by the hard-charging Bandits.

LSU drew first blood with 8:14 left in the second period when Hilliard used blocks by Mike Montz and Malcolm Scott to dash around left end 16 yards for a touchdown. He dragged two Alabama players with him across the goal line to cap an 11-play, 90-yard drive. Betanzos' PAT made it 7-0.

"I felt I had to get in the end zone," said Hilliard, who rushed for 30 first-half yards before sitting out all but one series in the second half with a bruised thigh and calf. "Against Alabama, you have to make each play a big one."

Hilliard made another big play in the drive, catching a swing pass from Risher and turning it into a 33-yard gain by running through three potential Tide tacklers. Only a shoestring stop at the 29 by Rocky Colburn kept Hilliard from going 62 yards and a score. Risher said it was a new play — a tailback delay pass in the flats.

LSU then got 10 quick points thanks to Alabama's uncharacteristic generosity. On Coley's first play from scrimmage, halfback Joe Carter fumbled and Liffort Hobley recovered at the Tide 27 with 5:37 left before intermission. Nine plays later,

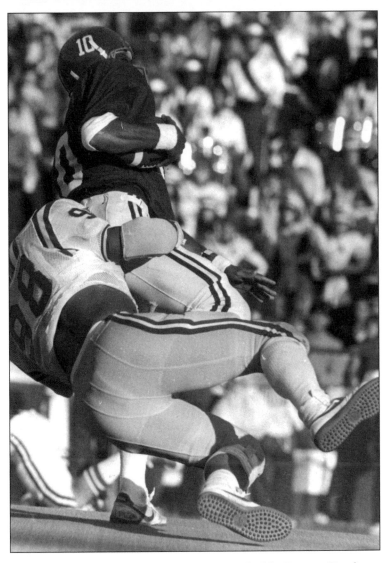

■ **Alabama quarterback Walter Lewis is sacked by Ramsey Dardar.**

Obviously embarrassed by its first half showing, Alabama came out with fire.

After Parker's 33-yard punt on another low snap, the Tide marched to the LSU 5. But on third-and-four, Lewis was hit by linebacker Lawrence Williams and fumbled out of bounds at the 14. Peter Kim was called on to kick a 31-yard field goal with 8:08 left in the third period to cut the gap to 17-3.

On LSU's next possession, Hilliard fumbled a pass from Risher and Al Blue recovered at the LSU 28. On the next play, Lewis then fired a 28-yard scoring pass to Joey Jones, whose post-corner route had cornerback James Britt beaten by a step. Kim's PAT made it 17-10 and gave the Tide its second score in 26 seconds.

It had all the makings of a typical Alabama comeback.

"Yes, there was little bit of fear," said LSU outside linebacker Tim Joiner. "They scored 10 quick points and I started to wonder."

"I was thinking we'd have to play a little bit harder," said defensive tackle Leonard Marshall. "And that's what we did."

LSU answered with a 9-play, 37-yard drive. Although it didn't produce any points, it cut off the Tide's wave of momentum.

When the Tigers got the ball back, they went 63 yards in 13 plays to set up Betanzos' ninth field goal of the year — a 20-yarder with 10:41 left to play to make it 10-10. The drive consumed 5:55 and was highlighted by Risher completions of 13, 6, 5 and 11 yards.

The Tigers finally put the game away when tackle Bill Elko sacked Lewis, forcing a fumble which linebacker Gregg Dubroc recovered at the Tide 48 with 4:57 remaining.

"I was just thinking, 'Please don't throw that damn ball,' " Elko said of his rush on Lewis. "I was hoping he wouldn't. I got a good clean hit and the ball popped out."

And when Dubroc pounced on it, he had more than just the football. He had a piece of LSU history. When the Tigers proceeded to run out the clock by marching to the 9, it snapped a dozen years of sometimes bitter frustration.

"This is the highlight of my football career," said Elko, a transfer from Arizona State who was plagued by injury last season. "Hopefully, it won't be the last."

Nose guard Ramsey Dardar hopes Elko is correct.

"Right now we are tasting Sugar," said Dardar. But he knows LSU must not only beat Mississippi State next week to gain a Sugar Bowl berth. He knows Auburn must beat Georgia for LSU to win the SEC.

That, of course, hasn't happened in 11 years. Which leaves Risher with a few more chains to unbuckle and another cage to open.

Risher fired a 3-yard bullet to Scott on a third down play-action pass with 58 seconds showing.

Betanzos' ensuing sky-kickoff was fumbled by Craig Turner — one of four Tide turnovers — and Alvin Thomas recovered at the Alabama 30. Risher's 12-yard rollout moved the ball to the 11, and two plays later Betanzos kicked a 23-yard field goal with five seconds left. His boot came after consecutive timeouts by LSU, then Alabama. It sent LSU into the dressing room with a 17-0 cushion to the delight of some 12,000 Tiger fans who made the trip.

Unlike the second half against Florida last month, when LSU became conservative in an effort to protect a 24-5 lead, Brown continued with a wide open attack.

"We felt like we could not sit on the ball," said Brown. "We told our kids at the half to play like it was 0-0. We knew Alabama, with their tradition and athletes, had a chance to score every time they had the football."

It looked that way at the beginning of the third quarter.

The Tigers' Domination was Total

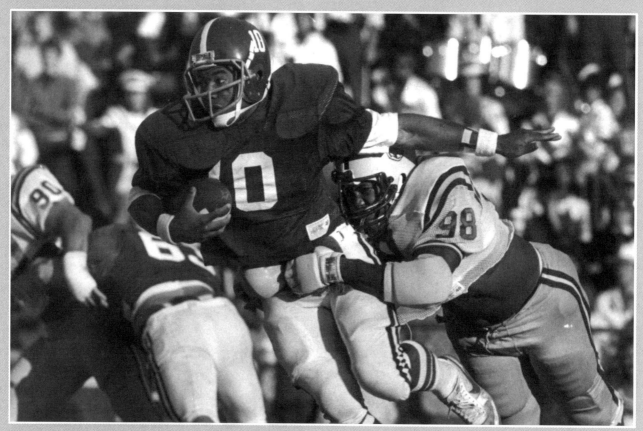

■ The relentless pressure of LSU's defense shut down Alabama's wishbone attack.

BY JOHN ADAMS
The Advocate

Birmingham, Ala. — *Nov. 6, 1982*

There was a twin killing here this afternoon. Two long-time LSU tormentors bit the artificial turf at Legion Field.

The wishbone was the first to go. It was buried somewhere between the 20s.

And don't tell Alabama quarterback Walter Lewis about the wishbone's triple options. He'll tell you there are no options at the bottom of a pile, which is where he found himself too many times today.

Having broken — make that shattered — the wishbone, the rest was easy.

Let quarterback Alan Risher go to work on a Tide secondary that didn't include its best player — injured strong safety Tommy Wilcox. Then give them a little fancy footwork —

Dalton Hilliard — and watch the Tide defense look as befuddled as Oregon State, Florida and all the others that have tried to bring Hilliard to his knees.

That's how it was when it mattered today as LSU remained unbeaten with a 20-10 victory.

"They made the big plays," said Alabama defensive end Mike Pitts. "That's what college football is all about."

Risher has been making big plays all season. But he's never made so many big plays in a game that was so big.

He completed 20 of 26 passes for 182 yards. And when he wasn't shooting holes in the Tide secondary, he was outsmarting the folks up front with scrambles and bootlegs.

Although Hilliard only gained 30 yards rushing, he dazzled the Tide in LSU's 90-yard touchdown drive in the second quarter. Go back to the 40-yard line near the north end of the field, and you'll probably find two defenders kneeling in wonderment over a three-way collision that grounded everybody but Hilliard on a 33-yard pass-run play.

But this game was won by LSU's defense. Because to beat Alabama, you need to stop the wishbone. The Tigers did more than stop it. They shook it until it rattled.

Ask Lewis what the Tigers took away from the wishbone, and you'll draw a pause. His look said, "Everything."

"Let me think," he said. "I'm too tired to think. Oh, I'm tired ... They gave us very little."

That's a little as in no first downs in the first half, 45 yards rushing for the game, 119 yards total offense. And this was no pop-gun outfit. This was an Alabama offense that had been cranking out 300 yards per game rushing this season. In fact, the Tide has been producing outrageous rushing statistics ever since Bryant borrowed Texas' wishbone in the spring of 1971.

LSU hasn't beaten Alabama since then. From Terry Davis to Ken Coley, it seems like LSU has been forever chasing the wishbone into the end zone.

This time, it didn't have to catch the wishbone. There was never a take-off, just a few occasional gasps and sputters.

When Lewis took a snap, his whole offensive line seemed to collapse under the weight of Bill Elko, Ramsey Dardar, Leonard Marshall, Albert Richardson and Lawrence Williams. It happened so many times, it looked choreographed.

After that, Lewis was running naked, calling on his athletic talents — which are considerable — for survival. In other games — such as against Penn State — Lewis has turned such odds topsy-turvy.

But Lewis couldn't run clear of outside linebackers Rydell Malancon and Tim Joiner. They were too fast for him and his blockers, who were often nothing more than embarrassed spectators.

"They're so quick," Alabama center Danny Holcombe said of the Tigers' front seven. "You go to block them over there, and when you get there, they're gone. Yes, they're definitely the quickest defense we've played."

Even down 17-0 at halftime, there's a reluctance to dismiss Alabama as a threat. You think about all that tradition and all those comebacks. Just three years ago, Tennessee had the same lead at halftime. Final score: 27-17, Alabama.

But LSU was playing with too much confidence to let this one slip away. You can almost imagine Lawrence Williams, rather than an official, rapping on the Tide's dressing room door at halftime: "Time to come out, boys."

Alabama cut the lead to 17-10 because its defense hit hard enough to knock the ball loose from Hilliard and because Lewis had just enough time to hurl a marvelous pass to a speeding Joey Jones, a step ahead of James Britt in the LSU end zone.

But neither could turn the game Alabama's way. After the Tide cut the lead to 17-10, LSU converted on four of eight third-down conversions — and another time on fourth — in subtracting vital minutes from the clock and adding three precious points to the scoreboard.

Throughout the game, LSU made the plays that Alabama usually makes. It forced seven fumbles and recovered four, two of which set up scores.

Conversely, Alabama appeared stupefied at times. When the ball squirted free from halfback Joe Carter in the second quar-

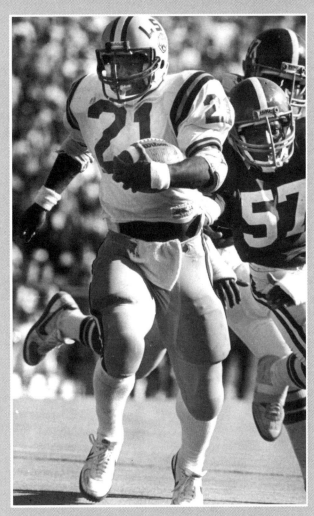

■ **Dalton Hilliard scoots 16 yards for a touchdown in the second quarter.**

ter, offensive guard Mike Adcock never left his feet as the ball bounced and bounced until it found the welcome arms of Liffort Hobley. His recovery set up LSU's second TD.

Midway in the fourth quarter Lewis broke from the pocket and began running wide in hopes of converting a third-and-13. He all but begged fullback Ricky Moore to scrap the pass play and pick up an oncoming defender. Moore never responded to Lewis' signal, and the deserted quarterback was dropped 9 yards short of a first.

"I think that's the best beating we've had since the 1960's," said Bryant, who talked as though the Alabama football program was in the hands of an incompetent leader.

While Bryant was hinting at retirement, the slower moving fans were in for another shock as they filed out of Legion Field. A whiskey bottle came sailing over the top of the stadium and crashed in the middle of five fans.

Seconds later, another bottle hit the pavement. Then a third. There were no victims, just scattered glass in the parking lot.

But inside the stadium, Alabama football had just been victimized. And if you didn't mind digging for evidence, there were pieces of a wishbone buried beneath Legion Field.

LSU Mauls Seminoles, 55-21

By John Adams
The Advocate

Baton Rouge, La. — *Nov. 20, 1982*

When you have Dalton Hilliard and Alan Risher pointing the way, Baton Rouge to Miami is an easy trip. Just make sure you don't trip over the oranges or get lost in the fog.

The Tigers avoided the hazards with ease as they roared to a 55-21 victory over the Florida State Seminoles tonight before 76,637 fans in Tiger Stadium. The victory earned the Tigers, 8-1-1, a berth in the Orange Bowl, and put Florida State, 8-2, in the Gator Bowl.

While today was the first day for officially extending bowl bids, LSU and Florida State entered the game knowing the winner would meet the Big Eight champion in the Orange Bowl New Year's night in Miami, and the loser would be paired against West Virginia in Jacksonville, Fla., Dec. 30.

There was no doubt which bowl the Tiger fans preferred. While no one threw an alligator onto the field, the sidelines were littered with oranges before the game ever began.

More were soon to fall as LSU broke open a 14-14 game with two touchdowns in the final 38 seconds of the first half. The 12th-ranked Tigers then overwhelmed the seventh-ranked Seminoles, 27-7, in the second half.

"I haven't seen any better team than LSU this year," Charles Kimbrell, the president of the Orange Bowl's team selection committee, said of the Tigers' performance. "And I think

Score by Periods

Florida State	7	7	0	7 —	21
LSU	7	21	14	13 —	55

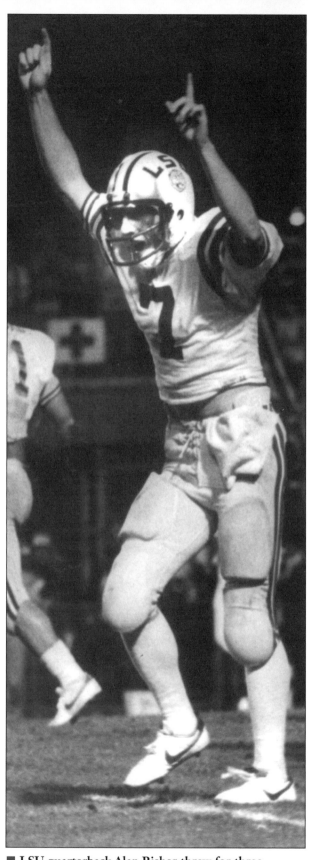

■ LSU quarterback Alan Risher threw for three touchdowns against Florida State.

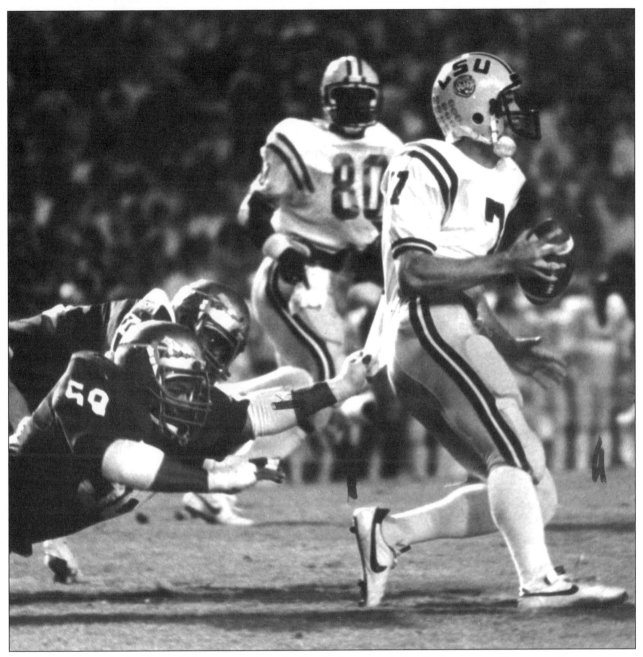

■ **Alan Risher (7) had an incredible game against the Seminoles, completing 8 of 12 passes for 212 yards.**

Hilliard is a Heisman Trophy candidate in the years ahead."

Speaking of the Heisman, Hilliard produced Herschel Walker-like figures tonight. He gained 183 yards on 36 carries and scored four touchdowns to break the NCAA touchdown record for freshmen.

The record of 15 was shared by Georgia's Walker (1980) and Lou Kusserow of Columbia (1945). The Tigers' freshman tailback has scored 16 touchdowns with one regular-season game remaining, next week against Tulane.

Hilliard said that kind of production was nothing more than his older teammates deserved. "We came into the season respecting our upperclassmen," he said. "And I felt we owed

them a lot. It wasn't easy.

"We had to establish our running game tonight. We were motivated both by last week's loss and thoughts of the Orange Bowl."

Hilliard rushed for three touchdowns and also caught a 40-yard TD pass from Risher, who completed eight of 12 passes for 212 yards and three touchdowns. Risher's other scoring passes went to Eric Martin and covered 34 and 70 yards.

That gave Risher 17 TD passes this season and 31 for his career. Bert Jones held the records of 14 and 28.

While the passing of Kelly Lowrey and Blair Williams helped the Seminoles pile up 425 yards against the Tigers' No. 2-ranked defense, Florida State couldn't keep pace with the

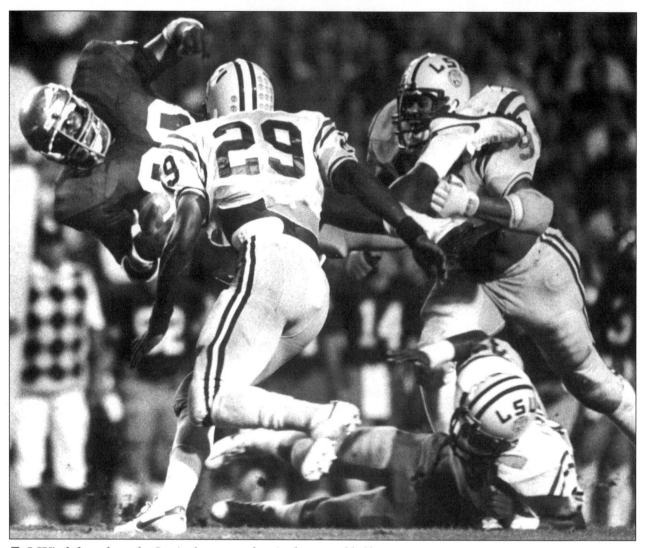

■ **LSU's defense kept the Seminoles wrapped up in the second half.**

Tigers in the final minutes of the first half.

The Tigers, who gained 20 yards total offense, broke the 14-14 tie on a 2-yard run by Hilliard. They added another TD on a 34-yard Risher to Martin pass after Sean Moore recovered a fumble by Tony Smith on the ensuing kickoff.

That left the Seminoles staggering, and they never regained their balance in the second half.

The victory means LSU will play the winner of this week's game between fourth-ranked Nebraska and Oklahoma. But at this point, head coach Jerry Stovall wasn't interested in the opposition.

"It doesn't matter," he said when asked about Nebraska-Oklahoma. "These little ragamuffins are looking forward to going to Miami and playing.

"Our team was prepared emotionally to play. A great deal of credit should be give to the young men who worked last spring and this year in preparation for a good year.

"I can't say enough about what our coaches and young men have done. The staff gave them a lot of confidence. Before the season, nobody wanted the young men so they gave them back to me. Tonight they made us — not only the coaches, but the state of Louisiana — extremely proud."

Tonight's victory highlighted LSU's turn-around from 3-7-1 a year ago. Not since 1973 has LSU won as many as nine games in a season, a feat the Tigers can accomplish with a triumph over Tulane next Saturday.

"We knew what was at stake," said senior offensive guard Mike Turner, who missed last season with a broken leg. "At 3-7-1, nobody loved us. It's been a dogfight to overcome that."

The oranges came first tonight. Then the

■ **It was a long night for FSU coach Bobby Bowden.**

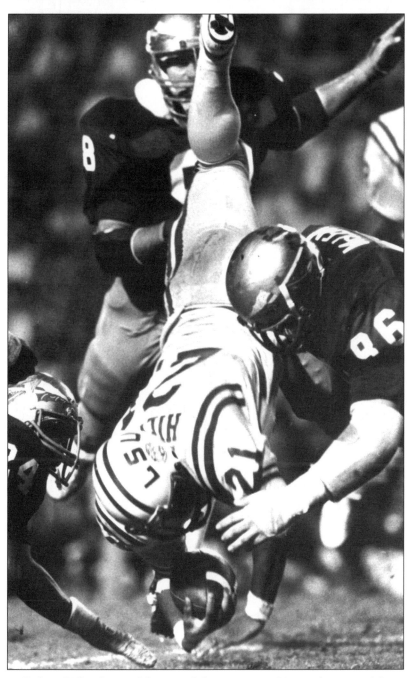

■ **Dalton Hilliard scored four touchdowns — 3 rushing and one receiving.**

On a third-and-five, Risher ignited the Tigers' first scoring drive with a 12-yard completion to tight end Malcolm Scott against an inside blitz.

After another completion to Scott, Risher spotted Hilliard behind linebacker Tommy Young and pitched a strike to the Seminoles' 26. Hilliard then eluded Gary Henry and Brian McCrary and raced into the end zone to complete the 46-yard play with 3:31 left in the quarter.

Florida State responded with a 56-yard drive in seven plays. The Seminoles lost one touchdown when Jessie Hester, a step ahead of Eugene Daniel, dropped a pass deep in the end zone.

Following the long miss, Lowrey went short to Tony Smith in the right flat and he rambled 25 yards to the Tigers' 5-yard line. After a timeout, Lowrey faked to Greg Allen, who executed a high dive over the middle without the ball. With the ball on his hip, Lowrey rolled around left end for the touchdown with 2:05 left in the quarter.

Florida State, which ranks second in the country in total offense, came roaring back from its 21 to the Tigers' 33. But Lowrey was called for intentional grounding when pressured by Leonard Marshall on second down, and tight end Zeke Mowatt fumbled after receiving a Lowrey pass on third down. Richardson made the hit and Daniel recovered.

Risher countered quickly with a pass to Martin over the middle for 17 yards to the Seminoles' 44. Two runs by Garry James gained one first down and helped set up the Tigers' second TD.

On a second-and-1 at the Seminoles' 23, James took a Risher pitch, rolled right and hurled a touchdown pass to Herman Fontenot deep in the end zone behind Henry and McCrary. Juan Betanzos' extra-point kick put LSU on top, 14-7, with 9:43 left in the half.

Then came the oranges. And more oranges. Fifteen yards worth, in fact. The penalty for unsportsmanlike conduct came after the LSU fans had been warned repeatedly by the public-address announcer.

Kicking off from his 25-yard line, Betanzos booted the ball out on the 9, and tried again from his 20. Billy Allen, who returned a kickoff 97 yards for a TD against LSU last year returned the kick 47 yards to the LSU 30.

After a 4-yard loss on first down, Lowrey caught the defense off guard with a short pass in the right flat to Smith, who made

passes. It was enough to keep the cheerleaders and the defenses ducking for cover in the first half.

"I didn't think a whole lot about it," center Mike Gambrell said of the flying fruit, which cost LSU two 15-yard penalties for unsportsmanlike conduct. "I didn't want anything to keep me from going to Miami."

On the field, LSU's throwing paid off first, but only after the Tigers had turned back a Florida State threat on the 17-yard line midway through the first half. Lowrey fumbled when he was sacked by Jeffery Dale, and Albert Richardson recovered on the Tigers' 23.

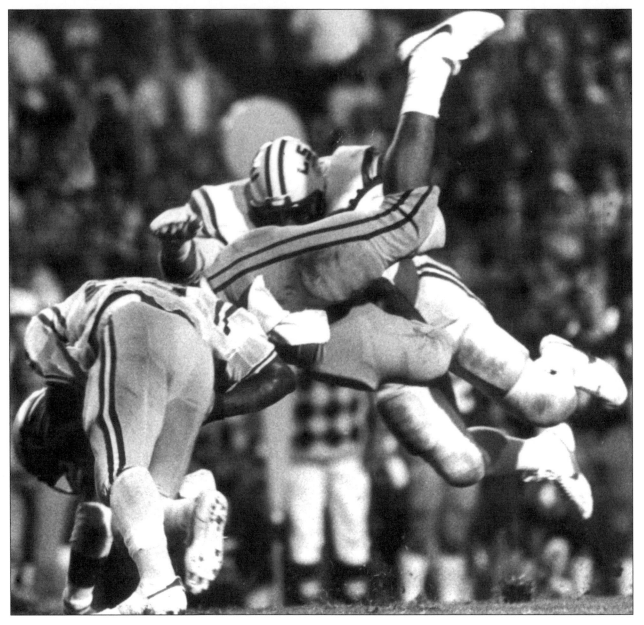

■ **FSU tailback Greg Allen was sent soaring by a pair of LSU defenders.**

the reception on the 28, dodged Lawrence Williams, and sprinted for the right corner of the end zone. Phillip Hall's extra-point kick evened the count at 14-all.

The last 9:16 of the half belonged to the Tigers, however. And it began to go their way after Scott Watson downed Clay Parker's punt on the Seminoles' 6-yard line.

Beginning their next series from the 50, the Tigers moved for the go-ahead score in 11 plays. With LSU's front six taking control at the line, Hilliard carried eight times for 46 yards in the drive.

"We started running our basic offense, that's all," Turner said of the drive. "We knew we had to score some points. As many times as the defense has pulled us through this year, we knew we had to come through tonight."

On second down-and-2, Hilliard came through, diving into the end zone as he was hit by Harry Clayton at the goal line with 38 seconds left. The Tigers then got two breaks. First, the fans didn't throw oranges. Second, Smith fumbled the kick over to the Tigers' Moore on the Florida State 34.

One play and six seconds later, LSU had a two touchdown lead. Risher passed to Martin, who beat Clayton across the middle, and dashed 34 yards for a touchdown.

"The two touchdowns they scored right before the half threw the whole game out of whack," said Florida State coach Bobby Bowden, whose team had beaten LSU the last three years in Tiger Stadium. "They were able to come out in the second half and beat us by keeping the ball on the ground."

The last minute of the first half was the beginning of the end

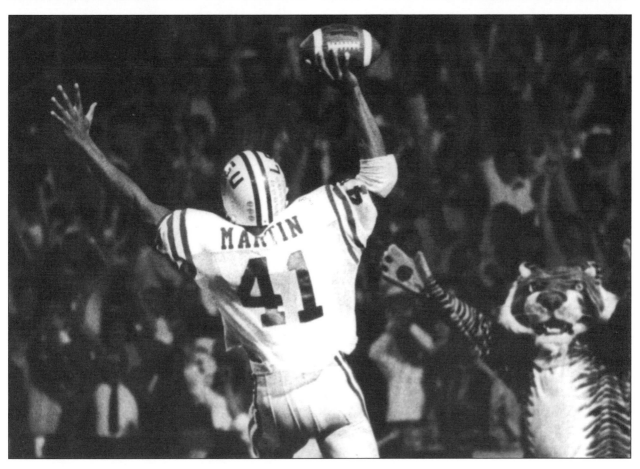

■ Eric Martin had touchdown receptions of 34 and 70 yards.

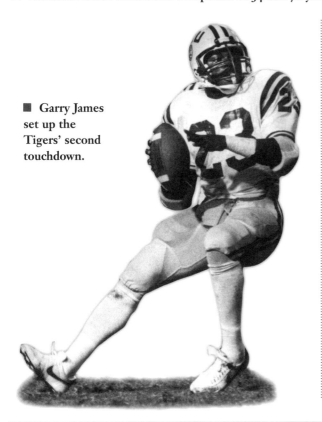

■ Garry James set up the Tigers' second touchdown.

for the Seminoles, who found themselves in a fog before the natural haze settled over Tiger Stadium late in the third quarter.

A massive dose of Hilliard dimmed the lights on the Seminoles. He carried 14 times in a 16-play, 80-yard scoring drive to open the second half. Hilliard, who accounted for all but 15 yards in the drive, scored on a 1-yard run with 6:16 left in the period.

Four minutes later, it was Risher's turn. He scrambled away from Alphonso Carreker behind the line and unleashed a 69-yard scoring pass to Martin.

A dazed Seminole defense was subjected to more Hilliard early in the fourth quarter as Stovall stuck with his first unit despite the 42-14 lead.

Following a 16-yard completion from Risher to Scott and a 14-yard gain by Mike Montz, Hilliard broke free around right end for a 28-yard scoring run.

The second team didn't fare badly either. Freshman quarterback Jeff Wickersham directed a 75-yard, 13-play drive after Florida State had scored on a 21-yard pass from Blair Williams to Hester. Wickersham capped the scoring with a 12-yard run around left end.

But that didn't end the throwing. Fans showered the field with oranges at the end of the game. In fact, the oranges were so thick, you almost couldn't see the fog.

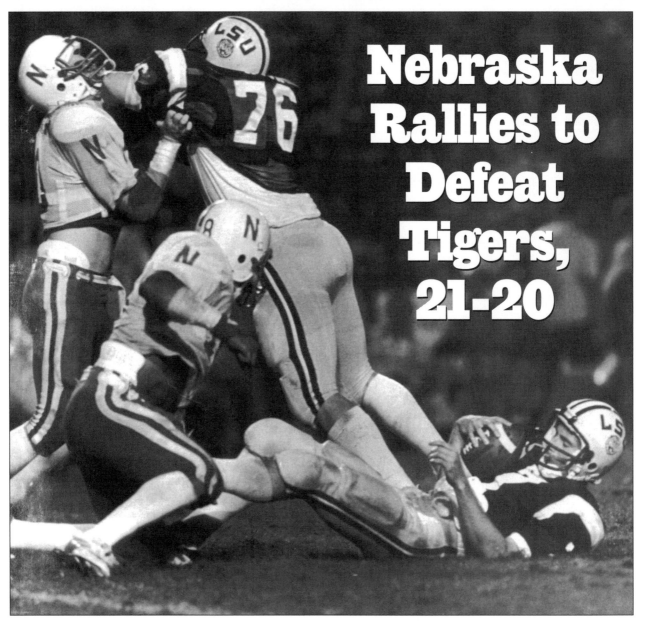

Nebraska Rallies to Defeat Tigers, 21-20

■ Nebraska's defense kept pressure on Alan Risher all evening in the Orange Bowl.

BY JOHN ADAMS
The Advocate

Miami, Fla. — *Jan. 1, 1983*

The No. 3-ranked Nebraska Cornhuskers, who couldn't hold on to the football for two and a half quarters, never let go of it in the final five minutes to nail down a 21-20 come-from-behind victory over the LSU Tigers in the 49th annual Orange Bowl here tonight.

Trailing, 7-7, midway through the third quarter, Nebraska cranked out touchdown drives in the third and fourth period, and then controlled the ball for the last 5:05 after Juan Betanzos' 49-yard field goal had pulled the Tigers to within a point.

Before Nebraska's late surge, it appeared the 10-point underdog Tigers were about to pull off the biggest upset of the new year before a disappointing crowd of 54,407 — the Orange Bowl's smallest in 36 years. LSU slowed down a Nebraska offense that averages 41.1 points and 518 yards per game with an alert defense that claimed five turnovers — four fumbles and an interception. Three turnovers in the first half and a pair of 1-yard TD runs by freshman tailback Dalton Hilliard had given the Tigers a 14-7 halftime lead. Betanzos upped the advantage to 17-7 with a 28-yard field goal with 6:04 left in the third quarter.

But Nebraska, which outscored its opponents 169-28 in the fourth period, began to roll. Quarterback Turner Gill and tailback Mike Rozier teamed up to spark scoring drives of 80 and 47 yards as Nebraska claimed its 12th victory in 13 games.

Gill, who completed 13 of 22 passes for 184 yards, tossed an 11-yard TD pass to Rozier to cap the first march, then scored on a 1-yard dive to put Nebraska on top with 11:14 left.

LSU, 8-3-1, had one more chance at winning the game, following a 20-yard interception by Lawrence Williams. Beginning at the Nebraska 37, LSU gained 9 yards in three plays — a 5-yard pass reception by Hilliard and two short runs.

On a fourth-and-one, Hilliard was stopped for no gain. But the play was negated by a delay-of-game penalty — flagged before the snap — against LSU. Betanzos then booted a 49-yard field goal to cut the lead to one with 5:05 left.

Nebraska never let go of the ball afterwards.

On its possession, Nebraska showed no signs of the frustrations to come in the first half. The nation's No. 1-ranked offense proved that. It advanced from its 20 to the LSU 37 on nine straight running plays before Gill completed a 13-yard pass to Irving Fryar on third-and-10. Nebraska then needed only two more plays to run out the clock.

"I told my players all week we were going to win the football game with 30 seconds left on a field goal," said LSU coach Jerry Stovall. "We would have to beat those suckers if we had got the ball back."

Asked about not going for the TD on fourth-and-6, Stovall said, "We kick a field goal and we still have five minutes to get the ball back. We get it back, Juan was kicking well, and it would have been 23-21.

"I wouldn't trade this football team for any other one in America tonight. They showed more strength and more character than any team I've ever been associated with."

The Nebraska offense was as good as advertised on a six-play, 51-yard touchdown drive.

Following a 25-yard Clay Parker punt, quarterback Turner Gill opened up with a 22-yard pass to wingback Irving Fryar, who was run out of bounds on the LSU 29. Nebraska then followed Gill's quick feet to inside the Tigers' 10-yard line.

Gill broke runs of 6- and 14-yard options around left end, then kept over left guard for 3 yards to the 5. A crushing block by All-America center Dave Rimington cleared the way for reserve fullback Mark Schellen's 5-yard scoring run on the next play with 10:57 left in the first quarter.

LSU responded quickly, moving from its 38 to the Nebraska 29 on two pass receptions by tight end Malcolm Scott and an alert play by Dalton Hilliard. After Scott caught a

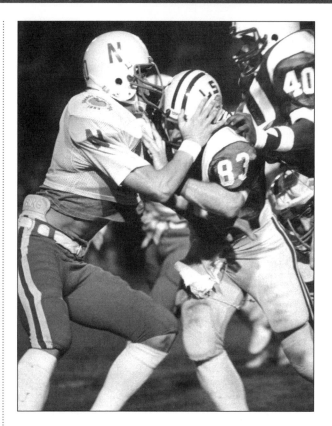

■ LSU held a 14-7 halftime lead, then Nebraska caught fire in the second half and won, 21-20.

21-yard pass from Alan Risher, he fumbled when hit by Bill Weber. Hilliard dove on the loose ball to keep the drive alive.

After an illegal-procedure penalty, Hilliard left a pair of Nebraska defenders spinning following a short pass from Risher, Hilliard gained 18 yards to the Cornhuskers' 16.

When the defense stiffened, LSU turned to Juan Betanzos, who kicked a 35-yard field goal. Coach Jerry Stovall decided he wanted more, however, after Allen Lyday was flagged for a late hit on Betanzos.

A 10-yard penalty gave LSU a first down on the 9, but the Tigers came up empty handed two plays later when tackle Toby Williams deflected a Risher pass and caught the ball on Nebraska's 10.

Then the Nebraska turnovers began to fall LSU's way. Rozier fumbled when he was rocked by Ramsey Dardar, and Liffort Hobley recovered on Nebraska's 11. After Hilliard sliced over left tackle for 8 yards, it took three plays — the last a 1-yard sneak by Risher — to produce a first down at the 1.

From there, Hilliard took two shots wide right. He scored the second time following a lead block by fullback Mike Montz.

Nebraska looked as though it would have little trouble breaking the deadlock. Gill completed three passes — two to Todd Brown — and Fryar gained 9 yards on an inside reverse as the Cornhuskers rolled from their 30 to the LSU 13.

On the first play of the second quarter, an LSU defense that recovered 23 fumbles during the regular season came up with

Score by Periods

LSU	7	7	3	3	— 20
Nebraska	7	0	7	7	— 21

its second of the game. Schellen lost the ball in the middle of the line and Rydell Malancon fell on it at the Tigers' 15.

Nebraska got its hands on the ball four plays later, but once again it couldn't hold on. Fryar fumbled before he was ever hit on a punt return and Gene Lang recovered at Nebraska's 45.

The Tigers' scoring drive was Hilliard and more Hilliard. He handled the ball by running or passing on all nine plays in a 45-yard scoring drive.

Twice, he turned short passes into big gainers with those darting moves that bedeviled so many defenders during the regular season. One gained 24 yards to the Nebraska 21. The second was on third-and-six from the 17. He made the catch on the 12 and raced to the 3-yard line.

He needed four plays to cover the next 3 yards. On fourth down, he received a pitch from Risher and swept wide left for one yard and the go-ahead touchdown. Betanzos' extra point gave the Tigers a 14-7 lead with 9:32 left in the half.

On its next try, Nebraska failed by an inch converting on a fourth-down fake punt at midfield. But after fullback Doug Wilkening was tackled short of the first down, LSU moved no further than the Cornhuskers' 39.

Nebraska had a chance to tie the game before halftime after a 33-yard Parker punt to the Tigers' 42. Gill connected with Fryar for a 17-yard completion on first down, but on third-and-five Malancon intercepted Gill's pass at the LSU 13. Gill was pressured on the play by strong safety Jeffrey Dale.

Nebraska was also frustrated on its first possession of the second half. A 20-yard kick return by Jeff Smith set the Cornhuskers on their 49.

Rozier gained 7, then broke three tackles on a 12-yard run to the 30. Facing a fourth-and-three at the 22, Kevin Seibel was four-for-four before the 39-yard field goal try.

Nebraska's fifth turnover in the game enabled LSU to up its lead to 10 points. Gill pitched wildly when hit by Dale and Lawrence Williams recovered on the Nebraska 41 with 8:17 to play in the third quarter.

On second down, Risher completed a 15-yard pass to Hilliard. Eric Martin then made a spectacular one-handed diving-catch on the Nebraska 7.

Montz carried to the Cornhusker 1 on the next play, but an illegal procedure penalty pushed LSU back to the 12. After Risher threw three straight incompletions, Betanzos kicked a 28-yard field goal with 6:40 left in the quarter.

Before the quarter ended, Nebraska showed what it can do when it doesn't drop the football. The Cornhuskers, who averaged 41.1 points per game during the season, marched 80 yards in 12 plays for their second TD.

The Tigers helped Nebraska along with a late hit that was worth 15 penalty yards to the Cornhuskers' 35. Gill gained 14 yards on an option to the LSU 44. And on fourth-and-one, Gill faked a handoff into the middle before completing an 18-yard pass to Brown on the LSU 17.

Three plays later, Rozier caught a swing pass from Gill in the right flat and ran down the sidelines untouched until he

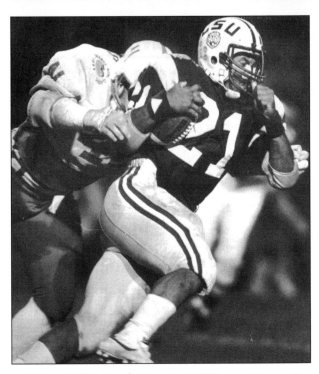

■ **Dalton Hilliard scored both of LSU's touchdowns in the first half.**

reached the end zone. Seibel's extra-point kick trimmed LSU's lead to 17-14, with 1:25 left in the half.

Nebraska's offensive momentum proved contagious. The Cornhuskers sacked Risher twice on LSU's next series to set up a fourth-and-19. When Parker was rushed on fourth down, he elected to run. Running with one foot bare, he went to the LSU 47, but was 8 yards short of a first down.

Once again, an LSU penalty got the Cornhuskers started. James Britt was flagged for pass interference on Brown at the 36. Two plays later, Gill hit Fryar cutting over the middle at the 25. He dashed to the LSU 5 before he was knocked off his feet.

Rozier slammed through the middle for 4 yards to the 1. Then Gill leaped over center for the go-ahead touchdown.

Nebraska almost added to its margin on its next possession. Fryar, who ranks third in the country in punt returns, eluded three LSU tackles on a 42-yard return to the Tigers' 25.

On a fourth-and-two at the 17, Nebraska, which is famous for trick plays, caught LSU off guard with a fake field goal but botched the execution. Tim Brungardt appeared to be running off the field before the ball was snapped. But when Gill took the snap and stood up from his holder's position, Brungardt cut down the left sidelines. Gill's pass was on target, but Brungardt dropped the ball at the 5.

LSU narrowed the gap to 21-20 following an interception by Williams, who returned the ball to the Nebraska 37. On a fourth-and-one, LSU was called for delay of game. Stovall then elected to go for a field goal, and Betanzos had room to spare on a 49-yard kick with 5:05 remaining.

Gill's Ball Control Spoils Stovall's Dream

BY JIMMY HYAMS

The Advocate

Miami, Fla. — *Jan. 1, 1983*

Jerry Stovall had a premonition earlier this week, but Nebraska quarterback Turner Gill foiled his dreams.

"I told the team all week we'd win the ballgame in the last 30 seconds with a field goal," said LSU's head coach. "It was set up perfectly . . . ."

Except for Gill.

After LSU had pulled to within 21-20 on Juan Betanzos' 49-yard field goal with 5:05 left in the fourth period, Gill faced a third-and-10 from his own 37 with 1:23 to play. The junior then hit Irving Fryar for a 13-yard gain allowing Nebraska to hold on for a 21-20 victory over the Tigers in the Orange Bowl tonight.

"We'd have beaten those suckers if we'd gotten the ball back," Stovall said.

Betanzos, who also kicked a 28-yard field goal and had a 35-yarder wiped out by a penalty, felt the same way.

"All we needed to do was cross the 50," said the sophomore sidewinder, "because I was kicking real good tonight. But we never got the ball back."

Nebraska, now 12-1, drove from its 20 to the LSU 16 before time expired, dropping the Tigers' record to 8-3-1.

"It was frustrating," Betanzos said of waiting on the sidelines in the final minutes hoping the Bandits would stop the nation's No. 1-ranked offense. "I couldn't do anything about it."

LSU punter Clay Parker tried to do something about it earlier, but his move backfired.

Facing a fourth-and-19 from his 36 one minute into the final quarter, Parker eluded a rusher, looked upfield, and instead of punting took off running. He was stopped eight yards shy of a first down.

Nebraska then marched 47 yards on seven plays, with Gill scoring from the 4 on a quarterback sneak with 11:14 to play. A pass interference call against cornerback James Britt and Gill's 28-yard pass to Fryar which carried the ball to the LSU 5 were the key plays.

"The snap was to the left and pressure was coming from the left," said Parker, a sophomore from Columbia. "I faked the guy coming from the left, and when I looked up field, it was wide open. I knew I had a long way to go for a first down. I just didn't think they would react that quickly. I realized I was six or seven yards short.

"It was one of those plays where if I get the first down, everybody says what a great play it was. But the way it turned out, I should have punted."

While it was a break which led to the Cornhuskers' winning score, LSU took advantage of breaks to score all 20 of its points. Fumble recoveries at Nebraska's 11 and 45 in the first half led to a pair of 1-yard TD runs by sensational freshman Dalton Hilliard, who played all but a couple of series since Garry James was suffering from a pulled groin.

In the second half, LSU's two field goals resulted from a Lawrence Williams fumble recovery at the Nebraska 41, and a Williams interception which he returned 20 yards to the Nebraska 37.

Following Williams' first fumble recovery, LSU marched to the Cornhusker 7. But fullback Mike Montz's run to the 1-yard line was nullified by illegal procedure, forcing the Tigers to eventually settle for a field goal.

"They said our split end (Eric Ellington) wasn't on the line of scrimmage," said LSU quarterback Alan Risher, who completed 14 of 34 passes for 173 yards. "We had an opportunity to win the game. If we go up, 21-7, we probably would have won."

Risher said the two key plays which went against LSU were the illegal procedure and Parker's failure to get a first down on the run from punt formation.

Risher said he "respected" Stovall's decision to go for the field goal on fourth-and-six in the final five minutes. "Give Nebraska credit," he said, "they held the ball and didn't give it back to us."

Risher said he thought Nebraska's defensive line played "excellent" and he said the Cornhuskers' secondary made it difficult for him to find open receivers, especially during the first half.

Stovall called Nebraska the "best team I've seen in my three years at LSU."

LSU nose guard Ramsey Dardar, who was matched against Nebraska's All-American center Dave Rimington.

Asked about the matchup, Dardar said, "I think I got the best out of the deal. The only thing was on passes, he held his butt off. I was telling the refs, but they just laughed."

But in the final minutes, there was nothing to laugh about on the LSU sidelines.

Stovall's dream on this New Year's Day was shattered when Gill played ball-hog in the final minutes.

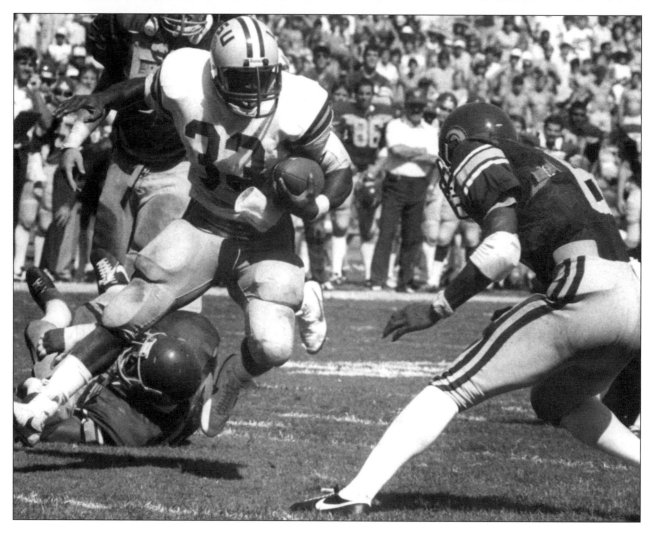

■ **Garry James (33) meets up with USC's Tim McDonald (6) en route to setting up LSU's second touchdown.**

Tigers Trample USC in Coliseum, 23-3

BY BRUCE HUNTER
The Advocate

Los Angeles, Calif. — *Sept. 29, 1984*

The University of Southern California mascot, Travellor III, took his traditional gallop around the Coliseum just before kickoff today, but was never heard from again.

The Trojan horse makes a triumphant trek around the famous Olympic track to celebrate touchdowns and other big plays for Southern Cal. LSU didn't give the Trojans a chance for any such pleasure in a 23-3 victory in front of a crowd of 60,128.

"We gave the game ball to the defense for the shutout," said LSU head coach Bill Arnsparger.

Of course, it wasn't technically a shutout. USC scored a field goal after LSU's only turnover of the game early in the first quarter.

The Tiger defense, however, stole the show for the final 56 minutes of the game. It produced five turnovers and went through a pair of USC quarterbacks.

"I thought it was a great win for the team," said Arnsparger. "I was proud of the defense with the shutout. It's hard to lose when you have a shutout. It was a real tough hitting game and that was the type of game we expected."

LSU remains undefeated, improving its record to 3-0-1 with a three-game winning streak. It has a week off before returning to Southeastern Conference play against Vanderbilt Oct. 13 for homecoming in Tiger Stadium.

The win will certainly boost the Tigers in the rankings. They entered the game ranked 18th by the United Press International and USC was ranked 14th by UPI and 15th in The Associated Press poll.

LSU bounced USC from the unbeaten ranks after it had won its first two games. This was the first time LSU had ever played in the Coliseum and the victory will go down as one of the greatest in school history. LSU was a slight favorite entering the game, but played its finest game of the season to totally devastate the Trojans.

"We knew about the USC tradition," said LSU tackle Lance Smith. "It's great to be in California. It's a great win for us."

Linebacker Ricky Chatman called it the best game the Tigers have played in his five years on the team. It was even more important to Chatman that the Tigers won because he almost went to USC.

"It's a thrill for me to come out here and win," he said. "To come out and win in their backyard makes me feel great.

"Right now it's the biggest win of my career. But hopefully, there will be a bigger win coming up."

Sophomore defensive end Karl Wilson, who had another big game up front, also had a reason to treasure this victory.

"I wasn't an LSU fan the last time LSU played USC," said Wilson. "I had a dream about playing in the Rose Bowl for USC, but I guess this is my Rose Bowl."

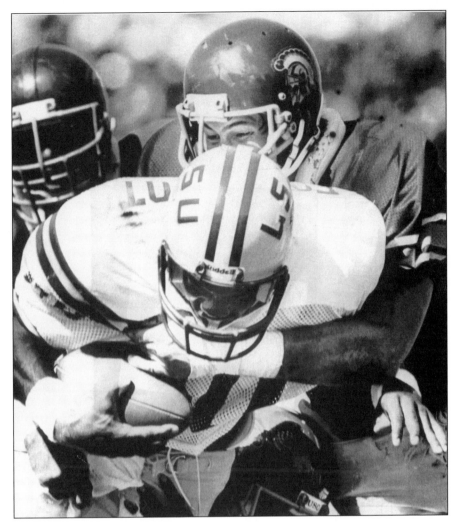

■ LSU's Herman Fontenot is stopped by USC cornerback Darrel Hopper after a 24-yard reception in the first quarter.

LSU's only other meeting with USC came in 1979 when the Trojans rallied in the closing minutes to win, 17-12.

The Tiger defense never let the Trojans get established and the offense played a near-perfect game, especially in the first half.

It was actually the defense that did the most severe damage in the half.

Trailing, 3-0, LSU set up its first touchdown when linebacker Michael Brooks separated USC quarterback Kevin McLean from the football. Wilson covered the fumble to give the Tigers possession at the USC 15.

"We had the eagle (blitz) on," said Brooks. "I just read the play and made the tackle. Nobody touched me."

Tailback Garry James carried twice, giving the Tigers a first-and-goal at the 2, and Dalton Hilliard went behind Smith at right tackle to score on his feet. Juan Betanzos added the extra point to give LSU a 7-3 lead and all the points it would need.

Early in the second quarter, USC had switched tailbacks and backup Zeph Lee was met head-on by Tiger linebackers Gregg Dubroc and Shawn Burks. The ball was dislodged and

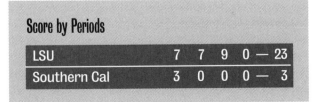

Score by Periods

LSU	7	7	9	0	— 23
Southern Cal	3	0	0	0	— 3

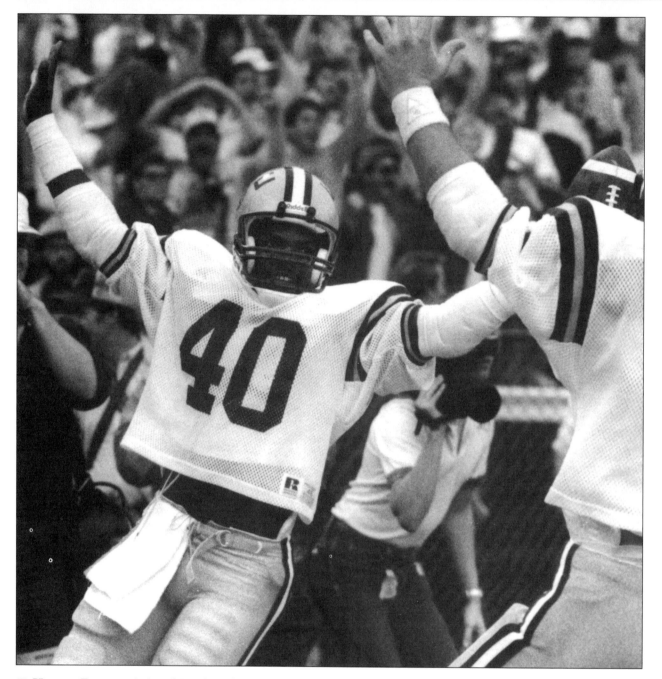

■ **Herman Fontenot (40) and Mitch Andrews celebrate after Fontenot's 2-yard touchdown reception.**

Burks recovered to stop a USC drive, setting the stage for LSU's only sustained scoring drive of the game.

Quarterback Jeff Wickersham marched the Tigers on a 16-play, 79-yard drive with Hilliard scoring on another 2-yard run. He got blocks from flanker Herman Fontenot and tailback Craig Rathjen and scored standing up to put the Tigers ahead, 14-3.

Wickersham, who completed 14-of-27 passes for 171 yards and a touchdown, completed passes to James, Mitch Andrews, Eric Martin and Rogie Magee on the expertly engineered drive.

The Tigers needed a little help, though. On fourth-and-1 from the USC 44, Clay Parker dropped back to punt, grabbed an errant snap and raced down the left sidelines for 16 yards and a first down.

"No, it wasn't planned that way," said Parker, who had his best game of the season. "It was open and I ran for it."

The Tigers had an excellent scoring opportunity taken away on the next series of downs. Freshman cornerback Kevin Guidry picked off a McLean pass at midfield and raced all the way down to the USC 14. But a clipping penalty on the play set the Tigers back to their own 37.

The LSU defense didn't get any more turnovers in the first half and neither team threatened to score as the half ended with

LSU in front, 14-3.

Tiger lightning struck again in the third quarter when reserve safety Steve Rehage made a diving interception of another pass by McLean, giving LSU the ball at the USC 30.

"I looked up and the tight end was coming across the middle. He tried to get it to him," Rehage said. "It looked like somebody must have hit the ball."

This time, LSU couldn't move the ball after the turnover. Betanzos came in to kick a 46-yard field goal to put the Tigers ahead, 17-3, with 4:39 remaining in the third quarter.

USC head coach Ted Tollner decided McLean, who replaced injured starter Sean Salisbury, wasn't getting the job done. So Tollner called on senior quarterback Tim Green. He wasn't any more effective against a defense which pressured the quarterback all afternoon.

"They (LSU) came in here to win. I think they're a real good football team," said McLean. "Our defense played well, but our offense has to get it together. LSU is going to go to a bowl game."

After Green failed to move the Trojans on his first try, they punted and gave LSU good field position at its own 49. Wickersham didn't need any help from his own defense this time.

The junior quarterback, who had his best game since the opener with Florida, completed his longest pass of the season, a 34-yard touchdown play to freshman receiver Glenn Holt, who fooled the Trojan defense and was wide open at the 10-yard line. It was Holt's first college reception.

"We spread it out and the safety bit on Herman (Fontenot) going across the middle," said Wickersham. "He (Holt) was wide open."

Betanzos missed the extra point, but the Tigers still led, 23-3, with 1:35 left in the game.

The Tigers almost added to their large margin of victory in the fourth quarter when Liffort Hobley made his second interception in two games, collecting a bad throw by Green. Hobley returned the ball 10 yards to the USC 34.

"It was just an overthrown pass," said Hobley, who set up the winning touchdown with an interception last week against Arizona. "I was just in the middle waiting for it and I tried to get as far downfield as I could. I made sure I was deep enough."

The Trojans pressured Wickersham with blitzes and he missed an open James at the goal line. So the Tigers punted from their own 32 after a penalty for delay-of-game. They probably would have kicked a field goal if the game was close. Also, Betanzos was erratic, missing an extra point and a 25-yard field goal on the day.

LSU went conservative in the closing minutes to run down the clock and USC never mounted a serious threat.

After the first few minutes of the second quarter, the Trojans never penetrated beyond the LSU 40.

Their only offense was the running of tailback Fred Crutcher, who gained 97 yards on 22 carries and was the game's leading rusher. Hilliard rushed for 81 yards on 28 carries for LSU.

Crutcher had a long run of 15 yards, but never really hurt LSU. He was stopped in all the critical situations.

"My initial reaction is that the turnovers finally caught up to us," said Tollner, whose team had been bothered by turnovers in its first two games, too. "It's obvious there's more to it than that, but it's critical for us to play our style. That's running the ball and not falling behind."

The Trojans had a chance to take a significant lead early in the game after Martin fumbled the ball over to the Trojans at the LSU 42 on the opening series. Crutcher ran the ball four times as the team moved inside the 10.

But on third down, McLean missed split end Hank Norman in the end zone. Norman beat Guidry on the play and was open. USC settled for a 22-yard field goal by Steve Jordan for its only points of the game.

USC had one more scoring chance in the first half when it moved from its own 43 to LSU's 23 behind the running of Lee. But Dubroc and Burks forced Lee to fumble, ending the threat.

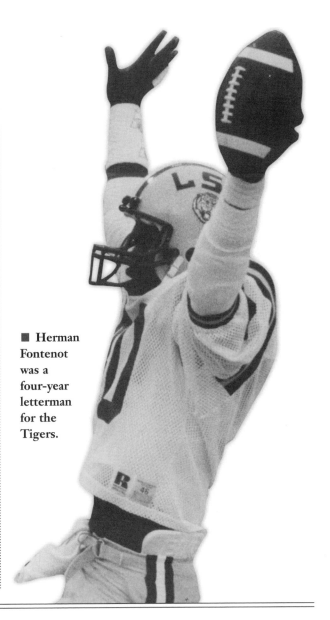

■ Herman Fontenot was a four-year letterman for the Tigers.

Tigers Send the Tide Tumbling

By Bruce Hunter
The Advocate

Birmingham, Ala. — *Nov. 10, 1984*

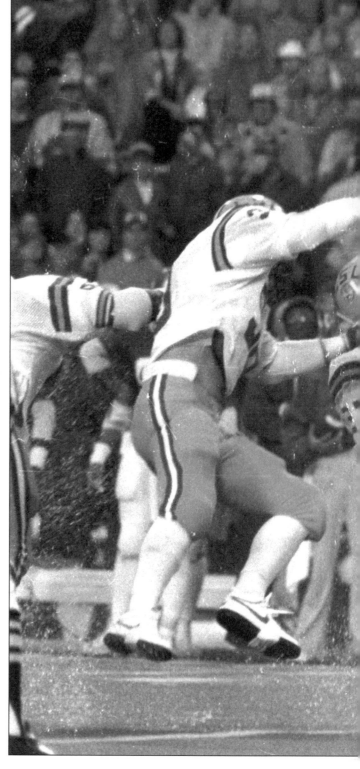

The Alabama Crimson Tide threw a giant road block in LSU's path to the Southeastern Conference football championship.

But the Tigers used a block of their own to salvage a 16-14 victory in Legion Field on this stormy afternoon.

Sophomore Michael Brooks led a 10-man rush and blocked a punt by Alabama's Terry Sanders to set up the winning touchdown early in the third quarter. The Tide was punting from its own 45 when Brooks broke through for the block and the ball bounded toward the end zone with Kevin Guidry recovering for the Tigers at the Tide 12.

Three plays later, Dalton Hilliard broke through the right side of the line to score a touchdown from 7 yards away and put the Tigers ahead for good, 16-14, with 7:53 left in the third quarter.

"That's the first time that we've worked on the all-out rush in practice," said Brooks, who pressured Alabama quarterback Mike Shula all afternoon on pass rushes. "We felt they had a breakdown in their punt protections and we felt we could get to them."

Brooks lined up on the right side of the line and found an opening between center and guard. "I just went right through and we made the big play," he said.

There were several other Tigers in position to make the critical block if Brooks wasn't able to do so.

"We brought some faster, specialized people up there," said LSU safety Jeffery Dale. "We brought in (Kevin) Guidry and Liffort (Hobley) and they had never been there before."

LSU head coach Bill Arnsparger said the Tigers tried the 10-man punt rush against Ole Miss last week. This was the first time the Tigers have come close to blocking a punt this season.

"It looked like Terry was slow getting the punt away," said

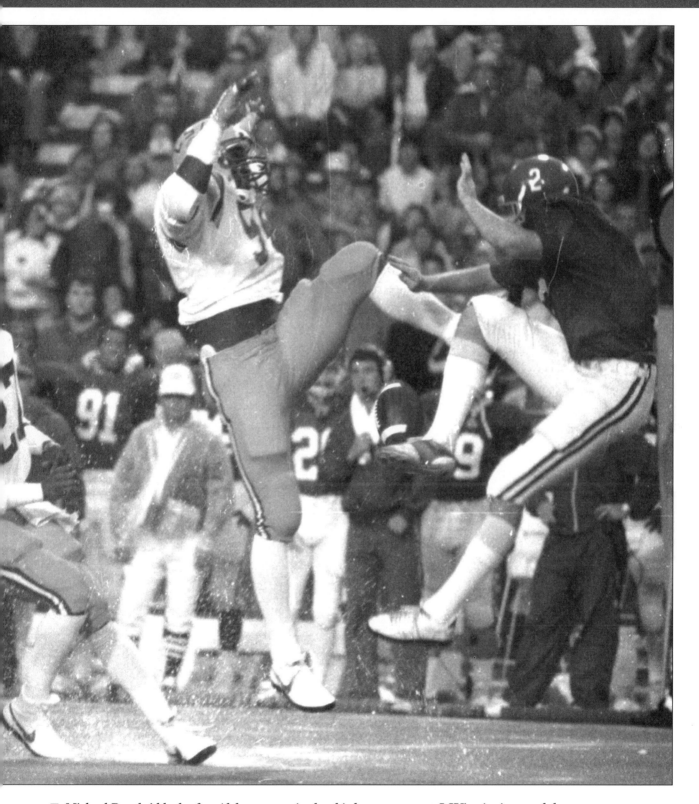

■ **Michael Brooks' block of an Alabama punt in the third quarter set up LSU's winning touchdown.**

Alabama head coach Ray Perkins. "I'd have to look at the films though. It could have been a combination of both."

The blocked punt and several outstanding returns on kick-offs and punts were the only bright spot for the Tigers, who improved to 7-1-1 overall and 4-0-1 in the SEC. With Florida's win over Georgia today, the Tigers can clinch at least a share of the SEC crown and a possible Sugar Bowl berth with a victory at Mississippi State next Saturday.

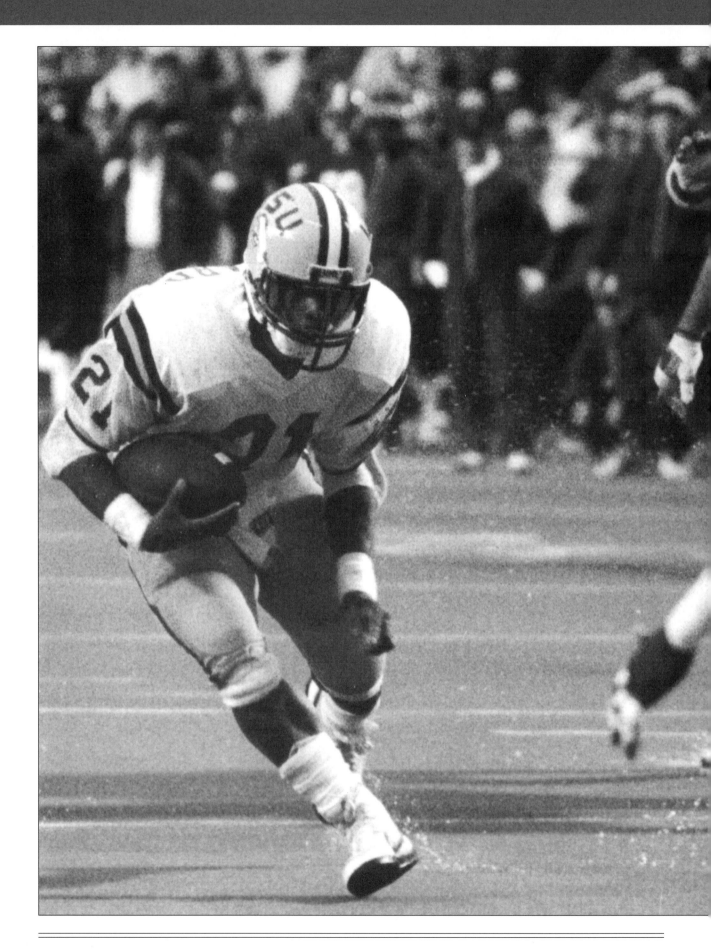

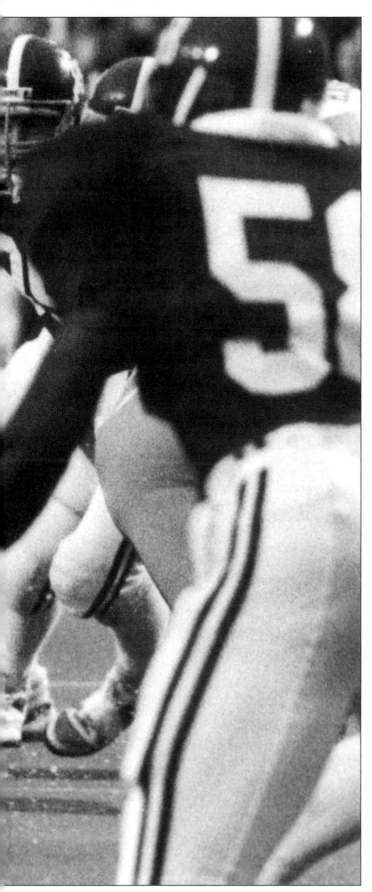

The Tigers haven't won the SEC title since 1970 and haven't gone to the Sugar Bowl since 1968.

Following the blocked punt, tailback Garry James ran over right guard to get down to the Alabama 10 on first down. Hilliard went over the left side for 3 yards on second down, breaking the 1,000-yard rushing mark for the season and joining Charles Alexander and Terry Robiskie as the only Tigers ever to accomplish the feat.

Hilliard's next carry was even more important. On third-and-five from the Tide 7, the Tigers surprised Alabama with a draw to Hilliard, who slid through the right side and fought his way into the end zone.

"I got a good block from Tommy Campbell at center," said Hilliard, who rushed for 78 yards on 17 carries to bring his season total to 1,055. "I was reading on Campbell's block, and tight end Mitch Andrews got a good block to get me into the end zone."

The Tigers elected to go for two points after the touchdown, but flanker Herman Fontenot dropped Jeff Wickersham's pass in the end zone. LSU didn't want to be left in a position where a field goal would tie the game because a tie would have knocked the Tigers out of title contention.

Alabama fell to 3-6 overall and 1-4 in the SEC, and is assured of it first losing season since 1957. But the Tide, which had won 12 of the previous 13 meetings with LSU, thoroughly dominated every phase of the game except special teams play.

The final statistics read like a horror story for the Tigers. They gained only eight first downs and 161 yards of total offense for their worst offensive showing of the season, while Alabama more than doubled their output with 22 first downs and 332 yards of total offense.

LSU's ball-control philosophy went out the window after its opening drive of the game.

The most telling factors in the game are Alabama's 85-49 advantage in offensive plays and an overwhelming edge in time of possession, 40:49 to 19:11.

The Tigers' longest drive was seven plays and they had to punt eight times.

Alabama had four drives of at least 10 plays, controlling the game from start to finish. The Tide built a 14-10 lead at halftime and had two prime opportunities to win the game in the second half with long marches.

■ **Dalton Hilliard rushed for 78 yards and became the third LSU back to rush for more than 1,000 yards in a season.**

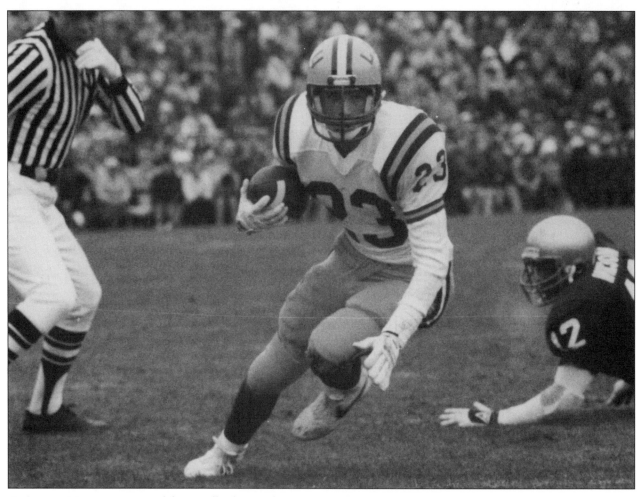

■ **Sammy Martin (23) moved from tailback to wide receiver and caught eight passes for 75 yards.**

LSU Grabs First Win Ever in Irishland

By Bruce Hunter

The Advocate

South Bend, Ind. — *Nov. 23, 1985*

On an afternoon when conference championships and major bowl bids were being decided all over the country, the happenings on the hallowed grounds of Notre Dame Stadium seemed rather insignificant, attracting representatives from only one bowl.

Yet, for traditional powers Notre Dame and LSU, today's game was a collision of a program fighting for its life and another one fighting for its dignity. LSU's struggle for respect prevailed in climactic fashion, 10-7, for the Tigers' first victory ever in the shadows of the Golden Dome.

"It's history," said Garry James, who scored the winning touchdown on a 2-yard run with 3:26 left. "We made history. Put it in the books. I wish we were at home, so we could put it up on the wall. Where's a wall? We'll put it up here."

James couldn't find an appropriate wall in the visitors' locker room on which to display the 10-7 score, but LSU's come-from-behind triumph in a game dominated by defense probably brought the walls down on Gerry Faust's five-year stay here. Faust began his career here at with a 27-9 win over LSU in 1981.

The Fighting Irish, who are more accustomed to playing for national championships in November, fell to 5-5 and must beat fourth-ranked Miami Saturday to salvage a winning season. LSU, ranked 17th, improved to 7-1-1 and kept alive its slim hopes of returning to the Sugar Bowl.

The Tigers' only hopes of going to the Sugar Bowl rest in a Tennessee loss to Vanderbilt in those teams' season final Saturday. However, if the Vols win, LSU is headed for a Liberty Bowl date with Baylor on Dec. 27 in Memphis, Tenn.

Baylor accepted its bid to the Liberty Bowl after losing 17-10 to Texas after falling from Cotton Bowl contention.

"If I am retained, that's fine," said Faust. "If I'm not, that's part of life. I never even thought about this being my last time walking off the field at Notre Dame. And that's the honest to God truth."

Most of the afternoon it appeared the Fighting Irish would extend their six-game winning streak at home and possibly Faust's career at Notre Dame. The Irish scored on their first possession with an impressive, 64-yard drive to go ahead, 7-0, with less than six minutes expired. But that was the end of such offensive prowess for the next three quarters, during which LSU's Henry Thomas blocked two field goals and forced John Carney to miss a third try.

The Irish maintained their 7-0 lead until the last play of the first half when LSU got a field goal by Matt DeFrank, subbing for Ron Lewis. Then the 7-3 advantage lasted until the closing minutes of the game at which time the Tigers rallied for their first victory in three games here.

"I have to compliment my players for hanging in there,"

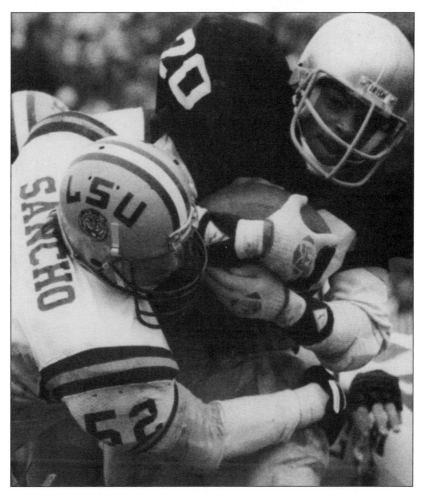

■ **LSU linebacker Ron Sancho wraps up Irish tailback Allen Pinkett.**

said LSU coach Bill Arnsparger. "They really worked hard to win this football game. It was one of those games where I don't imagine anyone turned off their TV sets. It was close and kept everybody hanging until the end."

LSU quarterback Jeff Wickersham, who set a record for the most completions (31) ever against a Notre Dame team, directed the Tigers on a pair of fourth-quarter drives. The first one didn't produce any points, but worked to set up the winning drive.

With 11:31 left in the game, LSU started at its own 14 and worked down to the Notre Dame 42. Wickersham completed 5 of 7 passes on the drive, including a couple of 11-yard passes to Dalton Hilliard and Rogie Magee.

Arnsparger gambled early on the drive when the Tigers came up six inches short on a third-down pass from Wickersham to tight end Mitch Andrews. The ball was just inside the LSU 35, but Wickersham sneaked a yard and a half on fourth down to maintain possesion. Several plays later, Wickersham hit tailback James for a first down at the Irish 42, but the drive stalled and DeFrank had to punt.

DeFrank's punt landed around the 15 and rolled to the 6 to pin Notre Dame deep in its territory. Irish tailback Allen

Score by Periods

LSU	0	3	0	7 —	10
Notre Dame	7	0	0	0 —	7

Pinkett, who went over 4,000 yards for his career in the game, could manage only 4 yards on two carries and quarterback Steve Beuerlein threw incomplete on third down, forcing Dan Sorensen to kick from his end zone.

LSU took over at its own 48 with 4:53 remaining in the game and Wickersham went straight to work. He connected with Andrews for a 9-yard gain on second down and found a weak spot in Notre Dame's defense to hit Hilliard for 18 yards on third down, going to the Notre Dame 25.

"It was a blitz read," said Wickersham, who completed 31 of 42 for 244 yards and moved into third place on the all-time Southeastern Conference list for total offense. "They brought their strong safety in, and Dalton and I read it. We were able to hit it for a big gain."

The Tigers came right back with another long gainer when Andrews turned a routine short-yardage pass from Wickersham into a 21-yard pickup, setting up a first-and-goal at the 4.

"I ran inside for an 8-yard hook route," said Andrews. "The linebackers went after our running backs and Jeff made a good read. He hit me and I broke a tackle. I smelled the goal line and I wanted to get in."

Notre Dame linebacker Tony Furjanic wrestled down Andrews before he could break into the end zone, but it only delayed the touchdown. James got half of the necessary yards on first down by powering over the left side for 2 yards.

Then James hit the same hole on second down and dashed through untouched behind the blocks of left tackle Curt Gore and guard Keith Melancon to score the winning touchdown. DeFrank added the extra point for a 10-7 lead with 3:26 left.

"I got excellent blocking by the offensive line," said James. "They wanted it more than anyone. They've been taking a lot of stuff from everyone." James' TD run concluded the scoring in the game, but the action was far from over. Three of the afternoon's four turnovers came in the final two minutes.

Beuerlein tried to rally the Irish for a tying field goal or winning touchdown, but his pass to split end Reggie Ward was tipped and intercepted by LSU linebacker Ron Sancho at the LSU 31 with 1:50 left.

The Tigers tried to run out the clock, but Hilliard's second straight carry ended in a fumble. Notre Dame tackle Eric Dorsey dislodged the ball from Hilliard, then recovered the fumble at the LSU 36 with 1:35 still to play.

"I thought that was going to be it because it aroused so much motivation and at such a critical point in the game," said Dorsey. "It seemed like it could be like one of the famous Notre Dame comeback stories."

The story ended abruptly for the Irish. Beuerlein attempted to pick up a large chunk of territory on first down by going to flanker Tim Brown across the middle, but Brown couldn't handle the hard pass and it was deflected into the hands of LSU safety Steve Rehage.

This time Hilliard held on to the ball and LSU ran out the clock successfully to clinch the school's second win in five games against Notre Dame.

The fifth game between the two schools was very similar to the inaugural meeting in 1970 when Notre Dame took a 3-0 victory here on a field goal late in the game.

As this contest developed, it seemed Notre Dame's first touchdown might stand as the winning margin. Each team had several long drives that ended in a big defensive play or a missed field goal. LSU was 1 of 4 in field-goal tries and the Irish missed all three, due to Thomas' ability to break through the line.

On the opening series of the second half, Notre Dame staged a beautiful, 18-play march with Pinkett, who rushed for 103 yards on 30 carries, getting the call 10 times.

The senior tailback gained only 25 yards on this circuit, but made a clutch run on fourth-and-2 from the LSU 23. He broke a tackle by cornerback Kevin Guidry and powered down to the 30 for the first down. The rest of the work was done by Beuerlein, who completed two passes to Brown and another one to Ward for a total of 48 yards.

From the 20, Beuerlein connected with fullback Frank Stams for 9 yards and on the next play, Stams rushed 2 yards for a first-and-goal at the 9. The Irish couldn't punch it in, though, as Thomas threw Stams for a loss on second down and linebacker Michael Brooks pressured Beuerlein into throwing an incompletion on third down, setting up a 23-yard field-goal try by Carney that was blocked by Thomas. Guidry picked up the ball in the end zone and returned it 17 yards.

LSU's offense responded with a long drive of its own, going 71 yards in 11 plays. Wickersham was 6 of 6 for 34 yards and Notre Dame helped the Tigers' cause with two 15-yard penalties for a late hit and facemasking.

But a 26-yard run by James to the Notre Dame 2 was nullified by a holding penalty. Notre Dame finally stopped the drive on a tackle by Furjanic that left Wickersham short of a first down at the 12. On fourth down, DeFrank tried a 29-yard field goal, but missed wide to the right, leaving the score at 7-3 with 1:19 left in the third quarter.

Once the Irish got the ball back, Pinkett had runs of 5 and 6 yards to go over the 1,000-yard mark for the third year in a row. Pinkett had several more gains as the fourth quarter opened. Notre Dame's deepest penetration was to the LSU 48, following a 4-yard gain by Pinkett, but Rehage tipped away a third-down pass from Beuerlein to Miller, which left the Irish in a punting situation.

LSU got the ball again and Wickersham engineered the two crucial possessions that led to James' touchdown run.

The Tigers' defense prevented the Irish from mounting any offense, which enabled LSU's offense to get the necessary field position to get on the scoreboard. Linebacker Toby Caston led the Tigers with 10 tackles and four others, Karl Wilson, Shawn Burks, Thomas and Sancho, had nine tackles each. Wilson had the Tigers' only sack.

Thomas, Tigers Got Respect

BY BRUCE HUNTER
The Advocate

South Bend, Ind. — *Nov. 23, 1985*

Henry Thomas tried not think about those painful memories.

A year ago the LSU nose guard was on his way to leading the Tigers to a national championship, as far as he was concerned. Thomas had developed into one of the premier defensive linemen in the Southeastern Conference and LSU had climbed to No. 6 in the nation.

But it all came crashing down on top of him Oct. 27 in Tiger Stadium, where Notre Dame dealt LSU a 30-22 loss and Thomas a season-ending knee injury.

"I wanted to keep my mind off that," said Thomas. "I didn't want it to affect me today."

Obviously it didn't. Thomas led a defensive effort that resulted in LSU beating Notre Dame, 10-7, today in Notre Dame Stadium. He more than made up for last year's disappointment by making numerous key plays to help the Tigers win for the first time here.

Thomas really came through on field-goal rushes, blocking two attempts by Notre Dame's John Carney and forcing him to kick wide into "Never Never Land" on another try. Thomas also had nine tackles, including one behind the line.

"I figured they owed me something," said Thomas, a 6-2, 255-pound junior from Houston. "They owed our team some respect. I think they lost some respect for us after they beat us last year."

The Fighting Irish manhandled LSU's makeshift defense, riddled with injuries on the line, in last year's triumph. It was a completely different story today, however.

Notre Dame scored on its first possession of the afternoon, but couldn't produce anything on its next 11 tries as LSU's defense took control. The closest the Irish got to scoring was the field-goal attempts by Carney, who had made 30 of 36 attempts (.829) for a school record before he ran into Thomas.

Thomas received plenty of assistance from his defensive teammates who felt Notre Dame "took something away from us" last year. Inside linebackers Toby Caston and Shawn Burks combined for 19 tackles, and outside linebacker Ron Sancho and Karl Wilson had nine tackles each. Sancho also had an interception and broken up pass, while Wilson added a sack.

"It just took a lot of determination," said Sancho. "Our defense has been playing with a lot of determination and pride

all year. It was gut-check time and we just slugged it out."

Outside linebacker Michael Brooks, a finalist for The Butkus Award for the outstanding linebacker in the country, finished with five tackles and one hit behind the line. He made an important play on Notre Dame quarterback Steve Beuerlein to force him to throw an incompletion on a third-and-goal play.

LSU's defense was ranked second in the nation in points allowed (9.0 average) going into the game. The Tigers had shutouts against Kentucky and Ole Miss, but this may have been an even stronger defensive showing.

"We came out here thinking that we had to earn some respect against Notre Dame," said cornerback Norman Jefferson, who had four tackles. "They were more physical and a lot of people thought they would dominate us. We had to prove today that we're one of the best teams in the country."

Both Thomas and Darrell Phillips had blocked kicks in earlier games this season. It's something that the defensive linemen really work on with Coach Pete Jenkins. Thomas said he learned something on Carney's extra point after the first-quarter touchdown that enabled him to break through on three straight field-goal rushes.

"We had an outside block on for the extra point," said Thomas. "Karl (Wilson) came over to me and said 'I think we can get this guy.' So he ran the outside block and I just went through the line."

Thomas had more than enough time to get in position to block Carney's first try from 52 yards in the second quarter. The kicker seemed to hesitate slightly, which made Thomas' job that much easier.

When Carney went back in to try another 52-yarder before halftime, Thomas was in the backfield, causing Carney to kick way off to the left.

"I came through and it went off the other way," said Thomas. "It went into Never, Never Land."

The final kick by Carney was a 23-yard attempt, coming at the end of an 18-play drive to open the second half. The Irish came away with nothing as Thomas got his hands on the ball again.

LSU had some kicking problems of its own, making only 1 of 4 attempts. Ron Lewis missed from 49 and 26 yards, which brought his season's stats to 4 of 15. So the Tigers went with Matt DeFrank as their kicker for the first time.

DeFrank made a 27-yard field goal at the end of the first half, but missed a 29-yard try in the third quarter.

"What I was trying to do was just punch it through," DeFrank said. "I just got under it too much the first time, but it went through. The second one I hit it good. It was just two feet wide."

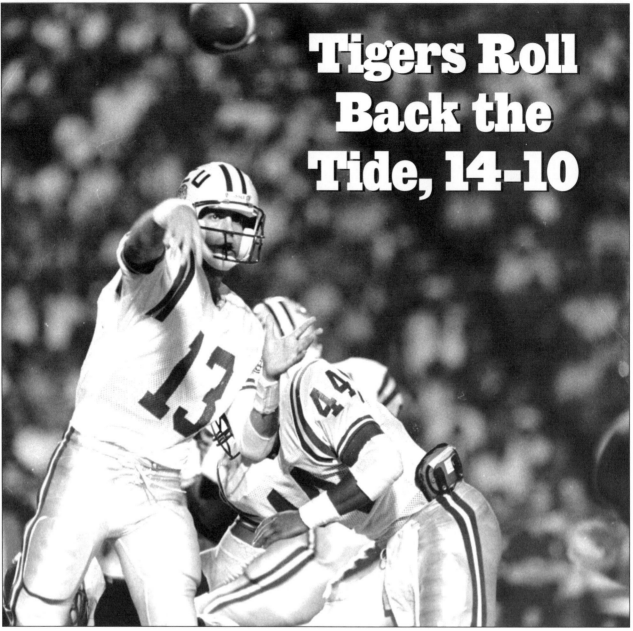

Tigers Roll Back the Tide, 14-10

■ Tommy Hodson completed 9 of 21 passes for 68 yards and one touchdown.

BY BRUCE HUNTER
The Advocate

Birmingham, Ala. — *Nov. 8, 1986*

For the third straight time, LSU's defense captured Legion Field. The determined Tiger defenders stopped Alabama twice in first-down situations inside their own 14 and came away with three fourth-quarter turnovers to hang on for a 14-10 victory tonight before 75,808 in Legion Field and a national television audience on ESPN.

"It doesn't matter how many times you win here. It feels great every time," LSU senior defensive end Roland Barbay said.

The victory was LSU's third straight in Legion Field and each time it's been the Tigers' defense leading the charge against their arch-rivals, who have held the upper hand in their long series.

The 18th-ranked Tigers, 6-2 overall, moved into a first-place tie with Alabama in the Southeastern Conference, both at 4-1, and can assure themselves of at least a share of the conference crown with a victory against Mississippi State next Saturday night in Jackson. The sixth-ranked Crimson Tide fell to 8-2 overall and finishes its SEC season here against Auburn on Nov. 29.

In 1982, the Tigers won, 20-10, here and salvaged a 16-14 decision in 1984. Both games were won by staunch defensive efforts by LSU, as was the case tonight.

"A couple of guys on this team and I are very fortunate to be able to make the statement that we've been able to beat Alabama three times here," said another LSU senior defensive end, Karl Wilson. "I don't think anybody else in SEC history could say that."

LSU scored all its points in the second quarter to build a 14-7 lead at intermission. Then its defense went to work in the second half, limiting Alabama to a 22-yard field goal by Van Tiffen early in the third quarter.

The Crimson Tide was in scoring position throughout the fourth quarter, but the Tigers wouldn't relent. Linebacker Eric Hill stripped the ball from halfback Bobby Humphrey just outside the goal line and cornerback Kevin Guidry recovered in the end zone to halt Alabama's best chance.

"The offense got the points in the first half and it was up to us to do it in the second half," Barbay said. "We almost shut them out in the second half. It was a great team effort by the defense."

In addition to causing a fumble, Hill intercepted a Mike Shula pass late in the fourth quarter to seal the outcome. Strong safety Greg Jackson accounted for the Tigers' other two takeaways with an interception in the third quarter and fumble recovery in the fourth quarter.

The Tigers had scoring drives of 80 and 62 yards in the second quarter to rally from a 7-0 deficit. Reserve quarterback Mickey Guidry scrambled 4 yards for the first touchdown. Later, starter Tommy Hodson, who completed 9 of 21 for 68 yards and two interceptions, threw a 6-yard touchdown pass to Wendell Davis for the other score. Davis had just three catches in the game.

Alabama scored first on a 3-yard touchdown pass from Shula to tight end Angelo Stafford in the first quarter, but that was the Crimson Tide's only touchdown, even though it crossed into LSU territory five more times, including three times in the final period.

"Our guys gave a real fine effort," said Alabama coach Ray Perkins. "They fought hard. We lost to a real fine team in LSU. That was not the same team that played Miami of Ohio and Ole Miss."

The Tigers were coming off a 21-19 upset loss to Ole Miss, but added Alabama to their own list of upset victims, which includes Texas A&M and Florida. They're 3-0 as the underdog this season.

Early in the third quarter, the Tigers gave the Crimson Tide

Score by Periods

LSU	0	14	0	0	— 14
Alabama	7	0	3	0	— 10

a prime scoring opportunity after an offensive pass interference call against Davis forced Matt DeFrank to punt from deep in his own territory. Greg Richardson fielded the punt at the LSU 49 and got down to the 44.

From there, Humphrey had a pair of 13-yard runs, both around right tackle. On first-and-goal from the 9, Humphrey tried going to the left side. He broke a tackle at the 5 and fought his way into the end zone. But a holding call against the Crimson Tide spoiled it and moved the ball back to the 19.

Shula, who completed 16 of 27 for 190 yards, a touchdown and two interceptions, gained a couple yards on first down and threw a screen to fullback Doug Allen that went for 12 yards to the LSU 5. Then Shula's third-down pass to Stafford was thrown out of the end zone, forcing Alabama to settle for a 22-yard field goal by Tiffen that made it 14-10 with 9:23 left in the quarter.

Soon after, the Tigers had a chance to add to their four-point lead. Tailback Harvey Williams had consecutive gains of 6, 7 and 6 yards to lead LSU into Alabama's side of the field at the 37.

But the Tigers weren't able to go much farther and tailback Sammy Martin was stopped on an option play on third down, forcing DeFrank to punt from the Alabama 36. His soft, low kick was downed by Chris Carrier at the 6.

The Crimson Tide got a break when LSU was called for a personal foul penalty that gave Alabama a first down out to its 27. Alabama overcame a third-and-11 situation with Shula connecting with flanker Al Bell for a 24-yard gain to the LSU 39.

On the first play of the fourth quarter, Alabama jumped offsides to set up a first-and-15 from the 44. Humphrey, who rushed for 134 yards on 24 carries to set a school record with 1,138 yards this season, got loose on a draw play and was fighting for extra yardage when the ball came free and LSU's Jackson recovered at the 18.

The Tigers moved quickly in the wrong direction and had to punt. Then Shula went to work completing a 12-yard pass to Richardson, and on third-and-12, he threw deep to tight end Howard Cross for a 29-yard play to the LSU 31.

Humphrey had run the ball three times for a first-and-goal at the 5. But on his next run, he made it to just outside the end zone when Hill jolted the ball loose and Guidry recovered in the end zone for a touchback with 8:26 left.

"I almost broke my back trying to get the ball," Guidry said. "It was in the end zone. If anyone else would have fallen on the ball, it would have been a touchdown."

Trying to control the ball and run off some time, Hodson threw a third-down pass from deep in his own territory and it was intercepted by safety Kermit Kendrick, who returned it to the LSU 15, but was later ruled out of bounds at the LSU 41.

The Tiger defense made another stand in its territory and nearly came up with an interception on a tipped pass on third down. On fourth-and-5 from the 36, Alabama tried a reverse with Bell going around right end, but linebacker Ron Sancho wasn't fooled and stopped the play.

Starting at its own 38 with 4:51 left, LSU immediately crossed into Alabama territory on a 13-yard run by Williams. But a procedure call against the Tigers eventually cost them dearly and they had to punt again from the Alabama 43. DeFrank punted into the end zone, giving the Crimson Tide possession at their 20 with 2:12 left.

But Alabama's last chance went astray when Shula's pass was tipped at the line and intercepted by Hill, who returned the ball 4 yards to the Alabama 28. The Tigers were able to get down to the 15 as they ran out the clock successfully.

"We had to make them put the ball in the air," Hill said. "We knew we couldn't win if they kept the ball on the ground all night."

In the first half, Alabama controlled the action offensively and defensively at the outset, building a 7-0 lead. But the LSU defense began to stiffen and the Tiger offense came to life with two touchdown drives.

Even with Hodson knocked out of the game for two plays, the Tigers moved the ball on the opening series of the night. They completed three passes, including one by Guidry, to march from their own 20 to the Alabama 46.

A personal foul penalty against the Tide sent LSU deeper into Alabama territory at the 35. But cornerback Freddie Robinson stepped in front of Rogie Magee to intercept a Hodson pass and end the scoring threat at the 27.

On its first possession, Alabama engineered a ball-control drive that went 46 yards in 12 plays with Shula completing three passes and Humphrey gaining 25 yards on the ground. But LSU stopped Humphrey for no gain on third-and-1 from the LSU 27 and Tiffen missed a 44-yard field goal.

LSU had penalty problems on its next series. DeFrank had to kick three times before he finally got off one that counted. Penalties for illegal procedure and holding moved the Tigers back to their 11 before DeFrank was finally able to make a legal punt. It went only 37 yards and gave Alabama great field position at the LSU 44 after a short return.

Using just six plays, Alabama capitalized on the LSU mistakes by punching it in for the first points of the game. Allen took a screen pass and bolted 21 yards and Shula came right back to pass to Bell for 9 yards.

An Allen run gave the Crimson Tide a first-and-goal at the 8, but it took three more plays before Shula found Stafford over the middle for a 3-yard touchdown pass. Tiffen's point-after made it 7-0 with 1:20 left in the quarter.

Early in the second quarter, Guidry came in for his usual relief stint and passed to Davis for 10 yards to get the initial first down of the drive.

Then Garland Jean Batiste broke a draw play for 21 yards all the way to the Alabama 24. Williams got them even closer with a 14-yard pickup on an option play. On first-and-goal,

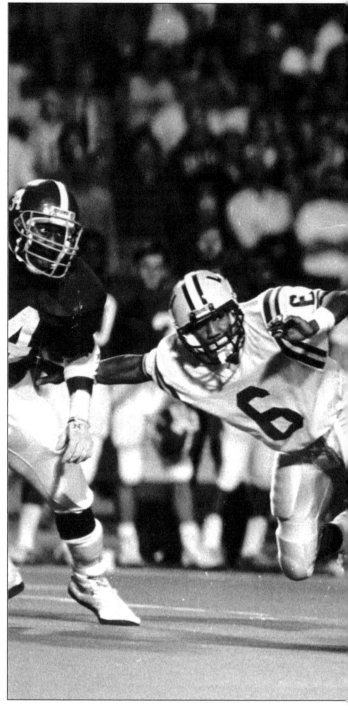

■ **Garland Jean Batiste drags two Alabama defenders with him at the end of a 25-yard run.**

Williams gained 5 more yards to the 5, but was held to just a yard on his next carry.

Guidry wanted to throw to Williams on third down, but he was covered. So Guidry tucked the ball away and found the left side wide open, dashing into the end zone with the ball raised high in the air. David Browndyke kicked the extra point for a 7-7 tie with 9:12 left in the half.

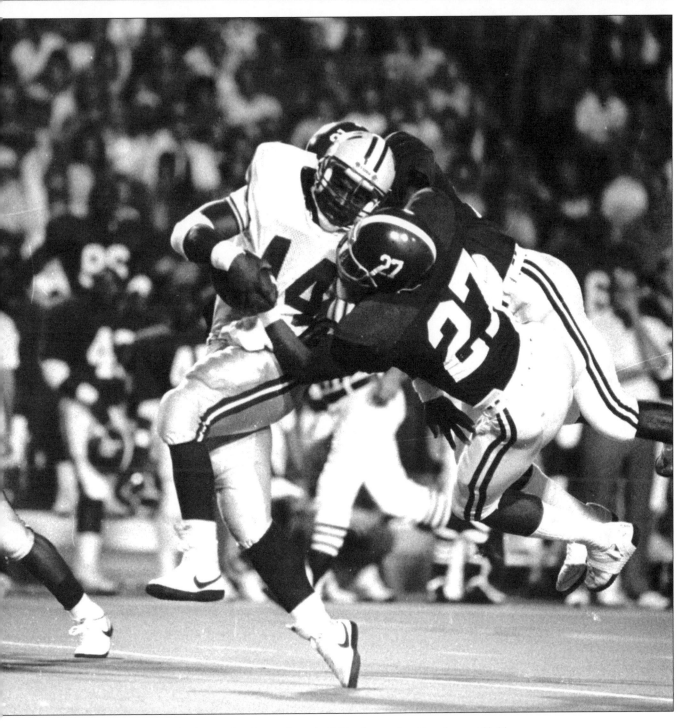

The Crimson Tide went back to work and swept down the field on a 67-yard drive. Shula threw a couple of short passes to get Alabama out to midfield and then unleashed a bomb to Richardson, who beat the LSU secondary for a 33-yard gain to the LSU 13.

But Shula was off target in trying to throw into the end zone to Stafford and Jackson picked it off just in front of the back line of the end zone.

Working with just 5:30 remaining, Hodson was perfect in the ensuing series, completing all four of his passes for 39 yards. He threw to Martin for 12 yards and to Brian Kinchen for another 8 yards to midfield.

Jean Batiste gained 7 yards to get into Alabama territory. On the next play, Hodson had to scramble when he couldn't find anyone open, picking up just a yard. But a late hit by the Crimson Tide moved the ball 15 yards farther.

Two plays later, Hodson found Davis on a short crossing route and the split end struggled for 13 yards for a first-and-goal at the 5. Tailback Eddie Fuller lost a yard on first down, but Hodson hit Davis in the back of the end zone for a 6-yard touchdown pass with just 25 seconds left.

Win Gives Tigers Share of SEC Lead

By Dave Moormann
The Advocate

Birmingham, Ala. — *Nov. 8, 1986*

Cornerback Willie Bryant and wide receiver Rogie Magee did an impromptu end-zone dance.

Six LSU players knelt on the Legion Field artificial turf in prayer.

Usually taciturn LSU coach Bill Arnsparger concluded an interview by hugging a group of cheerleaders. His players already had carried him off the field.

Nearly everyone associated with LSU whooped and hollered in celebration of the Tigers' stunning 14-10 victory over sixth-ranked Alabama here tonight.

"We put that on at the end as a means of expression," Bryant said of the dance orchestrated in front of the LSU end-zone crowd. "Celebration — that's what it's all about."

Better yet, it's about a victory that put 18th-ranked LSU at 6-2 overall and into a first-place tie with Alabama at 4-1 in the Southeastern Conference. Alabama is 8-2 overall. Auburn and Ole Miss are each a half-game back with 3-1 league records.

It's about a victory that saw an opportunistic defense recover two fumbles, including one in the end zone, and intercept two passes, including one in the end zone.

It's about sophomore strong safety Greg Jackson, who had one interception and one fumble recovery. It's about sophomore linebacker Eric Hill, who helped force one fumble and intercepted a pass.

It's about an entire team banding together after it lost to Ole Miss last week, 21-19, and fell behind early to Alabama, 7-0.

"All week long we practiced harder than we've ever practiced," Jackson said. "We knew we could win if we didn't make any mistakes. Coach told us all week that we had to gang tackle and try to strip the ball."

Jackson had that on his mind as Alabama sophomore halfback Bobby Humphrey neared the goal line midway through the fourth quarter. Jackson stuck his head into Humphrey, and that hit, combined with one from Hill, jarred the ball loose and into the end zone. Senior cornerback Kevin Guidry made the recovery.

"I didn't know the ball was loose," Guidry said. "Then I looked around and the ball was rolling by my leg. I thought, "What's that doing there?' "

It was there for the taking, and so Guidry took it with 8:26 remaining and LSU ahead, 14-10. But there were still some tense times before LSU won its third straight game at Legion Field.

LSU had to stop speedy wide receiver Al Bell on a fourth-and-five reverse play, and the Tigers had to face the threat of

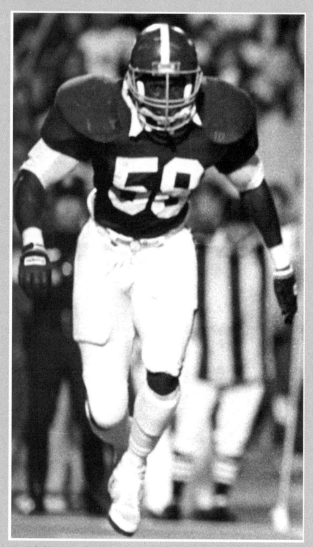

■ **Alabama's defense kept the game close, but Shula & Co. couldn't clinch the win.**

Alabama senior quarterback Mike Shula directing Alabama with 2:19 remaining and the ball on the Crimson Tide 20-yard line. LSU senior nose guard Henry Thomas tipped Shula's first pass attempt, and Hill intercepted to all but clinch the victory.

"We had to play good defense and shut them out in the second half," Arnsparger said, "and we did."

LSU limited Alabama to Van Tiffin's 22-yard field goal in the third quarter. The Tigers blanked Alabama in the fourth period, in part because weak safety Mike Dewitt forced Humphrey to fumble after a 25-yard gain, and Jackson recovered at the LSU 17-yard line.

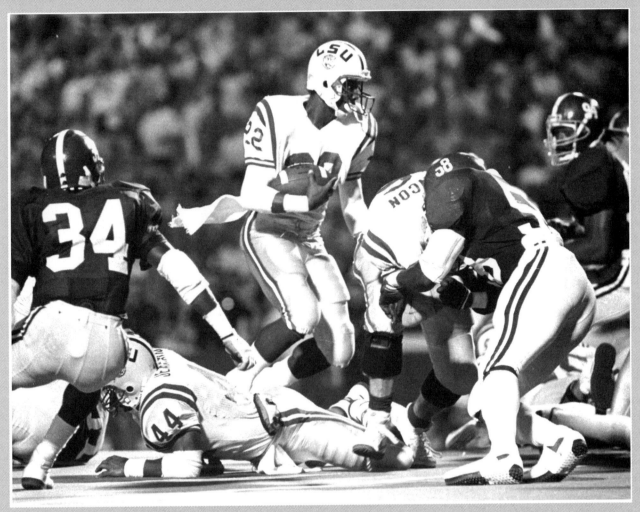

■ **Harvey Williams (22) hunts for an opening in the Tide defense.**

LSU has allowed only six fourth-quarter points this season.

"We came in at halftime and said, 'We're a better second-half team and we've already played a pretty good first half,' " Hill said, "... We made (Shula) make some bad decisions."

One of the worst came in the second quarter after Alabama had marched from its 20 to the LSU 13-yard line. A 33-yard pass to tight end Angelo Stafford put Alabama into position to break a 7-7 tie. Stafford had scored Alabama's only touchdown on a 3-yard reception at 1:20 of the first quarter.

But this time Shula overthrew Stafford and Jackson intercepted in the end zone.

"I read Shula's eyes all the way," Jackson said. "I knew where he was going to throw it, and I turned around and it was there."

The interception set up the game-winning 80-yard touchdown drive that took 12 plays and 5:05 to complete. It ended with quarterback Tommy Hodson's 6-yard pass to wide receiver Wendell Davis 25 seconds before halftime.

With primary receiver Sammy Martin covered in the right side of the end zone, Hodson said he saw Davis "running free" across the middle of the end zone. "I put it on him," said

Hodson, who had to throw the pass over Alabama cornerback Freddie Robinson. "I kind of dropped it in."

But Hodson didn't find things all that easy against a tenacious Alabama defense that sent him to the sidelines on the first series with a slightly twisted knee and limited him to 9 of 21 with two interceptions for 68 yards. Alabama also intercepted one Mickey Guidry pass.

"They did a heck of a job," Hodson said of the Alabama defense. "They took away a lot and limited us as to what we could do."

But they couldn't stop the LSU triumph and the victory celebration. "This is awesome," tight end Brian Kinchen said. "It's a great feeling."

Kinchen participated in the post-game prayer service with linebackers Darren Malbrough and Ron Sancho, safety Chris Carrier and defensive linemen Karl Wilson and Darrell Phillips. Shula also took part. Kinchen said the practice began three years ago after they met through the Fellowship of Christian Athletes.

"There's usually more out there," Kinchen said of the Alabama players. "I guess a lot of them were down."

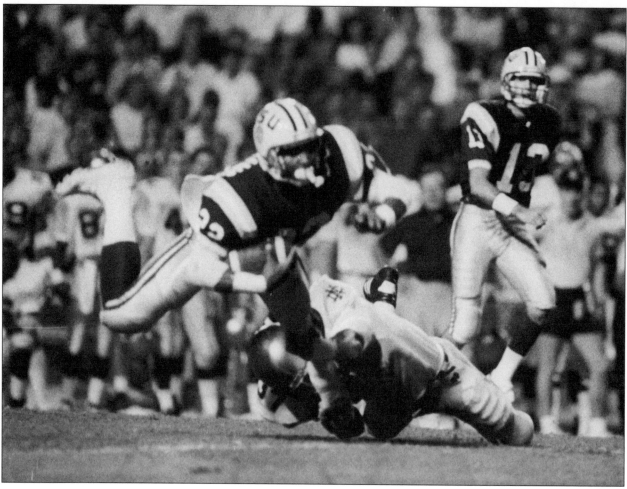

■ Harvey Williams (22) stretches for extra yardage on a pass reception across the middle.

Tiger Defense Turns Away Irish, 21-19

By Bruce Hunter
The Advocate

Baton Rouge, La. — *Nov. 22, 1986*

The LSU Tigers stood up Notre Dame inches from the goal line and staked their claim to a Sugar Bowl berth with a drama-filled, 21-19 victory tonight.

Quarterback Tommy Hodson threw three touchdown passes and the LSU defense gallantly fended off Notre Dame's second-half charge to earn a close, but never-the-less, gigantic triumph in front of a sellout crowd of 78,197 in Tiger Stadium and a national television audience on ESPN. LSU is 3-0 on ESPN this season.

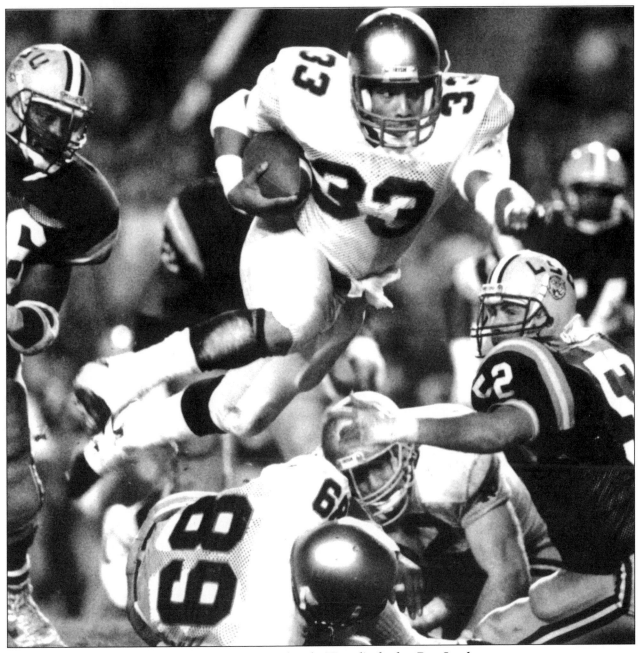

■ **Notre Dame's Hiawatha Francisco (33) is tripped up by Tiger linebacker Ron Sancho.**

But the crowd the Tigers were really trying to impress was the Sugar Bowl executive committee members at the game and watching on television.

"The only team that can catch us (Alabama) is the team we beat," LSU coach Bill Arnsparger said.

Taking a more direct approach to the matter, many of Arnsparger's players said they've already earned the right to represent the Southeastern Conference in the Sugar Bowl against Big Eight runner-up Nebraska. Sugar Bowl officials said they will wait until Nov. 30 to make the final choice in the event of a tie between LSU and Alabama.

"We put a bug in the Sugar Bowl committee's mind," said

Score by Periods

Notre Dame	7	0	3	9	— 19
LSU	14	0	0	7	— 21

LSU nose guard Henry Thomas. "We gave them something to think about. We wanted to show them 'Invite us to your bowl and we won't let you down.' "

Thomas helped lead the Tigers to two defensive stands in the second half, including a first-and-goal situation from the 2.

Then LSU turned back a two-point conversion attempt by the Fighting Irish that would have tied the game with 3:32 left.

By beating Notre Dame, the eighth-ranked Tigers, who earned a share of the SEC title last week, moved closer to assuring themselves of the Sugar Bowl invitation. The school announced after the game it's accepting ticket applications for the Sugar Bowl on a conditional basis. Bowl officials said the decision won't be made until after the Alabama-Auburn game next Saturday.

LSU is 8-2 overall and 5-1 in the SEC. Its only remaining game is against non-conference rival Tulane next Saturday. Alabama, idle on Saturday, is ranked ninth with a record of 9-2 overall and 4-1 in the SEC going into its finale.

Meanwhile, Notre Dame fell to 4-6 and is assured of its second straight losing season. The Irish, who never led in the game, went out with a valiant, comeback effort like they've done so many times this season. They've lost five games by a total of 14 points.

"This is absolutely unbelievable," Notre Dame coach Lou Holtz said. "What more can you tell kids after a game like this? You have to give LSU all the credit in the world. I congratulate them and Bill on a fine job. But these are getting painful and maybe our day will come."

Trailing, 14-7, at halftime, Notre Dame got a pair of field goals by John Carney and a 14-yard touchdown pass from backup quarterback Terry Andrysiak to D'Juan Francisco to rally in the second half. The Tigers managed only a 4-yard touchdown pass from Hodson to tight end Brian Kinchen, which proved to be the winning play.

In the first half, Hodson was accurate on 10 of his first 12 passes and led the Tigers on long touchdown drives the first two times they touched the ball. He threw touchdown passes of 13 yards to Wendell Davis and 4 yards to Rogie Magee in the first quarter. Both LSU's David Browndyke and Carney missed a field goal in the first half.

In between LSU's scores, Notre Dame's Tim Brown broke a kickoff return 96 yards for a touchdown to provide the Irish with their only points of the half.

With Andrysiak at the helm late in the game, the Irish needed only 1:34 to go 80 yards. A 25-yard pass from Andrysiak to split end Tony Eason moved them to the LSU 33.

Andrysiak completed two more passes before he found Francisco open in the back of the end zone. He pulled in the 14-yard pass just in front of the back line and just behind linebacker Toby Caston, bringing the Irish to 21-19 with 3:32 left.

They went for two points, but Andrysiak was pressured by linebacker Ron Sancho and threw out of the end zone.

LSU was able to clinch the victory when Hodson hit Davis and Magee on third-and-long situations in the closing minutes.

Hodson completed 20 of 28 passes for 248 yards and two interceptions. His primary receiver, Davis, collected seven catches for 121 yards and set the LSU record for most receiving yards in a season with 1,161 yards.

Running back Garland Jean Batiste gained 62 yards on 13 carries and tailback Harvey Williams added 52 yards on 20 carries. The Tigers outgained the Irish in total yards, 387 to 270.

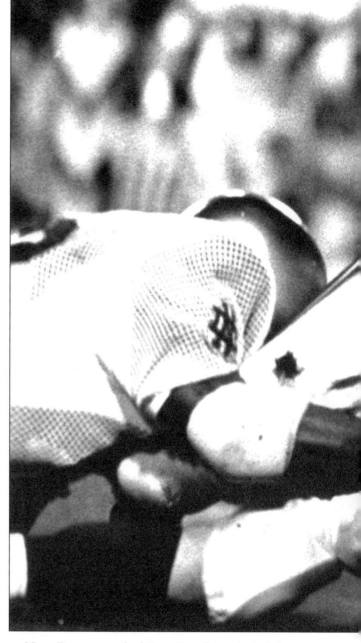

Notre Dame quarterback Steve Beuerlein, who had thrown for nearly 1,000 yards in his last four games, completed just 7 of 18 passes for 50 yards and an interception. Andrysiak came on in relief to complete 6 of 8 for 83.

Early in the second half, LSU's defense had a couple of golden opportunities slip away with weak safety Chris Carrier and linebacker Nicky Hazard coming close to interceptions.

The Irish were able to keep the drive alive when Beuerlein scrambled 15 yards, converting the first of three straight third-down plays. But cornerback Kevin Guidry came up to throw Aaron Robb for a 3-yard loss on a pass in the flats and the Irish couldn't convert again, having to settle for a 31-yard field goal by Carney that made it 14-10 with 5:50 left in the quarter.

Notre Dame free safety Steve Lawrence picked off a

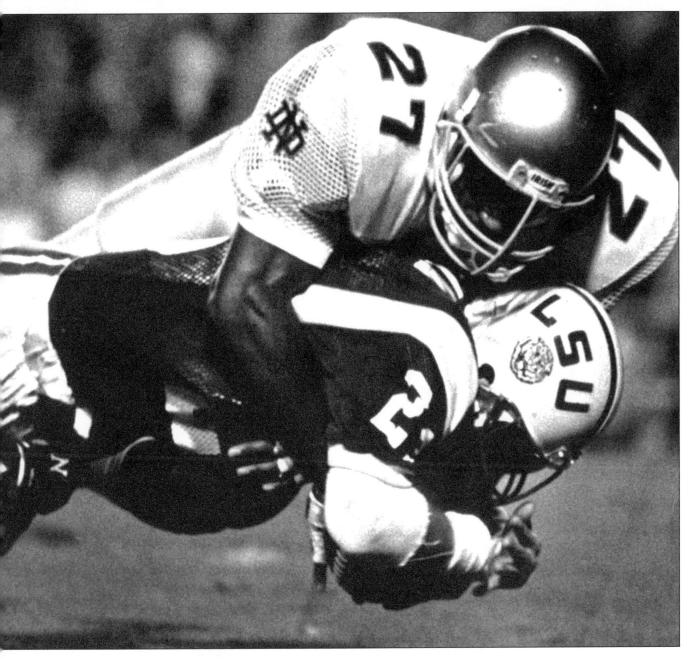

■ Notre Dame's George Streeter and Steve Lawrence force down Sammy Martin (23) after a short gain.

Hodson pass at the LSU 30 and was on his way to a touchdown before Williams bumped him out of bounds on the 2.

Spurred on by the crowd, the Tiger defense made its 10th goal-line stand of the season and one of its most crucial. Fullback Pernell Taylor plunged into the middle of the LSU line two straight times and came within inches of the goal line on his second run.

Then the Irish let tailback Anthony Johnson have a crack at the Tigers, but he was thrown back by Caston to just outside the 1. Going on fourth-and-goal, Beuerlein ran the option to the left side and was forced to pitch to Brown. Weak safety Steve Rehage was there to turn the play in and Brown went down at the 5, ending the threat.

"We have a play that we just try to beat the other team off the ball," said LSU defensive end Roland Barbay. "We try to penetrate and establish a new line of scrimmage. We take a lot of pride in our goal-line defense."

Unable to move the ball, LSU sent in punter Matt DeFrank, who fumbled the snap from center but was able to get off the kick that went for 45 yards to the Notre Dame 46.

But the Irish didn't take long to get into position to challenge for the lead again. Notre Dame, switching running backs in and out, got a couple of 10-yard runs and powered down for a first down at the LSU 13. Then Brown was thrown for an 8-yard loss by safety Greg Jackson on second down and defensive end Karl Wilson sacked Beuerlein for a 6-yard loss to the 27.

Carney still was good on a 44-yard field-goal effort, though, cutting the margin to 14-13 with 11:34 left.

The Tigers' offense awoke on their next possession. Hodson threw for 27 yards on three completions, Williams gained 20 yards on five carries and Jean Batiste added a 14-yard run.

Hodson capped the 11-play march with a 4-yard touchdown pass to Kinchen and Browndyke booted the point after for a 21-13 advantage with 7:45 left.

Then Carrier picked off a Beuerlein pass at the LSU 26 as he tried to find Brown in a crowd and the Tigers went on the move again, making the longest offensive play of the game. Hodson threw long to Davis, who beat the coverage on a streak route down the sidelines for 45 yards.

On the next play, Hodson tried to finish off the drive and threw to Magee in the end zone. Instead, cornerback Troy Wilson intercepted the pass and gave the Irish new life with 5:06 remaining.

In the first half, LSU controlled the action in every phase of the game, except special teams. Notre Dame had just four plays in the first quarter and didn't get its initial first down until midway through the second quarter.

Hodson engineered a pair of ball-control drives of 82 and 71 yards in the first quarter. On their first series, the Tigers moved steadily down the field with Jean Batiste picking up 19 yards on three carries and Hodson doing the rest through the air. He completed 4 of 5 for 57 yards on the march.

A 23-yard completion to Kinchen may have gone for a touchdown if Hodson's pass hadn't been so high, forcing him to leap into the air to pull it down at the Notre Dame 17. Hodson capped it off by hitting Davis on a curl pattern at the 1 and he fell back into the end zone for the score and a 7-0 lead after Browndyke's kick.

LSU's Ron Lewis booted a high kick to Brown at the 4 and the Irish speedster picked out a hole on the right side, sprinting through the Tigers and breaking into the clear. His 96-yard touchdown return took just 12 seconds and, with Carney's kick, tied the game at 7-7 with 9:36 left.

Undaunted by the touchdown, LSU regained control of the game with yet another sustained drive, which turned out to be its longest of the season.

Williams checked in at tailback and gained 15 yards on his first two carries. Hodson connected with Jean Batiste and Davis for 19 yards and a first down at the LSU 46. Then freshman flanker Tony Moss took a short pass from Hodson, broke a tackle and scooted 17 yards.

As they closed for the score, the Tigers had a bad break when Williams slipped and was ruled down on a run that would have gone to the 5, but actually went for a 3-yard loss. Jean Batiste finally dove for 2 yards over right guard on fourth-and-inches to get to the 4.

After Jean Batiste was held for no gain and Hodson threw incomplete, Magee broke open in the end zone on third down and pulled in a 4-yard touchdown pass with 49 seconds left in the quarter. Browndyke's kick put the Tigers back on top, 14-7.

When they kicked off for the second time, Matt DeFrank came in and squibbed it down field. But Brown still came up

with it at the 9 and returned it 22 yards. The Irish got their initial offensive play of the game with 42 seconds left in the quarter and couldn't keep the ball long enough to run out the quarter.

A 23-yard punt by Dan Sorenson gave LSU excellent field position at its own 41 and Hodson's 16-yard pass to Davis helped the Tigers moved down the Notre Dame 29. They picked up another first down, but had to settle for a 36-yard field-goal attempt from the right hash mark. Browndyke kicked the ball wide right, ending the threat with 3:20 remaining in the half.

On Notre Dame's third possession, it finally came up with a first down. Andrysiak scrambled 22 yards out to the Irish 48, but fumbled the ball away two plays later when Barbay delivered a hit on him. The fumble was recovered by Thomas at the LSU 49.

Although the Tigers couldn't move the ball, DeFrank was able to pin the Irish at their own 15 with a 36-yard punt.

Working with 4:17 left before halftime, Andrysiak led the Irish on their best drive of the half. The play that started the march was a 20-yard pass to split end Milt Jackson.

The Irish continued to move until LSU finally held and forced them to go for a 49-yard field goal by Carney. He made the kick, but LSU was offsides before the snap.

So Carney had to try again, this time from 43 yards out. His kick went off to the left with 17 seconds left.

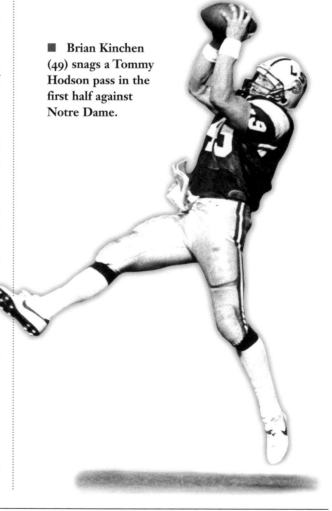

■ **Brian Kinchen (49) snags a Tommy Hodson pass in the first half against Notre Dame.**

Everything Went Right For Tigers' Dramatic Win

BY DAVE MOORMANN
The Advocate
....

Baton Rouge — *Nov. 22, 1986*

LSU defensive teammates Steve Rehage and Ron Sancho found themselves in the right place at the right time Saturday night, and senior linebacker Toby Caston is glad they did.

Caston also thought he was in the right place in the end zone. But his timing wasn't right, as Notre Dame quarterback Terry Andrysiak lofted a 14-yard touchdown pass to D'Juan Francisco with 3:32 remaining in the Irish's game against LSU in Tiger Stadium. Caston was covering on the play that went for the first fourth-quarter touchdown against LSU's defense this season.

"I don't know how the guy caught it," Caston said. "I bumped him and then looked, and saw he still had the ball and his toes were in bounds."

The score narrowed LSU's lead to 21-19, and Caston felt responsible for allowing a play that might have resulted in a tie for LSU. But on the ensuing two-point conversion try, Sancho hurried Andrysiak into throwing an incompletion in the end zone. Caston was relieved.

"I would have been crushed," Caston said of what a tie would have meant to him. "After we stopped the two-point conversion, I felt good."

Sancho did, too. And with good reason, for it was pressure from the sophomore linebacker that forced Andrysiak to throw incomplete for Joel Williams in the end zone.

Sancho said LSU had an "inside defensive play" called before Andrysiak dropped to pass. When Sancho saw that, he said he "aborted what I was doing and ran" after Andrysiak, who hurried his pass and threw it out of bounds.

Defensive coordinator Mike Archer said LSU had called the same blitz it had used on the preceding touchdown. "You live by the blitz and die by the blitz," he said.

Eighth-ranked LSU survived with a 21-19 victory that improved its overall record to 8-2 and its chances of appearing in the Sugar Bowl on New Year's Day. Should Alabama and LSU tie for the Southeastern Conference title at 5-1, Sugar Bowl officials said they will decide upon the SEC representative on Nov. 30.

Alabama must play Auburn on Nov. 29. LSU ends its regular season that same day at home against Tulane.

LSU coach Bill Arnsparger said again he believes his team belongs in the Sugar Bowl because "the only one who can catch us, we beat."

Notre Dame found itself trying to catch LSU the entire game. The Irish did once, when Tim Brown returned a kickoff for a 96-yard touchdown that tied the score, 7-7, at 9:48 of the

first quarter. LSU had taken the opening drive 71 yards, with quarterback Tommy Hodson throwing a 13-yard touchdown pass to Wendell Davis.

Davis, who finished with seven catches for 121 yards, became LSU's single-season yardage leader with 1,161 yards. Eric Martin set the old record of 1,064 in 1983. Davis has a school-record 75 catches. He was named the ESPN-TV Player of the Game and Coach Bill Arnsparger said he has "invited ESPN back for next week's game." LSU is 3-0 on ESPN this season and 5-0 overall.

"It was one of those football games where things went well for awhile and things didn't go well for awhile," Arnsparger said.

Things looked bleak for LSU in the third quarter when Notre Dame free safety Steve Lawrence intercepted Hodson's pass and returned it 28 yards to the LSU 2-yard line. But two runs up the middle by fullback Pernell Taylor gained only 1 yard, and Anthony Johnson gained nothing on a third-down play over the top, where he was met by Caston, who participated on all three tackles.

On fourth-and-1, Notre Dame quarterback Steve Beuerlein rolled left on an option and pitched to Brown. But Rehage shed a blocker and dropped Brown for a 4-yard loss.

"I knew the whole way," said Rehage. "I figured they had run three times to the middle and then were going to try either a toss sweep or the option ... I knew they were going to go to Brown. He's their horse."

But Rehage didn't even know if he was going to get in the game. Rehage returned to action briefly last week after missing three games with a knee injury. And up until Notre Dame reached the 2-yard line with 5:33 remaining in the third quarter and LSU ahead, 14-10, Rehage wasn't sure if he would play against the Irish. Then Archer sent him in for the goal-line series.

Archer said he intended to insert Rehage because sophomore Greg Jackson had begun to tire. Rehage figured he was in on only about 10 plays and Archer said Rehage's left knee "still isn't 100 percent."

But Rehage was feeling fine after he shed a blocker and tackled Brown. Rehage said he was assigned to the pitch man and senior cornerback Norman Jefferson was to take the quarterback.

"The last three weeks we've played option teams," Rehage said, "and Coach Archer does a great job of telling us what he wants us to do."

After sitting on the bench with an stretched knee ligament, the intense Rehage was ready to vent his emotions.

"A game like tonight is three-fourths frustration coming out," he said. "The whole first half I was wondering when I would come in."

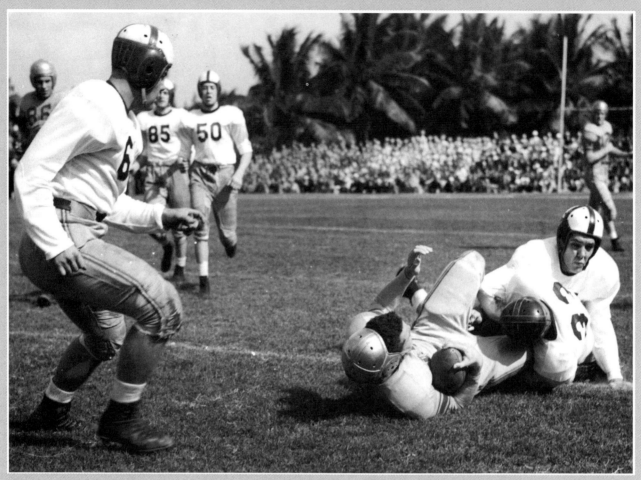

■ Texas A&M's gang-tackling finally brought down this Tiger on the loose.

Van Buren Stars in 19-14 Orange Bowl Win

By Maurice McGann
The Advocate

Miami — *Jan. 1, 1944*

Striking swiftly in the first and third quarters, the Louisiana State Tigers piled up three touchdowns and scored a well-earned 19-14 victory over the Texas Aggies here today before an overflowing crowd. Steven Van Buren was the big gun for the Bengals, sprinting 13 and 62 yards for touchdowns and tossing a scoring pass to Burt Goode.

Bernie Moore had put in some special plays for this game and he lost little time in seeing that they were made the most of. After the Tigers had worked the ball down to the Aggies' 12 the second time they got their hands on it, Van Buren caught the Aggies by surprise on a delayed double reverse and he sped over the goal without a hand being laid on him.

The Tigers failed on the extra-point attempt, but they lost little time in moving further out in front when Charley Webb recovered a punt fumbled by Jess Burditt on the Aggies' 22. Two running plays gained only two yards and then Van Buren passed neatly to Goode who stepped across the goal line for the score. Van Buren's extra-point attempt failed.

The Aggies quickly got back in the game, however, when they took the following kickoff and marched 70 yards for their first touchdown. Babe Hallmark had his pitching arm in fine

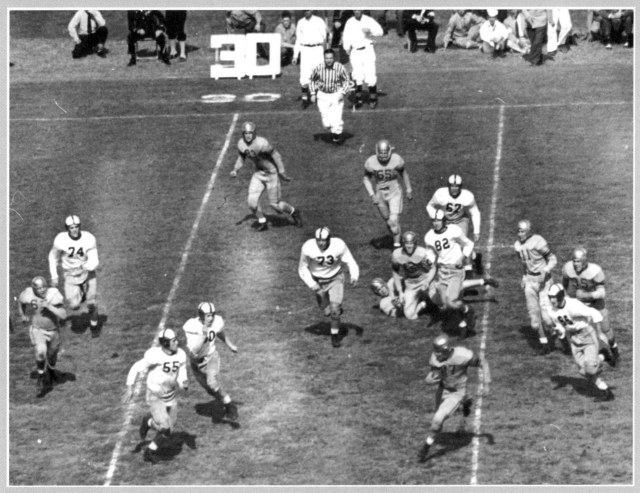

■ **Steve Van Buren raced for 13-yard and 62-yard touchdowns and passed for a third touchdown.**

trim and aided by a 15-yard roughness penalty the Aggies passed their way to the Tigers' 21.

The Bengals stopped a couple of Aggie running plays, but Hallmark found his mark, passing to Burditt for 11 yards and a touchdown. Stan Turner booted the extra point and the scoreboard read, LSU 12, Aggies 7.

The Tigers had three fine scoring chances in the second period but lacked the punch to add to their total. Van Buren faked a punt and raced 40 yards only to stumble and fall from exhaustion when he had a clear field. On another occasion, the Tigers made a first down on the Aggies' 5-yard line, but four smashes failed to put it over.

The Bengals came back strong at the start of the second half and within a few minutes, Van Buren showed his all-American form by breaking loose from scrimmage for 62 yards through the entire Aggie team and the third LSU touchdown. This time he converted the extra-point kick and the Bengals held a 19-7 advantage.

But the Aggies weren't through by any means and they went all out with their aerial game. Making the most of a stiff breeze at their backs, the Aggies worked the Bengals into a hole, and made the most of a break when they got it — recovering Joe Nagata's fumble on the LSU 25.

Score by Periods

Texas A&M	7	0	7	0	— 14
LSU	12	0	7	0	— 19

E.G. Beesley passed to Burditt for seven yards and then Hallmark shot a neat one to Marion Settegest on the LSU 5-yard line and he raced over for the score. Turner booted the point-after kick which reduced the Tigers' lead to five points, 19-14.

The Bengals held on gamely to their small lead and until the closing minutes of the game it was a defensive battle. In the final minutes, fumbled pass interceptions and laterals thrilled the fans of both teams, but failed to produce a score. The Bengals were in possession of the ball on the Aggies' 22 when the game ended.

The victory was especially sweet to the Tigers because they had been defeated, 28-13, by these same Aggies earlier in the year. It was even sweeter to LSU coach Bernie Moore since it marked his first bowl victory in four trips.

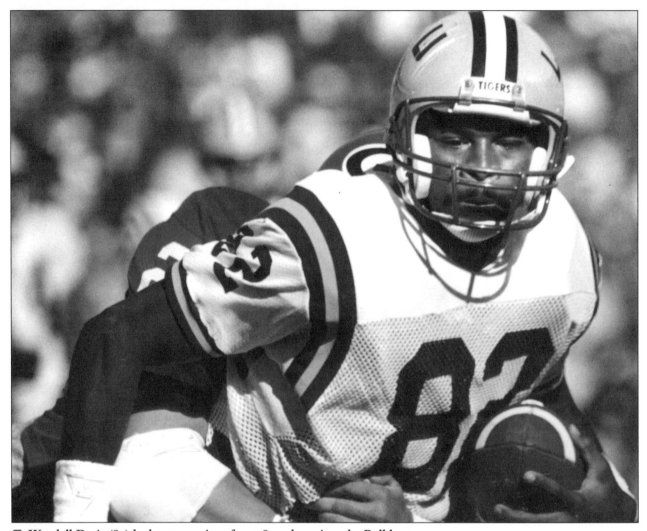

■ Wendell Davis (82) had 11 receptions for 128 yards against the Bulldogs.

Tigers Outduel Stubborn Georgia, 26-23

BY BRUCE HUNTER
The Advocate

Athens, Ga. — *Oct. 10, 1987*

LSU and Georgia lived and died by the big play, of which there were many on this wild afternoon.

The final two — a leaping touchdown catch by Brian Kinchen and a diving interception by Kevin Guidry — went LSU's way, allowing the Tigers to escape with a 26-23 victory before a thunderous, sold-out crowd of 82,122 in Sanford Stadium and national television audience on ESPN.

"I feel like I'm 34 years old going on 60," said LSU coach Mike Archer. "I was really feeling my age that last drive. We let them back into the game with the big plays, but our kids showed a lot of heart and desire. I can't say enough about our players and coaching staff and how we hung together."

LSU, leading 16-3 at halftime, had to come from behind in the final minutes after the Bulldogs, as they have done so often in 24 seasons under Vince Dooley, found a way to get back in the game and make it close. But Georgia's 20-point comeback with three long touchdown plays in the second half was completely out of character for the Bulldogs.

Quarterback Tommy Hodson connected with Kinchen for a 5-yard TD pass to provide LSU with the winning margin with 3:36 left to play. But the explosive Bulldogs weren't out of it until a James Jackson pass deflected off tailback Rodney Hampton and into the hands of Guidry, who caught the ball just off the grass. Guidry's interception Georgia's final drive at the LSU 28 with 1:01 left and atoned for a touchdown pass that he surrendered earlier in the second half.

"I felt like the difference in the two halves was big plays," Dooley said. "In the second half, we had the long catch by (John) Thomas, then (Cassius) Osborn got loose by breaking a tackle and scored on the long run. We also had a big play on Vince Guthrie's interception. It was a great game for everybody involved, but unfortunately someone had to lose. And this time it was us."

Engaging in close games like this one was nothing new for either team. The seventh-ranked Tigers have found ways to survive these tests, while the 16th-ranked Bulldogs continue to falter in the clutch.

LSU, 5-0-1, moved into sole possession of the Southeastern Conference lead, going to 2-0 in defense of its league championship. The Tigers went to the wire for the third straight Saturday, including a 13-10 decision over Florida last week and 13-13 tie with Ohio State two weeks ago. All three opponents were nationally ranked.

Georgia, on the other hand, hasn't won the crucial SEC

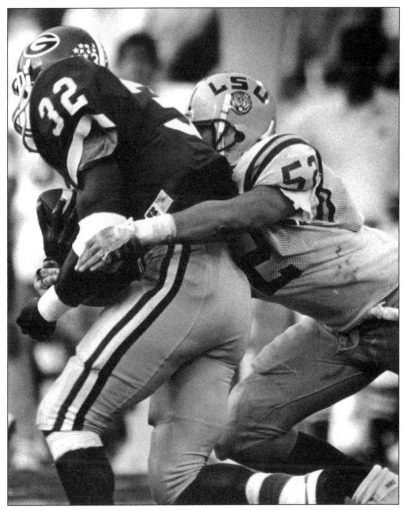

■ Georgia's Lars Tate (32) is wrestled down by Ron Sancho (52).

games since Herschel Walker left school after leading the Bulldogs to conference titles from 1980-82. The Bulldogs, 4-2 overall and 1-1 in the SEC, have lost twice this season by a combined total of just four points.

"It was a great win today," Kinchen said. "It seems like every week it gets closer and closer. But this was better because it was in their backyard."

Georgia, which lost for just the sixth time at home in the 1980s, appeared to be on its way to another miracle "Between the Hedges" that surround the 58-year-old stadium.

Jackson, who passed for 170 yards and rushed for 85 more in the game, threw touchdown passes of 31 yards to Thomas and 74 yards to Osborn. Then Hampton raced 14 yards for the go-ahead points, giving the Bulldogs a 23-19 lead with 6:58 left.

LSU's first-half points came on a 36-yard touchdown pass from backup quarterback Mickey Guidry to Tony Moss and three field goals by David Browndyke. Another Browndyke field goal early in the fourth quarter enabled him to tie his own school record of four in a game and set the stage for the final offensive fireworks.

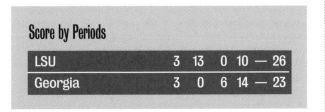

Score by Periods

LSU		3	13	0	10 —	26
Georgia		3	0	6	14 —	23

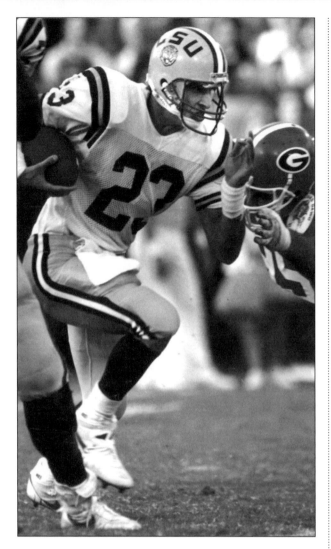

■ **Tailback Sammy Martin (23) finds a seam in the Georgia defense.**

After Georgia went in front, the Tigers responded with a 39-yard kickoff return by Eddie Fuller that led to a nine-play scoring drive. Even with Hodson knocked out of the game for two plays on a late hit by Georgia's Ben Smith, LSU was relentless on its 61-yard touchdown march that used up 3½ minutes.

"I was really confident," Hodson said. "It was kind of like Kentucky last year (when he rallied LSU to a 25-16 victory after being knocked out of the game). I really felt confident then and I was confident today that we could drive down and score."

Although Hodson was dizzy on the sidelines, he spelled Mickey Guidry at quarterback and completed four passes, including two 11-yard strikes to split end Wendell Davis, who had 11 catches for 128 yards. Davis' second reception left the Tigers with a first-and-goal at the 7, a position from which they've been unsuccessful in the last three games.

This time Fuller picked up 2 yards on a first-down carry around left end. On the next play, Hodson faked a handoff and dropped back to pass, looking for tailback Sammy Martin or

tight end Willie Williams. Instead, he had enough time to find Kinchen going all the way across the field.

"He got out of the pocket and just happened to roll my way," Kinchen said. "I think Willie picked off my man and it left me open. It was kind of a fluke play."

Kinchen's touchdown sent LSU back on top, but left plenty of time for the Bulldogs. Hampton returned the kickoff out to the 24 and Jackson quickly tossed first-down passes to Troy Sadowski and Lars Tate, sending Georgia to midfield.

Staying in the air, the Bulldogs advanced into LSU territory on a 19-yard reception by Osborn over the middle with 1:50 remaining. But Georgia's comeback bid ended two plays later when Jackson's pass slipped away from Hampton and was corralled by Kevin Guidry.

"We were in zone coverage and my primary responsibility was to come up and make the tackle," Guidry said. "I just think the Lord that the guy bobbled the ball. ... I had some breakdowns early in the game, but I did something to get the respect of my teammates back."

Guidry, a fourth-year starter at cornerback, walked off the field with tears welling in his eyes. "This was the biggest game of my life," he said later.

The interception provided Guidry with a memorable ending to what had been a nightmare of a second half. It began with Thomas sprinting down the left sidelines and Guidry running with him step-by-step.

However, Thomas caught Jackson's 31-yard pass over his left shoulder in the end zone before Guidry could even get his hands up. The Georgia touchdown, coming three plays after Bill Goldberg recovered a Harvey Williams fumble, pulled the Bulldogs to within 16-9 after Steve Crumley missed the extra point with just four minutes gone in the third quarter.

Almost 10 minutes of hard-knocks defense went by before either team threatened. And it was Thomas who put Guidry in an awkward position again.

The junior split end was 15 yards behind Guidry on a flea-flicker pass from Jackson late in the third quarter. Thomas, the fourth Georgia player to touch the ball on the reverse-pitch-back pass, was pulling it down with the official signaling a touchdown, only to let it slide through his hands in the end zone, spoiling a 48-yard touchdown pass.

Another incomplete pass forced the Bulldogs to punt back to LSU, which seemingly was motivated by the near miss. The Tigers, starting at their 14, were quickly off to the races with a 41-yard run by Martin, who rushed 13 times for 84 yards and caught six passes for 55 yards in the game.

Martin and Fuller kept gaining large chunks of ground against the Georgia defense, leading the Tigers to a first-and-goal at the 2. Then a delay-of-game penalty stymied the march and Browndyke came on to kick a 21-yard field goal, increasing the margin to 19-9 with 11:17 left in the game.

Backed up against the wall, the Bulldogs broke loose with consecutive scoring drives. Osborn was running a basic down-and-out pattern on third down, but cornerback Willie Bryant

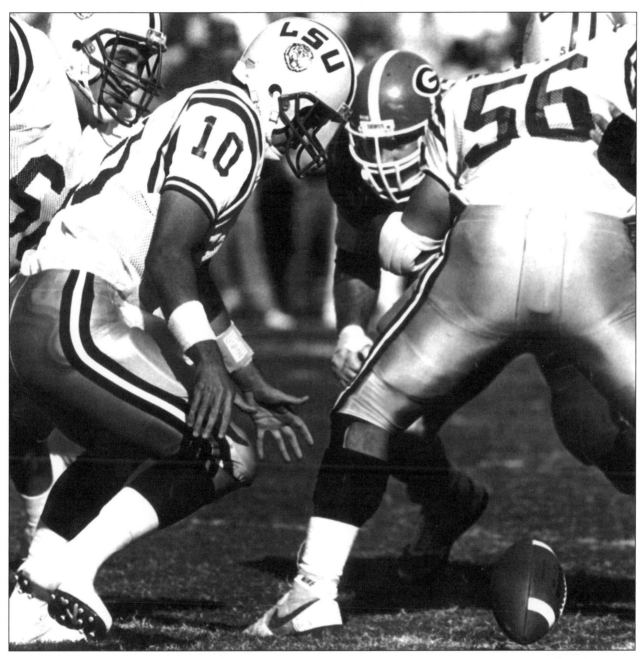

■ **LSU quarterback Mickey Guidry (10) attempts to recover his fumble, which is between the legs of Nacho Albergamo (56).**

missed the tackle, giving Osborn room to run away from the pack down the right sidelines.

Osborn's 74-yard touchdown play sliced the Bulldogs' deficit to 19-16 with 9:45 left and Guthrie put them back in business with an interception of Hodson, who completed 21 of 31 for 209 yards with just one turnover. The Georgia linebacker returned the interception 28 yards to the LSU 17 before being tripped up by Rogie Magee, the intended receiver.

The Bulldogs needed just two plays to take their first lead since early in the game. Tate gained 3 yards around left end and Hampton dashed the remaining 14 yards, breaking two tackles

to get across the goal line. Crumley's kick put the Bulldogs in front by more than a field goal at 23-19, putting LSU in a position to play for a touchdown.

The Tigers were up to the test, just as they were in the first half when they scored on four of their six possessions in taking a 13-point lead.

After Browndyke kicked a 27-yard field goal to match Crumley's 34-yarder earlier in the first quarter, LSU dominated the rest of the first half, scoring on its final three offensive series. Mickey Guidry, seeing his first action at quarterback in two weeks, engineered the only touchdown drive of the half by completing 4 of 5 for 72 yards and a TD strike to Moss.

Hodson Rallies Tigers in Win over Georgia

By Dave Moormann

The Advocate

Athens, Ga. — *Oct. 10, 1987*

It was shades of Kentucky.

An injury. A trip to the sidelines. A re-entry into the lineup. The need for a rally. The game-winning points.

So how did LSU quarterback Tommy Hodson feel about this sense of deja vu?

"It was Georgia," he said, the ringing of a late tackle still fresh in his ears.

Georgia it was. Hodson hadn't lost his senses. Nor had he lost his flair for the dramatic. His Bulldog-induced headache kept him on the bench for two plays. Upon returning, Hodson took six plays to push LSU into the end zone, hitting tight end Brian Kinchen with a 5-yard pass that rallied LSU to a 26-23 victory.

"It (the pain) was like Kentucky," said Hodson, shaken up today when Georgia cornerback Ben Smith hit Hodson, who was out of bounds, "only not as bad."

Against Kentucky last year, Hodson bit through his tongue, requiring five stitches. He missed most of the first half. Upon his return LSU trailed, 7-0. Hodson promptly rallied LSU to a 12-7 halftime lead and a 25-16 victory.

Against Georgia, Hodson didn't feel as bad, but the situation was worse. LSU trailed, 23-19, with 6½ minutes left and the ball 42 yards from the end zone. Hodson had just run 3 yards and out of bounds and Smith's personal-foul penalty added 15 yards to the play.

Smith said he couldn't tell if he was out of bounds, but he had committed himself and made a mistake. He also said LSU coach Mike Archer grabbed him and berated him but apologized on the next play.

"I lost my cool in that situation," Archer said. "I apologized. That was uncalled for."

Hodson was more restrained.

"That's all part of the game, it happens," said Hodson, who admitted he was still somewhat woozy when he re-entered the game.

Hodson had a handful of Tylenol packages next to him in his locker-room stall.

"I'm sure he's (Smith) a nice guy," Hodson said. "He probably didn't mean it."

Hodson vented his frustration on the field, hitting 3 of 4 passes before Eddie Fuller gained 2 yards. Then came the play that eased whatever pain Hodson felt, excited a faithful LSU throng in sold-out Sanford Stadium, and brought Kinchen his second touchdown of the season.

It was the second time this season that LSU ran its "Cougar Route."

"We name all our goal-line stuff after animals," Kinchen said.

The first time, Kinchen, who is not the primary receiver, wasn't involved in the play. This time, with wide receiver Rogie Magee running a deeper route in the end zone and tight end Willie Williams running a crossing pattern underneath Kinchen, Kinchen found himself free. After a play-action fake and a rollout to his left, Hodson located Kinchen.

"It wasn't a dead spiral," said Kinchen, who jumped to make the catch. "Anytime it's a little wobbly, there's a chance you could drop it."

Despite an injury to his right hand, which Kinchen said has ached for two weeks and was reaggravated today when someone stepped on his two outside fingers, Kinchen clutched Hodson's 31st pass attempt with 3:36 remaining. Hodson completed 21 passes for 209 yards. Junior Mickey Guidry, who replaced Hodson for a second-quarter series and again when Hodson was sidelined, hit 4 of 5 passes, including a 36-yard touchdown toss to Tony Moss.

The pass to Kinchen was designed for a touchdown. The sideline pass to Moss was meant only to gain a first down. But Moss turned the third-down pass into a touchdown with nifty footwork along the sideline, as he avoided three potential tacklers. It was Moss' first collegiate touchdown.

"I was just trying to get to the outside for more yardage," Moss said. "I was trying to get away from 15 (Mark Vincent). All of the sudden I had one man to beat. I really like a one-on-one situation."

In a game featuring two defenses with reputations for preventing big plays, numerous one-on-one confrontations developed. Georgia's Cassius Osborn raced for a 74-yard touchdown catch-and-run after cornerback Willie Bryant missed a tackle. The Bulldogs' John Thomas slipped behind cornerback Kevin Guidry to make an over-the-shoulder 31-yard touchdown catch, later dropping an apparent 48-yard touchdown pass after the ball changed hands three times in the Georgia backfield.

Finally, Guidry found himself one-on-one against freshman Rodney Hampton, who earlier had scored Georgia's go-ahead touchdown on an 14-yard run. Following Kinchen's touchdown, Georgia had driven 45 yard to the LSU 31-yard line when quarterback James Jackson passed to Hampton.

"My primary goal is to make the tackle and keep him to a 4- or 5-yard gain," Guidry said. "The guy bobbled the ball."

And Guidry made the interception, securing the victory for LSU, which improved to 5-0-1 and 2-0 in the Southeastern Conference. Georgia, losing for only the sixth time in 47 home

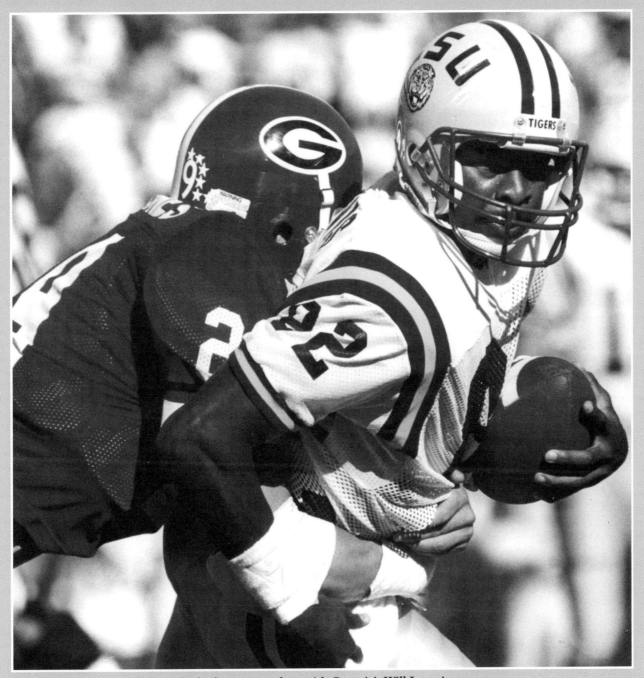

■ **LSU receiver Wendell Davis looks for extra yardage with Georgia's Will Jones in tow.**

games this decade, fell to 4-2 overall and 1-1 in the SEC. Guidry, a senior, left the field in tears.

"That's something I can't explain," he said. "That's the first time I've ever cried at LSU. To know you made the deciding factor in winning the game is a great feeling."

"It was a total team effort," Archer said. "We need all the people."

No one was more valuable then sophomore place-kicker David Browndyke, who kicked four field goals, matching a school record he tied twice last season. Browndyke has made eight straight field goals. He began his career with seven consecutive kicks.

Browndyke's success also pointed to LSU's growing frustration around the goal line. One LSU drived stalled when the Tigers lost yardage on third-and-1 at the Georgia 2. Another drive fizzled after a delay penalty on first-and-goal from the 2.

"We made two or three glaring errors," LSU offensive coordinator Ed Zaunbrecher said. "We thought we had corrected those things. It's a matter of concentration."

Hodson concentrated. But no matter how hard he thought, the latest drama didn't remind him of Kentucky.

It was Georgia.

Hodson's 4th Down Strike Clinches Win Over Auburn

By Bruce Hunter
The Advocate

Baton Rouge, La. — *Oct. 8, 1988*

I t will go down in the LSU record book as Tommy Hodson's 40th touchdown pass. He's never thrown a more important one at a more crucial moment in a more exciting football game.

His 11-yard pass, coming on fourth down with 1:41 left, was pulled down by tailback Eddie Fuller in the back of the end zone, almost in the same spot where he had been ruled out of bounds only three plays earlier.

The dramatic touchdown pass, along with David Browndyke's extra point, lifted LSU to a 7-6 victory over fourth-ranked, previously unbeaten Auburn tonight in Tiger Stadium.

"That was the only throw I had left in me," Hodson said. "If football had five downs, I don't know if I would have had it left in me."

Hodson, who was 17 of 38 for 167 yards, led LSU on a last-ditch drive that went 75 yards on 15 plays. All but one of those plays were passes, including a fourth-down throw to tight end Willie Williams that set up the game-winning pass.

It was only the second time all night that LSU had crossed midfield. It also broke a string of seven quarters without a touchdown.

When Fuller came down with the touchdown catch, the LSU players on the field, those on the sidelines and the majority of the 79,431 fans in the stands exploded in celebration.

"I've been around a lot of college football games," LSU coach Mike Archer said. "But I've never been around a bunch of kids that have made a gutsier effort than our players just have. They never got down on themselves."

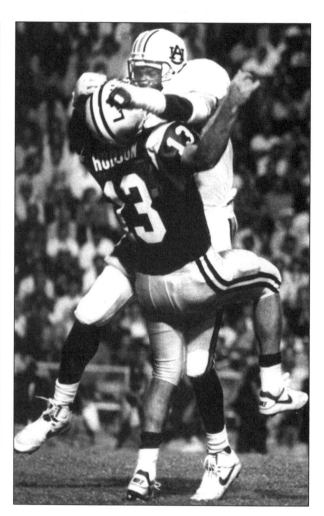

■ **It was a night of hard knocks for LSU quarterback Tommy Hodson, whose late pass won the game.**

In the nationally televised game on ESPN, Auburn built a 6-0 lead on field goals of 41 and 33 yards by Win Lyle. And its defense had held LSU to just nine first downs until the fateful final march.

To start that drive, Hodson threw over the middle to flanker Tony Moss for a 17-yard gain out to the 42. Then he hit Williams for 12 yards to move into Auburn territory.

A third-down reception by Moss went for 20 yards to the Auburn 21. And then the excitement really started.

Fuller dropped a possible touchdown pass. It was a high throw from Hodson, but definitely catchable.

Faced with fourth-and-9, Hodson rolled out under pressure

Score by Periods

Auburn	0	3	0	3 —	6
LSU	0	0	0	7 —	7

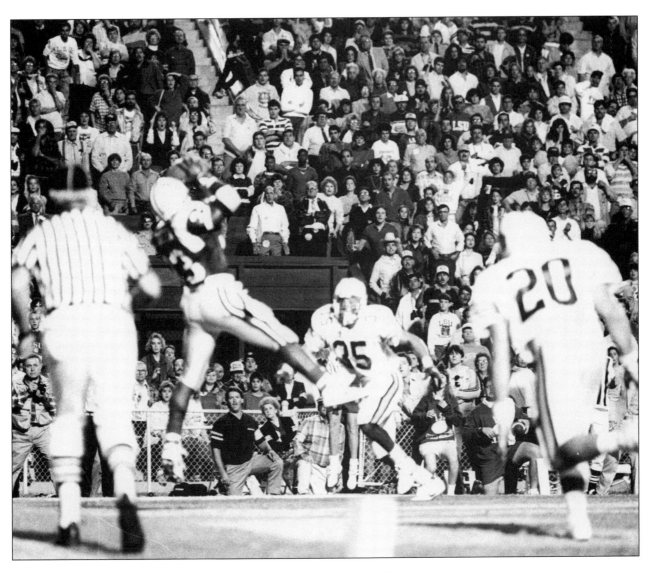

■ **Eddie Fuller's touchdown leap gave the Tigers a come-from-behind victory.**

and connected with Williams on an out route. The 6-6 tight end fell forward to reach the first-down marker. LSU was still alive.

On first down, Fuller, missing a second chance to score, was ruled to have come down out of the end zone on an apparent touchdown reception. It was the same route he would soon run again.

Then Hodson misfired on his next two attempts. That set up fourth-and-10 and in all likelihood LSU's last shot.

"I didn't know if I was going to get the ball again," Fuller said. "I'm just glad Tommy had enough confidence in me to come back to me."

Although Fuller wasn't the primary choice, Hodson had enough time to find him over the middle and behind the Auburn secondary.

"The (line)backer kind of lost him," Hodson said. "And the free safety moved over to cover the wide receivers. And it left a little seam in there for Eddie."

Fuller caught the pass and immediately looked down to see where his feet had landed this time. He didn't need to look. The crowd gave him the answer.

"This is beyond me," he said afterwards. "I can't even describe this feeling."

LSU, 3-2 overall, broke a two-game losing streak, its longest since 1983, and climbed back into the Southeastern Conference race at 2-1. Auburn fell to 4-1 and 2-1 in the SEC.

"You've got to give LSU an awful lot of credit because they didn't have a lot of success driving the ball until that last drive of the game," Auburn coach Pat Dye said. "When it came down to winning and losing, they did what they had to do to win the football game."

Up until those closing minutes, defense had ruled the battle of the SEC's Tigers, their 25th meeting overall and first since 1981.

The defensive war consumed most of the game. The second half started with LSU failing to move beyond its 23 and Rene' Bourgeois punting for the eighth time.

Auburn quarterback Reggie Slack, throwing to Alexander Wright and Walter Reeves, directed Auburn down to the LSU 24. After an illegal motion penalty, Slack tried to hit Wright again, but cornerback Mike Mayes tipped the pass and weak safety Greg Jackson intercepted it at the 18.

What ensued was LSU's longest drive to that point. Hodson connected with Ronnie Haliburton for 17 yards and then went to Moss for back-to-back receptions for 32 yards. Moss got most of it on his own, taking a quick out 23 yards to the Auburn 33.

A defensive holding call against cornerback Carlos Cheattom gave LSU another first down at the 23. But Auburn held and was helped by a third-down clipping penalty that pushed LSU back to the 40 and out of field-goal range.

Brian Griffith, LSU's pooch punter, narrowly missed the coffin corner. His punt went into the end zone, and Auburn took over at the 20.

Neither offense could mount an attack the rest of the quarter. LSU got the best of the punt exchanges, however.

"I love that kind of game," LSU outside linebacker Eric Hill said. "It was a tough, physical game. I wish they were all like that."

Auburn finally put together a 71-yard drive that took 15 plays and almost six minutes.

Tailback James Joseph rushed 3 yards for a first down to the 25. Then Slack threw to Freddy Weygand for a 21-yard completion to midfield.

After that, Slack converted on two third-down plays. On third-and-18, he found Lawyer Tilman on a deep out that went for 19 yards. Then on third-and-10, he connected with Greg Taylor on a crossing pattern that gained 19 yards to the LSU 20.

LSU's defense held Stacy Danley to 3 yards on back-to-back carries, and fullback Vincent Harris picked up a yard on a third-down reception. Lyle finished off the drive with a 33-yard field goal for a 6-0 lead with 10:12 left.

Mickey Guidry took his second turn at quarterback for LSU. Despite a personal foul against Auburn, Guidry couldn't mount a drive and LSU punted back to Auburn.

After LSU's defense held, the homestanding Tigers got another opportunity with 6:07 left and Hodson back at quarterback. He completed six passes on the march and saved his biggest throw for last.

In the first half, Slack's third pass was well behind Wright and was picked off by cornerback Jimmy Young at the LSU 20.

LSU wasted the opportunity when Haliburton dropped a pass over the middle at the LSU 48.

Auburn had the first scoring threat, driving from its own 34 to the LSU 33. Harris had two carries for 15 yards to lead the way.

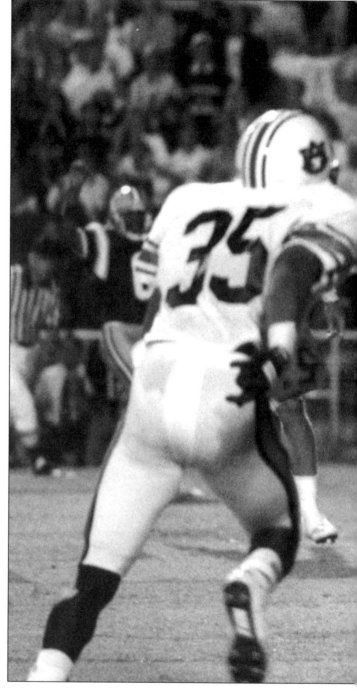

But on third down, defensive end Clint James batted Slack's pass into the air. Slack caught the ball, but was thrown for a 2-yard loss by Ron Sancho. Auburn chose to punt, rather than attempt a 52- yard field goal.

Ironically, LSU had an identical play on its next series. Hodson's pass was deflected by inside linebacker Brian Smith, and he caught his own pass, but was thrown for a 4-yard loss by Tracy Rocker.

Hodson hit Alvin Lee on a third-down pass over the middle that went for 21 yards. But on LSU's next third-down play, Fuller was stopped a yard short on a pass reception to the LSU 41, forcing a Bourgeois punt.

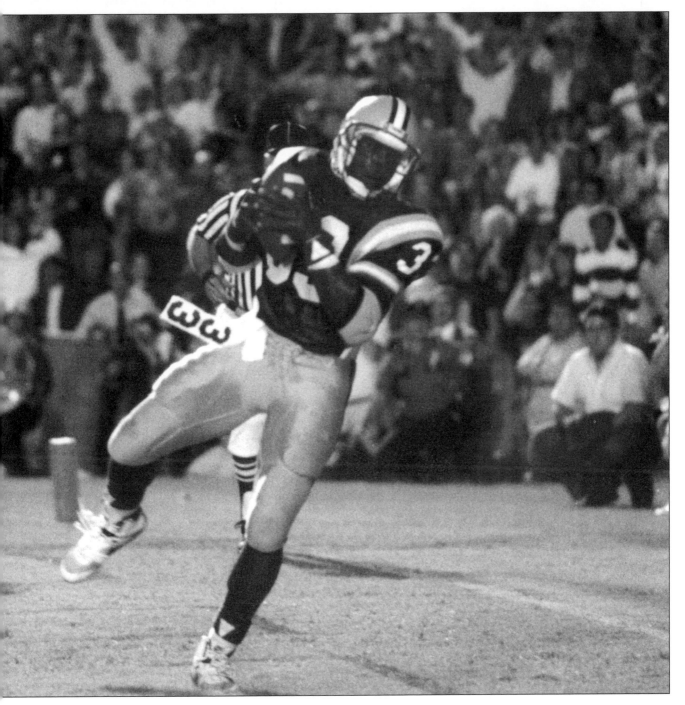

■ **Eddie Fuller missed his first two possible touchdown receptions, but the third one made the difference.**

Once again, Auburn drove into LSU territory. Slack threw to Joseph on third down, connecting on a deep out that went for 20 yards. He went right back to the air and hit Wright over the middle for 19 yards to the LSU 37.

But major infractions for clipping and a personal foul pushed Auburn all the way back to its 46, spoiling another scoring chance.

Auburn's defense came up with a big play to get the ball right back. Outside linebacker Craig Olgetree blitzed on third down and threw Hodson for a 7-yard loss, breaking LSU's

seven-game streak without allowing a sack.

Then Bourgeois shanked the punt. It rolled only 24 yards to the LSU 38, giving Auburn its third opportunity to get on the scoreboard.

Slack threw three straight incomplete passes, two that were broken up by LSU. Hill delivered a a hard hit to dislodge the ball from Danley on a third-down pass. And Auburn's Brian Shulman punted for the third time.

On LSU's first possession of the second quarter, Guidry

took a turn at quarterback and completed his first pass to Fuller. But he couldn't move LSU, either. Bourgeois came on and punted 42 yards.

LSU's defense finally prevented Auburn from crossing midfield, and Shulman punted only 29 yards to LSU 34.

With Hodson back, LSU picked up one first down, but was hurt by an illegal prodecure call and stalled out at its own 36.

That led to three more punt exchanges before Auburn finally broke the scoreless tie with a 45-yard march. Starting at its own 33, Auburn got two first-down runs by Harris and a personal foul call against LSU to move down to the LSU 28.

Wright gained nothing on a reverse, and Harris netted only 6 yards on back-to-back carries. That brought on Lyle to score the first points with 1:41 left in the half.

A 26-yard kickoff return by Slip Watkins set up LSU at its 33. But the third illegal procedure penalty against LSU backed the offense into a second-and-12. Hodson connected with tight end Willie Williams for 10 yards, but overthrew Lee on third down. Bourgeois made his seventh appearance and booted a 54-yarder to the Auburn 5 with 11 seconds to play.

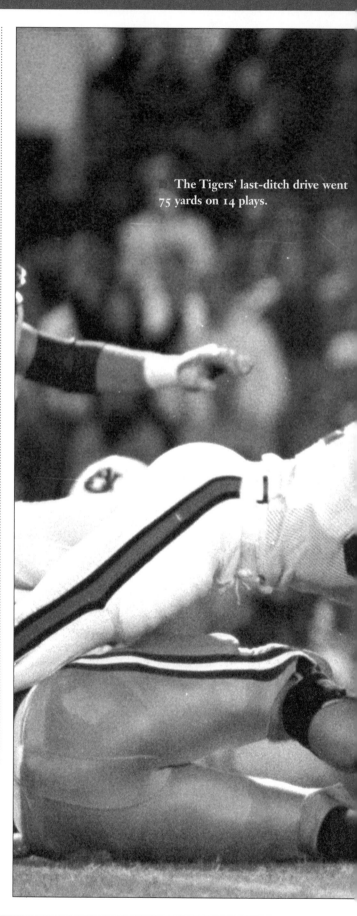

The Tigers' last-ditch drive went 75 yards on 14 plays.

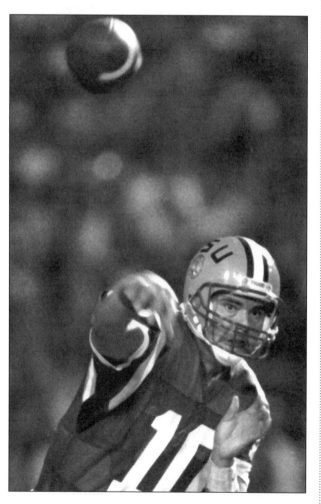

■ **Mickey Guidry wasn't able to kick-start the LSU offense in relief of Tommy Hodson.**

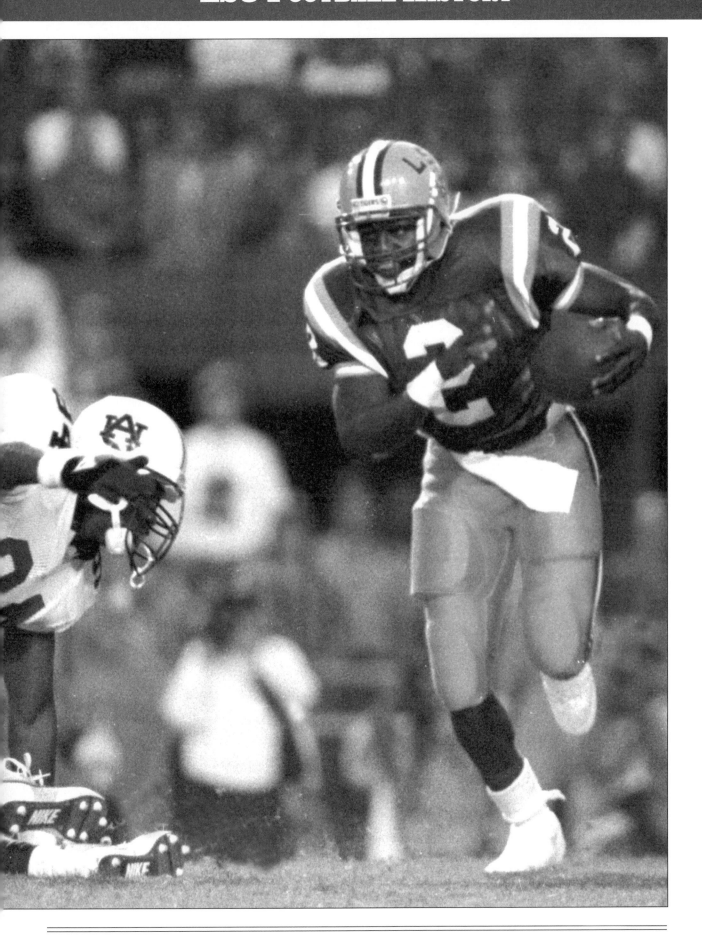

LSU & Razorbacks Can't Break 0-0 Tie

By Dan Hardesty

The Advocate

Dallas, Tex. — *Jan. 1, 1947*

The Tigers of LSU shoved the Arkansas Razorbacks all over the rain and sleet-swept Cotton Bowl gridiron here this afternoon but couldn't breach the Porkers' Red line when the chips were down and had to settle for a scoreless tie in what was probably the coldest game in college football history.

The bayou Bengals piled up 15 first downs and three times had first downs inside the Arkansas 10, but great defensive play aided by the impossible weather halted the attack each time as an estimated 38,000 half-frozen fans sat in snow, ice, rain and freezing temperature.

Arkansas made a first down on an 18-yard smash by its terrific fullback, Leon Campbell, four minutes after the opening kickoff, and that was the only time during the afternoon that the defense-minded Razorbacks succeeded in gaining 10 yards on one series of downs.

Throughout the contest it was all LSU, but down near the goal line, it just wasn't LSU's day. They stormed down the field several times on powerful marches but always the rugged Arkansas defense halted them in time. Three times penalties nullified plays on which the Tigers had made first downs in scoring territory, and at least two more times frozen fingers couldn't hang on to passes which might have meant touchdowns.

There will probably be a lot of second-guessing on LSU's quarterbacking near the goal line, but under those playing conditions it's a wonder the teams could even line up to put the ball in play. The Arkansas line — one of the most vicious faced by the Tigers all season — had a lot to do with the Tigers' lack of success on some of those crucial plays. The Razorbacks charged hard and tackled for keeps.

Score by Periods

LSU	0	0	0	0 —	0
Arkansas	0	0	0	0 —	0

An account of today's game wouldn't be complete without first describing the contest's weather conditions.

The snow stopped falling yesterday and this morning everything was frozen solid. But a sudden thaw at midmorning sent the temperature slightly above the freezing mark. When the Tigers reached the stadium, the ice and snow were slightly melting. The big tarpaulins were rolled back and the field was in almost perfect condition.

The LSU board of strategy had 40 bales of hay delivered to the Tigers' bench. This was piled along the sideline and stacked deep in front of the bench. Most of the players stuck their feet in the hay to keep them warm, but there were at least a dozen people simply buried in it with their heads sticking out.

The Tigers were enthusiastic about the condition of the playing field itself before the game, got into grid togs and went on into the dressing room.

And then it happened.

First, it was just a light sprinkle. Gradually, it increased to a steady drizzle, and then it turned to sleet. Throughout the entire game, either sleet or freezing rain was falling. The spectators, who turned out in surprising numbers, huddled in snow-covered seats.

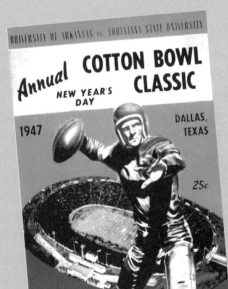

LSU kicked off and after an exchange of punts, Arkansas took over on its own 20. Campbell, who played a tremendous defensive game for the Porkers, pounded through center, bounced off Buck Ballard and churned 18 yards for the one and only first down made by Arkansas all afternoon. Then Aubrey Fowler got off a great quick kick to the Tiger 3-yard line.

Red Knight punted back to the LSU 45 and Fowler returned to the 37. The Tigers dug in and forced Arkansas to punt.

Starting at their 20, Dan Sandifer circled left end for 11 yards and Ray Coates and Rip Collins pounded out

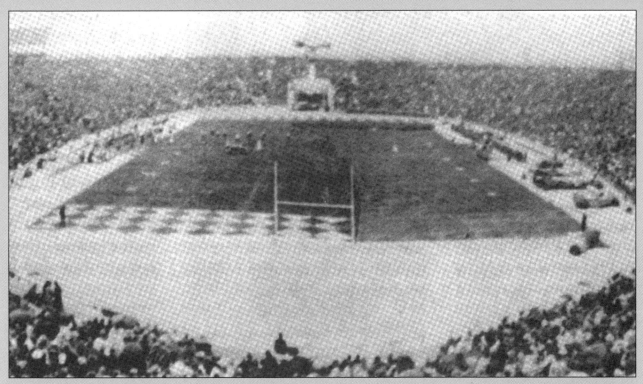

■ **LSU and Arkansas battled to a 0-0 tie on the icy field of the Cotton Bowl.**

yardage for another first down on the Arkansas 49. Two plays lost three yards. Y.A. Tittle flipped a screen pass to Collins who gained almost 13 yards but it was inches short of a first down.

Knight fumbled trying to plunge on fourth down and John Hogman recovered for Arkansas on the Porkers' 42.

Hogman promptly fumbled back and Tittle grabbed the ball on the LSU 43. Knight got off a great punt which rolled to the Arkansas 3, but Jeff Adams raced in and fell on the ball, thus making it an automatic touchback and pulling the Porkers out of a big hole in the opening minutes of the second quarter.

Knight broke through the middle for 16 yards a few minutes later, and then ran for another first down but LSU was penalized for backfield in motion. Knight's fourth-down punt was blocked by tackle Charles Lively and end Alton Baldwin scooped up the ball and took off for the Tiger goal line, but little Jim Cason dove right over a blocker and pulled him down from behind on the LSU 43 to save a probable touchdown.

Later, Tittle intercepted a Porker pass at the Arkansas 23 and returned it to 16. Two passes failed and two running plays lacked a foot of 10 yards. Unable to move the ball, Fowler punted to the Arkansas 42 and Cason returned it to the 19 with three minutes left in the half. In four plays, the Tigers moved to a first down at the Porkers' 8, with only 40 seconds remaining. In one running play, which lost two yards, and an incomplete pass the Tigers failed to score before the clock ran out.

The second half was completely LSU — except that the Tigers didn't score.

Taking a punt on their eight, LSU staged a powerful drive with Ray Coates smashing through the middle of the line for 18 yards and then for 17 more. Sandifer picked up 19 yards over the middle as the Porkers continued to play their linebackers wide. Coates and Knight pounded for a first down at the Arkansas 21. Then the attack bogged down and the Porkers took over on the 18.

Early in the fourth quarter, the Bengals began a drive from the Arkansas 42 — and this time they almost made it. Almost — but not quite.

Sandifer picked up six yards and Collins swept through left tackle and churned for 16 yards to the Arkansas 19. Coates roared through right guard for 10 yards and another first down at the Porkers' 9. Collins made another yard, then Tittle whipped a pass to Adams who was knocked out of bounds just as he caught the ball on the 1-yard line by Clyde Scott. The entire Arkansas lineup ganged up to stop Zollie Toth, the expected ball carrier, on the plunge — and stop him they did. A couple of feet from the goal line.

The Bengals got another chance again on the next series with six minutes left in the game. Dale Gray returned a Fowler punt from the Arkansas 29 to the 20. Gray made 3 yards, then Willard Landry blasted through the line for a first down at the Arkansas 20. Landry carried two more times to pick up a first down at the Porkers' 9.

Gray added 3 yards and Toth picked up two more to the Porkers' 4. Landry then lost a yard. The Tigers' field goal attempt never worked due to a botched center snap.

In the final three minutes, both Arkansas and LSU failed to get a drive started.

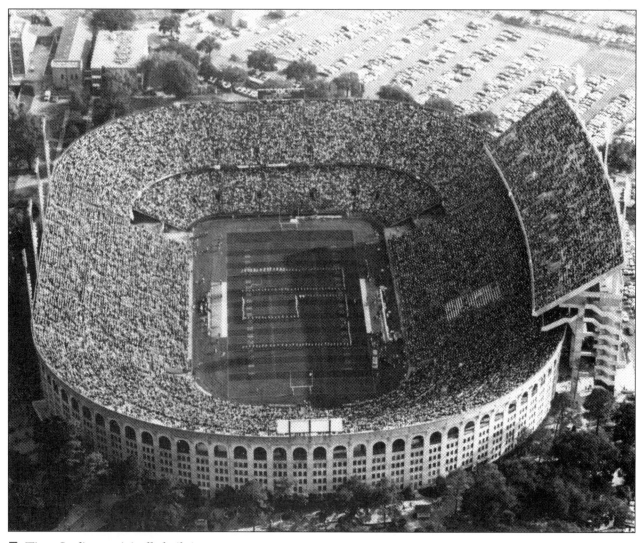

■ Tiger Stadium, originally built in 1924, now seats 79,940.

The Mystique of Tiger Stadium

By Sam King
The Advocate

How dare you call it a mere football stadium. It is the heart of a university — the cornerstone of a community — the focal point for a state. It has stood as a shrine for 105 years of football ... a temple for Tiger faithful to pay homage to the team and to the program in which they so strongly believe. It is the body, soul and spirit of a football program laden with rich tradition and glory.

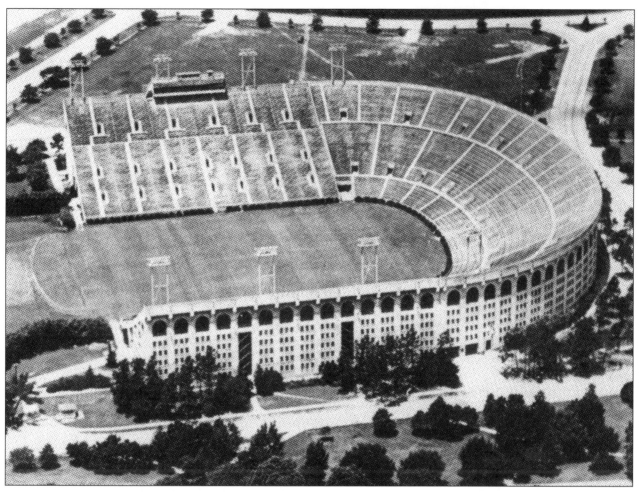

■ **Tiger Stadium before the north end zone was completed in the 1950s.**

The mystique that has enveloped Tiger Stadium going into this its 75th year has become unforgettable for those — coaches, players and fans — who have experienced it.

There's something about this home of LSU's football warriors that makes men rise past their capabilities, play to heights they never dreamed possible.

"Running into Tiger Stadium was an enormous uplift — the people hollering and the crowd roaring," recalled former Tiger Hart Bourque. "We would go running out on the field five feet off the ground.

"Nothing could get your adrenaline going quicker than having 60,000 fans screaming to try and get you to do something. It rejuvenates you and makes you want to do something. In a few games it made me play way, way above my skills," said Bourque.

"It did things to a guy like Bert Jones who came into the game from out of nowhere and threw three touchdowns passes," said former LSU player and coach Jerry Stovall of the future pro who starred from 1970-72.

"It did something to a little kid like (running back) Dalton Hilliard, who comes from out of nowhere to play great.

"They were both good players, but 70,000 to 80,000 people

had something to do with that. It excites you to another degree of excellence."

It is no wonder that in a recent poll conducted by ESPN, Death Valley is deemed the greatest site anywhere for a college football game. The TV network noted, "for the college football fan, there is no better place to be on planet Earth on Saturday than LSU's Tiger Stadium."

It's a mystique you can't explain. You have to be there. Tiger Stadium, you see, is much more than a football stadium. It has been home for 118 All-Southeastern Conference performers, 38 All-American selections, one Heisman Trophy winner and one national championship team.

It is the birthplace of the legendary Chinese Bandits, a heroic bunch of defensive demons who played far, far above their heads. The specially-written Chinese Bandits song was played and hundreds of fans would don coolie hats as their Bandits took the field. That explosion of roars, music and excitement lifted third-team players to heights unknown.

"I don't know what it did to them, but they went wild," recalled former LSU coach Charles McClendon.

"It made them play exceptionally well," said Dietzel. Both coaches concurred: "they really weren't that good, but no one told them."

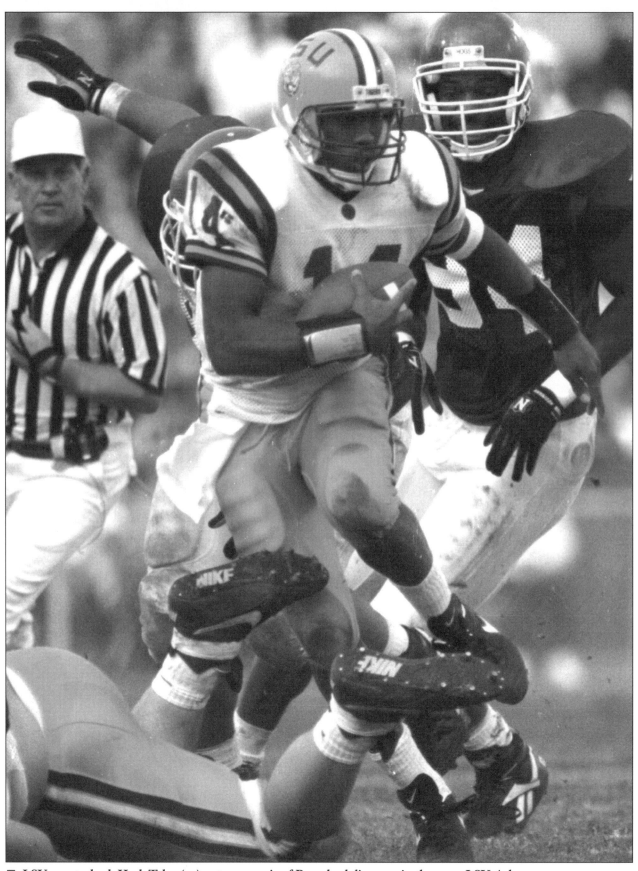

■ LSU quarterback Herb Tyler (14) outruns a pair of Razorback linemen in the 1995 LSU-Arkansas game.

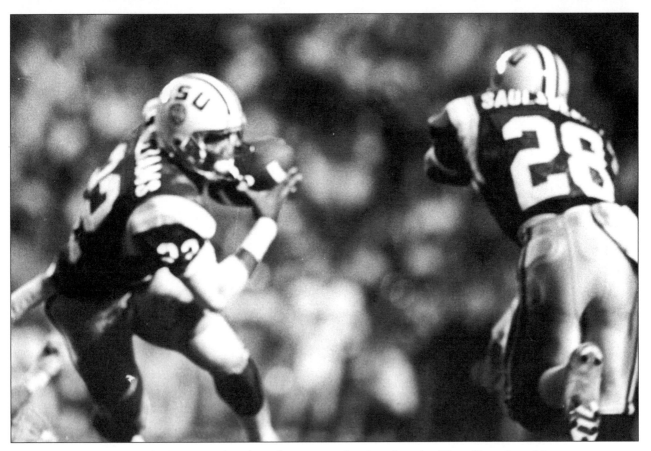

■ **Harvey Williams (22) rushed for 52 yards and caught two passs for 18 yards against Notre Dame in 1986.**

In fact, thousands told them just the opposite every week. Death Valley has seen its great plays, few — if any — causing a bigger roar from the Tiger loyal than when Tommy Hodson's touchdown pass to Eddie Fuller defeated Auburn, 7-6, in 1988, in the game dubbed "the night the Tigers moved the earth." It registered a reading of earthquake proportions on a seismograph machine in the geology department.

The most famous of all plays here, though, was "The Run" — that 89-yard, Halloween night return of a punt by Billy Cannon in 1959 that lifted LSU to a 7-3 victory over Ole Miss and won Cannon the Heisman Trophy.

Almost every year on the eve of the Ole Miss-LSU game you will hear a replay of the run. For 30 years after the run you heard it two, three or four or more times.

This great series, especially in the 1950's and early 60's, produced some great moments.

How many games the mystique of Tiger Stadium helped the Tigers win, with goal line stands, final second plays, in the LSU-Ole Miss series is unbelievable — Cannon's run, the ensuing goal line stand, so many other goal line stands in so many other games and Billy Ezell's Halloween night, two-point pass to Doug Moreau in 1964.

And, what a deafening place it was when LSU managed to run two plays in eight seconds in their 1972 game. LSU defeated the Rebs, 17-16, on the PAT after Bert Jones' TD pass to Brad Davis as regulation time expired. What a setting for such a fierce rivalry. Getting inside Death Valley wasn't always cheap and sometimes it was almost impossible.

But, Jackson, Miss., native Bill Rogers did to watch Cannon make his great run. Rogers was a high school official in Jackson, caught a ride down to go to the game but could not find a ticket — not one that he could afford. He came prepared, though. He also brought his official's uniform. So, he went to work, so to say. Rogers said he dressed and managed to file through the gate where the game officials entered without attracting any special attention. Once in the stadium he said he went to the sideline and was finally seated on the Ole Miss players' bench.

Just prior to the kickoff, however, Rogers said one of the game officials wanted to know what he was doing out there. He confessed, but pleaded with the official not to kick him out. They didn't. Few people ever noticed him — until near the end of the game and then thousands saw him and cheered.

If you notice the end of Cannon's run, Rogers — a car salesman — is standing on the 30-yard line. He is the first to signal a touchdown for Cannon.

And this writer, a part-time LSU student who played basketball against Cannon in high school, was the only one to outrun him down the east sideline.

The traditions are many in Tiger Stadium, none more unbelievable than the number of goal line stands at the south

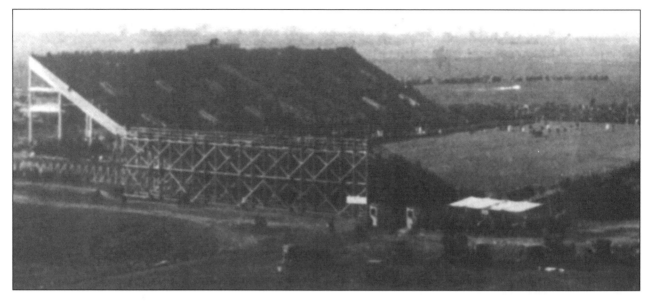

■ **Tiger Stadium on Opening Day against Tulane in 1924.**

end zone. So many opponent drives, so few points.

Mike the Tiger is paraded around the stadium in a cage topped by cheerleaders prior to the game, bringing Tiger fans to a standing roar, but sometimes making opponents feel uncomfortable.

Tradition has it, LSU will score one touchdown for each time Mike roars.

But the tradition starts much earlier in the week than at kickoff. The fans start gathering in motor homes, campers and the like as early as Thursday or Friday. They party and let the good times roll. They're up well before game time, cooking, partying and getting the proper attitude adjustments to cheer their Tigers to victory.

The mystique of Tiger Stadium has been most valuable to football teams playing so great, to players rising to the occasion. However, Cannon when asked about the mystique of Tiger Stadium, questions back, "Mystique? What mystique? It was the people.

"We played as freshmen in 1956 and would draw like 15,000 people. In '57 we lose four games in a row and we're playing to 30,000 empty seats. We had to beat Tulane to finish 5-5.

"Jimmy Taylor was an All-American, a great player, but you didn't feel any mystique," said Cannon. "But, in '58, we're going 11-0 — and now it's full of mystique," said Cannon. "But, let me tell you, there's always something special about a night game in Tiger Stadium.

"Playing in there in the evening helped the mystique even back then," said Cannon.

Stovall remembers his days as a player and said the tradition of goal line stands didn't come about accidentally.

"It started in practice. Coach (Paul) Dietzel and (Charles) McClendon, in spring practice, would go into the stadium to scrimmage. They would put the Chinese Bandits on defense and give us first and goal at the nine. It seemed like we never

got it in.

"They would make it first-and-goal at the three — and we never got it in," said Stovall. "The tougher it got, the more adamant the coaches and players got.

"I think the fans picked up on that in the south end zone," said Stovall, noting the fans were not only louder and more aggressive, but closer to the field.

"It seemed like they could reach out and touch you. I remember when LSU stopped Ole Miss four downs near the end zone. They were trying to stick it down our throats. Here we were sitting there fixing to lose a national championship — but (Warren) Rabb, Cannon and 30,000 people in the end zone stopped them."

The mystique of this stadium that has earned the nickname of Death Valley is indisputable. It cannot be denied. As easily as it can strike fear into the heart of an opponent, it can send goose bumps up the backs and necks of Tigers, spur them on to do things on a football field that they are not capable of doing.

It's an emotional place where women have wept and grown men cried. Countless are the number of times when those Saturday evening heroes felt a lump in their throat and tears in their eyes when they made that final trip through the north end zone chutes.

Or, the mystique of this great arena could leave you in awe as you entered your first time.

Stovall gave his recollections.

"I was being recruited from West Monroe in 1958. I was standing in the tunnel, came out and there were more people in there (Tiger Stadium) than in it was in my whole home town — and so much noise," said Stovall. "It made the hair stand up on the back of my neck. The initial impression was awesome."

His first time out the chute as a player was as a sophomore against Texas A&M.

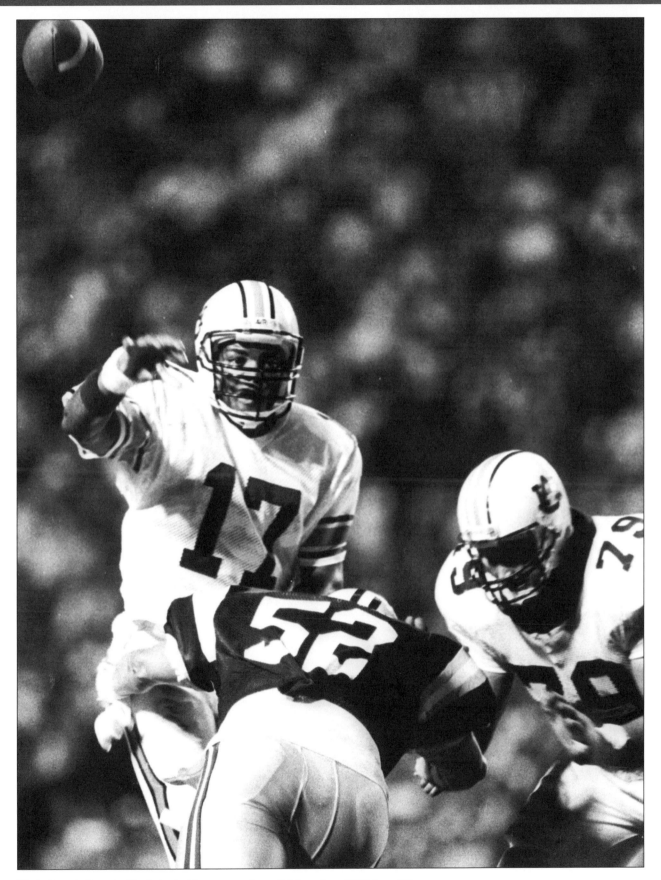

■ Auburn's Reggie Slack (17) rifles a pass downfield against LSU in 1988.

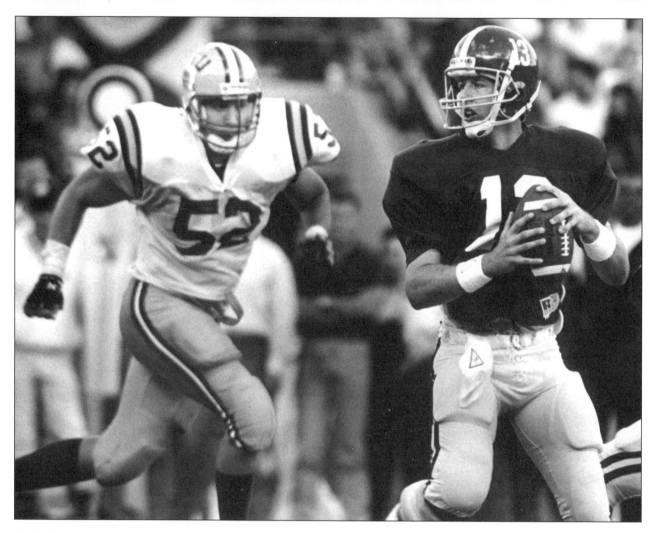

■ Alabama quarterback David Smith, while looking downfield, doesn't see Ron Sancho (52) closing in for the sack.

Archer's Tongue-Lashing Inspires Tigers To Win

BY BRUCE HUNTER
The Advocate

Tuscaloosa, Ala. — *Nov. 5, 1988*

With less than six minutes left in the first half today, LSU was in near-desperate straits. The Tigers had no points and no first downs and were headed nowhere.

Alabama, on the other hand, had scored on four consecutive possessions and secured a 15-0 lead at home in Bryant-Denny Stadium.

It could have been much, much worse.

By halftime, LSU had pulled to within 15-7. But LSU coach Mike Archer was furious with his team's "lackadaisical" play, especially on defense. He gave the players a tongue lashing during the break.

"I told them, 'We're very lucky to be down 15-7. We've got to go out in the second half and be patient offensively and create some turnovers,' " Archer said. "And that got us some points."

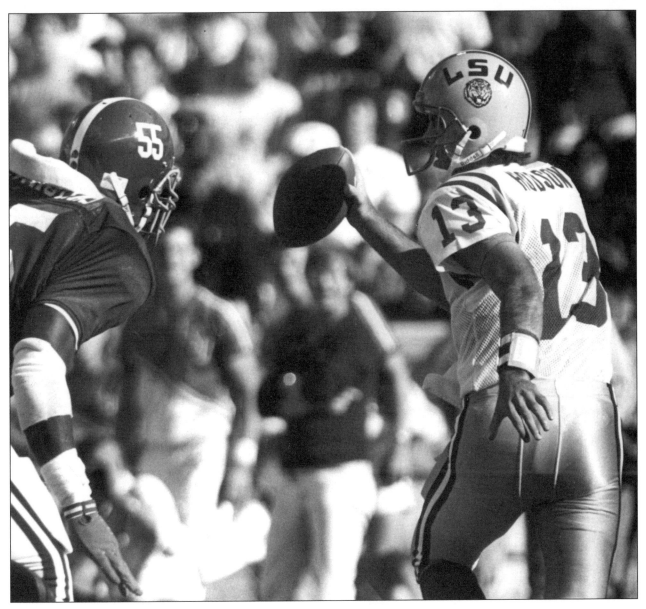

■ **Tommy Hodson (13) tries to escape from Alabama linebacker Derrick Thomas.**

The game was played in two segments with a frantic finish to cap it off.

Alabama totally dominated the first 25 minutes in mounting the 15-0 lead. LSU took over and rallied for 16 unanswered points over the next 27 minutes. Then it was up for grabs in the thrill-a-second final minutes.

LSU finally prevailed, 19-18.

"I think the key thing was the drive Mickey (Guidry) put together to bring us back in the ballgame," Archer said. "And we came out in the second half and made some things happen."

Guidry, spelling Tommy Hodson on LSU's last series of the first half, completed three straight passes for 37 yards, including a 21-yard strike to Alvin Lee. That led to a 3-yard touchdown run by Jay Egloff.

"That's the number one job of the second-string quarter-

Score by Periods					
LSU	0	7	9	3 —	19
Alabama	6	9	0	3 —	18

back, to change the tempo of the game," Guidry said. "The problem was field position."

Alabama had excellent field position in the first half, starting twice inside the LSU 45. Meanwhile, the Tigers didn't get outside their own 33 until the closing minutes of the half.

Hodson was just two of five for 9 yards in the first half and failed to lead the Tigers to a single first down. He was sacked twice for losses of 28 yards.

"I think we started mixing it up (in the second half)," Hodson said, explaining the turnaround. "You can mix it up with better field position. I think Mickey came in and got them off balance. Then we got some field position and things started to work."

Despite three interceptions, Hodson completed 10 of 18 for 213 yards and a touchdown in the second half.

The Hodson-Tony Moss combination ignited the Tiger offense. Moss turned a 4-yard pass into a 48-yard touchdown and totaled four catches for 124 yards in the second half. He finished with six catches for 133 yards.

"That's my main goal, just to improve each week," said Moss, who had six catches for 128 yards and two touchdowns against Ole Miss last week. "I just want to help my team as much as I can and I'll be happy."

Moss was indeed a happy young man as dusk approached today. He caught two passes for 41 yards on the Tigers' final drive.

Hodson, rebounding from an interception and fumbled snap, was three of four for 63 yards on the march.

"Tommy did a good job of fighting back," LSU offensive coordinator Ed Zaunbrecher said. "He made some mistakes, but he came right back. He made some great throws."

It marked the third time in the Tigers' last four games that Hodson rallied them to victory. He threw fourth-quarter touchdown passes to beat Auburn and Kentucky.

"I think it has a lot to do with experience," Hodson said. "Hopefully, it has a lot to do with my personality. I want the ball in clutch situations."

David Browndyke's 34-yard game-winning field goal came with the help of Mike Hebert, who was making his first college snap.

Jim Hubicz snapped on Browndyke's first two kicks, a field goal and extra point. But the snaps rolled to holder Chris Moock, who had to make nifty plays to get the ball on the tee.

"I did not worry about having to change snappers during the week," Browndyke said. "As a kicker, if I would have let that bother me, it would have affected my kicking. I thought Hebert did a good job of snapping."

LSU's snapping problems resulted from Pat O'Neill quitting the team on Thursday. His departure was not announced by LSU. Archer said he didn't want to give anything away to Alabama.

"It was just a tremendous effort by our players and coaches," Archer said. "I've been around some good things, but nothing like this on the road, for what the game meant, playing for the opportunity to win the Southeastern Conference against a very good football team."

The Tigers, tied with Georgia for the SEC lead, can clinch a share of the title by winning at Mississippi State on Saturday. They were in a similar situation in 1984 and lost to the Bulldogs, 16-14.

"What you've got to do is know what you're playing for," Guidry said. "In '84, we hadn't played for a championship in about 14 years. It's different now. We have our goals now. We know what we're striving for."

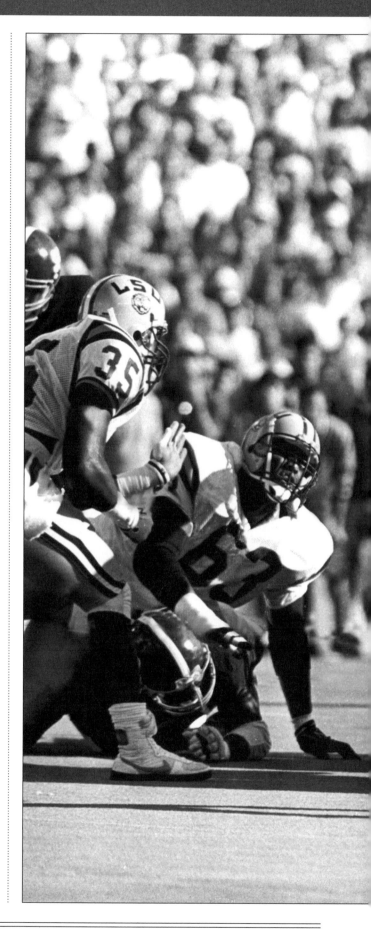

■ **Alabama halfback David Casteal (28) attempts to hurdle the LSU defense.**

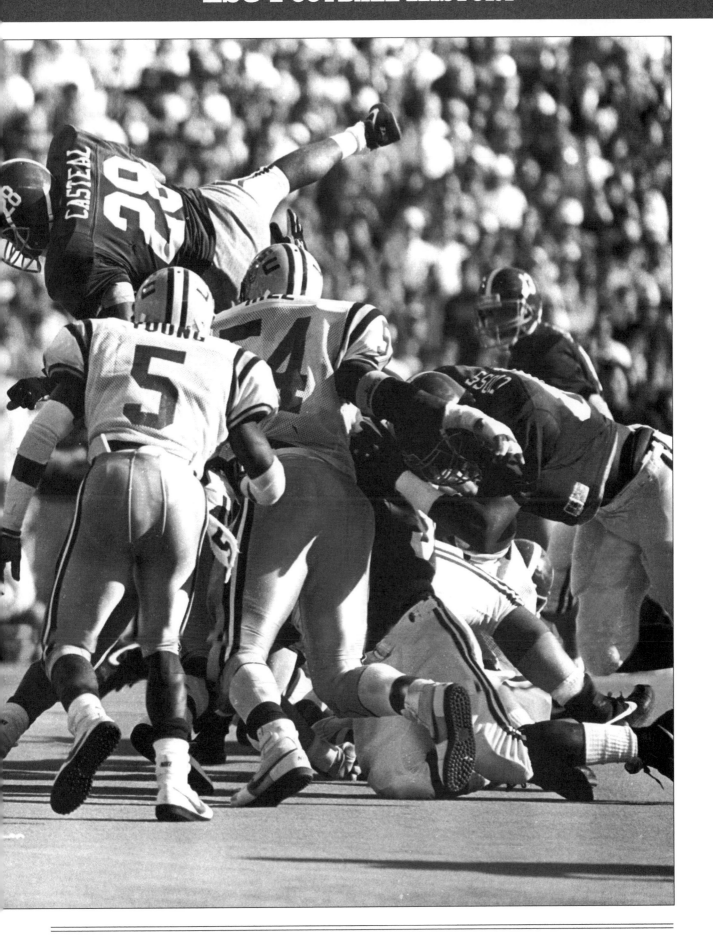

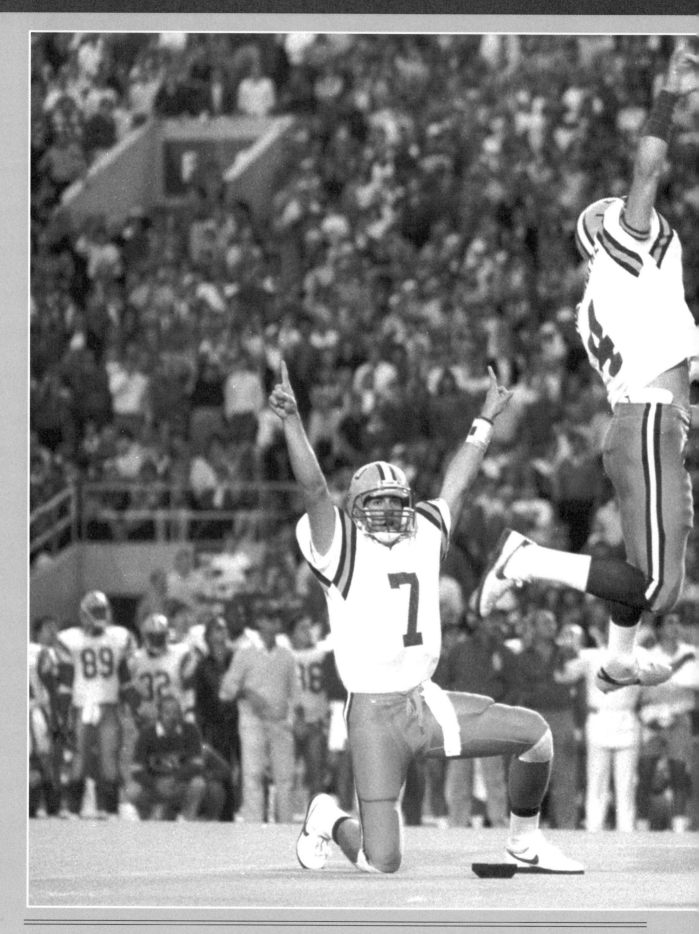

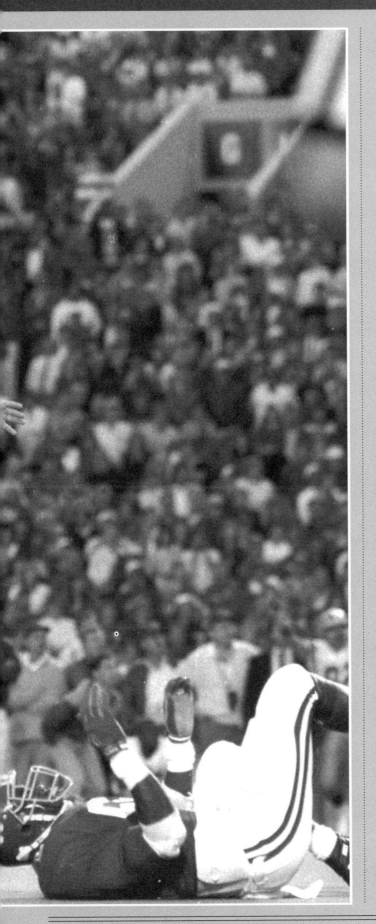

Bronwndyke's 34-yard FG Stuns Alabama

By BRUCE HUNTER
The Advocate

Tuscaloosa, Ala. — *Nov. 5, 1988*

They just don't get any closer. They don't often matter any more.

As the final four seconds ticked off, Alabama place-kicker Philip Doyle's 54-yard field-goal attempt faded just right, a mere foot outside the uprights.

LSU, by virtue of David Browndyke's 34-yard field goal with 28 seconds left, survived a rare trip to Bryant-Denny Stadium, 19-18, this afternoon.

It was a fitting finish to a Southeastern Conference showdown that was as glorious as the scenic fall setting in the Capstone. A sellout crowd of 70,123 and a split-national audience on CBS-TV were treated to a classic, matching two teams with three-game winning streaks and championship hopes.

The 13th-ranked Tigers, overcoming a 15-0 first-half deficit and four second-half turnovers, made enough crucial plays to move within a game of clinching a share of the SEC championship. LSU, 6-2 overall, is tied with Georgia for the league lead at 5-1.

"The bottom line is we just wouldn't give up," LSU offensive guard Ruffin Rodrigue said. "We knew we would come back. We did it against Georgia and Florida last year. We did it against Auburn earlier this year. And now we've done it against Alabama. We're a team of pride. We never give up."

LSU split end Tony Moss caught six passes for a career-high 133 yards, including a 48-yard touchdown catch and two fourth-quarter receptions that put Browndyke in position for the game winner.

Outside linebacker Ron Sancho led the Tigers' defense with nine unassisted tackles, two sacks and a pass deflection, helping LSU hold Alabama to only a field goal in the second half. And Mike Hebert, in his first attempt as a kick snapper, made a perfect delivery to Chris Moock on Browndyke's final field goal.

But 18th-ranked Alabama, 6-2 and 4-2, had its own heroes in this hotly contested rivalry that has had a direct bearing on the SEC title for the last five years.

■ **Kicker David Browndyke (4) goes airborne as he and holder Chris Moock (7) celebrate LSU's winning field goal.**

Quarterback David Smith was almost flawless in completing 22 of 34 passes for 241 yards. Middle linebacker Willie Shephard charged up the Tide defense with 12 tackles, an interception and a 23-yard loss on a sack.

"It was a great effort by both teams," Alabama coach Bill Curry said, "but the little fine details, the kind that win championships, were not there. The great catch, the great kick, the great run — we didn't have them."

To many, it appeared the Tide had its great kick. Doyle's attempt soared into the cool, early-evening air with plenty of distance. It just didn't have quite enough accuracy.

Alabama's dreams for its first title since 1981 faded with Doyle's miss.

"It just wasn't it for us today," said Doyle, who tied a school record with four field goals, but missed three times from outside 50 yards in the final 19 minutes.

Doyle kicked field goals of 35, 24 and 33 yards and David Casteal scored on a 2-yard run to stake Alabama to its 15-0 lead. LSU backup quarterback Mickey Guidry led the Tigers to their only first-half score, a 3-yard touchdown run by fullback Jay Egloff. It was 15-7 at halftime.

Moss' touchdown and two Browndyke field goals enabled LSU to outscore the Tide 12-3 in the second half.

LSU quarterback Tommy Hodson completed 12 of 23 for 222 yards and a touchdown, but lost a fumble and was intercepted three times in the second half, twice by Lee Ozmint.

But Hodson took charge on LSU's final drive. After Doyle hit a 20-yard field goal to put the Crimson Tide ahead, 18-16, with 7:13 left, there ensued a wild finish with three turnovers in a span of less than two minutes.

Starting at its own 15 with 2:57 left, LSU drove to the Tide 17 with Hodson connecting on three passes for 63 yards. Tailback Eddie Fuller dropped a potential touchdown catch. But Browndyke finished off the drive.

"During the drive, I tried to keep to myself on the sidelines," Browndyke said. "I tried to relax before going in. When I was called on, I wanted to prove that I could kick it through in the last seconds."

Browndyke's squib kickoff was returned by John Cassimus to the Alabama 31 with 22 seconds remaining and the Tide out of timeouts.

Making a daring effort to rally, the Tide picked up 18 yards on a Smith pass to flanker Marco Battle. Then tight end Lamonde Russell found an opening near the left sidelines and caught a 14-yard pass to the LSU 37 with four seconds to play.

That brought on Doyle for his seventh field-goal try.

"I thought it was going through," Browndyke said of his counterpart's attempt.

After the kick missed, LSU broke out in celebration. It must still win at Mississippi State on Saturday to get at least a share of the title.

For most of the first half, it didn't look like LSU would ever get started offensively, while Alabama lived in LSU territory.

Casteal and Smith keyed the Tide's first drive. Casteal had a 12-yard run and Smith completed two passes for 24 yards. On third-and-2 from the LSU 18, Smith was pressured by Clint James and Karl Dunbar and threw incomplete. Doyle put the Tide on the board with a 35-yard field goal.

Alabama's defense made its first big play of the day when Shephard came on a blitz and threw Hodson for a 23-yard loss back to the LSU 2. Rene Bourgeois punted out to the LSU 49, but Murry Hill returned it to the 35.

On first down, Hill rushed for 9 yards, but sustained a lower back injury on a tackle by Greg Jackson. He was taken off on a stretcher. The injury was later determined to be only a bad bruise.

With Hill out, Casteal ran 10 yards on a sweep around right end to the 7. A procedure penalty cost the Tide, and Doyle kicked a 24-yard field goal for a 6-0 lead still in the first quarter.

After Hodson was sacked by Derrick Thomas, Bourgeois punted from just outside his end zone. Cassimus returned the 39-yard kick to the LSU 41.

Smith threw a swing pass to Casteal who bolted 16 yards to the 25. Smith connected with Russell for a 6-yard gain, setting up first-and-goal at the 4.

Casteal went the final 2 yards around left end, running over cornerback Mike Mayes to get into the end zone. On a two-point conversion attempt, Casteal was stopped short by Sancho, but the Tide led, 12-0.

After LSU punted a fourth time, Smith engineered another scoring drive. Defensive facemask and pass interference calls helped Alabama.

But when it appeared the Tide was about to pull away, Sancho came up with back-to-back key plays. He sacked Smith and stopped Robert Stewart on a run up the middle. That led to Doyle's 33-yard field goal and a 15-0 lead.

Guidry finally gave the Tigers an offensive spark. The drive's key play was Guidry's 21-yard pass to Alvin Lee.

On second-and-goal from the 3, Fuller went in motion to left, and Guidry handed off to Egloff up the middle. The fullback scampered through a massive hole to score standing up. Browndyke, despite a poor snap by Jim Hubicz, kicked the extra point to make it 15-7 with 2:52 left.

In the second half, Hodson returned to the game and led the Tigers to two first downs out to the 44. Then he was pressured and forced into an intentional grounding that sent the ball back to the 21.

He came back to throw to Fuller for 16 yards over the middle, but his third-down pass was intercepted by Ozmint at the Alabama 25.

LSU's defense held the Tide to three plays and a punt, and Hodson had another chance from the LSU 26. His first-down pass went to Moss for 35 yards.

From Alabama 39, Hodson tossed a short pass to Darrell Williams, who rambled for 17 yards. A holding penalty stalled the Tigers, and they settled for Browndyke's 36-yard field goal, again coming on a poor snap by Hubicz, that made it 15-10.

Alabama kept the ball just one play. Smith threw over the middle to Russell who made the catch but was hit and fumbled away to Jimmy Young at the LSU 46.

After two running plays, Moss made the play of the day. He lined up in the slot left and came across the field in motion. Then he ran a short crossing route, making the catch at the 44

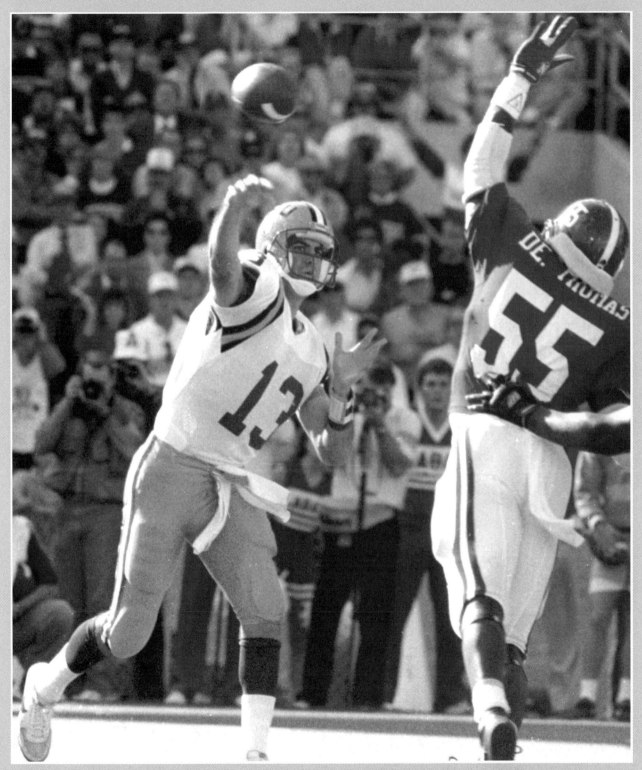

■ Tommy Hodson (13) airs out a deep pass against the fierce Crimson Tide rush, led by Derrick Thomas.

in front of linebacker Vantreise Davis.

Running hard to the left, Moss changed directions to fake out Ozmint and Charles Gardner on his way to a 48-yard touchdown. On a two-point try, Hodson was sacked by Thomas, but the Tigers still led, 16-15, with 5:19 left in the third quarter.

Alabama came up empty on field-goal attempts from 59 and 55 yards. But in the fourth quarter, Smith completed 6 of 7 passes to set up Doyle's 20-yard field goal, putting the Tide back on top, 18-16.

The rash of turnovers followed before Browndyke and Doyle each had a final kick.

LSU Holds Off No. 5 Crimson Tide, 17-13

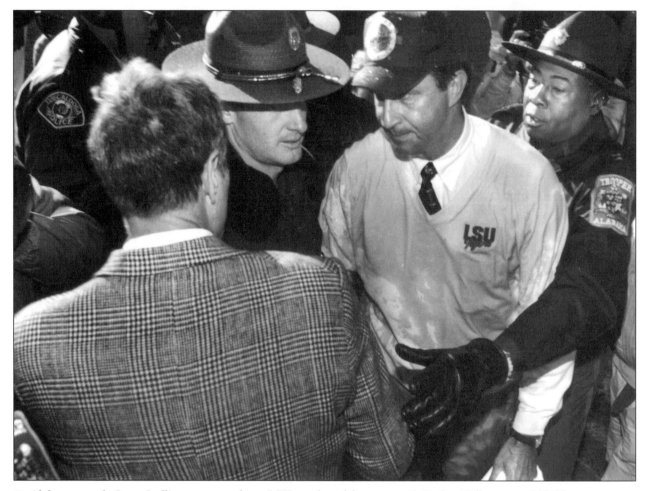

■ Alabama coach Gene Stallings congratulates LSU coach and former pupil Curley Hallman at midfield.

By Dave Moormann
The Advocate

Tuscaloosa, Ala. — *Nov. 6, 1993*

From bowled over to bowl gazing. Imagine that.

How the tide has turned.

In one afternoon, LSU went from an uncertain football team to one toying with the possibility of postseason plans.

A centennial season that produced the worst loss in school history featured perhaps its most improbable victory when LSU stunned fifth-ranked Alabama, 17-13, today.

Looking more like the defending national champion than Alabama, LSU intercepted four passes, recovered a fumble and turned to backup quarterback Chad Loup en route to the dramatic upset.

The verdict touched off a celebration among LSU fans in

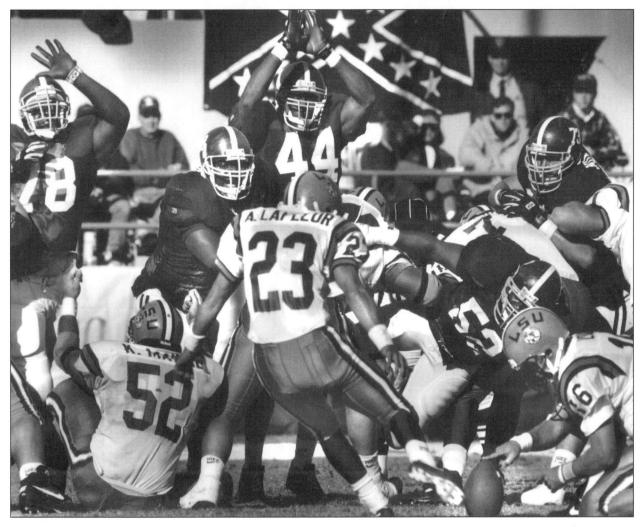

■ **Tiger kicker Andre Lafleur boots a 36-yard field goal in the fourth quarter to ensure LSU's 17-13 win.**

Bryant-Denny Stadium, and numerous players rushed over to join in an impromptu singing and dancing.

It was sweet vindication for third-year coach Curley Hallman, who returned home as an embattled figure and will leave buoyed by the memorable triumph.

"I love my hometown ... I have a lot of ties here ...," said Hallman, who grew up about five miles away in Northport. Looking back, its hard to imagine LSU rose above the ashes of a 58-3 loss to Florida and the other mistakes that have characterized much of the season.

But LSU surprised Ole Miss last week, 19-17, and in beating Alabama put together two Southeastern Conference victories for the first time since beating Kentucky and Ole Miss in 1991.

More than that, LSU snapped the nation's longest unbeaten streak at 31 games in a feat reminiscent of the 22-game victory string LSU ended when it beat Arkansas, 14-7, in the 1966 Cotton Bowl.

Alabama had defeated LSU twice in fashioning its 30-0-1 mark. But by winning in Tuscaloosa for only the third time

Score by Periods						
LSU	0	0	14	3	—	17
Alabama	0	0	0	13	—	13

ever, LSU halted a four-game losing streak.

LSU also improved to 4-5 overall and 3-4 in the Southeastern Conference and put itself in contention for its first bowl berth since 1988.

Victories over Tulane and Arkansas in its last two games will likely send LSU to the Peach Bowl as the fourth-seeded SEC team in the bowl coalition, or to the Carquest Bowl as the fifth-seeded team.

LSU is idle next week.

Alabama, which clinched the SEC Western Division title by virtue of LSU's victory over Ole Miss, fell to 7-1-1 and 4-1-1 in the SEC. Alabama entertains Mississippi State next week.

"Yesterday (Friday), we came to the stadium and walked through just to clear our minds and visualize what would happen," LSU senior center Kevin Mawae said.

"I pulled the team together on the 50-yard line and told them we were playing for a bowl game tomorrow.

"It's the best win I've ever had. I've always dreamed about beating Alabama, and I did it today. There's no better time to do it than your senior year."

LSU battled Alabama to a scoreless halftime tie, just as it had against Texas A&M, then ranked fourth, in the season opener.

But unlike before, when LSU wilted under an Aggie onslaught, 24-0, the Tigers erupted in the second half.

Alabama tried three quarterbacks, including David Palmer to no avail, as LSU intercepted all three and scored after three of the interceptions.

Alabama sophomore Brian Burgdorf started his second straight game for Jay Barker, who remains sidelined with a shoulder injury.

Burgdorf was ineffective, though, and threw Alabama's first interception to end the opening series of the third quarter.

Anthony Marshall's theft and 4-yard return left LSU on Alabama's 38-yard line at 12:48. Five plays later, sophomore tailback Jay Johnson took a pitch 2 yards into the end zone for a 7-0 lead at 10:41.

Sophomore fullback Robert Toomer carried four times for 27 yards during the drive and finished with a 18 carries for a career-high 72 yards. Johnson gained a game-high 83 yards on 14 carries.

LSU finished with 227 yards against the SEC's best defense. Alabama gained 341, but its three quarterbacks completed only 14 of 27 passes for 189 yards and were sacked four times. LSU had only seven sacks in its first eight games.

"This is the biggest victory for me," said Marshall, a product of Mobile, Ala., who returned to his home state for the first time in eight months.

Loup, a senior who has played sparingly the last two years, kept the victory in perspective despite the thrill of helping to contribute to a victory again.

"We've got two games left to worry about," he said. But the prospect of a bowl is compelling.

"It'd be fun," he said. "I've never been associated with one."

It's been a long time between wins for Loup, who found himself taking over for starter Jamie Howard, who completed only 3 of 10 passes for 16 yards, at 8:21 of the second quarter and LSU on its 9-yard line.

LSU punted after the two series Loup played in the quarter, but he returned in the second half and was the beneficiary of LSU's stingy defense. Loup finished 4 of 9 for 45 yards.

After Marshall's theft, Alabama coach Gene Stallings inserted freshman quarterback Freddie Kitchens. LSU junior strong safety Ivory Hilliard intercepted Kitchens on two straight series with the first swipe resulting in Toomer's 2-yard touchdown run and a 14-0 lead at 4:38.

"We couldn't get any continuity going, we had penalties at critical times and turnovers at critical times," Stallings said.

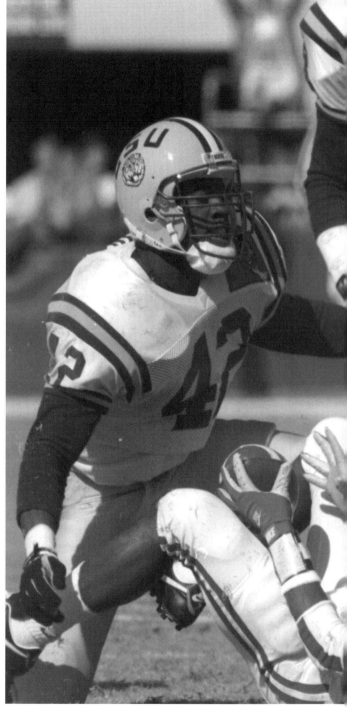

"We couldn't stop them. When it came down to it, we didn't perform like a championship-caliber team."

Stallings finally went with Palmer at 3:16 of the third quarter, and although Palmer staged a furious rally, it wasn't enough to offset the Tigers' defense.

Palmer narrowed the deficit to 14-7 on a 3-yard touchdown pass to fullback Tarrant Lynch with 14:14 remaining, and he tacked on the final six points with a 22-yard touchdown pass to Kevin Lee with 2:41 left.

But in between, LSU junior cornerback stole a Palmer pass

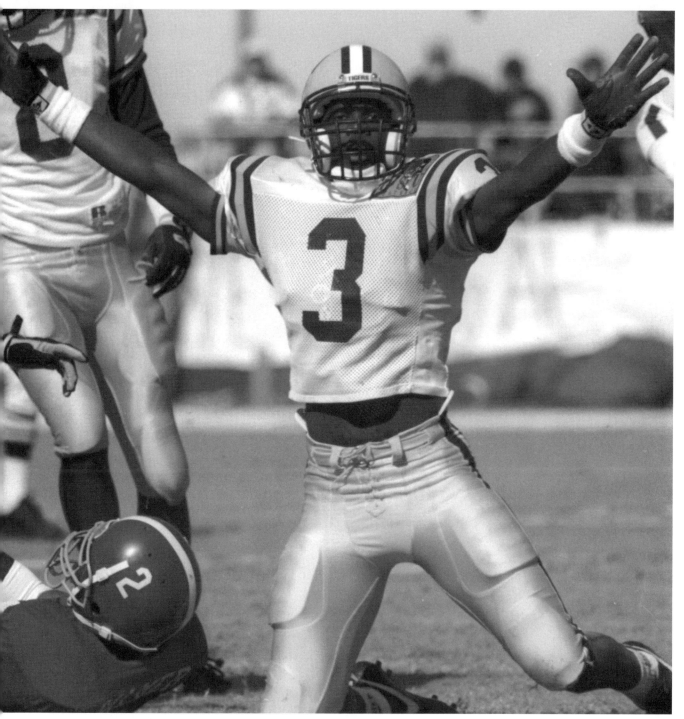

■ LSU's Ivory Hilliard (3) celebrates after tackling Alabama's David Palmer (2).

intended for Lee and returned it 23 yards to LSU's 47-yard line with 9:04 left.

Loup then directed a 10-play, 47-yard march that resulted in Andre Lafleur's 36-yard field goal and a 17-7 advantage with 4:22 remaining.

After Alabama's last score, Palmer was stopped on a two-point conversion run and LSU recovered the ensuing onside kick with 2:41 left.

LSU ran out the clock, as Johnson scampered 11 yards for a critical first down in the middle of the possession.

Harking back to Mawae's earlier comments, sophomore defensive end Gabe Northern said LSU has renewed vigor.

"He said we had a chance to win our last three, and if we did we'd go to a bowl," Northern said. "He said he didn't know if everybody felt the same. It's good to know everybody is on the same page."

It is a page of history.

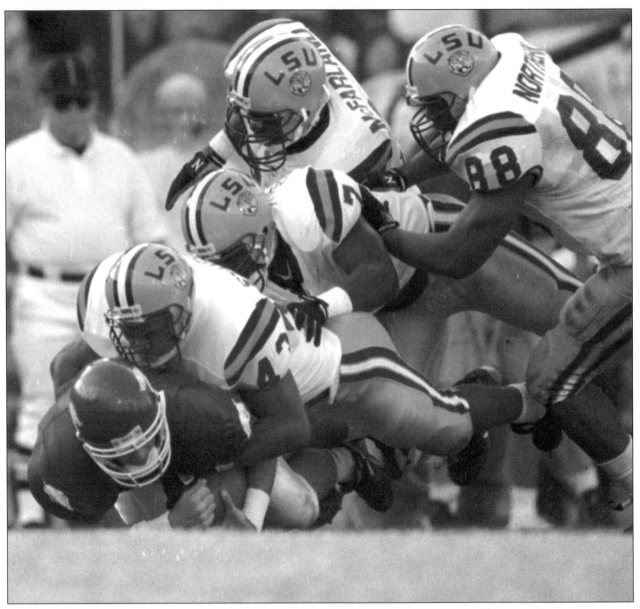

■ A group of LSU defenders team up to bury Arkansas quarterback Barry Lunney Jr. in the second quarter.

Tigers Stun Arkansas, 28-0

By Dave Moormann

The Advocate

Baton Rouge — *Nov. 18, 1995*

No need to call a psychic hot line. Junior linebacker Pat Rogers has seen the future of LSU football. Rogers relied on LSU's 28-0 victory over 14th-ranked Arkansas to clue him in about impending events. "In coming years that's going to be LSU, as long as Gerry DiNardo is the head coach at the school," Rogers said.

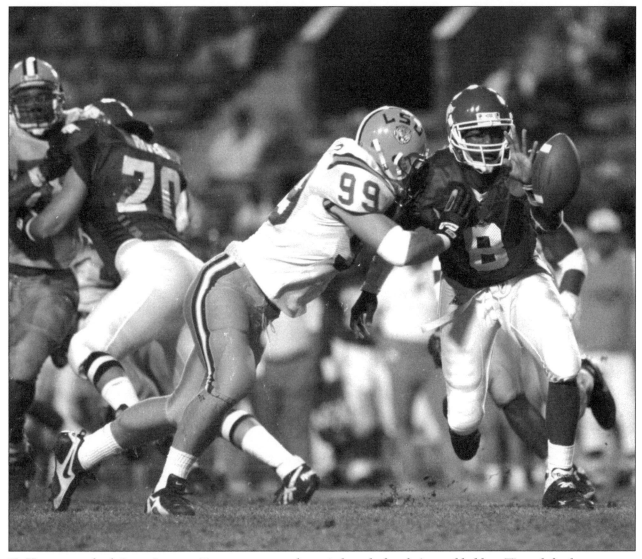

■ Hog quarterback Barry Lunney (8) attempts to make a pitchout before being tackled by a Tiger defender.

If so, that will mean more bowl games and more winning seasons. But, perhaps, nothing short of a championship will match the magnitude of today's victory before an announced crowd of 66,548 in Tiger Stadium.

LSU took out its frustrations of six losing seasons on an Arkansas team that offered little resistance against a Tiger onslaught that featured Kendall Cleveland's three touchdown runs and first 100-yard game.

"We gave Kendall an inch," senior offensive guard Mark King said, "and he made it a mile."

Actually, it was more like a game-high 102 yards on 24 carries, but it went a long way toward securing the victory in LSU's regular-season finale. After Sheddrick Wilson's 9-yard touchdown catch at 5:05 of the first quarter, Cleveland rushed for first-half touchdowns of 4, 20 and 1 yards. It didn't matter that LSU failed to score in the second half. The damage was complete.

The redshirt freshman tailback did it, too, against an SEC defense that ranked second overall and first against the run.

Score by Periods

Arkansas	0	0	0	0 —	0
LSU	7	21	0	0 —	28

"I don't see how they're only 6-4-1," said Arkansas senior quarterback Barry Lunney, who was sacked five times. "That blows my mind that they're only that."

LSU blew Arkansas away to reach that point and a likely Independence Bowl invitation. The fact that LSU finally realized those once unobtainable goals is mind-numbing, in itself. Two years ago, Arkansas denied LSU, 42-24.

"I can't tell you how happy I am for the players," said DiNardo, who when hired last December promised to "bring back the magic" to Tiger Stadium. "It's been a hard year for them ... For the guys who stayed, it's a chance to play in anoth-

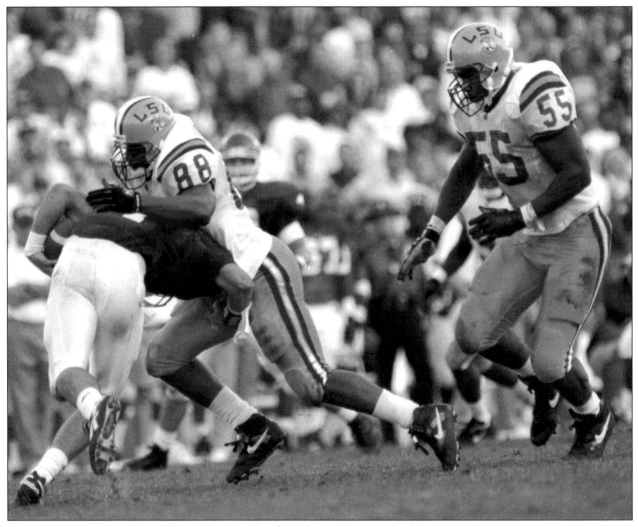

■ **NOWHERE TO RUN: This was the story for the Arkansas offense all afternoon.**

er game. That makes it all worth it."

Arkansas, the Southeastern Conference Western Division champion, has two games ahead of it. The Razorbacks will meet Florida in the SEC Championship Game before finishing in a bowl game. Wilson would have none of the notion that LSU caught Arkansas at a time when the Tigers' had more at stake.

Arkansas fell to 8-3 overall and 6-2 in the SEC. LSU hiked its SEC record to 4-3-1.

"All I can tell you is that we went out and did our job to the best of our ability, and things worked out," said Wilson, a senior flanker who caught a game-high eight passes for 81 yards. "To say they were flat takes away from what we did tonight."

Wilson ignited the explosion with his 9-yard touchdown catch on third down. That helped LSU atone for an illegal-motion penalty on first down at the one. It also completed a 19-play, 80-yard march to begin the game.

"I knew from there, there was no stopping us," freshman quarterback Herbert Tyler said. "We could only stop ourselves."

With Tyler in control, there was none of that. Tyler won his third game in as many starts in replacing senior Jamie Howard,

who remains sidelined with a bruised right shoulder. Howard stood on the sidelines with his right arm in a sling.

Tyler completed 12 of 17 passes for 188 yards with a touchdown and an interception. He also accomplished what Wilson deemed important to the Tigers' welfare.

"All we wanted to do was come out and get points early because we knew the defense would hold them," Wilson said.

Even at that, Wilson said he didn't expect a shutout. But LSU cast Arkansas away at every turn in recording its first shutout since a 27-0 victory over Texas A&M in 1988. LSU held Arkansas to 21 yards on 20 first-half plays and a season-low 144 for the game. LSU registered 348 yards.

"The defense got together and said we were going to stop the run," LSU sophomore defensive tackle Chuck Wiley said. "That was the main focus."

In so doing, LSU held tailback Madre Hill, the SEC's second-leading rusher, to 64 yards on 22 carries. Lunney completed 10 of 28 passes for 78 yards with an interception.

"We kind of caught on to his checks," Rogers said of how the Tigers managed to contain Lunney and his teammates.

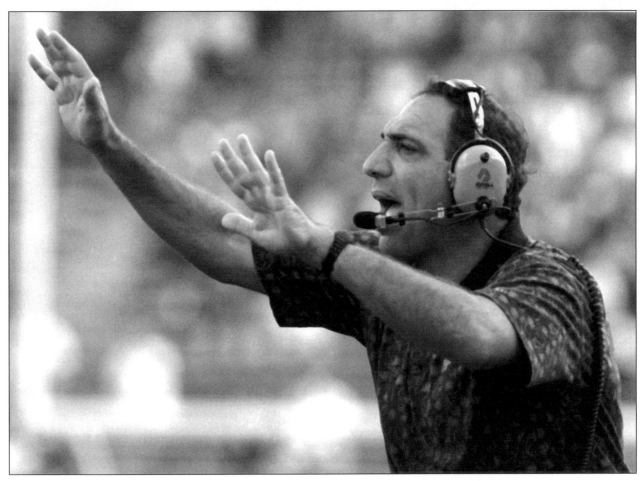

■ **Tiger head coach Gerry DiNardo signals in an offensive play.**

Stansberry said Lunney's audibles usually had Arkansas running away from LSU's strong safety.

Stansberry took advantage of it to share the team lead in tackles with eight, including 1½ quarterback sacks. Rogers intercepted a second-quarter pass and returned it 37 yards to the 1-yard line. Cleveland scored on the next play just 2:37 before halftime.

Cleveland first scored on a 4-yard run at 13:17 of the second quarter. That completed LSU's second possession after 10 plays, 58 yards and 4:16. Cleveland's 20-yard touchdown run at 3:50 was highlighted by his twists and turns and what Cleveland said was Wilson's critical block.

"It was great blocking by the offensive line, mostly," Cleveland said in assigning credit for his overall success. "It felt real good to get the win. It means a lot to me because last year I didn't play. I look at it as the start of a good trend."

Not only did Cleveland upstage Hill, but he also compensated for the thigh bruise that slowed teammate Kevin Faulk to 18 yards on eight carries. And Tyler overshadowed Lunney, despite losing two fumbles, throwing two interceptions and getting sacked three times. Only one of Tyler's turnovers came in the first half when he completed 8 of 10 passes for 121 yards.

"His composure and competitiveness are two of Tyler's finer attributes," DiNardo said. "I like a lot of things about him."

Despite the game's significance, Tyler said he felt no different than he did before any of his other starts. Tyler has opened three of the last four games and played briefly in a 10-3 loss to Alabama.

"There's pressure every week," Tyler said. "You just have to take each week one at a time."

LSU now will have several weeks to prepare for a bowl game, which DiNardo said will help to fortify the Tigers.

"I think that helps you as a program," said DiNardo, who will be coaching in his first bowl since Colorado with DiNardo as offensive coordinator won the Orange Bowl to clinch the 1990 national championship. "The strong get stronger ... It helps the development of the younger players."

It also represents a reward for the older players, whose dream finally came true. King celebrated by helping to dump a bucket of ice water on DiNardo's head with less than 90 seconds left. King said he was on the sidelines as freshman Ryan Thomassie played in an effort to earn a letter.

"That had to be the worst part of the evening," a smiling DiNardo said of the dousing.

But for the most part, the Tigers found it to be an exquisite affair.

"I think it's the best game I've ever played in," Wilson said. "It was the best thing I've ever been a part of. I love the guys for what they did for the senior class tonight."

Determined Tigers Were on a Mission

By Sam King
The Advocate

Baton Rouge, La. — *Nov. 18, 1995*

LSU was not to be denied.

Focused, intent and determined, it was obvious from the outset, LSU came to win.

It would settle for nothing less.

It dominated offensively.

It destroyed defensively.

It manhandled Southeastern Conference Western Division champion Arkansas like no one else has been able to do this year.

Piling up 115 yards rushing on the league' best defense against rushing and 236 yards of offense against the SEC's second-best total defensive team, LSU scored four first-half touchdowns en route to its 28-0 victory.

The Tigers' sixth win of the season against four losses and a tie not only provides them with the school's first winning season since 1988, but puts LSU in a bowl game, most likely the Poulon Weed Eater Independence Bowl at Shreveport.

The chips were down and LSU responded in a fashion seldom seen in six previous seasons in which the Tigers lost 41 (of 66) games, two head coaches and a score of assistants.

It was LSU's first shutout since a 27-0 win over Texas A&M in 1988 and the first SEC shutout since a 47-0 rout of Mississippi State in 1986.

It showed just what this team is capable of doing. That was not a bad football team on the other side of the ball, although LSU left it standing in an upright position only on a few occasions.

It wasn't just the offense that dominated in the first half, although scoring 28 points speaks awfully good for it. The defense was a bit unreal, maybe a little unbelievable, allowing the Razorbacks only 21 yards on 20 plays.

Sooey Pigs!

When the Tigers' offense faltered in the third quarter, the defense again rose to the occasion. Freshman quarterback Herbert Tyler fumbled the ball away twice and threw two interceptions, but the Razorbacks were stymied despite getting great possessions on the LSU 21 and 31 and Arkansas' 46.

It was obvious the Tigers were determined to deny a repeat of 1993 when they were routed by Arkansas (42-24) in this same stadium in an identical situation — a winning season and

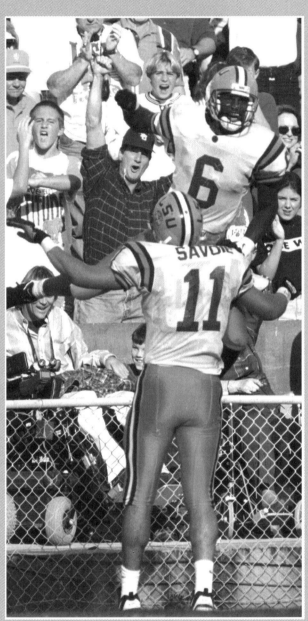

■ **LSU's 28-0 shutout of Arkansas gave Tiger players and fans a lot to shout about.**

bowl bid awaiting.

LSU quite likely played its best ball of the year.

"I think so, considering the pressure," said a happy Gerry DiNardo, who is headed to his first bowl ever as a head coach. "We probably played a more complete game last week (in beating Ole Miss), but I think the fact that we needed a win for a winning season and to go to a bowl game makes it much better.

"Although it may not look as good statistically as last week because we didn't score points in the second half, I still think it was best of the year because of what was at stake," said DiNardo.

Admittedly, it was DiNardo's finest hour as a head coach.

"This is my fifth year I've been a head coach and the first bowl we've gotten and the best team we've had," he said. "I've had fun since I've had this job ... all the obvious things and the locker room scene after the game."

Appropriately, DiNardo was doused with a barrel of "Power Aid" drink by celebrating players at the end of the game. It was a fitting, even if chilling, climax to an up-and-down season in which players were left by the wayside as the Tigers continued to improve and get on with the DiNardo program.

"That'll give you a heart attack," he said of the sudden and unexpected dousing just prior to the end of the game.

But, DiNardo maintained he was not surprised that LSU had a winning season.

"I thought we had enough talent to do something like this, but I didn't think it was automatic," he said. "I think talent just gives you a chance."

Despite a surprising 3-1 start, LSU faltered and eventually stood at 4-3-1 with Alabama, Ole Miss and Arkansas remaining.

"Before the Alabama game we were talking about playing the last 12 quarters the best we could," said DiNardo. "I think our defense probably did, but our offense struggled against Alabama."

At 4-4-1, the season was on the brink. LSU could have finished at 4-6-1 as easily as it did 6-4-1.

DiNardo thought not.

"I thought we could win the last two," he said. "We played exceptionally well in the last two. They really came back strong.

"I didn't think we would win this game 28-0 or last week would be the way it was, but I thought we could win the last two."

The victory was vitally important in rebuilding the Tiger program.

It broke the losing streak and got rid of the albatross which has been around LSU's neck for six years.

Now the Tigers can start a winning streak.

"I think that's big time, but we will still have a lot of work to do as you go through it. Look what happened to South

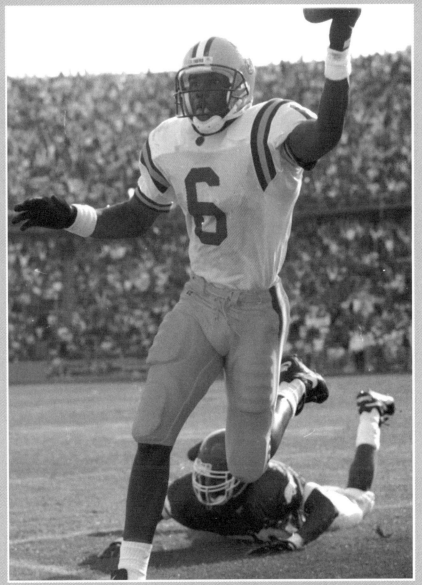

■ LSU wide receiver Sheddrick Wilson (6) high steps it into the end zone after his 9-yard touchdown catch.

Carolina," he said of a team which went to a bowl under a new coach last season but finished 4-6-1 this season. "We can't have that happen to us. In the second year of a program you can't take a step back."

He admitted the victory was good to build on next year, but noted, "It's not automatic."

On Jan. 1, 1966, LSU defeated a highly-favored Arkansas team 14-7, in the Cotton Bowl in one of the Tigers' greatest wins.

Almost 30 years later, 47 players and coaches on that team sat in the stands to watch another LSU team defeat Arkansas in a game which could surpass that one in greatness.

Twenty or thirty years from now, fans may look back to 1995 as the year, Nov. 18 as the day and this 28-0 win as the victory which brought back the magic to LSU football.

Green Wave's Jinx Continues, LSU Wins 7-6

By Bud Montet

The Advocate

New Orleans, La. — *Dec. 1, 1956*

The Bengal Tigers of LSU continued their jinx over the Tulane Green Wave and grabbed a 7-6 victory from the Billow before 60,000 fans here this afternoon.

Today's victory assured LSU its dominance over the Greenies, a victory pact that has held good since 1949. The last time Tulane handed the Tigers a setback was in Baton Rouge in 1948 when they bested the Tigers, 46-0.

Since that time, LSU has won all the games with the exception of two ties.

Tulane, who was favored in today's game, scored first when they picked up a touchdown in the second quarter with Ronnie Quillian, the Baton Rouge youth, going two yards for the score.

LSU came back to dominate play in the second half as they took advantage of Tulane fumbles to get their score with Jimmy Taylor going over from the Tulane 1 for the touchdown and kicking the extra point to secure the victory.

A succession of Tulane fumbles in the second half kept the Bengals in Tulane's backyard during the second half of the game.

Prior to their scoring drive, LSU had driven to the Tulane 3-yard line where a fourth-down pass from M.C. Reynolds to Billy Hendrix failed. But on the first play after this attempt, Tulane's quarterback fumbled and LSU's Durwood Graham recovered the ball on the Tulane 3. Taylor scored two plays later.

For the rest of the game, the Tigers dominated play although they failed to score after reaching the Tulane 1-yard line early in the fourth quarter.

A few minutes later, Earl Leggett's recovery of a Green Wave fumble on the Tulane 30 gave the Bengals a chance which they muffed as they drove to the Tulane 13, where

Taylor fumbled and Tulane recovered.

The Green Wave dominated the statistics as they picked up 202 yards rushing to the Bengals' 128 and added 32 yards in the air while completing two of 12 passes. LSU failed to connect on any of the half dozen they attempted.

For the Bengals, the hard running of big Taylor sparked their ground attack as the Baton Rouge native picked up 86 yards in 26 carries.

J.W. Brodnax, the Tiger halfback, picked up 28 yards in 15 tries.

For LSU, the game was one of capitalizing on breaks as they received them.

After a scoreless first quarter, the Green Wave got a break as Brodnax fumbled on the LSU 36 and the Green Wave recovered. Freddie Wilcox rambled for five yards, then Boo Mason raced around the Tiger left end for 16 yards and a first down at the Bengal 16. Mason added three yards as the first period ended and on the first play of the second quarter Willie Hoff picked up two yards to the Bengal 11.

After Eugene Newton missed on a pass in the end zone, he kept for eight yards to the Bengal 3 and then Quillian raced over right guard for the first score of the game.

Emmet Zelenka failed to kick the extra point, but the Green Wave trotted off the field at the end of the first half leading, 6-0.

LSU scared the Green Wave fans midway in the second quarter when Taylor intercepted a Newton pass on the Bengal 4-yard line and ran it back 44 yards before being hauled down. However, the Bengals' threat was halted as a 15-yard penalty stymied the Bengals.

LSU took control of the game in the second half, playing most of the remaining game in the Tulane territory.

Driving from their 39 — after Paul Ziegler recovered a Green Wave fumble — to the Tulane 3, where they ran out of steam after being stopped on fourth down.

However, Graham's recovery of a Green Wave fumble on the Tulane 3 a few plays later gave LSU the chance they needed. LSU pushed the ball over with Taylor carrying on two plays.

Tulane made a bid to get back in front midway in the fourth period when they moved from midfield to the Bengal 20-yard line, but John Caruso missed on two long passes.

The victory gave the Bengals their third win of the season, their first SEC triumph of the 1956 season and their first win over Tulane for young Paul Dietzel.

LSU has six of their last eight games with the Green Wave. Their have been two ties, in 1950 and 1955. Today's victory saved them from one of the worst seasons ever suffered by a Tiger eleven.

Score by Periods

LSU	0	0	7	0 —	7
Tulane	0	6	0	0 —	6

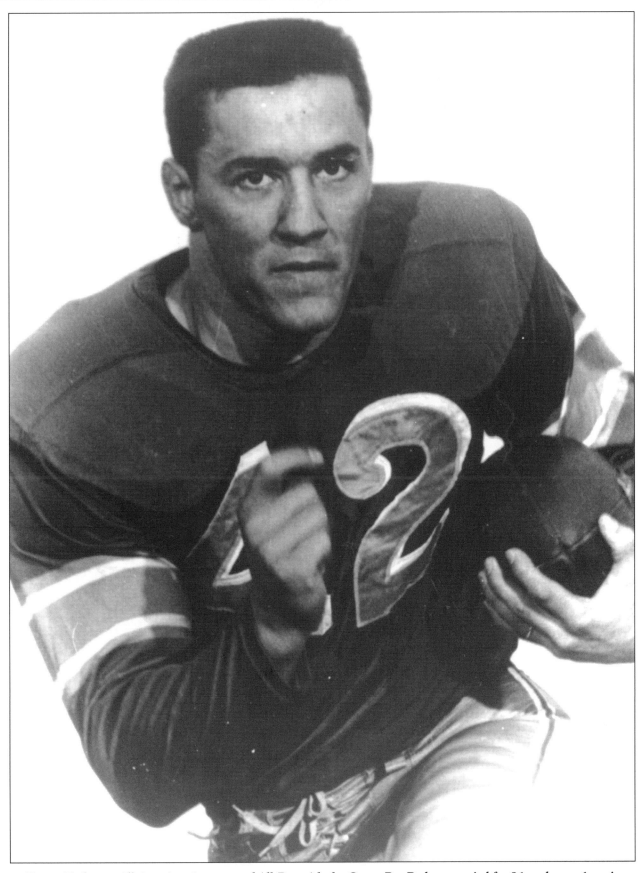

■ Jimmy Taylor, an All-American in 1957 and All-Pro with the Green Bay Packers, carried for 86 yards on 26 carries.

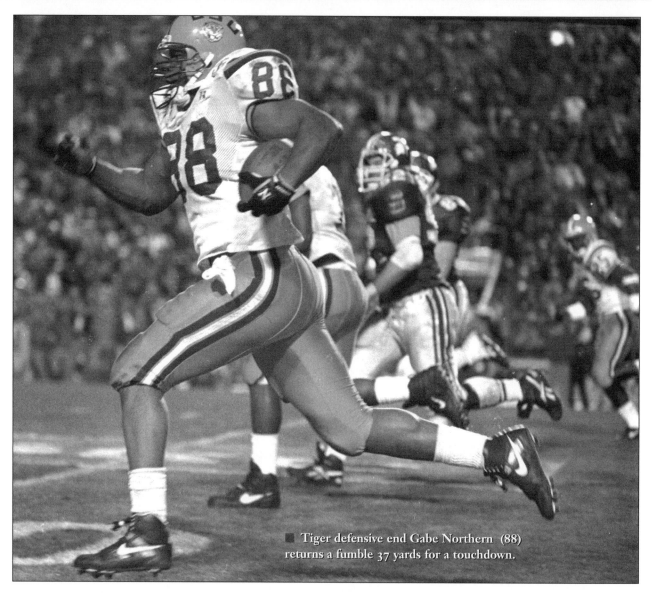

■ Tiger defensive end Gabe Northern (88) returns a fumble 37 yards for a touchdown.

LSU Routs Spartans In Independence Bowl, 45-26

By Dave Moormann

The Advocate

Shreveport, La. — *Dec. 29, 1995*

Michigan State scored on the game's second play from scrimmage. LSU scored on the second play of the third quarter.

LSU's Eddie Kennison returned a kickoff for a record 92-yard touchdown. Michigan State's Derrick Mason followed with a record 100-yard kickoff return.

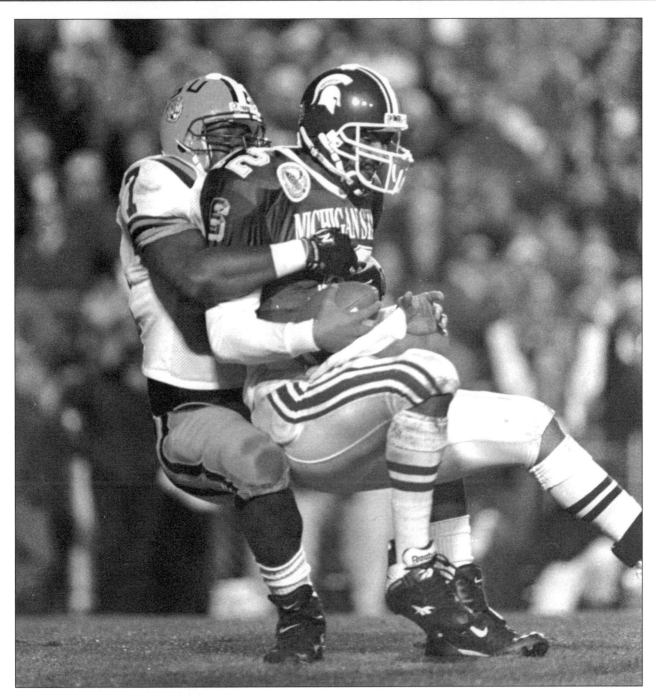

■ **James Gillyard (7) bulldogs Michigan State quarterback Tony Banks (12) for a loss.**

If Michigan State produced the bizarre in the Poulan Weed Eater Independence Bowl, LSU answered with the unusual Friday.

Finally, about the time defensive end Gabe Northern recovered a third-quarter fumble and returned it for a 37-yard touchdown, LSU put an end to the counterpunching and walloped Michigan State, 45-26.

"That turned the game around," said LSU freshman quarterback Herb Tyler, who completed 10 of 20 passes for 164 yards and one touchdown.

Score by Periods

	1	2	3	4	
Michigan State	7	17	0	2 —	26
LSU	7	14	21	3 —	45

Maybe so, but freshman tailback Kevin Faulk certainly pointed LSU in the right direction in rushing 25 times for 234 yards, including touchdown runs of 51 and 5 yards.

Faulk was named the game's offensive most valuable player. Northern won the defensive award in LSU's first Independence Bowl appearance.

"At halftime we talked about, 'Let's just forget about the results of the game, let's just make sure we play with great intensity,' " LSU coach Gerry DiNardo said.

And so it did, as LSU claimed one of the most electrifying Independence Bowls in its 20-year history. LSU capped its first winning season and bowl appearance in seven years with a 7-4-1 record.

LSU won its second bowl in seven tries and its first since the 1987 Gator Bowl. Michigan State, playing its first football game against LSU, fell to 6-5-1.

LSU also scored on Kennison's 27-yard catch, freshman tailback Kendall Cleveland's 6-yard run and sophomore Wade Richey's 48-yard field goal. Kennison collected 249 all-purpose yards, including a team-high five catches for 124 yards.

"From the start of the game, I thought we had the better team," DiNardo said.

That was hard to tell, though, given the first-half fireworks that gave Michigan State a 24-21 halftime lead. At one point, four touchdowns were scored in a 93-second span of the second quarter.

"I didn't know when it was going to stop," DiNardo said. "I still thought we had the better team."

LSU finally showed it by dominating the second half in scoring 24 unanswered points before the sellout crowd of 48,835 at Independence Stadium. The Spartans' only second-half score came with 5:57 left when punter Chad Kessler took a safety in running time off the clock.

Michigan State managed just 125 of its 448 total yards in the second half. LSU amassed 436 total yards, including 201 in the second half.

"That was a wakeup call," LSU junior linebacker Pat Rogers said of the manner in which the Spartans scored against a defense that led the Southeastern Conference in allowing just 14.6 points per game.

LSU forced six turnovers overall, including an interception by junior linebacker Allen Stansberry, who made an Independence Bowl-record 18 total tackles. But no turnover was more prominent than the first fumble return for a touchdown in school history.

Northern and freshman strong safety Greg Hill forced a fumble from Michigan State quarterback Tony Banks. Northern scooped up the loose ball and raced into the end zone to give LSU a 35-24 lead at 9:20 of the third quarter.

"I just had some kind of determination that I was going to do something to put the team over the top," said Northern, who noted that he told someone on the ride from Baton Rouge that he would be defensive MVP. Northern and fellow senior defensive end James Gillyard each had an Independence Bowl-record three quarterback sacks.

Tyler said he sensed LSU would win when it scored early in

■ **Freshman Kevin Faulk (3) led the Tigers with 234 yards rushing on 25 carries and two touchdowns.**

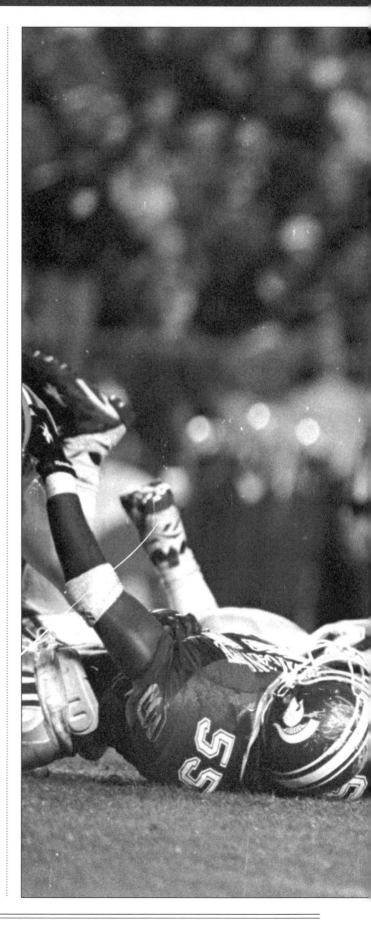

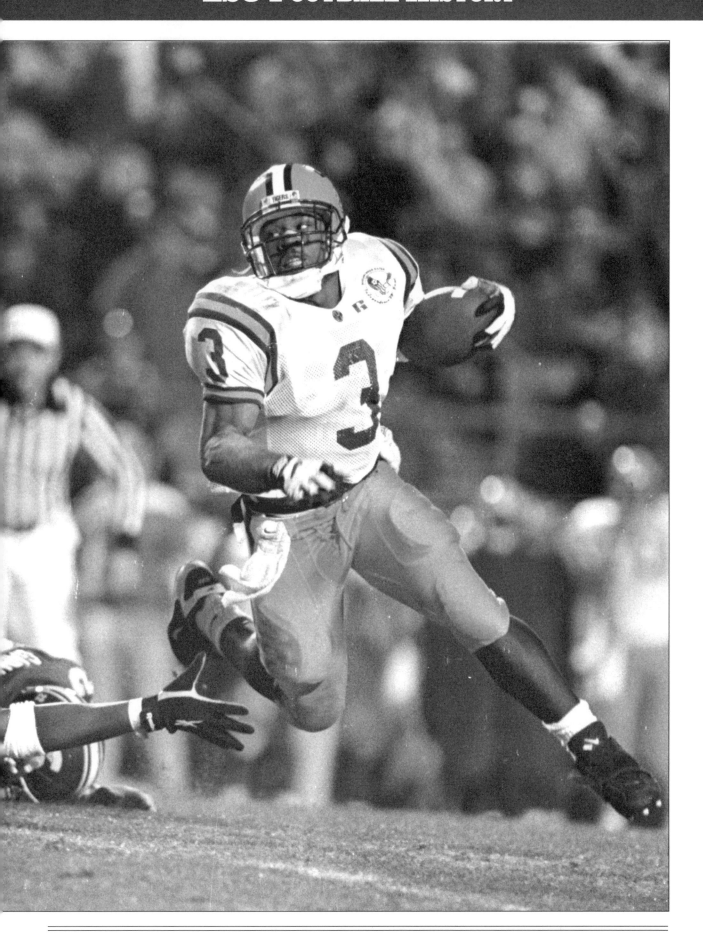

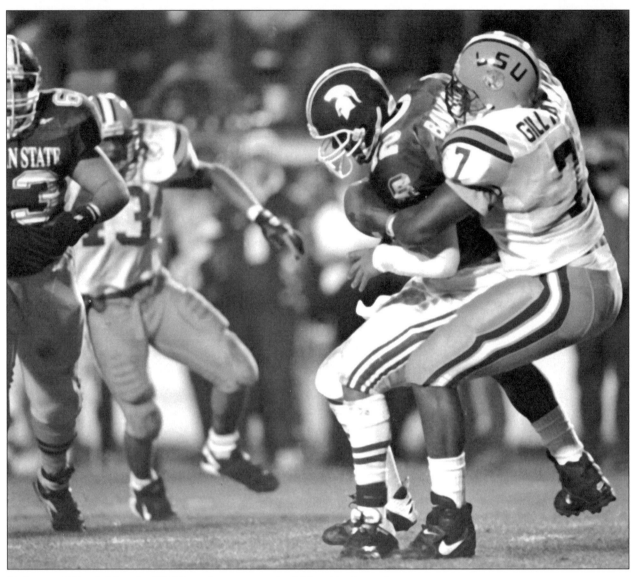

■ **James Gillyard (7) sacks Michigan State quarterback Tony Banks again.**

the second half to take a 28-24 lead, and again on Northern's fumble return. Tyler highlighted the second half's opening possession that resulted in Faulk's 5-yard touchdown run at 14:29 of the third quarter.

After the Spartans were penalized for roughing Tyler, Kennison caught a 49-yard pass from Tyler on the first official play from scrimmage. Faulk followed with his score.

"In the locker room, I was telling my cousin (Derrick Beavers), I was going to cause a catastrophe with my feet," Faulk said.

Faulk did just that, as he rushed for the most yards by an LSU freshman, the most in LSU bowl history, and the second-most ever by an LSU player. LSU does not count bowl statistics in its record book.

In addition to his 51-yard touchdown run that tied the score, 21-21, at 13:11 of the second quarter, Faulk had a 40-yard run on LSU's first scoring drive and a 68-yard run in the second quarter that was the longest nonscoring run in

Independence Bowl history.

"I thought it was an outstanding and exciting football game in the first half," said Michigan State coach Nick Saban, who's in his first year as is DiNardo. "We just came out in the second half and seemed to be a little flat off the bat. For what reason, I don't know."

The first half surely didn't give an indication that either team would cool down. Michigan State scored on its second play when Banks fired a 78-yard touchdown pass to Muhsin Muhammad at 14:13. LSU retaliated with an 80-yard drive that ended in Cleveland's 6-yard run at 12:07.

The most explosive portion of the game began when Michigan State's Carl Reaves intercepted a pass and returned it 17 yards to the LSU 3-yard line to begin the second quarter. Fullback Scott Greene, who was benched for the first quarter because he missed curfew early Thursday morning, scored from there at 14:44.

Michigan State missed the extra point, but the scoring frenzy had begun. Kennison picked up a bouncing kickoff, slipped

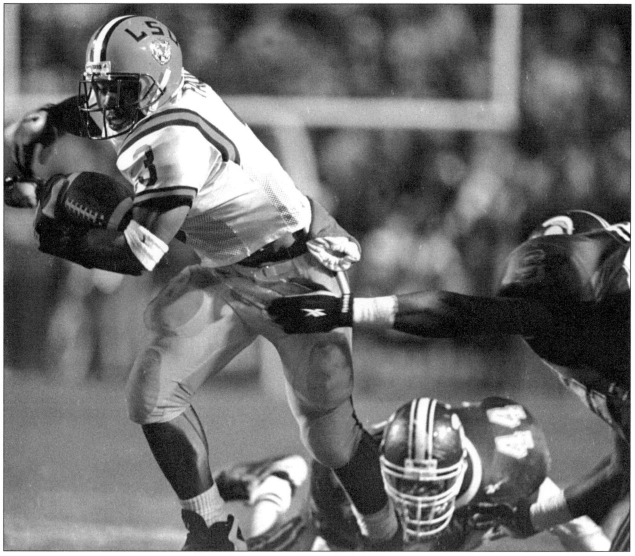

■ **Kevin Faulk (3) escapes a pair of diving Michigan State defenders.**

a tackle in the middle of the field and outran two defenders down the right sideline to score at 14:30. Mason retaliated with his bowl-record 100-yard scamper at 14:17 in becoming the Big Ten Conference career leader in kickoff returns. Greene scored on a 2-pointer to put Michigan State ahead, 21-14.

Faulk's 51-yard dash came 66 seconds later, and although LSU fell behind one second before halftime on Chris Gardner's 37-yard field goal, the Tigers were to continue the assault in the second half.

"They say you practice like you play," Kennison said. "We played like we practiced."

Meanwhile, Saban blamed himself for what he said were Michigan State's poor practices this week.

"He's nice to have around," Tyler said of Kennison. "I hope

he's around next year."

Kennison said he hasn't made a decision on whether to enter the NFL draft or return for his senior year.

Kennison's 27-yard touchdown catch at 7:13 of the third quarter gave LSU a 42-24 lead. The Tigers had a chance for even more points, but Andre Lafleur missed field-goal attempts of 37 and 38 yards in the third and fourth, quarters, respectively. That led Richey, with 8:45 left, to kick his first career field goal on his only try this season.

That ended LSU's scoring, but it only added to the heightened expectations that DiNardo knows exist now.

Asked what the Tigers must do in the future, DiNardo said, "Win more than seven games next year."

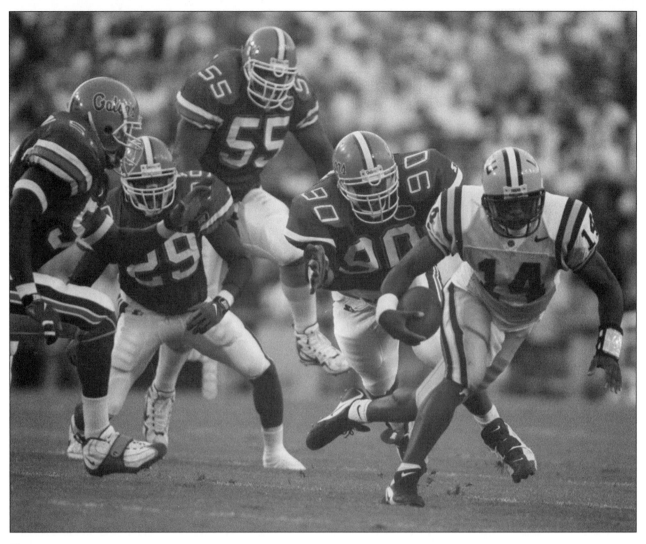

■ Herb Tyler ran past Florida's defense for two touchdowns, finishing with 50 yards rushing.

Pandemonium Reigns After Tigers Defeat No. 1 Florida

By Dave Moormann
The Advocate

Baton Rouge, La. — *Oct. 11, 1997*

Stunning isn't strong enough. Unthinkable, maybe. Pandemonium, for sure.

In an upset unlike any before in LSU's proud 104-year football history, the 14th-ranked Tigers shocked top-ranked Florida, 28-21, tonight and set off a wild, exhilarating scene in Tiger Stadium.

Many in LSU's second-largest paid crowd of 80,677 stormed the field and ripped down the goal posts in celebration of the monumental triumph.

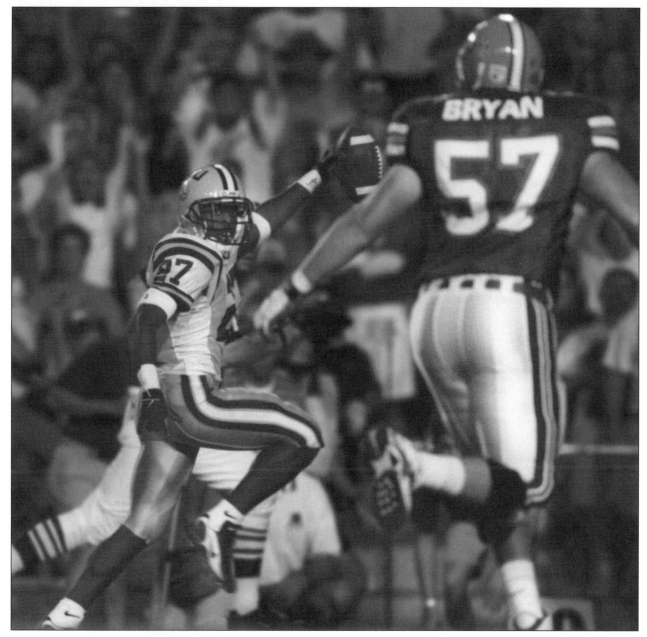

■ **LSU's Cedric Donaldson returns a 31-yard interception for a touchdown which put LSU in front to stay.**

Never before had LSU beaten a No. 1 team, having gone 0-7-1 in such games, including losses to Florida in two of the previous three seasons.

"Other than getting a bill from (LSU Athletic Director) Joe Dean for the goal posts, it was a great night," LSU coach Gerry DiNardo said.

LSU took immediate control in bolting to a 14-0 first-quarter lead. The Tigers became the first team to score a first-quarter touchdown against Florida this season.

LSU also ended Florida's Southeastern Conference winning streak at 25 games, two short of the league record. In the process, it snapped Florida's SEC road win streak at a record-tying 19 games.

Florida's first loss of the season dropped them to 5-1 overall and 3-1 in the SEC, where it shares first place in the Eastern Division with Tennessee. LSU, which owns the same records, trails Auburn by one-half game in the West.

"The first drive set us off mentally," sophomore left offensive tackle Al Jackson said.

LSU established itself with a 58-yard march, even if the possession ended with Rondell Mealey's fumble. The Tigers stormed back with a pair of one-play touchdown drives to stun the Gators.

After Florida punted, LSU junior quarterback Herb Tyler sped around the right side on an option for a 40-yard touchdown that gave LSU a 7-0 lead at 8:42 of the first quarter.

Score by Periods

Florida	7	0	7	7	— 21
LSU	14	0	0	14	— 28

Tyler added an 11-yard rushing touchdown that proved to be the difference on another option run around the right side to put LSU ahead, 28-14, with 11:40 left.

"We just had the attitude of playing hard and executing and winning the game," said Tyler, who had been criticized in recent weeks for his erratic play. Tyler improved his career record as a starter to 19-3.

Tyler's second touchdown allowed LSU to weather Fred Taylor's 3-yard TD run with 6:44 to play. It was the last of Taylor's three touchdowns.

LSU ended Florida's last possession when junior strong safety Raion Hill came up with LSU's fourth interception of the night.

Senior cornerback Cedric Donaldson already had intercepted two passes, returning one for a 31-yard touchdown that put LSU in front, 21-14, at 13:13 of the fourth quarter.

Donaldson's first theft and 68-yard return set up freshman fullback Tommy Banks for a 7-yard touchdown run that put LSU ahead, 14-0, at 7:44 of the first quarter.

"(Florida sophomore quarterback Doug) Johnson is not as accurate as (Danny Wuerffel)," Donaldson said of the current New Orleans Saints quarterback who helped defending national champion Florida past LSU last season, 56-13. "He throws the ball all over the place. We knew he was going to mess up and throw one (interception). I ran out of gas (on the 68-yard return)."

Taylor slowed the Tiger express with a 2-yard touchdown run that cut the early deficit to 14-7 at 2:14 of the first quarter. LSU took that lead into halftime before Taylor tied the score, 14-14, on his 1-yard touchdown run at 12:17 of the third quarter.

But LSU broke the deadlock with Donaldson scoring on his team-best sixth interception of the season, and Tyler adding the decisive touchdown on his scamper. Florida's Bo Carroll fumbled a kickoff return to put LSU in position for Tyler to score.

"They just outplayed us, outcoached us, and they deserved to win," said Florida coach Steve Spurrier, who had guided the Gators in seven of the nine consecutive games they had won against LSU.

"We just got beat tonight," Johnson said. "They were the better team and more prepared."

LSU ended Florida's NCAA-record string of regular-season games with a touchdown pass at 62.

LSU will return to action Saturday at home against Ole Miss. Florida must visit eighth-ranked Auburn.

LSU rushed for 158 yards after gaining 28 yards on the ground last year at Florida. Kevin Faulk rushed 22 times for 78

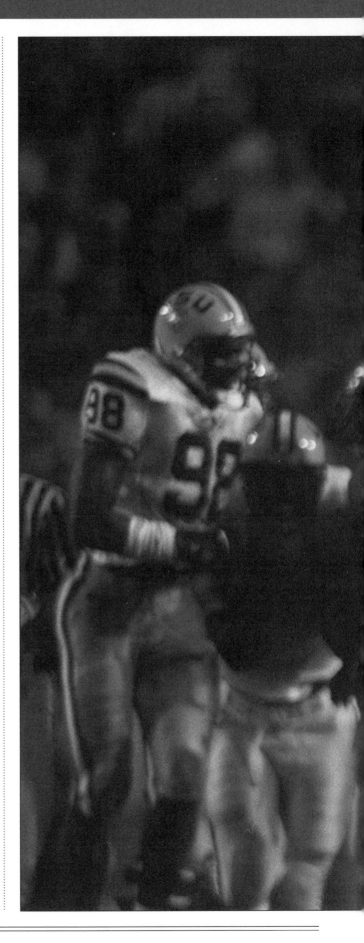

■ **Mark Roman (8) celebrates after teammate Chris Cummings blocked a Florida field goal.**

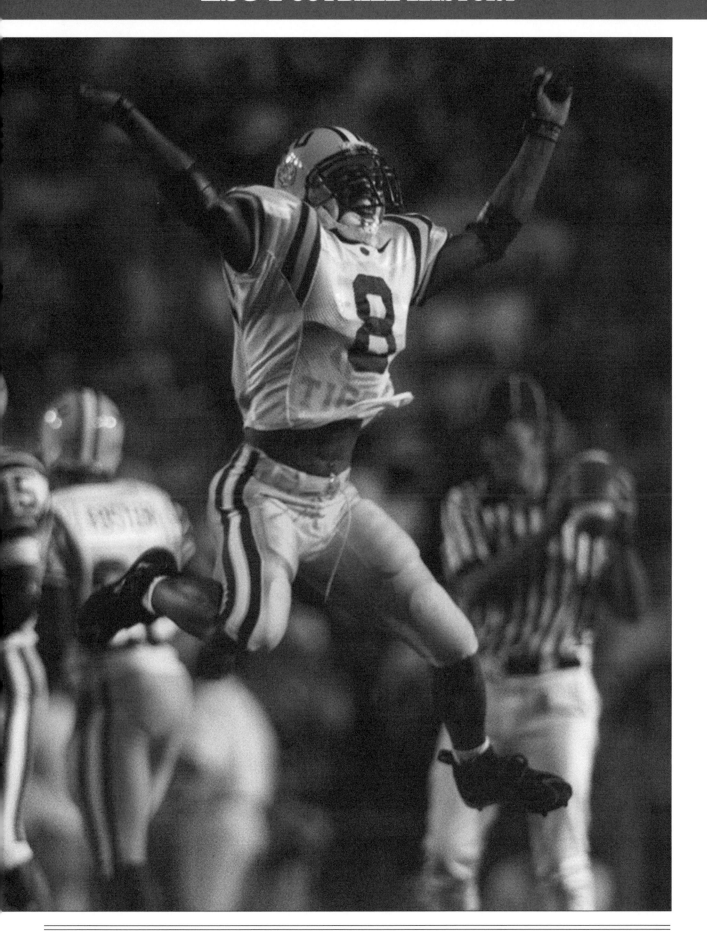

yards; a year ago he gained 26 yards. Florida outgained LSU, 391-330, but it wasn't enough.

"It hit me as soon as the clock had 50 seconds on it," Faulk said. "It's really exciting."

It was a measure of vindication both for LSU and Tyler, with LSU coming off a 31-28 loss to Auburn on Sept. 20 and a 7-6 lackluster victory against Vanderbilt last week.

Tyler hadn't played particularly well in either game, and LSU was a decided underdog against Florida. He completed 10 of 17 passes for 172 yards without an interception Saturday.

"I don't know what the critics are going to say now," Jackson said.

"We wanted to hit them in the mouth," LSU junior defensive tackle Anthony McFarland said. "We wanted to play physical ... There's nothing like Saturday night in Tiger Stadium."

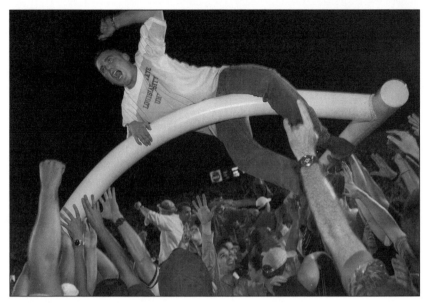

■ **LSU fan Bryan Allen leads the postgame celebration by tearing down one of the goalposts.**

LSU surprised Florida with an unusual defensive scheme that it branded "The Bandit" package in taking the name from the defensive group that played during LSU's 1958 national championship season.

When it went to that formation, LSU used a 3-3-5 alignment with backup players. LSU normally lines up in a 4-2-5 set.

After LSU opened up its 14-0 lead, Florida responded with an 80-yard scoring drive. Taylor capped it with his 2-yard scoring run into the right corner of the end zone.

Copying how LSU began the game, Florida started the second half by marching downfield for a touchdown that tied the score, 14-14, on Taylor's 1-yard run.

Taylor not only scored to end the seven-play, 80-yard drive, but he also figured prominently into the march.

Florida opened with Taylor's 53-yard reception and run. Taylor also rushed for 19 yards in moving into fifth-place on Florida's all-time rushing list.

LSU threatened on its next drive, but Florida blocked Wade Richey's 44-yard field-goal attempt. Richey finished with three failed field-goal tries, missing also from 37 and 39 yards out.

In scoring on its two one-play touchdown drives in the first quarter, LSU became the first team to take a lead on Florida this season.

Florida entered the game with a composite 91-3 first-quarter lead over its opponents. But LSU shocked the Gators.

Not only did LSU win the pregame coin toss, but it elected to receive and embarked on an impressive seven-play, 58-yard drive that began at its 20-yard line.

However the drive ended when Mealey, in what would be his only first-half carry, fumbled the football. After everyone was slow to react as it rolled backward, Willie Rodgers finally recovered and returned it on the Florida 25-yard line.

LSU forced Florida to punt after three plays, and on first down from the Florida 40-yard line, Tyler ran an option around right end.

He stumbled just past the line of scrimmage before recovering his balance and racing into the end zone to put LSU ahead, 7-0.

"A lot of people had talked about him," junior center Todd McClure said, "but we need Herb Tyler. He showed the quarterback he is."

Carroll's 44-yard kickoff return put Florida in good field position on its 45-yard line. Taylor gained 14 yards on first down before Johnson threw incomplete to Green. Johnson followed with his worst pass of the half, which Donaldson intercepted.

Some nifty running and strong blocking allowed Donaldson to return it 68 yards to the Florida 7-yard line. Donaldson didn't score, but Banks zipped up the middle on first down for a 7-yard touchdown. Banks' second touchdown of the season gave LSU a 14-0 lead.

Florida responded with a 13-play, 80-yard scoring drive that Taylor capped with his 2-yard run.

Both teams tried second-quarter field goals with futile results. A snap that rolled to the holder didn't help Richey, who missed a 39-yarder at 9:41.

Florida came back with a methodical 16-play, 51-yard drive. LSU's defense stiffened when Florida reached the Tigers' 27-yard line, and rather than go for the first down on fourth-and-12, the Gators had Collins Cooper attempt a 44-yard field goal.

Chris Cummings blocked the kick, giving LSU its third block in as many games. Kenny Mixon blocked an extra-point attempt on the final play to preserve LSU's one-point victory over Vanderbilt the previous week. Before that, Arnold Miller batted down a field-goal try in LSU's 56-0 victory over Akron.

In leading 14-7 at halftime, LSU led a top-ranked team after two quarters for the first time since jumping ahead of Florida State, 16-7, in 1991. FSU came back to win, 27-16.

Not only did LSU hold on this time, it made its way into history.

Beating Gators Tops the List

BY SAM KING

The Advocate

Baton Rouge, La. — *Oct. 11, 1997*

Go ahead, call it The Greatest.

The 999,999 people who will swear they were in Tiger Stadium on Oct. 11, 1997, to witness football's Mission Impossible will call LSU's 28-21 triumph over defending national champion and No. 1-ranked Florida the greatest victory, the greatest victory in Tiger Stadium and the greatest game every played by an LSU team.

It is all debatable.

Certainly LSU's 14-7 upset of No. 2-ranked Arkansas in the Jan. 1, 1966, Cotton Bowl was great. There is also the Heisman Trophy-winning run of Billy Cannon in a 7-3 victory over Ole Miss in this same stadium in 1959.

As for the greatest game in between these walls, you can't forget Charles McClendon's last year in 1979 when No. 1 Southern Cal needed the benefit of generous officials to get out alive. And even Bear Bryant and his No. 1 Tide won by only 3-0 the same year, although it was probably the most lopsided 3-0 rout these eyes ever witnessed.

How great it was when they had a sign to set our clocks back four seconds when you crossed the Louisiana-Mississippi state line after the Tigers recorded what many Rebel fans emphasized was a post-game, 17-16 victory in 1972.

The band played late. The fans swarmed the field. The crowd was wild.

It was also a similar scenario after a 61-17 rout of Ole Miss in 1970 with oranges filling the sky and field as LSU prepared to go to the Orange Bowl, the same as against Florida State, 55-21, in 1982.

But, on this humid October night in Tiger Stadium, there was a little of it all — plus the element of surprise.

It was a completely, shocking, stunning upset. It had the offensive and defensive thrills that would send a wave of pandemonium throughout the second-biggest crowd (80,677) in Tiger Stadium history.

Oh, how they relished the sweet taste of victory — those who weren't wearing that gaudy Orange and Blue stuff.

And, for the record, there was no porch for these football Tigers. They proved they can run with the biggest of dogs in college football. It is they who put the bite on No. 1. It is this team that became the first LSU club to defeat a top-ranked team.

They call it history.

You can also call Florida's 25-game SEC winning streak history. The Gators' string of 19 consecutive triumphs away from Florida Field are also gone with the win — LSU's win, that is.

Remember this night when a determined, battling team waged a total team effort to make this one of the most unforgettable nights, games and victories in Tiger football history.

The goal posts came down, the students stormed the field — wild, screaming and running with reckless abandon.

Damn, we of the media found out quickly how Florida quarterback Doug Johnson must have felt as LSU sent wave after wave of charges at him all night. They wrecked the poise and confidence of this team that had won the national championship only a year ago — after it virtually obliterated this same group of Tigers, 56-13. That's a 50-point swing. That's a big deal.

But, this was not the same LSU team, by any stretch of the imagination, that escaped the wrath of being upset by Vanderbilt a week ago — thanks only to Vandy's own inability to run a simple play.

Please welcome back the Tigers.

Welcome back Clarence LeBlanc — a defensive back out since the second game with an injury. What a comeback, what a heck of a game.

Don't welcome Cedric Donaldson back. He's not been anywhere. Just tell him thanks for two interceptions, one that he returned 31 yards for the Tigers' third TD.

Welcome back Herb Tyler ... wherever you have been. Why did you stay away so long? What was it you had, 10 completions in 17 attempts for 172 yards and scrambling for 50 on the ground, including touchdown runs of 40 and 11 yards. Superb ... just superb.

Believe me, Kevin Faulk's stats can't tell you what he meant. Seventy-eight yards on 22 carries never seemed so much. He's probably never faced a night so long — nor ever enjoyed one quite as much.

Give Carl Reese and Morris Watts, the coordinators much credit. Guess those guys can really give a clinic now on how to beat Florida now.

Give the fans also much credit for the never-ending roar.

After the triumph, Gerry DiNardo said, "I know I've never seen anything like it in my years here."

And I'm not sure I have either.

It was one for the history book.

Call it The Greatest.

You may as well.

Mostly everyone else will — especially the 999,999 other people who were in Tiger Stadium when LSU finally beat No. 1.

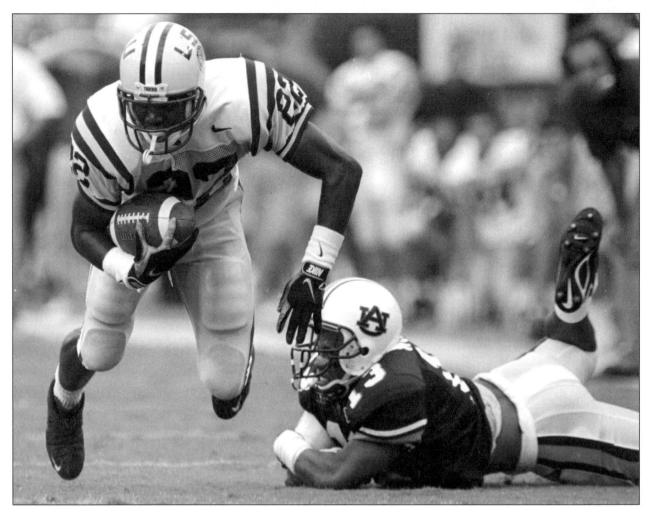

■ Larry Foster (22) scored on a 29-yard touchdown reception in the third quarter.

Tyler & Daring Tigers Destroy Auburn, 31-19

By Scott Rabalais
The Advocate

Auburn, Ala. — *Sept. 20, 1998*

If the Auburn Tigers thought LSU quarterback Herb Tyler couldn't beat them with his throwing arm, they were right. The LSU senior needed more than that. He required nimble feet, a head full of big-game experience and a throwing arm that has rarely been more on target.

With all of those things working for him near peak efficiency, Tyler threw for three touchdowns and ran for another, leading No. 7-ranked LSU to a crucial 31-19 victory in its SEC opener at Jordan-Hare Stadium.

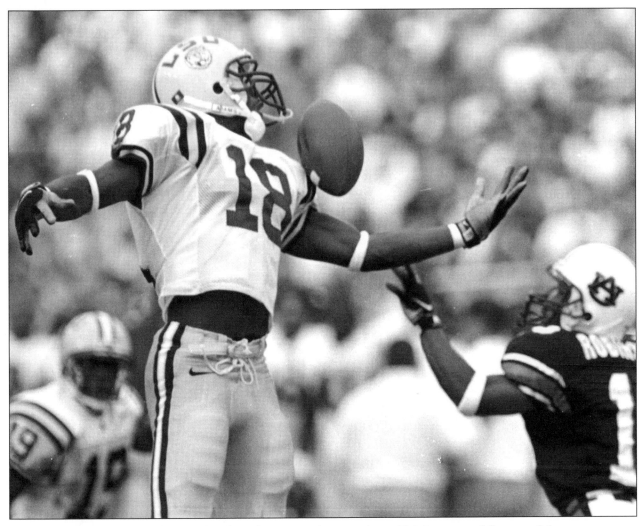

■ **LSU's Clarence LeBlanc (18) reaches for a first-quater interception, which he returned for a touchdown.**

"You're supposed to save your best for the big games," said Tyler, his right (throwing) hand heavily bandaged afterward, courtesy of a helmet he banged into in the first quarter. "We came out on top."

LSU improved to 2-0, 1-0 in the SEC and won the game that has meant so much to these two teams in recent SEC Western Division races. The Tigers now have the early half-game lead and tiebreaker on Auburn (1-2, 1-1 in the SEC), the team picked in the preseason to be LSU's closest SEC West pursuer.

"It was a great win," tailback Rondell Mealey said. "It was our first step in reaching our goals."

In this series marked by "earthquakes," interceptions, great comebacks and even a burning building outside Jordan-Hare two years ago, this game will add another quirky chapter. LSU won despite seemingly being unable to stop Ben Leard's third-down passing the entire first half and its seeming inability to ever convert an extra point opportunity.

But as LSU coach Gerry DiNardo pointed out, "When you come on the road in the SEC looking good is winning. At times we didn't look as good as we can.

Score by Periods

LSU	19	0	6	6 —	31
Auburn	7	10	2	0 —	19

"After the game I told the team we played hard for 60 minutes. I guess we'll be ranked No. 6 in the morning because someone (No. 2 Florida or No. 6 Tennessee) has to lose. I told them there's a lot of responsibility in being No. 6."

There's a lot of responsibility going into being an LSU quarterback, especially with a defense like Auburn's geared to stop the Tigers' most notorious weapon, tailback Kevin Faulk.

Auburn did limit Faulk to 21 carries for 88 yards. But time and again it was Tyler doing the damage: scrambling away from a rush or hitting Abram Booty and Larry Foster with touch sideline patterns.

"Their quarterback was totally the difference in the game," Auburn defensive coordinator Bill Oliver said. "I don't think

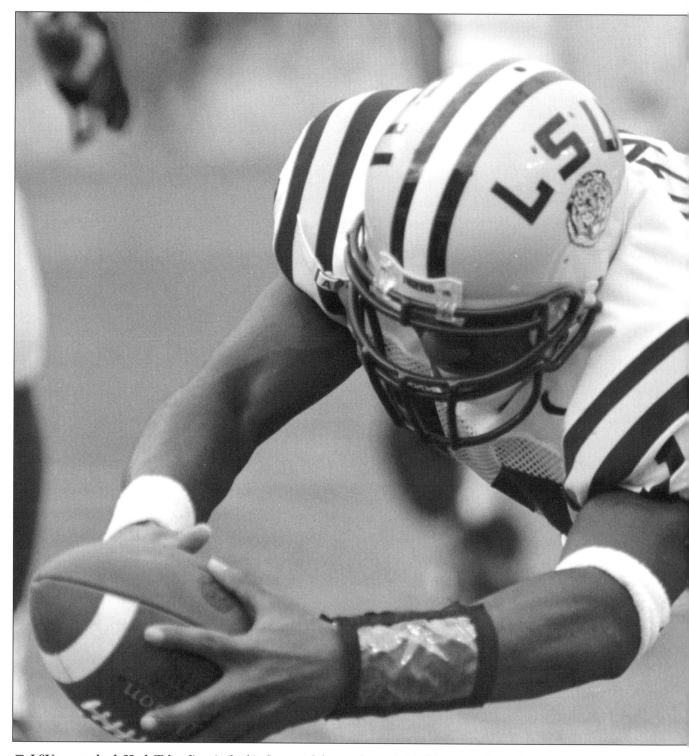

■ **LSU quarterback Herb Tyler dives in for his first touchdown, after twisting his way to the end zone.**

we got a sack."

No they didn't, but not for lack of opportunities. Tyler scrambled around for a net 12 yards on 11 carries and a touchdown. He passed 20 times, completing 16 for 174 yards and three touchdowns.

"It was typical Herb Tyler," said DiNardo, who ran to the

10,000 or so LSU fans in the north end zone after the game and acknowledged them by pumping his fist in the air. "He found a way to win."

Tyler improved to 25-5 as a starter, tying Warren Rabb for second-most victories in LSU history for a quarterback behind Tommy Hodson's 31.

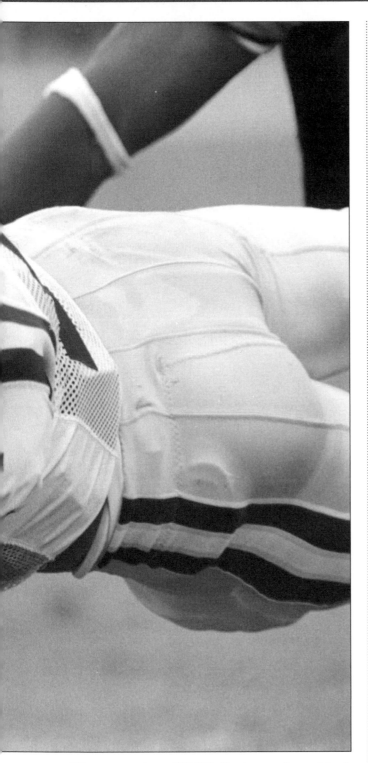

"His maturity showed," LSU offensive coordinator Morris Watts said. "He never got down or bothered the entire game."

It looked as if this would go down as Auburn's self-destruction game in the first 5½ minutes. Turnovers on Auburn's first two plays led to a 13-0 LSU lead on a one-handed interception and 21-yard return by strong safety Clarence LeBlanc on Auburn's first offensive play and Tyler's juking 5-yard quarterback draw. That score was set up when linebacker Aaron

Adams stripped Auburn tailback Michael Burks of Kenner, the ball recovered by inside linebacker Thomas Dunson.

"That's what Herb offers you," said Watts, describing a run in which Tyler zig-zagged around strong safety Rob Pate and dived into the end zone. "It's not a run everyone could make."

After the interception, LSU struggled to contain Auburn quarterback Ben Leard the rest of the half. Without much help from his running game but plenty from a confused-looking LSU defense, Leard completed 16 of 22 passes for 221 yards, including a 54-yard TD pass to wide-open fullback Heath Evans and a 10-yard TD pass to wide receiver Karsten Bailey.

After Evans' score, LSU went up, 19-7, late in the first quarter on a 19-yard Tyler-to-Faulk scoring pass with Faulk working out of the slotback position. Auburn pulled within 19-14 on Bailey's grab then made it 19-17 at halftime on a 29-yard Robert Bironas field goal as time expired.

Their early big lead all but gone, some LSU players began to worry.

"After we got up 13-0 some of them started to panic when Auburn came back," nose guard Anthony McFarland said. "But we knew it would be a 60-minute game."

LSU dominated field position in the third quarter but struggled to score. Tyler struggled, too, unable to get a first down on fourth-and-inches at the Auburn 18 and a fumble that Pate recovered at his 7.

But LSU took over at the Auburn 41 late in the third and finally produced some points. After three straight runs, Tyler rolled right to give an option fake, dropped back and found wide-open flanker Larry Foster streaking across the middle for a 29-yard score.

Auburn pulled within 25-19 after Charles Dorsey blocked his second Danny Boyd extra-point try and Brad Ware returned it 88 yards for two points. But LSU's defense continued to harass Leard in the second half. He completed 5 of 16 for 64 yards in the second half and was sacked five times.

"In the second half they were one step ahead of us offensively," Auburn coach Terry Bowden said. "When you are trying to keep the run in and it's not working too well, you're asking Ben to do a lot of things."

A diving interception by cornerback Chris Cummings at the LSU 46 gave the Tigers the ball with 10 minutes left. With Faulk running and Tyler passing, LSU reached the 1 but was pushed back to the 6 by a procedure penalty.

In last Saturday's 42-6 win over Arkansas State, Tyler overthrew tight end Kyle Kipps in the right flat of the end zone on fourth down. This time he rolled right and found the big tight end left open by an Auburn defender who came up to stop Tyler's run for the clinching points with 5:27 remaining.

"Last year Herb kind of struggled," against Auburn, said Faulk, recalling a bitter 31-28 loss in Baton Rouge. "This year he was hurt and continued to play his heart out."

Halftime Made All the Difference

By Sam King
The Advocate

Auburn, Ala. — *Sept. 20, 1998*

Two years after the great Barn Fire in Auburn, LSU's secondary was caught practicing fire drills in the midst of a game.

Or, at least that's what the confusion in the secondary looked like.

Ben Leard looked like Dameyune Craig.

LSU's great season looked like history.

The Tigers looked a gift horse in the mouth and squandered most of a charitable 13-point as Leard passed for 221 first-half yards and two touchdowns that left LSU holding a slim 19-17 lead.

Now, the rest of the story.

Let Auburn coach Terry Bowden tell you.

"I thought they changed in the second half," said Bowden. "I thought they did. I got a little frustrated, too. I'm going to have to go back and look.

"They changed some things and got me out of sync — I say me, because I was calling the plays. They got us out of sync.

"They did a great job. I was getting blitzed at different times," continued Bowden. "In the first half we kind of got momentum (on offense). We stayed one step ahead of them. But, in the second half, they were one step ahead of us."

That, in a nutshell, is why LSU left here with a 31-19 victory.

That is why the No. 7-ranked Tigers are 2-0 and have a good start on their quest of winning the Southeastern Conference Western Division.

One of the greatest assets of any coaching staff is being able to adjust at halftime.

It meant everything this afternoon.

Leard managed only five completions in 16 attempts for 64 yards and the Auburn rushing game that had managed only 16 yards in the first half ended with a net 21 yards for the game. That's big-time, major-college defense — although Leard was sacked for losses totaling 50 yards.

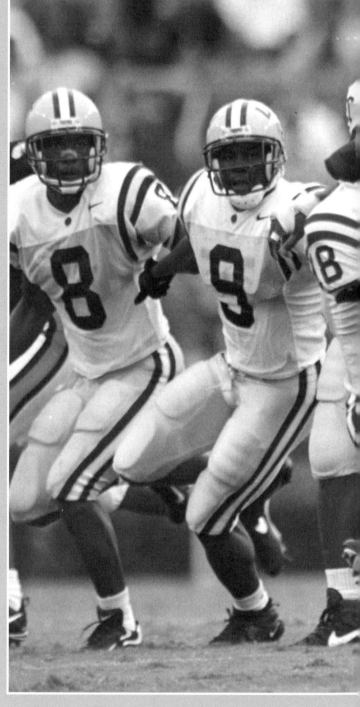

"We just turned it up a little bit," is what Anthony McFarland said of the second-half surge. "We made a few switches.

"We were getting in their face the first half, but they were throwing the ball. In the second half, we were able to get there a little quicker," continued McFarland. "We just tried to run a few more stunts up front and were able to get home."

He admitted, however, that Leard finding an open receiver — sometimes no defender even close — was getting to some of the players.

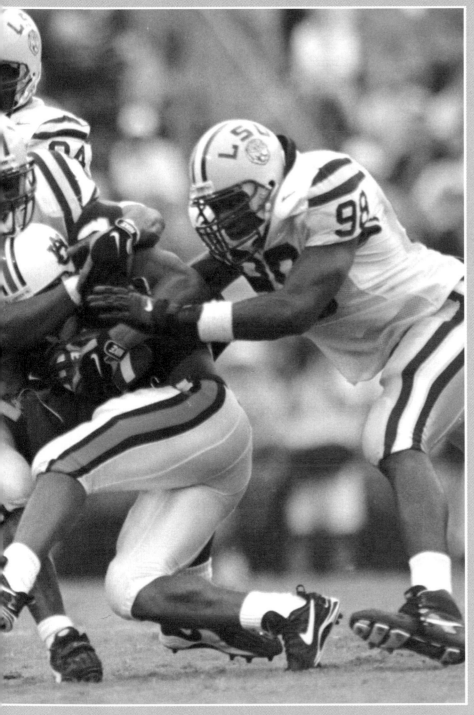

■ LSU defenders Mark Roman (8), Robert Davis (9) and Anthony McFarland (94) close in to help as Joe Wesley (48)and Arnold Miller (98) wrap up Auburn running back Michael Burks. LSU held Auburn to 21 total yards rushing.

In this wild and wacky series anything happens and it seems this year it was a case of turnabout being fair play. Last year Craig put two quick first-quarter scores on the board. This time, on Auburn's first offensive play of the game, Leard was intercepted by Clarence LeBlanc who raced into the end zone after less than three minutes of play.

On Auburn's next offensive play, Michael Burks fumbled with linebacker Thomas Dunson recovering. LSU capitalized and led by 13-0 with 9:34 still remaining.

The lead came almost too quickly and too easily.

But, if you've kept up with this series, you know no lead is ever completely, totally safe.

LSU's defense answered the challenge in the second half. The Tigers maintained field position most of the half and threatened, only to be repelled by an Auburn defense that was anything but poor.

As expected the battle in the trenches was big time and it wasn't until LSU's defensive front started making its stand with strong pressure on Leard that the Tigers were able to take control.

Not enough can be said of the very key, clutch and vital play of quarterback Herb Tyler, who connected with receivers on critical third-down plays or ran, scrambled and dazzled with some moves to get a first — or a touchdown as he did on the second TD of the game (from 5 yards out).

Flanker Larry Foster had the best game of his career with 10 catches, some absolutely astounding, in picking up 111 yards.

Abram Booty had three catches, two for first downs.

The defense was remarkable in adjusting and LSU continues its great ability to win on the road — all of which should help lead to better things.

"I got up and told the guys to just stay calm, that it isn't the worst thing for someone to be driving," said McFarland. "I told them to stay calm. We knew it was going to be a 60-minute game and later on the game would come to us.

"I said, 'Don't get in a frenzy. Stay calm. The game will come to us,' and eventually it did."

Color this one a big victory.

Although one game is not a season, this was a major decision the Tigers had to have to be able to achieve some lofty goals this season.

Now, it's up to them to make sure they don't squander such a good start.

Early Errors Cost Auburn

By Sam King
The Advocate

Auburn, Ala. — *Sept. 20, 1998*

"You can't spot the No. 7 team 14 and beat them," Auburn coach Terry Bowden said, mistakenly referring to the quick 13 points the hosts helped dish out to LSU in today's 31-19 loss.

"Spot 'em 14 and lose by 12 — that's as close as you're going to come."

To Bowden, you had to look no farther than the Tigers' veteran four-year starting quarterback Herb Tyler for the difference in the game.

"That experienced quarterback just made so many plays," Bowden said of Tyler, who not only completed 16 of 20 passes for three touchdowns and 174 yards, but came up with some critical scrambles for vital first-down yardage. "You've got to have a guy who, on every little third-and-four situation makes 4½ yards.

"I saw that over and over again. It's what we saw in Dameyune Craig last year."

Despite spotting LSU a two-touchdown lead, Auburn played some outstanding offense to get back in the game and trail by only 19-17 at half. Quarterback Ben Leard sparkled by completing 16 of 22 passes for 221 yards and two touchdowns, although two were intercepted, one returned by Clarence LeBlanc for the game's first touchdown.

"We were one step ahead," Bowden said of the first-half surge. "I guess we were doing some things they weren't expecting. We were one step ahead.

"We did well in the first half, but they made the adjustments necessary. They made some sacks in long yardage situations," he said.

Something else he pointed out: "They are a team that doesn't give up the naked bootleg like Ole Miss. Their style is not

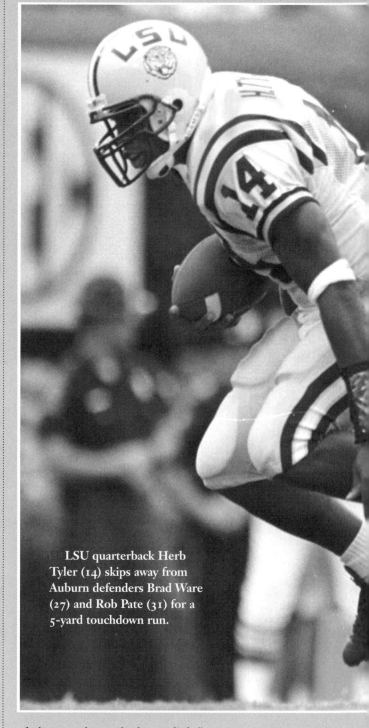

LSU quarterback Herb Tyler (14) skips away from Auburn defenders Brad Ware (27) and Rob Pate (31) for a 5-yard touchdown run.

of a bump-and-run, play loose a little."

Bowden pointed out Auburn had a problem preparing for LSU since it had only played Arkansas State and they had nothing else to evaluate the new defense by.

"They did a good job of playing their base (defense), but they were also giving us some things we didn't know about," Bowden said.

For the second time in three games, Auburn finished with paltry rushing yardage: Auburn gained a net 18 against Virginia

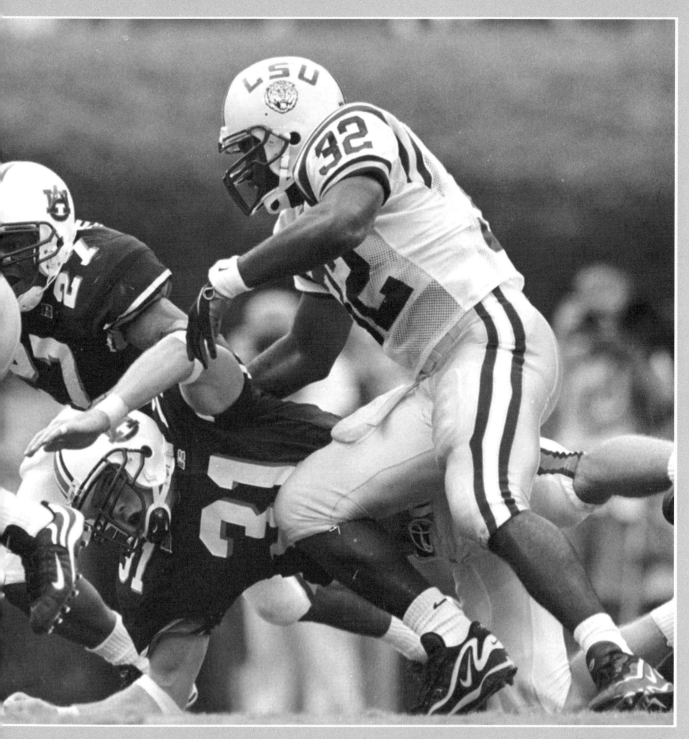

and was limited to 21 by LSU — although that includes 50 yards of losses when Leard was sacked.

"We have got to run the ball," Bowden said. "Last year (with Craig), I could debate if we needed to run when we could throw like we did. But now what we've got to do is get past the line of scrimmage (rushing) a few more times."

Bowden was especially complimentary of LSU's passing game.

"Take (Abram) Booty and (Larry) Foster, I thought they both played good," Bowden said. "Booty is just so depend-

able. He came to our camp in high school. He's a lot better football player than he gets credit for being. He has good speed, runs perfect routes and sometimes makes some unbelievable catches.

"On third-and-ten, he catches for 12 — right at the line, I mean."

With LSU's passing game, their running game has to get tougher.

"Foster can really hurt you a lot," he said of the Tiger flanker, who snared 10 passes for 111 yards and one TD.

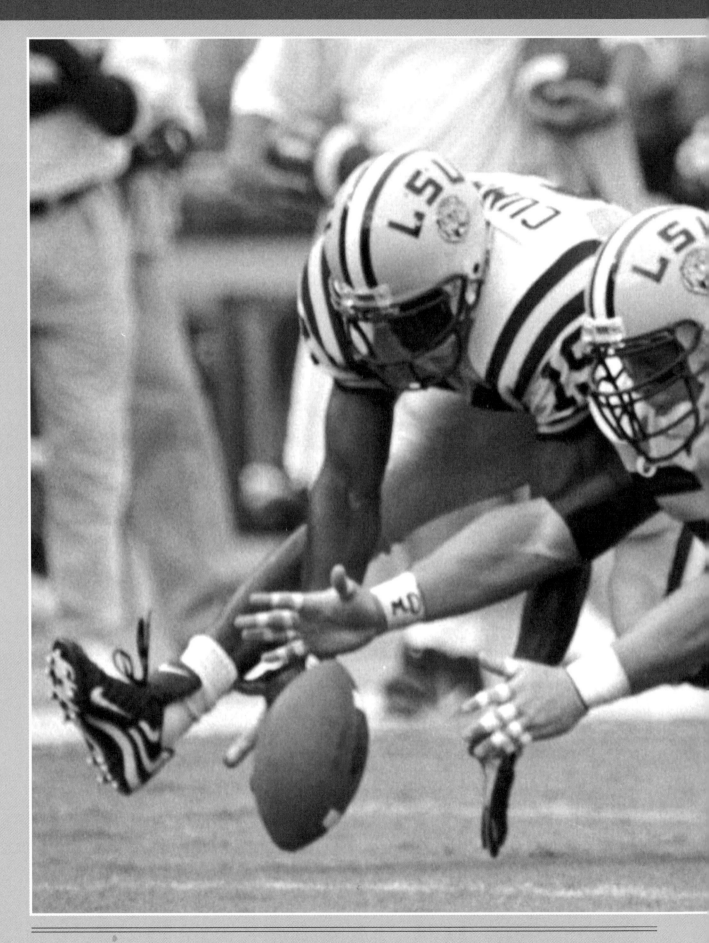

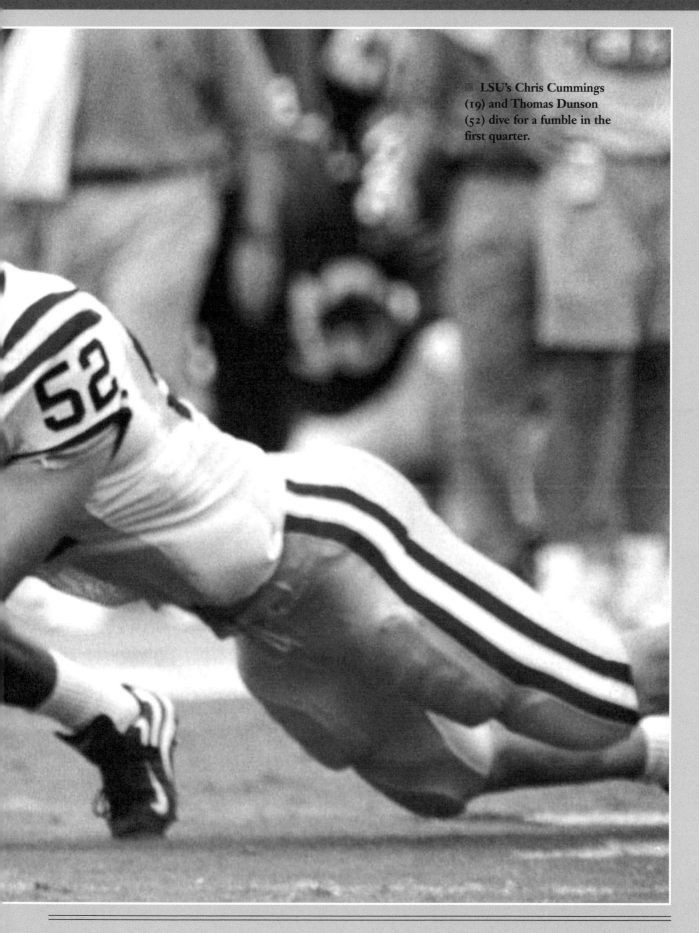

LSU's Chris Cummings (19) and Thomas Dunson (52) dive for a fumble in the first quarter.

PHOTO CREDITS